W9-ALV-141

Alternative Medicine

The Definitive Guide

Compiled by
The Burton Goldberg Group

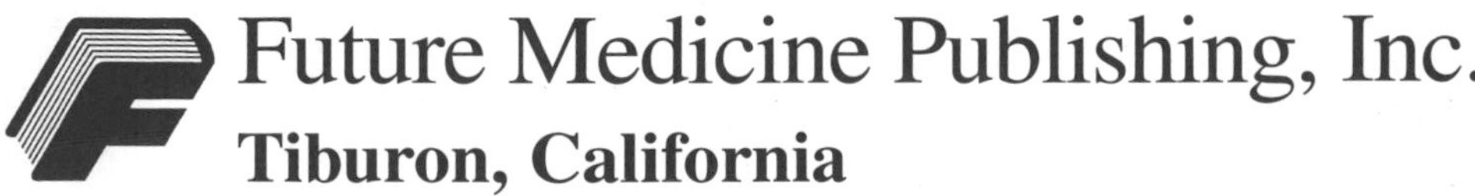
Future Medicine Publishing, Inc.
Tiburon, California

Copyright © 1993, 1999
by Future Medicine Publishing, Inc.
All rights reserved.

ISBN: 1-887299-33-5

Library of Congress Catalogue Card Number: 93-74059

Publisher's Cataloging in Publication Data

Alternative medicine: the definitive guide / compiled by
The Burton Goldberg Group.
p. cm.
Includes bibliographical references and index
Preassigned LCCN: 93-74059

1. Alternative medicine Popular works. I. Burton Goldberg Group (Firm)

R733.A484 1994 615.5
QBI94-176

Cover design by Janine White

No part of this book may be reproduced in any form without the expressed written consent of the publisher, except by a reviewer, who may quote brief passages in connection with a review.

Printed in the United States of America.

9 8 7 6 5 4 3 2 1

Future Medicine Publishing, Inc.
1640 Tiburon Blvd., Suite #2
Tiburon, CA 94920

This book is *interactive.*

Use these symbols to find more information and get the most out of this book.

Turn to another place in this book for more information on the same subject.

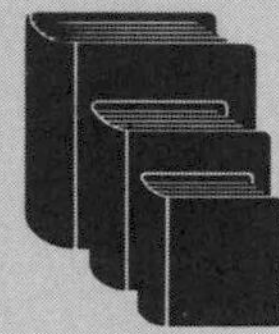

Here are more books on the same subject worth reading.

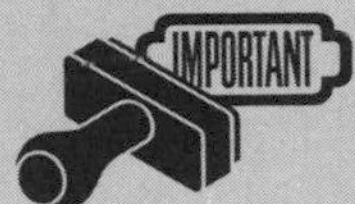

Please give this point your special attention.

CAUTION This sign tells you there may be some risks, uncertainties, side-effects, or special contraindications regarding a procedure or substance.

Telephone numbers and addresses of organizations, publications, or professionals whom you can contact immediately.

Alternative medicine has many self-help techniques for you. When you see this icon, it means here is a self-help exercise you can practice today.

This means it is advisable to contact a professional health care practitioner for more information or treatment.

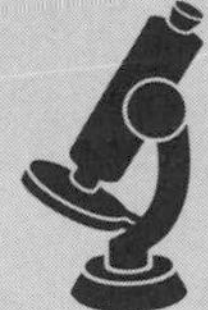

This indicates a promising area that needs more scientific research and medical testing.

Alternative medicine saves money; here is another example of its cost-savings ability.

INDEX Use our extensive index to look up your health condition and appropriate treatments.

If this book has helped you get over an illness, we would love to hear from you. Please contact us at 800-333-4325 or write to 1640 Tiburon Blvd., #2, Tiburon, CA 94920 or fax us at 415-435-9448. Visit us at our website http://www.alternativemedicine.com.

Mission Statement

Future Medicine Publishing was created to help alleviate our present medical crisis by informing the public of effective and affordable alternatives in health care and promoting freedom of choice in medicine.

Responding to a growing consumer demand for alternatives to conventional medicine, we have produced *Alternative Medicine: The Definitive Guide,* the most comprehensive and authoritative work of its kind. This landmark work is the result of a global effort spanning four years, a two million dollar budget, and involving over 400 leading alternative health professionals.

As the "Voice of Alternative Medicine," our goal is to help bring about a rebirth of health care in America. We seek to unite the most successful approaches to health maintenance, disease prevention, and the treatment of chronic illness from both conventional and alternative medicine. We envision this integration as the hallmark of future medicine and the catalyst for the dawning of a new Health Age in America.

Dedication

Recently, my five-year-old son, Blake, came to me and said, "Daddy, you should tell them about my 'dee-dee' in your book." Blake's 'dee-dee' is his security blanket and whenever he doesn't feel good he wraps himself in it and immediately feels better.

Although conventional physicians tend to dismiss the positive results of alternative medicine as simply being 'a placebo effect,' my son's observation captures a simple truth that too many of us have forgotten. Like my son's security blanket, there is a magical and intangible element in the healing process which cannot be scientifically measured—the role of the mind and the emotions.

This book is dedicated to my son Blake, my grandchildren, Margaux Star, Allen, Ryan, and Brittany, and to all the children of the world: may you not forget the wonder of healing.

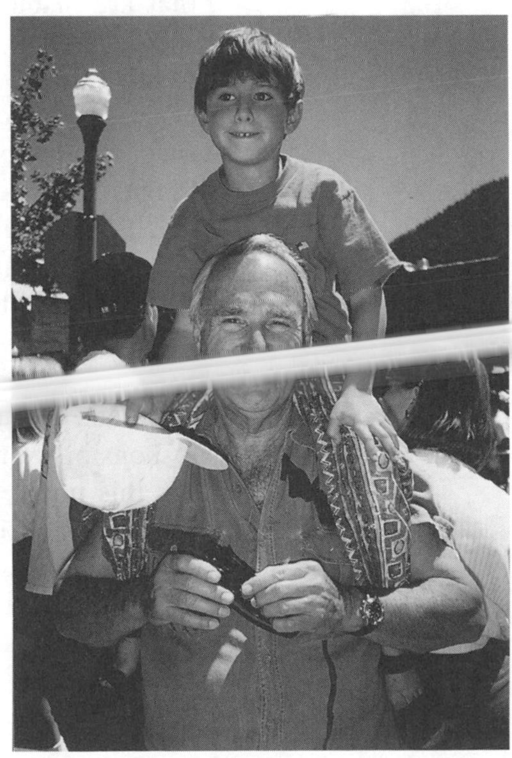

An Important Message

This book is intended as an educational tool to acquaint the reader with alternative methods for the maintenance of good health and the treatment of illness. The publisher hopes the book will enable the reader to improve his or her well-being and to better understand, assess, and choose the appropriate course of treatment for an illness or health condition. Because the methods described in this book are, by definition, **alternative** methods, many of them have not been investigated and/or approved by any government or regulatory agency. National, state, and local laws vary regarding the use and application of many of the treatments that are discussed. Accordingly, this book should not be substituted for the advice and treatment of a physician or other licensed health professional, but rather should be used in conjunction with professional care. Pregnant women in particular are especially urged to consult with their physician before using any therapy.

Your health is important. Use this book wisely. Discuss the alternative treatment options described herein with your doctor. Ultimately, you, the reader, must take full responsibility for your health and how you use this book. The publisher expressly disclaims responsibility for any adverse effects resulting from your use of the information contained herein.

Table of Contents

Part One: The Future of Medicine

Part Two: Alternative Therapies

Part Three: Health Conditions

Quick Reference Guide to Additional Health Conditions

To the Health Professional:

The nearly 400 health professionals who contributed to this book have performed an invaluable service. You now have a single, authoritative source of information on diet, and nutrition, herbal medicine, homeopathy, acupuncture, chiropractic, Ayurveda, Traditional Chinese Medicine, environmental medicine, chelation therapy, and the other disciplines of alternative medicine.

This reference volume is just a beginning, however. We hope that you, along with your fellow health professionals, will continue to pioneer the field of alternative medicine, and keep us informed of your findings, in order to allow this book to evolve and continue to be an up-to-date and useful tool.

We hope this book is a beginning in a larger sense, as well. We look forward to a Health Age, a time of wellness and freedom from disease. This age will arise as alternative medicine permeates and invigorates Western medicine, so that physicians no longer view themselves simply as rescuers of their patients when illness occurs, but as daily providers of their well-being.

Our goal is to have the knowledge contained in this book spill over into our health practices, research, conferences, medical school curricula, and into our nation's health plan. We welcome your contributions, and critical feedback. With your help, we look forward to the dawning of the Health Age.

Credits

Publisher: Burton Goldberg

Executive Editor: James Strohecker

Senior Editor: Larry Trivieri

Associate Editor: Doug Lewis

Managing Editor: Mari Florence

Research Editor: Steve Hart

Editor, Quick Reference Guide: Lisa Bonnice

Medical Editor: Leon Chaitow, N.D., D.O.

Senior Contributing Editors: Sue Astrum, Ph.D., D. Lindsey Berkson, M.A., D.C., Paul Duran, Celia Farber

Contributing Editors: Alex Demyanenko, Susan Deutsch, Neal Dublinsky, J.D., Michael Duncan, Karin Elstad, Danny Feingold, Dennis Haig, Jane Vernon Lewis, Natalie Nichols, Sara Prejean, Molly Siple, Mark Waldman

Copy Editor: Gina Misiroglu

Research: Cathleen Alexander, Dena Allen, Pilar Alessandra, Mary Ann Bendel, Chris Breyer, Nayoon Cho, Denise Domb, Melinda Gordon, Deborah Grandinetti, Merdyce McClaran, Tana March, Teri Neville, Richard Ortega, Patrick Polk, Jonathan Steigman, Bill Zide

Assistants to Executive Editor: Marcia Hirsh, Mark Kotlyar

Illustrator: Jeanne Hayden

Production: John Coyle, Lori Jerome, Jonathan Pepper, Heidi Schmitt, Andy Simon

Design: 3DMARK, Inc.

Editorial Board

Ed Arana, D.D.S., Co-founder and President of the American Academy of Biological Dentistry, Carmel Valley, California

Robert C. Atkins, M.D., Founder and Medical Director, The Atkins Center for Complimentary Medicine, New York, New York

Rudolph M. Ballentine, M.D., Director, Center for Holistic Medicine, New York, New York; Author; Board of Trustees, Medical Staff, Himalayan Institute

Abram Ber, M.D., Founding Member, American Holistic Medical Association, Phoenix, Arizona

Mark Blumenthal, Executive Director, American Botanical Council; Editor, *HerbalGram,* Austin, Texas

Joan Borysenko, Ph.D., President, Mind-Body Health Sciences, Inc., Boulder, Colorado

David E. Bresler, Ph.D., L.Ac., Director of Program Development, Los Angeles Healing Arts Center; Co-director, Academy for Guided Imagery, Mill Valley, California

William Michael Cargile, B.S., D.C., F.I.A.C.A., Chairman of Research, American Association of Acupuncture and Oriental Medicine (AAAOM); Gulfcoast Medical Arts Center, Daphne, Alabama

Leon Chaitow, N.D., D.O., Director, Nutrition and Health Research Associates, London, England; Editor, *Journal of Alternative and Complementary Medicine*

Perry A. Chapdelaine Sr., M.A., Executive Director/Secretary, Rheumatoid Disease Foundation, Franklin, Tennessee

Emmanuel Cheraskin, M.D., D.M.D., Editoral Board, Journal of Advancement in Medicine; Professor Emeritus, University of Alabama Medical Center, Birmingham, Alabama

Deepak Chopra, M.D., Author of *Quantum Healing*; Executive Director, Sharp Institute for Human Potential and Mind Body Medicine, San Diego, California

Trevor Cook, Ph.D., D.I.Hom., President, United Kingdom Homeopathic Medical Association, Middlesex, England

William Lee Cowden, M.D., International Health Guard, Dallas, Texas

Elmer M. Cranton, M.D., President, American College of Advancement in Medicine; Mount Rogers Clinic, Troutdale, Virginia

Samuel Epstein, M.D., Professor of Occupational and Environmental Medicine, School of Public Health, University of Illinois Medical Center, Chicago, Illinois

Charles Farr, M.D., Ph.D., Medical Director, International Bio-Oxidative Medicine Association; Medical Director, Genesis Medical Center, Oklahoma City, Oklahoma

Alan R. Gaby, M.D., President-Elect, American Holistic Medical Association, Baltimore, Maryland

Garry F. Gordon, M.D., (H.) Founder, American College of Advancement in Medicine; President, Get Healthy, Inc., Tempe, Arizona

Jay N. Gordon, M.D., F.A.A.P., Medical Consultant to ABC, CBS, NBC; private practice, Santa Monica and Malibu, California

Dick Gregory, comedian, nutrition advocate and internationally acclaimed Health Educator, Washington, D.C.

Jane Heimlich, Author of *What Your Doctor Won't Tell You,* Cincinnati, Ohio

Roger C. Hirsh, O.M.D., L.Ac., Dipl. (NCCA), Doctor of Oriental Medicine; Director, Metamedical Group, Santa Monica, California

Philip Jay Hodes, Ed.D., Holistic Health Enrichment, Detoxification and Orthomolecular Nutrition to Combat Aids, Learning Disorders, Alcoholism and Alzheimers

Abram Hoffer, M.D., Ph.D., President, Canadian Schizophrenia Foundation; Editor-in-Chief, *Journal of Orthomolecular Medicine*, Victoria, British Columbia, Canada

David Hoffmann, B.Sc., M.N.I.M.H., past President, American Herbalist Guild, Sebastopol, California

Sir Jay M. Holder, M.D., D.C., Ph.D., 1991 Winner, Albert Schweitzer Prize in Medicine; Founder, Medical Director, Exodus Treatment Center and Holder Research Institute, Miami, Florida

Hal A. Huggins, D.D.S., M.S., Director, Huggins Diagnostic Center, Colorado Springs, Colorado

Bernard Jensen, D.C., lecturer; Author of *Nature Cures;* Founder and Director, Valley Ranch, Escondido, California

Konrad Kail, N.D., President, American Association of Naturopathic Physicians, Phoenix, Arizona

Vasant Lad, M.A.Sc., Ayurvedic Physician; Director, The Ayurvedic Institute, Albuquerque, New Mexico

Susana Alcázar Leyva, M.D., President of the Albert Szent-Gyorgy Gerontological Center; Vice-President of the Hans Selye Institute of Scientific Research, Mexico City, Mexico

Evarts Loomis, M.D., F.A.C.S., Founder, Meadowlark Holistic Health Retreat, Hemet, California; Co-founder, American Holistic Medical Association

Wolfgang Ludwig, Sc.D., Ph.D., Director, Institute for Biophysics, Horb, Germany

Marshall Mandell, M.D., F.A.C.A.I., F.A.A.E.M., Medical Director, New England Foundation for Allergic and Environmental Diseases, Norwalk, Connecticut

Gaston Naessens, Director, Center for Experimental Research and Biologics, Rock Forest, Quebec, Canada

Maoshing Ni, D.O.M., Ph.D., L.Ac., Vice-President, Yo San University of Traditional Chinese Medicine, Santa Monica, California

Patricia A. Norris, Ph.D., Director, Biofeedback and Psychophysiology Clinic, Menninger Clinic, Topeka, Kansas

Richard Passwater, Ph.D., Director of Research, Solgar Nutritional Research Center, Berlin, Maryland

Linus Pauling, Ph.D., Two-time Nobel laureate: Chemistry-1954, Peace-1962; Director, Linus Pauling Institute of Science and Medicine, Palo Alto, California

Kenneth R. Pelletier, Ph.D., M.D. (hon), Senior Clinical Fellow, Stanford Center for Research in Disease Prevention, Department of Medicine, Stanford University School of Medicine, Palo Alto, California

Joseph E. Pizzorno, N.D., President, Bastyr College, Seattle, Washington

John Powers, past President, Prentice Hall, Aspen, Colorado

Theron G. Randolph, M.D., President, Human Ecology Research Foundation, Batavia, Illinois

Martin L. Rossman, M.D., Founder, Academy for Guided Imagery, Mill Valley, California

Anthony Scott-Morley, D.Sc., Ph.D., B.A., B.Ac., M.D. (Alt. Med.), Director, Institute of Bioenergetic Medicine; Member of the World Research Foundation, Dorset, England

Hari Sharma, M.D., F.R.C.P.C., Professor of Pathology, Director, Cancer Prevention and Natural Products Research, The Ohio State University College of Medicine, Columbus, Ohio

C. Norman Shealy, M.D., Ph.D., Co-founder, American Holistic Medical Association; Director, the Shealy Institute for Comprehensive Health Care; Professor of Psychology, Forest Institute of Professional Psychology, Fairgrove, Missouri

Bernie Siegel, M.D., Founder of ECaP (Exceptional Cancer Patients), New Haven, Connecticut

Carl Simonton, M.D., Board Certified, Director, Simonton Cancer Center, Pacific Palisades, California; Director, Psychoneuroimmunology Counseling Program, Cancer Treatment Centers of America, Brea, California

Lendon H. Smith, M.D., Author of thirteen books including *Feed Your Kids Right,* Portland, Oregon

Virender Sodhi, M.D. (Ayurveda), N.D., Founder and Director, American School of Ayurvedic Sciences, Bellevue, Washington

Hector Solorzano Del Rio, M.D., D.Sc., Coordinator, Alternative Medical Studies Program; Professor of Pharmacology, University of Guadalajara, Mexico; President of the Society of Investigation of Acupuncture and Oriental Medicine, A.C.

William Tiller, Ph.D., Professor, Stanford University, Palo Alto, California

John E. Upledger, D.O., O.M.M., Medical Director, Upledger Institute, Upledger Foundation, Palm Beach Gardens, Florida

Melvyn R. Werbach, M.D., Director, Biofeedback Medical Clinic, Tarzana, California; Author of *Nutritional Influences on Illness* and *Nutritional Influences on Mental Illness*

Julian Whitaker, M.D., President, American Preventive Medical Association; Editor, *Health & Healing;* Director, Whitaker Wellness Institute, Newport Beach, California

Harold Whitcomb, M.D., Director, Aspen Clinic for Preventive and Environmental Medicine, Aspen, Colorado

Jonathan Wright, M.D., Director, Tahoma Clinic, Kent, Washington

Contributors and Consultants

Ernesto Adler, M.D., D.D.S., Clinica Dental, Lloret de Mars, Spain

Lauri Aesoph, N.D., medical writer, Sioux Falls, South Dakota

Moses Albalas, O.D., O.M.D., H.M.D., Ph.D., L.Ac., Los Angeles, California

Majid Ali, M.D., DIPL., Consulting Physician, Institute of Preventive Medicine, Denville, New Jersey; Associate Professor, (Adj.), Columbia University Medical School; Director, Department of Pathology, Immunology, and Laboratories, Holy Name Hospital, Teaneck, New Jersey

Ted Allen, M.D., private practice, Nassau, the Bahamas

Connie Allred, President, International Association of Colon Therapy, Los Angeles, California

Connierae Andreas, Co-director, NLP Comprehensive, Boulder, Colorado

Nancy Appleton, Ph.D., Santa Monica, California

Judith Aston, M.F.A., Founder and Director, The Aston Training Center, Incline Village, Nevada

Laurence Badgley, M.D., Foster City, California

Steven Bailey, N.D., Graduate Assistant Professor, National College of Naturopathic Medicine, Portland, Oregon; Director, North West Naturopathic Clinic

Julian Barnard, Author of *Guide to the Bach Flower Remedies* and *Healing Herbs of Edward Bach,* Hereford, England

Beatrice Barnett, N.D., D.C., Director, Lifestyle Institute, Margate, Florida

John Baron, D.O., Director, Baron Clinic Inc., and Associates, Cleveland, Ohio

Richard Barrett, N.D., Associate Academic Dean, National College of Naturopathic Medicine, Portland, Oregon

Dr. Guy Berard, E.N.T., Les Ollieres, France

D. Lindsey Berkson, M.A., D.C., nutritionist and educator, Santa Fe, New Mexico

Ann Berwick, B.S.C., Founder and President of the National Association for Holistic Aromatherapy, Boulder, Colorado

Rita Bettenburg, N.D., Research Director, Clinical Faculty, National College of Naturopathic Medicine, Portland, Oregon

David R. Bierman, L.Ac., President, Safe Environments, Berkeley, California

Harvey Bigelson, M.D., Medical Director, Center for Progressive Medicine, Scottsdale, Arizona

Robert Bingham, M.D., Medical Director, Desert Arthritis and Medical Clinic, Desert Hot Springs, California

Timothy C. Birdsall, N.D., licensed midwife, Technical Director, Thorne Research, Inc., Sandpoint, Idaho

Leyardia Black, N.D., Past Member, Drugless Therapeutics Exam Committee, State of Washington; Former Professor of Gynecology, Bastyr College, Lopez Island, Washington

Robert Blaich, D.C., D.I.B.A.K., Diplomate, International Board of Applied Kinesiology, Los Angeles, California

Jeffrey Bland, Ph.D., President, HealthComm, Inc., Gig Harbor, Washington

Dean Bonlie, D.D.S., President, MagnetiCo Inc., Calgary, Alberta, Canada

Helen L. Bonny, Ph.D., R.M.T., Director, The Bonny Foundation, Philadelphia, Pennsylvania

Mary Bove, N.D., L.M., Chair, Botanical Medicine Department, Bastyr College, Seattle, Washington

Randall Bradley, N.D., D.H.A.N.P., private practice, Lincoln, Nebraska

James Braly, M.D., Medical Director, Immuno Labs, Inc., Fort Lauderdale, Florida; President and Medical Director, Doctor's Best, San Clemente, California; Medical Director, Biometrics, Inc., Newbury Park, California; Medical Editor, *Immuno Review*

Eric Braverman, M.D., Director, Princeton Associates for Total Health (PATH), Princeton, New Jersey

Arline and Harold Brecher, Co-authors of *Forty-Something Forever*, Health Savers Press, Herndon, Virginia

Phyllis J. Bronson, Nutritional biochemical consulting, Aspen Clinic for Preventive and Environmental Medicine, Aspen, Colorado

Donald J. Brown, N.D., Natural Product Research Consultants, Seattle, Washington

Erma Brown, B.S.N., P.H.N., Co-director, Foundation for Environmental Health Research, Beaverton, Oregon

Annemarie Buhler, The Phyto-Aromatherapy Institute, South Pasadena, California

Helen Varney Burst, C.N.M., M.S.N., D.H.L.(Hon), F.A.C.N.M., Professor, Nurse Midwifery Program, Adult Health Division, Yale University School of Nursing, New Haven, Connecticut

Dwight Byers, President, Ingham Publishing, Inc., International Institute of Reflexology; Author, *Better Health with Foot Reflexology*, St. Petersburg, Florida

Cherie Calbom, M.S., C.N., Author of *Juicing for Life, Cooking for Life,* and *Nutrition and Cancer,* Kirkland, Washington

Don G. Campbell, B.M.E.D., Director of the Institute for Music, Health & Education, Boulder, Colorado

Eve Campanelli, Ph.D., Nutritional Consultant, Master Herbalist, Beverly Hills, California

Patricia Cane, Ph.D., Research Associate in Ob. Gyn., Cedars Sinai Hospital, Los Angeles, California

James A. Carlson, D.O., F.A.O.A.S., Musculo-skeletal and Athletic Medicine, past President, American Association of Orthopedic Medicine, Knoxville, Tennessee

James Carter, M.D., Professor of [illegible] University School of Public Health and Tropical [illegible], Louisiana

Nalini Chilkov, Lic. Ac., O.M.D., private practice, Santa Monica, California

Walter Jess Clifford, M.S., President and Director, Clifford Consulting and Research, Colorado Springs, Colorado

Drew Collins, N.D., Director, Oasis Naturopathic Medical Clinic, Prescott Valley, Arizona

Vaughn Cook, L.Ac., Dipl. Ac. (NCCA), Director, Utah Acupuncture Clinic, Salt Lake City, Utah

Ignacio Coronel, M.D., Mexico City, Mexico

Harris L. Coulter, Ph.D., Center for Empirical Medicine, Washington, D.C.

William Crook, M.D., F.A.A.P., F.A.C.A., F.A.C.A.I., President, International Health Foundation, Jackson, Tennessee

Pat Culliton, M.A., Dipl. Ac. (NCCA), Director, Acupuncture and Alternative Medicine, Hennepin County Medical Center, Minneapolis, Minnesota

Michael Cummings, D.O., F.N.T.O.S., London, England

Ralph Alan Dale, Ed. D., Ph.D., C.A., Dipl. Ac., Director, Acupuncture Education Center, North Miami Beach, Florida

Katie Data, N.D., private practice, Fife, Washington

Stephen Davies, M.A., B.M., B.Ch., Biolab Medical Unit, London, England

Don G. Davis, D.C., Director, Davis Chiropractic Group, Hayward, California

Rena Davis, M.S., President, Davis Nutritional Consultants, St. Helens, Oregon

Christopher Day, M.A., Vet. M.B., M.R.C.V.S., Vet. F.F.Hom., Alternative Medicine Veterinarian, Veterinary Dean to the Faculty of Homeopathy, Oxon, England

Martin Dayton, M.D., D.O., B.S., H.M.D., F.H.F.P., Director, Medical Center Sunny Isles, Miami Beach, Florida

Sandra C. Denton, M.D., Alaska Alternative Medicine Center, Anchorage, Alaska

Kathleen DesMaisons, M.Ed., President, Radiant Recovery, Burlingame, California

Ravi Devgan, M.D., Toronto, Canada

Subhuti Dharmananda, Ph.D., Director, Institute for Traditional Medicine, Portland, Oregon

W. John Diamond, M.D., Medical Director, Triad Medical Center, Reno, Nevada; Medical Director, BHI-Heel, Albuquerque, New Mexico; Medical Editor, *Biological Therapy*

Darius Dinshah, S-CN., President, Dinshah Health Society, Malaga, New Jersey

Roy Dittman, L.Ac., O.M.D., Director, Bodymind Systems Medical Center, Santa Monica, California

Patrick Donovan, R.N., N.D., Fellow, Health Studies Collegium Academic Faculty, Bastyr College, Seattle, Washington, private practice, Seattle and Tacoma, Washington

John Downing, O.D., Ph.D., Director of Light Therapy, Preventive Medical Center of Marin, San Rafael, California

Suzannah L. C. Doyle, Certified Fertility Educator, Director of Fertility Awareness Services, Corvallis, Oregon

James Duke, Ph.D., Economic Botanist, United States Department of Agriculture (USDA), Beltsville, Maryland

Nancy Dunne, N.D., President, Montana Association of Naturopathic Physicians, private practice, Missoula, Montana

Charmane Eastman, Ph.D., Director, Biological Rhythms Research Laboratory; Associate Professor, Psychology Department, Rush Presbyterian, St. Lukes Medical Center, Chicago, Illinois

Gary Emerson, D.C., Opti Health, Santa Ana, California

Donald Epstein, D.C., Originator of Network Chiropractic; Founder and President of Association for Network Chiropractors, Boulder, Colorado

Robert Erdman, M.A., Ph.D., Kent, England

William Faber, D.O., Director, Milwaukee Pain Clinic, Milwaukee, Wisconsin

Steven Fahrion, Ph.D., Director, Center for Applied Psychophysiology, The Menninger Clinic, Topeka, Kansas

J. Herbert Fill, M.D., private practice, former New York City Commissioner of Mental Health, New York, New York

Ray Fisch, N.D., Ph.D., C.H., Los Angeles, California

Richard Fischer, D.D.S., F.A.G.D., F.I.A.O.M.T., Executive Vice-President, International Academy of Oral Medicine and Toxicology, Annandale, Virginia

Bob Flaws, Dipl. Ac., Dipl. C.H., F.N.A.A.O.M., Iris Acupuncture Health Associates, Boulder, Colorado

Bill Flocco, Director, American Academy of Reflexology, Burbank, California

David Frawley, O.M.D., Director, American Institute of Vedic Studies, Santa Fe, New Mexico

Joyce Frye, D.O., F.A.C.O.G., Founder, The Women's Group, Chairman, Gynecology Department, Presbyterian Medical Center, Philadelphia, Pennsylvania

Charles Gabelman, M.D., Diplomate, American Board of Allergy and Immunology, Director, Comprehensive Medical Center, Encinitas, California

Michael Reed Gach, Ph.D., Director, The Acupressure Institute, Berkeley, California

Daniel Gagnon, Medical Herbalist, Botanical Research and Educational Institute, Inc., Santa Fe, New Mexico

Stuart Garber, D.C., Director, Westside Chiropractic Center, West Los Angeles, California

Zane Gard, M.D., Co-director, Foundation for Environmental Health Research, Beaverton, Oregon

Larrian Marie Gillespie, M.D., Assistant Professor, Urology and Urogynecology; Director, The Pelvic Pain Treatment Center and the Women's Clinic for Interstitial Cystitis, Beverly Hills, California

Jochen Gleditsch, M.D., D.D.S., Hon. President of German Acupuncture Association, Munich, Germany

George Goodhart, D.C., F.I.C.C., D.I.B.A.K., Research Director, International College of Applied Kinesiology, Grosse Point Woods, Michigan

James Gordon, M.D., Clinical Professor, Departments of Psychiatry and Community and Family Medicine, Georgetown Medical School; Director, The Center for Mind-Body Studies; Chair, National Advisory Council to the Office of Alternative Medicine, National Institutes of Health

Ray Gottlieb, O.D., Ph.D., private practice, Madison, New Jersey

Robert N. Grove, Ph.D., Medical Psychologist, Center for Neurofeedback, Culver City, [illegible]

Scott J. Gregory, O.M.D., private practice, Pacific [illegible]

Warren S. [illegible] Director, Laser Research and Technology Development, Cedars [illegible] Center, Los Angeles, California

H.C. Gurney, Jr., D.V.M., Veterinary Clinical Research, Alternative Health Care, Conifer, Colorado

Elson M. Haas, M.D., Director, Marin Clinic of Preventive Medicine and Health Education, San Rafael, California

Leonard Haimes, M.D., Medical Director, Medicine and Lifestyle, Environmental and Internal Medicine, Chelation Therapy, Boca Raton, Florida

Tim Hallbom, M.S.W., Partner, Western States Training Associates, NLP of Utah LC, Salt Lake City, Utah

Steven Halpern, Ph.D., President, SOUND Rx Records and Tapes; Director, Sound Health Research Institute, San Anselmo, California

Jeff Harris, N.D., Seattle, Washington

Joseph Hattersley, M.A., Self-employed researcher, Olympia, Washington

Christopher J. Hegarty, Health researcher; author, Novato, California

Joseph Heller, Founder and Director, Hellerwork, Mt. Shasta, California

Eileen Henry, L.Ac., Director, Institute of Psycho-Structural Balancing, Santa Monica, California

Silena Heron, N.D., R.N., Sedona, Arizona

John Hibbs, N.D., Natural Health Clinic, Seattle, Washington

Joy Holm, Ph.D., University of California at Santa Cruz, Extension Division

Mark Holmes, O.M.D., L.Ac., Dip. Acupuncture and Herbal Medicine, (NCCA), Director, Center for Regeneration, Beverly Hills, California

Susanne Houd, M.D., midwife (Denmark), Program Director, Department of Midwifery, The Michener Institute, Toronto, Canada

Tori Hudson, N.D., Academic Dean, National College of Naturopathic Medicine, Portland, Oregon

Richard P. Huemer, M.D., Medical Director, Cascade Park Health Center, Vancouver, Washington

Vicki Hufnagel, M.D., Beverly Hills, California

David Hughes, D.Sc., Hyperbaricist, The Hyperbaric Oxygen Institute, San Bernardino, California

Bonnie Humiston, R.N., M.S., Director, The Feldenkrais Guild, Albany, Oregon

Karl Humiston, M.D., retired holistic psychiatrist, Albany, Oregon

Corazon Ibarra-Ilarina, M.D., H.M.D., Biomedical Health Institute, Reno, Nevada

Christine Jackson, Editor, *Explore* magazine, Mt. Vernon, Washington

Jennifer Jacobs, M.D., M.P.H., Evergreen Center for Homeopathic Medicine, Edmonds, Washington

Robert H. Jacobs, N.M.D., D. Hom. (Med), Society for Complimentary Medicine, London, England

Terry S. Jacobs, N.M.D., D.Hom. (Med), Director, College of Homeopathy, Santa Monica, California, U.S.A. Registrar, British Institute of Homeopathy

Roger Jahnke, L.Ac., O.M.D., Director, Health Action, Santa Barbara, California

Philip A. Jenkins, D.D.S., Los Gatos, California

Carol Jessup, M.D., El Cerrito, California

Kris Johnson, Director of Public Relations and Marketing, Western States Training Associates, NLP of Utah, Salt Lake City, Utah

Eric Jones, N.D., Dean of Academic Affairs, Bastyr College, Seattle, Washington

Deane Juhan, Author of *Job's Body*, Trager Instructor, Mill Valley, California

James J. Julian, M.D., Medical Director, Chelation Research Foundation, Los Angeles, California

Jon Kabat-Zinn, Ph.D., Associate Professor of Medicine; Director, Stress Reduction Clinic, University of Massachusetts Medical Center, Worcester, Massachusetts

Jon Kaiser, M.D., private practice, San Francisco, California

Harvey Kaltsas, Ac. Phys. (FL), D. Ac. (RI), Dipl. Ac. (NCCA), Sarasota, Florida

Leslie J. Kaslof, researcher, writer, educator in the field of holistic health and preventative medicine; Author of *Wholistic Dimensions in Healing*.

Richard Kaye, D.C., Director, Quantum Healing Center, San Diego, California

Julian Kenyon, M.D., M.B., Ch.B., Southhampton, Hampshire, England

Robert King, past President, American Massage Therapy Association; Co-director, Chicago School of Massage Therapy, Chicago, Illinois

Patrick Kingsley, M.B.B.S., L.R.C.P., D.Obst., R.C.O.G., Leicestershire, England

Dietrich Klinghart, M.D., Ph.D., President, American Academy of Neural Therapy, Santa Fe, New Mexico

Janet Konefal, Ph.D., M.P.H., C.A., Associate Professor, University of Miami, School of Medicine, Miami, Florida

Constantine A. Kotsanis, M.D., Grapevine, Texas

Evgenij Kozhevnikov, M.D., St. Petersburg, Russia

A .M. Krasner, Ph.D., Founder and Director, American Institute of Hypnotherapy, Santa Ana, California

Dolores Krieger, R.N., Ph.D., Professor Emeritus, New York University; Founder of Therapeutic Touch, Port Chester, New York

Daniel F. Kripke, M.D., Department of Psychiatry, University of California at San Diego, San Diego, California

Fredi Kronenberg, Ph.D., Director, Richard & Hinda Rosenthal Center for Alternative/Complementary Medicine, Columbia University College of Physicians and Surgeons, New York, New York

Tom Kruzel, N.D., Associate Professor of Medicine, National College of Naturopathic Medicine, Gresham, Oregon

Paul J. Kulkosky, Ph.D., Professor of Psychology, University of Southern Colorado

Richard A. Kunin, M.D., Orthomolecular Medicine and Psychiatry, San Francisco, California

Roy Kupsinel, M.D., Editor and Publisher, *Health Consciousness*, Oviedo, Florida

Marc LaBel, O.M.D., L. Ac., private practice, Los Angeles, California

Gary LaLonde, C.Ht., President, Premiere Performance Inc., Wales, Michigan

Raymond W. Lam, M.D., Department of Psychiatry, University of British Columbia

Susan Lange, O.M.D., Co-director, Meridian Health Center, [illegible]

Susan Lark, M.D., [illegible] PMS Self-Help Center, Los Altos, California

[illegible] R. Lee, M.D., physician, educator, Sebastopol, California

Lita Lee, Ph.D., Enzyme Therapist, Eugene, Oregon; Author of *Radiation Protection Manual*; Editor, *Earthletter*, a quarterly newsletter

Martin Lee, Ph.D., Director, Great Smokies Diagnostic Laboratory, Asheville, North Carolina

Buck Levin, Ph.D., R.D., Assistant Professor of Nutrition, Bastyr College, Seattle, Washington

Emil Levin, M.D., Medical Director, Holistic Medical Center, West Hollywood, California

Warren Levin, M.D., F.A.A.F.P., F.A.C.N., F.A.C.A.I., Medical Director, World Health Medical Group, New York, New York

Stephen Levine, Ph.D., Founder and President, Allergy Research Group, San Leandro, California

Douglas C. Lewis, N.D., Chairperson of Physical Medicine, Bastyr College Natural Health Clinic, Seattle, Washington

Jacob Liberman, O.D., Ph.D., Director, Aspen Center for Energy Medicine, Aspen, Colorado

John Limehouse, D.V.M., Holistic Veterinary Clinic, North Hollywood, California

Molly Linton, N.D., L.M., private practice, licensed midwife, Seattle, Washington

Andrew H. Lockie, M.R.C.G.P., M.F. Hom., Dip. Obst., R.C.O.G., Guildford, Surrey, England

Nancy Lonsdorf, M.D., Medical Director, Maharishi Ayurveda Medical Center, Washington, D.C.

Howard F. Loomis, D.C., Forsyth, Missouri

Nicholas J. Lowe, M.D., Clinical Professor, Department of Dermatology, UCLA School of Medicine; Director, Skin Research Foundation of California

Jeff Maitland, Faculty Chair, The Rolf Institute, Boulder, Colorado

Sir Peter Guy Manners, M.D., D.O., Ph.D., Director, Bretforton Hall Clinic, Worcestershire, England

Rick Marinelli, N.D., M.Ac.O.M., President, Naturopathic Physicians Acupuncture Association, Beaverton, Oregon

Hugh McGrath, Jr., M.D., Associate Professor, Department of Rheumatology, Louisiana State University Medical Center, New Orleans, Louisiana

Paul McTaggart, nutritional researcher, technologist, President, and Founder, Progressive Nutrition, Ventura, California

Faizi Medeiros, N.D., Director, Upper Valley Naturopathic Clinic, Norwich, Vermont

Bruce Milliman, N.D., Associate Professor of Medicine, Bastyr College, Seattle, Washington

Robert D. Milne, M.D., private practice, Las Vegas, Nevada

Gerald Montgomery, M.D., Director, New Mexico Orthopedic Medicine and Pain Treatment Clinic, Albuquerque, New Mexico

Warwick L. Morrison, M.D., Associate Professor of Dermatology, Johns Hopkins University, Baltimore, Maryland

Richard Moskowitz, M.D., Watertown, Massachusetts

Robin Munro, Ph.D., Director, Yoga Biomedical Trust, Cambridge, England

Margaret Naesser, Ph.D., Associate Research Professor of Neurology, Boston University School of Medicine; licensed acupuncturist, Massachusetts, Dipl.Ac. (NCCA)

Rex E. Newnham, Ph.D., D.O., M.D., Director, Arthritis and Rheumatism Natural Health Association, North Yorkshire, England

Robert Norett, D.C., Director, Stillpoint Health Center, Venice, California

Christiane Northrup, M.D., F.A.C.O.G., past President, American Holistic Medical Association, Yarmouth, Maine

Gary R. Oberg, M.D., F.A.A.P., F.A.A.E.M., Medical Director, The Crystal Lake Center for Allergy and Environmental Medicine; past President, American Academy of Environmental Medicine, Crystal Lake, Illinois

Katherine O'Hanlan, M.D., Associate Director of Stanford University's Gynecologic Cancer Section; Co-author of *Natural Menopause: Guide to a Woman's Most Misunderstood Passage*

David W. Orme-Johnson, Ph.D., Chairman, Department of Psychology, Maharishi International University, Fairfield, Iowa

Humphrey Osmond, M.D., M.R.C.P., F.R.C., Psy., Bryce Nova Program, Tuscaloosa, Alabama

Frank Ottiwell, Director, Alexander Training Institute, San Francisco, California

Tonis Pai, M.D., Kivimae Hospital, Tallin, Estonia

Hazel Parcells, N.D., D.C., Ph.D., Founder and Director, Parcells System of Scientific Living, Albuquerque, New Mexico

Terry Patten, President, Tools for Exploration, San Rafael, California

David Paul, M.D., Medical Director, Vail Valley Medical Center, Vail, Colorado

Larry Payne, Ph.D., Director, Samata Yoga Center, President, International Association of Yoga Therapy, Los Angeles, California

Meyrick J. Peak, Ph.D., Argonne National Laboratory, Center of Mechanistic Biology, Argonne, Illinois

Raymond Peat, Ph.D., President, International College, Eugene, Oregon

Gene Peniston, Ed.D., A.B.M.P., Chief, Psychology Service, Sam Rayburn Memorial Veterans Center, Bonham, Texas

Marvin Penwell, D.O., Director, Linden Medical Center, Linden, Michigan

Erik Peper, Ph.D., Associate Director, Institute for Holistic Healing Studies, San Francisco State University

Janice Keller Phelps, M.D., author, *The Hidden Addiction and How to Get Free From It,* Sagle, Idaho

William H. Philpott, M.D., Chairman, Bio-Electro-Magnetic Institute Institutional Review Board, Choctaw, Oklahoma

Richard Pitcairn, D.V.M., Ph.D., Eugene, Oregon

John Pittman, M.D., Medical Director, CURE AIDS NOW, Salisbury, North Carolina

Kent L. Pomeroy, M.D., F.A.A.P.M., & R., Founder, past President, American Association of Orthopedic Medicine, Scottsdale, Arizona

Michelle Pouliot, N.D., Torrington, Connecticut

Marvin Prescott, D.M.D., private practice, Los Angeles, California

Joan Priestley, M.D., private practice, Anchorage, Alaska

James Privitera, M.D., Medical Director, NutriScreen, Inc., Covina, California

Gus J. Prosch, Jr., M.D., Biomed Associates, P.C. [illegible]

Bonnie Prudd[illegible], [illegible], Institute for Physical Fitness and Myotherapy, Stockbridge, Massachusetts

Karl Ransberger, M.D., Medizinische, Enzymeforschungsgesellschaft, Geretstried, Germany

Doris J. Rapp, M.D., F.A.A.A., F.A.A.P., F.A.A.E.M., Clinical Assistant Professor of Ped., State University of New York at Buffalo; Past President, American Academy of Environmental Medicine, Buffalo, New York

Harold Ravins, D.D.S., private practice, Los Angeles, California

William Reed, M.D., Center for Health, Santa Monica, California; Vice-President, California Homeopathic Medical Association

Bernard Rimland, Ph.D., Director, Autism Research Institute, San Diego, California

Hugh D. Riordan, M.D., Director, Center for the Improvement of Human Functioning International, Wichita, Kansas

Berndt Rohrmann, M.D., Heidelberg, Germany

Terry Rondberg, D.C., President, World Chiropractic Alliance, Chandler, Arizona

Harvey M. Ross, M.D., private practice, Los Angeles, California

Jonathan Rothschild, President, Cardiovascular Research, Concord, California

Robert Jay Rowan, M.D., Director, Omni Medical Center, Anchorage, Alaska

F. Fuller Royal, M.D., Medical Director, The Nevada Clinic, Las Vegas, Nevada

Theodore Rozema, M.D., F.A.A.F.P., President, Great Lake Association of Clinical Medicine; Secretary, American Board of Chelation Therapy, Landrum, South Carolina

Dante Ruccio, N.D., Adjunct Professor, La Salle University, private practice, Newark, New Jersey

Mary Kay Ryan, N.C.C.A., Dipl. Ac., Co-founder, AIDS Alternative Health Project and Northside HIV Treatment Center, Chicago, Illinois

Debra Nuzzi St. Claire, M.H., Boulder, Colorado

Trevor K. Salloum, N.D., naturopathic physician, Kelowna, British Columbia

Mary Pullig Schatz, M.D., President, Medical Staff, Centennial Medical Center, Nashville, Tennessee

Alexander Schauss, Ph.D., Executive Director, Citizens for Health, Tacoma, Washington

Luc De Schepper, M.D., Ph.D., Lic. Ac., C. Hom., D.I. Hom., private practice, Santa Fe, New Mexico

Michael A. Schmidt, B.S., D.C., C.C.N., Director, Brookview Health Sciences, Anoka, Minnesota

Kurt Schnaubelt, Dr. (rer.nat.), Director, Pacific Institute of Aromatherapy, San Rafael, California

Allen Schoen, D.V.M., M.S., Director, Veterinary Institute for Therapeutic Alternatives (V.I.T.A), private practice, Sherman, Connecticut

Therese Schroder-Sheker, Executive Director, The Chalice of Repose Project; Professor of Music-Thanatology, St. Patrick Hospital, Missoula, Montana

Deane Shapiro, Ph.D., Professor in Residence, Department of Psychiatry and Human Behavior, California College of Medicine, University of California, Irvine, California

David Shefrin, N.D., private practice, Beaverton, Oregon

John Sherman, N.D., Portland Naturopathic Clinic, Portland, Oregon

Benjamin Shield, Ph.D., Certified Rolfer, Craniosacral Therapist, Pacific Health Resources, Santa Monica, California

Charles Siemers, Certified Rolfer, Manhattan Beach, California

Penny Simkin, P.T., Seattle, Washington

Solomon Slobins, O.D., Director, College of Syntonic Optometry, Fall River, Massachusetts

Marian Small, N.D., L.Ac., Seattle, Washington

C. Tom Smith, M.D., Ph.D., H.M.D., D.Hom. (Med.), Director, International Clinic of Biological Regeneration (North American Office) Florissant, Missouri

Michael Smith, M.D., Medical Director, Lincoln Hospital, Substance Abuse Division, New York, New York

Nick Soloway, L.M.T., D.C., L.Ac., Portland, Oregon

Anne H. Spencer, Ph.D., Founder and Executive Director of the International Medical and Dental Hypnotherapy Association, Inc.

Ralph Sprintge, M.D., Head, Interdisciplinary Pain Clinic and Music Medicine Research Labs at Sportkrankenhaus Hellersen; Executive Director, International Society for Music in Medicine, Germany

William H. Stager, M.S., D.O., The Upledger Institute, Palm Beach Gardens, Florida

Leana Standish, N.D., Ph.D., Director of Research, Bastyr College, Seattle, Washington

Jill Stansbury, N.D., Assistant Professor of Botanical Medicine, National College of Naturopathic Medicine, private practice; Battle Ground, Washington

John Steele, Aromatic Consultant, Lifetree Aromatix, Sherman Oaks, California

Joanne Stefanatos, D.V. M., Animal Kingdom Veterinary Hospital, Las Vegas, Nevada; President, American Holistic Veterinary Medical Association, Las Vegas, Nevada

Peter M. Stephan, M.D. (hom.), M.Sc., Kt. Comm., O.S.J.J., Principal, The Stephan Clinic, London, England

Michael Stern, D.C., private practice, Minneapolis, Minnesota

Ralph Strauch, Ph.D., certified Feldenkrais practitioner, Los Angeles, California

Gerard V. Sunnen, M.D., Associate Clinical Professor of Psychiatry at the New York University-Bellevue Hospital Medical Center, New York, New York

Murray R. Susser, M.D., Medical Director, Omnidox Medical Group, Santa Monica, California

Roy Swank, M.D., Ph.D., Director, Swank Multiple Sclerosis Clinic, School of Medicine, Oregon Health Sciences University, Portland, Oregon

Jon M. Sward, Ph.D., Director of Counseling, Center for the Improvement of Human Functioning International, Inc., Wichita, Kansas

Glen M. Swartwout, A.B., O.D., F.I.C.A.N., F.S.C.O., Founder, Achievement of Excellence Research Academy International; President, Starfire International, Hilo, Hawaii

Joyal Taylor, D.D.S., President, The Environmental Dental Association, San Diego, California

Michael Terman, Ph.D., Director, Light Therapy Unit, New York State Psychiatric Institute, New York, New York

Dick Thom, D.D.S., N.D., Senior Staff Physician, Portland Naturopathic Clinic, Portland, Oregon

Billie M. Thompson, Ph.D., Director of Sound, Listening and Learning Center, Phoenix, Arizona

Kay Thompson, D.D.S., Pittsburgh, Pennsylvania

Carvel Tiekert, D.V.M., Executive Director of the American Holistic Veterinary Medical Association, Bel Air, Maryland

Robert Tisserand, author; Editor, *International Journal of Aromatherapy*, Hove, East Sussex, England

Desmond Tivy, M.D., Lee, Massachusetts

Marjorie K. Toomim, Ph.D., Director, Biofeedback Institute of Los Angeles, Los Angeles, California

Joseph Trachtman, O.D., Ph.D., Brooklyn, New York

Elias Tsambis, M.D., A.B.P.N., Director of Medicine, New York Institute of Medical Research, Nyack, New York

Dennis Tucker, Ph.D., L.Ac., Sierra Acupuncture Clinic, Nevada City, California

Dana Ullman, M.P.H., Director, Homeopathic Educational Services, Berkeley, California

Joseph F. Unger, Jr., D.C., D.I.C.S., Chairman of the Board, Sacro Occipital Research Society International, SORSI, Prairie Village, Kansas

Matt Van Benschoten, O.M.D., M.A., C.A., private practice, Reseda, California

Joseph Vargas, Ph.D., Founder and Director, Wholistic Health Center, Houston, Texas

Gary Verigan, D.D.S., private practice, Escalon, California

George Von Hilsheimer, Ph.D., Neuropsychologist; Diplomate of the American Academy of Pain Management, Maitland, Florida

Dietrich Wabner, Dr. (rer. nat.), Hon. I.F.A. and Forum Essenzia; President, Natural Oils Research Association, Windsor, England; Professor, Technical University, Munich, Germany

Charles Wallach, D.Sc., Ph.D., President, Behavioral Research Association; Chairman, California Review Board; Director, AIDS Policy Research Center, Canoga Park, California

William Walsh, Ph.D., Carl Pfeiffer Treatment Center, Naperville, Illinois

Dale Walters, Ph.D., Director of Education, Center of Applied Psychophysiology, Menninger Clinic, Topeka, Kansas

Gunther M. Weil, Ph.D., clinical psychologist, private practice, Aspen, Colorado

Toni Weschler, M.P.H., Founder, FACTS (Fertility Awareness Counseling and Training Seminars), Seattle, Washington

Bill Wesson, D.D.S., private practice, Aspen, Colorado

Richard S.Wilkinson, M.D., Director, Yakima Allergy Clinic, Yakima, Washington

Sharon Willoughby, D.V.M., D.C., Founder, American Veterinary Chiropractic Association, Port Byron, Illinois

Jacquelyn J. Wilson, M.D., D.Ht., past President, American Institute of Homeopathy, Escondido, California

Rex Wilson, N.D., private practice, Beverly Hills, California

Honora Lee Wolfe, Dipl. Ac., Iris Acupuncture Health Care Associates, Boulder, Colorado

Helen M. Wood, L.M.T., Director, Wood Hygenic Institute, Inc., Kissimmee, Florida

Jing-Nuan Wu, O.M.D., L.Ac., President, Taoist Health Institute, Washington, D.C.

Ray C. Wunderlich, Jr., M.D., Preventive/Nutritional Medicine, St. Petersburg, Florida

Leon Young, D.V.M., Young's Veterinary Clinic, Thomasville, Georgia

Jared L. Zeff, N.D., Naturopathic physician, Portland, Oregon

Qingcai Zhang, M.D. (China), Lic. Ac., New York, New York

Zheng Rong-rong, M.D., Director of Research Department, Qi-Gong Institute of Shanghai Academy of Traditional Chinese Medicine, San Francisco, California

Michael F. Ziff, D.D.S., Foundation for Toxic-Free Dentistry, Orlando, Florida

Sam Ziff, Ph.D., Foundation for Toxic-Free Dentistry, Orlando, Florida

John Zimmerman, Ph.D., Diplomate, American Board of Sleep Medicine; Laboratory Director, Washoe Sleep Disorders Center; Director, Bio-Electro-Magnetics Institute, Reno, Nevada

Contributors and Consultants by Chapter

Part I: The Future of Medicine

Contributing Writers: John R. Lee, M.D.; Leon Chaitow, N.D., D.O.

Consultants: Mark Blumenthal; Alan R. Gaby, M.D.; Garry F. Gordon, M.D.; Jay Geller; Elson Haas, M.D.; Konrad Kail, N.D.; Warren Levin, M.D.; Stephen Levine, Ph.D.; Robert Jay Rowen, M.D.; Alexander Schauss, Ph.D.; Julian Whitaker, M.D.; Jonathan Wright, M.D.

Part II: Alternative Therapies

Acupuncture
Consultants: William Michael Cargile, B.S., D.C., F.I.A.C.A.; Jay Holder, M.D., D.C., Ph.D.; Maoshing Ni, D.O.M., Ph.D., L.Ac.; Dennis Tucker, Ph.D., L.Ac.

Applied Kinesiology
Contributing Writer: Robert Blaich, D.C.
Consultant: George Goodheart, D.C., F.I.C.C., D.I.B.A.K.

Aromatherapy
Consultants: Kurt Schnaubelt (Dr. rer. nat.); Robert Tisserand, Debra St. Claire, M.H.

Ayurvedic Medicine
Contributing Writer: Vasant Lad, M.A.Sc. (India)
Consultants: Virender Sodhi, M.D. (Ayurveda), N.D.; Deepak Chopra, M.D.; David Frawley, O.M.D.

Biofeedback Training
Consultants: Melvyn Werbach, M.D.; Stephen Fahrion, Ph.D.; Robert N. Grove, Ph.D.; Marjorie Toomim, Ph.D.

Biological Dentistry
Contributing Writer: Ed Arana, D.D.S.
Consultants: Ernesto Adler, M.D., D.D.S.; Walter Jess Clifford, M.S.; Richard D. Fischer, D.D.S., F.A.G.D., F.I.A.O.M.T.; Jochen Gleditsch, M.D., D.D.S.; Hal A. Huggins, D.D.S., M.S.; Harold Ravins, D.D.S.; Joyal Taylor, D.D.S.; Michael F. Ziff, D.D.S.

Bodywork
Contributing Writer: Eileen Henry, L.Ac.
Consultants: Judith Aston; Dwight Byers; Michael Reed Gach, Ph.D.; Joseph Heller; Bonnie Humiston, R.N., M.S.; Robert King; Dolores Krieger, R.N., Ph.D.; Frank Ottowell; Bonnie Prudden; Ralph Strauch, Ph.D.

Cell Therapy
Contributing Writers: Ted Allen, M.D.; Hector Solorzano Del Rio, M.D., D.Sc.
Consultants: C. Tom Smith, M.D., Ph.D., H.M.D., D.Hom. (Med); Peter Stephan, M.D. (Hom), M.Sc., Kt.Comm., O.S.J.J.

Chelation Therapy
Contributing Writer: Perry Chapdelaine, M.A.
Consultants: Elmer Cranton, M.D.; Charles Farr, M.D., Ph.D.; Garry F. Gordon, M.D.; James Julian, M.D.; Theodore Rozema, M.D., F.A.A.F.P.; Arlene and Harold Brecher

Chiropractic
Consultants: Robert Blaich, D.C.; William Michael Cargile, B.S., D.C., F.I.A.C.A.; Don Davis, D.C.; Donald Epstein, D.C.; Steven Hinkey, D.C.; Jay Holder, M.D., D.C., Ph.D.; Terry Rondberg, D.C.

Colon Therapy
Consultants: Connie Allred; Drew Collins, N.D.; Joseph Vargas, Ph.D.

Craniosacral Therapy
Contributing Writer: Robert Norett, D.C.
Consultants: Benjamin Shields, Ph.D.; Joseph F. Unger, Jr., D.C., F.I.C.S.; John Upledger, D.O., O.M.M.

Detoxification Therapy
Contributing Writer: Zane Gard, M.D.
Consultants: Erma Brown, B.S.N., P.H.N.; Leon Chaitow, N.D., D.O.; Rena Davis, M.S.; Elson Haas, M.D.; Evarts Loomis, M.D.; Marshall Mandell, M.D., F.A.C.A.I., F.A.A.E.M.; David Steinman, B.A., M.A.

[illegible]
Contributing Writer: Buck Levin, Ph.D.
Consultants: D. Lindsay Berkson, D.C., M.A.; John R. Lee, M.D.; David Steinman, B.A., M.A.

Energy Medicine
Contributing Writers: Anthony Scott-Morley, D.Sc., Ph.D., B.A., B.Ac., M.D. (Alt. Med.); William Tiller, Ph.D.
Consultants: Abram Ber, M.D.; Vaughn Cook, L.Ac., Dipl. Ac. (NCCA); Rena Davis, M.S.; Gary Emerson, D.C.; George Godfrey, M.D.; H.C. Gurney, Jr., D.V.M.; Robert Jacobs, N.M.D., D.Hom. (Med); Philip Jenkins, D.D.S.; Robert Milne, M.D.; Sir Peter Guy Manners, M.D., D.O., Ph.D.; F. Fuller Royal, M.D.; Joanne Stefanatos, D.V.M.

Environmental Medicine
Contributing Writer: Richard S. Wilkinson, M.D.
Consultants: Marshall Mandell, M.D., F.A.C.A.I., F.A.A.E.M.

Enzyme Therapy
Contributing Writers: Lita Lee, Ph.D.; Hector Solorzano Del Rio, M.D., D.Sc. (Mexico)
Consultants: Howard Loomis, D.C.; Karl Ransberger, M.D. (Germany)

Fasting
Consultants: Steven Bailey, N.D.; Leon Chaitow, N.D., D.O.; Elson Haas, M.D.; Evarts Loomis, M.D.; Trevor Salloum, N.D.

Flower Remedies
Consultants: Julian Barnard; Terrry S. Jacobs, N.M.D., D.Hom (Med); Leslie Kaslof; Susan Lange, O.M.D.; Harold Whitcomb, M.D.

Guided Imagery
Contributing Writer: Martin L. Rossman, M.D.
Consultants: David Bresler, Ph.D., L.Ac.; Patricia Norris, Ph.D.

Herbal Medicine
Contributing Writers: Mark Blumenthal; David L. Hoffmann, B.Sc., M.N.I.M.H.
Consultants: Donald Brown, N.D.; Mary Bove, N.D., L.M.; James Duke, Ph.D.; John Sherman, N.D.

Homeopathy
Consultants: Trevor Cook, Ph.D., D.Hom.; Terry S. Jacobs, N.M.D., D.Hom. (Med); Wolfgang Ludwig, Sc.D., Ph.D., (Germany); Robert D. Milne, M.D.; Dana Ullman, M.P.H.

Hydrotherapy
Contributing Writers: Nancy Shaw Strohecker; Douglas C. Lewis, N.D.
Consultants: Leon Chaitow, N.D., D.O.; Tori Hudson, N.D.

Hyperthermia
Contributing Writer: Douglas C. Lewis, N.D.

Hypnotherapy
Consultants: A.M. Krasner, Ph.D.; Gary LaLonde, C.Ht.; Anne H. Spencer, Ph.D.; Gerard V. Sunnen, M.D.; Kay Thompson, D.D.S.; Maurice Tinterow, M.D., Ph.D.

Juice Therapy
Consultants: Steven Bailey, N.D.; Cherie Calbom, M.S., C.N.; Elson Haas, M.D.

Light Therapy
Consultants: John Diamond, M.D.; John Downing, O.D., Ph.D.; Charmane Eastman, Ph.D.; Ray Fisch, N.D., Ph.D., C.H.; Warren Grundfest, M.D.; Daniel F. Kripke, M.D.; Richard W. Lam, M.D.; Jacob Liberman, O.D., Ph.D.; Nicolas J. Lowe, M.D.; Hugh McGrath Jr., M.D.; Warwick L. Morrison, M.D.; Meyrick J. Peak, Ph.D.; Marvin Prescott, D.M.D.; C. Norman Shealy, M.D., Ph.D.; Solomon Slobin, O.D.; Michael Terman, Ph.D.; Dennis Tucker, Ph.D., L.Ac.; John R. Zimmerman, Ph.D.

Magnetic Field Therapy
Contributing Writers: Wolfgang Ludwig, D.Sc., Ph.D. (Germany); William H. Philpott, M.D.
Consultants: Dean Bonlie, D.D.S.; John Zimmerman, Ph.D.

Meditation
Contributing Writer: Deane Shapiro, Ph.D.
Consultants: Joan Borysenko, Ph.D.; Jon Kabat-Zinn, Ph.D.; Patricia A. Norris, Ph.D.; David Orme-Johnson, Ph.D.

Mind/Body Medicine
Contributing Writer: Eric Peper, Ph.D.
Consultants: Joan Borysenko, Ph.D.; Steven Fahrion, Ph.D.; James S. Gordon, M.D.; John Sward, Ph.D.

Naturopathic Medicine
Contributing Writer: Jared Zeff, N.D.

Neural Therapy
Consultants: James A. Carlson, D.O., F.A.O.A.S.; William Faber, D.O.; Luis Guerrero, M.D., P.A.; Dietrich Klinghart, M.D., Ph.D.; Marvin Penwell, D.O.

Neuro-Linguistic Programming
Contributing Writer: Tim Hallbom, L.C.S.W; Kris Johnson.
Consultants: David Paul, M.D.; John Sward, Ph.D.; Janet Konefal, Ph.D.; Connierae Andreas

Nutritional Supplements
Contributing Writer: Jeffrey Bland, Ph.D.
Consultants: D. Lindsay Berkson, D.C., M.A.; Paul McTaggert

Orthomolecular Medicine
Contributing Writer: Nick Solway, D.C., L.M.T., L.Ac.
Consultants: Phyllis J. Bronson; Alan R. Gaby, M.D.; Abram Hoffer, M.D., Ph.D.; Richard P. Huemer, M.D.; Richard Kunin, M.D.; Jonathan Wright, M.D.

Osteopathy
Contributing Writer: Leon Chaitow, N.D., D.O.
Consultant: William Faber, D.O.

Oxygen Therapy
Consultants: Charles Farr, M.D., Ph.D.; Martin Dayton, M.D., D.O., B.S., H.M.D., F.H.F.P.; Jeff Harris, N.D.; David Hughes, D.Sc.; John Pittman, M.D.; Gerald V. Sunnen, M.D.; Jonathan Wright, M.D.

Qigong
Contributing Writer: Roger Jahnke, O.M.D.

Reconstructive Therapy
Contributing Writer: William Faber, D.O.
Consultants: James A. Carlson, D.O., F.A.O.A.S.; Kent Pomeroy, M.D.

Sound Therapy
Contributing Writer: Don Campbell, B.M.E.D.
Consultants: Helen L. Bonny, Ph.D., R.M.T.; Steven Halpern, Ph.D.; Sir Peter Guy Manners, M.D., D.O., Ph.D.; Ralph Sprintge, M.D.; Billie M. Thompson, Ph.D.

Traditional Chinese Medicine
Contributing Writer: Robert Flaws, Dipl.Ac., Dipl. C.H., F.N.A.A.O.M.
Consultants: Roger Hirsh, O.M.D., L.Ac., Dipl. NCCA; Roger Jahnke, O.M.D.; Maoshing Ni, D.O.M., Ph.D., L.Ac.

Veterinary Medicine
Consultants: Christopher Day, M.A., Vet.M.B., M.R.C.V.S., Vet.M.F.Hom.; H.C. Gurney, Jr. D.V.M.; John Limehouse, D.V.M.; Richard Pitcairn, D.V.M., Ph.D.; Joanne Stephanatos, D.V.M.; Carvel Tiekert, D.V.M.; Sharon Willoughby, D.V.M., D.C.; Leon Young, D.V.M.

Yoga
Consultants: Rudolph Ballentine, M.D.; Robin Munro, Ph.D.; Mary Pullig Schatz, M.D.

Part III: Health Conditions

Addictions
Contributing Writer: Lauri Aesoph, N.D.
Consultants: James Braly, M.D.; William Michael Cargile, B.S., D.C., F.I.A.C.A.; Leon Chaitow, N.D., D.O.; Pat Culliton, Dipl. Ac. (NCCA); Steven Fahrion, Ph.D.; Jay Holder, M.D., D.C., Ph.D.; Corazon Ilarina, M.D.; Paul Kulkosky, Ph.D.; Maoshing Ni, D.O.M., Ph.D., L.Ac.; Gene Penniston, Ed.D.; Janice Keller Phelps, M.D.; Michael Smith, M.D.; Virender Sodhi, M.D. (Ayurveda), N.D.; Dale Walters, Ph.D.

AIDS
Contributing Writers: Jon Rappaport; Celia Farber; Leon Chaitow, N.D., D.O.
Consultants: Robert Atkins, M.D[illegible]wrence Badgley, M.D.; Herb [illegible], N.D.; William Michael Carg[illegible], D.C., F.I.A.C.A.; Subhuti Dh[illegible]anda, Ph.D.; Charles Farr, M.D., Ph.D.; [illegible]ay Holder, M.D., D.C., Ph.D.; Jon Kaiser, M.D.; Janet Konefal, Ph.D.; Joan Priestley, M.D.; Leanna Standish, N.D., Ph.D.; Quingcai Zhang, M.D. (China), Li.Ac.

Allergies
Consultants: James Braly, M.D.; William Michael Cargile, B.S., D.C., F.I.A.C.A.; Leon Chaitow, N.D., D.O.; Charles Gableman, M.D.; Michael Reed Gach, Ph.D.; Marshall Mandell, M.D., F.A.C.A.I., F.A.A.E.M.; Theron G. Randolph, M.D.; F. Fuller Royal, M.D.; Virender Sodhi, M.D. (Ayurveda), N.D.; Dick Thom, D.D.S., N.D., Richard Wilkinson, M.D., Ray C. Wunderlich, Jr., M.D.

Alzheimer's Disease and Senile Dementia
Contributing Writer: Angeline Vogl
Consultants: William Crook, M.D., F.A.A.P., F.A.C.A., F.A.A.E.M.; Sandra C. Denton, M.D.; Charles Farr, M.D., Ph.D.; Abram Hoffer, M.D., Ph.D.; David L. Hoffmann, B.Sc., M.N.I.M.H.; Hal Huggins, D.D.S., M.S.; Maoshing Ni, D.O.M., Ph.D., L.Ac., Gary Oberg, M.D., F.A.A.P., F.A.A.E.M.; Joseph E. Pizzorno, N.D.; Virender Sodhi, M.D. (Ayurveda), N.D.

Arthritis
Contributing Writer: Perry Chapdelaine, M.A.
Consultants: F. Batmanghelidj, M.D.; Robert Bingham, M.D.; James Braly, M.D.; William Michael Cargile, B.S., D.C., F.I.A.C.A.; Hal Huggins, D.D.S., M.S.; Marshall Mandell, M.D., F.A.C.A.I., F.A.A.E.M.; Raymond Peat, Ph.D.; Virender Sodhi, M.D. (Ayurveda), N.D.; Julian Whitaker, M.D.

Autism
Consultants: Leon Chaitow, N.D., D.O.; Bernard Rimland, Ph.D.; Constantine Kotsanis, M.D.; William H. Stager, M.S., D.O.; Billie Thompson, Ph.D.; John E. Upledger, D.O., O.M.M.

Back Pain
Consultants: Robert Blaich, D.C.; David Bresler, Ph.D., L.Ac.; Leon Chaitow, N.D., D.O.; Eugene Kozhevnikov, M.D., O.M.D. (Russia); Douglas C. Lewis, N.D.; Maoshing Ni, D.O.M., Ph.D., L.Ac.; Melvyn R. Werbach, M.D.

Cancer
Contributing Writer: Neal Dublinsky, J.D.
Consultants: Harvey Bigelson, M.D.; Bri[illegible] Briggs; Arlin J. Brown; Stanislaw [illegible]ynski, M.D., Ph.D.; Ernesto Cont[illegible] M.D.; Wayne Martin; Charl[illegible], M.D., Ph.D.; Wayne Garl[illegible] Gard, M.D.; Nicholas Gonzalez, [illegible]D.; Richard Huemer, M.D.; Jacinte Levesque, O.M.D.; Renato Martinez, M.D.; Neil Nathan, M.D.; Lorraine Rosenthal; Geronimo Rubio, M.D.; Dante Ruccio, N.D.; Francisco Soto, M.D.; David Steenblock, D.O.; Wolfgang Woppel, M.D.; Richard Shames, M.D.

Candidiasis
Contributing Writer: Leon Chaitow, N.D., D.O.
Consultants: Layardia Black, N.D.; James Braly, M.D.; William Michael Cargile, B.S., D.C., F.I.A.C.A.; Elson M. Haas, M.D.; Lita Lee, Ph.D.; Virender Sodhi, M.D. (Ayurveda), N.D.; Murray R. Susser, M.D.

Children's Health
Contributing Writers: Lendon Smith, M.D.; Lauri Aesoph, N.D.
Consultants: Eric Jones, N.D.; Richard Moskowitz, M.D.; Virender Sodhi, M.D. (Ayurveda) N.D.; Maoshing Ni, D.O.M., Ph.D., L.Ac.; David L. Hoffmann, B.Sc., M.N.I.M.H.; Harris Coulter, Ph.D.; Jacquelyn Wilson, M.D.; Randall Bradley, N.D.

Chronic Fatigue Sydrome
Contributing Writer: Leon Chaitow, N.D., D.O.
Consultants: William Michael Cargile, B.S., D.C., F.I.A.C.A.; Bruce A. Cunha, M.D.; Bruce Milliman, N.D.; Maoshing Ni, D.O.M., Ph.D., L.Ac.; Virender Sodhi, M.D. (Ayurveda), N.D.; Murray Susser, M.D.; Matt Van Benschoten, O.M.D., M.A., C.A.; Bill Wesson, D.D.S.

Chronic Pain
Contributing Writer: David Bresler, Ph.D., L.Ac.
Consultants: Dean Bonlie, D.D.S.; James Braly, M.D.; Leon Chaitow, N.D., D.O.; William H. Philpott, M.D.; Gerald V. Sunnen, M.D.; George Von Hilsheimer, Ph.D.; Jon Kabat-Zinn, Ph.D.

Colds and Flu
Contributing Writer: John Hibbs, N.D.
Consultants: Mary Bove, N.D., L.M.; Marian Small, N.D., L.Ac.; William Michael Cargile, B.S., D.C., F.I.A.C.A.; Virender Sodhi, M.D. (Ayurveda), N.D.

Constipation
Consultants: James Braly, M.D.; Donald Brown, N.D.; Leon Chaitow, N.D., D.O.; Patrick Donovan, N.D.; John Hibbs, N.D.; Vasant Lad, M.A.Sc.; Maoshing Ni, D.O.M., Ph.D., L.Ac.; Virender Sodhi, M.D. (Ayurveda), N.D.

Diabetes
Consultants: Abram Ber, M.D.; William Michael Cargile, B.S., D.C., F.I.A.C.A.; Charles Farr, M.D., Ph.D.; Garry F. Gordon. M.D. (H.); David L. Hoffmann, B.Sc., M.N.I.M.H.; Maoshing Ni, D.O.M., Ph.D., L.Ac.; William H. Philpott, M.D.; Virender Sodhi, M.D. (Ayurveda), N.D.; Jonathan Wright, M.D.

Female Health
Contributing Writers: John R. Lee, M.D.; Lauri Aesoph, N.D.
Consultants: Patricia Cane, Ph.D.; Nailini Chilkov, Lic.Ac., O.M.D.; Roy Dittman, L.Ac., O.M.D.; Suzzanah Doyle; Joyce Frye, D.O.; Larrian Gillespie, M.D.; Silena Heron, N.D., David L. Hoffmann, B.Sc., M.N.I.M.H.; Tori Hudson, N.D.; Vickie Hufnagel, M.D.; Jennifer Jacobs, M.D., M.P.H.; Fredi Kronenberg, Ph.D.; Susan Lark, M.D.; Nancy Lonsdorf, M.D.; Christiane Northrup, M.D.; Katherine O'Hanlon, M.D.; Toni Weschler, M.P.H.; Honora Lee Wolfe, Dipl. Ac.; Jonathan Wright, M.D.; Jing-Nuan Wu, L.Ac., O.M.D.

Gastrointestinal Disorders
Consultants: James Braly, M.D.; William Michael Cargile, B.S., D.C., F.I.A.C.A.; Patrick Donovan, N.D.; David L. Hoffmann, B.Sc., M.N.I.M.H.; Virender Sodhi, M.D. (Ayurveda), N.D.

Headaches
Consultants: James Braly, M.D.; David Bresler, Ph.D., L.Ac.; Donald Brown, N.D.; William Michael Cargile, B.S., D.C., F.I.A.C.A.; Leon Chaitow, N.D., D.O.; Michael Reed Gach, Ph.D.; Robert Milne, M.D.; James Privitera, M.D.; Harold Ravins, D.D.S.; Julian Whitaker, M.D.

Hearing Disorders
Consultants: William Crook, M.D., F.A.A.P., F.A.C.A., F.A.A.E.M.; Katie Data, N.D.; John Hibbs, N.D.; Roger Hirsh, O.M.D., L.Ac., Dipl. NCCA; David L. Hoffmann, B.Sc., M.N.I.M.H.; Constantine Kotsanis, M.D.; Robert D. Milne, M.D.; Michael Schmidt, B.S., D.C., C.C.N.; Virender Sodhi, M.D. (Ayurveda), N.D.; Billie M. Thompson, Ph.D.

Heart Disease
Contributing Writer: Joseph Hattersley, M.A.
Consultants: Harvery Bigelson, M.D.; William Lee Cowden, M.D.; Alan R. Gaby, M.D.; Charles Farr, M.D., Ph.D.; Abram Hoffer, M.D.; David L. Hoffmann, B.Sc., M.N.I.M.H.; Margaret Naeser, Ph.D.; Maoshing Ni, D.O.M., Ph.D., L.Ac.; Richard Passwater, Ph.D.; James Privitera, M.D.; Hari Sharma, M.D.; Virender Sodhi, M.D. (Ayurveda), N.D.

Hypertension
Consultants: Eric R. Braverman, M.D.; Leon Chaitow, N.D., D.O.; William Lee Cowden, M.D.; David L. Hoffmann, B.Sc., M.N.I.M.H.; Mark Holmes, O.M.D., L.Ac., Dipl. Acupuncture and Herbal Medicine (NCCA), Harvey Kaltsas, Ac. Phys. (FL), D.Ac. (RI), Dipl. Ac. (NCCA); Virender Sodhi, M.D. (Ayurveda), N.D.; Jonathan Wright, M.D.

Male Health
Contributing Writer: Tom Kruzel, N.D.
Consultants: Bruce McFarland, Ph.D.; Rick Maranelli, N.D., O.M.D.; Virender Sodhi, M.D. (Ayurveda), N.D.; Dana Ullman, M.P.H.

Mental Health
Consultants: Leon Chaitow, N.D., D.O.; Richard Kunin, M.D.; Harvey M. Ross, M.D.; Karl Humiston, M.D.; Doris Rapp, M.D.; Hugh Riordan, M.D.; Harvey M. Ross, M.D.; William Walsh, Ph.D.

Multiple Sclerosis
Contributing Writer: Judy Graham
Consultants: Stephen Davies, M.A., B.M., B.Ch. (England); Hal Huggins, D.D.S., M.S.; Patrick Kingsley, M.B.B.S., L.R.C.P., D.Obst., R.C.O.G. (England); Gary R. Oberg, M.D., F.A.A.P., F.A.A.E.M.; Hector Solorzano Del Rio, M.D., D.Sc. (Mexico); Roy Swank, M.D., Ph.D.

Obesity and Weight Management
Contributing Writer: Lauri Aesoph, N.D.
Consultants: Majid Ali, M.D.; Timothy Birdsall, N.D.; Erma Brown, B.S.N., P.H.N.; Nancy Dunne, N.D.; Zane Gard, M.D.; Elson M. Haas, M.D.; Susan Kano; Joseph Pizzorno, N.D.; Michelle Pouliot, N.D.; Gus Prosch, M.D.; David Shefrin, N.D.; Virender Sodhi, M.D. (Ayurveda), N.D.; Richard J. Wurtman, M.D.

Osteoporosis
Contributing Writer: John R. Lee, M.D.
Consultants: Nancy Appleton, Ph.D.; Alan R. Gaby, M.D.; David L. Hoffmann, B.Sc., M.N.I.M.H.; Andrew H. Lockie, M.R.C.G.P., M.F. Hom., Dip. Obst., R.C.O.G. (England); Katherine O'Hanlan, M.D.; Honora Lee Wolfe, Dipl. Ac.

Parasites
Contributing Writer: Mariel Tennison
Consultants: Steven Bailey, N.D.; Rita Bettenberg, N.D.; Maoshing Ni, D.O.M., Ph.D., L.Ac.; Virender Sodhi, M.D. (Ayurveda), N.D.; Murray R. Susser, M.D.

Pregnancy and Childbirth
Contributing Writer: Lauri Aesoph, N.D.
Consultants: Timothy Birdsall, N.D.; Helen Burst, R.N., M.Sc.; Roy Dittman, L.Ac., O.M.D.; Susanne Houd; Molly Linton, N.D., L.M.; Lendon H. Smith, M.D.

Respiratory Conditions
Contributing Writer: John Sherman, N.D.
Consultants: Richard Barrett, N.D.; James Braly, M.D.; William Michael Cargile, B.S., D.C., F.I.A.C.A.; Leon Chait[illegible] Alan R. [illegible] David L. Hoffmann, B.Sc., M.N.I.M.H.; Doug Lewis, N.D.; Joseph E. Pizzorno, N.D.

Sexually Transmitted Diseases
Contributing Writer: Tori Hudson, N.D.
Consultants: David L. Hoffmann, B.Sc., M.N.I.M.H.; Tom Kruzel, N.D.; Faizi Medeiros, N.D.; Jill Stansbury, N.D.

Sleep Disorders
Contributing Writer: John Zimmerman, Ph.D.
Consultants: Leon Chaitow, N.D., D.O.; William Lee Cowden, M.D.; Katie Data, N.D.; Steven Fahrion, Ph.D.; John Hibbs, N.D.; Roger Hirsh, O.M.D., L.Ac., Dipl. NCCA; David L. Hoffmann, B.Sc., M.N.I.M.H.; Konrad Kail, N.D.; John R. Lee, M.D.; Robert D. Milne, M.D.; Anthony Scott-Morley, D.Sc., Ph.D., B.A., B.Ac., M.D. (Alt. Med.); Virender Sodhi, M.D. (Ayurveda), N.D.; Richard S. Wilkinson, M.D.; Jonathan Wright, M.D.

Stress
Contributing Writer: Konrad Kail, N.D.
Consultants: William Lee Cowden, M.D.; Steven Fahrion, Ph.D.; Daniel Gagnon, Medical Herbalist; John Hibbs, N.D.; Jon Kabat-Zinn, Ph.D.; Maoshing Ni, D.O.M., Ph.D., L.Ac.; Harvey M. Ross, M.D.; Martin L. Rossman, M.D.; Hari Sharma, M.D.; Virender Sodhi, M.D. (Ayurveda), N.D.

Vision Disorders
Consultants: Moses Albalas, O.D., Ph.D., L.Ac.; John Downing, O.D.; Steven Fahrion, Ph.D.; Alan R. Gaby, M.D.; Ray Gottleib, O.D., Ph.D.; David L. Hoffmann, B.Sc., M.N.I.M.H.; Maoshing Ni, D.O.M., Ph.D., L.Ac.; Joseph E. Pizzorno, N.D.; Virender Sodhi, M.D. (Ayurveda), N.D.; Glen Swartwout, O.D.; Gary Todd, M.D.; Joseph Trachtman, O.D., Ph.D.; John E. Upledger, D.O., O.M.M.; Jonathan Wright, M.D.

Quick Reference A-Z Section of Health Conditions and Treatments

Senior Editor Quick Reference Section
D. Lindsey Berkson, M.A., D.C., Nutritionist and Educator, Santa Fe, New Mexico

Acupuncture
Consultant: Maoshing Ni, D.O.M., Ph.D., L.Ac., Vice-President, Yosan University of Traditional Chinese Medicine, Santa Monica, California

Applied Kinesiology
[illegible] George Goodheart, D.C., of Groose Pointe Woods, Michigan, Research Director, International College of Applied Kinesiology

Aromatherapy
Consultant: Ann Berwick, of Boulder, Colorado, Founder and President, The National Association of Holistic Aromatherapy

Ayurveda
Consultant: Dr. Vasant Lad, M.A.Sc., Director of The Ayurvedic Institute in Albuquerque, New Mexico

Biofeedback Training
Consultant: Marjorie Toomim, Ph.D., Director, Biofeedback Institute of Los Angeles

Bodywork

- ***Acupressure*:**
  Consultant: Michael Reed Gach, Ph.D., Director, The Acupressure Institute, Berkeley, California
- ***Alexander Technique*:**
  Consultant: Frank Ottowell, Alexander Training Institute, San Francisco
- ***Aston Patterning*:**
  Consultant: Judith Aston, Founder and Director, The Aston Training Center, Incline Village, Nevada
- ***Feldenkrais:***
  Consultant: Bonnie Humiston, President, The Feldenkrais Guild, Albany, Oregon
- ***Hellerwork*:**
  Consultant: Joseph Heller, President of The Body of Knowledge/Hellerwork, Mt. Shasta, California
- ***Massage*:**
  Consultant: Eileen Henry, C.A., C.M.T., Director, Institute of Psycho-Structural Balancing (IPSB), Santa Monica, California
- ***Myotherapy:***
  Consultant: Bonnie Prudden, Founder and Director, Bonnie Prudden, Inc., Stockbridge, Massachusetts
- ***Reflexology:***
  Consultant: Dwight Byers, President, International Institute of Reflexology, St. Petersburg, Florida
- ***Rolfing:***
  Consultant: Jeff Maitland, Faculty Chair, The Rolf Institute, Boulder, Colorado
- ***Therapeutic Touch*:**
  Consultant: Dolores Krieger, R.N., Ph.D., Founder of Therapeutic Touch
- ***Trager*:**
  Consultant: Deane Juhan, Instructor, Trager Institue, Mill Valley, California

Cell Therapy
Consultant: Peter Stephan, M.D., Director, The Stephan Clinic, London, England

Chelation Therapy
Consultant: Elmer Cranton, M.D., of Troutdale, Virginia, past President, The American College of Advancement in Medicine

Chiropractic
Consultant: Stuart Garber, D.C., Director, Westside Health Clinic, Los Angeles, California

Colon Therapy
Consultant: Connie Allred, President, American Colon Therapy Association

Craniosacral Therapy
Consultant: Robert Norett, D.C., Director of Stillpoint Health Center, Venice, California

Detoxification Therapy
Consultant: Elson Haas, M.D., Director, Marin Clinic of Preventive Medicine and Health, San Rafael, California

Diet
Consultant: D. Lindsey Berkson, M.A., D.C., nutritionist and educator, Santa Fe, New Mexico

Environmental Medicine
Consultant: Marshall Mandell, M.D., F.A.C.A.I., F.A.A.E.M., Medical Director, New England Foundation for Allergic and Environmental Diseases, Norwalk, Connecticut

Enzyme Therapy
Consultant: Hector Solorzano, M.D., D.Sc., Coordinator of the Program for Studies of Alternative Medicine; Professor of Pharmacology at the University of Guadalajara in Mexico

Fasting
Consultant: Steven Bailey, N.D., Graduate Assistant Professor, National College of Naturopathic Medicine; Director of the Northwest Naturopathic Clinic in Portland, Oregon

Flower Remedies
Consultant: Julian Barnard, of Hereford, England, author of *Guide to the Bach Flower Remedies* and *The Healing Herbs of Edward Bach*

Guided Imagery
Consultant: Martin L. Rossman, M.D., Founder and Co-director, Academy of Guided Imagery, Mill Valley, California

Herbs
Consultant: David L. Hoffmann, B.Sc., M.N.I.M.H., past President, The American Herbalists Guild

Homeopathy
Consultant: Trevor Cook, Ph.D., D.I. Hom., President of the United Kingdom Homeopathic Medical Association; Director, British Institute of Homeopathy

Hydrotherapy
Consultant: Douglas Lewis, N.D., Chairperson, Department of Physical Medicine, Bastyr College, Seattle, Washington

Hypnotherapy
Consultant: A.M. Krassner, Ph.D., Founder and Director, American Institute of Hypnotherapy, Santa Ana, California

Juice Therapy
Consultant: Steven Bailey, N.D., Graduate Assistant Professor, National College of Naturopathic Medicine; Director, The Northwest Naturopathic Clinic in Portland, Oregon

Light Therapy
Consultant: Glen Swartwout, O.D., founder, Achievement of Excellence Research Academy International, Hilo, Hawaii

Magnetic Field Therapy
Consultant: William H. Philpott, M.D., Chairman, Bio-Electro-Magnetic Institute Institutional Review Board

Naturopathic Medicine
Consultant: Joseph E. Pizzorno, N.D., President of Bastyr College, Seattle, Washington

Neural Therapy
Consultant: James Carlson, D.O., of Knoxville, Tennessee, past President, American Association of Orthopedic Medicine

Nutritional Supplements
Consultant: D. Lindsey Berkson, M.A., D.C., nutritionist and educator, Santa Fe, New Mexico

Orthomolecular Medicine
Consultant: Abram Hoffer, M.D., Ph.D., Editor-in-Chief, *Journal of Orthomolecular Medicine*; President, Canadian Schizophrenia Foundation

Osteopathy
Consultant: Leon Chaitow, N.D., D.O., Editor, *Journal of Alternative and Complimentary Medicine*; Director, Nutrition and Health Research Associates, London, England

Oxygen Therapy

- ***Hydrogen Peroxide Therapy***
  Consultant: Charles Farr, M.D., Ph.D., Medical Director, International Bio-oxidative Medicine Association; Medical Director, Genesis Medical Center, Oklahoma City, Oklahoma
- ***Hyperbaric Oxygen Therapy***
  Consultant: David Hughes, D.Sc., Director, The Hyperbaric Oxygen Institute, San Bernardino, California
- ***Ozone Therapy***
  Consultant: Gerard V. S[illegible], Associ[illegible] Psychiatry, The New York University-Bellevue Hospital Medical Center

Qigong
Consultant: Roger Jahnke, L.Ac., O.M.D., Director, Health Action, Santa Barbara, California

Reconstructive Therapy
Consultant: William Faber, D.O., Milwaukee Pain Clinic, Milwaukee, Wisconsin

Traditional Chinese Medicine
Consultant: Roger Hirsh, O.M.D., L.Ac., NCCA, Doctor of Oriental Medicine, Director, Metamedical Group, Santa Monica, California

Yoga
Consultant: Rudolph Ballentine, M.D., author, Board of Trustees, Medical Staff, Himalayan Institute

Appendices

Antibiotics
Contributing Writer: Michael Schmidt, B.S., D.C., C.C.N., Director, Brookview Health Sciences, Anoka, Minnesota

Probiotics
Contributing Writer: Leon Chaitow, N.D., D.O., Director, Nutrition and Health Research Associates, London, England; Editor, *Journal of Alternative and Complementary Medicine*

Key to Professional Titles

Ac. Phys.	Acupuncture Physician
B.M.	Bachelor of Medicine
B.M.E.D.	Bachelor of Music Education
B.Sc.	Bachelor of Science
B.S.N.	Bachelor of Science in Nursing
C.A.	Certified Acupuncturist
C.C.N.	Certified Clinical Nutritionist
Ch.B.	Bachelor of Surgery
C.Ht.	Certified Hypnotherapist
C.N.	Certified Nutritionist
D. Ac.	Diplomate of Acupuncture
D.C.	Doctor of Chiropractic
D.D.S.	Doctor of Dental Science
D.H.A.N.P.	Diplomate of Homeopathic Academy of Naturopathic Physicians
D.Hom.(Med)	Diplomate of Homeopathic Medicine
D.I.B.A.K.	Diplomate of the International Board of Applied Kinesiology
D.I.Hom.	Diplomate of the Institute of Homeopathy
Dipl. Ac.	Diplomate of Acupuncture (NCCA)
Dipl. C.H.	Diplomate of Chinese Herbs
D.M.D.	Doctor of Dental Medicine
D.O.	Doctor of Osteopathy
D.O.M.	Doctor of Oriental Medicine
D.Sc.	Doctor of Science
D.V.M.	Doctor of Veterinary Medicine
F.A.A.E.M.	Fellow of the American Academy of Environmental Medicine
F.A.A.F.P.	Fellow of the American Academy of Family Practice
F.A.A.P.	Fellow of the American Academy of Pediatrics
F.A.A.P.M.	Fellow of the American Academy of Physical Medicine
F.A.C.A.	Fellow of the American College of Allergists
F.Ac.A.	Fellow of the Acupuncture Association (British)
F.A.C.A.I.	Fellow of the American College of Allergy and Immunology
F.A.C.N.	Fellow of the College of Nutrition
F.A.C.S.	Fellow of the American College of Surgeons
F.A.C.O.G.	Fellow of the American College of Obstetricians and Gynecologists
F.A.G.D.	Fellow of the Academy of General Dentistry
F.A.O.A.S.	Fellow of the American Osteopathic Academy of Sclerotherapy
F.I.A.C.A.	Fellow of the International Academy of Certified Acupuncturists
F.I.A.O.M.T.	Fellow of the International Academy of Oral Medicine and Toxicology
F.I.C.A.N.	Fellow of the International College of Applied Nutrition
F.I.C.C.	Fellow of the International College of Chiropractors
F.I.C.S.	Fellow of the International College of Surgeons
F.N.A.A.O.M.	Fellow of the National Academy of Acupuncture and Oriental Medicine
F.N.T.O.S.	Fellow of the Natural Therapeutic and Osteopathic Society
F.R.C.Psy.	Fellow of the Royal College of Psychiatry
H.M.D.	Homeopathic Medical Doctor
L.Ac.	Licensed Acupuncturist
L.C.S.W.	Licensed Clinical Social Worker
Lic. Ac.	Licensed Acupuncturist
L.M.T.	Licensed Massage Therapist
M.A.	Master of Arts
M.Ac.O.M.	Master of Acupuncture and Oriental Medicine
M.D.	Medical Doctor
M.F.Hom.	Member of the Faculty Homeopathy (British)
M.N.I.M.H.	Member of the National Institutes of Medical Herbalist (British)
M.P.H.	Master of Public Health
M.R.C.G.P.	Member of the Royal College of General Practitioners (British)
M.R.C.P.	Member of the Royal College of Physicians (British)
M.S.	Master of Science
NCCA	National Commission for the Certification of Acupuncturists
N.D.	Doctor of Naturopathy
N.M.D.	Naturopathic Medical Doctor
O.M.D.	Oriental Medical Doctor
O.M.M.	Osteopath Manipulative Medicine
P.H.N.	Public Health Nurse
R.C.O.G.	Royal College of Obstetricians and Gynecologists
R.D.	Registered Dietician
rer. nat.	Rerum Naturalium
R.M.T.	Registered Music Therapist
R.N.	Registered Nurse

Why This Book Was Written

My name is Burton Goldberg, and I've been a businessman for over forty years. My interest is in results, so let us get right to the point.

Two systems of health care are available in this country today: conventional Western medicine and alternative medicine. The first is the world of the American Medical Association; medical doctors who practice by the book, and who inadvertently align themselves with the multibillion dollar pharmaceutical industry. Conventional medicine is superb when it comes to surgery, emergency, and trauma.

But there's no question that alternative medicine works better for just about everything else, especially for chronic degenerative diseases like cancer, heart disease, rheumatoid arthritis, and for more common ailments such as asthma, gastrointestinal disorders, headaches, and sinusitis.

Alternative medicine has a lot to offer you. But our government is ignoring its well-established methods, and federal funds are not being sufficiently allocated to study them. We should all be asking, "Why?"

And that's the reason for this book. It represents the collective wisdom of thousands of alternative physicians and practitioners worldwide who are practicing the medicine of the future today.

The alternatives in this book are sound, based on science, and really work. Many are natural, as opposed to drug-based therapies. I've seen dramatic healing in a wide range of serious cases, without the disturbing side effects mainstream medicine so often creates. The damage of strokes can be reversed, if caught early enough. Even the symptoms of AIDS can be reversed. The procedures are available and being used now, but you won't hear about them from your doctor.

Alternative medicine is more cost-effective over the long term. Because it emphasizes prevention and goes after causes rather than symptoms, it doesn't trap people on the merry-go-round that begins with one drug, and ends up requiring them to take others to compensate for the side effects each one causes. Many alternative methods works by assisting your own body to heal itself instead of introducing strong drugs.

You probably know someone who has had the experience of getting rid of one illness, only to come down with another from the procedure used by the doctor. Maybe that someone is you. People I love, including my own son and both of my parents, have suffered through medical procedures that were unnecessarily traumatic because their physicians neglected the basics. And yes, that makes me angry. But rather than hold onto that anger, I'm going to work with you to change the system, by channeling our consumer medical dollars toward a more humane and effective medicine. Too many mainstream doctors today become so specialized they treat the body parts and forget they are treating a whole human being. Disease usually appears as a local symptom, but it is always related to the entire system. So you have to treat the whole person to cure the disease, and not just the symptom.

Naturally, you are thinking, if these methods were really any good, doctors would be using them. But it takes time for new ideas to be accepted. Back in Vienna in the 1800s, one doctor had the audacity to suggest to his colleagues that they wash their hands after they finish working on cadavers, rather than using their *unwashed hands* to deliver babies. He knew this would keep the women and their babies alive, by sparing them infections. But his colleagues ridiculed him. It took them thirty years to catch on and wash their hands. Imagine how many babies died because of such doctors who thought they knew it all?

I never expected the study of alternative medicine to become the passion of my life. But when the nineteen-year-old daughter of the woman I loved tried to commit suicide by slitting her wrists, I had to find a way to help. Most people would send her to a psychologist and figure that's the answer. But it wasn't the answer. Her therapist finally threw his hands up and suggested vitamin therapy, so we pursued it. We found out that the daughter's mental distress was caused by hypoglycemia, an imbalance created by food allergies, problems in her pancreas, and an overgrowth of bad bacteria in her gastrointestinal tract. When she was treated for hypoglycemia, her mental illness disappeared. That troubled nineteen-year-old is now a healthy mother of eight children—seven girls and a boy.

That's how it started for me—seeing people who had serious mental illness being cured just by changing their lifestyle and diet and taking nutritional supplements. The amazing success I saw got me hooked. One Connecticut doctor, Marshall Mandell, M.D., dramatically showed me how a person's state of mind could be affected when a substance to which they were allergic was placed under the tongue. He brought a very bright woman in and out of depression simply by placing different substances under her tongue. A single dose of one substance to which she was allergic caused her to put her head between her knees and cry. When she was given a relieving dose, she experienced instantaneous release.

This episode sparked my interest in environmental medicine, the study of how substances affect the body. From there I went on to study such alternatives as homeopathy, electromagnetic diagnosing and treatment, mind/body medicine, and the newest protocols for cancer and AIDS. After attending alternative medical conventions with a doctor who could explain doctor talk to me, my interest in new concepts in health care led me to Western Europe, Russia, and Israel. There I discovered people being cured of diseases, even the most serious, by methods never even heard of in our country. It is possible to reverse chronic disease. Many of the health problems you face can be solved simply, directly, and inexpensively without toxic side effects.

I keep checking out what's out there, what's new and what works. Your well-being—and that of every member of your family—depends upon knowing about these alternatives. That's why a team of over 350 medical doctors, naturopaths, osteopaths, homeopaths, chiropractors, acupuncturists, scientists, researchers, and reporters have been assembled under the auspices of Future Medicine, Inc. to produce this work. This story has never been told before.

In Part One we will lay out the new principles in medicine. You'll learn what causes disease, what you can do to counter it, why so much of this important information is being suppressed, and what steps you can take to help bring about change.You'll also learn how to find the best health care practitioners for you and your family.

In Part Two we'll introduce you to a wide range of alternative methods of treatment. Each chapter will tell you how each particular method of treatment works, what conditions it is best suited for treating, and how to use it yourself or locate a qualified practitioner.

In Part Three we describe how alternative medicine treats epidemic twentieth century diseases like AIDS, cancer, heart disease, and chronic pain. Over 30 conditions are covered in depth, with over 175 more cross-referenced alphabetically to provide you with information on the best self-care and professional treatments that deal with them. A more extensive cross-referencing of health conditions is provided in the index.

We've researched this in-depth, and now are ready to give you the straight story. Busy people don't like to waste their time. I've tried to give you the information as concisely as possible and in a way that is simple to understand. Our work is ongoing and we are committed to continuing our investigation and reporting the most current discoveries in alternative medicine.

Let me conclude by saying that I'm not against mainstream, conventional medicine. The Chinese have a saying about the wisdom of "walking on both feet," which means using the best of Eastern and Western procedures. That's what I want to see us do. There is no single approach that works for all people, or with all conditions. This goes for alternative medicine as well.

Experience shows that you're likely to get the best results with a practitioner who has trained in a number of different modalities. There may be many underlying factors influencing your health—nutritional deficiency, poor digestion, toxicity from environmental pollutants, or mental and emotional stress. You want a practitioner who is capable of determining exactly what needs to be done to help you regain health and vitality. You also want an open-minded practitioner who treats you as an individual. What's good for Harry is not necessarily good for Mary. You are biochemically unique.

Here is a most important, optimistic, and totally realistic thought to carry with you. Most everything is reversible. You need only to find the right therapies.

Be well!

Burton Goldberg

"My dear Kepler, what do you say of the leading philosophers here, to whom I have offered a thousand times of my own accord to show my studies, but who, with the lazy obstinacy of a serpent who has eaten his fill, have never consented to look at the planets or moon, or telescope? Verily, just as serpents close their ears, so do men close their eyes to the light of truth."

—Galileo in a letter to Johannes Kepler ca. 1630

Part One: The Future of Medicine

An Important Message

This book is intended as an educational tool to acquaint the reader with alternative methods for the maintenance of good health and the treatment of illness. The publisher hopes the book will enable the reader to improve his or her well-being and to better understand, assess, and choose the appropriate course of treatment for an illness or health condition. Because the methods described in this book are, by definition, **alternative** methods, many of them have not been investigated and/or approved by any government or regulatory agency. National, state, and local laws vary regarding the use and application of many of the treatments that are discussed. Accordingly, this book should not be substituted for the advice and treatment of a physician or other licensed health professional, but rather should be used in conjunction with professional care. Pregnant women in particular are especially urged to consult with their physician before using any therapy.

Your health is important. Use this book wisely. Discuss the alternative treatment options described herein with your doctor. Ultimately, you, the reader, must take full responsibility for your health and how you use this book. The publisher expressly disclaims responsibility for any adverse effects resulting from your use of the information contained herein.

A New Understanding of Alternative Medicine

"The doctor of the future will give no medicine, but will interest his patients in the care of the human frame, in diet, and in the cause and prevention of disease."

—Thomas Edison

In the face of an increasingly inadequate system of conventional medicine, a growing number of people are turning to alternative medicine to address their needs. The general public is starting to recognize the effectiveness of alternative medicine's approach to health, which blends body and mind, science and experience, and traditional and cross-cultural avenues of diagnosis and treatment. In fact, a recent study published in the *New England Journal of Medicine* found that over one-third of those surveyed chose alternative medicine over conventional methods, because of the medical establishment's emphasis on diagnostic testing and treatment with drugs without focusing on the patient as a whole.[1] It is obvious that what was once considered a "fringe" interest is now on its way to becoming the primary medical approach of the next millennium.

The Crisis in Modern Medicine

It is no secret that our contemporary United States medical system is in a state of terrible disarray. Though conventional medicine excels in the management of medical emergencies, certain bacterial infections, trauma care, and many, often heroically complex surgical techniques, it seems to have failed miserably in the areas of disease prevention and the management of the myriad new and chronic illnesses presently filling our hospitals and physicians' offices. In addition, as a nation we pay more for our medical care and accomplish less than most other nations of comparable living standards, while health care costs continue to spiral out of control.

Treatment of chronic disease currently accounts for 85 percent of the national health care bill.[2] This state of affairs is due to the fact that we spend almost nothing to treat the causes of chronic disease before major illness develops, according to a report from the American Association of Naturopathic Physicians. "We wait for it [illness] to develop and then spend huge sums on heroic measures, even then ignoring the underlying lifestyle-related causes. This is the equivalent of waiting for a leaky roof to destroy the infrastructure of a house and then repairing the damage without fixing the leak. This is naturally expensive and ineffective.

"Perhaps the greatest evidence of the depth of the crisis is that we have come to accept such levels of chronic disease as normal, despite evidence that much of it is preventable. [Former] Surgeon General C. Everett Koop, in his 1988 Report on Nutrition and Health, points out that 'dietary imbalances' are the leading preventable contributors to premature death in the U.S. and recommends the expansion of nutrition and lifestyle-modification education for all health care professionals."[3] This is borne out by the Centers for Disease Control, which state that 54 percent of heart disease, 37 percent of cancer, 50 percent of cerebrovascular disease, and 49 percent of atherosclerosis (hardening of the arteries) is preventable through lifestyle modification.[4]

The changes that are necessary, however, will not be implemented as long as physicians earn their living and win renown primarily by delivering rescue medicine (interventions that simply treat symptoms), since it is in this area and not prevention that they benefit most. If the United States is to be saved from catastrophic health care costs, it is time to take a good look at the wisdom and cost-effectiveness of alternative medicine.

"If the United States is to be saved from catastrophic health care costs, it is time to take a good look at the wisdom and cost-effectiveness of alternative medicine."

Doctors are confronted daily with patients suffering from illnesses for which conventional medicine offers only superficial treatment of symptoms. The magic of antibiotics is vanishing as a host of resistant infections emerge; diseases such as AIDS and chronic fatigue syndrome have shown us clearly that our present treatments are simply not effective and hint at new health problems which may lie ahead.

The metaphor of a modern plague may be appropriate. Growing numbers of people lack vitality and suffer from a host of complaints difficult to define. Most adults, and many children, today suffer from complaints including allergies, headaches, lack of energy, excessive fatigue, and various digestive and respiratory disorders, along with a variety of emotional states ranging from mild depression to mood swings and anxiety.

They are manifesting what Jeffrey Bland, Ph.D., of Gig Harbor, Washington, calls a state of "vertical ill-health." "They are not sick enough to lie down (in which case they would become 'horizontally ill') and yet consider themselves 'normal' because most of the people they know are equally unhealthy," explains Leon Chaitow, N.D., D.O., of London, England. "They derive only limited benefit from the flood of tranquilizers, antidepressants, analgesics, and anti-inflammatory drugs they are commonly prescribed, while the side effects they develop from these drugs just add to their list of woes."

Thoughtful physicians are becoming increasingly aware that something is wrong with their patients' immune systems, since they continue to suffer from illnesses which normal immune function should be able to deal with. Yet this decline in immune efficiency is something contemporary medical treatments seem unable to do anything about. Doctors and patients alike are perplexed by this failure of drug-based therapies to bring relief. As a result, patients often become trapped in a cycle of dependency on physicians to monitor and constantly adjust their medications rather than becoming empowered to change lifestyle factors that might allow their body to regain its healthful potential.

"Most over-the-counter and almost all prescribed drug treatments merely mask symptoms or control health problems, or in some way alter the way organs or systems such as the circulatory system work," states John R. Lee, M.D., of Sebastopol, California. "Drugs almost never deal with the reasons why these problems exist, while they frequently create new health problems as side effects of their activities.

"People realize that their headaches are not due to aspirin deficiency or that their hypertension is not being properly addressed by prescriptions of drugs that merely induce diuresis [excessive urine excretion]. They are seeking answers that address the root causes of their health problems and aid in restoring normal, healthy body function. This is not to say that treatment of the symptoms of a condition is wrong. What would be wrong would be to think that by eliminating the symptom we have dealt with the problem itself."

> *"Most over-the-counter and almost all prescribed drug treatments merely mask symptoms or control health problems or in some way alter the way organs or systems such as the circulatory system work. Drugs almost never deal with the reasons why these problems exist, while they frequently create new health problems as side effects of their activities."*
>
> —John R. Lee, M.D.

Roots of the Crisis

The underlying concepts of alternative medicine are not new. They represent a return to the principles that have been part of human understanding of health and disease for thousands of years. Over the centuries, medical wisdom evolved within a framework which linked health to a state of harmony or balance, and disease to a state of disharmony or imbalance, and took into account the factors that contributed to both.

"The genius of the ancient Greek physician Hippocrates, the father of Western medicine, was not in the drugs he used or his diagnostic skills," Dr. Lee points out, "but in his insight that the elements which were needed to produce and maintain health were natural, and that they included hygiene, a calm balanced mental state, proper diet, a sound work and home environment, and physical conditioning. In addition, he recognized the life forces that pervade all of nature, and which have multiple expressions—some known, some theorized, and many unknown. He taught that health depended upon living in harmony with these forces." Recognition of these life forces is also vital to Traditional Chinese Medicine and Ayurvedic medicine from India.

A Dangerous Detour

In the mid-nineteenth century, following the discovery of disease-causing microbes, a departure from this philosophy of health occurred due to rival theories concerning the cause of disease. One theory was that infecting microbes called germs (viruses, bacteria, and fungi) were the cause of illness. The opposing theory maintained that these microbes only became infectious if conditions inside the body were right for them. According to this theory, by keeping the internal environment of the body healthy, these potential agents of infection will remain dormant.

When the germ theory of disease became dominant, the birth of contemporary medicine, with its emphasis on infectious causes of diseases rather than physiologic balance or harmony, occurred. This provided medical science with the opportunity to greatly expand its role in the treatment of illness. This was followed by the rapid development of microscopy, bacterial cultures, vaccines, x-ray, and in the 1930s, the discovery of antibacterial drugs such as penicillin and sulfa drugs. However, the more that medical science embraced the germ theory of disease, the more it also superseded the individual's role in his or her own health.

The Purpose of Medicine: War or Repair?

The thrust of twentieth century medicine can be described by the metaphor of war. Disease is considered an invasion by an enemy and treatment is aimed at developing "magic bullets" in the form of drugs and vaccines to eliminate that enemy. We have seen, for example, a failed "war on cancer," a proliferation of antibiotics, and a growing number of surgical procedures, cell-killing radiation treatments, and chemical medications (such as chemotherapy), all of which do harm to the body, in one form or another, in their attempts to restore health.

Lost in this approach is the concept of repairing the imbalances which allow the illnesses to occur in the first place. Medical science has become one-sided in its focus, increasingly losing sight of the whole person in its attempt to treat the body's individual parts.

"A more useful metaphor for medicine would be repair, not war," says Dr. Lee. "If we think of the body as a house, we see that problems lie in the gaps and breakdowns that occur in the foundation, allowing various pests to make their way inside. The contemporary physician addresses this problem by selling you poisons or traps to kill or catch the pests. But this still doesn't prevent other undesirables from coming in through the gaps in the future. How much better it would be for your physician to learn where the holes are and help you to repair them, while teaching you how to prevent them from occurring again."

> *"As long as providers make their income and fame largely by delivering 'rescue' medicine, they will have less economic interest in prevention."*
> —Paul Mencel, *Medical Costs, Moral Choices*

Because the emphasis of conventional medicine remains upon war and not repair, it has led to the organization of medical schools with their various departments, such as cardiology, nephrology, neurology, dermatology, orthopedics, and psychiatry. This forces students to focus their study on one organ system at a time as if each bodily organ functioned independently of all the others; or to choose one for exclusive study in preparation for a career in medicine as a "specialist" in that organ system. "Our system of disease classification is based on specific organs as well," notes Dr. Lee. "We name our diseases by the organ that is being affected. Thus we have arthritis, tonsillitis, appendicitis, heart or gallbladder disease, colitis, prostatitis, and many other examples. We even name the cancer we get by the organ it affects. This diverts attention away from the intrinsic interrelatedness of all parts of our body and the complex dynamism of life forces. It is no wonder that our 'modern' doctors understand so little of holistic concepts of health."

WHY CONVENTIONAL DOCTORS THINK THE WAY THEY DO

When people first hear about alternative medical treatments they often ask the obvious question: "If this treatment is so effective, why doesn't my doctor know about it?"

According to John R. Lee, M.D., of Sebastopol, California, there are a number of reasons for this. "The first reason lies in the fact that the selection process of medical students depends in large part on college grades," says Dr. Lee. "Students get high grades when they simply repeat in their tests exactly what the teacher wants them to say. Students who question what they are being taught, on the other hand, usually do not get the higher grades. Medical schools therefore are filled with students who are good at adopting given 'wisdom', but not necessarily good at thinking and questioning, because they have learned to follow precepts handed to them by presumed authorities."

The second reason that accounts for the way many doctors think is that medical schools tend to be organized into organ-specific departments. "The idea of an underlying link between these different departmentalized diseases is nonexistent within this framework," Dr. Lee says. "Furthermore, the influence of nutrition on the way cells function is ignored or derided by many department heads who defend their own orthodox concepts."

The third reason is one of simple economics. "When leaving medical school, the young doctor finds him- or herself in a system that rewards what is called 'rescue' medicine, or interventions that treat symptoms," Dr. Lee explains. "There is no reward, and there may well be scorn from fellow doctors, for those who take the time and trouble to try and prevent illness or attempt to correct nutritional deficiencies which may be causing the patients' conditions. Medical record keeping and billing for insurance also require doctors to adhere to this superficial, organ classification of disease. Economic rewards follow only from sticking to this particular model of ill-health and treatment."

Malpractice is another great fear among doctors. "People should note that the definition of malpractice is not whether the practice is 'good' or 'bad' for the patient, but rather if the practice in question is what other doctors in the given locality normally do or prescribe," says Dr. Lee. He adds that doctors also, quite naturally, seek the professional and social approval of their peers. "Both of these factors conspire to 'keep the doctor in line', limiting the likelihood of a doctor adopting some unconventional practices techniques."

Why Are We Ill?

Health is far more than the absence of disease. When we are healthy all the bodily systems and functions are harmoniously balanced and integrated with each other and we are also in balance with our environment. In this state of equilibrium our defense mechanisms and our immune system can efficiently handle most of the hazards that life presents, whether these are pathogenic (disease-causing) organisms, toxic substances, or stress factors of various kinds.

Foundations of Health

According to Dr. Chaitow, positive health depends upon three factors, which are interconnected. The first of these is the body's structural system, including all of the muscles, bones, ligaments, nerves, blood vessels, and organs, and their functions. The second factor is the body's biochemical processes, which involve the absorption and utilization of nutrients, and the elimination of wastes, along with the complicated biochemical relationships which are the key to cellular function and health. The third factor comprises the mind and emotions, as well as the spiritual dimension of each person.

"When there is a balanced, energetic, interplay between these three components we have health," Dr. Chaitow says. "But when imbalances exist within any of these factors, or in their relationships with each other, ill-health occurs."

Homeostasis

In a state of health, if we cut ourselves, we heal. If we are bruised, strained, or suffer a broken bone, healing starts immediately. If we are exposed to infection our immune system deals with it. These examples are illustrations of the body's natural tendency towards repairing itself. This tendency is known as homeostasis, the maintenance of the body's internal organs and defenses to compensate for external health hazards.

When homeostasis is called into play to handle a "crisis," its activity is usually experienced as "symptoms." For example, when you are exposed to an infection your body will mount an aggressive defensive response which might result in fever. Or, should you injure yourself, the healing process which starts immediately might involve inflammation and swelling of the traumatized area. In other words, under normal conditions, the body will attempt to heal itself without help, and the symptoms produced will indicate what sort of healing process is going on. Unfortunately many people, including all too many physicians, rather than respecting these homeostatic processes and simply waiting for them to finish their tasks, will actively try to suppress the symptoms of self-repair, whether this be a raised temperature or inflammation in an injured area. When this occurs, we are in effect saying that we know more than our body's innate intelligence about what is good for it.

"It is more important to know what sort of person has a disease than to know what sort of disease a person has."
—Hippocrates (460-377 B.C.)

In order to maintain good health, therefore, it is important to recognize that many symptoms are actually evidence that healing is underway, and that, unless they are actually unbearable or dangerous, the symptoms should be left alone so that the repair processes can be completed.

Stress Adaptation

The late Canadian physiologist Hans Selye developed a model of how the body copes with stress which he called the general adaptation syndrome (GAS). The three stages of GAS offer a clear explanation of how and why nearly all forms of illness develop.

In Dr. Selye's model, the initial acute reaction to any irritant or stress factor is called the Alarm Stage. An example of this stage occurs when a muscle in the body is overworked. Soreness will follow, and the muscle may even become inflamed. In a state of health, such symptoms will quickly pass, and the muscle will return to its normal state within a day or two as the self-regulating, balancing mechanisms of homeostasis do their work.

However, if the muscle is continuously overworked, or exposed to additional strains from other stress factors, it will eventually start to adapt and accommodate itself to the repetitive stress factor in order to cope with the demands of the stress in ways beyond those of the Alarm Stage. Eventually, the body as a whole will also begin adapting itself in this same manner, at which point, the second, or Resistance Stage comes into play.

This stage is usually without symptoms at first, and it can last for many years. In fact, Resistance Stage adaptation lasts for as many years as the body's resources and reserves will allow, while the body continues its attempts to repair itself. Depending upon individual genetic makeup, as well as factors such as nutritional deficiencies, traumas, illnesses, medications, and surgeries which have been acquired in life, the ability to continue to adapt and resist will vary significantly from person to person. This explains why two people faced with apparently identical challenges will respond quite differently. One might meet the challenge with no sign of difficulty, while the other might collapse into serious ill-health.

Most people will display the collection of minor symptoms which seem to have become the norm of Dr. Bland's "vertically ill" as they cope with life's stresses, whether these be structural, biochemical, or emotional. It is at the end of the Resistance Stage, when a person's adaptive mechanisms begin to fail, that the final stage of GAS results, known as the Exhaustion Stage. At this point, the person's ability to cope with repetitive, and often multiple, stress factors will inevitably lead into actual disease, usually of a chronic nature.

See Stress.

Returning to the example of the overworked muscle, one can clearly see how each of these stages would progress. When a muscle is first overworked, the Alarm Stage reaction manifests as pain, stiffness, and perhaps inflammation. If this stress of overwork becomes chronic, during the Resistance Stage the muscle would become increasingly less elastic and more fibrous, placing stress on the points where it is anchored into bone. This creates additional problems of pain, coordination difficulties, and stress on the joints. Left untreated, the muscle will eventually enter into the Exhaustion Stage, with the fibrousness and inflammation possibly degenerating into fibrositis (muscular rheumatism), and the joints, due to the uneven wear and tear caused by muscular imbalances, would show signs of arthritis.

It is the interaction between what is being adapted to and the individual's reserves and resources which decides when, and at [illegible] health will result. To use another [illegible] high blood pressure by prescribin[illegible] would possibly be effective in momentarily lowering blood pressure, but if it is being caused by emotional stress or improper diet, the underlying causes would be unaffected and could soon result in additional problems elsewhere in the body. Helping the person learn to better deal with his or her emotions, or instructing him or her in the role proper diet and nutrition plays in overall health, would be far more effective long-term approaches.

"The same principles apply to all health problems," states Dr. Chaitow. "If we can remove the cause of the problem, increase the powers of adaptation and resistance, or, ideally, do both of these, we restore the opportunity for the self-regulating mechanisms of homeostasis to operate again and healing can begin."

Other Factors Contributing to Illness

As a growing number of patients struggle with illnesses involving depressed immune function and overstressed hormonal and nervous systems, physicians must cope with the fact that these illnesses simply do not respond to the types of treatments being offered by conventional medicine today. To better understand this situation, we must first look at some of the factors influencing our health.

Genetics: From our parents we receive our genetic inheritance, and are born with constitutional strengths and weaknesses over which we have no control. External factors provide additional layers of influence which act on our genetically acquired ability to adapt and cope.

See Diet, Nutritional Supplements.

Diet: Emmanuel Cheraskin, M.D., D.M.D., of Birmingham, Alabama, pictures the sick individual as a layered "onion" whose signs and symptoms serve as the onion's outer layers, with layers of biochemical imbalance laying underneath. At the core of the onion, according to Dr. Cheraskin's research, lies poor diet.

That diet is so essential to health is not surprising. The foods and liquids we consume, along with the air that we breathe, have a fundamental effect on our well-being. A healthy diet of pesticide-free fruits and vegetables, whole grains, seeds, and nuts, along with organically raised, free-range poultry and certain types of fish, can supply us with all of the essential nutrients our bodies require for optimum efficiency, energy, and freedom from disease. Such a diet is rare today, however, having been replaced by foods high in unhealthy levels of fat, preservatives, chemical additives, and, in the case of most of the meat available in the United States, antibiotics and hormones, due to the way our livestock is raised. These factors alone can contribute to much of the chronic ill-health conditions besetting people today.

See Mental Health.

Mental and Emotional Stress: Research in the field of mind/body medicine has revealed that there is a direct link between mental and emotional distress and the body's ability to resist illness. It has also been discovered that unresolved or unexpressed thoughts and feelings are translated in the body as neurochemicals. These chemicals communicate with other systems of the body, particularly the autonomic nervous system, causing the body to react in a manner similar to when physical stress is present. Fear, for example, arouses the nervous system and triggers a flood of adrenal hormones, causing an accelerated heart rate and intensified breathing. Under healthy conditions, such reactions soon subside, but chronic fear, anger, grief, and other powerful emotions can keep the nervous system in a constant state of arousal. This allows stress to build up in the body, eventually attacking the body's organs and resulting in depressed immunity.

Environmental Pollution: Pollutants in the air, water, soil, and the foods we eat can contribute to illnesses ranging from birth defects and cancer to Alzheimer's disease. They also can create a severe toll on the immune system, leading to many other chronic conditions, such as allergies.

See Detoxification Therapy, Environmental Medicine.

Dental Factors: The relationship between common dental silver amalgam fillings and chronic illness is now becoming recognized by a growing number of dentists, physicians, and researchers. The problem lies with the fact that calling the fillings silver is a misnomer because they are actually composed of 50 percent mercury, one of the metals most toxic to the human body. Over time, the mercury can slowly leech out of the fillings. When this happens, damage may occur to the nervous system, leading to symptoms resembling multiple sclerosis, chronic fatigue syndrome, and senile dementia. Infections in the gums can also diminish health by suppressing immune function and increasing the susceptibility of disease elsewhere in the body. The misalignment between the skull and jaw caused by temporomandibular joint syndrome can also create various types of stress that can result in depression, insomnia, headaches, fatigue, chronic pain, and low back pain.

See Biological Dentistry.

The Inappropriate Use of Antibiotics: Antibiotics are valuable drugs when they are used appropriately. But the evidence today points to massive overuse. Antibiotics are often prescribed for medical conditions that do not warrant them. For instance, they are routinely given for colds, but many colds are the result of viral infections, and while antibiotics kill bacteria, they have no effect on the viruses.

For a more in-depth discussion of the implications of antibiotics on health, see Antibiotics and Probiotics (in Appendix), as well as Candidiasis, Chronic Fatigue Syndrome.

The use of antibiotics can also result in a variety of side effects due to the way their powerful actions can interfere with the delicate balance of the body's systems. This can result in the destruction of the friendly bacteria in the body, leading to yeast overgrowth, both locally, such as in vaginal infections, and systemically, in the form of candidiasis; interference of nutrient absorption; the development of food allergies; recurrent ear infections; and immune suppression, as evidenced by the large percentage of adults suffering from chronic fatigue syndrome who have histories of recurrent antibiotic treatment as children or adolescents.[5]

Electromagnetic Fields: Electromagnetic fields (EMFs) are invisible yet active forces produced by electrical appliances (including computers, microwave ovens, and even electric razors), power lines, and wiring. Researchers have only recently begun to realize the effects EMFs can have on health. Recently, the Special Epidemiology Studies Program of the California Department of Health Services noted that EMFs can, in fact, change biological tissue, although the full range of their health effects remain unknown.[6] Additional studies by the United States Environmental Protection Agency have found that, in the last twenty years, possible associations have been found between EMFs and miscarriages, birth defects, leukemia, brain cancers, and lymphomas.[7]

For a more in-depth discussion of the implications of EMFs to health, see Energy Medicine, Magnetic Field Therapy.

Geopathic Stress: Geopathic refers to illnesses that are caused, or contributed to by [illegible] of harmful radiation from the earth itself. That such a possibility exists has been known to traditional cultures for thousands of years. The Chinese art of *feng shui* (the study of subtle earth energies and their relation to human life), for instance, takes into account the effects of harmful radiation from the earth to safeguard against building over the locations from which they emanate. According to Anthony Scott-Morley, D.Sc., Ph.D., M.D. (alt. med.), of Dorset, England, as many as 30 to 50 percent of the chronically ill exhibit some signs of geopathic stress. These include excessive sleeping, cold extremities, respiratory difficulties, and unexplained mood changes and depression. "While geopathic stress may not be the cause of these conditions, it certainly seems likely that it is a contributing factor," Dr. Scott-Morley says.

For a more in-depth discussion of the implications of geopathic stress to health, see Geopathic Stress in Cancer chapter, page 563.

All of these factors can contribute to a decline in organ and body system function, resulting in illness. Even so, the pathway back to health does exist.

The Return to Health

The vast majority of illnesses are self-limiting, meaning that they get better all on their own. Alternative medicine recognizes this fact, realizing that health will usually arise spontaneously when the conditions for health exist. Therefore, once you are ill, getting healthy again requires the very same inputs that were needed to keep you healthy in the first place.

This may seem obvious but it's a message worth restating. As Dr. Chaitow says, "To regain health once it has been lost we need to begin to reverse some, and ideally all, of those processes which may be negatively impacting us, and over which we have some degree of control. This includes taking responsibility for stopping those lifestyle choices which we know are harmful, whether this be smoking, excessive alcohol intake, or using drugs. In addition, we need to start to positively address the real needs that such behavior masks."

"To regain health once it has been lost we need to begin to reverse some, and ideally all, of those processes which may be negatively impacting us, and over which we have some degree of control."
—Leon Chaitow, N.D., D.O.

Depending on the nature of our health problems, this might involve starting to eat more nutritiously, sleeping and exercising in a more regular and balanced way, and making sure of receiving reasonable exposure to fresh air and sunlight. It may also include hygienic considerations, detoxifying and cleansing our bodies, addressing any structural or mechanical imbalances, as well as learning how to properly cope with stress, and deal with our mental and emotional needs.

"That sounds like a vast prescription," Dr. Chaitow says. "However, even if only some of it can be addressed, such as diet and relaxation, a remarkable phenomenon occurs as homeostasis begins to function more efficiently and health begins to return."

In beginning the journey back to health, we may require help, especially if our bodies have been overloaded and compromised for some time. According to Dr. Chaitow, the help should come from the treatment that is most appropriate for the individual. "This might involve alternative treatments aimed at helping restore nutritional balance, or treatments geared toward the removal of toxic burdens in the body. Or it might involve restoring normal nerve and circulatory supply by addressing structural imbalances. One of the advantages of alternative medicine is that it affords the individual the broadest range of health treatment options. Of course, preventive care is always a better choice than waiting to restore health once it has been lost."

Our bodies are not designed to become ill, they are designed to heal and become healthy. "Even if conventional medicine tells you that your condition is incurable or that your only option is to live a life dependent on drugs with troublesome side effects, there is hope for improving or reversing your condition," Dr. Chaitow says.

"Even if conventional medicine tells you that your condition is incurable or that your only option is to live a life dependent on drugs with troublesome side effects, there is hope for improving or reversing your condition."
—Leon Chaitow, N.D., D.O.

SELECTING AN ALTERNATIVE PRACTITIONER

The choice to explore alternative medicine can be a crucial turning point in one's life, affecting physical as well as mental and emotional health. With the help of an alternative practitioner, it is possible to take control of one's personal health, and thereby eliminate the sense of frustration and helplessness that many feel when dealing with conventional medicine.

But how does one go about selecting an alternative practitioner? Not surprisingly, many of the same criteria used to choose a conventional doctor are important in seeking out an expert in natural medicine. Yet because the very nature of the alternative approach is far more encompassing than the conventional one, there are a number of other critical factors that should be taken into account in the selection process.

The following suggestions offer basic guidelines for choosing an alternative practitioner:

• Educate yourself about the general principles of alternative health care. *The success of alternative care is dependent upon an informed patient as well as a knowledgeable practitioner. Even after selecting a practitioner, the education process must continue, becoming an ongoing aspect of a person's approach to alternative care. As Garry F. Gordon, M.D., co-founder of the American College of Advancement in Medicine, notes, "I encourage people to learn to become their own doctor, and use health practitioners as 'educators', realizing that we can learn something from everyone."*

• If you are selecting a general practitioner, choose someone with a diverse background an[illegible] expertise in a wide vari[illegible] dis-ciplines. *"I thi[illegible] want to find someo[illegible] has a relatively eclectic [illegible]kground," says Elson Haas, M.D., Director of the Center for Preventive Medicine in San Rafael, California. "A great limitation of conventional medicine is that the only choice is really drugs or surgery. Ideally, you want someone who can use both natural approaches as well as pharmaceutical ones, someone who can balance their rational approach with a more intuitive approach, so that they are not just operating from their own bias."*

• Find a practitioner with whom you can communicate openly and with whom you have a good rapport.

"If you do not have a doctor who will sit back and listen to what you have to say for twenty minutes to a half-hour," says John R. Lee, M.D., of Sebastopol, California, "you do not have a doctor who is going to find the cause." Adds Dr. Gordon: "If you don't feel you can communicate adequately and get your questions answered, you need to shop some more, because any anxiety over the doctor-patient selection puts a real negative damper on the healing process."

• Select a physician who is sensitive to your particular needs and circumstances. *Dr. Haas stresses the importance of what he calls "patient-centered" health care. "This means you really take the person as the primary mode and really work around what their needs are," he says.*

• Choose an alternative approach in which you have confidence. *In alternative medicine, the mental and emotional aspects of healing cannot be separated from the physical. It is vital, therefore, that one believe in the alternative method one has chosen. As Dr. Gordon explains, "If I could show you stacks of evidence about homeopathy, but you tell me that you will never understand how it works, I'm going to get half the effect from you than I wo[illegible] a person that had a [illegible]bor whose life was sa[illegible] homeopathy, was well-[illegible]ed about therapy, and was ready to take a homeopathic remedy when they walked in the door."*

There are numerous ways to locate alternative practitioners. In the "Where to Find Help" sections at the back of the chapters which follow, you will find listings of organizations that can provide nationwide referrals. Another valuable resource is the Alternative Medicine Yellow Pages (Future Medicine Publishing, 1994).

Treatment

When, for any of a variety of reasons, our homeostatic potential is limited, or when we are more vulnerable and susceptible because of a decline in immune system efficiency, it is time to seek treatment to encourage the recovery processes. The treatment chosen should ideally seek to eliminate causes, remove the obstacles to recovery, or encourage normal homeostasis.

> *"The treatments themselves do not 'cure' the condition, they simply restore the body's self-healing ability."*
> —Leon Chaitow, N.D., D.O.

"All alternative healing methods focus on one or more of these key elements," says Dr. Chaitow, "which explains why there are so many different forms of treatment in the field of alternative medicine. The treatments themselves do not 'cure' the condition, they simply restore the body's self-healing ability. Some treatments focus on biochemistry, others address structural imbalances, while some deal with a person's energetic or emotional requirements. Whatever treatment approach works will effectively help homeostasis to function more efficiently and will not have added to the body's burden by increasing toxicity or weakening any element of the body's ability to function."

Selecting the Appropriate Treatment: Many Roads to Rome

See Bodywork, Chiropractic, Craniosacral Therapy.

See Diet, Nutritional Supplements, Herbal Medicine, Enzyme Therapy.

See Biofeedback Training, Guided Imagery, Hypnotherapy, Mind/Body Medicine, Meditation, Neuro-Linguistic Programming.

See Acupuncture, Energy Medicine, Homeopathy, Magnetic Field Therapy, Neural Therapy.

Alternative medicine offers a wide variety of treatment options. Some of these, such as chiropractic, osteopathy, craniosacral therapy, and the various systems of bodywork, address structural imbalances within the body. Others focus on maintaining the body's biochemical balance of hormones, enzymes, and nutrients, in order to maintain proper cellular function. These include diet, nutritional supplements, herbal medicine, and enzyme therapy. Still others seek to restore mental and emotional balance, including mind/body medicine, biofeedback training, meditation, hypnotherapy, guided imagery, and neuro-linguistic programming. Finally, systems such as acupuncture, homeopathy, energy medicine, magnetic field therapy, and neural therapy address the energetic levels of the body.

Some systems of alternative medicine, such as Ayurvedic medicine, Naturopathic medicine, and Traditional Chinese Medicine, incorporate a wide range of these methods to offer complete systems of healthcare.

While the treatment methods of alternative medicine may vary in their approach, all of them are linked by a common philosophy that:

- Focuses on empowering the individual to accept responsibility for at least a part of the task of recovery and future health maintenance
- Emphasizes sound nutrition as a core requirement for health
- Recommends a balanced lifestyle, adequate and appropriate exercise, rest, sleep, and emotional tranquillity as prerequisites for a state of health
- Attempts to ensure detoxification and the efficiency of the organs and systems of the body
- Recognizes the importance of the musculoskeletal system as a potential source of interference with nerve transmission and the body's

energy pathways, and as a reflection of the individual's internal physical and emotional state
- Most importantly, treats the individual instead of his or her symptoms

See Ayurvedic Medicine, Naturopathic Medicine, Traditional Chinese Medicine.

Individuality

The late Roger Williams, Ph.D., of the University of Texas, showed that in any group of fifteen to twenty people there can be a range of nutritional requirements from person to person that varies by as much as 700 percent.[8]

"Your actual need for a particular vitamin is almost certain to be different from mine," says Dr. Chaitow, "and our requirements for this vitamin will also vary depending upon our age and any emotional, biochemical, or physical stresses which we may be coping with. What this illustrates is that there is no uniform prescription as to what any of us require nutritionally. Our bodies know what we need, however, and as long as they remain healthy and we supply them with the benefits of a healthy diet, in their own innate wisdom they will automatically take what they need from the food we eat."

Since, even in terms of nutritional requirements, each person is unique, it follows that what is required to return to health also can vary drastically from individual to individual. It is with this in mind that alternative physicians begin their diagnosis and subsequent treatments. Understanding all of the factors that play a role in both health and illness, their focus is on meeting the specific needs of each of their patients, rather than attempting to superimpose any one particular model or approach to health as the answer for every person.

"All too often, this understanding is lacking in conventional medicine, however," Dr. Chaitow says. "For example, the conventional doctor who has twelve patients with asthma will often provide each of them with the same recommendations and prescription drugs, in effect treating the condition and not the patients themselves.

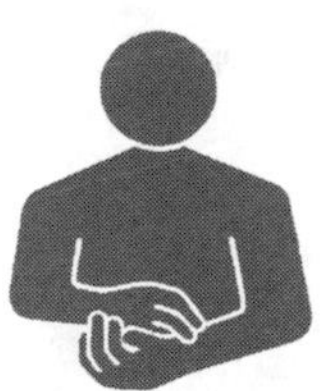

Alternative medicine also offers much in the way of self-help approaches, with therapies such as [illegible], guided imagery, flower remedies, aromatherapy, qigong, and yoga.

"An alternative practitioner, on the other hand, will realize that asthma has numerous causes. Some of his patients might be experiencing an allergic reaction to foods or something in their environment, others might have succumbed to a viral infection, while still others might be asthmatic because of diminished nerve supply due to a misaligned spine. Such a practitioner will therefore seek to determine the underlying cause for his patients' conditions, and treat each of them differently, using the method that will best stimulate their bodies to heal themselves. This distinction between approaches is a cornerstone of alternative medicine."

The return to health, therefore, is a road which each person must walk according to his or her own unique individuality. It is also a road that needs to address one's entire being, taking into account one's mental, emotional, and physical aspects, as well as the structural, biochemical, and energetic components that shape each of us. It is precisely because alternative medicine honors and understands these concepts, that it is now positioned to become a valuable and necessary pathway for meeting the medical crisis we, as a planet, are currently facing.

"Medicine is for the patient.
Medicine is for the people.
It is not for the profits."

—George Merck

Medical Freedom and the Politics of Health Care

"Unless we put medical freedom into the Constitution, the time will come when medicine will organize into an undercover dictatorship . . . To restrict the art of healing to one class of men and deny equal privileges to others will constitute the Bastille of medical science. All such laws are un-American and despotic and have no place in a republic . . . The Constitution of this republic should make special privilege for medical freedom as well as religious freedom."

—Benjamin Rush, M.D., Signer of
Declaration of Independence,
Physician to George Washington.
From *The Autobiography of Benjamin Rush*

Freedom is at the heart of American society. We have freedom of speech, freedom of worship, and freedom of the press. But Americans lack one freedom which seems increasingly more vital for a truly free society. The freedom to choose the health care of their choice. This basic freedom is being suppressed by state and federal agencies, as well as the vested financial interests of the "medical/pharmaceutical complex," comprised of the conventional medical establishment and the multinational pharmaceutical companies. Despite the fact that conventional treatments are often ineffective, simply mask symptoms, and are subject to troubling side effects, Americans who seek better and more effective medicine must struggle to win the right to open access to alternative practitioners and treatments.

In the last decade:

- There has been a concerted effort on the part of government regulatory agencies to punish and harass medical professionals who recommend or practice nutritional and herbal medicine, and other alternative therapies to maintain health and prevent and treat illness.
- State medical boards have censured and revoked the licenses of conscientious physicians who practice alternative medicine simply because their treatments are not conventional and do not conform to accepted "standards of care." These actions are taken despite the fact that many of these treatments work.
- Insurance companies have routinely refused to pay for alternative treatments such as acupuncture, chiropractic, homeopathy, and nutritional medicine, labeling them unapproved therapies, regard-

"State medical boards have censured and revoked the licenses of conscientious physicians who practice alternative medicine simply because these treatments are not conventional and do not conform to accepted 'standards of care'. These actions are being taken despite the fact that these treatments work."

less of the benefit received by the patients. This stance denies tens of millions of Americans their basic right to the health care of their choice.

- The general public has been denied free access to information concerning the documented health benefits of nutritional supplements and herbs by restrictive labeling regulations established by the Food and Drug Administration (FDA). This restriction of information flow comes despite the fact that large scale independent studies have shown that many Americans, especially the elderly, are suffering from nutritional deficits which could be corrected by dietary supplementation.
- Manufacturers of nutritional supplements and herbs, as well as health food stores, have been the target of FDA seizures in an attempt to block the manufacture and sale of numerous natural substances such as coenzyme Q10 and evening primrose oil, whose therapeutic effects have been scientifically validated.

These strong-arm tactics are being used despite the estimate of former Surgeon General C. Everett Koop that, out of 2.1 million deaths a year in the United States, 1.6 million are related to poor nutrition.[1]

The bias against alternative medicine on both the state and federal level has become clearly established and has links to the campaign of the medical establishment to squelch the emergence of alternative medicine in the United States.

The Food and Drug Administration: Medical Establishment Cops

The FDA's suppression of alternative medicine, and especially of nutritional supplements, constitutes a war for power with billions of dollars and American's health at stake, according to Julian Whitaker, M.D., President of the American Preventive Medical Association and editor of the successful alternative newsletter *Health and Healing*. "This is not a reasonable debate on public safety or honesty in labeling," says Dr. Whitaker. "It is an ugly struggle for power by FDA Commissioner David Kessler, and those who support giving the FDA more power over the nutritional supplement industry, that smacks of the tactics of Joe McCarthy in the 1950s. Whereas Joe McCarthy's witch hunt was based on the theory that communists were everywhere, today's persecution of innocent people by the FDA is based on the premise that nutritional supplements are a menace."

The FDA is a branch of the Department of Health and Human Services. It is funded annually through the United States Congress and has the authority to regulate foods, drugs, cosmetics, and medical devices that are sold between states or imported. The FDA is also responsible for ensuring that products are pure and unadulterated, and not misrepresented through false labeling, declarations of ingredients, or net weight statements. The FDA also regulates certain manufacturing processes, holding jurisdiction over a product from the initial shipment of its raw materials across state lines to the shipment of the finished product from a manufacturing distribution facility outside the state. In addition, some drugs, medical devices, food additives, and food coloring require premarketing FDA approval. If someone markets a product without such approval the FDA can take regulatory action.

PRICE GOUGING BY THE PHARMACEUTICAL INDUSTRY

The Food and Drug Administration's (FDA) process for approval of a drug costs as much as $250 million and five to ten years of development time. Yet the profits of pharmaceutical companies are among the highest of any industry in the world, and often come at the expense of human health. For example, a recent cancer drug, Levamisole, taken in combination with another drug, Fluorouacil, was shown to reduce the recurrence rate of advanced colon cancers by 41 percent when taken following surgery, according to a study conducted at the Mayo Clinic in Rochester, Minnesota. But this same drug, which costs $15 annually when used as a treatment for worms in animals, has a price tag of $1,200 when used to treat cancer patients for the same year period.[5]

American pharmaceutical prices are also much higher than those of other nations, especially those with national health insurance and centralized purchasing and price negotiation. And if drug companies wish to peddle their medicines in countries with national health insurance, they are told that they must lower their price.

In Mexico, for example, the price of the common prescription pain reliever, Naprosyn, is less than one-fourth of that in the United States. Indeed, many drug prices in the United States are much higher than in Mexico, as the following table demonstrates.

COMPARATIVE PRICES OF PHARMACEUTICAL DRUGS IN THE U.S. AND MEXICO[6]

Drug	Dosage in Milligrams	Quantity Tablets	U. S. Price	Mexico Price
Amoxil	500	30	24.40	17.80
Calan	240	100	108.90 - 125.57	37.98
Carizem	120	20	33.20	8.28
Ceclor	250	30	66.20	21.27
Lanoxin	.25	100	20.40	4.24
Mevacor	20	60	121.10	101.32
Naprosen	500	45	48.50	10.48
Premarin	.625	100	42.90	[illegible]
Procardia	10	20	12..20 - 15.[illegible]	2.14
Seldane	60	30	66.20	21.27
Synthroid	.125	[illegible]	32.30	34.09
Vasotec	5	100	90.55	30.09
Zantac	150	60	98.00	23.50

"The FDA has very wide-ranging regulatory powers that are restricted only by the courts. However, the FDA is rarely restricted by the courts because it is considered to be an agency of experts dealing with expert issues," notes attorney Jay Geller, of Santa Monica, California, an authority on FDA law and former employee in the general counsel's office of the FDA. This lack of restriction allows the FDA to persecute alternative medicine practitioners with a relative lack of accountability. "There are two ways that the FDA is able to harass alternative physicians," says Alan R. Gaby, M.D., of Baltimore, Maryland, President-elect of the American Holistic Health Association. "They can raid their clinics or restrict the availability of effective medicinal substances. Whether or not the FDA has overstepped their legal boundary is unclear, but I do believe that what they are doing is improper. If there were unbiased individuals running the FDA this would not be happening, as I think it has much to do with their own bias and attitudes."

Konrad Kail, N.D., past President of the American Association of Naturopathic Physicians, holds a similar view. "The FDA's plan right now is to remove the agents used by alternative physicians, such as supplements and herbs, since they cannot remove the physicians," he says. "They are using the brute force of their power to unfairly police a specific group of individuals who tend to practice alternative medicine. As far as I am concerned this is a politically motivated move by conventional medicine in order to remove the competition from the marketplace. They are using the FDA to accomplish their own political motivations."

> *"Prices of the twenty most popular prescription drugs jumped 80 percent on average from 1984 to 1991, four times the general inflation rate for the period."*
>
> —Report of Families USA Foundation

The FDA's bias in favor of conventional medicine may stem from the informal but very real connection it has with the pharmaceutical industry. One study, for instance, found that half of the high-ranking FDA officials have been formerly employed as key executives in pharmaceutical companies immediately prior to joining the FDA. In addition, the study found that half of these officials would then serve in an executive capacity in a pharmaceutical company immediately upon leaving the FDA.[2]

The FDA's bias is further shown by its selective implementation of policy directives. Its duty, by law, is to set standards for drug advertisements. Yet, according to a study done last year at the University of California and published in the *Wall Street Journal*, 60 percent of the pharmaceutical ads from medical journals violated FDA guidelines. But the FDA, to this day, has done nothing about these violations.[3]

Another connection between the FDA and the pharmaceutical industry is through the Pharmaceutical Advertising Council. In 1985, the Pharmaceutical Advertising Council teamed up with the FDA to solicit funds from the pharmaceutical industry for the purpose of combatting medical quackery. "The Pharmaceutical Advertising Council and the FDA also issued a joint statement addressed to the presidents of advertising and PR agencies nationwide asking them to cooperate with a joint venture antifraud and quackery campaign," according to Mark Blumenthal, Executive Director of the American Botanical Council. "The letter has joint letterhead from the FDA and the Pharmaceutical Advertising Council, and is signed by the directors of both organizations. On the surface it appears to be patently illegal. The FDA is supposed to regulate the pharmaceutical industry, but instead they are teaming up to work on an antifraud campaign against an industry that some could construe to be an economic competitor."

Further evidence of the FDA's bias toward drugs as opposed to nutritional supplements is demonstrated by the FDA's *Dietary Supplements Task Force Final Report*, which reads in part, "The Task Force considered various issues in its deliberations, including . . . what steps are necessary to ensure that the existence of dietary supplements on the market does not act as a disincentive for drug development.[4]

We thank you in advance for your participation in this important government-industry program. It is a project that is sure to be good for everyone.

Sincerely,

Frank E. Young, M.D., Ph.D.
Commissioner
Food and Drug Administration

Roger O'Neill
President
Pharmaceutical Advertising Council

Enclosure: Backgrounder

PAC
Pharmaceutical Advertising Council Inc.
342 Madison Avenue
Suite 1915
New York, N. Y. 10173
(212) 370-1701

Department of Health and Human Services
Food and Drug Administration
5600 Fishers Lane
Rockville, Md. 20857
(301) 443-3220

FDA

October 22, 1984

Dear Agency President:

The Pharmaceutical Advertising Council and the United States Food and Drug Administration have just announced a unique program and we are inviting you to join us.

The program is a nationwide campaign to warn the public of the dangers of quack medical products primarily through using public service announcements on television and radio and in newspapers, magazines and journals.

We are asking people like you to help [illegible] public service campai[illegible] will publish or broad[illegible]

A panel of industry and government leaders will choose the three [illegible] creative concepts from those submitted. All three will be released approximately four months apart.

The importance of this project is inestimable. First, this is an unusual opportunity for government and industry to work together for a common cause. Secondly, creators of the public service messages will get appropriate recognition and credit for their participation.

And not least, the subject of quack medicines is terribly important. U.S. consumers spend billions on quack medical products every year. Some of these so-called "health" products directly endanger lives; others are indirectly fatal as they distract people from getting proper and timely medical care.

The deadline for submission of creative concepts for our public service campaign against quack products is January 30, 1985. We'd like to hear from you by November 30 if you will participate. If you have any questions please feel free to call Mr. Paul Chusid, PAC coordinator for the project at (212) 546-1565.

Freedom of Information and FDA Regulation of the Manufacture and Sale of Nutritional Supplements and Herbs

"The FDA has always had a perceived bias against dietary supplements and has historically looked on them with a jaundiced eye," says attorney Geller. "The agency has expressed virtually no interest in trying to find a balance between the requirements necessary to approve prescription drugs and those appropriate to allow preventive health claims for naturally-occurring substances such as vitamins, minerals, enzymes, amino acids, and herbs. Even with the studies that have just come out on the potential benefits of vitamin E for preventing heart disease, the FDA's position is that there are not going to be any claims allowed to be made for dietary supplements that do not meet the standards applied to prescription drugs."

"A search of the Medlars' Data Base at the National Library of Medicine shows that, since 1966, there have been 12,896 studies on vitamin C, of which 5,546 deal with humans, and 7,043 studies on vitamin E, of which 3,205 deal with humans. In total, there probably have been more than 75,000 studies on nutrients now being consumed as dietary supplements. Many of these studies provide the kind of evidence that would persuade anyone—except, of course, the FDA—of the health benefits of dietary supplements."
—Saul Kent, President, The Life Extension Foundation

The FDA has also seized safe and effective natural remedies such as coenzyme Q10 and evening primrose oil from health food stores and distributors because they did not approve of the statements being made about these supplements, according to Dr. Gaby. "This, despite the fact that extensive scientific literature supports their use. Coenzyme Q10 has been shown to be valuable in treating congestive heart failure, cardiomyopathy [a disease of the heart muscle], and high blood pressure; and evening primrose oil has proven effective in the treatment of eczema, high blood pressure, and arthritis," he notes.

Dr. Gaby also finds that the policies of the FDA make it extremely difficult for consumers to learn about the health benefits of any natural substance, including nutritional supplements and herbs. "According to the FDA's interpretation of the law," he says, "any substance for which a health claim is made becomes a drug, subject to the same strict rules and regulations as prescription pharmaceuticals."

Dr. Kail feels that such rules are unnecessary. "We don't need to have more restrictions on supplements and herbs," he says. "This will only act to benefit the pharmaceutical companies and doctors who are already making enormous profits in this field and make it more expensive for people to take care of themselves. Health care will be taken out of the hands of the people and put back into the hands of institutions. People can do a lot to take care of themselves if they are taught how to do it."

One such example of FDA bias and its damaging effect on national health concerns the use of saw palmetto berries for prostate disease. "The extract of the saw palmetto berry has been shown by scientific studies to be about three times more effective than the Merck prostate drug, Proscar, for alleviating symptoms of prostate enlargement, such as poor urinary stream, urinary retention, and nightime urination," reports Dr. Whitaker. "Furthermore, saw palmetto extract has no toxicity."

On the other hand, Proscar causes impotence, ejaculation dysfunction, decreased libido, and is teratogenic (birth defect-causing).[7]

Yet, the FDA has recommended that saw palmetto berry be removed from the market while allowing Proscar to remain available. "As a result," says Dr. Whitaker, "ten million men have been robbed of a safer, more effective therapy."

The bias against natural cures is alarming. For example, according to summaries from the nation's poison control centers, one death was associated with the use of a nutritional supplement from 1983 to 1990, and that was due to regular overuse of niacin by a mentally-disturbed individual,. On the other hand, drug use causes fatal reactions in .44 percent of hospitalized patients. This translates to about 130,000 deaths a year, or roughly 356 deaths every day.[8]

"So as not to alarm the public or hurt the pharmaceutical industry, the FDA looks the other way when prescription drugs kill hundreds of thousands and harm millions," says Dr. Whitaker. "But if someone drinking Sleepytime tea has a restless night, the agency raids the health food stores, confiscates the tea, and dupes the TV networks into airing biased exposés on the dangers of nutritional supplements."

"We don't need to have more restrictions on supplements and herbs. This will only act to benefit the pharmaceutical companies and doctors who are already making enormous profits in this field and make it more expensive for people to take care of themselves."

—Konrad Kail, N.D., past President, American Association of Naturopathic Physicians

The Persecution of Dr. Jonathan Wright

One of the most outspoken critics of FDA policy has been Jonathan Wright, M.D. A widely publicized incident involving Dr. Wright and the FDA illustrates how ruthless the agency's regulatory action can be when directed against physicians practicing alternative medicine. On the morning of May 6, 1992, FDA agents, accompanied by ten officers from the King's County Police Department, broke down the door of Dr. Wright's Tahoma Clinic in Kent, Washington, wearing flak jackets and with guns drawn.

Prior to this raid, the clinic had never been subject to an official FDA inspection, nor received a request for an inspection. Yet during the subsequent fourteen-hour raid, FDA agents confiscated a truckload of items, including patient and employee records; banking statements; payroll data; injectable, preservative-free vitamins, mineral and glandular extracts; noninvasive allergy and sensitivity-testing equipment; instruction and training manuals; the entire printed contents of the hard drive on the clinic's central computer system; and even the clinic's supply of postage stamps.

One of the items confiscated in the armed raid was a vitamin B_{12} complex manufactured in Germany. Though the FDA claims that the sale of these vitamins is against the law, Dr. Wright argues that vitamins, minerals, and other nutrients are not drugs, but natural substances over which the FDA should not have jurisdiction. Because he treats many patients with allergies, Dr. Wright uses the German form of vitamin B_{12} because it is the only injectable vitamin he has found that does not contain preservatives or additives, both of which can cause adverse reactions in some of his patients. In addition, the German form of vitamin B_{12} is in use around the country, and stronger doses of the vitamin made in America are also available in numerous pharmacies.

FDA harassment of Dr. Wright, a former columnist for *Prevention* magazine who is considered one of the world's experts in nutritional biochemistry, began in 1991 when agents confiscated from his clinic a dispensary stock of L-tryptophan that had previously been verified as being uncontaminated.

L-TRYPTOPHAN: THE BANNING OF AN INVALUABLE NATURAL TREATMENT FOR ANXIETY AND INSOMNIA

Much has been said and written about L-tryptophan, an essential amino acid widely used for more than thirty years as a dietary supplement to treat depression, insomnia, premenstrual syndrome, stress, and hyperactivity in children. At its core, however, the L-tryptophan story is a textbook case in how the government and private industry conspire to keep safe and effective natural remedies out of the hands of the public.

In December 1989, the FDA, responding to an outbreak of a rare blood disorder among some individuals taking L-tryptophan, pulled the substance off the market pending investigation. The disorder, eosinophilia-myalgia syndrome (EMS), was linked to impurities in the supplements as well as immune system weaknesses that increased susceptibility to the illness. Among the 1,550 known cases in the United States as of May 1990, 24 deaths were reported.

The outbreak was traced to a contaminated batch of L-tryptophan produced by one Japanese manufacturer. Despite the fact that FDA and the Centers for Disease Control and Prevention have both conluded that virtually all EMS patients used L-tryptophan from the Showa Denko K. K. company of Japan, this amino acid conintues to be banned in capsules or tablets. The FDA's double standard continues, however, since this same substance is allowed to be freely added to baby foods, tube feedings, and pet products.

David Kessler, FDA Commissioner, under attack by his critics, told Congress, in July 1993, "Despite recent intense research, the exact cause of EMS and an understanding of how it develops have not been established."

"This is an obvious lie," counters Julian Whitaker, M.D., President of the American Preventive Medical Association. "You do not allow babies, the elderly, and the infirm to have access to a supplement that is too toxic for the healthy adult population."

According to Garry F. Gordon, M.D., co-founder of the American College of Advancement in Medicine, the agency's crusade against L-tryptophan dates back at least a decade. When Dr. Gordon served as a medical expert for the National Nutritional Food Association, which opposed the FDA's original effort to remove L-tryptophan from the market, he recalls that, "As we left the courtroom, they said, 'Well, you beat us this time, but we have lots of other avenues and we will get it stopped.'"

The FDA's ban on L-tryptophan, asserts Dr. Gordon, is directly linked to the power of the pharmaceutical industry. Because of L-tryptophan's effectiveness in combating insomnia, depression, and other health problems, it was impacting the pharmaceutical market for prescription drugs. "People didn't need their valium; they didn't need their librium; they didn't need their Prozac," says Dr. Gordon. "Therefore, physicians who use L-tryptophan, along with other dietary supplements, are harassed by the FDA acting on behalf of the pharmaceutical industry."

In August 1991, Dr. Wright sued for recovery of the L-tryptophan. Within three weeks, FDA investigators started systematic searches of the trash bin located in the parking lot of the office complex housing the Tahoma Clinic. Between December and March of the following year, they also visited the clinic posing as patients, leading up to the May raid.

As of this writing, the FDA has still not filed charges against Dr. Wright. Yet his practice is now the subject of a drawn-out, secret grand jury investigation. A Jonathan Wright Legal Defense Fund has been set up to help pay the doctor's legal costs. (P.O. Box 368, Tacoma, WA 98401)

Doctors and alternative care advocates say Dr. Wright was singled out because he has been outspoken about treatment methods that traditional practitioners deem unorthodox. Dr. Wright speculates the action is tied to a lawsuit he has pending with the FDA over the seizure of his stock of L-tryptophan. He also reports that when he and his wife have traveled abroad since the incident, they have been singled out in customs lines and their belongings meticulously searched, something that had never happened previously during his many foreign travels. Upon returning from a recent trip, his wife was even taken to a room and strip-searched. Dr. Wright, a prominent physician with over twenty years of experience in family practice and an international reputation for the safety and effectiveness of his practice, is being treated like a common criminal—simply because he has stood up for his right to practice alternative medicine.

The Harassment of Dr. Stephen Levine & NutriCology

Critics of the FDA have long asserted that the agency has unjustly waged health fraud campaigns against alternative treatments, products, or practitioners, while at the same time ignoring gross health violations by major pharmaceutical companies. For instance, when it was discovered that Pfizer, Inc. produced and sold a defective heart valve which resulted in 310 deaths, the heart valve was removed from the market but no fraud charges were filed. And when Bristol-Myers was caught selling unapproved cancer drugs through illegal promotions, they too escaped criminal charges. On May 9, 1991, however, Stephen A. Levine, Ph.D., learned of the FDA's selective practices firsthand.

Holding a temporary restraining order secured by the Department of Justice, U.S. Attorney's Office, and Attorney General on behalf of the FDA, a dozen FDA agents burst into the headquarters of Dr. Levine's small San Leandro, California company, NutriCology. To complete their exhaustive search of his offices and warehouse, they effectively shut the company's operations down for two full days. Although the FDA had not warned Dr. Levine of any serious noncompliance for three years prior to the raid, he was now accused of selling "unapproved new drugs" and slapped with a temporary restraining order on nine products. These products were coenzymne Q10, flaxseed oil, geranium, borage oil, OxyNutrients™, citrus seed extract, *Artemesia annua*, Ovalectin™ (an extract of hen egg yolks), and a natural antioxidant called pycnogenol. Dr. Levine maintained that the products were to be classified as foods and not "drugs," because they are reputable supplements that can be found in most health food stores in the United States.

In addition, in the government's memorandum Dr. Levine was compared to a "snake oil salesman" and the products in question termed "at best worthless." He was also threatened with criminal charges associated with the mail fraud act. Under this act the government can seize property, assets, records, and other belongings of the accused; thus the court was asked to also freeze Dr. Levine's company and personal assets.

Later, depositions of the FDA's two leading experts revealed that they had not read any of the scientific literature substantiating NutriCology's products, and that neither, in fact, had conducted any research personally. The basis of their action was based solely on the hearsay statements of others.

Perhaps one of the reasons the FDA targeted NutriCology, a small company with no history of customer complaints, was because of its leading scientific role in developing new products.

Furthermore, Dr. Levine has played a key role in successfully educating physicians regarding antioxidant therapies through his book, *Antioxidant Adaptation: Its Role in Free Radical Pathology*.

In response to this unprovoked attack, NutriCology submitted evidence from several expert witnesses, affidavits from sixty physicians, and a twelve-inch stack of scientific papers supporting the products under FDA attack.

On May 23, 1991, Federal Judge F. Lowell Jenson denied the government's request for a preliminary injunction on the nine products. In a twenty-page opinion, Judge Jenson held that the FDA had failed to provide evidence necessary to support its charges against NutriCology. The court even went so far as to state in its decision that to prevent the sale of products the FDA was targeting would "clearly threaten the viability of the [NutriCology] business itself, which, in light of the attestations of numerous physicians, health officials, and other experts, would constitute a real and potentially unnecessary loss to the health needs of the general public."

But the FDA filed for reconsideration and was again denied the motion for the same reasons. In December 1992, the FDA petitioned the 9th Circuit Court of Appeals for a fourth injunction. When the FDA was questioned as to why it was bringing the case to the appellate level after it had already been denied previous injunctions, it responded by saying that NutriCology was dangerous to the public. The court responded by citing that in the past ten years there were no complaints or injuries arising from NutriCology products, the majority of which cater to medical doctors and health care professionals. The injunction was again denied.

As of May 1993, NutriCology has accumulated over one thousand petitions from health care professionals supporting the company as it awaits the prospect of a full-scale trial in federal court. If the trial comes to pass, it will be the latest in a series of FDA tactics designed to discredit NutriCology, and an expensive campaign funded by taxpayer dollars.

The Medical Establishment and the Suppression of Unorthodox Research

The FDA is not the only force that practitioners of alternative medicine must contend with. In order to receive grants for medical research and be published in the major medical and scientific journals, physicians and researchers are compelled not to stray far from conventional views. Otherwise they run the risk of being shut out of the mainstream and find themselves without the funding they need to carry on their work. The American Society for Clinical Nutrition, for example, publishers of the *American Journal of Clinical Nutrition*, acknowledge at the front of each issue of their journal the "generous support" of certain organizations for selected educational activities of the society. Among the companies that provide this support are the Coca-Cola Company, General Foods Corporation, General Mills Foundation, Gerber Products Company, the Nutra-Sweet® Group, the Pillsbury Company, and numerous pharmaceutical companies. "Would these organizations support research about the damaging effects of the processed foods they are selling?" Dr. Gaby asks, pointing out the unlikelihood of such a scenario.

Furthermore, physicians who abide by a conventional Western medical perspective are more likely to publish papers and end up being on editorial boards of scientific journals than are their peers who hold to different philosophies. "There is kind of a self-selection process where physicians who are against alternative medicine end up being on the editorial boards of the journals," Dr. Gaby says. It's important to bear in mind, too, that a large percentage of medical journals receive a substantial amount of their revenue from the advertising dollars they get from the pharmaceutical industry, whose interests would not be served by articles and studies that recommended the use of alternative medicine over drugs and surgery.

The Case of Dr. Peter Duesberg

The bias against unorthodox medicine has never been more clear than in the case of Peter Duesberg, Ph.D., of the University of California at Berkeley, a specialist in the field of microbiology with impeccable credentials who is recognized internationally as an expert in retroviruses, an area he also helped to pioneer. Due to the quality of his research work, Dr. Duesberg was awarded a $250,000 federal research grant as an independent investigator, meaning he could choose his own area of research. But when Dr. Duesberg went against conventional wisdom to assert that HIV (human immunodeficiency virus) was not the cause of AIDS, as is commonly believed, but possibly only an incidental factor, the government took away his grant and his views were dismissed as out of hand. Now, however, some four thousand cases of AIDS have been discovered where no trace of the HIV virus exists, giving weight to Dr. Duesberg's position. In addition, research from the renowned Pasteur Institute in Paris, France, which was originally responsible for the discovery of HIV, has also shown that HIV is not the sole cause of AIDS and in fact requires co-factors for the disease to develop. Despite this, Dr. Duesberg continues to be discounted, and even vilified, by the medical establishment.

See AIDS.

Repression of a Cancer Drug that Works: Dr. Joe Gold and Hydrazine Sulfate

In the area of cancer, the National Cancer Institute (NCI) has shown an equal bias against alternative practitioners. Despite the apparent failure of the costly war on cancer, NCI continues to wage a campaign against nutritionally-based cancer treatments that may be one of the keys to halting and even reversing cancerous growths. An example of this can be found in the case of Joe Gold, M.D., of Syracuse, New York.

See Cancer.

A veteran of NASA's medical corps, Dr. Gold discovered that an easily synthesized substance called hydrazine sulfate could help cancer patients reverse their disease by preventing the wasting-away process that accompanies cancer and which inhibits the body's normal processing of nutrients. In fact, a significant percentage of cancer victims die of the malnutrition caused by this inhibition, rather than the cancer itself.

Hydrazine sulfate is inexpensive, and was first developed by Dr. Gold at the Syracuse Cancer Research Institute in the early 1970s. It has subsequently undergone more than fifteen years of controlled testing at both UCLA Harbor Hospital and at the Petrov Research Institute in St. Petersburg, Russia. Results showing that hydrazine sulfate is able to stop,

“I am personally convinced that many of these scientists and practitioners are not ‘quacks’ . . . but really are good scientists working on good scientific theories. Unfortunately, we have a society and a system which says that anybody doing anything new or different is a quack.”

—Berkeley Bedell, former Iowa congressman, Member of the National Institutes of Health Alternative Medicine Evaluation Panel

and even reverse, tumor growth in many cancer patients have been published in leading medical journals, including, *The Lancet, Cancer*, and the *Journal of Clinical Oncology*. And in a 1991 multi-institutional study, a team of scientists from the Petrov Institute reported that hydrazine sulfate stopped tumors in roughly half their patients, including those tumors which attack the breast, ovaries, cervix, endometrium, and vulva. A smaller but significant number of patients had even more profound results, with their tumors disappearing altogether.[9]

NCI has not followed up on the Russian study, which American cancer officials have dismissed as “poorly done work . . . not up to our standards.”[10] Compounding NCI’s omission is the fact that national U.S. clinical trials conducted in 1992 and 1993 were allowed to occur without heeding Dr. Gold’s warnings that hydrazine sulfate is not effective when used in conjunction with incompatible substances such as alcohol, sleeping pills, and tranquilizers. Patients were allowed to ingest these substances, in effect scuttling the test results, which were inconclusive.[11] Instead of initiating further tests and conducting them according to Dr. Gold’s established protocol, NCI officials continue to reject hydrazine sulfate as a viable cancer treatment, informing physicians that its use is little more than “quackery.”[12]

State Medical Boards: Does Conformity Equal Competence?

In 1847, the American Medical Association (AMA) was formed, ostensibly to protect the public from charlatans, since, at that time, anyone could offer medical services and drugs uncontested. For the remainder of the nineteenth century, the AMA successfully lobbied states to require licensing of all physicians. Eventually, the AMA set up a Council on Medical Education to oversee all medical schools. The AMA was so successful that the number of medical schools in the United States actually decreased by half between the early 1900s and 1944, going from 160 in 1904 to just 77 in 1940.[13] Today the AMA is able to prevent doctors who do not subscribe to its views from serving on hospital staffs, and it also controls medical boards on the state level.

The purpose of such medical boards is to protect the public against incompetent and unscrupulous doctors. But, as Dr. Gaby notes, “They often inappropriately extend that function to eliminating doctors that deviate from the arbitrary standards of care that are based on what they understand. The excuse for censuring a doctor or revoking his license is that he is incompetent, and the proof is that he deviates from the standards of care. Therefore, by definition, if you deviate, you are incompetent.”

The Persecution of Dr. Warren Levin

A telling example of the power of state medical boards to censure and harass competent physicians who deviate from conventional therapies is the case of Warren Levin, M.D., of New York City. The medical establishment so strenuously objected to Dr. Levin's effective use of chelation therapy, vitamin supplements, exercise, and counseling that it waged a sixteen-year campaign against him, at a cost of approximately 1 million dollars.

Despite its efforts, the Office of Professional Medical Conduct of the New York State Health Department was unable to come up with a single allegation of patient injury attributed to Dr. Levin. Nevertheless, the state medical board's hearing officers managed to ignore and insult a parade of highly respected physicians and scientists who came to Dr. Levin's defense, including two-time Nobel Prize-winner Linus Pauling.

At the same time, the hearing officers did accept and honor the testimony of a doctor who denounced chelation therapy as useless. And although the prosecution witness in question admitted under cross-examination that he had never read anything about chelation therapy, met a doctor who used it, or even seen a patient who received it, the panel found him to be a "credible and authoritative witness." The panel therefore recommended that Dr. Levin be stripped of his license to practice.

It is ironic that at the same time the government is searching for highly effective, lower-cost approaches to the nation's health care needs, a physician like Dr. Levin, who for years was providing his patients with exactly such an approach and achieving impressive results, could be prevented from practicing his profession.

Positive Developments in Protecting Your Medical Freedom of Choice

Since 1990, three states, Alaska, Washington, and North Carolina, have passed freedom of practice statutes, allowing physicians the freedom to practice alternative forms of medicine without fear of retribution from their state medical boards. The statutes state that failure to conform to standards of care shall not by itself be considered incompetence unless patients are harmed or exposed to unreasonable risk.

These new laws are paving the way for medical freedom in the United States, providing citizens with a true choice in their medical treatment. The United States Congress is also beginning to recognize the validity of alternative medicine. In 1992, Congress established the Office of Alternative Medicine at the National Institutes of Health (NIH), with an annual budget of two million dollars to be used to investigate the potential of promising alternative therapies. Although this is hardly adequate funding for such an important task, it is clearly a step in the right direction.

Both developments are in the spirit of the World Health Organization's call for the integration of the various forms of "traditional medicine," such as homeopathy, naturopathic medicine, Traditional Chinese Medicine, Ayurvedic medicine, and herbal medicine, with conventional modern medicine in order to help meet the global health care needs of the twenty-first century.

ROBERT JAY ROWEN, M.D. AND ALASKA'S LEGISLATIVE MIRACLE

When Robert Jay Rowen, M.D., took on a new patient in the spring of 1989, he did not know that he would soon be taking on Alaska's medical establishment as well. Little more than a year later, however, Dr. Rowen's battle would culminate in an historic victory for practitioners of alternative medicine.

A family practitioner based in Anchorage, Dr. Rowen founded the Omni Medical Center in 1986, which offers a range of alternative treatments, including acupuncture, homeopathy, and chelation therapy. Though he often publicly addressed the benefits of such treatments, he was anything but a political activist.

All this changed after a meeting with Patrick Rodey, Alaska's Senate majority leader, who came to Dr. Rowen as a patient. After a discussion about the dangers facing alternative physicians in this country, Senator Rodey agreed to sponsor a bill protecting freedom of choice in medicine.

With the help of another of Dr. Rowen's patients, former state attorney general Edgar Paul Boyko, a bill was drafted. But the state Medical Board and the Department of Occupational Licensing testified against the measure, and it languished in the Senate. When a similar version of the bill was attached to a piece of legislation in the House supported by the medical establishment, the House finance committee removed the entire provision protecting alternative medicine due to pressure from lobbies for the Alaska State Medical Association. But the bill was reintroduced as an amendment and passed in the House by a two-to-one margin. Despite additional pressure from the medical lobby, it finally passed the Senate and the governor signed the bill into law on June 14, 1990.

In order for change to take place in the practice of medicine in America, it is important to have alternative physicians on state medical boards. In fact, certain laws already on the books may help to put this into action. Vincent Speckhart, M.D., of Norfolk, Virginia, reports, for instance, that in dealing with the State Medical Board of Virginia, he discovered a one hundred year old state law that required that two homeopaths always sit on the board, a law that had been ignored for over twenty years.

The state of Alaska, meanwhile, is taking the lead in this area. On July 23, 1992, Alaska Governor Walter J. Hickel, appointed Robert Jay Rowen, M.D. to the State Medical Board. Dr. Rowen is an alternative physician from Anchorage, Alaska, whose dedicated effort led to the passage of the landmark legislation on freedom of practice, making Alaska the first state to adopt such a measure. Governor Hickel announced his bold move in the following press release:

"I am putting Dr. Rowen on the Medical Board not to be controversial but to be helpful. He is a strong advocate of prevention as the first line of defense. And as the costs of traditional medical care continue to go up, it will be those who care for themselves through prevention who will live better lives. He believes prevention simply costs society less."

The governor went on to proclaim, "Dr. Rowen has a sound medical background, yet he is open minded about new ideas that can help heal. I think we need that now more than ever. I believe a balanced perspective in this seven-member board is best for Alaskans, and best for the future of health care."

Actions We Can Take To Restore Our Medical Freedom

A combination of grassroots activity, market forces, and public awareness about the full benefits of alternative medicine will do much to restore medical freedom in America. Because people can feel powerless in the face of large, influential institutions such as the FDA or Congress, it is essential that they are able to find a common vehicle through which they can empower themselves and affect change.

Alexander Schauss, Ph.D., Executive Director of the non-profit health care advocacy groups Citizens for Health, and of the American Preventive Medical Association (APMA), cites the effect grassroots movements can have on legislation: "A United States Senator was trying to introduce an amendment that would delay restrictive labeling laws for dietary supplements. It was predicted to be defeated. Through our network, we were able to initiate a series of 1,800 phone calls through our national phone tree, and we reached an additional 15,000 people through a fax network. Within 48 hours, the United States Senate was receiving approximately 10,000 phone calls per hour. That helped the bill to be easily passed by a margin of ninety-four to one, and shows that people really can make a difference."

In North Carolina, grassroots forces also demonstrated their ability to affect change. Doctors statewide were losing their licenses as a result of alternative health care modalities which they incorporated into their standard practices. The movement started out as twelve people fed up with government interference in their freedom to make health choices, but soon grew to a core group of 3,000 people. The group ended up having a dramatic impact on state legislators.

As Dr. Schauss points out, people often underestimate the power of grassroots organizations. "The average congressional district has around 200,000 people and only about 10 or 15 percent of those people vote," he says. "So you only need half of those voters to keep a person in Congress."

Therefore, one of the most practical ways citizens can hasten the acceptance of alternative medicine is to organize letter-writing campaigns to Congress and the President demanding that research into these methods be conducted, and that persecution of practitioners, manufacturers and researchers of alternative medicine cease.

"We strongly urge concerned citizens to join Citizens for Health or the American Preventive Medical Association and donate money or volunteer time to this important cause."

It is important to note that this is not to imply that any new medicines should be approved without proper testing, as reasonable safeguards are always desirable. But in a time when some legislators are proposing that it be illegal to purchase vitamins without a prescription, it is essential to promote freedom of choice in both gaining access to information on new treatments, as well as access to the treatments themselves once they are established as viable alternatives.

"If everyone in this country wrote a truthful and honest letter to all their congressmen and senators at both state and federal levels expressing their feelings about the medical industry and demanding a choice in health care, we could see a big change," states Dr. Kail. "Tell them that you want to be able to choose your health practitioners—an acupuncturist, chiropractor, naturopath, or an M.D.—who can practice alternative therapies without fear of losing their licenses."

Citizens must also mobilize to overcome the refusal of insurance companies to pay for established alternative treatments such as nutritional medicine, chiropractic, acupuncture, naturopathic medicine, homeopathy, chelation therapy, and environmental medicine. Through both the American Preventive Medical Association and Citizens for Health, Dr. Schauss and grassroots organizations have been contacting major medical insurance companies, urging them to pay for preventive, nutritional, and exercise programs.

CITIZENS FOR HEALTH AND THE AMERICAN PREVENTIVE MEDICAL ASSOCIATION

Two organizations that exemplify the effectiveness of grassroots health movements are Citizens For Health and the American Preventive Medical Association (APMA).

Citizens For Health, founded in December 1991, was formed as a response to the government's repression of medical freedom of choice. Starting out with only thirty-five members, the Tacoma, Washington-based group now has chapters in all fifty states, in addition to 125 local chapters in virtually every major metropolitan area in the country. Over 40,000 people now receive the Citizens for Health National FAX Network News Update.

The group has played an important role in promoting or opposing bills on both the national and state levels, and its chapters conduct public forums throughout the country. For example, after the Midwife Bill failed to pass its first committee hurdle in California, Citizens For Health utilized its grassroots power not only to propel the bill through committee but also through the Senate. "That is what happens when people are willing to work together, who all feel powerless, but through a common purpose and association are empowered," says Alexander Schauss, Ph.D., the organizations' Executive Director "And that is the essence of Citizens For Health."

The American Preventive Medical Association is a non-profit health care advocacy organization whose nationwide membership includes physicians, other health practitioners, and the lay public. According to Julian Whitaker, M.D., President of the APMA, and editor of the highly successful alternative newsletter, Health & Healing, *the group's mission is "to insure that there exists a health care system in which practitioners can practice in good conscience with the well-being of the patient foremost in their minds without fear of recrimination."*

To that end, APMA encourages public and professional education in alternative medicine, and lobbies for the development of a health care system that affords patients with a wide range of therapies. The organization provides support to physicians and other health care providers whose practices are in danger of being curtailed simply because of their willingness to explore options outside of the mainstream of conventional medicine. Members are updated in the latest developments regarding their rights as health consumers, and linked to a nationwide news fax network.

We strongly urge concerned citizens to join Citizens for Health and APMA and donate money and/or time to this important cause. To join Citizens for Health, call (800) 357-2211 or (303) 417-0772. Or write to: Citizens for Health, P.O. Box 2260, Boulder, Colorado 80306. To join APMA, call (800) 230-APMA, or write to: American Preventive Medical Association, P.O. Box 211, Tacoma, Washington 98401-2111.

The grassroots effort has started to pay off. "We are real pleased to have learned that Mutual of Omaha, one of the major insurance companies in this country has indicated that they would reimburse people for Dean Ornish's program, which deals with exercise and dietary and lifestyle changes," reveals Dr. Schauss.

As alternative medicine continues to wage its battle against the seemingly unyielding forces of government and conventional medicine, grassroots organizations will play perhaps the most important role in raising public awareness and in initiating both legislative and societal change. If alternative medicine is to gain its proper place in preventing and alleviating health problems, citizens must organize, mobilize, and act.

An Open Letter To the President

To the President
The White House
1600 Pennsylvania Avenue, N.W.
Washington, D.C. 20500

Dear President:

To realize effective care with cost reduction requires unlocking the strangulation hold of the pharmaceutical companies, the AMA, and FDA on all forms of fully-effective, low-cost alternative medicine.

No group can be expected willingly to surrender a profitable monopoly position, even in national interests, unless forced to do so.

Nowhere has conventional western medicine produced more dismal results than in the quest to defeat cancer and AIDS. After more than fifty years of U.S. Government-sponsored research, the rate of cancer has increased in America while the death rate remains unchanged. Incredibly, the pharmaceutical-medical establishment is persecuting those who are succeeding at reversing these scourges. The Federal Republic of Germany sponsors alternative therapies and is having extraordinary success.

It didn't take fifty years to usher in the Atomic Age once President Roosevelt decided it should be done. It didn't take fifty years to usher in the Space Age once President Kennedy decided it should be done.

Beyond any plan for health care lies the **Health Age**. Rapid giant strides in improving health care and its costs can be made if you will:

- Put a strong leader, free of entanglements with any form of medicine, in charge of the fight against cancer and AIDS.
- Instruct that person allocate resources to those alternative approaches that produce the most objectively favorable results.
- Expand the NIH Office of Alternative Medicine and increase public funding for research into alternative medical therapies, especially for the treatment of cancer and AIDS.
- Curb the FDA from protecting the medical establishment by blindly attacking alternative medicine.
- Change FDA procedure so that cost effective natural compounds can win approval to make health claims, not just expensive, highly synthesized, often-toxic patentable drugs.
- Stop toxic chemicals and pollutants from getting into our air, water, food, homes, schools, workplaces, and Earth. Stop allowing the abundant studies [illegible] these toxins in cancer be silenced by those [illegible]

To bring [illegible] you will have to reclaim the many innovative [illegible] that have been driven underground by powerful forces. You will have to refocus the funds for research into areas that threaten these powerful forces.

We want you to go down in history as the President who ushered America into the **Health Age**.

For Medical Freedom,

Grassroots public pressure on the administration to incorporate legislation favoring alternative medicine is essential as health care reform is debated in the nation's capital. We urge every reader of this book to write to the White House to let the President know of your desire for medical freedom.

A personal letter is best, but you can also copy and send the President the letter here. Your doing so will make a difference.

"The highest ideal of cure is the speedy, gentle, and enduring restoration of health by the most trustworthy and least harmful way."[7]

—Samuel Hahnemann (1755-1844)
Founder of Homeopathy

Part Two: Alternative Therapies

An Important Message

This book is intended as an educational tool to acquaint the reader with alternative methods for the maintenance of good health and the treatment of illness. The publisher hopes the book will enable the reader to improve his or her well-being and to better understand, assess, and choose the appropriate course of treatment for an illness or health condition. Because the methods described in this book are, by definition, **alternative** methods, many of them have not been investigated and/or approved by any government or regulatory agency. National, state, and local laws vary regarding the use and application of many of the treatments that are discussed. Accordingly, this book should not be substituted for the advice and treatment of a physician or other licensed health professional, but rather should be used in conjunction with professional care. Pregnant women in particular are especially urged to consult with their physician before using any therapy.

Your health is important. Use this book wisely. Discuss the alternative treatment options described herein with your doctor. Ultimately, you, the reader, must take full responsibility for your health and how you use this book. The publisher expressly disclaims responsibility for any adverse effects resulting from your use of the information contained herein.

Acupuncture

Acupuncture alleviates pain and can increase immune response by balancing the flow of vital life energy throughout the body. It is a complete system of healing and provides effective treatment for numerous conditions, from the common cold and flus, to addiction and chronic fatigue syndrome. It is also effective as an adjunctive treatment for AIDS.

Acupuncture originated in China over five thousand years ago. It is based on the belief that health is determined by a balanced flow of *qi* (also referred to as *chi*), the vital life energy present in all living organisms. According to acupuncture theory, *qi* circulates in the body along twelve major energy pathways, called meridians, each linked to specific internal organs and organ systems. According to William Michael Cargile, B.S., D.C., F.I.A.C.A., Chairman of Research for the American Association of Acupuncture and Oriental Medicine, there are over one thousand acupoints within the meridian system that can be stimulated to enhance the flow of *qi*. When special needles are inserted into these acupoints (just under the skin), they help correct and rebalance the flow of energy and consequently relieve pain and/or restore health.

See Traditional Chinese Medicine.

How Acupuncture Works

In the 1960s, Professor Kim Bong Han and a team of researchers in Korea attempted to document the existence of meridians in the human body using microdissection techniques. They found evidence that there exists an independent series of fine ductlike tubes corresponding to the paths of traditional acupuncture meridians. Fluids in this system sometimes travel in the same direction as the blood and lymph, but at other times flow in the opposite direction. They realized that these ducts are different from the vascular and lymphatic systems that Western science had previously identified, and that the meridians themselves might exist within them.[1]

The existence of the meridian system was further established by French researcher Pierre de Vernejoul, who injected radioactive isotopes into the acupoints of humans and tracked their movement with a special gamma imaging camera. The isotopes traveled thirty centimeters along acupuncture meridians within four to six minutes. Vernejoul then challenged his work by injecting isotopes into blood vessels at random areas of the body rather than into acupoints. The isotopes did not travel in the same manner at all, further indicating that the meridians do indeed comprise a system of separate pathways within the body.[2]

The Electrical Properties of Acupuncture

Current research suggests that there is a specific relationship between acupuncture points, meridians, and the electrical currents of the body. Since the 1950s, numerous studies have been conducted using electrical devices to measure the galvanic skin response (GSR) of both meridians and specific acupoints. These studies not only verify the existence of the meridian systems, but also indicate that the acupoints themselves have a higher level of electrical conductance than non-acupuncture sites.[3]

In the 1970s, under a grant from the National Institutes of Health, Robert O. Becker, M.D., and Maria Reichmanis, a biophysicist, were able to prove that electrical currents did indeed flow along the ancient Chinese meridians and that 25 percent of the acupuncture points did exist along those scientifically measurable lines. They reasoned that these points acted as amplifiers to boost the minute electrical signals as they travelled along the body, and that the insertion of a needle could interfere with that flow and thus block the stimulus of pain.[4] The other acupuncture points, Dr. Becker suggests, "may be spurious; or they may simply be weaker, or a different link than the ones our instruments revealed."[5]

ACUPUNCTURE IN A WESTERN WORLD

Chinese immigrants brought acupuncture to America in the mid-1800s, but it was largely ignored until 1972, when James Reston, a respected New York Times *columnist, underwent an emergency appendectomy while in China. Reston reported on the amazing postsurgical pain relief he enjoyed via a few well-placed acupuncture needles. This report attracted the attention of the American medical community, and many physicians traveled to China to observe for themselves the use of acupuncture for pain relief. They discovered that acupuncture is part of a complex, integrated healing system that goes far beyond pain relief and can treat a variety of conditions, including diseases of the eyes, nerves, muscles, heart, and the organs of digestion and reproduction. By the end of the 1970s, acupuncture schools and practitioners could be found throughout America, supported by dozens of professional associations and publications.*

Conditions Benefited by Acupuncture

The World Health Organization has cited 104 different conditions that acupuncture can treat, including migraines, sinusitis, the common cold, tonsillitis, asthma, inflammation of the eyes, addictions, myopia, duodenal ulcer (damaged mucous membrane in a portion of the small intestine) and other gastrointestinal disorders, trigeminal neuralgia (a severe facial pain), Meniere's disease (ringing in the ears coupled with dizziness), tennis elbow, paralysis from stroke, speech aphasia (loss of language abilities due to brain damage), sciatica, and osteoarthritis.[6] Acupuncture has also been found to be effective in the treatment of a variety of rheumatoid conditions, and brings relief in 80 percent of those who suffer from arthrosis.[7] There is also evidence to suggest that acupuncture is valuable in the treatment of environmentally-induced illnesses due to radiation,[8] pesticide poisoning,[9] environmentally toxic compounds, and air pollution.

Maoshing Ni, D.O.M., Ph.D., L.Ac., Vice-President of Yo San University of Traditional Chinese Medicine in Santa Monica, California, treats many conditions with acupuncture, and reports, "Even in acute abdominal problems, acupuncture can be used before surgery to arrest the condition before it progresses further." Dr. Ni also treats hormonal imbalances that lead to menstrual- and menopause-related problems, and he helps many people with depression, anxiety, and schizophrenia without having to resort to psychiatric drugs.

Sir Jay Holder, M.D., D.C., Ph.D., Director of the Holder Research Institute in Miami, Florida, states that there are literally thousands of conditions that acupuncture is appropriate to treat. He recalls children in the emergency room on the verge of asthmatic asphyxiation being relieved in less than thirty seconds solely with the use of acupuncture. Dr. Holder believes that acupuncture should be considered an essential life support measure for emergency room medicine.

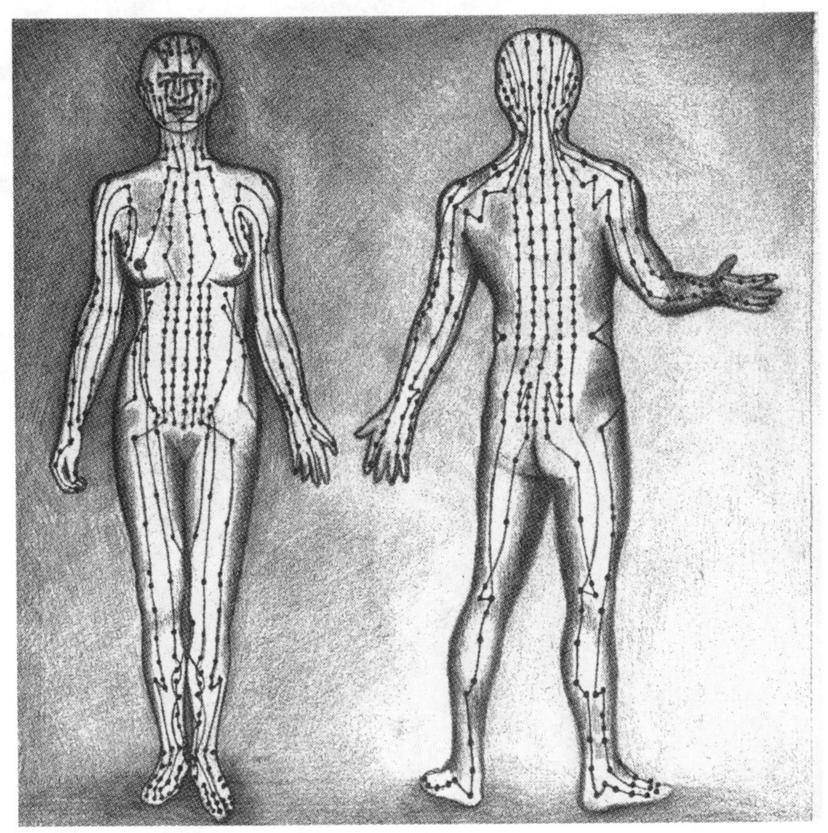

Front and back view of acupuncture meridians.

Pain

Acupuncture has proven to be a very successful treatment for pain relief, as it appears to stimulate the release of endorphins and enkephalins, the body's natural pain-killing chemicals.[10] David Eisenberg, M.D., Clinical Research Fellow at Harvard Medical School states that, "There is evidence that acupuncture influences the production and distribution of a great many neurotransmitters (substances that transmit nerve impulses to the brain) and neuromodulators (substances produced by neurons which affect neurotransmitters), and that this in turn alters the perception of pain."[11] In 1983, the medical journal *Pain* reviewed a number of studies that provide further evidence of acupuncture's im[illegible] alternative to convention[illegible] (pain-relieving) medication.[12] In one study of over [illegible],000 patients at the University of California at Los Angeles, acupuncture reduced both the frequency and severity of muscle tension headaches and migraines.[13] Another study, involving 204 patients suffering from chronic painful conditions, resulted in 74 percent experiencing significant pain relief for over three months after acupuncture treatment.[14] Other studies show that younger patients are particularly helped by acupuncture for the treatment of various types of pain.[15]

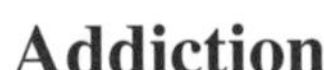

Addiction

In 1989, the British medical journal *The Lancet* documented a study noting that when acupuncture was added to the treatment program of chronic alcoholics, it significantly increased the percentage of those who completed the program. Furthermore, it reduced their need for alcohol, with fewer relapses and readmissions to a detoxification center.[16]

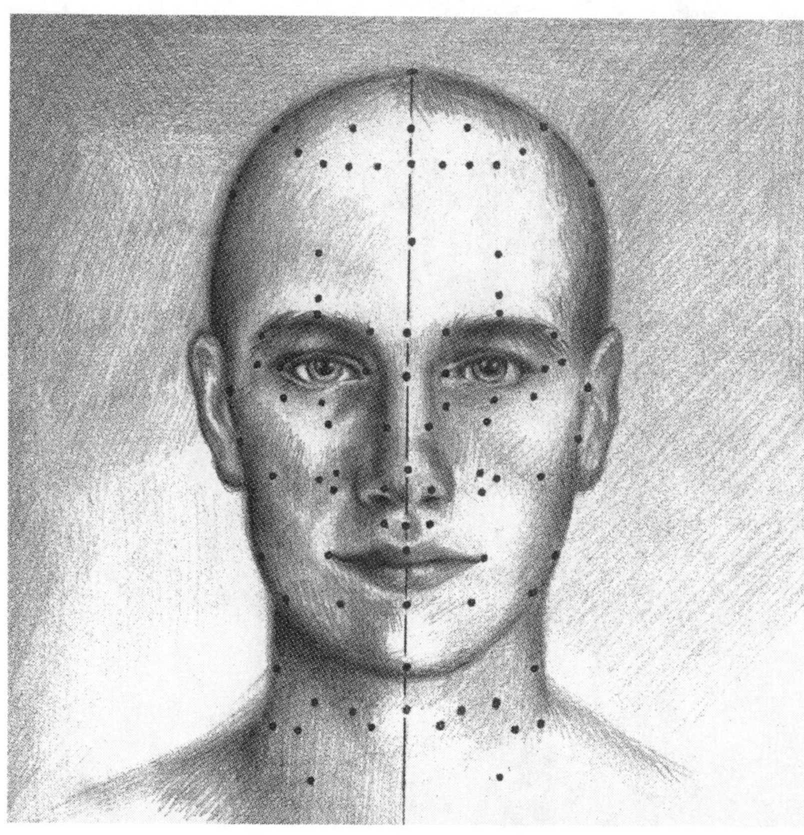

Acupoints on the face.

In another study conducted at the Lincoln Substance Abuse/ Acupuncture Clinic in New York City, sixty-eight pregnant women addicted to crack or cocaine participated in a program in which they received acupuncture treatments in conjunction with a detoxification regimen, counseling, and daily urinalysis tests. Those who attended the program for ten visits or more showed significantly higher infant birth weights than those who attended less than ten times.[17]

Other studies have documented the effectiveness of acupuncture in the treatment of opium and heroin addictions, with a 100 percent success rate in alleviating the symptoms of withdrawal.[18] "Acupuncture also claims good success rates with cigarette addiction, where a newly discovered acupoint called *Tien Mi* is used in conjunction with other traditional acupoints, particularly those located on the ear," says Dr. Ni.

Dr. Holder, who is also the founder and director of Exodus, a residential treatment hospital for addicts in Miami, Florida, has had success in the research and treatment of addictions relating to work, sex, gambling, food disorders, as well as substance abuse (chemical dependency), and has developed a form of auriculotherapy (ear acupuncture) for addiction treatment.

The government should examine the wealth of existing studies on the efficacy of acupuncture and fund further studies to speed the integration of this valuable form of treatment into America's health care system.

According to Dr. Holder, every addiction corresponds to a different set of ear acupoints. "Every drug of choice has a receptor site mechanism that is very specific. What we do is meet the needs of that receptor site by supplying and directing the endorphins or enkephalins through acupuncture." Using auriculotherapy, Dr. Holder reports success rates of over 80 percent for nicotine, alcohol, cocaine, heroin, and other mood-altering substances among addicts.[19] For this work, Dr. Holder was the first American to be awarded the Albert Schweitzer prize in medicine.

Today, there are approximately three hundred acupuncture-based substance abuse programs in the United States. In Portland, Oregon, four new acupuncture programs will address chronic mental illness, patients diagnosed with more than one chronic disease, and AIDS. The Rossano Clinic in Flint, Michigan, has recently begun a program at the Wayne

County jail in Detroit, Michigan. Because of the success of these programs, many state judiciary systems and legislators have encouraged their development. According to the National Acupuncture Detoxification Association:

- The United States House of Representatives and the Senate Appropriations Committee reported that the use of acupuncture for substance abuse recovery is cost-effective and should be more widely utilized.
- Several methadone programs in New York City noted that using acupuncture as a part of their treatment program resulted in major reductions in client tension and increased compliance with the program.
- In treatment programs begun in the state of Washington, acupuncture participation correlated with reduced drug use (as much as 50 percent compared with patients who did not use acupuncture).
- Women incarcerated in the Santa Barbara, California, county jail who received thirty-two or more acupuncture treatments while in custody had an overall reincarceration rate 26 percent lower than the control group that received no acupuncture. Those who received less than thirty-two treatments had a 17 percent lower rate of incarceration during the first four months after release from jail.[20]
- Acupuncture detoxification programs have also been established in countries around the world, including Canada, Mexico, Great Britain, Sweden, Germany, Hungary, Romania, Spain, Saudi Arabia, and Trinidad.

See Part III for listings of health conditions that can benefit from acupuncture.

ACUPUNCTURE: A SUBSTITUTE FOR SURGICAL ANESTHESIA

In 1979, David Eisenberg, M.D., was invited to the Beijing Neurosurgical Institute in China to witness and assist in a major surgical operation carried out using only acupuncture for the relief of pain. The patient was a fifty-eight-year-old university professor with a brain tumor located near his pituitary gland. The neurosurgeon, Dr. Wang Zhong-cheng, recommended acupuncture analgesia because it had significantly fewer side effects than other anesthetic treatments. Throughout a four-hour operation that included the removal of a portion of the skull to reach the tumor, the patient remained fully conscious, alert, and relaxed. He received only a mild preoperative sedative, and the acupuncture consisted of the insertion of five needles attached to a low-voltage battery. He felt no pain, and his pulse and blood pressure remained stable. When the surgery was completed, the patient stood up, thanked the surgeon, and walked out of the operating room without help.[21]

More than 90 percent of all head and neck surgeries performed at the Beijing Ne[illegible]surgical [illegible] performed using acupuncture analgesia. Dr. Eisenberg has also reported on its use for thyroid operations, where treatment consisted of inserting two needles in the hand. It has also been used successfully for open-chest surgery and tonsillectomies. It does not however, always provide adequate pain relief for abdominal, gynecological, or heart and lung surgery, according to the Beijing Institute. And because not all patients respond well to acupuncture analgesia, traditional anesthesia is kept available during all surgical operations.

Mental Disorders

P[illegible]ard of the Medical Faculty of Paris, France, and Dr. Ming Wong of the Medical Faculty of Rennes, report that acupuncture "is equivalent to the effect of tranquilizers in cases of depression, worry, insomnia, and nervous disorders, and its action is swift and lasting."[22]

In a six-month study conducted by Tom Atwood, M.S.W., Director of Mental Health Care Management at Heart of Texas Region Mental Health Mental Retardation Center in Waco, Texas, sixteen patients in a residential care home received auriculotherapy for a variety of conditions including paranoid schizophrenia and

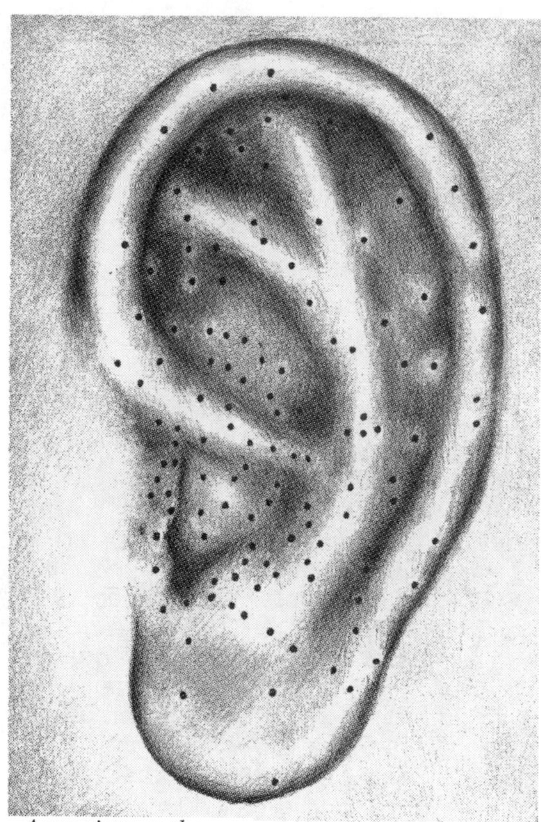
Acupoints on the ear.

borderline personality disorders. Hospitalization stays dropped from twenty-seven to eight days following the initiation of acupuncture, compared to records of the previous year. Hypertensive patients experienced reduced blood pressure, and patients generally reported sleeping better. In addition, they became more productive.[23] According to Atwood, other responses were:

- Less agitation and calmer behavior
- Improved clarity of thought
- Reduced aggression
- Improved social interaction
- Improvement in facial complexion

Atwood notes that, "These patients who are normally the most resistant, and the most likely to be readmitted for hospitalization, were also more willing to have acupuncture as opposed to other treatments offered at our center."

AIDS

Although acupuncture does not cure AIDS, it is often used with Chinese herbs to improve a patient's immune function and to reduce uncomfortable or dangerous symptoms, including night sweats, fatigue, and digestive disturbances.

At an international conference held by the European associations for acupuncture detoxification, Dr. Wu Bo Ping of China reported on his work in Tanzania where he treated 160 AIDS patients with Chinese herbology. In addition to noting considerable improvement among them, seven of the patients converted from HIV (human immunodeficiency virus) positive to HIV negative.[24]

Along with his associate, Harvey Grossbard, O.M.D., D.Hom., Dr. Holder has used acupuncture to significantly extend the life span and improve the quality of life in AIDS patients. Dr. Grossbard predicts that the final result of research in this area will be statistically significant and will establish acupuncture as beneficial in the treatment of HIV and AIDS patients. Drs. Holder and Grossbard describe the case of a man with AIDS, who was suffering from Kaposi's sarcoma, whose T-cell count returned to normal within three months of treatment with acupuncture and Chinese herbs. Additionally, the patient's lesions disappeared.

"I think that if we had more acupuncture and less AZT [an AIDS medication], we would see a qualitative improvement in these patients' health."
—William Michael Cargile, B.S., D.C., F.I.A.C.A.

Dr. Ni also cites research being conducted with HIV patients at the Kuan Yin Clinic in San Francisco, California, where preliminary studies show acupuncture to be beneficial in increasing immune function, white blood cell production, and T-cell production, as well as alleviating many of the symptoms relating to HIV infection and AIDS.

Dr. Cargile has worked with AIDS patients for many years, and has increased T-cell counts from 210 to 270 with just three acupuncture treatments. "One of these patients," adds Dr. Cargile, "had a T-cell count of 30 to 40. We eventually brought it up to 270, and although that is half the level a person needs, he's been doing great for the last six months." He adds that the key to understanding acupuncture's influence on blood values and cell counts lies in its ability to minimize stress and strengthen the body's adaptive mechanisms. "I think that if we had more acupuncture and less AZT [an AIDS medication], we would see a qualitative improvement in these patients' health."

A Typical Acupuncture Treatment

First-time patients generally fill out a questionnaire regarding their medical history and are then interviewed by the acupuncturist, who will study the patient, observing the color of the face and any coating on the tongue. Practitioners take into account body language and tone of voice, and will ask about urine color, the menstrual cycle, sensitivity to temperature and seasons, digestive problems, eating and sleeping habits, and emotional stress. Finally, the practitioner will use the wrist to diagnose and test the twelve radial pulses commonly used in Chinese medical diagnosis.

After diagnosis, specific needles are placed in any of over one thousand locations on the body. Acupuncture, however, calls for no more than ten to twelve needles per treatment. In fact, the more skillful the acupuncturist, the fewer the needles he or she will need to use. Essentially, acupuncture is painless. Although a slight pricking sensation may be felt when needles [illegible] inserted, [illegible] acupuncturist will cause no pain. Any slight tugging or aching sensation passes quickly. As a patient, it is important to tell the acupuncturist if any acupoint is uncomfortable, as a slight change of needle position or pressure can instantly eliminate the discomfort.

Acupuncture needles are of different lengths and gauges, but are generally hair-thin, solid, and made of stainless steel. To protect both the acupuncturist and patients from AIDS or hepatitis, most acupuncturists use presterilized, disposable needles.

Some treatments last only a few seconds, while others take forty-five minutes or longer. Sometimes, an ear needle is used that lies flush against the skin of the ear and, after being covered with tape, is allowed to remain in the ear for more than a week. Generally, however, needles are left in from twenty to thirty minutes.

Auriculotherapy (Ear Acupuncture)

Auriculotherapy, or ear acupuncture, was developed in France shortly after World War II by Paul Nogier, M.D. As a young physician in Lyon, Dr. Nogier observed a tiny peculiar scar in the auricula, or outer ear, of certain patients. The scar, he discovered, was the result of cauterization performed by a local healer as a treatment for sciatica. In most of the cases, Dr. Nogier learned, the procedure had cured the condition.

Dr. Nogier investigated this phenomenon and found that certain points on the outer ear formed a reflex system that could affect other areas when the points were properly stimulated. By 1957 he had worked out thirty basic auricular points that could neurologically affect the body's different layers of skin tissue. Dr. Nogier presented a paper on his discoveries at the Munich Acupuncture Convention. This led to further research on the subject in China and Japan that corroborated Dr. Nogier's findings. Today, Chinese ear acupuncture charts are adapted from Dr. Nogier's work and he has been officially recognized by the Chinese government as the father of modern ear acupuncture. In 1989, auriculotherapy was officially recognized by the World Health Organization as a viable medical modality.

Auriculotherapy is used in the treatment and control of pain, dyslexia, and other functional imbalances. It is applied through the use of acupuncture needles, ear massage, and, in certain cases, electrical stimulation or infrared treatment. In the United States, it has also become known as a successful treatment for alcohol, cigarette, and drug addiction and is used in treatment centers throughout the country.

Chinese herbs in the form of teas, pills, and capsules are often given to supplement acupuncture therapy. Finally, the acupuncturist may also recommend changes in diet, lifestyle, and physical activity.

Non-Needle Stimulation of Acupoints

In addition to the use of needles, other forms of treatment are applied to acupoints. Heat is used by burning an herb called moxa (mugwort, or *Artemisia vulgaris*) above the point to be treated. Studies from China have suggested that this particular herb is unique in that it stimulates acupoints and hastens the body's self-healing. The acupuncturist burns a pinch of moxa on a slice of ginger atop an acupoint, or alternatively, the moxa is placed directly on the point and removed as soon as it feels too warm to the patient. "There are certain points," says Dr. Cargile, "where a needle can't be used, for example, the navel, nipples, or penis."

Another traditional treatment, especially for large muscle pain, is cupping, which utilizes a glass or bamboo cup to create a suction on the skin above a painful muscle or acupuncture point.

In place of needles the acupuncturist may substitute electrostimulation, ultrasound waves, laser beams, or heat to acupuncture points. In China, experiments have included the use of synthetic needles, sonar rays, and injections of water or steroids into acupuncture points.

Acupuncture and Pet Care

H.C. Gurney, D.V.M., a Colorado-based veterinarian, is one of a growing number of veterinarians in the United States who has discovered the benefits of acupuncture for animals. Dr. Gurney has found it an effective alternative for conditions not amenable to conventional therapy, such as behavioral problems, chronic pain, allergies, and autoimmune diseases.

Dr. Gurney is a member of the International Veterinary Acupuncture Society (IVAS), under whose auspices veterinarians are trained to become pet acupuncturists. IVAS's director, Meredith Snader, D.V.M., reports using acupuncture to successfully treat dolphins, birds, monkeys, horses, and livestock, as well as dogs and cats.

Acupuncture is recognized as a valid veterinary medical procedure used mainly for surgical anesthesia and for the alleviation of chronic pain; it has been shown to be clinically effective in relieving symptoms in 84 percent of those animals suffering from arthritic pain and other degenerative joint diseases. It is also effective in eliminating certain forms of epileptic convulsions.[25]

The Future of Acupuncture

A growing understanding and greater respect for acupuncture, resulting from tests being conducted worldwide, leads Dr. Cargile to feel that acupuncture will increasingly be integrated into a system of overall health care in the United States. Dr. Cargile argues that, "Not only is acupuncture effective as a primary modality, it also can play a vital role as an adjunctive therapy due to how effective the meridian system is as a means of proper diagnosis. Because the meridians influence every cell in the body and pass through every organ and organ system, acupuncture provides health practitioners with an accurate and noninvasive means of determining health deficiencies, as well as a method of reestablishing balance. In short, it provides maximum benefits without the dangerous side effects associated with many of the approaches of conventional medicine."

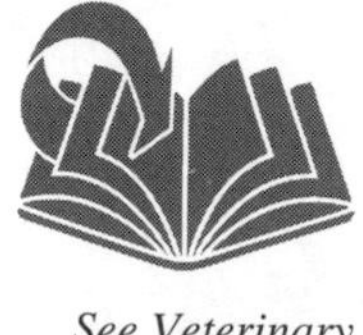

See Veterinary Medicine.

According to Dennis Tucker, Ph.D., L.Ac., of Nevada City, California, "While acupuncture represents a legacy of concepts that predate Western civilization, as a contemporary health care system it also represents a synthesis of continuously evolving scientific and technological developments which provides us with new tools to meet current clinical challenges. The future of acupuncture will to some degree depend upon our ability to reconcile the old and the new within a new science of energy medicine. This can only be accomplished if we honor both our traditional roots and the challenge of building on the foundation provided by scientific research."

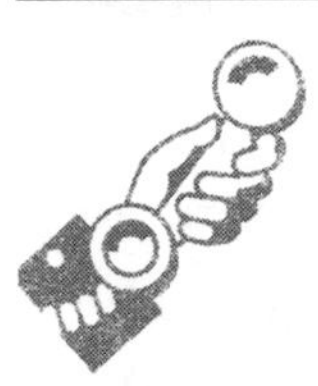

Where to Find Help

As with other forms of alternative health care, the legality of practicing acupuncture varies between states. In some states, there is no licensing, while others limit practice to physicians such as medical doctors and chiropractors. In other states, such as Maryland, nonphysician licensed acupuncturists are allowed to practice, provided their patients have been referred to them by a physician. In California and a few other states, acupuncturists are considered primary health care professionals and can see any patient without a physician's referral. Where acupuncture is legal, the acupuncturist must have graduated from an approved school and passed a state licensing examination. The following organizations will help you find a qualified acupuncturist:

American Association of Acupuncture and Oriental Medicine
4101 Lake Boone Trail, Suite 201
Raleigh, North Carolina 27607
(919) 787-5181

The AAAOM is a national professional trade organization of acupuncturists who meet acceptable standards of competency and can provide you with the names and locations of local members.

National Commission for the Certification of [illegible]
[illegible] Street NW, Suite 601
Washington, DC 20036
(202) 232-1404

The NCCA offers a test that some states use to verify basic competency in acupuncture.

The American College of Addictionality and Compulsive Disorders
5990 Bird Road
Miami, Florida 33155
(305) 661-3474

This is the official agency that board certifies doctors of all specialties in acupuncture treatment of addiction and compulsive disorders.

National Acupuncture [illegible]
3115 Broadway, Suite 51
New York, New York 10027
(212) 993-3100

NADA offers literature in eight languages, plus videotapes dealing with their program. Training is also provided for both practitioners and the lay public. Certification is available.

Recommended Reading

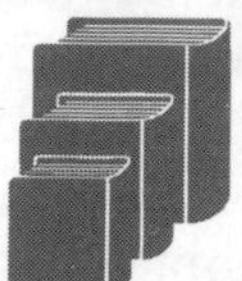

Acupuncture: Is It for You? Worsley, J. R. New York: Harper & Row, 1973.

An in-depth question and answer session with the founder of the College of Traditional Chinese Acupuncture (UK) and the Traditional Acupuncture Institute.

Between Heaven and Earth: A Guide to Chinese Medicine. Beinfield, Harriet, L.Ac.; and Korngold, Efrem, L.Ac., O.M.D. New York: Ballantine Books, 1991.

Combines Eastern tradition with Western sensibilities. The authors address three vital areas of Traditional Chinese Medicine: theory, therapy, and types, to present a comprehensive, yet understandable, guide to this ancient system.

Plain Talk About Acupuncture. Mitchell, Ellinor R. New York: Whalehall, Inc., 1987.

A book for prospective acupuncture patients who would like to learn what acupuncture can do for their health.

The Web That Has No Weaver: Understanding Chinese Medicine. Kaptchuk, Ted. New York: Congdon and Weed, 1992.

An excellent introduction to Acupuncture and Traditional Chinese Medicine for the layperson familiar with Western medicine. It contains detailed case histories comparing Acupuncture and Traditional Chinese Medicine with conventional Western medicine.

"It's supposed to be a professional secret, but I'll tell you anyway. We doctors do nothing. We only help and encourage the doctor within."

—Albert Schweizer

Applied Kinesiology

Applied kinesiology can determine health imbalances in the body's organs and glands by identifying weaknesses in specific muscles. By stimulating or relaxing these key muscles, an applied kinesiologist can diagnose and resolve a variety of health problems.

"Because of the close clinical relationship between specific muscle dysfunction and related organ or gland dysfunction, applied kinesiology can be used to identify and treat a wide variety of health problems, whether the problem originates in a muscle, gland, or organ," says Robert Blaich, D.C., of Los Angeles, a leading expert in applied kinesiology. "In applied kinesiology, the muscle-gland-organ link can indicate the cause of the health problem and lead to further diagnostic tests for confirmation. Once the problem is identified, it can be treated by a variety of techniques to strengthen the muscles involved and restore health."

How Applied Kinesiology Works

An applied kinesiologist studies the activity of muscles and the relationship of muscle strength to health. To illustrate this relationship, Dr. Blaich contrasts the approach taken by applied kinesiology with that of conventional medicine in treating asthma. Conventionally, asthma is treated with adrenal hormones or their [illegible] is still considered to be a problem [illegible] the lung. By contrast, an applied kinesiologist looks for a weakness in specific low back and leg muscles which, although normally associated with low back pain or knee problems, also share a connection with the adrenals. The applied kinesiologist would both strengthen these muscles and help the adrenal glands produce their own bronchodilators (chemicals that relax or open the air passages in the lungs).

"Muscle testing is often the key to balancing mechanically opposed muscles, since a muscle spasm usually exists secondary to and opposite a weak muscle," says Dr. Blaich. "If you want to bend your elbow, the bicep muscle must 'turn on' and the tricep muscle 'turn off'. If both muscles are either 'on' or 'off' the elbow will not bend. When you realize

THE ORIGIN OF APPLIED KINESIOLOGY

George Goodheart, D.C., of Detroit, Michigan, a chiropractic physician and the founder of applied kinesiology, first observed in 1964 that in the absence of skeletal deformity, postural distortion is often associated with muscle dysfunction.

A delivery boy who frequently came to Dr. Goodheart's office exhibited "winged scapulae" (flaring of the shoulder blades). This deformity occurs if a specific muscle is weakened by being slightly separated from the bone and is not doing its job of holding the shoulder blades in their proper position. Dr. Goodheart was aware of the development and utilization of manual muscle tests for the purpose of disability evaluation (developed at Johns Hopkins University in the 1940s), and he experimented with the boy by doing a manual procedure of firm, goading pressure on the attachment points of the weak (serratus anterior) muscles. An immediate response was that the muscles "turned on" and the boy's shoulder blades adopted a normal position.

Dr. Goodheart saw that these noninvasive, manipulative treatments restored neuromuscular function, and today they are the core approach to a therapy that encompasses joint manipulation and mobilization, myofascial (muscle sheath) therapies, cranial adjustments, meridian therapy, clinical nutrition, dietary management, and various reflex procedures.

Over the years, Dr. Goodheart discovered and developed many other procedures that returned injured, strained, or otherwise disabled muscles to their normal state. He taught his techniques to others, and eventually applied kinesiology was born. In 1974, a group of practitioners founded the International College of Applied Kinesiology, and today applied kinesiology is a widely practiced method of diagnosis and treatment.

that muscles turn 'on' and 'off' during all normal activities, it is easy to understand how an injury may leave a particular muscle stuck 'on' or 'off'.

"For example," Dr. Blaich explains, "when you step forward with your left leg, the right arm also goes forward because the extensor muscles that pull back on the right arm are 'turned off.' This 'turning off' is controlled by and dependent upon getting the correct messages from the nerve endings in the left foot. When you step down on the left foot, the joint receptors there send a message that shuts off the right shoulder. So, if a patient comes to me with a right shoulder problem, it may actually be due to a misaligned bone in the left foot that is causing the shoulder to be stuck 'on' or 'off.' The person's nervous system is acting as if he's taking a step with his left foot when, in fact, he is not.

"A muscle that is stuck 'on' acts like a tense muscle spasm, such as a 'charlie horse'. A muscle that is stuck 'off' may appear flaccid. Diagnostic evaluation by the applied kinesiologist determines whether muscles are 'on' or 'off' as they should be during normal activity." Dr. Blaich adds that, "This knowledge gives us an entirely new mechanism for the understanding of muscle spasm."

Muscle dysfunction in an otherwise healthy person can be corrected through the use of various reflexes or by performing a manual procedure on the muscle, such as deep massage, goading pressure on the attachment points, or realignment. By this method, according to Dr. Blaich, muscles can be reset to function smoothly.

The goals of applied kinesiology are to:

- Determine patient health status, and correlate findings with standard diagnostic procedures
- Restore postural balance, correct gait impairment, improve range of motion
- Restore normal nerve function
- Achieve normal endocrine, immune, digestive, and other internal organ functions
- Intervene early in degenerative processes to prevent or delay pathological conditions

Strong and Weak Muscles

Recent research has demonstrated a neurologic difference between "strong" and "weak" muscles, as identified through applied kinesiology testing.[1] Weak muscles will commonly exhibit as much actual force as normal muscles. However, there are other dynamics to a weak muscle besides the actual force it generates. Studies suggest at least part of this other quality lies in the timing of the electrical activity in the muscle. A weak muscle, notes Dr. Blaich, will often have a delayed reaction to stimulus.

Muscles become weak for many reasons, including immobility (such as when an arm is in a cast), lack of exercise, poor posture, gland or organ dysfunction, or injury. According to Dr. Blaich, some of the common internal causes of muscle weakness are:

- Dysfunction of the nerve supply (nerve interference between the spine and the muscles)
- Impairment of lymphatic drainage
- Reduced blood supply
- Abnormal pressure in the cerebrospinal fluid affecting the nerve-to-muscle relationship
- Blockage of an acupuncture meridian
- Chemical imbalance
- Organ or gland dysfunction

If one or more of these conditions exists, a muscle may exhibit abnormal function when tested. The abnormality usually manifests as muscle weakness. The bones that should be supported by that muscle may be misaligned or inflamed, or may exhibit signs of premature wear and tear, commonly in the form of osteoarthritis.

Conditions Benefited by Applied Kinesiology

Muscles perform the critical function of supporting and moving the bones. According to George Goodheart, D.C., the founder of applied kinesiology, if a muscle is not functioning properly, the bones and joints that it supports will function poorly, or not at all. This is why people with structural imbalances, musculoskeletal imbalances, and joint problems can benefit from applied kinesiology, and why applied kinesiology is so popular with the chiropractic profession, which many patients consult because of physical pain or dysfunction.

Muscle/Organ Relationships in Applied Kinesiology

While developing his theory and practice of applied kinesiology, Dr. Goodheart concluded that specific muscles are universally related to specific organs. Because of this relationship, a wide variety of nonmuscular conditions (problems with organs or systems, e.g. digestive) are often benefited. For example, because the deltoid muscle in the shoulder shares a relationship to the lungs, the muscle test can be an indicator of the state of the lungs, and can serve as an excellent monitor of their condition.

Reflex areas that stimulate either the deltoid or the lungs stimulate both. If an individual has a lung infection or an abnormal function in one or both lungs, he or she will probably exhibit weakness of one or both deltoid muscles. Not only would there be a lung infection, but because of deltoid weakness a problem may develop in the shoulder. Under normal circumstances, once the lung infection clears, or if the body adapts to the infection, the deltoid muscle will return to its normal state. However, if a chronic, low-grade infection lingers, the patient can be left with a weakened deltoid muscle. The applied kinesiologist evaluating the patient will likely need to stimulate the nerve and blood supply, as well as lymphatic drainage and acupuncture energy to the lungs in order for them to clear. Once the lung problem is resolved, deltoid muscle function can return to normal.

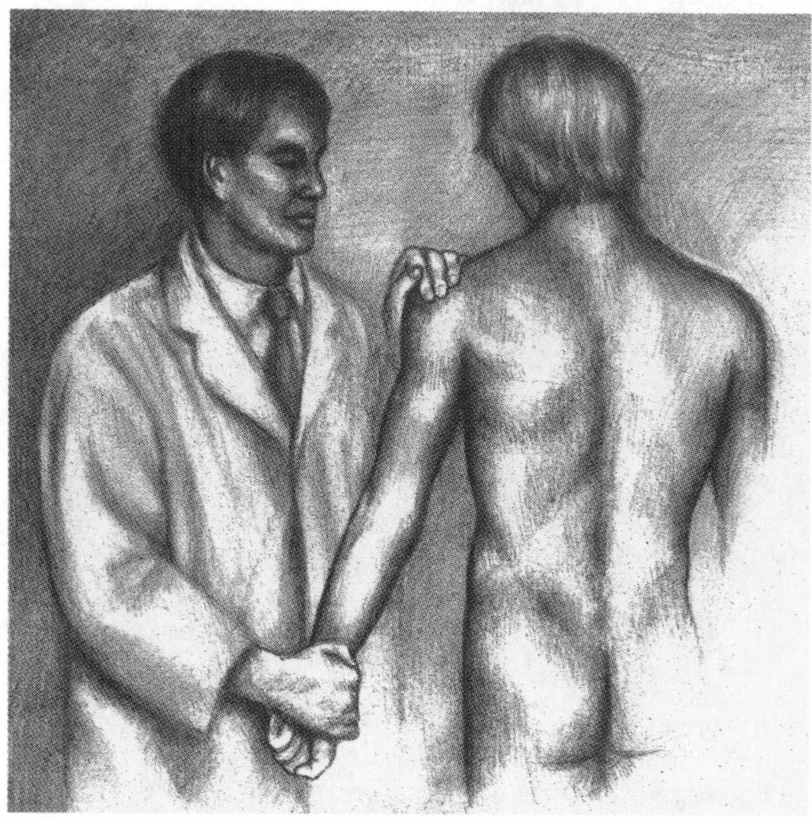

Doctor and patient performing applied kinesiology procedure.

Interestingly, toxic fumes inhaled into the lungs can conceivably stimulate the brain to produce an immediate weakening of a deltoid muscle, as its link to the lung can serve to monitor lung toxicity. Inhalation of the same fumes may also weaken a muscle related to the liver, such as the pectoralis major (a large fan-shaped muscle of the upper chest that acts to flex and rotate the arm), because of the increased demands placed on the liver to detoxify the harmful substances.

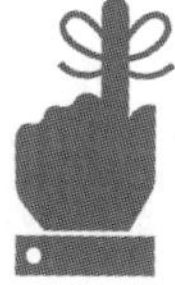

Applied kinesiology procedures are not intended to be used as a single method of diagnosis. They should enhance standard diagnosis, not replace it.

Nutrition in Applied Kinesiology

Specific vitamins or nutrients are sometimes needed to help a patient with a particular condition, such as an upper respiratory tract infection. One way to identify nutritional substances of value to this specific ailment is to test the patient's weak deltoid muscle while putting the substance on the tongue to stimulate nerve endings, which, in turn trigger certain areas in the brain to make changes in the body. If the correct nutrient is applied, there should be an immediate strengthening of the deltoid muscle.

Dr. Blaich tells of a conductor who came to him because severe pains in his shoulder were inhibiting his ability to conduct. After four hours in front of the orchestra, he could not raise his shoulder. Dr. Blaich evaluated the shoulder area and determined the main problem to be a specific muscle, the pectoralis major. He reset the muscle by correcting a specific cranial fault (minute manipulation of the bones in the head). The problem recurred, and through detailed testing, Dr. Blaich determined that the problem was caused by eating wheat. The patient was found to have a gluten allergy, and as long as he avoided eating wheat, he had no problems with his shoulder.

Applied Kinesiology and Sports

Because it deals so effectively with the interaction of muscles during activity, applied kinesiology is a superb approach to any type of athletic ailment or injury. It is so effective at improving muscle interaction and stabilization that it is often used not only for rehabilitation, but as a way to prevent injury and improve athletic performance.

A football player running down the field with a weak knee-stabilizing muscle is an "accident looking for a place to happen," notes Dr. Blaich. If he moves the wrong way, the knee joint could give out and conceivably cause serious injury. If he is evaluated and treated by an applied kinesiologist, the weak knee muscle will be recognized and treated, and serious injury avoided.

The muscle/organ link can be helpful in identifying "rate limiting factors," or "weak links," in the performance of top athletes. In 1983 and 1984, Dr. Blaich identified adrenal weakness accompanying other structural and chemical imbalances in a bicyclist named Alexi Grewal. Alexi was a talented young athlete, full of promise and motivation, but with a history of asthma. He was treated by Dr. Blaich, who worked to improve Alexi's adrenal gland and diaphragm muscle function as well as structural balance. Alexi's health and performance improved enough to win a gold medal in the 1984 Olympics.

A TYPICAL VISIT TO AN APPLIED KINESIOLOGIST

What happens on a visit to an applied kinesiologist depends entirely on the particular problem, and whether it is acute or chronic. Patient history is recorded, including diet and lifestyle. Inquiries are made about changes in either that could relate to the problem. The patient's posture, gait, and any obvious physical problems such as a dropped shoulder, a limp, or a lean to one side are carefully examined. In addition, before muscle testing is performed, blood tests may be ordered if organ dysfunction or infection are suspected.

The results of muscle testing may indicate the need for stimulation of acupuncture points or it may indicate the need to test nutrients on the tongue to see if these strengthen the weak muscle. The spine may be adjusted and reflexes may be stimulated to aid in the lymphatic drainage to a particular organ. Further blood tests may be indicated, or specific therapies suggested to strengthen a particular organ.

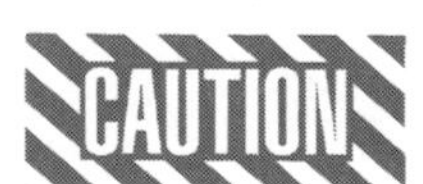

***Caution**: Applied kinesiology is a highly [illegible] and should only be [illegible] health professional trained in differential diagnosis (a systematic method for diagnosing a disorder that lacks unique signs or symptom). There have been many sincere attempts to teach lay people to use manual muscle testing as a method of home health care, but there are definite limitations to diagnostic conclusions made by someone not properly trained in manual muscle testing. For example, the skill of the practitioner in the accuracy of performing manual muscle testing, and the diagnostic conclusions that one makes regarding the outcome of a muscle test, are very significant. A manual muscle test can be a valuable indicator of some function in the body, but the interpretation of the test is complex, and should be handled by trained professionals.*

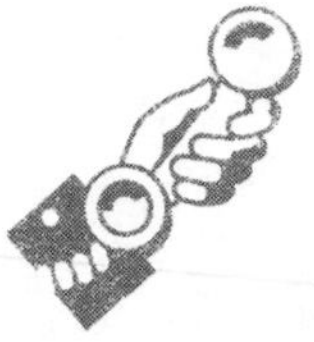

Where to Find Help

For more information on applied kinesiology, or for help in locating an applied kinesiology professional, contact:

International College of Applied Kinesiology
P.O. Box 905
Lawrence, Kansas 66044-0905
(913) 542-1801

Referral service for those seeking an applied kinesiologist. Supplies written information on various aspects of health and nutrition as well as public newsletter on request.

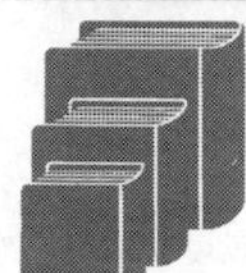

Recommended Reading

Applied Kinesiology: Muscle Response in Diagnosis, Therapy and Preventive Medicine. Valentine, Tom and Carol. Rochester, VT: Inner Traditions, 1989.

This book is a clearly written layperson's description and explanation of applied kinesiology principles and how they are used.

Everyone Is an Athlete. Maffetone, Philip. Mahopac, NY: David Barmore Productions, 1990.

Written by a leading applied kinesiology practitioner who has trained and treated some of the world's top athletes. The theme is "how to achieve both health and fitness." Applied kinesiology procedures are used to monitor body function in their development.

You'll Be Better, The Story of Applied Kinesiology. Goodheart, George, Jr., D.C. Geneva, OH: AK Printing, 1989.

Explanations, stories, and a history of applied kinesiology firsthand from the originator and developer. The book contains many insights and great practical information in natural health care. Distributed by Dr. George Goodheart, (313) 881-0662.

"The physician is nature's assistant."

—Galen, 2nd Century A.D.

Aromatherapy

Aromatherapy uses the essential oils extracted from plants and herbs to treat conditions ranging from infections and skin disorders to immune deficiencies and stress. Essential oils are widely used throughout Europe and a system of medical aromatherapy is currently practiced in France.

Aromatherapy is a unique branch of herbal medicine that utilizes the medicinal properties found in the essential oils of various plants. Through a process of steam distillation or cold-pressing, the volatile constituents of the plant's oil (its essence) are extracted from its flowers, leaves, branches, or roots. According to Dr. (rer. nat.) Kurt Schnaubelt, Director of the Pacific Institute of Aromatherapy, the term "aromatherapy" is somewhat misleading, as it can suggest an exclusive role for the aroma in the healing process. "In actuality," says Dr. Schnaubelt, "the oils exert much of their therapeutic effect through their pharmacological properties and their small molecular size, making them one of the few therapeutic agents to easily penetrate bodily tissues."

See Herbal Medicine for a description of pharmacological properties.

Aromatherapy is very effective for bacterial infections of the respiratory system,[1] immune deficiencies such as Epstein-Barr virus (a form of herpes virus believed to be the causative agent in infectious mononucleosis), and numerous skin disorders.[2] It is also useful for other infections such as cystitis[3] and herpes simplex.[4] The immediate and often profound effect that essential oils have on the central nervous system also makes aromatherapy an excellent method for stress management.[5]

How Aromatherapy Works

According to Dr. Schnaubelt, "The chemical makeup of essential oils gives them a host of desirable pharmacological properties ranging from antibacterial, antiviral, and antispasmodic, to uses as diuretics (promoting production and excretion of urine), vasodilators (widening blood vessels), and vasoconstrictors (narrowing blood vessels). Essential oils act on the adrenals, ovaries, and the thyroid and can energize or pacify, detoxify, and facilitate the digestive process." The oils' therapeutic properties also make them effective for treating infection, interacting with the various branches of the nervous system, modifying immune response, and harmonizing moods and emotions.

The Physiological Effects of Fragrance

Aromatic molecules that interact with the top of the nasal cavity give off signals that are modified by various biological processes before traveling to the limbic system, the emotional switchboard of the brain.[6] There they create impressions associated with previous experiences and emotions. Because the limbic system is directly connected to those parts of the brain that control heart rate, blood pressure, breathing, memory, stress levels, and hormone balance, scientists have learned that oil fragrances may be one of the fastest ways to achieve physiological or psychological effects.

John Steele, Ph.D., of Sherman Oaks, California, and Robert Tisserand, of London, England, leading researchers in the field of aromatherapy, have studied the effects on brain wave patterns when essential oils are inhaled or smelled. Their findings show that oils such as orange, jasmine, and rose have a tranquilizing effect and work by altering the brain waves into a rhythm that produces calmness and a sense of well-being. In the same way, the so-called "stimulating" oils—basil, black pepper, rosemary, and cardamom—work by producing a heightened energy response.[7]

How aromas affect the limbic system.

Inhaling the fragrance of certain essential oils can help clear sinuses or free congestion in the chest, as well as alter the neurochemistry of the brain to produce changes in mental and emotional behavior. Even aromas too subtle to be consciously detected can have significant effects on central nervous system activity, sometimes to the point of cutting in half the amount of time needed to perform a visual search task.[8]

How to Use Aromatherapy

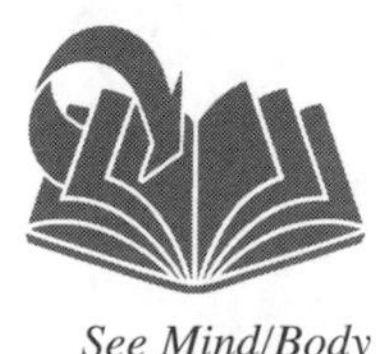

See Mind/Body Medicine.

Aromatherapy uses essential oils to affect the body in several ways. The benefits of essential oils can be obtained through inhalation, external application or ingestion.

- **Through a diffusor:** Diffusors disperse microparticles of the essential oil into the air. They can be used to achieve beneficial results in respiratory conditions, or to simply change the air with the mood-lifting or calming qualities of the fragrance.
- **External application:** Oils are readily absorbed through the skin. Convenient applications are baths, massages, hot and cold compresses, or a simple topical application of diluted oils.[9]

Essential oils in a hot bath can stimulate the skin, induce relaxation, and energize the body. According to Debra Nuzzi St. Claire, M.H., an aromatherapist and herbalist from Boulder, Colorado, using certain essential oils, such as rosemary in the bath, can stimulate the elimination of toxins through the skin. In massage, the oils can be worked into the skin and depending on the oil and the massage technique, can either calm or stimulate an individual. When used in compresses, essential oils soothe minor aches and pains, reduce swelling, and treat sprains.

- **Floral waters:** These can be sprayed into the air or sprayed on skin that is too sensitive to the touch.
- **Internal application:** For certain conditions (such as organ dysfunction/disorder), it can be advantageous to take oils internally. It is essential to receive proper medical guidance for internal use of oils. However, such professional guidance is difficult to obtain in the United States.

CAUTION

In their pure state, certain oils, such as clove and cinnamon, can cause irritation or skinburn. These oils call for careful and expert application.[16] It is recommended that they be diluted with a less irritating essential oil before being applied to the skin. Essential oils can cause a toxic reaction if ingested. Consult a physician before taking any oils internally.

Conditions Benefited by Aromatherapy

The value of aromatherapy in the treatment of infectious diseases has gained increased attention in recent years. Its use for this purpose is widespread in France, where a system of aromatherapeutic medicine has been developed.[10] French physicians routinely prescribe aromatherapy preparations, and French pharmacies stock essential oils alongside the more conventional drugs. In England, aromatherapy is used mainly for stress-related health issues. Hospital nursing staffs administer essential oil massage to relieve pain and to induce sleep.[11] This type of massage has proven particularly effective in relieving stress associated with surgery, terminal cancer,[12] and AIDS. English hospitals also use a variety of vaporized essential oils (including lemon, lavender, and lemongrass) to help combat the transmission of airborne infectious diseases.[13] Essential oils are also used topically on wound sites to counter infection.

“English hospitals also use a variety of vaporized essential oils (including lemon, lavender, and lemongrass) to help combat the transmission of airborne infectious diseases.”

Bacterial and Viral Infections

Essential oils are powerful antimicrobial (microbe-fighting) agents.[14] They lack the negative side effects (kidney toxicity, anemia, lowered white cell count, deafness) of conventional antibiotics and do not destroy intestinal bacteria, the loss of which can lead to secondary infections.

In a hallmark study conducted in 1973, a blend of the essential oils clove, cinnamon, melissa, and lavender was found to be as effective in treating bronchial conditions as were commercial antibiotics.[15] “Because the oils work in a different way from antibiotics, they do not have the usual side effects, and they tend to stimulate the immune system instead of depressing it,” says Tisserand. “Oils of cinnamon and eucalyptus are as powerful against some microorganisms as conventional antibiotics, and are especially effective against flus. Sandalwood oil from Mysore, India, is not only a classic perfume oil but is also a traditional remedy for sore throats and laryngitis. Lavender oil, so often used in toilet waters and scented sachets, has a dramatic healing action on burns."[16]

> *"Due to their strong antiviral properties, many essential oils are highly effective against the herpes simplex virus, according to a study presented at the 1st Congress on Aromatherapy in Cologne, Germany, in 1987."*

Herpes Simplex

Due to their strong antiviral properties, many essential oils are highly effective against the herpes simplex virus, according to a study presented at the 1st Congress on Aromatherapy in Cologne in 1987.[17] Jean Valnet, M.D., a French physician, recommends a blend of lemon and geranium[18]; Tisserand suggests *Eucalyptus radiata* and bergamot. Dr. (rer. nat.) Dietrich Wabner, a professor at the Technical University of Munich, reports that a one-time application of either true rose oil or true melissa oil led to complete remission of herpes simplex lesions.

The most effective treatment is to apply the oil(s) at the first sign of an outbreak. If herpes lesions have already appeared, the oil(s) is applied directly on the lesions and, in most cases, the lesions dry within a day or two and are in complete remission within three to five days. If the drying process creates discomfort, a 10 percent dilution of the essential oil(s) is mixed in a high quality vegetable base oil. "We have documented this pattern of remission in almost all the cases we were able to observe over the years," reports Dr. Schnaubelt. "Whenever the specific pain indicating the recurrence of the lesions occurs, oils are applied before the outbreak of the lesion and more often than not the outbreak is prevented. After repeating this procedure three to four times, herpes simplex typically stops recurring."

History of Aromatherapy

Plants and their essential oils have been used therapeutically from ancient times in countries as diverse as Egypt, Italy, India, and China.[19] In most of the world, plant essences remain popular as therapeutic agents and are utilized in everything from antiseptic creams and skin ointments to liniments for arthritic pain.

The term aromatherapy was coined in 1937 by the French chemist René-Maurice Gattefossé. While working in his family's perfume laboratory, Dr. Gattefossé burned his hand. He knew lavender was used in medicine for burns and inflammation, and immediately immersed his hand in a container of pure lavender oil he had on his workbench. When the burn quickly lost its redness and began to heal, he was impressed enough by the oil's regenerative ability to begin researching the curative powers of other essential oils. This marked the beginning of the modern-day science of aromatherapy for the treatment of common ailments. In the United States, the popularity of aromatherapy has grown rapidly over the last ten years, fueled by the increasing demand for nontoxic and nonthreatening restorative therapies.

Shingles (Herpes Zoster Infection)

"Another effective use of essential oils is the topical treatment of shingles, a painful skin virus," says Dr. Schnaubelt. "Our greatest success in the treatment of shingles is by applying a blend of 50 percent *Ravensera aromatica* and 50 percent *Calophyllum inophyllum* (related to St. John's Wort). Drastic improvements and complete remission occur within seven days."

Skin Conditions

Essential oils are also utilized for skin problems based on their skin-friendly properties. Examples are thyme oil, whose highly antiseptic properties are non-irritating; neroli oil, whose rejuvenating properties produce an effect similar to hormones (neroli is also utilized to prevent stretch marks); rosemary oil, known to regenerate cells and improve metabolic activity in the inner layer of the skin; and everlast, possibly the most effective anti-inflammatory agent in aromatherapy. Thyme-linalol and rosewood oil are effective when used topically for acne. Other effective essential oils for skin conditions are carrot seed oil (an effective tissue revitalizer excellent for use on the face), and eucalyptus oil (commonly used to regulate overproductive sebaceous glands—which help to retain body heat and prevent sweat evaporation). In cases of bites or stings, Dr. Valnet points out that the essential oils basil, cinnamon, garlic, lavender, lemon, onion, sage, savory, and thyme are effective due to their antitoxic and antivenomous properties.[20]

Muscular Disorders

There have been many studies outlining the effects of various essential oils on the nervous system and their ability to relieve muscle spasm.[21] Combinations of essential oils with high proportions of ester compounds (clary sage, roman chamomile, and lavender) are especially effective in this regard, and are used in massage as well as in advanced spa treatments.

Arthritis

Studies by Dr. Hildebret Wagner, Chair of the Institute of Pharmaceutical Biology at Ludwig Maximilian University in Munich, Germany, show that the essential oils that stimulate, such as clove, cinnamon, and thyme, can have anti-inflammatory effects in treating arthritis. Dr. Wagner suggests that the irritation caused by these oils stimulates the adrenal glands and triggers the release of anti-inflammatory corticoid substances, the body's natural cortisone-like material.[22] The more practical and effective application of everlast and eucalyptus to relieve arthritis pain comes out of French medical aromatherapy. "Because of their very strong local anti-inflammatory action, these oils often reduce arthritis symptoms within moments of application," says Dr. Schnaubelt.

Some Essential Oils and Their Applications

According to Dr. Schnaubelt, the following essential oils are among the most widely used therapeutically:

Eucalyptus *(Eucalyptus radiata)*: This particular form of eucalyptus, also called *Eucalyptus australiana*, is a classic antiviral and expectorant agent.[23] It is best used through a diffusor, or topically as a chest rub.

Everlast *(Helichrysum italicum)*: Skin care professionals use everlast in dilutions of 2 percent or lower for its tissue-regenerating qualities on scars. Applied topically, it is a powerful anti-inflammatory agent, and can prevent hemorrhaging and swelling after sports injuries or bruising. Because of its ketone (an organic chemical derived by oxidation of alcohol) content this oil should only be used topically and in concentrations not exceeding 2 percent.

Geranium *(Pelargonium x asperum)*: A fragrant oil with antifungal[24] and antiviral properties. It is gentle on the skin and gives body to the fragrance of many essential oil compositions.

Lavender *(Lavandula angustifolia)*: The classic oil of aromatherapy. It can be used undiluted on burns, small injuries, and insect bites. A high ester content gives it a calming, almost sedative quality.

Mandarin *(Citrus reticulata)*: Mandarin's calming properties and universally pleasing fragrance make this oil a top choice to release anxiety. It is typically dispersed in a room with a diffusor.

Niaouli *(Melaleuca quinquenervia viridiflora)*: Niaouli calms respiratory allergies, is a vitalizing, balancing agent for overactive and oily skin, and helps with hemorrhoids (in the nonacute stage).

Palmarosa *(Cymbopogon martinii)*: A staple in many different homemade aromatherapy compositions, palmarosa's pleasant fragrance and excellent antiseptic/antiviral activity have uses in skin care and in the treatment of herpes.

Peppermint *(Mentha piperita)*: A drop on the tongue of this oil provides excellent relief for nausea and travel sickness. It is also effective for irritable bowel syndrome. In France, small doses of peppermint oil (fifty milligrams) are given three times a day as a stimulant for the liver during convalescence.

Roman Chamomile *(Anthemis nobilis)*: Recommended to calm an upset mind or body. A drop rubbed on the solar plexus can bring rapid relief of mental or physical stress.

Rosemary *(Rosmarinus officinalis)*: There are a number of varieties of rosemary which have different chemical compositions. The softest and most expensive type is rosemary verbenon, which is a staple in aromatherapy skin care compositions, as it activates the metabolism in the outer layer of the skin and improves cell regeneration.

Spikenard *(Nardostachys jatamansi)*: This oil is from the root of a plant from the Himalayan mountains. It has an open life cycle and a theoretically endless life span. One belief is that the spikenard oil embodies the life energy of

PURCHASING OILS

Selecting essential oils from the many different offerings in the marketplace can be confusing. Vast differences in price exist for what seems to be one and the same oil. Inquiries are practically always met with a universal assurance that the oil is absolutely pure and natural. This is not always the case. Many suppliers do not verify the purity of the oils they distribute. When purchasing essential oils, it is important to take note of their purity, quality, and price.

"Pure essential oils are expensive," according to Dr. (rer. nat.) Kurt Schnaubelt, Director of the Pacific Institute of Aromatherapy. "Often one thousand pounds of plant are needed to produce one pound of essence. This process involves manpower to cultivate and harvest the plant, and the energy cost for distillation. Because of the variations in these factors, the prices of essential oils can differ. If every oil in a line carries the same price tag, this is a sure sign of large-scale homogenization and adulteration for the production of sheer fragrance oils as opposed to essential oils.

"Essential oils should be called 'essential oils'. If names are used that sound evasive, such as 'pure botanical perfume' or 'pure fragrance essence', this is an indication that the supplier is aware that the oils are not true essential oils," adds Dr. Schnaubelt.

Oil essences are most commonly produced to create fragrances and to process food. The quality requirements of these oils are substantially lower than those used for aromatherapy. Companies that concern themselves solely with aromatherapy will go to great lengths to ensure purity.

While pure, natural essential oils may seem expensive, the smallest amounts will go far, and this makes them cost-effective. In contrast, the effectiveness of lower grade oils, or oils that are diluted, drastically diminishes over time due to a loss of their essential properties.

The best way to purchase essential oils for aromatherapy applications is from a supplier who specializes in essential aromatherapy oils.

the plant.[25] For that reason it is often used at the core of aromatherapy blends that are aimed as much toward benefiting the psyche as they are the skin.

Tea Tree *(Melaleuca alternifolia)*: A nonirritating antiseptic, tea tree has antibacterial, antiviral, and antifungal properties. Applied topically, It is useful in healing pus-filled wounds and for treating many types of mild or chronic infections.

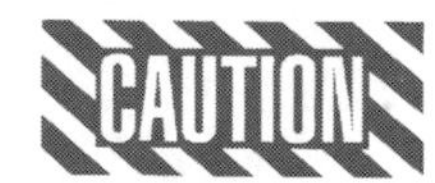

Caution: *Certain essential oils, such as those derived from thuja, wormwood, mugwort, tansy, hyssop, and sage, can cause a toxic reaction if taken internally. However, their toxicity is much lower when applied externally. Other essential oils with high phenol (disinfectant) content, such as oregano and savory, should not be taken internally for any prolonged period of time (exceeding ten to twenty-one days). Doing so might have negative implications on certain aspects of the liver metabolism. Clove and cinnamon should also be used with caution, as they are known allergenics. Approximately 5 percent of the population will exhibit a dermatitis reaction to these two oils when they are applied to the skin. Interestingly, the toxicity of these oils is a factor when applied to the skin, but comparatively low when ingested (in moderate doses).[26] Occasionally irritation can also occur from overuse of a certain oil. This is not hazardous, and will disappear when use of the oil is discontinued.*

Aromatherapy in the Home

Aromatherapy is ideally suited for home use. While it is true that irresponsible or ignorant use of essential oils may pose certain risks, these risks are small compared to the potential gain. Typical problems are caused by excessive use of potentially irritating or allergenic oils such as clove, cinnamon, oregano, or savory, but with proper knowledge these pitfalls are easily avoided. Most health food stores now carry essential oils, and many even carry "starter kits" with selections of the most widely used essential oils. Following are some typical applications of essential oils in the home:

- **Daily hygiene:** Gentle antiviral essential oils, such as *Eucalyptus radiata*, *Ravensera aromatica*, and niaouli can be spread over the skin before, during, or after the morning shower. This practice strengthens the body's resistance to sickness during the cold or flu season.
- **Digestive and stress-related discomfort:** A drop of anise seed oil, taken on a spoon of honey (or by itself) helps to release gastrointestinal cramping. Tarragon stimulates digestion and calms a nervous digestive tract.
- **Bruises and sports injuries:** Everlast relieves pain after injuries, and prevents hemorrhaging and swelling.
- **Mosquito and other insect bites:** Lavender is unsurpassed in treating itching or stinging from mosquito bites or bee stings.
- **Burns:** The restorative powers of lavender oil on burnt skin inspired the very emergence of aromatherapy.

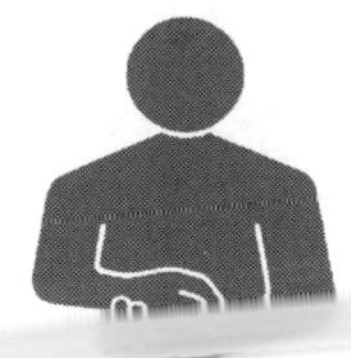

Aromatherapy is uniquely suited to self-care and can easily become part of your personal health maintenance program.

- **Energy:** Essential oils of black spruce and peppermint are effective stimulants that work by strengthening the adrenal cortex.[27]
- **Relaxation:** Essential oils like citronella and *Eucalyptus citriodora* can be diffused in the air, or rubbed on the wrists, solar plexus, and temples for quick and effective relaxation. Mandarin is a fragrance favored by children, and its calming qualities can slow down highly active children. Lavender oil added to the bath or sprayed on the bed sheets reduces tension and enhances relaxation.[28]
- **Nausea:** Peppermint is the classic oil for alleviating nausea and travel sickness. Its beneficial uses for irritated colon are clearly documented.[29]

The Future of Aromatherapy

"While aromatherapy is practiced by medical doctors in France, this has not been the case in England and the United States," says Tisserand. "With the increasing demand for holistic health care and the 'green revolution', the demand for aromatherapy will increase, and hopefully we will reach the point where medical doctors incorporate it into their repertoire. It will become routine for doctors to send culture samples to the pharmacist for testing, and identify the relevant aromatherapy for the patient. The stress-relieving properties associated with aromatherapy make it an indispensable part of health care."

"For many common infectious diseases aromatherapy offers more effective and more wholesome solutions than conventional medicine."

—Dr. (rer. nat.) Kurt Schnaubelt

Dr. Schnaubelt also believes that the use of aromatherapy will become increasingly widespread. "For many common infectious diseases aromatherapy offers more effective and more wholesome solutions than conventional medicine," he says. "If aromatherapy was allowed to compete only on its merit it would be a great competitor for a variety of aspects of conventional medicine. Much of the future of aromatherapy will be determined through political processes. The powers in place in the medical 'market' will try to keep aromatherapy out because it threatens profits to the conventional medical establishment. However, the demand of the consumer for more and better access to alternative methods will continue to offset such vested interests and should do much to make aromatherapy more popular as a healing modality."

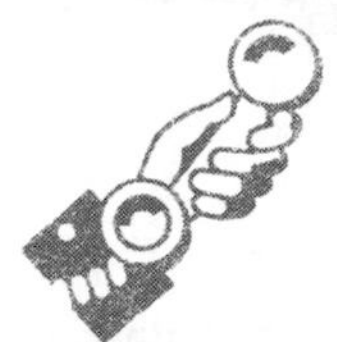

Where to Find Help

For more information on aromatherapy, or help in locating aromatherapy products, contact:

The Pacific Institute of Aromatherapy
P.O. Box 6842
San Rafael, California 94903
(415) 479-9121

The Pacific Institute of Aromatherapy offers courses to individuals and companies interested in learning about, or becoming certified in, the practice of aromatherapy. Call for a brochure and course listing.

National Association for Holistic Aromatherapy
P.O. Box 17622
Boulder, Colorado 80308-0622
(303) 258-3791

NAHA offers aromatherapy courses, and they distill and sell their own aromatherapy products. NAHA also acts as a referral service for aromatherapists.

Aromatherapy Seminars
3379 S. Robertson Boulevard
Los Angeles, California 90034
(800) 677-2368
(310) 838-6122

Provides programs to become a certified aromatherapist, locally or through a correspondence course. They offer specialty classes for those already certified and have available videotapes, audiotapes and blending materials.

Lotus Light
P.O. Box 1008
Wilmot, Wisconsin 53170
(414) 889-8501

Provides mail order distribution of aromatherapy videotapes, books, and materials.

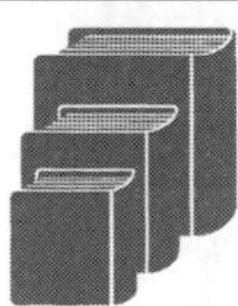

Recommended Reading

The Aromatherapy Book: Applications and Inhalations. Rose, Jeanne. Berkeley, CA: North Atlantic [illegible].

[illegible] Rose has been writing on herbs for over twenty years. Her book thoroughly covers the healing qualities of herbal aromatherapy, and is considered a bible for those interested in incorporating aromatic cures into a healthy life.

Aromatherapy for Common Ailments. Price, Shirley. New York: Simon & Schuster, 1991.

Explains aromatherapy, with emphasis on its practical and medicinal uses, as well as how to blend your own oils.

Aromatherapy, to Heal and Tend the Body. Tisserand, Robert. [illegible], 1988.

This book explains the history of aromatherapy, how it is applied and what to expect from treatment. It also includes detailed case studies, psychological and physical results and monographs on a number of oils.

Aromatherapy Workbook. Lavabre, Marcel. Rochester, VT: Healing Arts Press, 1990.

A practical guide to essential oils, including the history, chemistry, application and treatments of aromatherapy. Over seventy oils are classified by botanical family and a section is provided on the blending of oils.

The Art of Aromatherapy. Tisserand, Robert B. Rochester, VT: Destiny Books, 1987.

A classic reference book on essential oils and their uses. Includes tables on evaporation rates and odor intensity, recipes, and detailed information on Swedish, shiatsu, *and neuromuscular massage techniques.*

The Complete Aromatherapy Handbook: Essential Oils for Radiant Health. Fisher-Rizzi, Suzanne. New York: Sterling Press, 1991.

An illustrated handbook that describes the history of aromatherapy, its herbs, and essential oils. Includes drawings and recipes in the informative chapters that outline physical, mental, and cosmetic applications of aromatherapy.

The International Journal of Aromatherapy
P.O Box 746
Hove, East Sussex
BN3 3XA, UK

The International Journal of Aromatherapy *is edited by Dr. Robert Tisserand and can be obtained by writing to the above address.*

The Practice of Aromatherapy. Valnet, Jean. Rochester, VT: Inner Traditions, 1990.

One of the classic books on aromatherapy and its many applications.

"Man is ill because he is never still."
—Paracelsus

Ayurvedic Medicine

Practiced in India for the past five thousand years, Ayurvedic medicine (meaning "science of life") is a comprehensive system of medicine that combines natural therapies with a highly personalized approach to the treatment of disease. Ayurvedic medicine places equal emphasis on body, mind, and spirit, and strives to restore the innate harmony of the individual.

The first question an Ayurvedic physician asks is not 'What disease does my patient have?' but 'Who is my patient?' " explains Deepak Chopra, M.D., a Western-trained endocrinologist who has introduced Ayurvedic medicine to the general reader through a number of popular books. "By 'who,' " adds Dr. Chopra, "the physician does not mean your name, but how you are constituted."

"Constitution" is the keystone of Ayurvedic medicine, and refers to the overall health profile of the individual, including strengths and susceptibilities. The subtle and often intricate identification of a person's constitution is the first critical step in the process. Once established, it becomes the foundation for all clinical decisions.

To determine an individual's constitution, Ayurvedic doctors first identify the patient's metabolic body type. A specific treatment plan is then designed to guide the individual back into harmony with his or her environment, which may include dietary changes, exercise, yoga, meditation, massage, herbal tonics, herbal sweat baths, medicated enemas, and medicated inhalations.

The Three Metabolic Body Types: *Vata*, *Pitta*, and *Kapha*

Ayurvedic medicine is founded on the concept of metabolic body types, or *doshas*. The three metabolic body types are known as *vata*, *pitta*, and *kapha*. They include distinctions of physique similar to the Western view of body types as thin, muscular, and fat, but Ayurvedic medicine considers them to have far greater influence on a person's health and well-being than do physical attributes alone.

Dr. Chopra describes the Ayurvedic body type as a blueprint which outlines all of the innate tendencies built into a person's system. One's *dosha* and the characteristics which reveal it, clarify why one person, for example, will have no reaction to milk, chili, loud noise, or humidity, while another will not be able to tolerate them.

Most people are a mixture of *dosha* characteristics (such as *vata-pitta*), with one usually more predominant than another. Each of the body types flourishes under a specific diet, exercise plan, and lifestyle.

The *Vata* Body Type

According to Dr. Chopra, the primary characteristic of the *vata* metabolic type is changeability. Unpredictability and variability—in size, shape, mood, and action—is the *vata* trademark. *Vatas* tend to be slender with prominent features, joints, and veins, with cool, dry skin. Moody, enthusiastic, imaginative, and impulsive, the *vata* type is quick to grasp ideas and is good at initiating things but poor at finishing them. *Vatas* eat and sleep erratically and are prone to anxiety, insomnia, premenstrual syndrome, and constipation. *Vata* energy fluctuates, with jagged peaks and valleys.

The *Pitta* Body Type

The *pitta* metabolic body type is relatively predictable. The *pitta* person is of medium build, strength, and endurance. He or she is well-proportioned and easily maintains a stable weight. Often fair, the *pitta* type will frequently have red or blond hair, freckles, and a ruddy complexion. *Pittas* have a quick, articulate, biting intelligence, and can be critical or passionate with short, explosive tempers. Efficient and moderate in daily habits, the *pitta* type eats and sleeps regularly, eating three meals a day and sleeping eight hours at night. *Pitta* types tend to perspire heavily and are warm and often thirsty. They suffer from acne, ulcers, hemorrhoids, and stomach ailments.

CHARACTERISTICS AND TENDENCIES OF AYURVEDIC METABOLIC BODY TYPES

Vata

- *Thin*
- *Prominent features, joints*
- *Cool, dry skin*
- *Hyperactive*
- *Moody*
- *Vivacious*
- *Eats and sleeps at all hours*
- *Imaginative*
- *Nervous disorders*
- *Constipation*
- *Enthusiastic, infectious energy*
- *Intuitive*
- *Cramps*
- *Anxiety*

Pitta

- *Medium build*
- *Fair, thin hair*
- *Warm, ruddy, perspiring skin*
- *Orderly, efficient*
- *Intense*
- *Short temper*
- *Doesn't miss a meal*
- *Lives by the clock*
- *Intelligent*
- *Ulcers, heartburn*
- *Hemorrhoids*
- *Warm, loving*
- *Passionate*
- *Articulate*
- *Acne*
- *Perfectionism*

Kapha

- *Heavyset*
- *Thick, wavy hair*
- *Cool, thick, pale, oily skin*
- *Slow, graceful*
- *Relaxed*
- *Slow to anger*
- *Eats slowly*
- *Sleeps long, heavily*
- *Affectionate*
- *Obesity*
- *Allergies, sinus*
- *Forgiving and tolerant*
- *Compassionate*
- *High cholesterol*
- *Procrastination*

The *Kapha* Body Type

"The basic theme of the *kapha* metabolic type is relaxed," says Dr. Chopra. The *kapha* body type is solid, heavy, and strong. With a tendency to be overweight, *kaphas* have slow digestion and somewhat oily hair, and cool, damp, pale skin. Everything *kapha* is slow—*kapha* types are slow to anger, slow to eat, slow to act. They sleep long and heavily. *Kaphas* tend to procrastinate and be obstinate. A *kapha* body type will be prone to high cholesterol, obesity, allergies, and sinus problems.

The Three *Doshas* and Health

Although each person's metabolic type is determined by a predominant *dosha*, all three *doshas* are present in varying degrees in every cell, tissue, and organ of the body.

According to Vasant Lad, M.A.Sc., an Ayurvedic physician and Director of the Ayurvedic Institute in Albuquerque, New Mexico, the *doshas* are located in specific areas of the body:

- ***Vata*** is motion that activates the physical system and allows the body to breathe and circulate blood. The seats of the *vata* are the large intestine, pelvic cavity, bones, skin, ears, and thighs.
- ***Pitta***, the metabolism, processes food, air, and water and is responsible for charging the hundreds of enzymatic activities throughout the body. The seats of *pitta* are the small intestine, stomach, sweat glands, blood, skin, and eyes.
- ***Kapha***, the structure of bones, muscle, and fat that holds the body together, offers nourishment and protection. For example, [illegible] surrounding the spinal cord are the seats of *kapha* in the body.

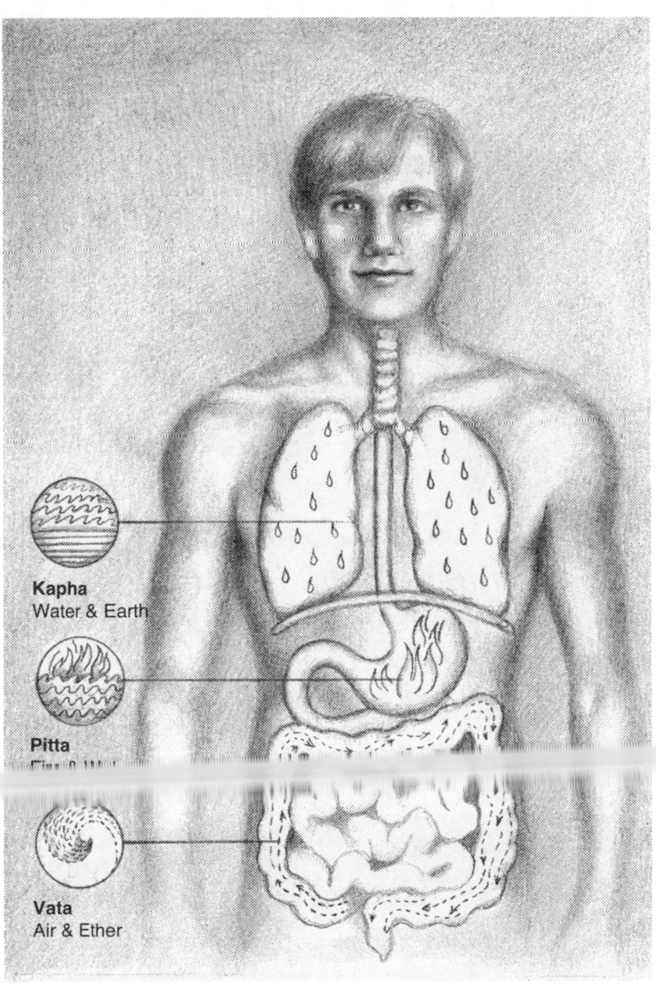

The seat of the three doshas *in the body.*

When the *doshas* are balanced in accordance with an individual's constitution, the result is vibrant health and energy. But when the delicate balance is disturbed, the body becomes susceptible to outside stressors, which may range from viruses and bacteria to poor nutrition and overwork. Imbalance in the *doshas* is the first sign that mind and body are not perfectly coordinated, notes Dr. Chopra. He points out that once people understand the characteristics and qualities ascribed to their body types, they can take appropriate measures, through changes in diet, lifestyle, and environment, to restore *dosha* balance, which will prevent disease and ensure continued good health.

The Disease Process According to Ayurvedic Medicine

Ayurveda defines health as a soundness and balance between body, mind, and soul, and an equilibrium between the *doshas*. According to Ayurvedic medicine, there are seven major factors that can disrupt physiological harmony—genetic, congenital, internal, external trauma; seasonal, natural tendencies or habits; and magnetic and electrical influences. Virender Sodhi, M.D. (Ayurveda), N.D., Director of the American School of Ayurvedic Sciences in Bellevue, Washington, says that "disease is the result of a disruption of the spontaneous flow of nature's intelligence within our physiology. When we violate nature's law and cannot adequately rid ourselves of the results of this disruption, then we have disease."

There are pathologies recognized as being genetically based. For example, when placed in a particular environment, a predisposed individual may have a tendency to develop a health problem prompted by his or her surroundings. This genetic susceptibility can be triggered in the womb by the mother's lifestyle, diet, habits, activities, and emotions. Accordingly, individuals possess natural tendencies to adopt certain habits, such as overeating and smoking.

From birth, stressors—both inner and outer—challenge an individual's health. For example, hot, spicy food can induce an ulcer or damage the liver. Disease can also have an emotional cause, such as deep-seated, unresolved anger, fear, anxiety, grief, or sadness. External traumas and injuries can also play an influential role.

"Ayurvedic medicine takes into account how the seasons and time of day influence health. Dietary and other therapeutic suggestions are often prescribed with this in mind."

Ayurveda also takes into account how the seasons and time of day influence health. Dietary and other therapeutic suggestions are often prescribed with this in mind. To say that summer is a *pitta* season means that *pitta* qualities are at their height during this time. Summer's bright light and heat can induce inflammatory conditions such as hives, rash, acne, biliary disorders, diarrhea, or conjunctivitis in *pitta* individuals. *Vata's* season is autumn, and because autumn reflects windy, dry, and cold qualities, *vata* people tend to develop neurological, muscular, and rheumatic problems such as constipation, sciatica, arthritis, and rheumatism. Winter's deep cold and biting wind brings out more *kapha* characteristics, and stresses the *kapha* respiratory system with colds, hay fever, cough, congestion, sneezing, and sinus disorders. Spring is both *pitta* and *kapha*; the coolness, budding leaves, and beautiful flowers of early spring enhance *kapha's* constitution; late spring promotes *pitta*.

The Art of Ayurvedic Diagnosis

Ayurvedic physicians have traditionally relied on the powers of observation rather than equipment and laboratory testing to diagnose disease. Diagnosis is based on physical observation, questioning the patient as to personal and family history, palpation (feeling the body), and listening to the heart, lungs, and intestines. This approach is changing, however, as physicians integrate Ayurvedic traditions with modern diagnostic methods.

Ayurvedic physicians pay special attention to the pulse, tongue, eyes, and nails. Whereas Western medical doctors use the pulse to determine heart rate, Ayurvedic doctors describe three distinct types of pulses: *vata*, *pitta*, and *kapha*. They can distinguish twelve different radial (or wrist) pulses: six on the right wrist (three superficial and three deep) and, similarly, six on the left wrist. By focusing on the relationship between the pulses and the internal organs, a skillful practitioner can feel the strength, vitality, and normal physiological tone of specific organs at each of the twelve sites.

"Ayurvedic physicians pay special attention to the pulse, tongue, eyes, and nails."

The tongue is another diagnostic site. By observing the surface of the tongue and looking for discoloration and/or sensitivity of particular areas, an adept practitioner can gain insight into the functional status of internal organs. For example, a whitish tongue indicates a disruption of *kapha* and accumulation of mucus; and a black to brown discoloration indicates a *vata* disturbance. A dehydrated tongue is symptomatic of a decrease in the plasma, while a pale tongue indicates a decrease in red blood cells.

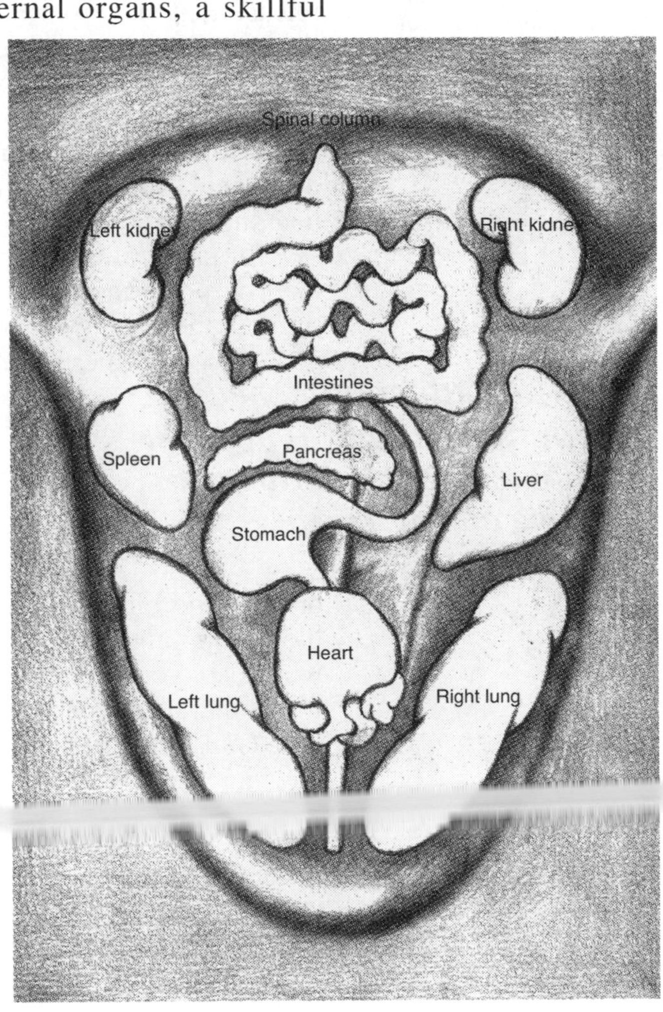

Tongue diagnosis in Ayurvedic medicine.

Ayurvedic physicians routinely perform urine examinations to help them diagnose doshic imbalance in a patient. An early morning midstream sample of urine is collected, and its color observed. Blackish-brown indicates a *vata* disorder; dark yellow, an imbalance with *pitta*. If the urine is cloudy, there is a *kapha* disorder. When a person is constipated or is not drinking adequate amounts of water, his or her urine will be dark yellow. Red urine indicates a blood disorder.

Normal urine has a typical uremic, or musty, smell. A foul odor, however, indicates toxins in the system. Acidic urine, which creates a burning sensation, indicates excess *pitta*. A sweet smell to the urine indicates a diabetic condition. An individual with this condition may experience goose bumps on the skin surface while passing urine. Gravel in the urine indicates stones in the urinary tract.

Disease Management in Ayurvedic Medicine

Ayurvedic medicine holds that in order to restore health one must first understand and correctly diagnose the disease or bodily imbalance. After diagnosis, there are four main methods by which an Ayurvedic physician manages disease: cleansing and detoxifying, palliation, rejuvenation, and mental hygiene.

With its strong emphasis on prevention and education, Ayurvedic medicine can help to provide long-term savings to consumers.

Cleansing and Detoxifying (*Shodan*)

Cleansing in Ayurvedic medicine takes on a far more encompassing role than in Western medicine, where a physician rarely has a patient release material from the stomach, nasal sinuses, or bowels. In contrast, the purifying techniques of vomiting, bowel purging, enemas, blood cleansing, and nasal douching, collectively called *pancha karma*, are commonly used by Ayurvedic physicians to remove toxins from different areas of the body. In Ayurvedic medicine, toxins are considered the root of disease, and are often the result of undigested, unabsorbed, and unassimilated food.

In preparation for cleansing, notes Dr. Sodhi, an herbal-oil massage may be performed. The oil is a liquid form of fat that is well absorbed through the skin. Once in the system, it can pick up various toxins such as pesticides, as well as viruses and bacteria. These toxins are eventually disposed of through normal channels of elimination. To further elimination, a herbal steam sauna often follows the massage treatment.

“Like all enlightened healing methods, Ayurveda emphasizes prevention above curing disease.”

Once cleansing begins, purgative therapy eliminates *vata*, *pitta*, and *kapha* impurities from the body.

Blood cleansing is accomplished by removing blood or donating blood to the blood bank, and by using certain cleansing and blood thinning herbs. “It’s a known scientific fact,” says Dr. Sodhi, “that whenever you give blood the bone marrow gets stimulated. They have found that the blood volume is restored in thirty to forty-five minutes.”

Ghee (clarified butter) and yogurt buttermilk are used to reestablish intestinal flora, especially if it has been washed away during the cleansing process.

Inserting herbs through various routes other than the mouth (such as the nose, anus, and skin), ensures that the medicinal qualities are not broken down by stomach enzymes. Certain herbal concoctions, medicated oils, and *ghee* are often administered into the nose to increase mental clarity.

Palliation (*Shaman*)

The next step in Ayurvedic disease management is palliation, or *shaman*, used to balance and pacify the bodily *doshas*. *Shaman* focuses more on the spiritual dimension of healing, and uses a combination of herbs, fasting, chanting, yoga stretches, breathing exercises, meditation, and lying in the sun for a limited time. These techniques are useful for people with dysfunctional immune systems, or for those who are too ill or emotionally weak to undergo the more strenuous forms of physical cleansing noted in *pancha karma*. Because of its curative and preventative aspects, *shaman* can also be utilized by the healthy person. Like all enlightened healing methods, Ayurveda emphasizes prevention above curing disease.

One method of *shaman*, called "kindling the fire," is absolutely necessary in *kapha* and *vata* disorders with patients who have low gastric fire. The patient consumes honey with certain herbs like pippili (long pepper), ginger, cinnamon, and black pepper. (This should be done cautiously with *pitta* people, however.)

Rejuvenation (*Rasayana*)

After the cleansing regimen, a program of tonification called *rasayana* (ra-sigh'-ana) begins. Tonification means enhancing the body's inherent ability to function, and *rasayana* is similar to a physiological tune-up. It is used to restore virility and vitality to the reproductive system, countering sterility and infertility, bringing forth healthier progeny and improving sexual performance. In addition, it is said that *rasayana* extends longevity by slowing down the biological clock and retarding the aging process.

Ayurvedic medicine uses three subcategories of *rasayana* treatments to rejuvenate and restore the body's tissues and organs: special herbs prepared as pills, powders, jellies, and tablets; mineral preparations specific to a person's condition and *dosha*; and exercises, specifically, yoga positions and breathing exercises.

Mental Hygiene and Spiritual Healing (*Satvajaya*)

Satvajaya (sat-va-j-eye'-a), is a method of improving the mind to reach a higher level of spiritual/mental functioning, and is accomplished through the release of psychological stress, emotional distress, and unconscious negative beliefs.

The categories of *satvajaya* include *mantra* or sound therapy to change the vibratory patterns of the mind; *yantra*, or concentrating on geometric figures to take the mind out of ordinary modes of thinking; *tantra*, to direct energies through the body; meditation, to alter states of consciousness; and gems, metals, and crystals for their subtle vibratory healing powers.

TREATMENTS IN AYURVEDIC MEDICINE

Some of the primary Ayurvedic treatments are:

Diet: *Prescribed according to dosha and season. The taste of the food (sweet, sour, salty, pungent, bitter, or astringent), its hot- or cold-producing abilities, and whether the food is light or heavy, solid or liquid, or oily or dry are primary considerations. Certain foods should also not be eaten together.*

Exercise: *Vigorous exercise and yoga stretching are encouraged in Ayurveda to kindle the internal fire, improve circulation, stimulate metabolism, and sharpen the mind. Exercises are prescribed according to an individual's constitution.*

Meditation: *Considered a form of mental cleansing, meditation enhances both self-awareness and awareness of one's environment, family, friends, and business.*

Herbs: *Ayurvedic physicians use an extensive number of herbs in treating conditions. Depending on their innate qualities, herbs are used to rebuild and rejuvenate the body and its various systems.*

Massage: *Massage that uses herbal oils is an important part of Ayurvedic treatment. Upon absorption through the skin, the medicated oils help to remove toxins from the system.*

Sun: *Ayurvedic philosophy states that the sun is not only a source of heat and light, but also of higher consciousness. It improves circulation, aids absorption of vitamin D, and strengthens the bones. Each of the three dosha constitutions benefit from different lengths of* [illegible] *and care is a must. Because of the risk of developing skin cancer, no one who has multiple moles should lie in the sun for extended periods of time.*

Breathing: *Breathing exercises, or pranayama can be learned from an experienced teacher. Depending on the dosha type, pranayama can bring a sense of tranquility and peace, and alleviate the stress of a hectic day.*

A CASE HISTORY—THE AYURVEDIC APPROACH

"The most common disease in the United States is heart disease," says Virender Sodhi, M.D. (Ayurveda), N.D., Director of the American School of Ayurvedic Sciences in Bellevue, Washington. Of the many heart cases he sees each year, one of the most interesting involved a fifty-five-year-old Asian male with chest pain so severe that he could not walk more than ten steps before having to sit down. He came to Dr. Sodhi's office after receiving word from the local hospital that he needed immediate bypass surgery. Refusing the surgery, doctors told him, would mean certain death.

Before beginning treatment, Dr. Sodhi ordered a battery of tests. "I do lab tests before and after a cleansing program," asserts Dr. Sodhi. Angiographic studies showed that his patient's coronary arteries were blocked—the left main coronary artery was 90 percent narrowed, the anterior descending was 80 percent narrowed, and the right coronary was 30 percent blocked. Blood tests indicated elevated cholesterol levels at 278 and decreased HDL (good cholesterol) at 38. Dr. Sodhi determined that his patient was a pitta-kapha *individual and started him on a appropriate cleansing program that included a change of diet, and appropriate herbs.*

After three months, the man's cholesterol levels dropped more than 30 percent and HDL's rose to 48. More importantly, though, his exercise tolerance had dramatically improved. "He was doing the treadmill exercise," reports Dr. Sodhi, "at the speed of five miles per hour for forty-five minutes without any angina." More than two years later, Dr. Sodhi says his patient "is doing fine": he now jogs up and down hills with no symptoms, and his EKG (electrocardiogram) readings have shown improvement. "There is a hospital in Bombay," continues Sodhi, "which has done about 3,300 cases with this method for [treating] coronary heart diseases. All of them with about 99 percent success."

"*Satvajaya* can decondition the mind so we can see things fresh, like with the eyes of a child," says David Frawley, O.M.D., Director of the American Institute of Vedic Studies in Santa Fe, New Mexico. "*Satvajaya* techniques rid us of negative emotions, thought patterns, and prejudices that may weigh us down like undigested food."

The Future of Ayurvedic Medicine

Although the advent of Western medical practices temporarily loosened the roots of Ayurvedic medicine in India, Ayurveda has since that time made a comeback in its country of origin and has spread around the world to Europe, Japan, and North and South America. There are 108 Ayurvedic colleges in India that grant degrees after a five-year program, and three hundred thousand Ayurvedic physicians are represented by the All India Ayur-Veda Congress. Ayurvedic conferences, sponsored by governments and/or medical associations, have taken place in Brazil, Poland, Czechoslovakia, and Hungary. In the Soviet Union, the Soviet Research Center for Preventive Medicine oversees the Institute of Maharishi Ayur-Veda. Furthermore, in the United States, the National Institutes of Health is researching Ayurveda and its integration with other healing practices, such as naturopathic, chiropractic, and allopathic medicines.[1]

Dr. Sodhi devotes much of his time to seeking out medical studies that support Ayurvedic treatments. He observes that "considerable modern research has proven the efficacy of Ayurvedic herbal preparations, and research has now moved to elucidating their mechanisms and sites of action."[2] In Dr. Sodhi's opinion, combining modern medical diagnostic procedures with traditional methods makes for more effective use of Ayurvedic treatments.

Groups outside of the Ayurvedic community have also taken steps to recognize this established healing tradition. The World Health Organization recognizes Ayurvedic medicine, and supports research and the integration of the Ayurvedic system of health care into modern

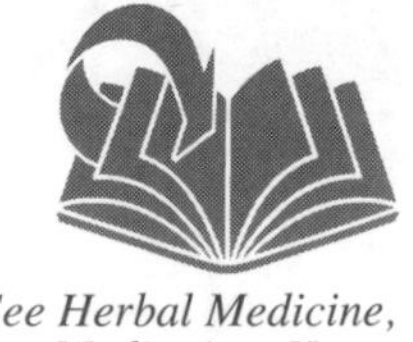

See Herbal Medicine, Meditation, Yoga.

medicine. Even the *Journal of the American Medical Association* has printed a short article on Ayurveda, followed by a lively response—both pro and con—from its readers.[3]

In light of this renewed interest, Dr. Lad reminds us of all that Ayurvedic medicine has to offer. "According to Ayurvedic principles, by understanding oneself, by identifying one's own constitution, and by recognizing sources of *doshic* aggravation, one can not only follow the proper guidelines to cleanse, purify, and prevent disease, but also uplift oneself into a realm of awareness previously unknown."

Ayurveda stresses the need for full patient participation and provides many self-care strategies such as diet, exercise, hygiene, yoga, meditation, and breathing exercises that can be incorporated into a personal health maintenance program.

Where To Find Help

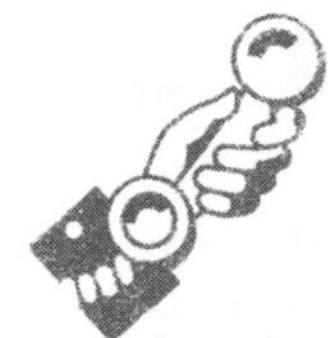

For more information on Ayurvedic treatments, or to locate an Ayurvedic physician, contact the organizations below. Other Ayurvedic medical centers throughout the United States often are associated with yoga institutes. Check the phone listings for other sources of Ayurvedic medical care.

American School of Ayurvedic Sciences
10025 NE 4th Street
Bellevue, Washington 98004
(206) 453-8022

This college provides medical training for physicians and health care practitioners, as well as individual courses for lay people. Dr. Virender Sodhi's Ayurvedic, Naturopathic Medical Clinic is also located at this address.

Ayurvedic Institute
11311 Menaul NE, Suite A
Albuquerque, New Mexico 87112
(505) 291-9698

The institute, directed by Dr. Vasant Lad, trains people from all walks of life in most of the [illegible]

The College of Maharishi Ayur-Veda Health Center
P.O. Box 282
Fairfield, Iowa 52556
(515) 472-5866

The center provides referrals to health centers, which offer methods for prevention and the treatment of a broad range of illnesses. They also train practitioners and provide information to the lay public.

Invincible Athletics
P.O. Box 541
Lancaster, Massachusetts 01523
(508) 368-1818

This organization teaches how to incorporate Ayurvedic training principles—releasing stress and building a feeling of well-being—and chiropractic methods into athletic conditioning.

Sharp Institute for Human Potential and Mind-Body Medicine
8010 Frost Street, Suite 300
San Diego, California 92123
(800) 82-SHARP

The Sharp Institute for Human Potential and Mind-Body [illegible] components. 1) Patient care at the Center for Mind-Body Medicine where Ayurvedic and other complementary therapies are offered in outpatient and residential settings; 2) Courses in Mind-Body and Ayurvedic Medicine for the general public and health care providers; 3) Research to validate the effectiveness of Ayurvedic therapies.

Canadian Association of Ayurvedic Medicine
P.O. Box 749 Station 'B'
Ottawa, Ontario
Canada K1P 5P8
(613) 837-5737

This professional organization maintains a referral list of Canadian Ayurveda doctors, supports university-based research, and submits proposals to provincial and federal governments advocating the research and practice of Ayurveda. CAAM provides training in Ayurveda for physicians and the general public. It also offers primary courses in French.

The Maharishi Ayur-Veda Health Center, RR #2
Huntsville, Ontario
Canada P0A 1K0
(705) 635-2234

This residential treatment center offers Ayurvedic treatments and education.

Recommended Reading

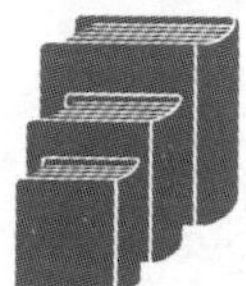

Ageless Body, Timeless Mind. Chopra, Deepak, M.D. New York: Harmony Books, 1993.

An examination of the mind/body connection in respect to the aging process, this book challenges conventional perceptions on growing old and discusses the concept of immortality.

Ayurvedic Healing. Frawley, David, O.M.D. Salt Lake City: Morson Publishing, 1990.

Detailed Ayurvedic methods of constitution balancing and treatment of common disease. Both general information for the layperson and specific knowledge of diet, herbs, oils, aromas, gems, and mantras.

Ayurveda: The Science of Self-Healing. Lad, Vasant, M.D. Wilmot, CA: Lotus Light Press, 1984.

The principals and practical applications of Ayurveda, along with fifty concise charts and illustrations.

Perfect Health. Chopra, Deepak, M.D. New York: Harmony Books, 1991.

A practical guide to harnessing the healing power of the mind. A useful, personalized daily plan for the "total perfect health" using the principles of Ayurveda.

Quantum Healing. Chopra, Deepak, M.D. New York: Bantam Books, 1990.

This book compares elements of healing the human body with quantum mechanics and shows that Ayurvedic medicine is a fully articulated model of the quantum-mechanical human body.

For a complete list of Dr. Deepak Chopra's books and audiotapes contact the following:

Quantum Publications
P.O. Box 598
South Lancaster, Massachusetts 01561
(800) 858-1808
(508) 368-1810

Biofeedback Training

Biofeedback training teaches a person how to change and control his or her body's vital functions through the use of simple electronic devices. Biofeedback is particularly useful for learning to reduce stress, eliminate headaches, control asthmatic attacks, recondition injured muscles, and relieve pain.

The idea that a person can learn to modify his or her own vital functions is relatively new. Before the 1960s, most scientists believed that autonomic functions, such as heart rate and pulse, digestion, blood pressure, brain waves, and muscle behavior, could not be voluntarily controlled. Recently, biofeedback, along with other methods of self-regulation, such as guided imagery, progressive relaxation, and meditation, has found widespread acceptance among physiologists and psychologists alike.

Biofeedback training is a method of learning how to consciously regulate normally unconscious bodily functions (such as breathing, heart rate, and blood pressure) in order to improve overall health. It refers to any process that measures and reports back immediate information about the biological system of the person being monitored so he or she can learn to consciously influence that system.

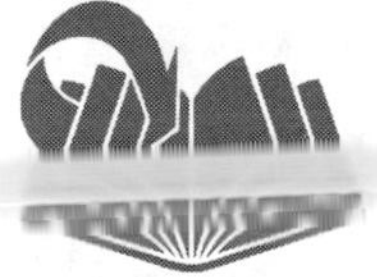

See Guided Imagery, Meditation, Mind/Body Medicine.

How Biofeedback Works

A person seeking to regulate his or her heart rate would train with a biofeedback device set up to transmit one blinking light or one audible beep per heartbeat. By learning to alter the rate of the flashes and beeps, the subject would be subtly programmed to control the heart rate. "The self-regulation skills acquired through biofeedback training are retained by the individual even after the feedback device is dispensed with," explains Patricia Norris, Ph.D., Clinical Director of the Biofeedback and Psychophysiology Clinic at the Center for Applied Psychophysiology at the Menninger Clinic in Topeka, Kansas. "In fact, with practice, biofeedback skills continue to improve. It is like taking tennis lessons. If you stop taking the lessons but continue playing, your game will improve. With biofeedback, it works the same way. The more you practice, the better you get."

The effects of biofeedback can be measured in a variety of ways: monitoring skin temperature (ST) influenced by blood flow beneath the skin; monitoring galvanic skin response (GSR), the electrical conductivity of the skin; observing muscle tension with an electro-myogram (EMG); tracking heart rate with an electro-cardiogram (EKG); and using an electroencephalogram (EEG) to monitor brain wave activity. Electrodes are placed on the patient's skin (a simple, painless process). The patient is then instructed to use various techniques such as meditation, relaxation, and visualization to effect the desired response (muscle relaxation, lowered heart rate, or lowered temperature). The biofeedback device reports the patient's progress by a change in the speed of the beeps or flashes.

> *"The self-regulation skills acquired through biofeedback training are retained by the individual even after the feedback device is dispensed with."*
>
> —Patricia Norris, Ph.D.

Normal, healthy, "relaxed" readings include fairly warm skin, low sweat gland activity (this keeps the skin's conductivity low), and a slow, even heart rate. Biofeedback technologies utilize computers to provide a rapid and detailed analysis of activities within the complex human system. Biofeedback practitioners interpret changes in these readings to help the patient learn to stabilize erratic and unhealthy biological functions.

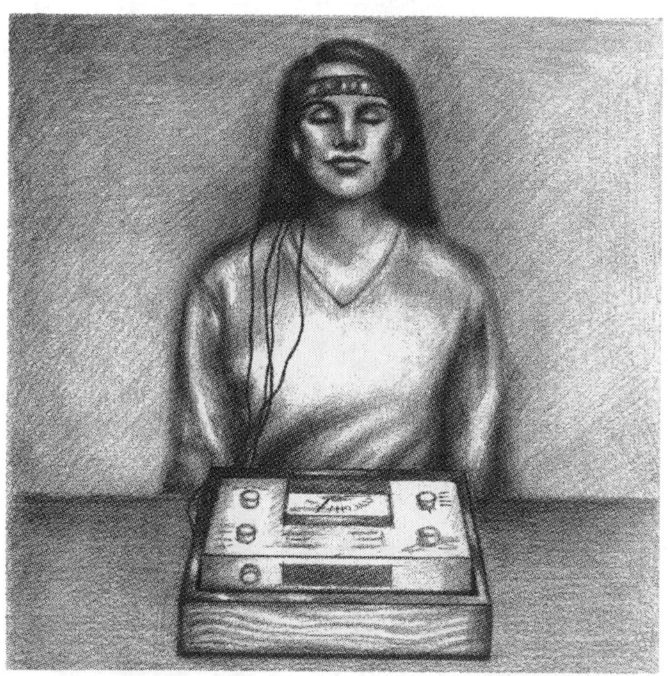

Using a biofeedback device for relaxation.

Conditions Benefited by Biofeedback Training

Biofeedback training has a vast range of applications for health and prevention, particularly in cases where psychological factors play a role. Sleep disorders, hyperactivity in children, and other behavioral disorders respond well to biofeedback training, as do dysfunctions stemming from inadequate control over muscles or muscle groups. Incontinence, postural problems, back pain, temporomandibular joint syndrome (TMJ), and even loss of control due to brain or nerve damage have all shown improvement when patients undergo biofeedback training.

Biofeedback has also been shown to help other problems such as heart dysfunctions, gastrointestinal disorders (acidity, ulcers, irritable bowel syndrome), difficulty swallowing, esophageal dysfunction, ringing in the ears, twitching of the eyelids, fatigue, and cerebral palsy. Severe structural problems like broken bones and slipped discs are among the only conditions that don't respond to biofeedback.

Stress-Related Disorders

One of the most common uses for biofeedback training is the treatment of stress and stress-related disorders, including insomnia, TMJ, migraines, asthma, hypertension, gastrointestinal disorders, and muscular dysfunction.

By teaching self-regulation skills biofeedback can allow patients to take more control of their health and help prevent disorders that can result in costly medical procedures.

Insomnia: Biofeedback can often successfully treat insomnia as long as the appropriate form of biofeedback is used with the specific, corresponding type of insomnia. "Biofeedback is appropriate when insomnia is due to overactivation of the autonomic nervous system," says Melvyn Werbach, M.D., Assistant Clinical Professor at the UCLA School of Medicine and Director of the Biofeedback Medical Clinic in Tarzana, California. "In this case we use biofeedback of muscle tension and skin dampness in conjunction with general relaxation techniques.

"EEG biofeedback, however, seems useful when insomnia is due to a mental/emotional problem, not a physical problem. I use it particularly with people who have a problem with obsessive thinking when they try to go to sleep. Their bodies relax very nicely, but they just can't get their minds off of whatever it is that their minds go to. This is when EEG biofeedback is most effective."

Temporomandibular Joint Syndrome: Dr. Werbach also reports using biofeedback to successfully treat TMJ. "The most dramatic case I can think of," he says, "is a patient who came to the UCLA Pain Control Unit after using bite plates in his mouth to stop the teeth from grinding together. His last bite plate had been a metal one, prescribed by a dentist who thought it would finally solve the problem. Instead, he bit through the metal. He had severe pain in all the typical areas associated with TMJ, and was quite depressed about the whole thing. He had tried everything. Working with him, we took biofeedback readings from the masseter muscle (the muscle involved in closing the jaw) and using them, trained him to relax his jaw. Since he was so preoccupied with his mouth, we also worked on reducing general muscle tension in the rest of his body by teaching him relaxation techniques through control of his breathing and surface finger temperature. It was strikingly effective."

Migraines: The use of biofeedback to treat migraines began as a chance discovery at the Menninger Clinic (previously Menninger Foundation) in the early 1960s. Elmer Green, Ph.D., and Alyce Green were measuring a woman's skin temperature to track her physiological changes while undergoing a series of relaxation exercises. They noticed a sudden ten-degree increase in the woman's hand temperature. When asked, she reported that a headache she had been experiencing had disappeared at that very moment.

The Greens pioneered a biofeedback temperature device and went on to teach patients how to alleviate migraines simply by using relaxation techniques to elevate the temperature of their hands. Biofeedback can also reduce the dosages of drugs needed to combat migraines, and sometimes eliminate them altogether, according to a report by Steven L. Fahrion, Ph.D., Director of the Center for Applied Psychophysiology at the Menninger Clinic.[1]

Asthma: Asthma responds especially well to biofeedback training. A recent fifteen-month follow-up study of seventeen asthmatics, trained with biofeedback to increase their inhalation volume, found that all of the participants reported fewer emergency room visits, a lowered need for medication, and decreased instance and severity of wheezing attacks. The authors of the study, Erik Peper, Ph.D., and Vicci Tibbets of San Francisco State University, concluded, "By learning to increase their inhalation volume the subjects knew they had control over their breathing. This experience reduced their fear so that they could continue to exhale and inhale air during the onset of wheezing. As one participant reported: 'It gave me a sense of control and hope that I never had before.'"[2]

HISTORY OF BIOFEEDBACK

Instrumented biofeedback was pioneered by O. Hobart Mowrer in 1938, when he used an alarm system triggered by urine to stop bed-wetting in children. But it was not until the late 1960s, when Barbara Brown, Ph.D., at the Veterans Administration Hospital in Sepulveda, California, and Elmer Green, Ph.D., and Alyce Green of the Menninger Foundation in Topeka, Kansas, used EEG biofeedback to observe and record the altered states/self-regulation of yogis, that biofeedback began to attract widespread attention.

"The Greens' work with yogis, and the work of Joe Kamiya to teach subjects to experience a 'drugless high' is what really brought biofeedback to public notice," says Dr. Werbach. "There started to be tremendous interest, articles on biofeedback in national newspapers and magazines, and the idea of higher states of consciousness being related to something that could be scientifically measured really caught on."

Hypertension: Biofeedback training is an effective tool for teaching people self-regulation and relaxation to help lower blood pressure.[3] The greatest successes in controlling hypertension are with patients who combine biofeedback training with other forms of relaxation, visualization, exercise, and a low-salt diet.

Gastrointestinal Disorders: Robert Grove, Ph.D., of Culver City, California, is a specialist in the application of biofeedback to gastrointestinal disorders. He reports great success in treating irritable bowel syndrome, colitis, a wide variety of eating disorders (including bulimia and anorexia), heartburn, and functional dyspepsia (a digestive disorder marked by stomachache, heartburn, or nausea). Dr. Grove uses motility (movement) retraining, wherein special sensors are able to pick up movement in the digestive tract and train it. "Gastrointestinal disorder is a specialty area," explains Dr. Grove, "and other forms of biofeedback will fail under these conditions. For one thing, gastrointestinal disorder patients seem to be hyper-reactive to all types of stimuli such as a light being turned on or a telephone ringing—things that normally don't bother other patients. The gastrointestinal tract responds to these stimuli by shutting down, and biofeedback helps focus in on protecting or creating a protection from the arousal." The Menninger Clinic also successfully treats many people for gastrointestinal disorders, including Crohn's disease (a chronic inflammatory condition affecting the colon and/or terminal part of the small intestine) and ulcerative colitis.

See Back Pain, Gastrointestinal Disorders, Headaches, Hypertension, Respiratory Disorders, Sleep Disorders, Stress.

Muscular Dysfunctions: Marjorie K. Toomim, Ph.D., Director of the Biofeedback Institute of Los Angeles, uses EMG biofeedback to detect muscle imbalances in order to prevent and correct injuries. For example, a runner with problem knee muscles was hooked to the EMG, and Dr. Toomim was immediately able to see that the runner was placing a disproportionate amount of her weight to one side. The muscles on the inside of the leg were diagnosed as stronger than those on the outside. To correct the imbalance the patient needed to exercise only the outer thigh muscles. While hooked up to the EMG feedback device, the patient could see exactly when the weaker outside muscles were exercising and when the stronger inner muscles were at rest. Says Dr. Toomim, "In this case, the EMG gave us information we couldn't have gotten in any other way, and it empowered the patient to take control of her own muscular re-education."

Dr. Werbach believes biofeedback training is sometimes more effective than surgery for patients with back problems. By teaching patients both relaxation techniques and control over their muscle spasms, biofeedback helps them reduce or eliminate back pain.

Psychologist Bernard Brucker of the University of Miami Medical School uses EMG biofeedback to teach patients with serious spinal injuries to walk again. Sophisticated EMG feedback replaces the sensation of motion lost by spinal cord injury, reduces muscle spasm, detects activity in muscles mistakenly believed to lack energy, and strengthens muscles so they function once again.[4]

Yale University research affiliate and Professor Emeritus at Rockefeller University, Neal E. Miller, along with Barry Dworkin, Ph.D., of Penn State University, developed a small biofeedback device worn on the body to treat curvature of the spine. When the wearer slouches forward, a soft beep is emitted; if he or she does not straighten up, a piercing alarm goes off. Several studies have shown it to be especially effective in treating kyphosis, a front to back curvature.[5]

AN UNUSUAL SUCCESS STORY

Melvyn Werbach, M.D., former Assistant Clinical Professor at UCLA Medical School and director of the Biofeedback Medical Clinic in Tarzana, California, was once approached by a woman whose husband had been in a coma for several months. Dr. Werbach and an associate arranged to hook the man up to various biofeedback devices in an attempt to communicate with him. While Dr. Werbach monitored the biofeedback equipment, his associate asked the comatose patient to concentrate on specific areas of his body. To everyone's surprise, the galvanic skin response monitor began to move with the request. Although he was in a coma, the patient was able to hear. At the end of the session, the family and staff were shocked to hear him moan loudly.

Perhaps catalyzed by the biofeedback communication, the patient came out of his coma within a month of this initial session. Almost two years later, Dr. Werbach got a call from the patient. Says Dr. Werbach, "Hearing his voice was one of the most rewarding moments I have ever had in the practice of medicine."[8]

Biofeedback can successfully treat incontinence, as well. A $13 billion a year problem among institutionalized elderly, it results when people lose the ability to control the muscles used for urination or defecation.[6] A recent report from the Department of Health and Human Services analyzed twenty-two different studies and concluded that muscular reeducation through biofeedback training had a success rate ranging from 54 to 95 percent, depending on the patient group.[7]

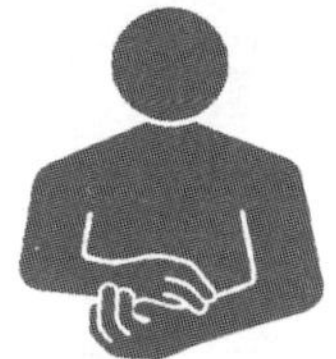

Biofeedback equipment is a valuable aid in learning self-regulation skills and can be easily used in the home.

Biofeedback Training as a Visualization Tool

Because biofeedback training empowers patients by teaching them to control one or more of their body processes, it is proving a useful adjunct to conventional therapies for cancer and other chronic diseases. Dr. Norris uses biofeedback training to teach cancer patients and patients with AIDS and other immune system disorders to reduce stress. Using imagery and visualization, she helps patients to become confident in the capacity for self-regulation of their bodies. Her first cancer patient, nine-year-old Garrett Porter, overcame an inoperable brain tumor with the help of biofeedback-assisted visualization.[9]

Now more than a decade later, upwards of three hundred cancer patients have been studied at the Menninger Clinic with results ranging from increased comfort and reduced stress to a complete recovery from cancer.

The Future of Biofeedback

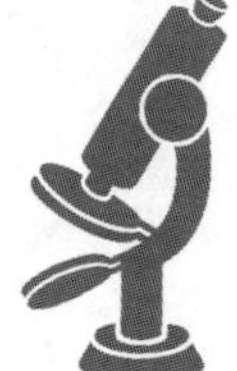

Additional research into biofeedback could help people better understand mind/body interaction and its importance in maintaining health.

The latest developments in biofeedback concern the self-regulation of bodily functions that, until now, were considered inaccessible. "The most exciting innovation in biofeedback would be to provide people with moment-to-moment feedback of changes in the levels of chemicals within the bloodstream," says Dr. Werbach. "In other words, to have equipment that can monitor, for example, hormone levels as they are at the moment and give feedback that will, in turn, enable a person to learn to influence his or her hormonal levels. Now that has incredible potential."

Clearly, as technology advances and biofeedback devices become more affordable and accessible, people can look forward to increasingly widespread use of biofeedback in the home along with an increased awareness of our innate ability to regulate themselves and influence their health.

Where to Find Help

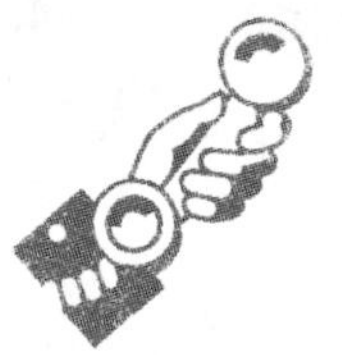

When undertaking biofeedback training it is important to find a qualified practitioner with a firm grasp of both physiology and psychology. Practitioners should be certified by the Biofeedback Certification Institute of America (see below). Most major cities have a biofeedback association. Check your local phone book or contact:

Association for Applied Psychophysiology and Biofeedback
10200 West 44th Avenue
Suite 304
Wheat Ridge, Colorado 80033
(303) 422-8436

Provides names and phone numbers of chapters in your state. (Formerly Biofeedback Society of America.)

Biofeedback Certification Institute of America
Same address as above.
(303) 420-2902

Runs the major certification program for biofeedback practitioners and provides information about certified local practitioners.

Center for Applied Psychophysiology
Menninger Clinic
P.O. Box 829
Topeka, Kansas 66601-0829
(913) 273-7500 Ext. 5375

One of the pioneering groups in biofeedback. This organization has research, treatment, and workshops in all areas of mind/body medicine, including extensive work with biofeedback, which includes the biofeedback and psychophysiology clinic.

Micro Straight, Inc.
2709 Cherry Street
Kansas City, Missouri 64108
(816) 474-0144
(800) 238-2225 (Outside Missouri)

Manufacturers of the Micro Straight Orthosis, the biofeedback device to train people out of their curvature of the spine. Available by doctor's prescription only.

Tools for Exploration
4460 Redwood Highway, Suite 2
San Rafael, California 94903
(415) 499-9050

Carries home biofeedback devices. Call for catalog.

Recommended Reading

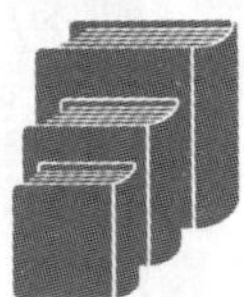

Biofeedback: An Introduction and Guide. Danskin, David G.; and Crow, Mark. Palo Alto, CA: Mayfield Publishing Co., 1981.

An excellent, but somewhat technical, introduction to the field.

The Future of the Body: Explorations into the Further Evolution of the Human Species. Murphy, Michael. Los Angeles: Jeremy P. Tarcher, Inc., 1992.

An exhaustive examination of the author's thirty-year investigation into mind/body research. Includes a chapter on biofeedback.

Third Line Medicine. Werbach, Melvyn, R. New York: Third Line Press, 1988.

Suggests a "new line" of thought to produce a more humane, more caring, and more therapeutically effective professional community.

Why Me? Harnessing the Healing Power of the Human Spirit. Norris, Patricia; and Porter, Garrett. Walpole, NH: Stillpoint Publishing Co., 1985.

An uplifting account of a nine-year-old's biofeedback-assisted struggle against cancer.

Biological Dentistry

Biological dentistry stresses the use of nontoxic restoration materials for dental work, and focuses on the unrecognized impact that dental toxins and hidden dental infections can have on overall health.

There is a growing recognition among alternative dentists and physicians that dental health has a tremendous impact on the overall health of the body. European researchers estimate that perhaps as much as half of all chronic degenerative illness can be linked either directly or indirectly to dental problems and the traditional techniques of modern dentistry used to treat them. The well-publicized dangers associated with the use of silver/mercury fillings (amalgams) are only the tip of the iceberg as far as the negative impact that dentistry can have on a person's health.

"Dental problems such as cavities, infections, toxic or allergy-producing filling materials, root canals, and misalignment of the teeth or jaw can have far-reaching effects throughout the body."

—Hal Huggins, D.D.S.

"One of the big problems in the United States," says Gary Verigan, D.D.S., of Escalon, California, "is that dentists are trained to practice with only the most meager of diagnostic equipment. These instruments, consisting primarily of x-rays, are incapable of detecting enough about the tooth and its surrounding environment, giving the dentist only a superficial understanding of the problem and the impact it may be having on the patient's overall health. People often go through many doctors and therapies in search of answers for their problems, never realizing that their chronic conditions may be traceable to dental complications."

In contrast, biological dentistry treats the teeth, jaw, and related structures with specific regard to how treatment will affect the entire body. According to Hal Huggins, D.D.S., of Colorado Springs, Colorado, a pioneer in this field, "Dental problems such as cavities, infections, toxic or allergy-producing filling materials, root canals, and misalignment of the teeth or jaw can have far-reaching effects throughout the body."

How Dental Problems Contribute to Illness

"Dental infections and dental disturbances can cause pain and dysfunction throughout the body," states Edward Arana, D.D.S., President of the American Academy of Biological Dentistry, "including limited motion and loose tendons, ligaments, and muscles. Structural and physiological dysfunction can also occur, impairing organs and glands."

Dr. Arana cites several major types of dental problems that can cause illness and dysfunction in the body:

- Infections under and around teeth
- Problems with specific teeth related to the acupuncture meridians and the autonomic nervous system
- Root canals
- Toxicity from dental restoration materials
- Bio-incompatability to dental restoration materials
- Electrogalvanism and ion migration
- Temporomandibular joint syndrome (TMJ), a painful condition of the jaw, usually caused by stress or injury

Some of the more common causes of these dental problems are unerupted teeth (teeth that have not broken through the gum), wisdom teeth (both impacted and unimpacted), amalgam-filled cavities and root canals, cysts, bone cavities, and areas of bone condensation due to inflammation in the bone. These conditions can be diagnosed using testing methods such as blood tests, applied kinesiology, electro-acupuncture biofeedback, and, in some cases, x-rays. A thorough review of the patient's medical and dental histories is also essential.

Infections Under the Teeth

Pockets of infection can exist under the teeth and be undetectable on x-rays. This is particularly true for teeth that have had root canals, as it is very difficult to eliminate all the bacteria and toxins from the roots during this procedure. These infections may persist for years without the patient's knowledge.

When infections are present, toxins can leak out and depress the function of the immune system, leading to chronic degenerative diseases throughout the body. Once the infection is cleared up, many of the symptoms of disease will disappear.

See Acupuncture, Applied Kinesiology, Energy Medicine.

Infections near the root of the tooth can also travel into the bone and destroy it, according to Harold Ravins, D.D.S., of Los Angeles. "One way to detect this is to stick a needle into the bone. If it is too soft, there is infection," he says. "Another way is with neural therapy. Neural therapy involves the injection of anesthetic around a suspected tooth. If this relieves the problems in other parts of the body, it means there is a disturbance under the tooth," says Dr. Ravins.

Some dentists use applied kinesiology testing to identify these hidden infections. Applied kinesiology employs a simple strength resistance test on a specific indicator muscle that is related to the organ or part of the body that is being tested. If the muscle tests strong, maintaining its resistance, it indicates health. If it tests weak, it can mean infection or dysfunction.

ELECTROACUPUNCTURE BIOFEEDBACK

Developed by Reinhold Voll, M.D., of Germany in the 1940s, electroacupuncture biofeedback makes use of the acupuncture meridian system to screen for infections and dysfunctions in the body. Today it is employed as a screening tool by alternative health practitioners worldwide, including biological dentists. As employed in biological dentistry, it involves placing an electrode on an individual tooth, then applying a small electrical current and recording the response. Any deviation from the normal reading indicates that there is an infection or disturbance in the vicinity of that particular tooth.[2] This deviation can also indicate a similar unhealthy state in the organ that shares the same meridian as the tooth. Any determinations using electroacupuncture biofeedback should always be confirmed by a physician.

Acupuncture points can also be used to diagnose infection. Dr. Ravins noticed that one of his patients showed sensitivity on his liver acupuncture point. This led him to an infection under the corresponding upper bicuspid.

Electroacupuncture biofeedback is another method used to screen for hidden dental infections. Philip Jenkins, D.D.S., of Los Gatos, California, uses electroacupuncture biofeedback testing to find infections, identify them, and then determine the appropriate homeopathic remedies with which to treat them.

Relationship between Specific Teeth and Illness

In the 1950s, Reinhold Voll, M.D., of Germany, discovered that each tooth in the mouth relates to a specific acupuncture meridian. Using his electroacupuncture biofeedback technique, he found that if a tooth became infected or diseased, the organ on the same meridian could also become unhealthy. He found that the opposite held true as well, that dysfunction in a specific organ could lead to a problem in the corresponding tooth.

For example, Dr. Ravins has observed that people who hit their front teeth too hard often have kidney disturbances, as there is a specific relationship between the kidneys and the front teeth.

Ernesto Adler, M.D., D.D.S., of Spain, reports that many diseases can also be caused by the wisdom teeth, which have a relationship to almost all organs of the body. When wisdom teeth are impacted, Dr. Adler points out, they press upon the nerves of the mandible (the large bone that makes up the lower jaw), which can result in disturbances in other areas of the body, including stammering, epilepsy, pain in the joints, depression, headaches, and heart problems. He adds that the upper wisdom teeth can cause calcium deficiency, resulting in muscle cramps.

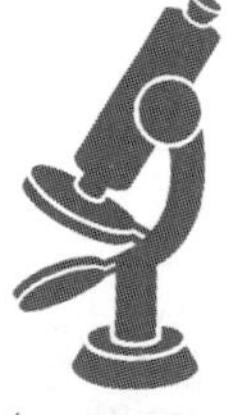

Although electroacupuncture biofeedback is used worldwide today, especially in Europe, it is approved in the United States only as an experimental device. More studies need to be undertaken to verify its importance in the field of biological dentistry and as a general diagnostic tool for all health practitioners.

Root Canals as a Cause of Illness

The late Weston Price, D.D.S., M.S., F.A.C.D., former Director of Research for the American Dental Association, made the astonishing claim that if teeth that have had root canals are removed from patients suffering from kidney and heart disease, these diseases will resolve in most cases. Moreover, implanting these teeth in animals results in the animals developing the same kind of disease found in the person from whom the tooth was taken. Dr. Price found that toxins seeping out of root canals can cause systemic diseases of the heart, kidney, uterus, and nervous and endocrine systems.[1]

Michael Ziff, D.D.S, of Orlando, Florida, points out that research has demonstrated that 100 percent of all root canals result in residual infection. This may be due to the imperfect seal that allows bacteria to penetrate. The oxygen-lacking environment of a root canal can cause the bacteria to undergo changes, adds Dr. Huggins, producing potent toxins that can then leak out into the body. Nutrient materials are also able to seep into the root canal through the porous channels in the tooth, allowing this bacteria growth to flourish. Susceptibility to these types of reactions is usually genetic, but stresses to the system (abuse of alcohol, drugs, caffeine) can induce them in normal individuals. Pregnancy and influenza also increase susceptibility to leakage of toxins from root canals, according to Dr. Huggins.

He adds that when a tooth with a root canal is removed, the periodontal ligament that attaches the tooth to the underlying bone should also be removed, otherwise a pocket of infection can remain. Full removal of the tooth and ligament stimulates the old bone to produce new bone for healing.

According to Dr. Ziff, however, there are cases where root canal teeth should not be pulled. It can be difficult to chew without certain teeth intact, and problems can arise if the teeth surrounding the extracted one become misaligned. "The best approach is a conservative one," says Dr. Ziff. "Try other measures first and only remove the tooth as a last resort."

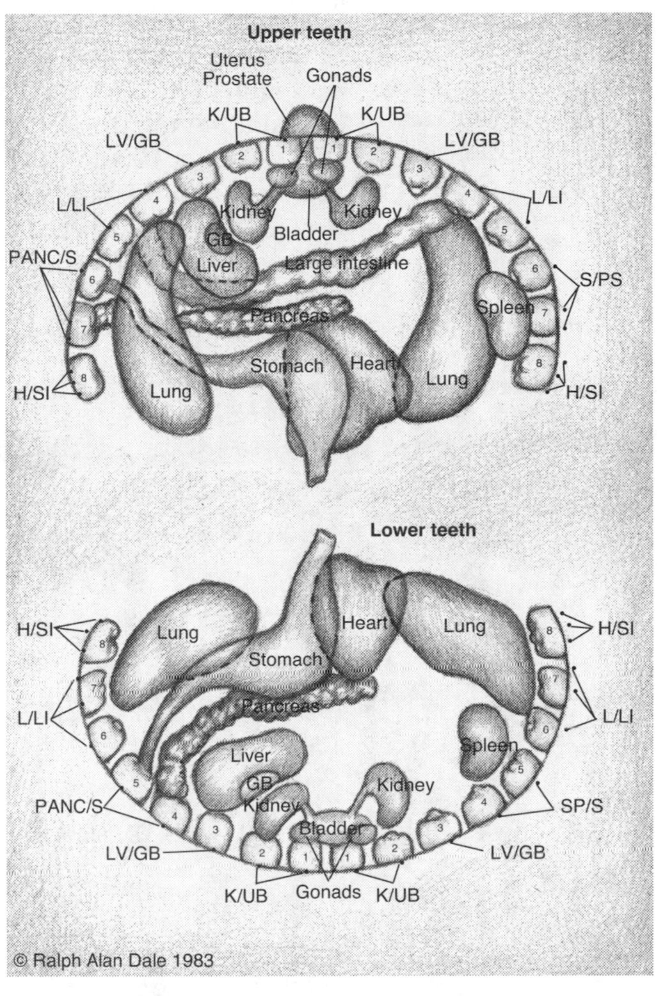

Correspondence of teeth acupuncture points.

Toxicity from Dental Restoration Materials

"Dental amalgam fillings can release mercury, tin, copper, silver, and sometimes zinc into the body," says Dr. A[illegible]. All of [illegible] [illegible] of toxicity and when placed as fillings in the teeth can corrode or disassociate into metallic ions (charged atoms). These metallic ions can then migrate from the tooth into the root of the tooth, the mouth, the bone, the connective tissues of the jaw, and finally on into the nerves. From there they can travel into the central nervous system, where the ions will reside, permanently disrupting the body's normal functioning if nothing is done to remove them.

> *"Research has demonstrated that 100 percent of all root canals result in residual infection due to the imperfect seal that allows bacteria to penetrate."*

Other types of metal-based dental restorations can similarly release toxic metals into the body. According to David E. Eggleston, D.D.S., of the Department of Restorative Dentistry at the University of Southern California in Los Angeles, a patient undergoing dental work developed kidney disease due to nickel toxicity from the dental crowns that were being placed in the patient's mouth. As each successive crown was placed, the disease intensified, verified by blood and urine tests, and physical examination. Once the nickel crowns were removed, the patient gradually became symptom free.[3]

Theron Randolph, M.D., of Batavia, Illinois, founder of the field of environmental medicine, believes that both the medical and dental professions have become too lax in dealing with the scope and potential danger of toxic metals. "Although it is not clear whether dental amalgams and other metals used in dental work are the primary or secondary cause of many health problems," he says, "both doctors and dentists have to be concerned with evaluating the clinical implications of using toxic metals in the human body." Dr. Randolph believes part of the problem stems from American dental schools ignoring the mounting evidence on toxicity from dental restorations, especially amalgams, despite clear documentation shown in European studies.

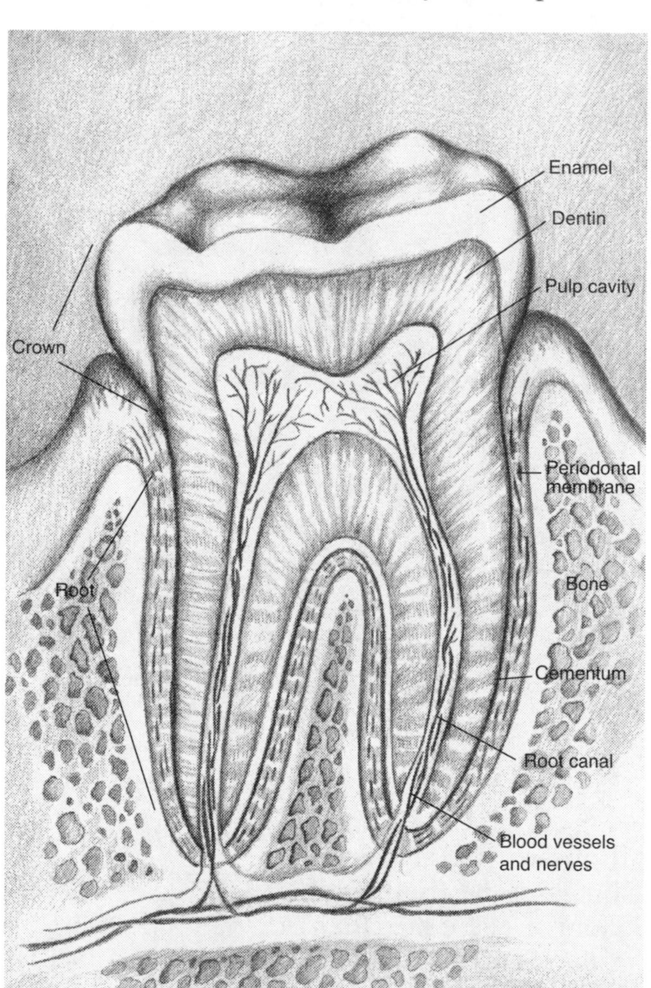

Diagram of a healthy tooth.

In September, 1992, California governor Pete Wilson requested that the State Board of Dental Examiners develop a fact sheet on dental materials to be distributed to dentists. California is the first state to pass such legislation, notes Joyal Taylor, D.D.S., of Rancho Santa Fe, California, President of the Environmental Dental Association. He hopes this will pave the way for a total ban on the use of mercury in dental restorations, adding that two to three thousand dentists across the country are now calling for such a ban on mercury dental amalgams.

Mercury Dental Amalgams: While all metals used for dental restoration can be toxic, the most harmful are the mercury dental amalgams (silver/mercury) used for fillings. According to Dr. Taylor, "These so-called 'silver fillings' actually contain 50 percent mercury and only 25 percent silver."

Mercury has been recognized as a poison since the 1500s, and yet mercury amalgams have been used in dentistry since the 1820s. They are still being used today even though the Environmental Protection Agency (EPA) declared scrap dental amalgam a hazardous waste in 1988. Even the American Dental Association, which has so far refused to ban amalgams, now instructs dentists to "know the potential hazards and symptoms of mercury exposure such as the development of sensitivity and neuropathy," to use a no-touch technique for handling the amalgam, and to store it under liquid, preferably glycerin or radiographic fixer solution, in unbreakable, tightly sealed containers.[4]

For some dentists, such as Richard D. Fischer, D.D.S., of Annandale, Virginia, these measures are not enough. Since becoming aware of the health risk amalgams pose, he has refused to work with them and has had his own silver fillings removed. "I don't feel comfortable using a substance designated by the EPA to be a waste disposal hazard," he says. "I can't throw it in the trash, bury it in the ground, or put it in a landfill, but they say it's okay to put it in people's mouths. That doesn't make sense."

According to the German Ministry of Health, "Amalgam is considered a health risk from a medical viewpoint due to the release of mercury vapor."[5] Everyday activities such as chewing and brushing the teeth have been shown to release mercury vapors from amalgams.[6] Amalgams can also erode and corrode with time (ideally they should be replaced after seven to ten years), adding to their toxic output.

Studies by the World Health Organization show that a single amalgam can release three to seventeen micrograms of mercury per day,[7] making dental amalgam a major source of mercury exposure.[8] A Danish study of a random sample of one hundred men and one hundred women showed that increased blood mercury levels were related to the presence of more than four amalgam fillings in the teeth.[9] American, Swedish, and German scientists examining cadavers have also found a clear relationship between the number of fillings and the mercury count in the brain and kidneys.[10]

In Germany the sale and manufacture of amalgams has been prohibited since March 1992,[11] and in Sweden, after a special commission determined that amalgam was a toxic material, that country's Social Welfare and Health Administration issued an advisory against its use in the dental treatments of pregnant women. Furthermore, Sweden has promised to ban amalgams entirely as soon as a suitable replacement is found.[12] Until then the government pays 50 percent of the cost for removal of amalgams. In the United States, however, little is being done to deal with the effects of mercury amalgams because most dentists still maintain that they are safe. They continue to place mercury in their patients' mouths even though the metal is more toxic than arsenic.[13]

> *"I don't feel comfortable using a substance designated by the Environmental Protection Agency to be a waste disposal hazard. I can't throw it in the trash, bury it in the ground, or put it in a landfill, but they say it's okay to put it in people's mouths. That doesn't make sense."*
>
> —Richard D. Fischer, D.D.S.

The problem is so widespread that Dr. Taylor now devotes his entire practice to the removal of amalgams. "There have been no studies [in the United States] on the safety of mercury in dental work, but when it leaks from the teeth it can cause both physical and mental problems," he states.[14] Dr. Arana adds that "numbness and tingling, paralysis, tremors, and pain are just some of the symptoms of chronic metal intoxication associated with the use of mercury dental amalgams."

Though the ideal replacement for mercury amalgams has not yet been found, there are some less toxic alternatives that biological dentists are working with. The best one so far is the so-called "composite amalgam," which is a combination of metals that are less toxic than mercury and slower to break down.

Dr. Huggins recommends that people who choose to have their amalgams removed ask their dentists to use a rubber dam, a thin sheet of rubber that slips over the teeth. "Dams prevent over 95 percent of the mixture of mercury and water produced by the drilling out of old fillings from going down your throat," he says. "They also reduce the amount of mercury that you might absorb from your cheeks and under your tongue." Dr. Huggins also suggests that people consider early morning appointments for amalgam removal, rather than later in the day, because the mercury vapor from other patients' sessions can linger in the air for hours and be absorbed by breathing. Some dentists use mercury vapor filter systems, he points out, but those who do are rare.

Charles Gableman, M.D., of Encinitas, California, a leader in the field of environmental medicine, always advises the removal of his patients' amalgam fillings. According to Dr. Gableman, patients with chronic fatigue syndrome, or with a lack of resistance to infections, allergies, and thyroid dysfunction, all improve after their fillings are properly removed. He believes it is possible that these patients have suffered from basic allergies their entire lives, and that the mercury toxicity from the fillings simply adds to the body's toxic load and "pushes them over the edge," resulting in chronic medical problems.

> *"Although it is not clear whether dental amalgams and other metals used in dental work are the primary or secondary cause of many health problems, both doctors and dentists have to be concerned with evaluating the clinical implications of using toxic metals in the human body."*
>
> —Theron Randolph, M.D.

Extensive clinical evidence based on patient case histories attests to the effects of mercury amalgam toxicity. Dr. Taylor cites an example of a woman who came to him suffering from rheumatoid arthritis. After having her amalgam fillings removed, she not only had relief from her arthritis, but her allergies abated to a large extent.

Another patient of Dr. Taylor was suffering from numerous symptoms of environmental illness. She exhibited multiple sclerosis–type symptoms, could only tolerate four or five foods, and developed sensitivities to chemicals, noise, light, and electromagnetic radiation. She also had jaundice and had been diagnosed with candida overgrowth. After having her amalgam fillings removed, she found that she was able to eat many different foods again, enabling her to put back on the sixty pounds she lost. Her sensitivities to noise, light, and electromagnetic radiation also diminished and her candida and jaundice cleared up.

A woman in Palm Beach, Florida, for years endured fatigue, mononucleosis (for which she was hospitalized at age sixteen), bladder infections, and, eventually, Epstein-Barr virus, candida, food allergies, and muscle spasms. Finally, her own investigation led her to consider the possibility of mercury poisoning and consult with Dr. Huggins. He found a tooth with a root canal that had been filled with dental amalgam. Once the amalgam was removed, her symptoms abated.

Bio-incompatibility to Dental Restoration Materials

In the same way that some people have adverse reactions to prescription drugs, some people also react negatively to specific dental materials. A person can already have been sensitized to dental restoration materials through previous exposure from the environment and foods.

Selected Health Symptom Analysis of 1,569 Patients Who Eliminated Mercury-Containing Dental Fillings[15]

The following represents a summary of 1,569 patients in six different studies evaluating the health effects of replacing mercury-containing dental fillings with non-mercury fillings. The data was derived from the following sources: 762 Patient Adverse Reaction Reports submitted to the FDA by patients; and 807 patients reports from Sweden, Denmark, Canada, and the United States.

% of Total Reporting	Symptom	Number Reporting	Number Improved or Cured	% of Cure or Improvement
14	Allergy	221	196	89
5	Anxiety	86	80	93
5	Bad temper	81	68	84
6	Bloating	88	70	80
6	Blood pressure problems	99	53	54
5	Chest pains	79	69	87
22	Depression	347	315	91
22	Dizziness	343	301	88
45	Fatigue	705	603	86
15	Intestinal problems	231	192	83
8	Gum problems	129	121	94
34	Headaches	531	460	87
12	Insomnia	187	146	78
10	Irregular heartbeat	159	139	87
8	Irritability	132	119	90
17	Lack of concentration	270	216	80
6	Lack of energy	91	88	97
17	Memory loss	265	193	73
17	Metallic taste	260	247	95
7	Multiple sclerosis	113	86	76
8	Muscle tremor	126	104	82

This bio-incompatibility, or incompatibility of the body, to the dental material can lead to severe allergic reactions including food allergies, and can contribute to chronic fatigue syndrome, chronic sinusitis and headaches, and can cause intractable pain syndrome. However, dentists often don't test for sensitivity to dental restoration materials before placing them in their patients' mouths.

The most common reactions are found to be produced by the mercury amalgams used for fillings, and by the various metal components that make them up, including mercury, copper, tin, zinc, and silver.[16] According to Dr. Arana, some of the symptoms caused specifically by amalgam fillings are:

- Chronic fatigue syndrome and lack of energy
- Tendency to chronic inflammatory changes (including rheumatoid arthritis, phlebitis, and fibromyalgia)
- Chronic neurological illnesses, especially when numbness is one of the leading symptoms
- Lowering of the pain threshold
- Disturbances of the immune system

Patients can be screened for sensitivity by a simple blood test, known as the Clifford Materials Reactivity Testing, after its developer, Walter

Jess Clifford, M.S., R.M., of Colorado Springs, Colorado. In this test, the patient's serum is exposed to the various components and by-products of dental materials to see if they provoke an immune reaction (antibody production). This makes it possible to determine which materials the body will be sensitive to. This information is then matched through a computer database to various dental products, enabling the dentist or physician to select which products are safe for each patient. "By using this form of testing," Clifford says, "it is possible to check the patient for an enormous number of dental product suitabilities without having to examine the finished dental product. One only needs to know what the dental restorative material contains and what it will give off when it breaks down." Bio-incompatible and toxic materials already in the mouth can then be replaced with those materials that have proven to be nonreactive. Applied kinesiology can also be used to test all materials and anesthetics before using them on patients.

After any dental material is removed, Dr. Huggins always recommends a thorough detoxification. According to Dr. Huggins, simply removing the fillings is not enough to rid the body of the toxic materials that may have built up over time, and may continue to cause allergic reactions. He places his patients on a detoxification regimen which can include nutritional support, acupressure, and massage treatments. Chelating agents, such as EDTA (ethylenediaminetetraacetic acid) and vitamin C, can be used intravenously or in tablet form as well. He cautions that any detoxification therapy should only be administered under the supervision of a qualified health professional.

Mercury Poisoning

Because mercury is a cumulative poison, building up in the body with repeated exposure,[17] its effects can be devastating. It can prevent nutrients from entering the cells, and wastes from leaving. Mercury can bind to the DNA (deoxyribonucleic acid) of cells, as well as to the cell membranes, distorting them and interfering with normal cell functions.[18] When this happens, the immune system no longer recognizes the cell as part of the body and will attack it. This can be the basis of many autoimmune diseases such as multiple sclerosis and arthritis.

Mercury poisoning can also lead to symptoms such as anxiety, depression, confusion, irritability, insecurity, and the inability to concentrate. It can cause kidney disease and cardiac and respiratory disorders. Multiple sclerosis patients have been found to have eight times higher levels of mercury in their cerebrospinal fluid (the fluid that surrounds the brain and spinal cord) as compared to neurologically healthy patients.[19]

Mercury poisoning often goes undetected for years because the symptoms presented do not necessarily suggest the mercury as the initiating cause. For example, it is capable of producing symptoms indistinguishable from those of multiple sclerosis,[20] and can mimic the symptoms of Lou Gehrig's disease (a syndrome marked by muscular weakness and atrophy due to degeneration of motor neurons of the spinal cord, medulla, and cortex).

Mercury can also produce allergic reactions with symptoms such as urticaria (an itchy rash), eczema, headaches, asthma, and digestive problems. The Environmental Protection Agency states that women chronically exposed to mercury vapor experience increased frequencies of menstrual disturbances and spontaneous abortions. A high mortality rate has also been observed among infants born to women who displayed symptoms of mercury poisoning.[21]

Electrogalvanism

Due to its mineral content, the saliva in the mouth is electrically conductive. As a result, when saliva in a person's mouth interacts with a dental restoration containing metal, a battery is created, causing an effect known as electrogalvanism. "Electrogalvanism is literally the electricity generated by a person's fillings," says Dr. Arana. "The saliva acts as a conductant and the dissimilar metal fillings then try to neutralize each other to balance out the electrical charge. This has the effect of causing toxic material from the fillings to erode, like the terminals of a battery, and leak out into the body." Dr. Arana points out that even two similar-looking amalgam fillings, if they were not placed on the same day, are likely to be of different compositions and therefore generate an electrical current between them. Even gold fillings or crowns are usually put over old fillings of a different metal, so electrogalvanism can even occur within a single tooth.

Since the teeth, the mouth, and the bone root all contain fluid, there are a variety of combinations that can determine where this electrical current flows. "It can go from a tooth to a muscle, tooth to a joint, tooth to an organ, and even a tooth to part of the brain, to the point where it can change the permeability of the blood-brain barrier," Dr. Arana states.

"Electrogalvanism is frequently the cause of lack of concentration and memory, insomnia, psychological problems, tinnitus, vertigo, epilepsy, hearing loss, and eye problems, to name but a few," says Dr. Arana. "Since high dental currents lead to erosion of the restoration materials, this problem rarely exists without coexisting problems of heavy metal toxicity, which can act synergistically with multiple chemical sensitivities to cause environmental illness."

> *"Electrogalvanism is frequently the cause of lack of concentration and memory, insomnia, psychological problems, tinnitus, vertigo, epilepsy, hearing loss, and eye problems, to name but a few."*
> —Edward Arana, D.D.S., President of the American Academy of Biological Dentistry

Electrogalvanism can be identified by an instrument known as an electrogalvanometer, which measures the electrical current and voltage generated by the dental amalgam in a tooth. Applied kinesiology can also be used to test for electrogalvanism between the upper and lower teeth. If the indicator muscle becomes weak when the patient gently touches the upper teeth to the lower teeth, then metal fillings from the top are forming a circuit with metal fillings on the bottom. Since high dental currents create neurological stress on the organism, the muscle becomes weak as soon as one metal touches another. Likewise, when the teeth are apart, and the circuit is broken, the indicator muscle will become strong again.

"We suspect that the reason why many dental splints, [illegible] a patient's TMJ dysfunction problem is that these splints are made out of plastic and work like a circuit-breaker whenever they are in place," notes Dr. Arana. "The TMJ dysfunction problems that improve are really not TMJ dysfunction problems, but problems created by the high dental currents."

Temporomandibular Joint Syndrome (TMJ)

TMJ dysfunction is caused by the malalignment of the teeth, jaws, and muscles. The symptoms of TMJ dysfunction vary, and include pain, clicking, or grating sounds when the mouth opens, and difficulty opening the mouth very wide.

See Chiropractic, Craniosacral Therapy, Osteopathy.

TMJ dysfunction can occur for three reasons. First, the patient loses teeth through decay or trauma, or looses height of some teeth through bruxism (grinding) or age. Second, there are iatrogenic (treatment-induced) problems such as dental restorations that make the teeth either too high or too low. The third cause can be developmental problems. "In the last two hundred years, developmental abnormalities of the upper and/or lower jaw have become very common. This has been shown to be directly linked to the intake of processed foods, especially sugar and flour," says Dr. Price.[22]

Because chewing is the primary mechanism necessary for supplying nutrients to the body, if the jaws or teeth are out of alignment, the entire cranium will distort in order to chew properly. The structural compensations necessary for this readjustment can be responsible for such varied symptoms as depression, loss of concentration, insomnia, headaches, neck pain, and low back pain—all caused by TMJ dysfunction.

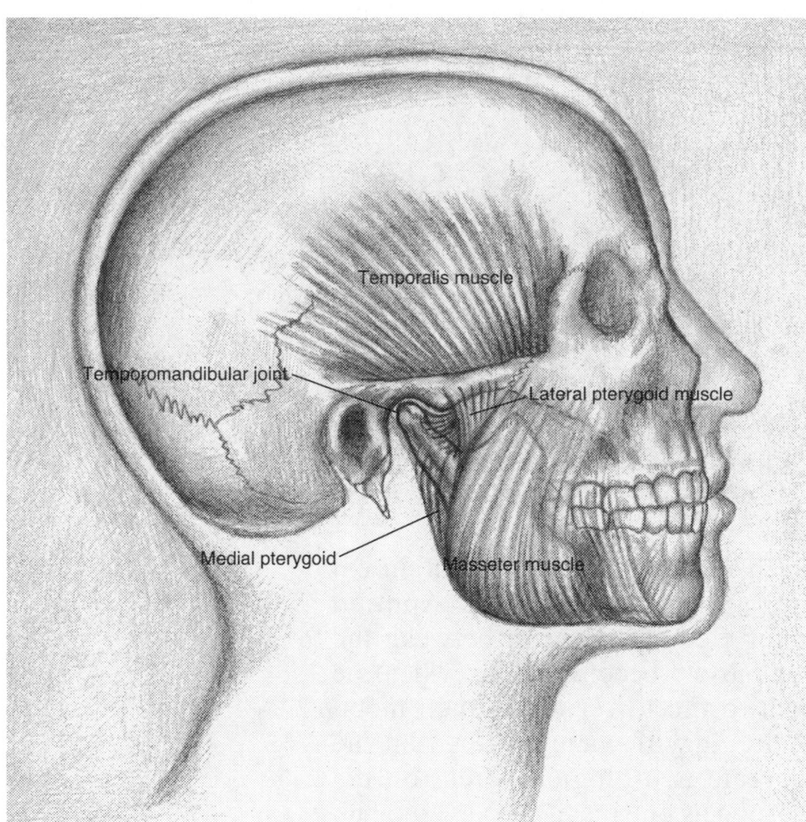

The temporomandibular joint.

TMJ dysfunction is diagnosed by observation of symmetry of facial features, midline shift of teeth, asymmetric wear of dental surfaces, asymmetry of jaw movement, tenderness over joints, and tenderness in associated muscles. It can also be diagnosed by x-rays, arthrograms (joint x-rays), MRI (magnetic resonance imaging), computerized motion studies, applied kinesiology testing, and electroacupuncture biofeedback.

Dr. Ravins believes balancing the jaw is essential to relieving TMJ dysfunction. Using computerized technology he can measure movements of the jaw and determine where irregularities lie. By using orthopedic appliances (similar to braces) worn in the mouth at night, he can realign the jaw and relieve the symptoms. Other dentists also use craniosacral therapy or cold laser therapy to help correct TMJ syndrome.

Biological Treatment of Dental Problems

Biological dentists treat dental problems in a variety of ways. They emphasize the conservation of all healthy tooth material and employ the latest techniques of bioenergetic medicine, including neural therapy, oral acupuncture, cold laser therapy, complex homeopathy, mouth balancing, and nutrition.

Neural Therapy

According to neural therapy, the body is charged with electricity or biological energy. This energy flows throughout the body, with every cell possessing its own specified frequency range. As long as this energy flow is unimpeded and stays within its normal range, the body will remain healthy. However, if this balance breaks down, disruptions in the the normal function of cells can occur, eventually leading to chronic disorders.

When injury, inflammation, or infection is present in the mouth, there is usually a corresponding blockage in the body's normal energy flow. "Neural therapy allows the dentist to confirm if the problem in the tooth is causing illness elsewhere in the body," says Dr. Arana. The problem may lie in the tooth itself, or in a distant organ on the same energy meridian as the tooth.

Injection of a local anesthetic such as procaine around the tooth to remove the energy blockage will often resolve the problem. Dr. Adler cites the example of a sports instructor suffering from "tennis elbow." When Dr. Adler injected the man's two upper right premolars with procaine, the instructor received immediate relief from his pain.

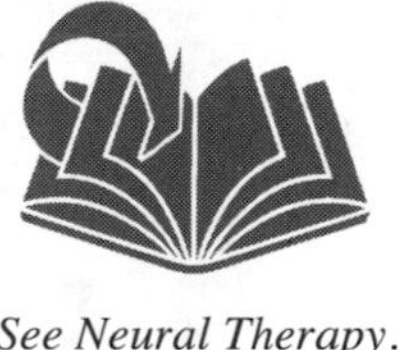

See Neural Therapy.

Dr. Arana conservatively estimates that one hundred dentists in the United States currently practice neural therapy. However, he adds, there are over four thousand dentists worldwide practicing neural therapy, including two to three thousand in Germany where it was developed.

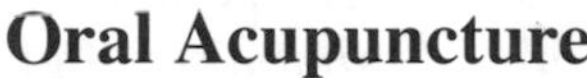

Oral Acupuncture

Oral acupuncture, according to Jochen Gleditsch, M.D., D.D.S., of Munich, Germany, has been taught to dentists since 1976, and its use is expanding rapidly. It involves the injection of either saline water, weak local anesthetics, or sterile complex homeopathics into specific acupuncture points of the oral mucous membrane. It can also be combined with neural therapy.

Both Dr. Arana and Dr. Ravins use oral acupuncture to relieve pain during dental procedures with great success. Some dentists also use it to relax patients before any dental procedure. Toothache, tooth sensitivities, jaw pain, gingivitis, and other local problems often respond to oral acupuncture.

Dr. Gleditsch discovered that there are specific oral acupuncture points related to each tooth. "The total of these oral acupuncture points form [illegible] "with a clear reference to the system of acupuncture meridians." When a particular acupuncture meridian is under stress, the corresponding oral acupuncture point(s) become very sensitive to localized pressure. This phenomenon can be used for both diagnostic and treatment purposes, according to Dr. Gleditsch. He commonly uses acupoints in the mouth to treat neuralgia, sinusitis, pain in distant parts of the body, acute, chronic, and allergic conditions, and digestive disorders. The oral acupuncture points in the retromolar area (the area behind the last molar in the upper and bottom jaw) are most valuable in treating shoulder and elbow complaints, pain and restricted movement of the neck, low back pain, and TMJ. Since needle acupuncture is impractical within the oral cavity due to the danger of choking, Dr. Gleditsch uses injections of saline or local anesthetic into the points. Laser stimulation can also be used.

Cold Laser Therapy

See Light Therapy.

Cold laser therapy is an alternative form of acupuncture that is especially useful for treating patients who object to the use of needles. The "cold laser" gets its name from the fact that its power output and the light spectrum it uses are incapable of causing any thermal damage to the body's tissues. This therapy kills bacteria, aids in wound healing, reduces inflammation, and helps to rebalance the flow of energy in the body's meridian system. It has also been used to treat TMJ dysfunction[23] and to promote healing and reduce muscle spasm after removal of impacted wisdom teeth, according to Dr. Ravins.

Homeopathy in Biological Dentistry

According to Dr. Fischer, "Homeopathic first aid remedies can help alleviate the pain or discomfort of dental emergencies, at least temporarily, until proper dental care can be received. They are not intended to replace regular dental care, but rather to serve as a safe and effective complement."

Abscesses can be treated with homeopathic dilutions of *Belladonna, Hepar sulph., Silicea, Myristica,* and *Calendula. Gelsemium, Aconite, Coffea cruda*, and *Chamomilla* can be used to allay the apprehension of a visit to the dentist. Postsurgical bleeding is treated with *Phosphorous*, and if accompanied by bruising and soreness, with *Arnica. Chamomilla* is good for a dry socket after an extraction. A toothache can be treated with *Belladonna, Magnesium phos., Coffea cruda*, or *Chamomilla*.

Mouth Balancing

Dr. Ravins specializes in "balancing" the mouth to improve a wide range of health problems, including TMJ dysfunction. He believes that structural deformities of the skull influence the entire body. "With the new computerized technology, I can diagnose muscle dysfunction and pick up vibrations from the jaw and movement of the mandible," he says. Often the misalignment has been caused by a prior accident. By analyzing this data and making special orthopedic braces to be worn in the mouth, Dr. Ravins can realign the jaw and remove pain and other symptoms such as headaches, shoulder pain, and back problems.

Many patients who come to Dr. Ravins complain of eye problems such as blurred vision (often occurring after eating), and pressure and pain behind the eyes. Since the bones around the eyes are close to those of the jaw, a misaligned jaw can easily put pressure on them, resulting in pressure on the eyes themselves. Stress in the mouth can also affect the nerves and blood supply to the eyes, and infections in the mouth can cause muscle spasms which will affect the eyes. According to Dr. Ravins, once any misalignments in the mouth are corrected with orthopedic braces, the eye problems usually dissipate. The problems often return though, when the appliances are removed. While eye problems should always be checked by an eye doctor first, if the problem is not uncovered by an eye examination, a biological dentist may be able to help.

Nutrition

Dr. Huggins, like many other biological dentists, makes nutritional supplementation part of his overall protocol for dealing with dental conditions, especially for the patient recovering from mercury amalgam toxicity. "There is a standard regimen we use to help correct basic chemistry problems," he says. "From there, we might use additional supplementation based on what the patient's chemistry dictates." According to Dr. Huggins, the basic supplementation program aids in the excretion of mercury from the cells, prevents the exacerbation of further symptoms, and provides the patient with a nutrient base for rebuilding damaged tissues.

Among the nutrients Dr. Huggins uses are magnesium, selenium, vitamin C, vitamin E, and folic acid, along with digestive enzymes. He cautions, however, that the nutrients need to be used in specific ratios, and that supplementation done without proper consultation can actually create further imbalances in the patient's system.

A proper diet is also important for patients suffering from mercury toxicity. Dr. Huggins recommends the avoidance of cigarettes, sugar, alcohol, caffeine, chocolate, soft drinks, refined carbohydrates, milk, cheese, margarine, fish, and excess liquids with meals.

THE POLITICS OF DENTISTRY

Although many new techniques of biological dentistry are available, only two to three thousand dentists across the United States are using them in practice. This is due to a deliberate effort by the American Dental Association (ADA) to suppress such practices, even to the point of rescinding the licenses of practitioners using them. Electroacupuncture biofeedback testing by dentists is not allowed in some states, and dentists may lose their license for using it, despite its proven effectiveness for screening hidden infections under teeth. For this reason most dentists are forced to use other methods for detecting hidden infections and other dental problems. Dental acupuncture is also banned in some states.

In 1987, the ADA wrote a provision into their code to declare the removal of clinically serviceable mercury amalgams from patients' teeth to be unethical, according to Michael Ziff, D.D.S., of Orlando, Florida. Any dentist doing so is in violation of the code, and the ADA is assisting state boards in prosecuting these dentists, despite all the evidence of the toxicity of mercury.

The financial and legal implications of an admission by the ADA that mercury is toxic and harmful to health may be a possible motive behind this move. If the ADA was to admit that mercury amalgams are toxic health hazards, insurance companies or the government would possibly have to foot the bill for the removal of mercury amalgams from practically the entire population of the United States.

Despite this ominous situation, the growing number of research studies on biological dental techniques, the information coming out of Europe and Canada on mercury toxicity[24] and [illegible] of the dangers of traditional dental practice are combining to build support for the small band of dentists risking their livelihood to practice safe dentistry in the United States.

The Future of Biological Dentistry

Mercury and other dental materials contribute to much of the degenerative diseases for which patients seek medical help today. Traditional dentistry and medicine have not yet recognized this growing danger, but biological dentistry is confronting it head-on. Using all the knowledge and skills of conventional dental medicine along with the disciplines of alternative, holistic health therapies, biological dentists are striving to provide individuals with biocompatible, aesthetic, comfortable, functional, and enduring dental and prosthetic replacements. While much research has already been done on mercury toxicity from dental amalgams, and on the creation of safe, nontoxic dental restoration material alternatives, much more still needs to be done, especially in the United States. Dr. Randolph believes that medicine and dentistry must

FLUORIDATION

Fluoride is commonplace today in toothpastes, mouthwashes, and drinking water. In the United States alone, over 121 million people are now drinking artificially fluoridated water. Many experts would argue that it poses a serious health risk. Fluoride is a known poison and has been classified as very toxic to extremely toxic by the National Library of Medicine's computerized data service on toxic substances. Numerous studies have demonstrated that fluorides are largely retained in the body and build up poisonous concentrations there.[25]

Drs. R. N. Mukherjee and F. H. Sobels of the University of Leiden in Holland found that fluoride increases the frequency of genetic damage in sperm cells of laboratory animals exposed to x-rays and inhibits the repair of DNA.[26]

Fluoride was first introduced into the public water systems in the United States in 1945 through an experiment, which grew out of research done by H. Trendley Dean, D.D.S. (the "father of fluoridation") for the Public Health Services. Dr. Dean was trying to determine the reason some people had higher than normal levels of staining of their teeth. His finding cited fluoride as the cause of the staining, but also credited fluoride as the reason these same people had fewer cavities.[27]

In 1950, the Public Health System recommended using artificial fluoridation in the public water systems to fight tooth decay. Since the time fluoride entered the water system in the United States, there have been many health-related problems while at the same time, no statistically significant reduction in tooth decay. Dr. Dean himself has twice been forced to admit in court that his original statistics favoring fluoridation were invalid.[28]

Christa Danielson, M.D., found an increased risk of hip fracture in men and women over age sixty-five who had been exposed to fluoride in their drinking water for about twenty years. At least 10 percent of fluoride in adults is deposited in bones, and studies have shown a positive correlation between higher fluoride intake and decreased bone mass and strength.[29]

In 1975, John Yiamouyiannis, M.D., and Dean Burk, M.D., compared ten large U.S. cities that fluoridated their water with ten cities that did not. They discovered a link between fluoride and a 10 percent increase in cancer deaths over a thirteen to seventeen-year period. As a result of these studies, tests were ordered by Congress that confirmed fluoride added to water causes cancer in laboratory animals.[30]

In spite of all the research and finding, fluoride is still commonplace in the United States today. It has, however, been banned in Austria, Denmark, France, Greece, Italy, Luxembourg, the Netherlands, Norway, and Spain.

come together to solve the mercury problem and make dentistry a health-enhancing endeavor that eliminates, instead of promotes, disease. "In the future," says Dr. Ziff, "I foresee bonding materials becoming much more biocompatible, along with new techniques being developed that will address the problems of modern dentistry."

"The emphasis must be more in the way of prevention," says Dr. Arana. "So when people in the anti-amalgam movement say we're going to have to retrain the dentists, they're right, but it can be done. I think the materials being used now are very close to being able to fix the teeth so they're white and beautiful without any danger of toxicity problems."

Toxic-free, biological dental treatment has the possibility of an overall stress reduction so great that patients could lose all or many of their distressing chronic disease symptoms. "The next great advancement in medicine will come from the dentists," says Dr. Arana. "Biological dentistry will, out of necessity, become the dental medicine of the twenty-first century."

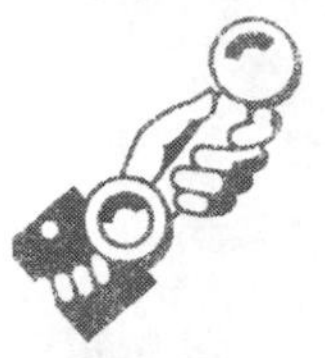

Where to Find Help

Many organizations and dentists are involved in promoting the practice of biological dentistry. Contact an organization below for more information.

American Academy of Biological Dentistry
P.O. Box 856
Carmel Valley, California 93924
(408) 659-5385
(408) 659-2417 (Fax)

The purpose of the AABD is to promote biological dental medicine, which uses nontoxic diagnostic and therapeutic approaches in the field of clinical dentistry. They publish a quarterly journal, Focus, *and hold regular seminars on biological diagnosis and therapy.*

International Academy of Oral Medicine and Toxicology
P.O. Box 608531
Orlando, Florida 32860-8531

A professional organization of dentists, physicians, and research scientists dedicated to scientifically investigating the bio-compatibility of materials used in dentistry. Members are worldwide.

Foundation for Toxic Free Dentistry
P.O. Box 608010
Orlando, Florida 32860-8010

A nonprofit group whose main goal is to educate and refer the general public to biological dentists all over the world. Send a self-addressed, stamped envelope for fifty-two cents and they will send you [illegible]

Environmental Dental Association
9974 Scripps Ranch Boulevard
Suite 36
San Diego, California 92131
(800) 388-8124/(619) 586-1208

The EDA is an organization of alternative dentists who are concerned about the potential toxic effects of various dental procedures and materials. Member dentists believe that the most important environment of all is the human body and that some dentistry can cause harmful side effects. The EDA provides a referral service for patients seeking alternative dentists in their area. It also offers books and products on alternative dentistry for the public. For a free packet of information call the EDA's toll-free number.

The Safe Water Coalition
West 5615 Lyons Court
Spokane, Washington 99208
(509) 328-6704

The purpose of this organization is to educate legislators and the public to the hazards of fluoridation.

DAMS
725-9 Tramway Lane Northeast
Albuquerque, New Mexico 87122
(505) 291-8239
(505)0294-3339 (Fax)

DAMS (Dental Amalgam Syndrome) is a support and educational organization, designed to help those suffering from mercury amalgam toxicity, to raise public awareness of the problem, and to provide documentation of the condition for the [illegible]

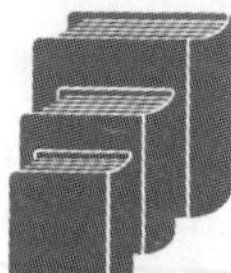

Recommended Reading

The Complete Guide to Mercury Toxicity from Dental Fillings. Taylor, Joyal. San Diego, CA: Scripps Publishing Co., 1988.

A step-by-step guide to help people evaluate themselves for mercury poisoning. Also included are anecdotes and nutritional information as well as alternatives to mercury fillings.

Dental Mercury Detox. Ziff, Sam and Michael. Orlando, FL: Bio-Probe Inc., 1993.

A book to help reduce mercury toxicity in your body.

Dentistry without Mercury. Ziff, Sam and Michael. Orlando, FL: Bio-Probe Inc., 1993.

An eighty-page book of the most recent scientific research and information on mercury toxicity.

Fluoride, The Aging Factor. Yiamouyiannis, John, Ph.D. Delaware, OH: Health Action Press, 1986.

A well-documented book that investigates the degenerative qualities of fluoride. It discusses the scientific, industrial, political, and moral aspects of fluoride exposure.

Infertility and Birth Defects—Is Mercury from Silver Dental Fillings a Hidden Cause? Ziff, Sam and Michael. Orlando, FL: Bio-Probe Inc., 1987.

A very accessible book that explains and documents the facts about mercury and lead and why mercury fillings may increase the risks of infertility and birth defects.

It's All in Your Head. Huggins, Hal, D.D.S. Colorado Springs, CO: Life Science Press, 1986.

Dr. Huggins analyzes the diseases and symptoms associated with mercury poisoning, as well as providing diagnostics and a nutritional guide to recovery.

Mercury Poisoning from Dental Amalgam—A Hazard to Human Brain. Stortebecker, Patrick, M.D., Ph.D. Orlando, FL: Bio-Probe Inc., 1986.

Dr. Stortebecker describes his principle of the shortest pathway with scientific evidence that mercury vapor released from fillings can travel directly to the brain.

The Missing Link. Ziff, Sam and Michael. Orlando, FL: Bio-Probe Inc., 1992.

A fully referenced book that scientifically explores the relationship of mercury with heart disease.

Silver Dental Fillings—The Toxic Time Bomb. Ziff, Sam. Santa Fe, NM: Aurora Press, 1986.

This book covers the history of the mercury controversy from 1819 to the present.

Bodywork

The term bodywork refers to therapies such as massage, deep tissue manipulation, movement awareness, and energy balancing, which are employed to improve the structure and functioning of the human body. Bodywork in all its forms helps to reduce pain, soothe injured muscles, stimulate blood and lymphatic circulation, and promote deep relaxation.

For centuries, the therapeutic use of touch has been applied to heal the body and reduce the tensions of daily life. There are literally hundreds of schools of bodywork, from therapeutic massage to the deep tissue bodywork therapies like Rolfing® and Hellerwork that aim toward a literal restructuring of the body. Movement therapies, such as the Feldenkrais Method™ and the Alexander technique, help realign the body through the correction of postural imbalances to promote a more efficient function of the nervous system. Energetic systems of bodywork, such as acupressure, polarity therapy, and Therapeutic Touch™, help balance energy in the body and bring about enhanced health and well-being. Today, the majority of bodywork practitioners employ a combination of bodywork methods.

Therapeutic Massage

Within the past decade, an overwhelming accumulation of scientific evidence has supported the claim that massage therapy is beneficial.[1] According to John Yates, Ph.D., author of *A Physician's Guide to Therapeutic Massage*, massage can benefit such conditions as muscle spasm and pain, spinal curvatures (lordosis, scoliosis), soreness related to injury and stress, headaches, whiplash, temporomandibular joint syndrome (TMJ), and tension-related respiratory disorders such as bronchial asthma or emphysema. Massage can also help reduce swelling, help correct posture, improve body motion, and facilitate the elimination of toxins from the body.[2] Lymphatic massage, for example, can move metabolic waste through the body to promote a rapid recovery from illness or disease. Other studies show that massage can be used as an adjunct in the treatment of cardiovascular disorders and neurological and gynecological problems, and can often be used in place of pharmacological drugs.[3]

According to the Quebec Task Force on Spinal Disorders, massage is the most frequently used therapy for musculoskeletal problems, and is particularly useful in controlling pain.[4]

Gertrude Beard, R.N., R.P.T., former Associate Professor of Physical Therapy at Northwestern University Medical School, summarizes the findings of numerous research studies on the therapeutic effects of massage. Studies indicate that massage:

- Has a sedative effect upon the nervous system and promotes voluntary muscle relaxation.
- Is effective in promoting recovery from fatigue produced by excessive exercise.
- Can help break up scar tissue and lessen fibrosis and adhesions which develop as a result of injury and immobilization.
- Can relieve certain types of pain.
- Provides effective treatment of chronic inflammatory conditions by increasing lymphatic circulation.
- Helps reduce swelling from fractures.
- Affects circulation through the capillaries, veins, and arteries, and increases blood flow through the muscles.
- Can loosen mucus and promote drainage of sinus fluids from the lungs by using percussive and vibratory techniques.
- Can increase peristaltic action (muscular contractions that move waste through the system) in the intestines to promote fecal elimination.[5]

Researchers have also found that certain massage techniques can trigger reflex actions in the body to stimulate organs. Beard adds that these should only be applied under the direction of a knowledgeable physician or physical therapist.

How Massage Releases Tension and Promotes Relaxation

Muscle tension, whether from normal activity or from awkward movement or stress, contributes to muscle fatigue and pain by compressing nerve fibers in the muscle. Prolonged contraction interferes

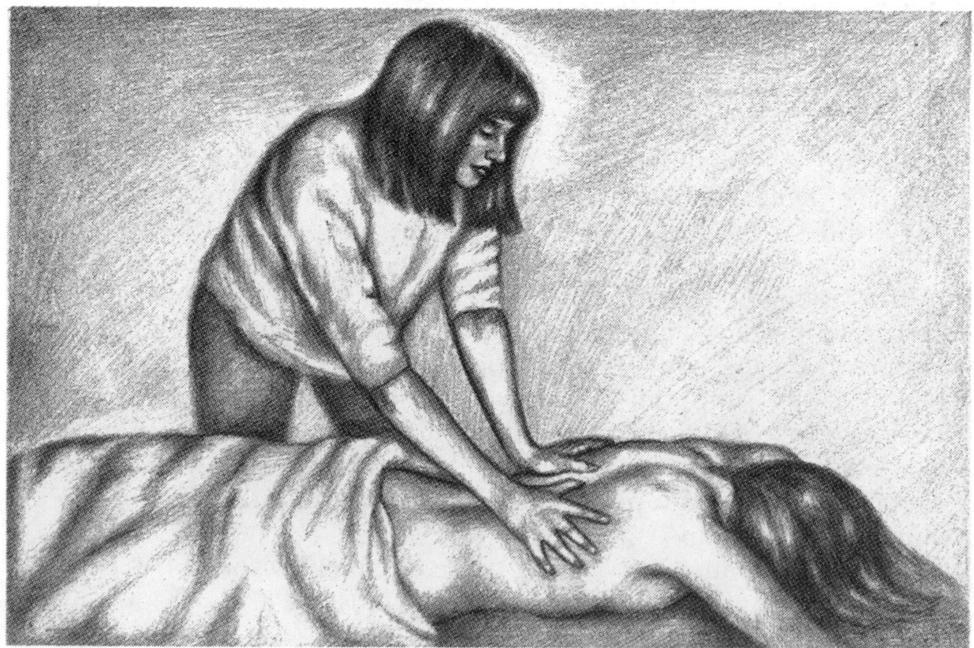

Traditional Swedish massage.

with the elimination of chemical wastes in the muscles and surrounding tissues, and can cause frequent nerve and muscle pain. If not properly addressed these body tensions have a tendency to build into chronic patterns of stress.

Prolonged tension can often cause pain in other parts of the body. For example, headaches are often caused by overly tense muscles in the neck, shoulders, and lower back. Even contracted abdominal muscles can trigger headaches in certain people (a common complaint of women with menstrual difficulties).

For these tension-related conditions, Robert D. Milne, M.D., of Las Vegas, Nevada, an expert on headache relief, finds that massage can break up muscular waste deposits and stimulate circulation. He adds that accumulated metabolic wastes often form "trigger points" within muscles. These are specific areas that are painful to the touch. "They feel like knots or ropes within the muscle and perpetuate muscle tension," explains Dr. Milne. By applying deep pressure to these points, the tension or spasm can often be eliminated.

Bodywork: A New Approach to Awareness and Physical Health

The contemporary systems of bodywork are as concerned with relaxation and physical therapy as are the traditional schools of massage. Terms such as neuromuscular therapy, connective tissue massage, myofascial therapy, trigger point massage, and soft tissue manipulation further distinguish these contemporary systems. However, the majority are based on one or more of the following principles or techniques:

- The use of pressure or deep friction to alter the muscular and soft tissue structures
- The use of movement to affect physiological structure and functioning
- The use of education and awareness to change or enhance physiological functioning
- The use of breathing and emotional expression to eliminate tension and to change physiological functioning

The following systems represent some of the most influential practitioners, theories, and techniques of contemporary bodywork.

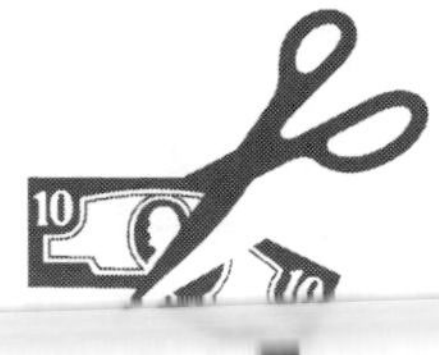

By addressing tension, stress, and structural imbalances in the body, the various forms of bodywork can be an important part of a health maintenance program and can reduce long-term health costs.

The Alexander Technique

Frederick Matthias Alexander was one of the first people to notice how faulty posture in daily activities (sitting, standing, moving) is connected with serious physical and emotional problems. Alexander pioneered a simple, effective approach to rebalancing the body through awareness, movement, and touch. A turn-of-the-century Shakespearean actor, Alexander began to experience a recurring loss of his voice while on stage. When he studied himself in a mirror, he discovered that he unconsciously and habitually moved his head back and down, tensed his neck and throat, and sucked in his breath whenever he thought of using his voice. From his observations Alexander developed a method that used his breath to alter this habitual muscular response, and he eventually recovered his voice. This marked the beginning of the development of the Alexander technique.

Alexander was aware that the correct relationship of one's head, neck, and back is essential for proper movement and functioning. He observed that people habitually "misuse" their bodies for such mundane activities as sitting or standing, and Alexander helped his students become conscious of these faulty habits and postures. He taught how to interrupt or inhibit familiar postural "sets" that corresponded to these recurring habits so that the body could be guided to allow improved motion, balance, and posture. Wilfred Barlow, author of the well-known book *The Alexander Technique*, states that, "Most people have lost good use of their bodies by the time they are past early childhood." Poor or inhibited use of the body can contribute to many diseases, including debilitating curvatures of the spine, rheumatism, arthritis, and a variety of gastrointestinal and breathing disorders.[6] According to Barlow, all of these can be positively affected by learning how to properly hold and use the body.

"Most people have lost good use of their bodies by the time they are past early childhood."

In the early 1970s, experiments conducted by Frank Pierce Jones at Tufts University concluded that Alexander's methods could effectively interrupt or inhibit habitual and learned responses that interfere with proper body functioning. By doing so, the techniques allow for a restoration of natural balance and responsiveness during movement.[7] In a typical session, a student may lie on a table, sit on a stool, or remain standing. The student may be given instructions such as, "Let your head move forward and up to allow your torso to lengthen and widen." While saying this, the teacher gently prevents the old habit and encourages a new improved response of the head/neck/back relationship. During this time, the student is instructed to "do nothing"; the student simply thinks the instruction given by the teacher. Eventually, the student constructs a new body image, and by doing so retrains and reorganizes the way he or she moves.

Over twenty-five hundred people worldwide have been trained in the Alexander technique. In Europe, it has been recognized by the Inner London Education Authority and many Alexander teachers at various colleges, particularly in the departments of drama, speech, dance, and music. Athletes find the Alexander technique helpful for improving their performance skills, and for the relief of chronic pain.

Alexander's work has influenced teachers, educators, and scientists. Nikolas Tinbergen, winner of the 1973 Nobel Prize in Physiology and Medicine, highly praised Alexander's contributions. And with chronic pain and back disorders on the increase, this gentle technique has much to offer.

The Feldenkrais Method

Moshe Feldenkrais was a physicist involved with nuclear radiation research and antisubmarine technology in France and England. Like Alexander, personal trauma in the form of a sports-related injury drove him to explore the functioning of the body. Rather than submitting to the recommended surgery, he sought an alternative solution through the study of the nervous system and human behavior. Applying his experience of martial arts, physiology, anatomy, psychology, and neurology, Feldenkrais succeeded in reversing his impairment and taught himself how to walk without pain.

The notion of "self-image" is central to the theory and technique of Feldenkrais and his method. According to Feldenkrais, "Each one of us speaks, moves, thinks, and feels in a different way, each according to the image of himself that he has built up over the years. In order to change our mode of action we must change the image of ourselves that we carry within us."[8]

Feldenkrais viewed the human organism as a complex system of intelligence and function in which all movement reflects the state of the nervous system and is also the basis of self-awareness. We become accustomed to our movements, be they good or bad, and this can lead to any number of physical and emotional problems. Feldenkrais reasoned that if the negative habitual patterns of movement are interrupted, the body will learn to function with greater ease, fluidity, and motion. This, in turn, improves one's self-image and simultaneously increases awareness and health.

> *"Each one of us speaks, moves, thinks, and feels in a different way, each according to the image of himself that he has built up over the years."*
> —Moshe Feldenkrais

Feldenkrais recognized the importance of breath and viewed it as an integral form of movement. Poor movement and poor functioning impairs the breathing and improper breathing interferes with the proper functioning of the body. He found that even the movement of the eyes could seriously interfere with how other parts of the body function.

Feldenkrais developed two approaches for working with students and clients; one implements group lessons (called Awareness through Movement®), and the other focuses on individualized hands-on touch and movement (called Functional Integration®). Participants of Awareness through Movement are guided through a slow and gentle sequence designed to replace old patterns of movement with new ones. As the client learns how to listen to these "lessons," he or she develops an awareness of subtle changes in habit and movement. Feldenkrais wrote that the lessons are designed to improve mobility, "to turn the impossible into the possible, the possible into the easy, and the easy into the elegant."[9]

With Functional Integration, learning occurs through touch. The practitioner actively directs the client's body through movements individualized to the client's particular needs. The Feldenkrais method differs from most other schools of bodywork in that there is no attempt to structurally alter the body. Instead, it is through touch that the practitioner attempts to communicate to the person a sense of improved self-image and movement.

Feldenkrais viewed forcefully imposed "posture" as rigid and inflexible, and shunned the idea of imposing rules of proper form and function. His teaching imparts a sense of exploration, experimentation, and innovation that allows each person to find his or her optimal style of movement.

The Feldenkrais method helps people move more easily. The method is also useful for those who have limitations of movement brought on by stress, accidents, back problems, other physically debilitating illnesses or diseases. "But," adds Ralph Strauch, Ph.D., a certified Feldenkrais practitioner, "our primary concern is with the person, not the disorder." Performers and athletes have attributed Feldenkrais for improving their levels of performance, and many have utilized the work as a means of enhancing personal growth.

Awareness Through Movement

Ralph Strauch, Ph.D., a certified Feldenkrais practitioner in Los Angeles, suggests the following simple method taken from a typical Awareness through Movement lesson. This particular lesson is designed to improve how the neck and head turn.

Sit comfortably with your body upright and your feet on the floor. Close your eyes and turn your head slowly to the right until it stops. Notice if the movement is smooth and fluid, or somewhat stiff and jerky. Open your eyes and notice how far you turned, then bring your head back to the center.

Repeat the movement slowly, another twenty to twenty-five times. Do not turn as far as you can, and do not "try" hard to do it; simply move slowly and easily, taking notice of what you feel. Pay attention to the parts of your body that take part in the turning; be aware of how far down your spine you feel the movement. Let your eyes move in unison with your head, looking to the right then coming back to the center. Allow your shoulders to take part in the movement as well.

Now sit quietly and notice how you feel. After a few moments, close your eyes and again turn your head to the right. Does it go farther this time? Has the quality of the movement changed?

Turn your head to both the left and the right, and notice any differences in movement or ease. Most people will notice an improvement in the quality of movement to the right.

This change is produced by the process of watching the movement, not by the movement itself. It is an increase in awareness that allows the movement to improve.

To test this, try the following: Close your eyes and imagine doing the same movement to the left. Imagine the movement becoming smoother and easier over ten to fifteen times. Feel the imaginary movement in the spine, the shoulders, and the eyes, just as if you had done the actual movement. Now actually turn the head to the left and the right, and notice how the movement has improved.

Rolfing

Biochemist Ida P. Rolf, Ph.D., gained her first exposure to therapeutic manipulation when, as a young woman, she was successfully treated by an osteopath for a respiratory condition. The doctor performed manipulations to reposition a rib that had been displaced by a kick from a horse. Dr. Rolf began to glimpse the operating premise that would become the cornerstone of her work: the body's structure profoundly affects all physiological and psychological processes.

Dr. Rolf was also influenced by her exposure to Hatha yoga, which led her to the principle that "bodies need to lengthen and be balanced, and a balanced body will give rise to a better human being."[10] She founded the Rolf Institute for Structural Integration in 1970, which has since trained nearly eight hundred people.

"Rolfing®," the popular name for Structural Integration, is based on the idea that human function is improved when the segments of the body (head, torso, pelvis, legs, feet) are properly aligned. Most people are not aware if and when their bodies are out of balance. For example, when standing, many people put most of their weight on their heels, but doing so throws the balance backward. In order to compensate, the upper body must lean too far forward, throwing the pelvis out of alignment. In addition, in order to see, the head has to be tilted back. In order to hold this position the muscles of the neck, back, and legs must remain overly contracted and stressed. After maintaining this posture for months or in some cases, years, the fascial tissues (fibrous layers covering muscles) of the body have to compensate to hold everything in this out-of-balance position. Movement becomes impaired, and this reduces mental clarity and increases emotional stress.

Dr. Rolf believed that balance and poise could be reestablished by manually manipulating and stretching the body's fascial tissues. The fascia is a thin, elastic, semifluid membrane that envelops every muscle, bone, blood vessel, nerve, and organ. It plays an integral role in maintaining posture and proper movement. Dr. Rolf defined fascia as the organ of change, and stated that injury, chronic stress, or other trauma can lead to its deterioration. According to Dr. Rolf, when fascia becomes increasingly more solid, rigid, and sticky, it begins to restrict the movement of muscles and joints.

Rolfers® use pressure applied with the fingers, knuckles, and elbows to release fascial adhesion. Doing so helps to reorganize the tissue back to its proper geometric planes by lifting, lengthening, and balancing the body segments. Balance is an essential fact in Rolfing: "If the head is supported and balanced by the shoulders, the shoulders by the chest, the chest by the pelvis," noted Dr. Rolf, "and so on, then gravity can only reinforce balance."[11]

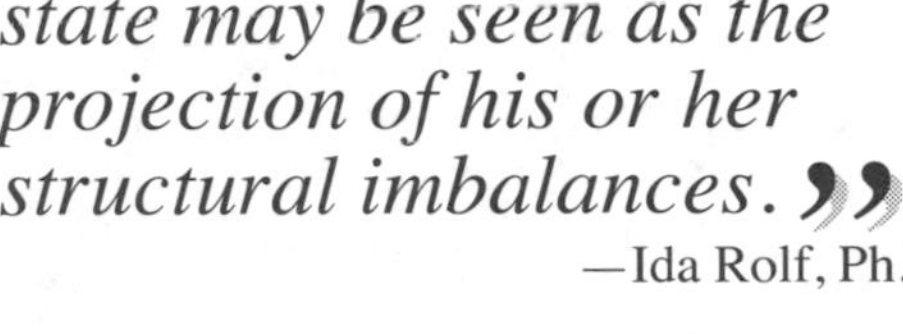
“A person's emotional state may be seen as the projection of his or her structural imbalances.”
—Ida Rolf, Ph.D.

Depending on the depth and degree of tissue adhesion, pain may be felt when pressure is applied. Dr. Rolf pointed out that it could hardly be expected that profound tissue changes such as changes in position or tone could be accomplished without a dramatic reaction. "People often call this reaction pain, but it is not the pain we associate with injury or hurt," she stated.[12]

Over the years, in order to enhance the effectiveness of the physical manipulations, a system of movement education called Rolfing Movement Integration has developed. Weekly sessions allow the teacher and client to explore the possibilities for developing freer, more balanced movements. These movements can then be applied to all aspects of daily living: sitting, standing, breathing, running, and housework.

Research on the effects of Rolfing have been conducted at UCLA's Department of Kinesiology by Valerie Hunt, Ed.D., and Wayne Massey. The study concluded that: movements were smoother, longer, [illegible]; there were less extraneous movements; body movements were more dynamic and energetic; carriage was more erect; and there was less obvious strain to maintain a held position.[13]

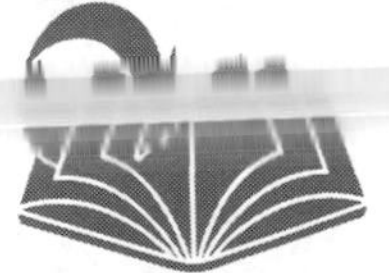

See Applied Kinesiology, Chiropractic, Craniosacral Therapy, Osteopathy.

A similar study conducted at the University of Maryland indicates that Rolfing reduces chronic stress, promotes changes in body structure, and enhances neurological functioning. In addition, those studied who suffered from lordosis, or sway back, experienced a reduction in the curvature of the spine.[14]

Ida Rolf's work has profoundly influenced contemporary bodywork. Her research into fascia and the role of gravity in determining balance has added tangible credibility to the structural approach to body therapy. Nearly everyone can benefit from Rolfing, and those who suffer from pain and stiffness related to mechanical imbalances and poor posture will be particularly rewarded.

Aston-Patterning

Several years after completing her graduate studies in dance and fine arts at UCLA, Judith Aston was involved in back-to-back car accidents that left her with debilitating injuries. After traditional medical treatment failed, a physician recommended that she see Ida Rolf. As a result of Rolf's technique, her condition improved dramatically. Because of Judith's background in teaching dance and movement, and her ability to train people to see and perform movement, Ida Rolf asked her to develop a movement education system for Rolfing in order to help maintain the structural alignment achieved in the sessions. This system was called Rolf-Aston Structural Patterning. She began training people in 1971, and during the next seven years, she trained Rolfers in movement analysis and in the basics of movement education.

Judith went on to develop Aston-Patterning® in its current form in 1977. Unlike Rolf's model and its focus on body symmetry and alignment, Aston noted that all movement is naturally asymmetrical, and that a healthy body develops asymmetrically through adaptation to the kinds of work, recreation, sports, and other daily activities it performs. In addition, she focuses on how to distinguish what is changeable, and what is a true asymmetrical limitation. Aston's work also has an individual focus, as she says, "people aren't recipes." Aston also teaches students a technique she calls "spiraling" to work the deep tissues without pain.

Aston's work focuses on four areas: movement reeducation, massage and soft tissue bodywork, fitness training, and environmental "design" (for example, altering the height of an office chair and furniture to suit a particular body). Participants learn to integrate Aston's principles of movement with specific methods for strengthening and stretching the body.

Neshama Franklin, a health journalist, describes a demonstration session she received from an Aston-Patterner: "We started with an evaluation of the way I walk. The practitioner noted that my weight distribution was off balance—heavy on the heels with my feet pointed at different angles. Then she explored my body with massage. Any

REICH, BODYWORK, AND EMOTIONAL RELEASE

People who undergo bodywork often experience powerful emotional releases. "All behavior is expressed through the musculoskeletal system" and "a person's emotional state may be seen as the projection of his or her structural imbalances," noted Ida P. Rolf, Ph.D., the developer of Structural Integration, or Rolfing.

In a similar way, Wilhelm Reich, M.D., realized that feelings and emotions are reflected in the body posture and behavior of the individual, and he developed a system of bodywork and breathing that is capable of bringing these often buried emotions to the surface. Although Dr. Reich, who was a former student of psychoanalyst Sigmund Freud, used his techniques for the purposes of psychological intervention, his work left a deep impression on many who later developed their bodywork techniques, including Dr. Rolf.

Dr. Reich's techniques were deceptively simple, foremost being the act of breathing. By asking his patients to breath deeply and continuously, he was able to unlock chronic physical tensions and release pent-up and unconscious feelings and memories. The power of the breath has led many bodywork practitioners to incorporate deep breathing techniques into their work.

Dr. Reich also gave close attention to how patients held themselves, and would occasionally apply deep pressure to tense muscle groups in the face, neck, back, torso, and legs. Additionally, he would ask his patients to kick, hit, or move in various ways that were designed to release the musculature and hidden emotions.

Today many bodyworkers have adapted Dr. Reich's techniques. Psychotherapists also recognize the importance the body plays in maintaining psychological health, and many have integrated bodywork and massage into their practices.

resistance or tension was dutifully marked on a chart. I liked the specific, graphic way the chart helped me see the patterns of tension in my body.

"After the massage, we returned to walking, and I explored ways to distribute my weight more evenly. The result was a new stride that felt springy and light. Six months later, I could still recapture that ease of movement when I focused on what I learned at the demonstration session."[15]

Aston-Patterning can be used to develop better movement and coordination, or for managing painful conditions such as backaches, headaches, and tennis elbow. Nancy Richardson, a registered physical therapist in Colorado, uses Aston-Patterning as an adjunct for clients suffering from neck and back pain, and for working with adolescents with postural dysfunctions.[16]

Hellerwork

Developed by Joseph Heller, who was the first president of the Rolf Institute, Hellerwork combines deep touch, movement education, and verbal dialogue. This approach works to structurally realign the body as well as facilitate an awareness of the mind/body relationship. Hellerwork specifically addresses the interwoven complexity of the mechanical, psychological, and energetic functioning of the human body. The mechanical aspect of Hellerwork is patterned after Rolfing, and is designed to properly align the body with the gravitational field of the earth. Heller felt that the physical changes achieved by manual manipulation were not sufficient to bring about permanent change in the body. He incorporated a thematic approach to each of the eleven Hellerwork sessions in order to provide for his clients a basis for organizing the emotional content of the work.

"Hellerwork can improve body alignment and flexibility, and can offer increased vitality and greater emotional clarity and freedom of expression."

For example, the first Hellerwork session is designed to unlock tension and unconscious holding patterns in the chest to allow for fuller and more natural breathing. The practitioner engages the client in a dialogue intended to call attention to emotions and attitudes that affect the physiological process of breathing.

Hellerwork works with movement and awareness to teach clients how to sit, stand, walk, lift, or run in ways that are appropriate to the natural design of their bodies. The process is designed to minimize mechanical stress and create more efficient use of the body's energy.

In a unique experiment, Hellerwork was administered to the staff of a computer software company in Portland, Oregon. At the completion of the series, employees were surveyed regarding their experiences. Every employee reported a reduction in physical stress and an improvement in his or her posture. Additionally, 84 percent noticed less back pain, 81 percent felt that their job effectiveness had increased, and 94 percent experienced an improvement in their work relationships and an improved ability to communicate.[17]

Hellerwork can improve body alignment and flexibility, and can offer increased vitality and greater emotional clarity and freedom of expression. It is beneficial for anyone suffering painful and stiff muscles due to structural imbalances, or for conditions that may be the result of injury, emotional trauma, or sustained stress. There are over three hundred trained Hellerwork practitioners in the United States.

The Trager Approach

Beginning in 1927, Milton Trager, M.D., developed this intuitive and playful approach to movement reeducation that uses a method of gentle, rhythmical touch combined with a series of movement exercises.[18] Although the techniques are very different from Feldenkrais work, the purpose is largely the same: to help the client recognize and release habitual patterns of tensions that are present in posture and movement. He established the Trager Institute with Betty Fuller in 1980.

Dr. Trager's approach uses no specific techniques of movement or massage. Instead, the practitioner is taught to feel how the client is holding his or her body, and by applying various rocking, pulling, and rotational movements to the client's head, torso, and appendages, the therapist gently loosens tense muscles and stiff joints.

"Dr. Trager takes a particular interest in applying his approach to people suffering from severe neuromuscular disturbances resulting from injury, disease, and aging, including disorders such as polio, muscular dystrophy, and multiple sclerosis."

"The concern of the Trager® approach," says Deane Juhan, an instructor at the Trager Institute, "is not with moving particular muscles or joints per se, but with using motion in muscles and joints to produce particular sensory feelings, namely positive, pleasurable feelings that enter the central nervous system and begin to trigger tissue changes by means of the many sensory-motor feedback loops between the mind and the muscles."[19] These gentle movements provoke a sense of deep relaxation and help increase flexibility and range of motion in the client's joints and limbs. Dr. Trager believes that the unconscious mind will always mimic movements that result in an improved sense of pleasure and freedom, and that it is the practitioner's responsibility to help plant this sense of well-being in the client's body.

Mentastics® is a term coined by Dr. Trager to mean "mental gymnastics." These exercises are free-flowing, dancelike movements designed to increase awareness of how the body moves for the purpose of learning how to move more effortlessly. An exercise may be as simple as letting the arms or legs drop to one side or the other, or adding a small shaking or swinging motion to a foot and leg while walking. Dr. Trager designed the exercises to reinforce the relaxation awareness established from the hands-on bodywork.

Dr. Trager takes a particular interest in applying his approach to people suffering from severe neuromuscular disturbances resulting from injury, disease, and aging, including disorders such as polio, muscular dystrophy, and multiple sclerosis. In addition, many athletes have found that the work has increased their efficiency of movement and stamina. To date, over seven thousand people have been trained in Trager's techniques, with nine hundred currently certified practitioners worldwide.

Bonnie Prudden Myotherapy

Bonnie Prudden is one of the world's leading authorities on physical fitness and exercise therapy. Her research helped create the President's

Council on Physical Fitness and Sports in the 1950s. From her experience, she developed a technique for relieving pain that is simple enough to be taught to a child.

Prudden's work is based on the application of manual pressure to sensitive spots known as "trigger points." Her work grew out of Janet Travell, M.D.'s pioneering medical discipline called trigger point injection therapy, where sensitive and often painful muscular spots are injected with a saline or procaine solution. In 1976, while working with Desmond Tivy, M.D., another advocate of trigger point injection therapy, Prudden discovered that a relatively deep pressure of between five and seven seconds applied to these same points could relieve pain for roughly 90 percent of all muscle-related pain without the use of invasive and often very painful injections. "At first, we worked mainly with backs," writes Prudden. "Instead of taking weeks to get rid of pain with exercise and injections, it was taking only a few sessions, often only one. Arm, shoulder, and neck pain all surrendered. We even had several stroke patients who . . . had severely contracted arm muscles. Soon they too were free of pain and their limbs free of contracture."[20]

Trigger points can be caused by any trauma at any age including prenatal injury, accidents, childhood and sexual abuse, any and all sports, the repetitive motions connected with occupation or hobbies, and any invasion of the body from injections, to hundreds of necessary and unnecessary operations. Trigger points are often exacerbated by disease, substance abuse, and aging. They are highly irritable spots that may lie quietly for years within a muscle, and can be "fired" as a result of certain physical or emotional conditions. Muscle spasm is the result. This in turn causes more pain and creates a spasm-pain-spasm cycle.

To relieve the pain the cycle must be broken. Although medication can interrupt the cycle, the underlying cause, the resident trigger point, remains. Once medication wears off, the pain is temporarily relieved. However, another bout with physical or emotional stress can reactivate the painful cycle. This is the cause of most recurring or chronic pain. Once a trigger point is created, others often form in the immediate and surrounding area. For treatment to be successful, these satellite points must also be addressed.

> *"If myotherapy can be safely developed for preliminary use before consulting a physician, or if physicians can feel safe prescribing it before engaging in a series of expensive diagnostic tests, then myotherapy could make a significant contribution toward solving the problem of the escalating costs of medical care."*
>
> —Desmond Tivy, M.D.

Prudden's two books on pain, *Pain Erasure* and *Myotherapy*, include charts for locating the major trigger points. These points can be easily found on yourself or somebody else by touch, as pressing on a trigger point can be relatively painful.

Press each muscle with your finger at one-inch intervals. When a tender spot is found, apply pressure until the first sign of discomfort. Anything more is counterproductive. Because the tension underlying these trigger points is of a chronic nature, several sessions will be needed to eliminate the trigger points and their satellites. This specific exercise, designed to reeducate the muscle to return to normal function, is the key to success with Bonnie Prudden Myotherapy™.

It is also important to do three-minute sessions five times a day to prevent old tensing habits from taking over. After the session, stretching exercises are needed to retrain the muscles to relax.

Bonnie Prudden Myotherapy can be effective in relieving muscle pain, strains, sprains, dislocations, tension headaches, and migraines. Numerous pain clinics now use the technique. Myotherapy also treats temporomandibular joint syndrome, and neck, shoulder, arm, hand, back, chest, and abdominal pain. Hemorrhoids, spasms in the muscles surrounding the prostate, as well as impotence and incontinence when resulting from spasms in the muscles of the pelvic floor, can also benefit. Myotherapy is invaluable in leg, lower leg, knee, and foot pain and cramps thought to be caused by aging. Diseases such as arthritis, lupus, and multiple sclerosis also respond, as they all affect muscles that house trigger points.

According to Desmond Tivy, M.D., myotherapy can also alleviate pain caused by a number of organic and structural diseases that are episodic in nature, and can sometimes be used diagnostically by physical therapists: "If myotherapy can be safely developed for preliminary use before consulting a physician, or if physicians can feel safe prescribing it before engaging in a series of expensive diagnostic tests, then myotherapy could make a significant contribution toward solving the problem of the escalating costs of medical care."

Reflexology

Bodywork provides a low-cost and effective way to reduce pain and improve the strength and overall functioning of the body.

Reflexology states that there are reflex areas in the hands and feet that correspond to every part of the body, including organs and glands, and that these parts can be affected by stimulating the appropriate reflex areas. Reflexology is used to relieve stress and tension, stimulate deep relaxation, improve the blood supply, and promote the unblocking of nerve impulses to normalize and balance the entire body.

Reflexology evolved out of an earlier European system known as zone therapy, and was introduced to America by William Fitzgerald, M.D., a laryngologist at St. Francis Hospital in Connecticut. Dr. Fitzgerald discovered he could induce numbness and alleviate certain symptoms in the body by applying finger pressure to specific points on the hands and mouth. Eunice Ingham, a physiotherapist, used Fitzgerald's work as the basis for what is known today as reflexology. Ingham mapped organ reflexes on the feet and developed techniques for inducing a stimulating, healing effect in those areas.

Reflexologists apply precise pressure to release blockages that inhibit energy flow and cause pain and disease. This pressure is believed to affect internal organs and glands by stimulating reflex points of the body. Practitioners often target the breakup of lactic acid and calcium crystals accumulated around the 7,200 nerve endings in each foot. "Perhaps this is why we feel so much better when our feet are treated," writes Ray Wunderlich, Jr., M.D., of Florida. "Nerve endings in the feet have extensive interconnection through the spinal cord and brain to all areas of the body." Dr. Wunderlich believes that even though reflexology is medically unproven, it still "deserves wide usage as a valuable adjunct to the medical care of patients in need."[21]

Modern reflexologists continue to witness startling effects from their treatments. Bill Flocco, founder of the American Academy of Reflexology, in conjunction with Terrence Oleson, Ph.D., Associate Professor of Research at the University of California at Los Angeles, conducted a study of the effects of reflexology in alleviating premenstrual syndrome (PMS). Results indicated a 62 percent reduction in the PMS symptoms of those undergoing reflexology treatment.[22] Dr. Wunderlich notes that reflexology is helpful for people with hypertension, anxiety, or painful conditions of the body.

Today, reflexology is practiced by nearly twenty-five thousand certified practitioners around the world. And since 1940, more than fifty thousand people have taken reflexology seminars. "In Denmark, reflexology is the number one alternative health modality," states Dwight Byers, President of the International Institute of Reflexology in St. Petersburg, Florida. "Even the Royal Family of Britain uses it," he adds. There's no question that reflexology is a safe and simple way to induce relaxation and a genuine sense of well-being.

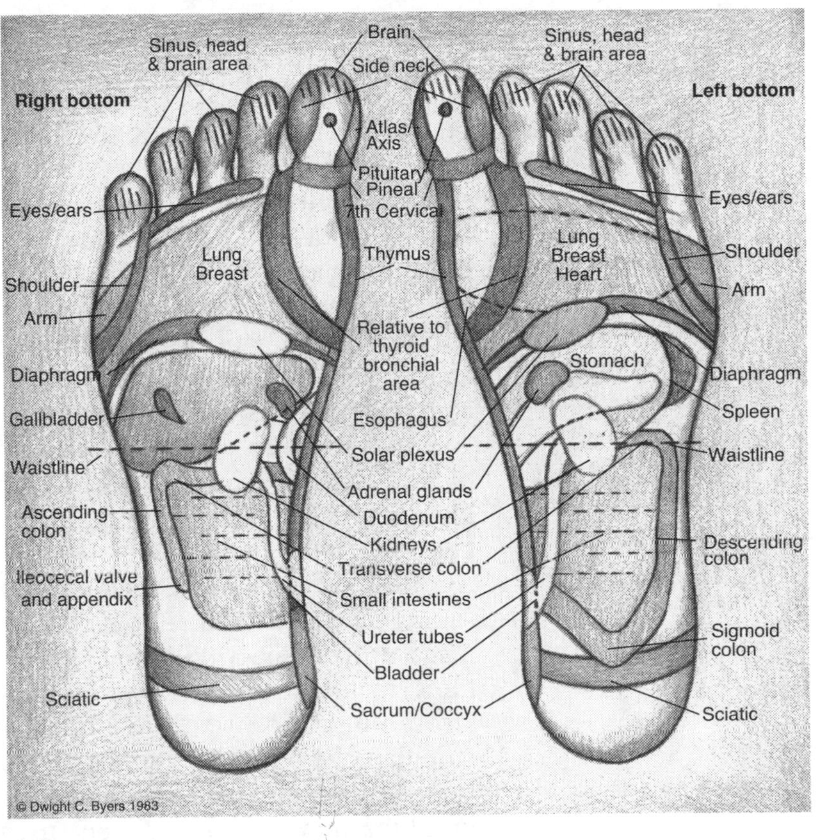

Foot reflexology charts.

Energy-Based Systems of Bodywork

Many systems of bodywork are based on various "energy" models. The oriental body therapies, for example, are primarily based on the concept of vital life energy, or *qi* (also referred to as *chi*), and although their concepts are not well understood in the West, modern research has documented their effectiveness.

Acupuncture and acupressure work on the principle that there are energy channels, called meridians, which run throughout the body and through which the *qi* flows. Different organs are associated with different energy meridians, and health problems in various organs show up as energy blocks in the meridians they are associated with.

Western energy therapies (such as polarity therapy), with their aim toward manipulating and balancing the client's energy flow through touch, often incorporate a variety of approaches gleaned from different cultures and traditions.

Therapeutic Touch™, a contemporary energy-healing system that is now widely used in American medical facilities and hospitals, is based on the premise that it is the healing force of the therapist that affects the patient's recovery and cure.

Acupressure and Oriental Bodywork Therapies

See Acupuncture, Qigong, Traditional Chinese Medicine, Yoga.

Over five thousand years ago, the Chinese discovered that when certain points on the body are pressed, punctured, or heated, certain ailments are relieved. The beneficial effects are thought to be due to the release of energy blocks in the meridians. As the art developed, more and more points were discovered that not only alleviated pain, but influenced the functioning of internal organs and body systems.

Whereas acupuncture uses needles, acupressure uses the pressure of the fingers and hands. Acupressure is the older of the two techniques, but was overlooked as the Chinese developed more "technological" methods for stimulating points, namely with needles and electricity. Still, acupressure continues to be an effective self-care and preventative health care treatment for tension-related ailments.

Acupressure considers symptoms as an expression of the condition of the whole person, and focuses on relieving pain and discomfort. It is also concerned with responding to tensions and toxicities in the body before they develop into illnesses.

Self-acupressure techniques such as Acu-Yoga and *Do-In* utilize the same points but teach effective methods for administering to oneself. Acu-Yoga utilizes the whole body for breathing, finger pressure, yogic postures, meditations, and stretches. *Do-In* also incorporates body awareness, stretching, and breathing, but focuses on vigorous techniques that stimulate the body through the points and meridians.

Acupressure massage techniques and practices (referred to as *Tui Na* in China and *Amma* in Japan) use rubbing, kneading, percussion, and vibration to improve circulation and to stimulate stale blood and lymph from tissues.

See Chronic Pain, Headaches, Stress.

Styles of Oriental Bodywork: Oriental bodywork has developed primarily through a combination of instinct and hands-on experience. Its principles and healing techniques integrate breathing meditations, herbal remedies, and massage. Contemporary practitioners continue to incorporate these traditional principles along with the discovery of new treatment protocols and bodywork styles.

While traditional points are common to all styles of Oriental bodywork, each style has distinctive characteristics that incorporate unique ways of touching and interacting with clients. The following descriptions focus on the primary styles or methods currently in practice.

- ***Shiatsu*** literally means "finger pressure" in Japanese. This well-known method uses a firm sequence of rhythmic pressure held on specific points for three to ten seconds and is designed to awaken the acupuncture meridians. Michael Reed Gach, Ph.D., Director of the Acupressure Institute in Berkeley, California, recalls a highly athletic patient, who often complained of pain in his back and leg muscles. He had found no relief with massage therapy, but *shiatsu* produced excellent results on his back and legs, the deep pressure releasing the stiffness and improving the muscle tone and circulation.

- ***Jin Shin Jyutsu*** was developed in Japan by Jiro Murai, who rediscovered the ancient *qi* flow in his own body and mapped a powerful system of healing points. Combinations of points are held with the fingertips for a minute or more, usually with the client lying on his or her back. Various schools of the *Jin Shin* style have evolved, including *Jin Shin Do*™ and *Jin Shin* acupressure.

All of these systems can positively regulate and harmonize the body, and can be used to relieve pain and muscular discomfort, correct imbalances, and prevent illness.

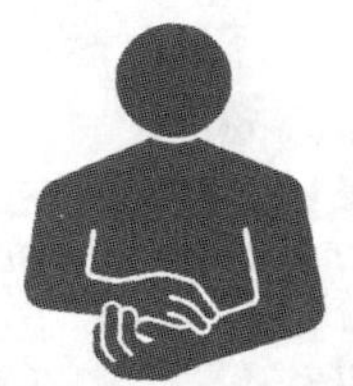

Several systems of bodywork are ideally suited to self-care and can easily become part of your personal health maintenance program.

Therapeutic Touch

Developed by Dolores Krieger, Ph.D., R.N., Professor Emeritus at New York University, and Dora Kunz, a healer, Therapeutic Touch™ is a contemporary interpretation of many healing practices, such as visualization, laying on of hands, and aura therapy. From its development in 1972, Therapeutic Touch has been taught in more than eighty American colleges and in sixty-eight countries.

In Therapeutic Touch there is a generally no physical contact between patient and practitioner. Occasionally, hands-on touching is employed when treating a fracture or other traumatically injured part of the body. A typical session begins with the practitioner centering or quieting him- or herself. A brief assessment period then takes place, where the practitioner places his or her hands two to six inches away from the patient and, with rhythmic and slow-hand motions, determines where the blockages in the patient's energy field lie. The practitioner then works to replenish the energy flow where necessary, release any congestion, and remove obstructions. The patient, who is in a relaxed comfortable state, can undergo a range of experiences, from a discharge of previously suppressed emotions to a quiet, gentle sense of well-being. A session usually lasts for twenty to twenty-five minutes.

"The effectiveness of Therapeutic Touch has been documented clinically, and its practice is accepted in many hospital situations."

Therapeutic Touch has proven effective in treating a variety of medical conditions. According to Dr. Krieger, Therapeutic Touch is "a contemporary interpretation of several ancient healing practices in which the practitioners consciously direct or sensitively modulate human energies."[23] The proper use of Therapeutic Touch can decrease anxiety, reduce pain, and ease problems associated with autonomic nervous system dysfunction.[24] This technique has been taught to more than 37,000 nurses, doctors, and health practitioners.

In clinical studies, Therapeutic Touch has been shown to have physiological effects. For example, it has altered enzyme activity, increased hemoglobin levels, and accelerated the healing of wounds.[25] However, the technique is primarily known for its ability to relieve pain and reduce stress and anxiety.[26] Studies have shown that patients receiving Therapeutic Touch experienced a significant reduction of headache pain.[27] Further evidence supports the use of this technique to calm crying babies, ease asthmatic breathing, reduce pain in postoperative patients, and reduce fever and inflammation.[28]

Therapeutic Touch has been used with pregnant women in connection with reducing anxiety and discomfort.[29] It is now commonly practiced and taught in Lamaze classes. Many people continue to use this healing technique with their infants and children, and it can be applied to one's own body to reduce pain and stress, or to heal injuries or increase relaxation.

Relieving Headaches

The following acupressure points are helpful for relieving most headaches. The point numbers are for identification and referencing in the acupressure and acupuncture professions.

Firmly press GB20: *With your thumbs, press underneath the base of your skull into the hollow areas on either side, two to three inches apart depending on head size. With your eyes closed, slowly tilt your head back, and press firmly up from underneath the skull for one to two minutes as you take long, deep breaths.*

Hold GV16 with B2: *Use the right thumb to press GV16 in the center hollow at the base of the skull. Use your left thumb and index finger to press B2 in the upper hollows of your eye sockets near the bridge of your nose. Again, tilt your head back and breathe deeply for one to two minutes.*

Firmly press LI4: *Place your right hand over the top of your left hand. Use your right thumb to press the webbing between the thumb and the index finger of your left hand. Angle the pressure toward the bone that connects with the index finger. Hold for one minute. Then press this point for one minute on your opposite hand. A note of caution: This point (known as* ho-ku*) is forbidden for pregnant women because its stimulation can cause premature contractions in the uterus.*

Polarity Therapy

Polarity therapy was developed by Randolph Stone, D.C., D.O., N.D., who was deeply interested in the electromagnetic energy currents of the human body. Dr. Stone explored the world's healing systems for an understanding of their underlying essence. He based his work on the Eastern concept that illness originates from blockages in energy flow.

Polarity hands-on techniques include manipulation of pressure points and joints, massage, breathing techniques, hydrotherapy, exercise, reflexology, and even simply holding pressure points on the body. Both hands are used (one is positive, the other negative) to release energy blockages in the body and help to restore a natural flow. Polarity bodywork is both invigorating and rejuvenating, and can result in positive changes on the physical, mental, and emotional levels.

The stretches and other exercises used in polarity therapy are simple techniques that anyone can employ to release energy blockages and restore a balanced energy flow in the body. These techniques, combined with dietary and nutritional counseling based upon Traditional Chinese Medicine's five element theory, as well as the emotional balancing work that is also part of polarity therapy, help clients achieve a heightened level of well-being.

The benefits of polarity therapy can include an enhanced sense of well-being, improvement in physical health, increased energy, and a deeper understanding of oneself. It is useful for all conditions, from excellent health to extreme disease, and Dr. Stone himself specialized in cases that others pronounced as hopeless.

Polarity therapy is taught by individuals and at various schools worldwide. In 1984 the American Polarity Therapy Association was formed to assist in networking, research, and maintaining quality of practice, and has certified 130 practitioners.

The Future of Bodywork

Numerous systems of bodywork have been reviewed in this chapter. Some are based on the physical manipulation of body structures, while others focus on the manipulation of the body's various energy fields. Others use awareness and learning as the basis for improving body movement and functioning. Importantly, most recognize the value of feelings and emotions and have integrated a mind/body philosophy into their practice.

According to Michael Murphy, author and co-founder of the Esalen Institute in Big Sur, California, these disciplines, when properly applied, have the potential for bringing about transformations of the human personality. He suggests that these systems of bodywork "promote attributes beyond those to which they are primarily addressed." These include increased somatic awareness and self-regulation, improvement of communication abilities, increased vitality, and an improved sense of self. "Somatic disciplines can contribute to balanced programs for growth," Murphy maintains, leading ultimately to extraordinary functioning and then to the possibility for self-transcendence. This, says Murphy, is the future of the body.[30]

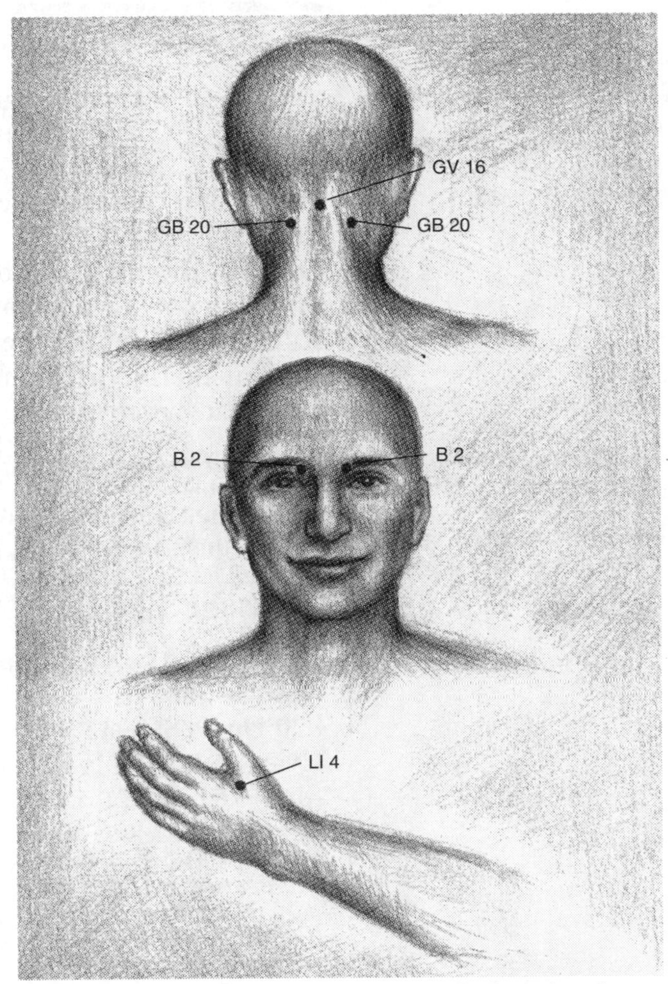

Headache points for acupressure.

Where to Find Help

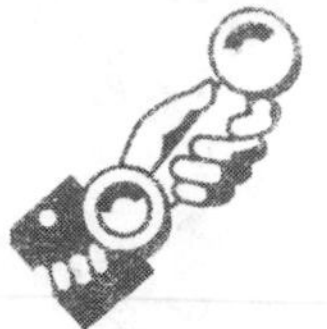

If you live in a large community, you should be able to find several alternative publications that list various bodywork and massage therapies. Other holistic practitioners are a good source for referrals. Information regarding the bodywork systems described in this chapter is listed below. Other schools of bodywork which may be of interest include: orthobionomy (a combination of neuromuscular and postural reeducation), Rubenfeld Synergy method (integrating Alexander, Feldenkrais, and Gestalt therapy), Hanna Somatic education, the Benjamin system of muscular therapy, postural integration (similar to Rolfing), and the Lomi School (combining both Western and Eastern bodywork techniques). Many massage therapy schools also offer training in various bodywork techniques and are a good source for information and referrals. Check your bookstore for literature on massage techniques.

Massage

American Massage Therapy Association
820 Davis Street, Suite 100
Evanston, Illinois 60201
(312) 761-2682

Offers comprehensive information on most areas of massage and bodywork, including an extensive review of scientific research. They also publish the Massage Therapy Journal, *available at many newsstands and health food stores.*

Massage Magazine
P.O. Box 1500
Davis, California 95617
(916) 757-6033

Published bimonthly, by NOAH Publishing Co. in Davis, California, Massage Magazine *covers the art and science of massage, bodywork, and related healing arts. A great resource for workshops and schools, including interviews with prominent people working in the field.*

Esalen Institute
Big Sur, California 93920
(408) 667-3000

Offers many weekend and extensive programs in holistic health. Many of the systems mentioned in this article were introduced and popularized at Esalen, which overlooks the Pacific ocean in Big Sur. Under the direction of Michael Murphy, Esalen offers a unique training program in integrative body therapy.

Alexander Technique

North American Society of Teachers of the Alexander Technique
(800) 473-0620

For information, referrals, and training.

The Feldenkrais Method

Feldenkrais Guild
P.O. Box 489
Albany, Oregon 97321
(503) 926-0981

For information, practitioner training, and certification.

Rolfing

International Rolf Institute
P.O. Box 1868
Boulder, Colorado 80306
(303) 449-5903

For information, practitioner training, and certification.

Aston-Patterning

The Aston Training Center
P.O. Box 3568
Incline Village, Nevada 89450
(702) 831-8228

Aston-Patterning is an integrated system of movement education, 3-D soft tissue work, environmental modification, and fitness training. The center trains people to become certified Aston-Patterning practitioners, offers classes to the health professionals, and provides a curriculum of courses to certify health care and physical training professionals.

Hellerwork

The Body of Knowledge/Hellerwork
406 Berry Street
Mt. Shasta, California 96067
(916) 926-2500

For information, referral directory, training, and certification.

Tragerwork

Trager Institute
33 Millwood
Mill Valley, California 94941
(415) 388-2688

For practitioner directory, information, training, and certification.

Bonnie Prudden Myotherapy

Bonnie Prudden Pain Erasure
3661 North Campbell, Suite 102
Tucson, Arizona 85719
(800) 221-4634

For a list of certified myotherapists, and those clinics where myotherapy is offered [illegible] nursing homes, industry, and for the handicapped.

Reflexology

International Institute of Reflexology
P.O. Box 12462
St. Petersburg, Florida 33733
(813) 343-4811

For information, seminars, publications, and referrals.

Acupressure and Oriental Body Therapies

Acupressure Institute
1533 Shattuck Avenue
Berkeley, California 94709
(510) 845-1059

For information, career trainings, and mail order catalog.

American Oriental Bodywork Association
6801 Jericho Turnpike
Syosset, New York 11791
(516) 364-5533

For information, professional membership, practitioner directory, and referrals.

Therapeutic Touch

Nurse Healers—Professional Associates, Inc.
175 Fifth Avenue, Suite 2755
New York City, New York 10010
(212) 886-3776

Cooperative among health professionals interested in healing.

Pumpkin Hollow Farm
Box 135, RR 1
Craryville, New York 12521
(518) 325-3583

Site of frequent Therapeutic Touch workshops.

Orcas Island Foundation
Box 86, Route 1
East Sound, Washington 98245
(206) 376-4526

Offers summer workshops on Therapeutic Touch.

Polarity Therapy

Polarity Wellness Center
10 Leonard Street, Suite A
New York, New York 10013
(212) 334-8392

For information, publications, and referral directory.

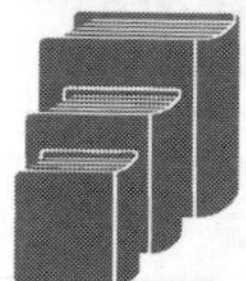

Recommended Reading

Massage

The Book of Massage. Lidell, Lucinda. New York: Fireside, 1984.

Excellent step-by-step instructional guide with extensive color illustrations on massage, shiatsu, *and reflexology.*

The Massage Book. Downing George. New York: Random House, 1972.

Considered the "classic book" on massage.

Massage for Common Ailments. Thomas, Sara. New York: Fireside, 1989.

A simple, comprehensive, step-by-step guide on how to alleviate a range of everyday health problems through massage and shiatsu *techniques. Extensive color illustrations.*

Alexander Technique

The Alexander Technique. Barlow, Wilfred. New York: Alfred A. Knopf, 1991.

The founder of the Alexander Institute shows how to reduce mental stress and muscular tension by becoming more aware of balance, posture, and movement in everyday activities.

The Alexander Technique. Gray, John. New York: St. Martin's Press, 1991.

This easy-to-follow guide allows everyone to learn the program with clear instructions for each exercise and helpful photographs that show the correct and incorrect positions to use for the exercises.

Body Awareness in Action. Jones, Frank P. New York: Schocken Books, 1976.

A presentation of F. M. Alexander's method by F. P. Jones, who studied the actual mechanics of the body in achieving awareness, providing scientific support for Alexander's ground-breaking discoveries.

The Feldenkrais Method

Awareness through Movement: Health Exercises for Personal Growth. Feldenkrais, Moshe. New York: Harper & Row, 1972.

This is a genuine self-help guide to improved posture, flexibility, breathing, health, and functioning through twelve easy-to-follow Awareness through Movement lessons. After an introduction emphasizing the importance of self-education and the primary relationships of movement to sensory, thinking, and emotional life, Feldenkrais shows us how to "use our skill, not our will" in order to improve.

The Potent Self: A Guide to Spontaneity. Feldenkrais, Moshe; and Kimmey, M. San Francisco, CA: Harper & Row, 1992.

The revolutionary theory behind the Feldenkrais method is explained, focusing on the underlying emotional mechanisms that lead to compulsive and dependent physical behavior that inhibits the individual from reaching full potential. Written for the general reader, anyone can apply Feldenkrais' secrets to his or her own life to achieve potency, self-realization, and spontaneity.

Rolfing

Rolfing: The Integration of Human Structures. Rolf, Ida, P. New York: Harper and Row, 1977.

The mother of Rolfing explains, "Once free of the muscular rigidity imposed by past experience, the body structure can be put back into natural alignment with the forces of gravity, a process necessary for physical well-being."

Hellerwork

Bodywise. Heller, Joseph; and Henkin, William. Berkeley: Wingbow Press, 1991.

Bodywise puts you on the path to restoring the "natural balance" of your body. By learning how to care for and carry it properly, and by following the unusual body awareness exercises in this book, you can begin to be conscious of and reduce stress, pain, and tension.

Tragerwork

Trager Mentastics: Movement as a Way to Agelessness. Trager, Milton; and Guadagno, Cathy. Barrytown, NY: Station Hill Press, 1987.

Trager explains the dancelike movements characterizing his largely intuitive method of mind/body healing.

Bonnie Prudden Myotherapy

Myotherapy. Prudden, Bonnie. New York: Ballantine Books, 1985.

Myotherapy, pain relief based on trigger points, is fully examined as a technique, requiring no special training or equipment, to do at home.

Pain Erasure. Prudden, Bonnie. New York: Ballantine Books, 1985.

This book explains Bonnie Prudden's method for pain relief using myotherapy. Her method has been hailed by doctors and patients.

Reflexology

Better Health with Foot Reflexology. Byers, Dwight. St. Petersburg, FL: Ingham Publishing, 1987.

This book is a practical guide that includes an introduction to each anatomical system of the body and step-by-step instructions in applying the tenets of reflexology.

Body Reflexology: Healing at Your Fingertips. Carter, Mildred. West Nyack, NY: Parker Publishing Co., 1986.

The author of several other books on foot and hand reflexology integrates the whole body. Shows safe and easy-to-use methods to relieve pain and discomfort and promote renewed health.

Hand and Foot Reflexology: A Self-Help Guide. Kunz, Kevin and Barbara. New York: Simon and Schuster, 1987.

A comprehensive, hands-on encyclopedia of personal reflexology. Informative, fully illustrated, with step-by-step procedures, including treatment plans for specific ailments from acne to whiplash.

Reflexology for Good Health: Mirror for the Body. Kaye, Anna and Matchan, Don. Hollywood, CA: Wilshire Book Co., 1980.

An approachable guide to reflexology answering the most commonly asked questions including things not to do.

Acupressure and Oriental Body Therapies

Acupressure's Potent Points. Gach, Michael, R. New York: Bantam Books, 1990.

Written in clear, accessible language with photographs and easy-to-follow line drawings, the book shows how to utilize acupressure on others as well as yourself.

Acu-Yoga: The Acupressure Stress Management Book: Developed to Relieve Stress and Tension. Gach, Michael, R. Tokyo & New York: Japan Publications, 1981.

A comprehensive, highly instructive handbook describing the origin, practice, and benefits of acupressure and yoga, with illustrations, diagrams, exercises, and self-help techniques designed to address a variety of health problems.

The Complete Book of Shiatsu Therapy. Namikoshi, Toru. Tokyo & New York: Japan Publications, 1981.

A thorough, scientifically-oriented text and guidebook on shiatsu.

Tsubo: Vital Points for Oriental Therapy. Serizawa, Toru, M. D. Tokyo & New York: Japan Publications, 1992.

A textbook on Tsubo, showing how to locate vital points and apply acupuncture and shiatsu. *Clear and straightforward enough for the layperson, yet contains charts and detailed information useful to medical professionals.*

Therapeutic Touch

Accepting Your Power to Heal: Personal Practice of Therapeutic Touch. Krieger, Dolores. Santa Fe: Bear and Company, 1993.

Dr. Krieger's most recent book, especially developed for use by lay people in the home as well as for professionals in health agencies. It gives in-depth details on the use of Therapeutic Touch in treating over two dozen ailments.

Living the Therapeutic Touch: Healing as Lifestyle. Krieger, Dolores. Wheaton, IL: Quest Books, 1988.

The original book on Therapeutic Touch practice, now in its twenty-seventh edition, has become a classic. This book teaches the reader how to do Therapeutic Touch starting with the simplest beginning steps through the intermediate phase.

Therapeutic Touch: A Practical Guide. McCrae, Janet. New York: Knopf, 1992.

A guide to using graceful sweeping movements of the hands, a few inches from the body, to scan the patient's energy flow, replenish it where necessary, release congestion, remove obstruction, and generally restore order and balance in the diseased system.

Polarity Therapy

A Guide to Polarity Therapy: The Gentle Art of Hands-on Healing. Seidman, Maruti. Boulder, CO: Elan Press, 1991.

An excellent introduction explaining the theory of polarity therapy and basic techniques.

***Polarity Therapy: The Complete and Collected Works.* Vols 1-2.** Stone, Randolph. Sebastopol, CA: CRCS Publications, 1987.

A gold mine of both energy-balancing principles and numerous therapeutic techniques that practitioners of all healing arts can employ.

Your Healing Hands: The Polarity Experience. Gordon, Richard. Santa Cruz, CA: Wingbrow Press, 1978.

A fully illustrated, hands-on approach to learning therapeutic touch and natural healing, specifically polarity balancing.

Cell Therapy

Cell therapy promotes physical regeneration through the injection of healthy cellular material into the body. It is used to stimulate healing, counteract the effects of aging, and treat a variety of degenerative diseases such as arthritis, Parkinson's disease, atherosclerosis, and cancer. Although not approved in the United States, cell therapy is used throughout Europe and in many countries worldwide.

Cell therapy was developed by the late Paul Niehans, M.D., a noted Swiss specialist in the field of gland and organ transplants. He discovered the process in 1931 while performing an emergency operation on a woman whose parathyroid glands had been damaged during thyroid surgery. Dr. Niehans intended to transplant fresh parathyroid glands from a steer calf (an accepted practice at the time), but as there was no time to perform a transplant, he mixed a finely minced portion of the gland with a saline solution and injected it into the patient. Her convulsions stopped and she recovered fully.

Following the success of this first procedure, Dr. Niehans administered cellular injections to thousands of people including Pope Pius XII, the Duke and Duchess of Windsor, Emperor Hirohito, and President Eisenhower.

What Is Cell Therapy?

The broadest definition of cell therapy includes the use of human blood transfusions and bone marrow transplants as well as injections of cellular materials. Cell therapy as it is discussed here refers to the injection of cellular material from organs, fetuses, or embryos of animals to stimulate healing and treat a variety of degenerative diseases.

Several schools of thought exist as to the ideal practice of cell therapy. The various methods include the use of live cells, freeze-dried cells (including whole cells and cell extracts), cells from specific organs, and whole embryo preparations. All of these techniques have been used successfully, with different methods targeting different conditions.

According to cell therapy expert Ted Allen, M.D., from Nassau, the Bahamas, "Initially live cells from organs of freshly killed sheep were used, but the time from the extraction of organs and cells to their subsequent injection was too short to allow for adequate sterility testing.

With live cells there is also the possibility of an immune reaction rejecting the transplant, as often happens with organ transplants."

In 1949, Swiss scientists at Nestlé developed the freeze-drying method of processing coffee. Professor Niehans worked with the Nestlé company to adapt this technique to conserve biological matter without damage. The result was a process in which sterility could be regulated and cell material could be conserved for longer periods of time. In this method, the injected cellular material contains a lesser amount of foreign protein than when an entire organ is transplanted, substantially reducing the rejection risk.

When whole cells are used in this freeze-drying procedure, the cell surface is still present. This surface is antigenic, meaning it may cause an immune response. For this reason, patients who receive freeze-dried whole cells should be warned of the possibility of an allergic reaction, although the likelihood of this occurring is rare.

The process of ultrafiltration (the fine filtering of homogenized whole cells down to cell components called ultrafiltrates) removes the cell surface coat and its antigenic material (a protein or carbohydrate substance, such as a toxin or enzyme) in order to reduce the risk of rejection. The use of freeze-dried cell ultrafiltrates also allows for better quality control and prolonged storage.

Another important aspect of cell therapy is the use of cells taken from embryos. Although once cells from mature animals were used, animal embryo cells are now the preferred choice. They do not induce immune sensitization or rejection because they do not yet bear the surface antigens.

Today most cell therapy employs embryonic tissues. However, in cases involving the parathyroid, adrenal, pituitary and sex glands, adult tissues are used, as these glands are too underdeveloped in the embryos. According to Dr. Allen, mature sheep have proven to be the best donor animals of organ cells as their proteins rarely trigger an allergic reaction in the recipient. More recently, cells from pigs have been found to work as efficiently, according to Peter Stephan, M.D., of the Stephan Clinic in London, England.

HUMAN FETAL CELL TRANSPLANTS

In 1988, former President Reagan placed a ban on any new research involving human fetal tissue. In 1993, President Clinton lifted the ban, enabling scientists to resume work in this field. A study published in the New England Journal of Medicine *in 1992 reported that the transplantation of human fetal cells has been successfully used to treat patients with Parkinson's disease. In the case of Parkinson's, cells that normally produce the neurotransmitter dopamine die off, resulting in a loss of muscle control. When fetal cells from a corresponding area of the brain are injected into the brain of a Parkinson's patient, many of the symptoms, such as tremors and paralysis, have been known to disappear, allowing the patient to lead a normal life. The studies cited marked constant improvement in the patients' motor skills and reported diminished symptoms and signs of Parkinson's as a result of these transplants.[1]*

Fetal cell transplants are also being investigated as a possible therapy for Alzheimer's disease, a chronic mental disorder involving progressive, irreversible loss of intellectual functions including comprehension, memory, and speech. Because fetal tissue is especially adaptive to transplantation, scientists are hopeful that transplanted fetal cells will be able to assume the functions of cells that have been destroyed or damaged.

The Practice of Cell Therapy

There are a variety of methods for employing cell therapy. According to Dr. Allen, "Cells injected into the body find their way to the patient's weak or damaged organ and stimulate the body's healing process. Cells do not actually travel whole, but are broken down to their molecular levels and incorporated in similar structures. This is supported by studies from the Universities of Vienna[2] and Heidelberg,[3] where the movement of cells labeled with dyes or radioactive material was traced after injection. Without fail, kidney cells migrated to the kidney, liver cells to the liver, and so forth."

Dr. Allen employs cell therapy mainly for revitalization purposes. He uses a combination of five different cell types: hypophysis (from the pituitary), liver, connective tissue, male or female gonads, and one which varies based on the needs of the patient. If the patient has problems with a certain organ, then additional cells specific to that organ can be used. Three to five injections are given in one session. For general revitalization purposes, the patient returns for further injections as necessary. This may continue for six months, one year, or even two years.

Dr. Allen believes cell therapy stimulates the immune system, helping it either to prevent disease or to fight it when necessary. In the case of cancer, Dr. Allen feels that cell therapy enhances the overall health of cancer patients and helps them withstand the rigors of chemotherapy and radiation.

"The main benefit of cell therapy is an overall stimulation of the body and its processes," says Tom Smith, M.D., Ph.D., H.M.D., D.Hom. He views cell therapy as an adjunct to other forms of therapy and feels it gives the body a basic support system that allows other therapeutic measures to work more successfully. At Dr. Smith's International Clinic for Biological Regeneration, which has branches in England and the Bahamas, patients are first screened to assess whether cell therapy is an appropriate treatment for them. Following this screening, an initial test injection is given to ensure that the patient will not suffer from an allergic reaction. For patients who exhibit a reaction, especially those with a history of allergies, cell therapy may not be advisable.

Dr. Smith uses injections of an omnigenic (whole embryo) ultrafiltrate. Two to five injections are normally given. This preparation stimulates the connective tissues and muscles, helps to retain fluids in the tissues, and retards aging. Because this ultrafiltrate preparation contains material from all areas of the embryo, it is effective as a total body stimulant. If a patient has problems with a particular area, such as the brain, liver, or kidney, he or she will be given an extract of that organ as well.

STAGES OF THERAPEUTIC EFFECT

According to Ted Allen, M.D., of Nassau, the Bahamas, the therapeutic effect of cell therapy appears in three stages. First, there is the immediate reaction in which the patient experiences increased vitality. For example, when Dr. Allen treated a patient with hepatitis, his blood and liver profile tests nearly returned to normal within thirty-six hours. His symptoms disappeared and follow-up tests confirmed a restored level of health.

In some cases this response is followed by an immune reaction that can cause slight fatigue and last for several weeks. The third stage is the long-term healing phase. Cellular and organ regeneration will take a minimum of four to six months, with the patient's condition continuing to improve over the next few years by way of increased stamina, better blood supply and skin tone, and an overall sense of well-being.

Dr. Stephan developed a form of cell therapy called Therapeutic Immunology, in which cell extracts are administered along with antibodies raised in animals. Therapeutic Immunology is distinguished from traditional cell therapy in that it is a gentler process and has no side effects. "It is more of a vaccination approach to regeneration," Dr. Stephan explains. "Cells of various organs, glands, and other parts of the body are taken from specially raised animals known to be healthy and free of disease. The cells are placed in solution and filtered to remove the unwanted protein elements, and then introduced into a secondary mammal. The injected antigens react with the cells of this mammal and produce antibodies, which appear in the mammal's bloodstream and can be measured. When the antibodies reach the desired level, blood is taken in the same way as it is for vaccines. The serum is then separated and the antibodies are prepared and tested for purity and effectiveness, before being given to the patient to regenerate various parts of the immune system."

"Dr. Niehans noticed that cancer rarely developed in the over one thousand women he treated for menopausal difficulties with ovarian follicular cells taken from sheep. Whereas the international number of registered deaths from cancer averaged 25 percent, the rate for Dr. Niehans' patients was 4 percent."

Strict control is exercised in matching the proper cells with the antibody preparations. In order to reduce patient stress and better enable the patient to tolerate the antibody serum, the preparation is introduced by injection and suppository in low doses over a longer period of time than other forms of cell therapy. Cell extracts containing RNA (ribonucleic acid) are also used to enhance the effects.

Dr. Stephan also uses a technique known as Bio-Nutritional therapy. In this therapy, cells, cell extracts, and antibodies are combined with nutrients and ATP (adenosine triphosphate, a compound involved in the storage and transfer of energy in cells), to promote cellular and tissue regeneration. The mixture is administered either under the tongue or via the nasal or rectal passage. This method of application helps to avoid side effects by allowing the body to absorb only as much as it needs.

Conditions Benefited by Cell Therapy

Although the reason cell therapy promotes healing is not fully understood, its practice has been successful with a number of health conditions.

Early in his practice Dr. Niehans noticed that cancer rarely developed in the over one thousand women he treated for menopausal difficulties with ovarian follicular cells taken from sheep. Whereas the international number of registered deaths from cancer averaged 25 percent, the rate for Dr. Niehans' patients was 4 percent. In the 1960s Dr. Stephan carried out a similar survey of his own patients and found the same 4 percent rate. Although these documented facts do not constitute a scientific study, these results suggest the need for further research.

Dr. Niehans considered cancer to be an immunological problem. He believed that cell injections from cancer-resistant animals could increase resistance to cancer in humans, and even induce regression of cancer cells in certain cases. This theory is gaining support due to several recent research projects that show that RNA from healthy cells injected into cancerous tissues retards cancer growth and reduces malignancy.[4]

Dr. Niehans used cell therapy to stimulate the regeneration of underdeveloped, diseased, and age-damaged organs. He was very successful at treating sexual dysfunction and discovered that sexual vitality could be restored through his therapy. His ultimate aim was "to give more years to life" and to "make all the organs struck by old age capable once more of functioning properly."[5] Dr. Stephan also uses cell therapy to treat male impotence. He has had great success with a combination treatment he developed consisting of erectile tissue and cells from the testicle, prostate, the pituitary gland, diencephalon (the area of the brain that includes the thalamus and hypothalamus), and the neurovascular system. A trial experiment using Dr. Stephan's protocol was conducted on thirty-five hundred people who had volunteered for help with sexual revitalization. The study found a 76 percent success rate among the patients, who ranged from twenty-two to seventy-six years old.

CELL THERAPY AND AIDS

Peter Stephan, M.D., of the Stephan Clinic in London, England, foresees cell therapy becoming more widely used to treat AIDS. "My belief is that the answer to the AIDS problem lies not with a specific vaccine or specific treatment," he says, "but with a therapy that improves the natural function of the total immune system. In cell therapy, this is accomplished by injecting new cells of the spleen, bone marrow, and lymph, together with those of the thymus. The injections improve the efficiency of these cell groups and thus increase the body's own ability to fight infection. This approach applies not only to AIDS but to other viral infections, since viruses have the ability to change form. A healthy immune system is able to adapt to this change by producing a whole range of antibodies to attack any viral form. Maintaining such health lies in the enhancement of the body's natural functions, not in overdosing it with unnatural chemicals."

Dr. Stephan has used cell therapy in the treatment of more than thirty thousand patients. Among the conditions he has treated are arthritis, heart and circulatory problems, menopause, painful menstruation, and infertility and sterility. Dr. Stephan's treatments have also been successful against cystitis, prostrate problems, herpes, lung and bronchial problems, and premature aging. He has also treated children with Down syndrome (a type of mental retardation) using Therapeutic Immunology and Bio-Nutritional therapy, and states that, "While it is not a cure for Down syndrome, it is possible to increase a child's intelligence using this therapy."

Hector E. Solorzano, M.D., D.Sc., Coordinator of the Program for Studies of Alternative Medicines and Professor of Pharmacology at the University of Guadalajara in Mexico, has researched cell therapy as a treatment for cancer, Parkinson's disease, epilepsy, Down syndrome, autoimmune diseases, and certain infant disorders. He tells of a child who underwent an extremely difficult birth. "At eighteen months, he could not hold his head up, nor could he crawl or concentrate on objects around him," says Dr. Solorzano. "Within two weeks of cell therapy treatment, he could hold his head up normally. By three weeks his attention span was normal, and after three months of therapy the child was performing as expected for someone his age."

CAUTION

Cell therapy is not recommended for those with severe kidney disease, liver failure, or acute (short-term) infections and inflammatory diseases. Patients who show an allergic reaction to the test injection should not receive the treatment.

Franz Schmid, M.D., of Aschaffenberg, Germany, reports on extensive studies with cell therapy in a wide range of diseases. In one study, seventy-two patients with arteriosclerosis were treated with a mixture of placenta, liver, and testes. Fifty-eight of them showed marked improvement with a lowering of cholesterol levels and improvement in walking distance.[6] In another study, one year after cell therapy, five of nine patients had improved EKG (electrocardiogram) readings and the remaining four were free of complaints.[7]

"Medical science and better food and hygiene have given us more years to our lives. Cell therapy is much more concerned with giving more life to those years."
—Peter Stephan, M.D.

For skin problems, particularly burns and scars, Dr. Schmid reports of the use of a recently developed topical cream prepared with cell extracts. In one case, a young child with second and third degree burns from a gas explosion showed almost complete healing within nineteen days. Eighteen months later, no scarring was visible. Certain skin problems may require cell therapy to be given intravenously.[8] Hepatitis is another disease successfully treated by cell therapy. Dr. Allen recalls a patient with hepatitis who refused hospitalization. "After about four weeks of conventional treatment at home, little progress was observed. Blood and liver profile tests were done and he was then injected with liver cells. Within thirty-six hours he became almost clinically normal. Fluid buildup in the abdomen and yellowing [of the skin] had disappeared. Repeat blood tests were all within normal limits. Today the patient remains well, with normal blood test values."

The Future of Cell Therapy

Dr. Stephan coined the phrase "body servicing" to explain his approach to medicine, because, according to him, people today service everything but their bodies.

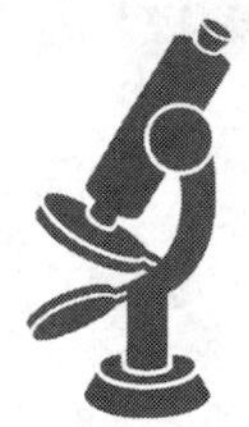

Additional research into cell therapy could provide valuable information on immunological disorders such as AIDS and cancer which, in time, could save many lives.

"We are living longer, but we are wearing out," he says. "Medical science and better food and hygiene have given us more years to our lives. Cell therapy is concerned with giving more life to those years. I feel that the future of this type of therapy has never been more secure, due to all of the recent research and development programs exploring the use of new tissues to repair worn out or damaged tissues in the human body. And obviously it is better to repair an organ than it is to replace it, since introducing new cells in the body is better tolerated than introducing whole new organs."

Cell therapy as a practice can contribute greatly to the servicing of the human body because of its ability to work in accordance with the body's natural system. "The process of the regeneration of the human system must be done within the laws of biological science," Dr. Stephan says. "It is a matter of helping things happen rather than forcing them upon the body."

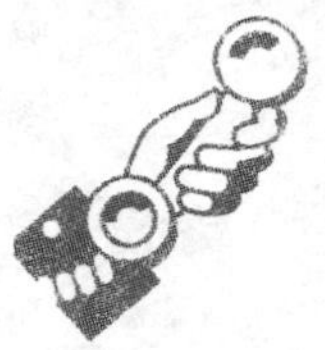

Where to Find Help

For more information on cell therapy, contact an organization below.

ICBR North American Information Office
P.O. Box 509
Florissant, Missouri 63032
(800) 826-5366
(314) 921-3997

International Clinic of Biological Regeneration has offices in England and the Bahamas. They also have an American information office where they can be reached for referrals and other information.

International Society for the Application of Organ Filtrates, Cellular Therapy, and Onco-Biotherapy
Robert Bosch Strasse, 56a
D-6906
Walldorf, Germany
06 2 276-3268
06 2 227-6330 (Fax)

A group of therapists whose aim is to unite worldwide the scientists and general practitioners in this field.

The Stephan Clinic
27 Harley Place, Harley Street
London, England W1N 1HB
071-636-6196
071-255-1626 (Fax)

The Stephan Clinic was founded in 1965 and since then more than thirty thousand patients have been treated. Dr. Stephan and his staff have been in the forefront of research and development of cell therapy and associated techniques.

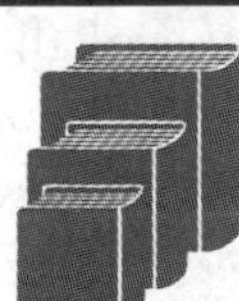

Recommended Reading

Forever Young: A Practical Guide to Youth Extension. Molnar, E. Michael. West Hartford, CT: Witkower Press, 1985. Chapter 11 [illegible] 1991.

An excellent pamphlet describing what cell therapy is, how it works, and what it can treat. To obtain this pamphlet call (800) 826-5366.

Introduction to Cellular Therapy. Niehans, Paul. Savage, MD: Cooper Square Publishers, Inc., 1960.

One of the fathers of cell therapy explains his theory. Though parts of the text are scientific, it is an excellent resource.

Options: The Alternative Cancer Therapy Book. Walters, Richard. New York: Avery Publishing Group, 1992.

A [illegible] and informative guide describing many alternative methods of treating cancer. A very accessible book for all, citing extra reading sources, clinical experiments, and doctors around the world.

Third Opinion. Fink, John M. New York: Avery Publishing Group, 1922.

An international directory to alternative therapy centers for the treatment and prevention of cancer. An excellent resource with an introduction describing guidelines to choose the right therapy.

Chelation Therapy

Chelation therapy is a safe and effective method for drawing toxins and metabolic wastes from the bloodstream. Chelating agents administered intravenously have been proven to increase blood flow and remove arterial plaque. Chelation therapy can help reverse atherosclerosis, can prevent heart attacks and strokes, and is used as an alternative to bypass surgery and angioplasty.

Chelation (key-LAY-shun) comes from the Greek word *chele* meaning "to claw" or "to bind." Chelation therapy is used to rid the body of unnecessary and toxic metals, and is employed by a growing number of physicians to reverse the process of atherosclerosis (hardening of the arteries). The reversal is accomplished in part through the removal of the calcium content of plaque from the artery walls through the injection of chelating agents. By restoring good circulation to all the tissues of the body, chelation therapy can help to avoid bypass surgery, reverse gangrene, alleviate intermittent claudication (cramps) of the legs, and restore memory. Due to its ability to remove toxic metal ions, chelation therapy reduces internal inflammation caused by free radicals (highly reactive destructive molecules), and as a result can ease the discomfort and disability from degenerative diseases such as arthritis, scleroderma (a hardening that occurs in skin and certain organs), and lupus.

"According to current drug safety standards, aspirin is about three and a half times more toxic than EDTA."

Chelation therapy has been used safely on more than five hundred thousand patients in the United States for the past forty years,[1] but EDTA (ethylenediaminetetraacetic acid), the drug used during the infusions, has yet to receive FDA (Food and Drug Administration) approval for anything other than lead and heavy metal toxicity. Still, there are over one thousand physicians who recommend and use chelation therapy for cardiovascular disease and related health problems. Following the treatment protocol set by the American College of Advancement in Medicine and the American Board of Chelation Therapy, FDA-approved studies are currently underway to establish the safety of EDTA.

How Chelation Therapy Is Administered

Chelation therapy is performed on an out-patient basis, is painless, and takes approximately three and a half hours. For optimal results, physicians who use chelation therapy recommend twenty to thirty treatments given at an average rate of one to three per week, with patient evaluations being made at regular intervals.[2]

The patient reclines comfortably and is given an intravenous solution of EDTA with vitamins and minerals. To monitor the patient's progress, James Julian, M.D., of Los Angeles, recommends that the following tests be taken before, during, and after chelation:

- Blood pressure and circulation
- Cholesterol and other blood components
- Pre- and postvascular
- Blood sugar and nutritional
- Kidney and organ function
- Tissue minerals, if indicated

A whole foods, low-fat diet, and appropriate exercise are normally recommended as part of a full treatment program. According to Garry Gordon, M.D., of Tempe, Arizona, a carefully tailored program of vitamin and nutritional supplements should also be part of the treatment, and can include ascorbic acid (vitamin C), heparin, selenium, chromium, copper, zinc, and manganese. Smoking is strongly discouraged, and alcohol should be consumed only in moderation. The cost per treatment can vary, depending in part on the nutritional ingredients the doctor may choose to use.

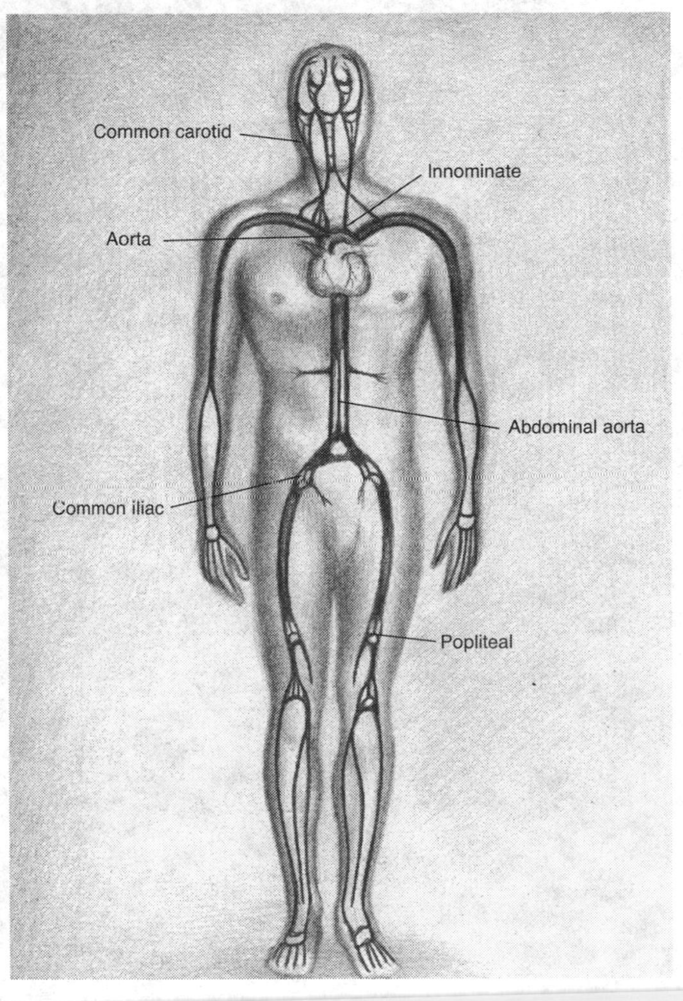

Sites of atherosclerotic lesions in the body.

Conditions Benefited by Chelation Therapy

By 1948 the U.S. Navy had begun using EDTA to safely and successfully treat lead poisoning. At the same time, EDTA was being used to remove calcium from pipes and boilers. Norman Clarke, Sr., M.D., Director of Research at Providence Hospital in Detroit, Michigan, hypothesized that because calcium plaque is a prominent component in atherosclerosis, EDTA would be an effective treatment for heart conditions. His experiments with EDTA chelation treatments for heart patients validated his theory. Patients with angina reported dramatic relief from chest pain. Healing was also reported by patients with gangrene. For many patients, memory, sight, hearing, and sense of smell improved, and most reported increased vigor.[3]

EDTA chelation therapy has since proven to be safe and effective in the treatment and prevention of ailments linked to atherosclerosis such as coronary artery disease (heart attacks), cerebral vascular disease (stroke), peripheral vascular disease (leading to pain in the legs and ultimately gangrene and amputation), as well as arterial blockages from atherosclerosis elsewhere in the body. According to current drug safety standards, aspirin is nearly three and a half times more toxic than EDTA.[4]

Warren Levin, M.D., of New York City, once administered chelation therapy to a psychoanalyst on the staff of a major New York medical center. "He was in his fifties and looked remarkably healthy, except that he was in a wheelchair. He had awakened that morning to discover his lower leg was cold, numb, mottled, and blue, with two black-looking toes. He rushed to his hospital and consulted the chief of vascular surgery, who recommended an immediate amputation above the knee. He asked this world-renowned surgeon about the possibility of using chelation in this situation, and was told, 'Don't bother me with that voodoo.'

"The ailing man decided to get a second opinion. This physician also urged him to have an immediate amputation. When asked about chelation therapy, the second doctor's response was, 'You can try it if you want, but it's a waste of time.'

"Through his own tenacity, the psychoanalyst showed up in my office. We started emergency chelation and after approximately nine treatments—one taken every other day—he was pain free and picking up. After approximately seventeen chelation treatments, he was walking on the leg again. He never had an amputation, and he lived the rest of his life without any further complications."

CHELATION THERAPY VERSUS BYPASS SURGERY AND ANGIOPLASTY

In 1988 nearly 1 million Americans died of cardiovascular disease, making it the number one killer in the United States. Each year nearly three hundred thousand bypass surgeries and two hundred-fifty thousand angioplasties are performed in the United States. Furthermore, nearly twenty thousand deaths occur each year as a result of these procedures.[5]

In 1992, Nortin Hadler, M.D., Professor of Medicine at the University of North Carolina School of Medicine, wrote that none of the two hundred-fifty thousand balloon angioplasties performed the previous year could be justified, and that only 3 to 5 percent of the three hundred thousand coronary artery bypass surgeries done the same year were actually indicated. Yet a cost comparison study prepared for the Great Lakes Association of Clinical Medicine in 1993 estimated that $10 billion was spent in the United States in 1991 on bypass surgery alone.[6] At a symposium of the American Heart Association, Henry McIntosh, M.D., stated that bypass surgery should be limited to patients with crippling angina who do not respond to more conservative treatment.[7]

Chelation therapy offers a viable alternative. In a 1988 study of 2,870 cases, Efrain Olszewer, M.D., and James Carter, M.D., head of nutrition at the Department of Applied Health Science, School of Public Health and Tropical Medicine at Tulane University, documented that EDTA chelation therapy brought about significant improvement in 93.9 percent of patients suffering from ischemic heart disease (coronary artery blockage).[8]

Elmer Cranton, M.D., of Troutdale, Virginia, estimates chelation therapy can help avoid bypass surgery in 85 percent of cases. He points out that during all the time that chelation therapy has been administered according to established protocol, not one serious side effect has been reported.

Anecdotal stories of patient success tend to mean little to a medical researcher like Morton Walker, D.P.M. "But," he writes, "what must an investigative medical journalist do when exposed to story after story of potentially imminent death, blindness, amputation, paralysis, and other problems among people, and upon visiting those people to check their stories, finds them presently free of all signs of their former health problems? About two hundred individuals who were victims of hardening of the arteries are . . . [now] vibrant, productive, youthful looking, vigorous, full of zest, and enthusiastically endorse chelation therapy as the cause of their prolonged good health. I have turned up not a single untruth."[9]

Medical journalists Harold and Arline Brecher, who have written extensively about chelation therapy, note that physicians who use it not only advise it for their patients, but use it for themselves, unlike many of their orthodox colleagues. "We have yet to find a physician who offers chelation to his patients who does not chelate himself, his family, and friends," they report.

Chelation therapy could save billions of dollars each year by preventing unnecessary coronary bypass surgeries, angioplasties, and other expensive procedures related to vascular disorders.

One study documented significant improvement in 99 percent of patients suffering from peripheral vascular disease and blocked arteries of the legs. Twenty-four percent of those patients with cerebrovascular and other degenerative cerebral diseases also showed marked improvement, with an additional 30 percent having good improvement. Overall, nearly 90 percent of all treated patients had marked or good improvement as a result of chelation therapy.[10]

A double-blind study in 1989 revealed that every patient suffering from peripheral vascular disease who was treated with chelation therapy showed a statistically significant improvement after only ten treatments.[11] In another study published in 1989, 88 percent of the patients receiving chelation therapy showed improvement in cerebrovascular blood flow.[12]

Other documented benefits of chelation therapy include:

- Normalization of 50 percent of cardiac arrhythmias[13]
- Improved cerebrovascular arterial occlusion[14]
- Improved memory and concentration when diminished circulation is a cause[15]
- Improved vision (with vascular-related vision difficulties)[16]
- Significantly reduced cancer mortality rates (as a preventive)[17]
- Protection against iron poisoning and iron storage disease[18]
- Detoxification of snake and spider venoms[19]

According to Elmer Cranton, M.D., of Troutdale, Virginia, chelation therapy has a profound effect on overall health. "In my clinical experience there is no doubt that intravenous EDTA chelation therapy to some extent slows the aging process," says Dr. Cranton. "Allergies and chemical sensitivities also seem to improve somewhat due to a better functioning of the immune system. All types of arthritis and muscle and joint aches and pains seem to be more easily controlled after chelation, although it is not a cure. In most cases, the progression of Alzheimer's disease will be slowed, and in some cases the improvement is quite remarkable and the disease does not seem to progress. Macular degeneration, a major cause of visual loss in the elderly, is often improved and almost always arrested or slowed in its progression by chelation therapy."

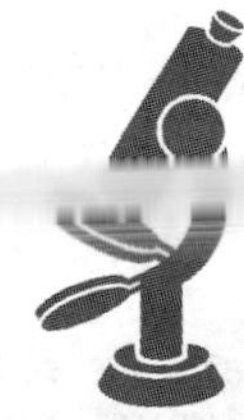

Research is needed to validate the effectiveness of chelation therapy in reversing atherosclerosis and related circulatory conditions. If approved by the FDA as a treatment for atherosclerosis, chelation therapy could save thousands of lives annually.

Oral Chelation

There are a variety of substances that act as oral chelating agents, according to Garry F. Gordon, M.D., of Tempe, Arizona. "Oral chelation is a well-documented, firmly established medical practice," he says. He points out that penicillamine, a drug used to treat heavy metal poisoning, rheumatoid arthritis, and Wilson's disease (a rare metabolic disorder resulting in an excess accumulation of copper in the liver, red blood cells, and the brain), works in a fashion very similar to EDTA. "Some of the benefits derived from penicillamine in the treatment of rheumatoid arthritis are undoubtedly related to the control and removal of excess free radicals. And EDTA itself, when taken orally, provides most of its chelating activities in the body even though only about 5 percent of it is actually absorbed. The chelating effects are less dramatic and slower than when received intravenously, but the oral approach has several major advantages, including convenience, potential long-term continuous health maintenance, and low cost."

CHELATION THERAPY AND CANCER

Beginning in 1958 a lengthy study was conducted in Switzerland on 231 adults who lived near a well-traveled highway and had a higher rate of cancer mortality than other people of the same city who lived in traffic-free areas. The study group also suffered from a higher incidence of nervous disorders, headaches, fatigue, gastrointestinal disorders, depression, and substance abuse. The researchers suggested that their symptoms might be due to a higher level of exposure to lead from automobile exhausts. Then in 1961, 59 patients from this group received ten or more EDTA chelation treatments plus vitamins C and B_1, while the remaining 172 members of the group were untreated and served as control subjects. An eighteen-year follow-up study of the group conducted by Walter Blumer, M.D., of Nestal, Switzerland, revealed that only one of the 59 treated patients died of cancer (1.7 percent) as compared to thirty deaths (17.6 percent) from cancer among the nontreated subjects. This is a 90 percent reduction of mortality from cancer. Dr. Blumer found that death from atherosclerosis was also reduced among the treated patients. His findings were based upon Swiss death certificates and statistical evidence showing that EDTA chelation therapy was the only significant difference between the control group and the treated patients.[20]

Commenting on Dr. Blumer's study, Garry F. Gordon, M.D., of Tempe, Arizona, says, "Anything that reduces your burden of toxic metals, which feeds the fire of free radicals, sufficiently safeguards your immune system so that your body can more efficiently handle early cancers." Dr. Gordon prefers to view chelation therapy in terms of cancer prevention and not as a treatment in itself. "Cancer has been linked to free radical pathology and EDTA chelation removes elements, such as iron, which can accelerate this pathology," he says. "Therefore, chelation treatments can minimize one's risk of developing cancer."

Dr. Gordon also uses many nutritionally based substances as oral chelators, such as garlic, vitamin C, carrageenan, zinc, and certain amino acids like cysteine and methionine. "Cysteine, for instance, is very effective in the treatment of nickel toxicity," he says, "and it seems to also increase glutathione in the body, which in turn helps to control free radicals."

In his patients who use oral chelation formulas, Dr. Gordon has consistently observed a reduction of serum cholesterol by an average of 20 percent or more, which he feels significantly decreases the likelihood of atherosclerosis. "The thousands of patients who visit my clinic each year and follow our recommended oral chelation program have all successfully avoided strokes, and heart attack rates were also greatly diminished," he says. "We've never had more than two heart attacks per year among all of our patients, even among those with a history of severe heart disease. I firmly believe that an oral chelation program can do more for your overall longevity than you can do even with the most prudent lifestyle possible because of the continuous nutritional protection chelation offers against a stressful and polluted world."

Dr. Gordon does not recommend oral chelation as a substitute for intravenous chelation therapy, however. "There is a significant difference in both the rapidity and degree of benefits achieved with intravenous chelation over any currently available oral chelation agents," he says. "And the intravenous approach is clearly the proper choice for patients who have only a few months to get well before facing surgery or worse." But for patients whose conditions are not as drastic, as well as for those who want to optimally safeguard themselves against free radicals and plaque buildup, Dr. Gordon views oral chelation as an effective, noninvasive, inexpensive choice.

EDTA should not be used during pregnancy, severe kidney failure, and hypoparathyroidism (low blood circulation).

How to Find the Right Doctor

Patients interested in chelation therapy should choose a doctor who follows the protocol of the American Board of Chelation Therapy or the American College of Advancement in Medicine (ACAM).

- Prior to chelation, a complete physical examination that includes a heart function test, hair mineral analysis, an electrocardiogram, a stress test, and doppler flow analysis should be conducted. Kidney function must also be checked.
- EDTA dosage should be individualized for each patient according to age, sex, weight, and kidney function, and should be administered slowly over a period of three or more hours.
- Treatments should be administered by well-trained staff members who are readily available to deal with any symptoms that might occur during the process, such as weakness or dizziness from low blood sugar levels.

If a patient decides to have chelation therapy, it should be performed by a doctor with several years experience, who has completed the training conducted by ACAM. If the therapy is administered by a nurse or nonphysician, a qualified physician must be on the premises at all times during the procedure.

"In my clinical experience there is no doubt that intravenous EDTA chelation therapy to some extent slows the aging process."

—Elmer Cranton, M.D.

The Future of Chelation Therapy

Patients interested in chelation therapy should choose a doctor who follows the protocol of the American Board of Chelation Therapy or the American College of Advancement in Medicine.

Because the patent for EDTA has expired, it is unlikely that any pharmaceutical company will invest the money necessary to fund studies for FDA approval of chelation therapy, despite the overwhelming evidence of its effectiveness. Robert Haskell, M.D., writes, "Of all the regimens you can use to help a patient combat degenerative disease and restore health, chelation therapy is the most powerful. It produces the greatest number of benefits to the body—far beyond those of improved blood flow. If you want to get your prescribed nutrition to those parts of the body in which they must work . . . chelation therapy is the way to do it."[21]

Where to Find Help

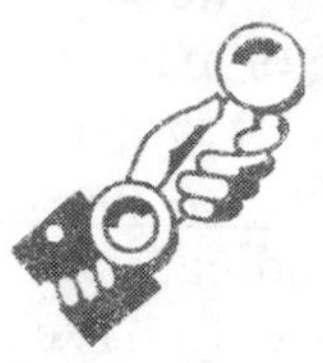

As in all the specialties of medicine, board certification assures that a particular physician has been trained, and his or her knowledge has been demonstrated to be at the highest level. For more information on chelation therapy, contact one of the following organizations:

American Board of Chelation Therapy
70 West Huron Street
Chicago, Illinois 60610
(312) 266-7246

ABCT established the protocol of chelation therapy in 1983, and has been certifying physicians trained in the specialty of chelation therapy. A letter or phone call will provide the names of board-certified physicians.

American College of Advancement in Medicine
P.O. Box 3427
Laguna Hills, CA 92654
(714) 583-7666

ACAM seeks to establish certification and standards of practice for chelation therapy. It provides training and education, and sponsors semiannual conferences for physicians and scientists. It provides referrals and informational material, including a directory listing of all physicians worldwide who have been trained in preventive medicine as well as in the ACAM protocol. The directory is updated monthly. The organization also provides a copy of the ACAM protocol for chelation to the public. For more information, send a stamped, self-addressed envelope.

Great Lakes Association of Clinical Medicine, Inc.
70 West Huron Street
Chicago, Illinois 60610
(312) 266-7246

Members of this association are M.D.'s and D.O.'s who practice preventive and nutritional medicine and offer chelation therapy. This association presents a biannual workshop in chelation therapy that eventually leads to certification by the ABCT.

The Rheumatoid Disease Foundation
5106 Old Harding Road
Franklin, Tennessee 37064
(615) 646-1030

This nonprofit, charitable organization has a listing of physicians who perform chelation therapy. Send a legal size, stamped, self-addressed envelope, along with a donation, when requesting information.

Recommended Reading

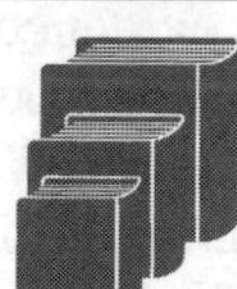

Bypassing Bypass. Cranton, Elmer. Troutdale, VA: Hampton Roads, 1990.

Dr. Cranton's book discusses metals, free radicals, and cross linking in relation to chelation therapy. His work on preventive medicine can enhance the benefits of surgery, as well as prevent surgery.

Chelation Extends Life. Julian, James, M.D. Hollywood, CA: Wellness Press, 1982.

This book shows you how to prevent and/or reverse arteriosclerosis. All medical terms are explained in the glossary at the beginning of the book before you meet them in the text.

The Chelation Way. Walker, Morten, D.P.M. Garden City Park, NY: Avery Publishing Group, Inc., 1990.

A complete how-to book on chelation, including over-the-counter chelation agents, where to find them, and how to use them.

40-Something Forever. Brecher, Harold, and Arline. N.Y.: Healthsavers Press, 1992.

A consumer's guide to chelation and a healthy heart.

The Healing Powers of Chelation Therapy. Trowbridge, John, P., M.D., and Walker, Morten, D.P.M. Stamford, CT: New Way of Life, Inc., 1992.

A primer for the layperson on IV chelation therapy.

The Scientific Basis of EDTA Chelation Therapy. Halstead, Bruce. Colton, CA: Golden Quill Publishers, Inc., 1979.

Provides the scientific basis of chelation therapy for the more technically oriented reader. This book includes detailed illustrations.

A Textbook on EDTA Chelation Therapy, Special Issue of Journal of Advancement in Medicine, Volume 2, Numbers 1 & 2. Cranton, Elmer, Ed. New York: Human Sciences Press, Inc., Spring/Summer, 1989.

This text is designed to provide pertinent clinical data and guidance on how to safely administer the therapy for professionals.

"I believe that you can, by taking some simple and inexpensive measures, extend your life and your years of well-being. My most important recommendation is that you take vitamins every day in optimum amounts, to supplement the vitamins you receive in your food."

—Linus Pauling, Ph.D., Two-time Nobel Prize Laureate

Chiropractic

Through adjustments of the spine and joints, chiropractors can influence the body's nervous system and natural defense mechanisms in order to alleviate pain and improve general health. Because of its effectiveness in treating back problems, headaches, and other injuries and traumas, chiropractic has become the second largest primary health care field in the world.

Chiropractic champions the idea of a holistic approach to health and illness, recognizing the body's inherent ability to heal itself during times of physical injury or mental and environmental stress.

Each year more than 15 million people turn to chiropractic physicians for a natural, drug-free approach to the treatment of pain, backaches, trauma, injuries, and certain internal disorders of the body. Since its formal introduction in 1895, chiropractic has gained worldwide acceptance, despite years of controversy within the medical community.

How Chiropractic Works

Chiropractic is concerned with the relationship of the spinal column and the musculoskeletal structures of the body to the nervous system. "The nervous system holds the key to the body's incredible potential to heal itself," explains Sir Jay Holder, M.D., D.C., Ph.D., of Miami, Florida, "because it coordinates and controls the functions of all the other systems of the body."

The reason that the proper alignment of the spinal column is essential for optimum health is because the spinal column acts as a "switchboard" for the nervous system, according to Donald M. Epstein, D.C., of Boulder, Colorado. When there is nerve interference caused by misalignments in the spine, known as subluxations, pain can occur and the body's defenses can be diminished. By adjusting the spinal joints to remove subluxations, normal nerve function can be restored.

The spinal column, or backbone, is made up of twenty-four bones called vertebrae that surround and protect the spinal cord. Between each vertebra, pairs of spinal nerves exit and extend to every part of the body, including muscles, bones, organs, and glands.

The nervous system itself is comprised of three overlapping systems:

- The central nervous system, which includes the brain and spinal cord

- The autonomic nervous system, which controls involuntary functions such as heart rate, digestion, and glandular function
- The peripheral nervous system, which connects the central nervous system to all the body tissues and voluntary muscles

Health relies upon the balance and equilibrium of these three interrelated nerve systems, which can be easily disrupted by spinal injury, malalignment, stress, or illness. When vertebrae get out of alignment, pressure is placed on the nerves in that area. As a result, the nerves cannot carry out their proper function and this can lead to dysfunction, disharmony, and eventually disease.

"The spine as a whole operates as a functional unit," says Don Davis, D.C., of Hayward, California. "Each vertebra can affect its neighbor and one portion of the spine may affect or damage other areas of the body." For instance, a lower back problem may force a person to bend forward, which can interfere with the movement of the ribs and restrict the functioning of the lungs. It may also cause the neck muscles to contract which, in some cases, could lead to muscle spasms, headaches, strained vision, or balance and coordination problems.

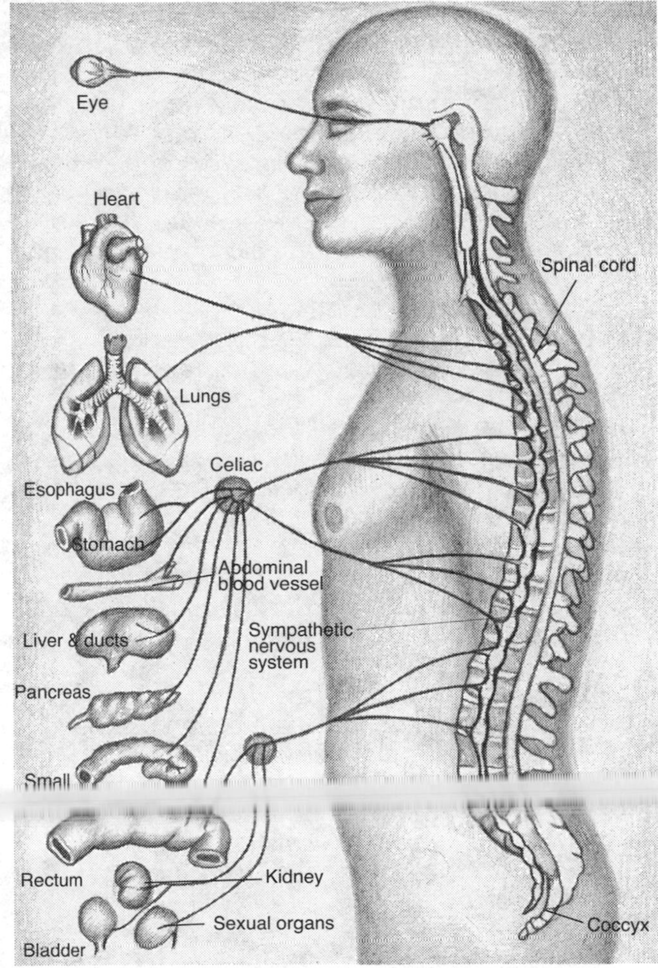

The spinal vertebrae and nerves.

Subluxations of the spinal vertebrae can also affect the body in less obvious ways. A subluxation can have a direct effect on an organ's function when it impedes the proper nerve flow to that organ. When the vertebrae are properly aligned, the spine remains mobile, allowing the electrical impulses from the brain to travel freely along the spinal cord to the organs, thus maintaining healthy function. However, when subluxations occur, they interrupt the normal flow in the nerve structures which, in turn, affects the normal functioning of the organ.

Robert Blaich, D.C., a chiropractic physician from Los Angeles, treated a woman with a long history of severe, almost monthly, bladder infections. The woman had already been through years of medical diagnosis but had yet to be treated successfully. In addition to her chronic infections, the woman also experienced severe bladder pain if she were under any stress at all, which indicated to Dr. Blaich a direct link to the nervous system.

"By identifying the subluxations of the lower vertebrae that were irritating the nerves to the bladder, and by correcting those subluxations, we were able to reduce the irritation to the bladder," states Dr. Blaich. "After only four treatments she got over the infections and had no more recurrences of either the infections or the pain."

The Benefits of Chiropractic Adjustments

Early chiropractors believed that subluxations were the cause of all disease. Today the profession understands much more clearly the multifactorial nature of health and illness. Yet, while subluxations may not be the sole cause of a given disease, they are still a major predisposing factor to it because they prevent the nervous system from working optimally to help keep the body healthy. By correcting vertebral subluxations, the chiropractic adjustment can help maintain the overall health of the nervous system and the body's organs.

The chiropractic adjustment is also helpful in preventing everyday wear and tear on joints and ligaments by maintaining the proper positioning of the joints. It can also help decrease accumulation of scar formation after serious injury, thus preventing later weakness or stiffness of the affected joints.

One of the most common complaints from patients seeking chiropractic care is low back pain. In a two-year study completed in 1990 by Britain's Medical Research Council, chiropractic treatment was found more effective than hospital outpatient care for low back pain. Years later, those patients treated with chiropractic care continued to suffer less pain than those treated by medical doctors.[1] Studies conducted by the Florida Department of Labor and the Rand Corporation in Los Angeles came to similar conclusions.[2] Furthermore, according to records from the 1986 Worker's Compensation Fund, the average medical patient was paid ten times more compensation than the average chiropractic patient for the treatment of low back pain. Even though the chiropractic patient tends to pay a little more for individual treatments than the medical patient, the medical costs were more extreme due to the fact that patients receiving medical care required more treatments.[3]

Along with these landmark studies, there is also a general shift of attitude within the medical community that supports chiropractic's new role and acknowledges the vital importance of the nervous system in relation to the normal functioning and relative health of the body.

According to Chester Wilk, D.C., of Chicago, author of several books on the subject, the following ailments have responded well to

HISTORY OF CHIROPRACTIC

Spinal adjustment has been practiced in every civilization, from the early Egyptians forward. In 1895 Daniel David Palmer, a longtime student of physiology and anatomy, founded the modern-day system and theory of chiropractic. Palmer had encountered a janitor who had been deaf for seventeen years, following an injury to his upper spine. While examining the janitor's spine, Palmer found a misaligned vertebra that corresponded to the spot the man had injured just prior to losing his hearing. By administering a specific thrust or adjustment to the vertebra, Palmer restored the janitor's hearing.

Fundamental to David Palmer's philosophy of health is the idea that all living beings are endowed with what he termed "innate intelligence." Palmer believed that this intelligence regulates all the vital functions of the body as it flows through the central nervous system.[4] Because of this belief, Palmer felt that the primary task of the chiropractor was not to treat conditions but to remove nerve interference caused by subluxations so that the innate intelligence could carry out its role of maintaining the body's health and equilibrium without obstruction.

In contrast to the growing popularity of medication and surgical intervention, Palmer's approach appealed to patients who had faith in natural methods of healing. Chiropractic, he said, embraces "the science of life, the knowledge of how organisms act in health and disease, and also the art of adjusting the neuroskeleton."

chiropractic care: respiratory conditions, gastrointestinal disorders, sinusitis (inflammation of a sinus), bronchial asthma, heart trouble, high blood pressure, and even the common cold.[5]

Dr. Davis recounts how a woman came to him suffering from shortness of breath, heart palpitations, fatigue, depression, and sharp pains radiating down her arm. These symptoms had begun three months before when she had felt a sharp twinge in her upper back and neck while putting away some sweaters on a high closet shelf. Prior to going to Dr. Davis, the woman had gone to an emergency hospital because she thought she might be having a heart attack, only to be released the next day with a clean bill of health and the suggestion that she relax.

Dr. Davis ascertained that her problems were not related to her heart, as spinal palpation revealed several subluxations of the vertebrae in her upper spine along with a compensating disrelationship in her neck vertebrae, which was forcing her upper back to bend forward in a humplike fashion. He diagnosed her condition as a common injury called cervical or thoracic angina, which can occur when lifting over the head or after suffering trauma to the upper back and neck. By using chiropractic adjustment, muscle stimulation, ultrasound, and hot packs, Dr. Davis was able to reverse the woman's symptoms after three visits and completely eliminate her pain after the fourth.

Patients visiting chiropractic physicians often discover that the underlying causes of their illnesses are not what they expected them to be. A man who had been experiencing extreme pain after ejaculation for a number of years came to Dr. Blaich. The man assumed that the problem stemmed from his vasectomy. The medical doctors he had seen hadn't been able to come up with any other conclusion. After a series of tests, Dr. Blaich was able to determine that the man's condition was actually caused by a misalignment in his lower back, which was affecting his prostate, and had nothing to do with his vasectomy. In a matter of three or four treatments with Dr. Blaich, the man's discomfort disappeared completely.

In a recent case published in the *Journal of Manipulative and Physiological Therapeutics*, a man whose speech was impaired due to a spastic constriction of his vocal chords, sought help from two university hospitals. When nothing could be found, he was prescribed psychiatric therapy. The man visited a chiropractor instead, who diagnosed a subluxation in the upper spine. His speech began to return after the second adjustment, and by the fifth adjustment, he was completely free of any speech impediments. When he became hoarse several months later, additional adjustments cleared up the problem, which never returned.[6]

Chiropractic has also been shown to be successful in treating various disturbances of the body, including peripheral joint injuries (hands, knees, elbows, hips, shoulders), sprains, arthritis, bursitis, menstrual difficulties, plus a wide range of emotional problems, from mild depression to schizophrenia. Evidence also shows that chiropractic adjustment combined with proper nutrition can improve, and in some cases reverse, osteoarthritis.[7]

When to See a Chiropractor

Subluxations rarely take care of themselves and, according to Dr. Blaich, most people have subluxations that are causing problems they aren't even aware of. "When someone takes a fall and ends up with a misalignment of the lower spine, typically he or she will just ignore it after a few days, when the pain has gone away," says Dr. Blaich. "Then the person finds out years later that the hip has been deteriorating more rapidly than it should have been."

Dr. Blaich laments that people often pay more attention to the maintenance of their cars than they do to the care of their bodies. "People can see the premature wear and tear on their car's tires that occurs if the wheels are misaligned, yet the same holds true for the human body if the spine is misaligned." A chiropractic examination can quickly show people where these subluxations are, and a chiropractic physician teaches how and when to recognize the warning signs that may eventually lead to serious health problems.

"It is essential for a person to have the spine aligned on a regular basis," contends Dr. Holder, "just as the person would go to a dentist to have his or her teeth cleaned to prevent disease. This keeps the spine free from subluxation and is the best preventative measure the person can take against disease." According to Dr. Holder, subluxations can be caused by five factors: physical, which includes trauma; mental, which includes stress; genetic, which includes genetic predisposition; chemical, which includes imbalance or toxicity; and thermal, which includes extreme changes in temperature.

Dr. Holder advocates that a person, on average, see a chiropractor "every month to a month and a half, though it really depends on how long an individual can hold the adjustment." Certain cases, adds to Dr. Holder, require more attention, such as alcohol and drug addiction, recurring injuries due to sports and work, and pregnancy. "If a woman is pregnant her needs are increased, because the nervous system of a woman directs the creation of the fetus and the embryo to begin with," says Dr. Holder. "When a woman receives adjustments during her pregnancy, there is also better delivery, less back pain, healthier children, and less chance of a miscarriage."

YOUR FIRST VISIT TO A CHIROPRACTOR

A typical first visit with a chiropractor begins with a discussion of your history—familial traits, dietary habits, work record, and previous health care. The chiropractic physician pays particular attention to the history of your current complaint and symptoms, along with your individual concerns. A thorough physical exam is then conducted, followed by palpation and analysis of the spine to determine any muscle imbalances and subluxations. Depending upon what is found, and the nature of your complaint, the doctor might feel that x-rays are needed. Following that, he or she explains the problem to you, and then proposes a treatment that will include a series of chiropractic adjustments.

Specific attention is also given to posture, work habits, and, if your complaint is an injury, the positioning of your body when the injury occurred. Examinations are oriented toward the problem at hand, and are focused on the various spinal and muscular factors concerning the injury or complaint, as well as your general state of alignment. However, the chiropractor also helps you improve body motion and coordination as part of an overall approach to reducing physical disability and/or disease. For the chiropractic physician, the proper function of the body is just as important as issues concerning pain. If necessary, a chiropractor may refer to an internist or neurologist for further diagnostic studies.

Dr. Holder's assertions are echoed by Terry A. Rondberg, D.C., President of the World Chiropractic Alliance. "By keeping the body as subluxation-free as possible through chiropractic adjustments and living a sensible, wellness-oriented lifestyle, we can significantly enhance the body's natural restorative powers," he says.

Types of Chiropractic Treatment

The primary feature of chiropractic treatment is the chiropractic adjustment. During an examination, if localized areas of dysfunction are apparent, treatment is begun specifically to increase spinal motion. The chiropractic physician may use a combination of touch (palpation), active motion (having the patient bend or stretch in different ways), and passive movement (in which the doctor assists the patient) to initiate a specific adjustment.

One type of adjustment is a maneuver in which the joint is gently and precisely stretched to just beyond its normal range of motion. An audible, painless click is often heard, which, according to Dr. Davis, is explained by the release of gases from the joint fluid. The patient will usually notice an increased range of movement, and any soreness should rapidly disappear.

Some chiropractors prefer to use "nonforce" techniques, applying gentle touch along the spine, skull, and pelvis. No forceful adjustment is used, and no "popping" sounds are heard when the vertebral subluxations are corrected.

Another option is the use of a hand held instrument called an Activator™, a small instrument with a rubber tip used to gently and painlessly move the vertebrae.

Still another method is applied kinesiology, which deals not only with the placement of bones, but with the muscles that hold them in position. Chiropractors employing applied kinesiology use special techniques to help balance opposing muscles attached to a misaligned bone. Their approach restores normal muscle function, in order to allow the adjustments to be more effective.

Network chiropractic is another recent development in the field of chiropractic. It was developed by Dr. Epstein, who observed from clinical experience that not all subluxations of the spine are the same. Network chiropractic combines a variety of chiropractic techniques to enable the practitioner to adjust subluxations with the precise amount and type of force suggested by clinical findings. "This is different from attempting to match the vertebra being adjusted to a specific technique," Dr. Epstein explains. "The difference lies in the sequence of the adjustments and the 'networking' of the various methods."

Just as there are several types of adjustments, there are also several types of chiropractic physicians. Though they are usually split into two groups, those who combine chiropractic with other modalities (mixers) and those who deal only with locating and removing subluxations (straight chiropractors), there are as many variations within the two groups as can be found within any medical profession.

According to Dr. Blaich, a mixer chiropractor uses a variety of adjunctive natural health care therapies (most commonly heat, cold, ultrasound, electrical stimulation, massage, exercise, and nutrition) in support of their adjustment therapy. Other mixers have nutritionally-based practices to holistically treat symptoms, and many of them often counsel on lifestyle choices to encourage wellness and the prevention of illness.

On the other hand, a straight chiropractor focuses on analyzing the spine for subluxations that impede the normal function of the nervous system, as opposed to diagnosing conditions and symptoms. "Their premise being," notes Dr. Blaich, "that if they can do that, the conditions themselves will disappear through the natural recuperative properties of the body."

Chiropractic and Addiction

Dr. Holder, working with the University of Miami School of Medicine and the Florida Chiropractic Society, is currently conducting the first large-scale human population study to prove the effectiveness of the chiropractic adjustment in dealing with chemical addiction. Dr. Holder, the first American recipient of the Albert Schweitzer Prize in Medicine, has already seen dramatic preliminary results from the triple-blind study showing that a person receiving chiropractic care is ten times more likely to complete a drug program. "This equates to about a 97 percent retention rate."

"The American College of Addictionology and Compulsive Disorders in Miami has chosen chiropractic as the profession of choice in training for board certification in addictionology."

Retention rate, or how long a person stays in a treatment program, is extremely important, Dr. Holder explains. "The longer a drug addict is in a treatment center, the better the end results will be, and the more likely the person will be successful staying drug-free the rest of his or her life.

"By removing subluxations that interfere with the normal functioning of the nervous system, a person in a drug treatment center is more likely to complete his or her term of stay because the person now can meet the needs of all the other modalities that are offered as treatment," continues Dr. Holder. "We have less people with drug detox or withdrawal symptoms. Their physical complaints are almost eliminated and they can now concentrate on dealing with their addiction."

The American College of Addictionology and Compulsive Disorders (ACACD) in Miami, Florida, has chosen chiropractic as the profession of choice in training for board certification in addictionology. "The ACACD targeted the chiropractic community because chiropractic is a drugless approach," states Dr. Holder. "People that are chemically dependant must stay away from mood-altering substances their entire lives. What type of primary care physician is going to be best able to meet the needs of the recovery community? Obviously someone who isn't going to use mood-altering substances."

Life Chiropractic College in Marietta, Georgia, has also started the first program to deal with chemical dependency in the professional training of chiropractic physicians, a training that doesn't yet exist in medical schools, according to Dr. Holder.

"It's very exciting," says Dr. Holder. "One day, hopefully, you'll have sixty-five thousand chiropractors trained to deal with the problem of addiction. This is a major chance for chiropractic to step forward and play a leading role in meeting one of the most serious problems facing our country."

The Future of Chiropractic

Chiropractic now enjoys wide acceptance by the medical community, with large increases in patient numbers. More and more chiropractors are on staff at hospitals, appointed to the workers' compensation medical examination boards, and commissioned to the armed forces as health care providers. Chiropractors are now used for expert testimony in the legal arena, and are often part of the physician team in sports medicine. The communication between chiropractic and medical physicians has greatly improved as well, and it is likely that these trends will continue to blossom in America and abroad.

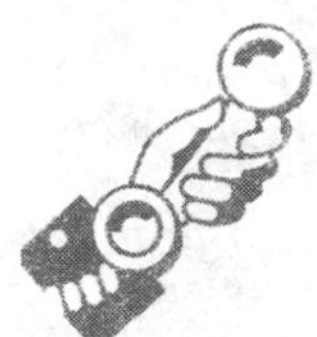

Where to Find Help

For more information on chiropractic and for referrals to chiropractic physicians in your area, contact one of the following organizations:

American Chiropractic Association
1701 Clarendon Boulevard
Arlington, Virginia 22209
(703) 276-8800

A major source for chiropractic information. Monthly publication and newsletter. Clinical councils with specialization in sports injuries and physical fitness, mental health, neurology, diagnosis and internal disorders, nutrition, [illegible] diagnostic imaging, and occupational health.

International Chiropractors Association
1110 North Glebe Road
Suite 1000
Arlington, Virginia 22201
(703) 528-5000

The original chiropractic association founded by B. J. Palmer, the son of the founder of chiropractic, Daniel David Palmer. Programs and services to meet the needs of chiropractors, patients, students, and the public. Concerned with legislation, health care policy, public relations, continuing education, skills development, publications, and interprofessional relations.

World Chiropractic Alliance
2950 N. Dobson Road, Suite 1
Chandler, Arizona 85224
(800) 347-1011

An international association of chiropractors with the purpose of promoting and advancing the profession. Offers guidance and assistance to [illegible] emphasis on vertebral subluxation correction. Provides public education and information. Publishes two newspapers for professionals and provides referrals for chiropractors nationwide.

Association for Network Chiropractic Spinal Analysis
P.O. Box 7682
Longmont, Colorado 80501
(303) 678-8086

Trains chiropractors in the art of network chiropractic. Focuses on the release of subluxations. Offers referrals and support through workshops, seminars, journals, newsletters, and other means.

International College of Applied Kinesiology
P.O. Box 905
Lawrence, Kansas 66044-0905
(913) 542-1801

Referral service for those seeking an applied kinesiologist. Public newsletter available upon request. Supplies written information on various aspects of health and nutrition.

The American College of Addictionology and Compulsive Disorders
5990 Bird Road
Miami, Florida 33155
(305) 661-3474

Trains and board certifies chiropractors as addictionologists. Also provides referrals of chiropractors certified as addiction specialists worldwide.

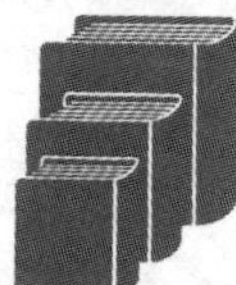

Recommended Reading

Chiropractic Speaks Out. Wilk, Chester. Chicago: Wilk Publishing Co., 1975.

A clear, concise book for both patients and doctors. To order send $2.50 to Dr. Chester Wilk, 5130 West Belmont, Chicago, Illinois 60641.

The Chiropractor's Adjuster. Palmer, Daniel David. Davenport, IA: Palmer College Press, 1992.

An excellent book written by one of the fathers of chiropractic medicine. It discusses the science, art, and philosophy of chiropractic.

Dynamic Chiropractic Today: The Complete and Authoritative Guide to this Major Therapy. Coplan-Griffiths, Michael. San Francisco, CA: Harper Collins, 1991.

An authoritative test that combines descriptions of chiropractic treatments, a history and philosophy, plus practice of this field of medicine.

Today's Health Alternative. Martin, Raquel. Tehachapi, CA: America West Publishers, 1992.

An easy-to-read overview with a short history of chiropractic medicine plus many anecdotes on emotional disorders, response of the immune system, insurance coverage, and professional training and techniques.

Colon Therapy

A healthy colon is essential for the absorption of vital nutrients and the natural elimination of bodily waste and toxins. Colon therapy promotes healthy colon function and can ease a range of problems from headache and backache to arthritis and hypertension.

The colon, along with the skin, kidneys, and lungs, is a major organ for eliminating bodily waste. The healthy function of the colon is essential for good digestion and the proper absorption of nutrients. If bowel movements are not consistent, waste products and toxins are not eliminated in a regular manner, and health can be compromised. Colon therapy uses a series of colonic water flushes to clean and detoxify the lower intestine and aid in the reconstitution of intestinal flora.

According to Drew Collins, N.D., of Prescott Valley, Arizona, "The therapeutic goals of colon therapy are to balance body chemistry, eliminate waste, and restore proper tissue and organ function." Ideally, says Dr. Collins, colon therapy also involves integration of appropriate diagnostic and therapeutic procedures. These include, along with the irrigation of the colon, an analysis of fecal structure and chemistry, an evaluation of environmental, immunological, and psychosomatic influences, and, often, a recommended program of exercise.

> *"The therapeutic goals of colon therapy are to balance body chemistry, eliminate waste, and restore proper tissue and organ function."*
> —Drew Collins, N.D.

The Colon's Role in Health and Disease

The colon (large intestine, rectum, and anus) is a key component of the gastrointestinal (GI) system, the largest system in the body. The length of the gastrointestinal tract is between twenty-eight and thirty feet, with a surface area of nearly six thousand square feet.

The proper functioning of the colon is essential to overall health. When the colon is unable to function efficiently, an accumulation of toxins can build up in the lymph, bloodstream, and intestines. Its proper function is dependent on:

- **A whole foods diet:** Especially recommended are such high-fiber foods as grains, legumes, vegetables, and fruit.
- **A balance of favorable bacteria:** A healthy GI tract contains nearly sixty varieties of bacteria or microflora which aid digestion,

promote the manufacturing of vital nutrients, help to maintain proper pH (acid-base) balance, and keep harmful bacteria in check.

See Constipation, Gastrointestinal Disorders.

- **Healthy colonic mucosa:** The mucosa, or surface cell layer lining the intestines, allows for the passage of nutrients into the bloodstream, secretes hormones and lubricants, and prevents the absorption of toxins.
- **Proper muscle tone:** Approximately fifteen contractive movements occur in the colon per minute. Known as peristalsis, this action moves food through the intestinal tract and helps to maximize absorption of valuable liquid and nutrients, while eliminating the stool.
- **Timely evacuation of waste:** Regular bowel movement and elimination prevents the buildup of toxic substances that result from putrefaction and excessive fermentation. According to Joseph Vargas, Ph.D., founder and Director of the Wholistic Health Center in Houston, Texas, "Bowel movements should be thorough and frequent, two or three daily, to prevent toxic residues and by-products from forming or remaining in the body."

Bowel Toxemia

Dr. Collins states, "When the colon becomes burdened with an accumulation of waste material—impacted feces, bacteria, fungi, viruses, parasites, and dead cellular material—the result is termed 'bowel toxemia'. This condition causes inflammation and swelling of the bowel surface, and can lead to a host of other health problems. Normal absorption of nutrients, secretory functions, and normal muscular function of the colon are disrupted. Irregular and inefficient bowel movement is the result, further suppressing recovery and encouraging other problems."

Bowel toxemia and improper digestion can cause a buildup in the intestines of pathological bacteria, viruses, and fermented and putrefactive gases that become dangerous to the body and can lead to other illnesses.

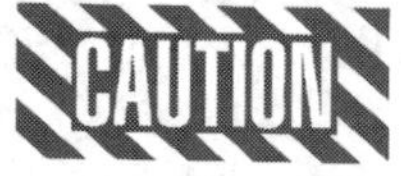

There are certain contraindications for colon therapy, including ulcerative colitis, diverticulitis, Crohn's disease (in the acute inflammatory state), severe hemorrhoids, and tumors of the large intestine or rectum. Patients in a weakened state should avoid colon therapy treatment without direct medical supervision.

Leaky Gut Syndrome

When toxic matter and undigested food, collected in the intestines as a result of bowel toxemia, are absorbed from the bowels into the bloodstream, the result is a recognized medical condition known as "leaky gut syndrome."

The undigested food molecules act as antigens, foreign substances that provoke an immune reaction. Many of these antigens are similar in structure to normal body components, and the antibodies produced to fight them can destroy healthy tissues. Recent studies suggest this immune reaction contributes to, or may cause, rheumatoid arthritis and other degenerative diseases.[1]

Bacteria and their toxic by-products can also be absorbed from the bowels into the bloodstream. A deficiency of secretory IgA, an antibody in the colon that binds food and bacterial antigens, can cause an influx of antigens from the bowels into the bloodstream. These antigens can induce autoimmune diseases such as thyroid disease, myasthenia gravis (a disease characterized by great muscular weakness), and some forms of meningitis, according to Patrick Donovan, N.D.[2]

Toxins that enter the bloodstream from the colon also burden the liver, circulatory system, lymphatic system, and excretory organs such as the lungs and kidneys. Because the liver plays such a vital role in clearing the blood of toxins, any impairment of liver function may aggravate the damage already done by bowel toxemia. "Foreign chemicals in the body, whether produced from ingestion or chemical interaction, chemical breakdown, or putrefaction of foodstuff in the fermentive processes, can alter RNA (ribonucleic acid) and DNA (deoxyribonucleic acid)," says Dr. Vargas. "RNA and DNA contain the blueprint for cellular manufacturing and, if tampered with, abnormal cell reproduction can occur. Many scientists believe this provokes cancer and other autoimmune diseases. All these factors make a properly functioning colon imperative to the maintenance of good health."

HISTORY OF COLON THERAPY

As a treatment for disease, colon therapy was recorded in the earliest known medical documents.[3] Eighty years ago, natural health pioneer John Harvey Kellogg, M.D., of Battle Creek, Michigan, used colon therapy to avoid surgery in all but twenty of forty thousand of his patients afflicted with gastrointestinal disease.[4]

The popularity of colon therapy reached its zenith in the United States in the 1920s and 1930s. At that time, colonic irrigation machines were a common sight in hospitals and physicians' offices. Although interest declined with the advent of pharmaceutical and surgical treatments, colon therapy is once more gaining in popularity and is now commonly used by alternative health practitioners.

A Typical Colon Therapy Session

In a typical session, a trained colon therapist gently guides an applicator, or speculum, into the anus. Filtered water, and occasionally herbs or oxygen (as prescribed by a physician), are gradually introduced into and released from the colon in order to remove fecal material and gas buildup. Colon therapy helps to dislodge fecal material trapped in the pockets and folds of the colon. In this way, conditions that favor normal flora are restored.

The colon.

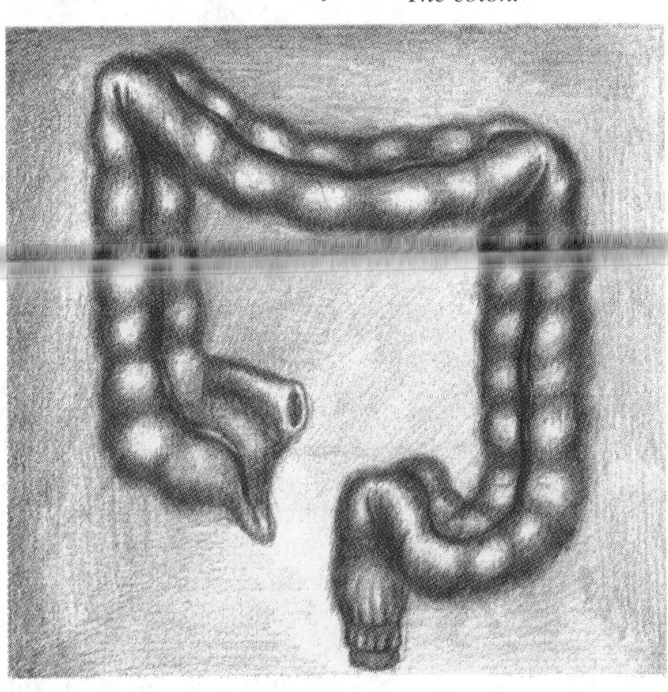

A single session lasts from thirty to forty-five minutes and uses two to six liters of water. Colonic irrigation cleans the entire five feet of the colon, unlike an enema which cleanses only the sigmoid colon, the lower eight to twelve inches of the bowel.

It is advisable to eat and drink lightly prior to colon therapy. An enema beforehand will empty the rectum and increase the efficiency of the colon therapy. After colon therapy, gentle, nourishing food should be taken, such as vegetable soups and broths and fruit and vegetable juices.

One colon therapy session may not be enough to produce major benefits. It may be necessary to have several if you have long-standing complaints or a serious problem with constipation.

Dr. Collins points out that very often toxic residues are released into both the bloodstream and the lumen (inside of the bowel) during colon therapy. Although colonic irrigation is usually a soothing and refreshing experience, a release of these toxins into the bloodstream can bring about a temporary "healing crisis."

There are certain contraindications for colon therapy, including ulcerative colitis (ulceration of the colon lining), diverticulitis (inflammation of a sac or pouch in the intestinal tract causing stagnation of feces), Crohn's disease (in the acute inflammatory state), severe hemorrhoids (spasms in the muscles surrounding the prostate), and tumors of the large intestine or rectum. Patients in a weakened state should avoid colon therapy treatment, without direct medical supervision.

Conditions Benefited by Colon Therapy

"Colon therapy releases toxins, cleanses the blood, stimulates the immune system, and aids in restoring the pH balance in the body," says Connie Allred, President of the American Colon Therapy Association. Colon therapy can help relieve a wide range of symptoms related to colon dysfunction, including:

- Backache
- Headache
- Bad breath
- Coated tongue
- Gas
- Bloating
- Indigestion
- Constipation
- Sinus and/or lung congestion
- Skin problems
- Loss of concentration
- Fatigue

Colon therapy also helps to reestablish regular bowel movements by restoring muscle tone and normal peristalsis. According to Dr. Collins, as the squeezing action of peristalsis moves the blood and lymph in the region of the colon, the cells lining the colon excrete toxins and waste products into both the colon and bloodstream for elimination.

Peristalsis also stimulates the liver to produce more bile. Increased bile production aids the absorption of lipids (liquid fats) and fat-soluble vitamins, aids in the removal of immune complexes (substances formed when antibodies attach to antigens), and assists in the breakdown of cholesterol. Increased bile production also induces proper blood clotting and helps prevent the production of gallstones.

Colon therapy is most effective when used in conjunction with special exercises and alternative therapies such as acupuncture and homeopathy, says Dr. Collins. He uses colon therapy as an adjunct treatment for a wide range of conditions, including hypertension, arthritis, depression, parasites, and lung problems.

In the case of hypertension, the muscular movements initiated by colon therapy help to control blood pressure by regulating the autonomic nervous system. Arthritis patients benefit because of the direct stimulation of the immune system, states Dr. Collins. This may help to remove immune complexes from the joints, a major factor in rheumatoid arthritis.

Colon therapy can also help rid the body of parasites without a need for the heavy drugs usually prescribed to treat them. Dr. Collins reports of a patient who had a case of giardiasis (a form of parasites). She received colon therapy treatments and an Ayurvedic oral flush with salt water. After several treatments that included pancreatic enzymes, she tested clear of the parasites.

Choosing a Colon Therapist

When choosing a colon therapist, be certain he or she has received proper training, and that the facility is clean and well cared for. Dr. Collins points out that because fecal matter can transmit disease, it is imperative that not only the equipment, but the facility be thoroughly sterilized. Disposable tubing and speculums have become the standard for modern colon therapy. Additionally, each operator is responsible for making sure that contaminated equipment is never used from one patient to the next. It is recommended that the therapist take test samples from various areas of the colonic machine to insure sterility. Colon therapy equipment manufacturers are currently addressing the dangers of disease carriers, including protozoa, viruses, and bacteria.

When choosing a colon therapist or facility, make sure that the administering therapist is certified and the facility appears clean and well maintained.

Where to Find Help

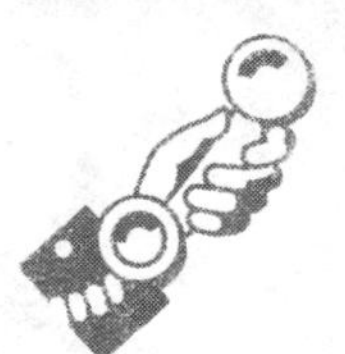

There are many sources of referral to a colon therapist: physicians, chiropractors, alternative practitioners and clinics, gastrointestinal specialists, naturopaths, health food stores, and your local phone directory. You may also contact the following organizations for a qualified colon therapist in your area:

American Association of Naturopathic Physicians
2366 Eastlake Avenue, Suite 322
Seattle, Washington 98102
(206) 323-7610

Refers to a nationwide network of accredited or licensed practitioners who are the only physicians trained in colon therapy in medical school. Publishes a quarterly newsletter for both professionals and the general public.

California Colon Hygienists Society
P.O. Box 588
Graton, California 95444
(707) 829-0984

Offers a complete apprenticeship and certification program in colon therapy. Provides education in cellular detoxification and cleansing. Refers to a nationwide network of colon therapists.

International Association for Colon Therapy
2051 Hilltop Drive, Suite A-11
Redding, California 96002
(916) 222-1498

Refers to a nationwide network of colon therapists. Holds seminars and trainings on colon therapy for both professionals and the general public. Funds a national certification panel for colon therapists.

Wood Hygienic Institute, Inc.
P.O. Box 420580
Kissimmee, Florida 34742
(407) 933-0009

Offers a complete certification program in colon hygiene. Refers practitioners in colon therapy and massage.

Recommended Reading

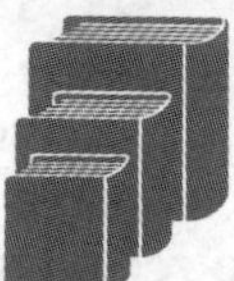

Colon Health: Key to a Vibrant Life. Walker, Norman. Prescott, AZ: Norwalk Press, 1979.

A layperson's textbook on colon health. Including how to's as well as a complete glossary of terms and index of professional referrals.

Colon Irrigation: A Forgotten Key to Health. Baker, Mark. St. Louis, MO: Mark Baker, 1989.

A helpful booklet, in easy-to-understand terms, about "autointoxification" and the role of colon irrigation in restoring vital health. This booklet can be ordered from the author for three dollars by writing to: Mark Baker, 11558 Saint Charles Rock Road, Bridgeton, Missouri 63044

A Doctor's Guide to You and Your Colon. Plaut, Martin. New York: Harper & Row, 1986.

An authoritative, easy-to-understand guide covering a variety of colon difficulties and treatments.

Tissue Cleansing through Bowel Management. Jensen, Bernard. Escondido, CA: Bernard Jensen, 1981.

A comprehensive look at detoxifying, cleansing, and maintaining better health through bowel management.

"A man may esteem himself happy when that which is his food is also his medicine."

—Henry David Thoreau

Craniosacral Therapy

Craniosacral therapy manipulates the bones of the skull to treat a range of conditions, from headache and ear infection to stroke, spinal cord injury, and cerebral palsy. For decades various forms of cranial manipulation have been used to improve overall body functioning, and today craniosacral therapy is gaining acceptance by health professionals worldwide as a successful treatment modality.

Every one of us is familiar with the body's cardiac rhythm (heartbeat) and respiratory rhythm (breathing). Yet there is a third and equally important rhythm known as the craniosacral rhythm that results from the increase and decrease in the volume of cerebrospinal fluid within and around the craniosacral system.

Cranio refers to the cranium, or head, and *sacral* refers to the base of the spine and tailbone. The craniosacral system is comprised of the brain and spinal cord (the central nervous system); the cerebrospinal fluid that bathes the brain and spinal cord; the surrounding meninges (membranes) that enclose the brain, spinal cord, and cerebrospinal fluid; and the bones of the spine and skull that house these membranes.

There is a rhythmical motion in the craniosacral system created by the rise and fall of cerebrospinal fluid pressure. An increase in this pressure occurs as cerebrospinal fluid filters from the bloodstream and enters the craniosacral system, causing a predictable movement of the cranial bones. The pressure diminishes as the cerebrospinal fluid is reabsorbed into the bloodstream through the inner membranes of the brain, allowing the bones to return to their original position. The cranial therapist monitors this wavelike motion to determine any restriction or dysfunction in the craniosacral system. This subtle rhythm ranges from six to ten cycles per minute, and is for the most part unaffected by the heart and respiratory rhythms.

“The craniosacral system has a profound effect on health and well-being.”

A cranial therapist is trained to “palpate,” or feel with his or her hands, the motion of the craniosacral system as a unified, integrated movement. The touch is extremely gentle and sensitive, and one is able to diagnose the movement of the system as a whole by locating critical points of restriction in the cranium.

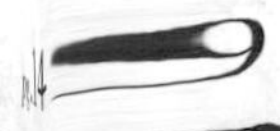

Restrictions that result from injury, inflexibility of the joints of the spine and cranium, or from dysfunctions in other parts of the body, can all cause abnormal motion in the craniosacral system. The abnormal motion

The craniosacral system.

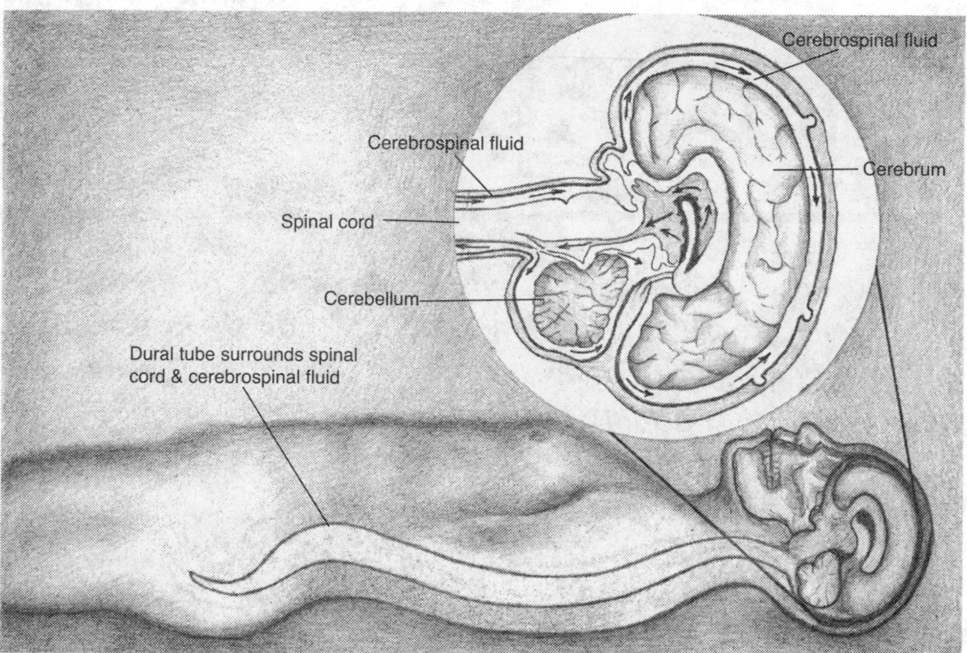

leads to stresses in the cranial mechanism which can contribute to dysfunction and poor health, especially in the brain and spinal cord. The purpose of craniosacral therapy is to enhance the functioning of this important system.

How Craniosacral Therapy Works

There are three major approaches to craniosacral therapy: sutural, meningeal, and reflex. Each differs slightly in its therapeutic approach and application.

The Sutural Approach

The sutural approach was popularized by Dr. William Garner Sutherland, an early twentieth century osteopathic physician. In this technique, the therapist manipulates the sutures of the skull (where the bones meet) in order to ease pressure and increase mobility of the cranial bones. By removing the stress between the cranial bones, the sutural approach normalizes the relationship of one bone to another. This allows for a remodeling of the entire craniosacral system, and an enhancement of its function and capacity for adaption.

While still a medical student, Dr. Sutherland observed that the bones of the skull are designed to move in accordance with one another. At the time, his theory was considered ridiculous, as prevailing scientific opinion stated that the bones of the skull become fused together around the age of thirty-five. Despite both scientific and clinical evidence to support Dr.

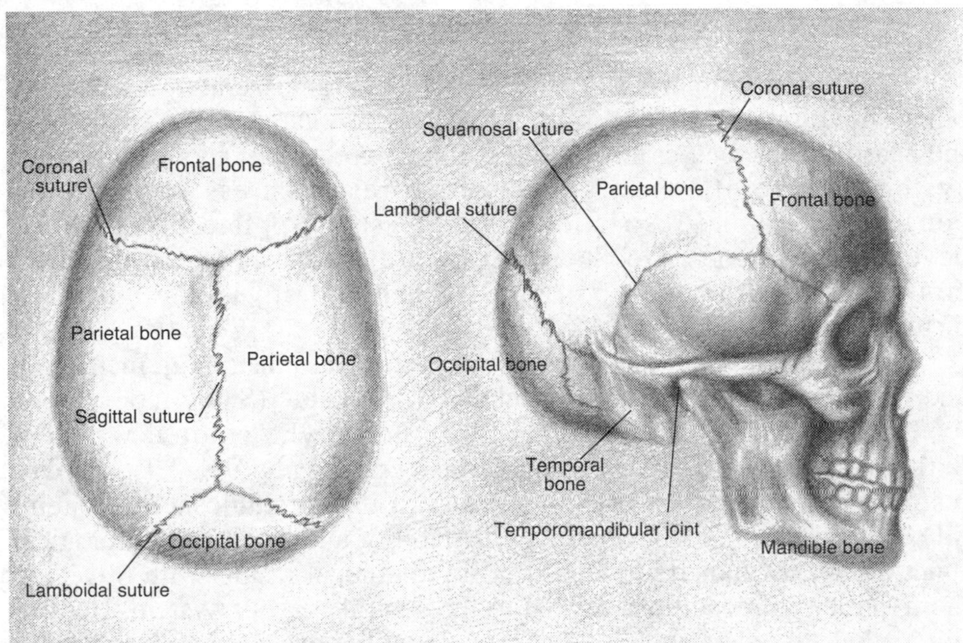

Top and side view of the cranium.

Sutherland's view,[1] debate continues to this day within the scientific community, and many anatomical texts still teach that the bones of an adult human skull are fused and immobile.

Dr. Sutherland spent years experimenting with his hypothesis, and eventually developed a sophisticated system of diagnosis and treatment known as cranial osteopathy.

The Meningeal Approach

In the late 1970s, John Upledger, D.O., O.M.M., an osteopathic physician, led a multidisciplinary research team of anatomists, physiologists, biophysicists, and bioengineers at Michigan State University in an attempt to determine the scientific basis of the craniosacral system. Their work produced a practical model of the dynamic movement of the cranium and craniosacral system. Dr. Upledger applied his research to develop CranioSacral Therapy™, an approach that focuses primarily on manipulating the underlying membranes, or meninges. He has taught this approach to thousands worldwide.

Tension or restriction in the meninges creates disturbances in the craniosacral system. A meningeal approach, such as Dr. Upledger's CranioSacral Therapy, focuses on releasing restrictions of the cranial sutures and the underlying membranes through gentle hands-on contact with the bones of the craniosacral system. The therapist monitors the rhythmical movement in the craniosacral system resulting from the increase and decrease in cerebrospinal fluid pressure. When abnormal motion is detected in the craniosacral system, the therapist locates the point of restricted movement and brings about a release by gently tractioning and elongating the meningeal membranes.

"The practical and theoretical significance of Dr. Upledger's therapeutic techniques, by the turn of the century, will be implemented in most hospitals and medical schools."

—Elmer Green, Ph.D.

The Reflex Approach

The reflex approach relieves stress in the craniosacral system and in other structures and organs of the body. By stimulating nerve endings in the scalp or between cranial sutures, this approach triggers the nervous system to turn off stress signals. As a result, stress patterns and consequent cranial restrictions are released. Applied kinesiology, developed by George Goodheart, D.C., utilizes the reflex approach in conjunction with specific cranial adjustments to locate and treat distortions in the craniosacral system.

See Applied Kinesiology.

A system of craniosacral therapy that combines the sacral, meningeal and reflex approaches is Sacro-Occipital Technique™ (S.O.T.), developed by Dr. Major B. DeJarnette, a chiropractor who studied with Dr. Sutherland in the 1920s. Also known as "craniopathy," S.O.T. removes restrictions between the cranial bones and in the craniosacral system. S.O.T. strives to reestablish structural stability and improve neurological function. Dr. DeJarnette produced positive clinical results with S.O.T. in the treatment of conditions related to the central nervous system. He also found that disorders such as diabetes, constipation, anxiety, impotence, asthma, cataracts, and inflammation, when associated with specific restrictions between sutures of the cranium, could be alleviated with a precise cranial technique.

Restrictions of motion of a particular cranial bone can pose serious consequences to the function of the body. Marc Pick, D.C., D.I.C.S., a widely acclaimed researcher and teacher of S.O.T., recalls a woman in her late seventies who had complete deafness in one ear for twenty-five years. After Dr. Pick corrected the restricted motion of the temporal bone (which houses the inner and outer ear on the affected side) the woman's hearing immediately returned.

Conditions Benefited by Craniosacral Therapy

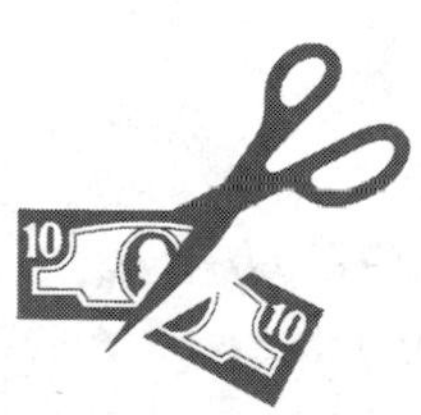

Through its ability to improve the general functioning of the central nervous system and address many difficult conditions, craniosacral therapy can offer substantial long-term cost savings to consumers.

Imbalances in the craniosacral mechanism often begin before birth. Inadequate prenatal nutrition can result in underdevelopment of the facial and jaw bones that can later impair smooth functioning of the craniosacral system. Difficult delivery, extended periods of engagement (the time the baby's head is in the birth canal), or the incorrect application of forceps, even suction, can produce severe stresses and distortion to the growing cranial tissues. This consequently can affect the baby's general health. Many of these stresses to the newborn's craniosacral system are normally considered untreatable by conventional medicine, and often go unnoticed.

Treating Infants and Children

Some of the most successful craniosacral treatments are performed on newborns and infants. At this stage the cranial bones are primarily cartilage and the membranes are growing and changing very rapidly, so they are very responsive to the gentle corrections of the therapist's fingers. Newborns can be treated immediately after birth.

For many years cranial osteopaths have successfully treated infants for common conditions such as earaches, sinus congestion, vomiting, irritability, and hyperactivity, using only craniosacral therapy. In these cases, craniosacral therapists commonly find compression at the base of the skull, which they maintain is related to the birthing process, and particularly the extreme backward extension of the baby's head during delivery.

“For many years cranial osteopaths have successfully treated infants for common conditions such as earaches, sinus congestion, vomiting, irritability, and hyperactivity, using only craniosacral therapy.”

Specific conditions that relate to the overall function of the craniosacral system also benefit from craniosacral therapy. Andrew Weil, M.D., writes about Bob Fulford, a retired osteopathic physician and instructor of craniosacral therapy who had great success in using craniosacral therapy to treat problems other doctors could not solve. “For instance, he [Fulford] regularly cured young children of recurring ear infections by simply, in his words, ‘freeing up their breathing and getting their tailbone [sacrum] unstuck’ so that it could get back into normal respiratory [craniosacral rhythm] motion. When this motion is restricted, fluid backs up in the ear, providing a perfect breeding ground for bacteria.”[2]

Effects on the Central Nervous System

Decreased efficiency of the central nervous system contributes to many chronic and nonspecific conditions, and problems within the craniosacral system are responsible for tremendous suffering and loss of potential vigor and health.

The proper functioning of the craniosacral system implies health for the central nervous system. The proper alignment of the craniosacral system allows the nervous system to rest at a more stress-free level. Individuals who experience craniosacral treatment describe profound states of relaxation, of feeling lighter and more integrated. “When there is synchronous movement in the craniosacral system, the physiology of the central nervous system functions more efficiently and the nerve tissue is, in general, healthier,” says Robert Norett, D.C., Director of the Stillpoint Health Center in Venice, California.

“When there is synchronous movement in the craniosacral system, the physiology of the central nervous system functions more efficiently and the nerve tissue is, in general, healthier.”

—Robert Norett, D.C.

Craniosacral therapy is used to evaluate and treat problems involving the brain and spinal cord, especially direct trauma to the head and spine. Other treatable conditions include chronic pain, headache, temporomandibular joint syndrome (TMJ), mood disorders, dyslexia, autism, stroke, epilepsy, cerebral palsy, dizziness, and tinnitus (ringing in the ear). Also benefited are systemic conditions such as edema (swelling), recurrent infections, hypertension, hypotension, and some types of muscular conditions.

According to Dr. Norett, the entrapments and compressions around the nerve and blood vessels that pass in and out of the cranium and spine can be alleviated through craniosacral therapy. Hundreds of small holes that carry these vessels can become thick with connective tissue and effectively “choke” the vessels. He cites the case of the owner and head chef of a French restaurant who had slipped and hit the back of his head against a stove. "As a result of the trauma, he lost his sense of smell, vital to his work as a chef," says Dr. Norett. "We found significant restriction of the area inside the cranium where the olfactory nerves (affecting the sense of smell) pass through, and within about five treatments, he had improved dramatically."

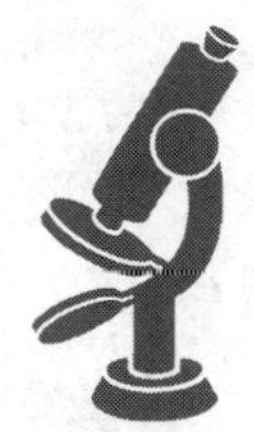

Research into the function of the craniosacral system could help provide a broader understanding of human anatomy, physiology, and the role of the craniosacral system in health.

Dr. Upledger has had great success treating chronic, severe, and disabling headaches. He reports that 80 to 85 percent of resistant long-term headache patients respond favorably to CranioSacral Therapy. The benefit of this treatment is that once the headaches are gone, they do not return, and the patient is not dependent upon a lifetime of periodic therapy sessions.[3]

Dr. Upledger cites the story of a United States naval officer on active duty during World War II. Recurring headaches accompanied by a loud noise in his ears began after he stood next to a cannon as it was being fired. Although he tried every kind of treatment available through the navy, he found no relief. When he visited Dr. Upledger, he had been living with the pain for twenty-five years. After evaluating his craniosacral system, Dr. Upledger found the skull bones on the left side of his head were jammed inward and stuck. Dr. Upledger manually released the compression of the cranial bones and the left side of the head expanded immediately. His pain vanished on the spot. By the third visit, his ear noise had stopped.[4]

Joseph F. Unger, D.C., F.I.C.S., reports of a patient in continual pain from a two-year-old radical mastectomy scar. She also had swelling and pains in the arm on the side of the surgery. Using one of Dr. Dejarnette's S.O.T. cranial techniques, Dr. Unger was able to eradicate the pain from the scar. Over the next two to three weeks, the swelling in her arm diminished almost to normal.

Craniosacral therapy is rapidly gaining acceptance among health practitioners and the public. This may be due in part to the nonintrusive nature of this therapy, and how it works with the entire structure, physiology, mind, and spirit.

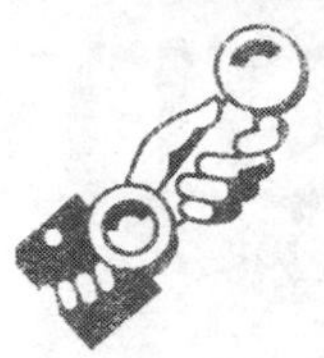

Where to Find Help

For further information about craniosacral therapy, and for referrals, contact:

Cranial Academy
3500 Depaw Boulevard
Indianapolis, Indiana 46268
(317) 879-0713

The Cranial Academy teaches cranial therapy to osteopaths according to the work of Dr. William Sutherland. Call for a referral to one of their international offices. Has approximately eight hundred members.

SORSI (S.O.T.)
P.O. Box 8245
Prairie Village, Kansas 66208
(913) 649-3475

SORSI teaches postgraduate courses and certifies chiropractors in Sacro-Occipital Technique according to Dr. Major B. DeJarnette. Trains and certifies chiropractors in craniopathy. Call for a referral to a certified chiropractor in craniopathy. Approximately five hundred members.

Upledger Institute
11211 Prosperity Farms Road
Palm Beach Gardens, Florida 33410
(407) 622-4706

The teaching arm of the Upledger Institute offers courses worldwide and teaches to cross-disciplinary health professionals. Offers information to public, and has a referral network of more than two thousand members.

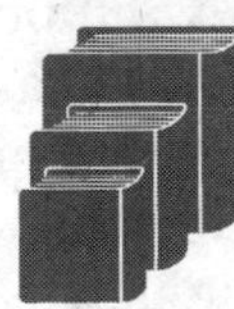

Recommended Reading

Craniosacral Therapy and SomatoEmotional Release: The Self Healing Body. Manheim, Carol J., M.S.C., P.T.; and Lavett, Diane K., Ph.D. Thorofare, NJ: SLACK Inc., 1989.

An in-depth coverage of the psychological and emotional perspectives of stored memory, craniosacral therapy, and SomatoEmotional Release. This book reviews types of patients and the process of craniosacral therapy, with technical references and an index.

Your Inner Physician and You: CranioSacral Therapy SomatoEmotional Release. Upledger, John E., D.O., F.A.A.O. Berkeley, CA: North Atlantic Books, 1992.

Ideal for the lay reader, this book explains CranioSacral Therapy—its philosophy, models of how it works, specific cases, and many different treatable conditions. Written in the first person by Dr. Upledger, it includes a chapter of questions and answers.

Detoxification Therapy

Each year people are exposed to thousands of toxic chemicals and pollutants in the earth's atmosphere, water, food, and soil. These pollutants manifest themselves in a variety of symptoms, including decreased immune function, neurotoxicity, hormonal dysfunction, psychological disturbances, and even cancer. Detoxification therapy helps to rid the body of chemicals and pollutants and can facilitate a return to health.

Detoxification is the body's natural process of eliminating or neutralizing toxins via the liver, the kidneys, the urine, the feces, exhalation, and perspiration. Yet, as a result of the industrial revolution and the post-World War II petrochemical revolution, toxins have accumulated in the human system faster than they can be eliminated. People now carry within their bodies a modern-day chemical cocktail derived from industrial chemicals, pesticides, food additives, heavy metals, anesthetics, and the residues of pharmaceutical drugs, legal drugs (alcohol, tobacco, caffeine), and illegal drugs (heroin, cocaine, marijuana).

> *"People now carry within their bodies a modern-day chemical cocktail derived from industrial chemicals, pesticides, food additives, heavy metals, anesthetics, and the residues of pharmaceutical, legal, and illegal drugs."*

Today people are exposed to chemicals in far greater concentrations then were previous generations: for example, over 69 million Americans live in areas that exceed smog standards;[1] most drinking water contains over seven hundred chemicals, including excessive levels of lead;[2] some three thousand chemicals are added to the food supply; and as many as ten thousand chemicals in the form of solvents, emulsifiers, and preservatives are used in food processing and storage, which can remain in the body for years.[3] To make matters worse, food and product labels do not always list every ingredient. When people consume these foods—especially seafood, meat, and poultry—they ingest all the chemicals and pesticides that have remained as contaminants accumulating in the food chain.

Everyday products such as gasoline, paint, household cleansers, cosmetics, pesticides, and dry cleaning fluid also pose a serious threat because the body cannot easily break them down. At the same time, ecological changes in the environment are occurring faster than the human organism can adapt to them. As the earth becomes more and more polluted, the body inadvertently becomes a filter that "traps" these pollutants.

"The current level of chemicals in the food and water supply and the indoor and outdoor environment has lowered our threshold of resistance to disease and has altered our body's metabolism, causing enzyme dysfunction, nutritional deficiencies, and hormonal imbalances," says Marshall Mandell, M.D., father of the field of bioecologic medicine.

According to Zane Gard, M.D., of Beaverton, Oregon, bioaccumulation (a buildup in the body of foreign substances) seriously compromises physiological and psychological health. Over the last ten years, hundreds of studies have demonstrated the dangers to health from toxic bioaccumulation.[4]

"A body with a healthy immune system, efficient organs of elimination and detoxification, and a sound circulatory and nervous system can handle a great deal of toxicity," states Leon Chaitow, N.D., D.O., of London, England. "But if they have been damaged from chronic exposure to environmental pollutants, restoring these functions, organs, and systems can be accomplished only through detoxification therapies, including fasting, chelation, and nutritional, herbal, and homeopathic methods, which accelerate the body's own natural cleansing processes. These therapies will dominate medical thinking in the years ahead."

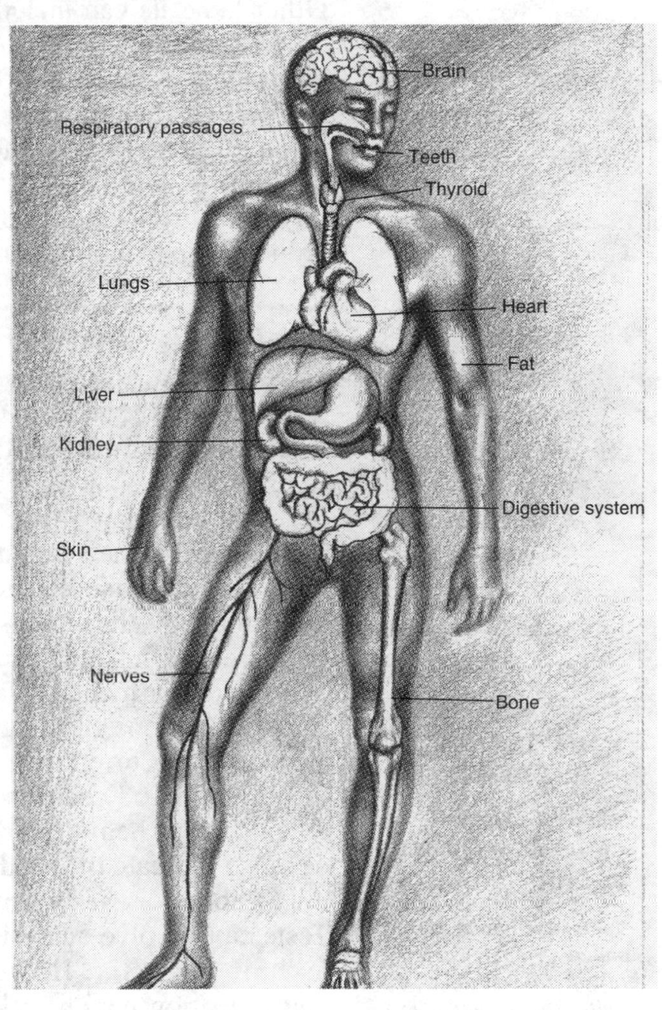

Sites of toxic accumulation in the body.

Benefits of Detoxification

"I believe that the process of detoxification through special cleansing diets as well as juice and water fasts is the missing link to rejuvenating the body and preventing such chronic diseases as cancer, cardiovascular problems, arthritis, diabetes, and obesity," says Elson Haas, M.D., Director of the Marin Clinic of Preventive Medicine and Health Education in San Rafael, California. "The modern diet with excess animal proteins, fats, caffeine, alcohol, and chemicals inhibits the optimum function of our cells and tissues. The cleansing of toxins and waste products will restore optimum function and vitality."

Dr. Haas has practiced juice fasting regularly for nearly twenty years, and advises his patients to undertake some form of detoxification periodically to clear wastes and dead cells and to revitalize the body's natural functions and healing capacities. He points out that along with greater mental clarity, the most important and longest lasting effect of detoxification therapy is the reduction of stress on the immune system. Other benefits can include increased vitality, reduced blood pressure and blood fats (cholesterol and triglycerides), and an improved assimilation of vitamins and minerals. Detoxification is instrumental for maintenance of the normal function and integrity of the intestinal flora, and can enhance the natural ability of the body to resist infections, allergies, and skin disorders. Dr. Haas adds that most people will feel mentally and physically rejuvenated after detoxification therapy, with a corresponding reduction in symptoms and disease.

How Do You Know if Your Body Requires Detoxification?

According to David Steinman, former representative of the public interest at the National Academy of Sciences, everyone has a specific level of tolerance that cannot be exceeded if good health is to be maintained. If the amount of toxins within the body stays below that level, the body can usually adapt and rid itself of these. "However," says Steinman, "when the system is overwhelmed, the body's defense mechanism malfunctions, and symptoms such as fatigue, confusion, aggression, or mental disorder may occur."

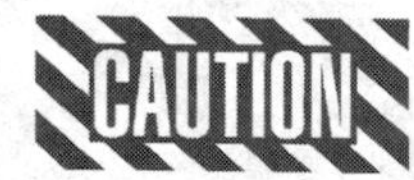

Great care must be taken to insure the safe and effective removal of toxins, and any detoxification therapy should be administered only after a consultation with a qualified health professional.

Indications that the body may need detoxification are headaches, joint pain, recurrent respiratory problems, back pain, allergy symptoms, insomnia, mood changes, and food allergies. Conditions such as arthritis, constipation, hemorrhoids, sinus congestion, ulcers, psoriasis, and acne can also indicate the need for detoxification.

Laboratory tests can also shed light on the need for detoxification. Tests can involve analysis of stool, urine, blood or liver function, as well as hair analysis. However, physicians who are not familiar with detoxification may be reluctant to perform such tests. People considering a detoxification program will want to find a doctor who understands the concepts of detoxification.

Some Preliminary Cautions

According to Dr. Chaitow, a key question to ask yourself is: am I well enough to undertake rapid and active detoxification or should I string the process out and do the job slowly? If a person is robust and vital, a more vigorous program may be required than if the person is unwell and somewhat fragile in health. Dr. Chaitow recommends that each individual seek the advice of a qualified health professional to help select the appropriate degree of intensity. People who are recovering drug users, alcoholics, diabetics, or who have eating disorders should not apply any method without strict medical supervision.

It is also important to note that detoxification may not be appropriate for individuals who are underweight or physically weak, or for those people with a hypothyroid or a hypoglycemic condition. Anyone with a cancerous condition, or who is just recovering from surgery, should always consult a qualified health professional before any detoxification program is carried out.

Finally, people should know what to expect during detoxification. Dr. Chaitow states, "Early on you could develop a headache and furred tongue. As the weeks pass your skin should become clearer, although it may be spotty for a while. Your eyes will become clearer, your brain sharper, digestion more efficient, energy levels high, and you may well regain a sense of youthful clarity."

Forms of Detoxification

Several methods of detoxification are currently available. These include fasting and specific diets, colon therapy, vitamin therapy, chelation therapy, and hyperthermia. It is advisable to seek professional advice when choosing a detoxification program.

Fasting and Diets

Fasting programs and specific dietary regimens are some of the easiest and most inexpensive and effective methods of detoxification. They involve very little cost other than the purchase of healthy food. Results depend upon both the patient and the length of the fast. Fasting is often combined with enemas and bowel stimulation for the purpose of ridding the body of bacteria and toxins trapped in the bowels. And while a detoxification program is not primarily concerned with weight loss, by introducing a more efficient and healthier way to eat, weight loss can be the result. It is important to note again that before embarking on any kind of fast or diet, one should always consult with a doctor or a qualified health professional.

Long fasts require medical supervision as well as prior assessment as to levels of nutrients, such as vitamins and minerals, to insure that deficiency does not occur. Short weekend fasts are safe for most people, although advice from an appropriate health care professional experienced in detoxification is advisable.

There are basically two types of fasts—water and juice:

Juice Fasting: Evarts G. Loomis, M.D., co-founder of the American Holistic Medical Association and founder of Meadowlark, America's first live-in health and growth retreat, prescribes vegetable juices (equal parts carrot—diluted with water 1:1—and celery) for detoxification. If desired, green vegetables such as green beans, zucchini, watercress, and parsley can be added. Dr. Loomis also prescribes a "detoxifying cocktail" that combines garlic, lemon juice, grapefruit juice, and olive oil. This is given at bedtime because the liver, a major organ for detoxification, is most active between 11:00 P.M. and 1:00 A.M., according to Traditional Chinese Medicine.

Dr. Haas recalls a man who, at five feet, nine inches and 231 pounds, had high blood pressure, an elevated cholesterol level and a marked inability to handle stress. After going on a ten-day juice cleansing diet supervised by Dr. Haas, he dropped eighteen pounds and was inspired to make major and permanent changes to his diet. He followed a vegetarian-oriented and whole foods regimen. Consequently, his blood pressure and cholesterol normalized and he found a more comfortable body weight of about 195 pounds.

Dr. Chaitow recommends a choice of two detoxification therapies that can be done over the weekend. He advises doing one or the other over every weekend for a few months to begin with.

DETOXIFICATION SUPPORT

A person undergoing detoxification therapy can do a number of things during the process to help aid the natural cleansing ability of the body, according to Dr. Chaitow. His suggestions include:

Hydrotherapy: *Epsom salts baths or wet sheet packs, once weekly.*

Skin brushing: *To assist the skin elimination function, daily.*

Stretching and relaxation exercises: *Practice daily.*

Aerobic exercise (if appropriate): *Brisk walking, jogging, dancing, etc., daily except during the fast period.*

Massage and manual lymphatic drainage: *As often as available, twice weekly if possible.*

Aromatherapy: *Use of appropriate (to your condition) essential aromatherapy oils, in baths or as part of massage.*

Breathing, relaxation, and meditation methods: *Daily for at least ten to fifteen minutes, twice if possible.*

Weekend Water Fast: A water only fast (twenty-four to thirty-six hours) starting Friday evening and ending Sunday morning (or as an alternative, just all day Saturday). Make sure that not less than four and not more than eight pints of water are consumed during the fast. On Sunday, have a day of raw foods (fruit/salad only, well chewed, plus the recommended amounts of drinking water).

Weekend Monodiet: A full weekend monodiet beginning Friday night and extending through to Sunday evening, relying on a single food such as grapes, apples, pears (best choices if you have an allergy history); papaya (ideal if digestive problems are present); or brown rice, buckwheat, millet, or potatoes (skin and all) boiled and eaten whenever desired.

Up to a pound (dry weight) of any grain such as rice or millet may be eaten daily; taste can be made palatable with the addition of a little lemon juice and olive oil. Or one may eat up to three pounds of potatoes daily.

According to Dr. Chaitow, "Whichever type of detoxification modality you choose, make sure you rest, keep warm, and don't have a very strenuous schedule; this should be a time in which you allow all available energy to focus on the cleansing and repairing processes of detoxification."

In between weekend detoxification intensives, Dr. Chaitow recommends a milder program of detoxification be employed:

- **Breakfast:** Fresh fruit (raw or lightly cooked—no sweetening) and live yogurt (with real yogurt cultures), homemade muesli (seeds, nuts, grains) and live yogurt, or cooked grains and yogurt (buckwheat, millet, linseed, barley, rice). Herbal tea is fine, especially linden blossom, chamomile, mint, sage, lemon verbena, or a lemon and hot water drink.
- **Lunch/Supper:** One of the meals should be a raw salad with potato or brown rice and either bean curd (tofu), low-fat cheese, nuts, or seeds. If raw food is difficult to digest, stir-fried vegetables and tofu or steamed vegetables eaten with a potato or rice and low-fat cheese, nuts, or seeds will suffice. The other main meal should consist of fish, chicken, or game, or be vegetarian (bean and grain combination and/or vegetables lightly steamed, baked, or stir-fried). Seasoning can include garlic and herbs, but avoid salt as much as possible.
- **Desserts:** Lightly stewed fruit with added apple or lemon juice (not sugar) or live natural yogurt is fine.

Remember, eat slowly, chew well, don't drink with meals, and consume at least two pints of liquid daily between meals. Also, take one high potency multimineral/multivitamin capsule daily and three garlic capsules, and a daily acidophilus supplement for bowel detox support.

When the tongue no longer becomes furred during detoxification and headaches no longer appear, these intensive detoxification weekends can be spaced apart—three a month and then two a month and then, as maintenance, once a month thereafter.

Alkaline-Detoxification Diet: Developed by Dr. Haas, this three- to four-week plan helps to detoxify the body tissues of protein and acid wastes that can create both inflammatory and degenerative changes when interacting in the body. "This diet plan is a gentle and safe way to detoxify," notes Dr. Haas, "and can also help to reduce weight, increase vitality, and promote healing."

Dr. Haas adds that when foods oxidize in the body, they leave a residue or ash. If the foods are acidic, they leave an acidic residue (i.e., acidic ash, sulfur, phosphorus, chlorine, or uncombusted acid radicals), which can be harmful. Success with this method is achieved by the elimination of acid-forming foods from your diet. This makes the question not what to eat, but *what not to eat*.

Essentially this diet consists of fruits and vegetables (mostly vegetables), plus fresh sprouts and millet. The diet also focuses on particular eating principles, including exceptional chewing (thirty to fifty times per mouthful), drinking quality water plus the steamed vegetable water, and eating all food prior to nightfall, advisedly before 6:30 P.M.

Dr. Haas recommends the following guidelines:

- Chew very well and take your time when you eat.
- Relax a few minutes before and after your meal.
- Eat in a comfortable sitting position.
- Eat primarily steamed fresh vegetables and some fresh greens.
- Take only herbal teas after dinner.

THE ALKALINE DETOXIFICATION DIET MENU

Morning (upon arising): *Two glasses of water (filtered, spring, or reverse osmosis)—one of these mixed with the juice of half a lemon. After a little stretching, have one serving of a fresh fruit such as apple, pear, banana, grapes, or citrus. Fifteen to thirty minutes later, eat one bowl of cooked whole grains—specifically millet, brown rice, amaranth, quinoa, or buckwheat. Flavoring can be two tablespoons of fruit juice for a sweeter breakfast taste, or use the "better butter" mixture (mentioned below) with a little salt or tamari for a deeper flavor.*

Lunch (12:00-1:00 P.M.) and dinner (5:00-6:00 P.M.): *One to two medium bowls of steamed vegetables; use a variety, including roots, stems, and greens. A seasoning—"better butter"—can be made by mixing a half cup of cold-pressed canola oil into a soft (room temperature) half-pound of butter; then place in dish, refrigerate. Use about one teaspoon per meal or a maximum of three teaspoons daily.*

11:00 A.M. and 3:00 P.M.: *One to two cups vegetable water, saved from steamed vegetables. Add a little seasalt or kelp and drink slowly, mixing each mouthful with saliva.*

Evening: *Herbal teas—peppermint, chamomile, pau d'arco, or blends.*

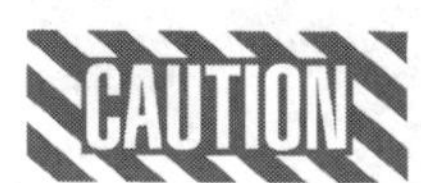

Caution: *Dr. Haas points out that you may feel a little weak or have a few symptoms the first couple of days, but notes that this will pass. "Clarity and a feeling of well-being should appear by day three or four, if not before. If during this diet, you start to feel weak or hungry, assess your water intake and elimination; if needed, you can eat a small portion of protein food (three to four ounces) in the midafternoon. This could be fish; free-range, organic chicken; or some beans, such as lentils,*

garbanzos, mung, or black beans." Remember that even in a clean and healthy body, the full effects of an alkaline diet do not begin to be felt for five to seven days.

Colon Therapy

Colonic irrigation is one of the most effective ways to cleanse the large intestine of accumulated toxins and waste products. It functions to draw toxins from the blood and lymph back into the colon for excretion. With the help of a trained professional and a colonic machine, purified water (which may contain vitamins, herbs, friendly bacteria, or oxygen) is introduced directly into the rectum. Colon therapy can be combined with massage, nutritional programs, and special diets to help cleanse the bowels and aid in the treatment of parasitic infections. It can be used prior to other detoxification programs, but is not recommended during the hyperthermic program described later.

Direction of lymph flow.

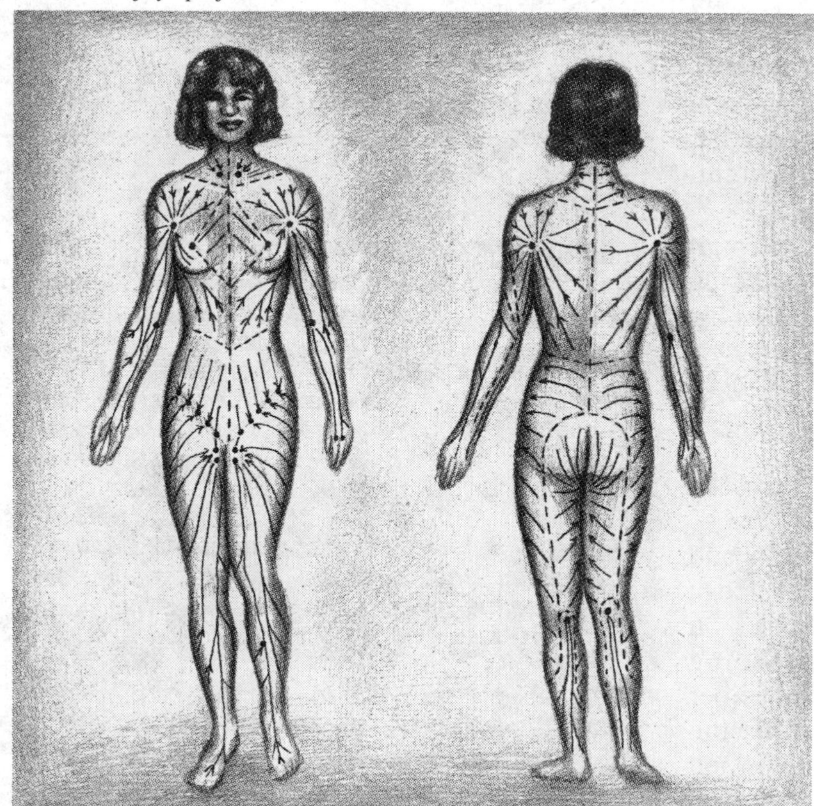

Vitamin C Therapy

Each year, more and more studies on vitamin C confirm its importance in healing and maintaining health. The relationship between vitamin C and body toxicity is complex. For example, if a person is deficient in vitamin C, he or she becomes far more susceptible to environmental pollutants. Conversely, exposure to various toxins, like lead or benzene, will deplete the person's vitamin C stores. Evidence also suggests that vitamin C deficiency hampers the body's own detoxification process.

As a detoxification agent, vitamin C combines with certain toxins in the body and destroys them.[5] According to Robert Cathcart, III, M.D., of Los Altos, California, vitamin C functions as a free-radical scavenger, neutralizing the immunosuppressive toxins produced by infectious diseases. Dr. Cathcart has successfully treated over eleven thousand patients with vitamin C therapy, and his results have been widely published in professional journals.

See Chelation Therapy, Colon Therapy, Hyperthermia.

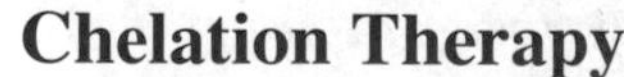

Chelation Therapy

In chelation therapy, a synthetic amino acid known as EDTA (ethylenediaminetetraacetic acid) is administered intravenously and binds to various toxic metals in the blood, such as lead, cadmium, and aluminum. The toxins are then flushed from the body through the kidneys.

Although it has been used primarily in the past to treat cases of lead poisoning, many doctors have found that EDTA can remove the calcium and plaque present in the walls of arteries in atherosclerosis, the major cause of heart disease. Chelation therapy has been tested and used safely for the past thirty years on an estimated five hundred thousand patients,[6] but has yet to receive FDA approval as a treatment for heart disease. However, several FDA-approved studies are currently being conducted. Over one thousand physicians offer chelation therapy in the United States.

Hyperthermia (Heat Stress Detoxification)

The only detoxification program that has proven successful in removing fat-stored toxins from the body is hyperthermia, or heat stress detoxification (saunas), according to Zane Gard, M.D., and Erma Brown, P.H.N. "Heat stress," says Dr. Gard, "can also remove calcium deposits from the blood vessels and break down scar tissue from their walls." Other studies demonstrate that hyperthermia can remove chemicals such as DDE (a metabolite of DDT), PCB's (polychlorinated biphenyls), and dioxin from fat cells.[7]

According to Dr. Gard, studies show that hyperthermia can affect numerous body systems, including the cardiovascular, endocrine, neurological, neuromuscular, bronchopulmonary, blood, skin, and immune.[8]

Hyperthermia can be combined with other detoxification therapies. However, proper medical supervision and laboratory evaluations are necessary because the removal of certain toxins can have a potentially adverse effect on the body, particularly on the kidneys and liver.

The BioToxic Reduction (BTR) Program: The BioToxic Reduction (BTR) Program™ created by Drs. Gard and Brown is a medically managed detoxification program designed to reduce the body's internal "toxic load" of chemicals, heavy metals, medical or street drugs, and alcohol.

Prior to starting the BTR detoxification program, it is necessary to have a complete evaluation by a physician. This includes a physical examination, health survey, immunologic profile, antibody level testing, toxic panel, and heavy metal analysis, as well as the usual CBC (complete blood count), blood chemistry panel, EKG

THE LYMPHATIC SYSTEM

Lymph is a clear fluid containing lymphocytes (T-cells and B-cells of the immune system) which circulate through the channels of the lymphatic system carrying waste away from all parts of the body to the lymph nodes. The lymph nodes filter out the wastes in the lymph, particularly bacteria, preventing it from entering the bloodstream, while at the same time allowing the lymphocytes to pass through.

Jack Shields, M.D., a lymphologist from Santa Barbara, California, conducted a study on the effects of breathing on the lymphatic system. Using cameras inside the body, he found that deep, diaphragmatic breathing stimulated the cleansing of the lymph system by creating a vacuum effect which sucked the lymph through the bloodstream. This increased the rate of toxic elimination by as much as fifteen times the normal pace.[9]

Lymphatic circulation can be enhanced by lymphatic massage as well as osteopathic and chiropractic lymphatic drainage techniques. According to Jared Zeff, N.D., L.Ac., Academic Dean of the National College of Natural Medicine in Portland, Oregon, "Any vigorous aerobic exercise causes lymphatic flow to accelerate." There are now devices which stimulate the lymphatic system such as the Light Beam Generator (LBG). An LBG puts out photons of light and a high-frequency electrostatic field to correct the electromagnetic charge on cells. Rena Davis, of Davis Nutrition Consultants in St. Helens, Oregon, believes that the Light Beam Generator stimulates the lymphatic system by breaking open sealed and calcified vessels, increasing blood circulation, reducing edema and carrying away waste products which have built up in the tissues, thereby inducing detoxification.

(electrocardiogram) readings, and personality and perception testing. Throughout the program, the patient meets weekly with the physician, and has additional laboratory follow-up if needed. Anyone with a heart condition needs to have frequent EKG monitoring and an authorization from a cardiologist to undergo BTR detoxification.

The BTR program should be undertaken for a minimum of two weeks, tailored to each patient and adjusted daily. It begins with therapeutic doses of vitamins, minerals, and oils, given in conjunction with exercise and dry sauna heat. The regimen consists of the following components:

- Daily doses of niacin
- Daily exercise routine prior to entering the sauna
- Sauna "sweat-out"
- Daily nutritional supplementation including replacement vitamins, minerals, trace elements, oil, and amino acids
- Pre- and post-program blood chemical analysis.

Drs. Gard and Brown note that most patients notice increased energy and mental clarity, and that many also report a decrease in body aches and pains, positive changes in hearing and vision, and changes in the texture of skin and hair. Most experience greater emotional stability and an overall sense of well-being.

Exercise, adequate fluid intake, and proper breathing are emphasized throughout this program. "But," says Dr. Gard, "it takes more than proper exercise and increased water intake to rid the body of the additional circulating toxins. We employ lymphatic massage at least three times weekly, and frequently give an intravenous infusion of five hundred milliliters of Lactated Ringers (a solution compatible with blood) with vitamin C, B-complex, and electrolytes." The BTR Program is currently available in Mexico.

Special Detoxification Baths

Hazel Parcells, N.D., D.C., Ph.D., a 103-year-old practicing naturopathic physician, recommends the following detoxification baths that she uses at The Parcells' System of Scientific Living in Albuquerque, New Mexico.

For poisoning from irradiated food (Cobalt 60): Dissolve two pounds of baking soda in a tub of very hot water, and sit in it. As the water begins to cool down, the toxins pass through the skin by osmosis.

For general radiation: Add one pound each of sea salt and baking soda to hot water and sit in the bath until the water has cooled down.

For heavy metals, insecticides, and carbon monoxide: Add one cup of Clorox™ to a hot bath and soak in it until the temperature cools down. This method can help eliminate environmental toxins such as lead, aluminum, insecticides, and the chemicals released from car exhaust.

The Future of Detoxification Therapy

"I believe that detoxification is a way to clear potential acute and chronic disease out of the body. It's a way to heal many early conditions," Dr. Haas states. Detoxification today has become a cornerstone for many doctors like Dr. Haas who stress preventative measures rather than just disease control.

"My idea is to create 'healing hospital environments,'" adds Dr. Haas. "People can check in and if they have a certain condition, still be provided with medicine or surgery if necessary. But it will also be a place where people can go to learn how to make changes in their life so they can clear up the problems that they already have and avoid those they don't." Detoxification is a major part of that process.

Dr. Chaitow states, "The need to tackle toxic burdens before they manifest themselves as disease has never been greater. It is clear to many who examine the problem that the future of health care will have at its very core an absolute requirement for safe and effective detoxification procedures—hopefully instituted before the individual's immune system and vital organs have ceased to operate adequately."

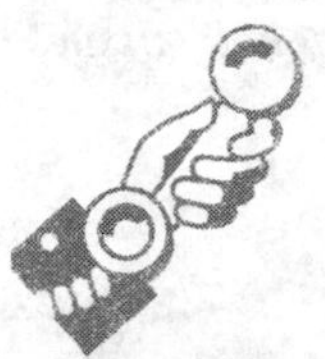

Where to Find Help

There are many modalities that address detoxification of the body. Contact the organizations below for information and referrals.

Chelation Therapy

American College of Advancement in Medicine
P.O. Box 3427
Laguna Hills, California 92654
(714) 583-7666

This pioneering organization seeks to establish certification and standards of practice for chelation therapy. They provide training and education, and sponsor semi-annual conferences for physicians and scientists. ACAM provides referrals and informational material, including a directory listing of all physicians worldwide who have been trained in preventive medicine as well as in the ACAM protocol for chelation therapy. The organization also provides a copy of the ACAM protocol for chelation to the public.

Colon Therapy

American Colon Therapy Association
11739 Washington Boulevard
Los Angeles, California 90066
(310) 390-5424

Refers to a nationwide network of colon therapists. Holds seminars and trainings on colon therapy for professionals and the general public. Funds a National Certification Panel for colon therapists. Publishes pamphlets.

Detoxification

Clinica del Lago
A. Postal PJ092
Provincia Juriquilla
C.P. 76230
Queretaro Qro. Mexico
011-52-429-40327

The clinic provides in-patient and out-patient Bio Toxic Reduction therapy using enzymatic potentiating desensitization. They treat all degenerative diseases and chemical toxic exposure, as well as street drug detox and silicone breast implant problems.

Fasting

International Association of Professional Natural Hygienists
Regency Health Resort and Spa
2000 South Ocean Drive
Hallandale, Florida 33009
(305) 454-2220

A professional organization of doctors who specialize in therapeutic fasting. They all follow the same protocol for fasting. Doctors in the United States, Canada, Australia, England, Greece, Israel, Japan, and Poland.

American Association of Naturopathic Physicians
2366 Eastlake Avenue, Suite 322
Seattle, Washington 98102
(206) 323-7610
(800) 206-7610

Provides referrals to a nationwide network of accredited or licensed naturopathic physicians for health professionals and the general public; supported by members and corporate sponsors. It hosts an annual convention, and works to move legislature and licensure in various states.

Hyperthermia

Bastyr College
144 NE 54th Street
Seattle, Washington 98105
(206) 523-9585

Offers postgraduate training in Naturopathic Medicine and supports teaching clinics. The physical medicine department of the Natural Health Clinic of Bastyr College uses hyperthermia treatment for detox and in conditions ranging from upper respiratory infection to chronic fatigue syndrome and HIV infection.

Laboratory Testing

Accu-Chem Laboratories
990 North Bowser Road
Suite 800
Richardson, Texas 75081
(800) 451-0116
(214) 234-5412 in Texas

This laboratory performs a complete array of pesticide and industrial chemical analyses on blood, urine and body tissues.

Pacific Toxicology
1545 Pontius Avenue
Los Angeles, California 90025
(310) 479-4911

This laboratory performs a complete array of pesticide and industrial chemical analyses on blood, urine, and body tissues.

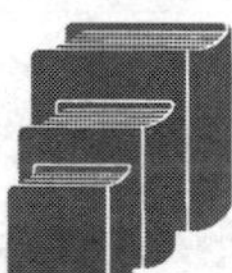

Recommended Reading

Body/Mind Purification Program. Chaitow, Leon, N.D., D.O. New York: Simon and Schuster/Gaia, 1990.

A holistic approach to enhance your physical, spiritual, and emotional well-being in a toxic world. Dr. Chaitow guides you through detoxification and introduces a clean nutritious diet, as well as exercises, stretches, massage, and other therapies. This book is only available from Educating Hands Bookstore, 261 SW 8th Street, Miami, Florida 33139, Phone (305) 285-6991, Fax: (305) 857-0298.

The Complete Guide to Health and Nutrition. Null, Gary. New York: Delacorte Press, 1986.

An authority in the field of nutrition—Gary Null clearly explains the use and importance of proteins, carbohydrates, fats, vitamins, and minerals.

Diet for a Poisoned Planet. Steinman, David. New York: Ballantine Books, 1990.

An in-depth guide for the consumer listing several foods and their contaminant levels.

Staying Healthy with Nutrition. Haas, Elson, M.D. Berkeley, CA: Celestial Arts, 1992.

Combining Eastern philosophies with his knowledge of Western medicine, Dr. Haas seeks to rejuvenate and cure using a mind/body approach to overall health. A comprehensive guide to diet and nutrition. Chapter 18 refers specifically to detoxification.

Diet

Conventional medicine has finally acknowledged the central role diet plays in a person's overall health. But achieving a good diet is not as simple as it sounds. Eating the right foods no longer insures proper health due to toxins contaminating the earth's food supply. Therefore, it is important to pay attention not only to what food to eat, but to where that food was grown or raised, and to what chemicals it might have been exposed to before it reaches the table.

The typical American diet of the past few decades has increasingly included more processed and contaminated foods than ever before. At the same time, Americans now suffer from more degenerative diseases, causing many physicians to suggest a strong link between what one eats and how one feels.

Over the years medical research has shown that saturated fats, white flour, refined starches, red meat, and chemical additives and pesticides, all common elements of the American diet, are major contributors to poor health and disease.

The 1988 Surgeon General's Report on Nutrition and Health acknowledged, "What we eat may affect our risk for several of the leading causes of death for Americans, notably, the degenerative diseases such as: atherosclerosis, coronary heart disease, strokes, diabetes, and some types of cancers. These disorders, together, now account for more than two-thirds of all deaths in the United States."

Toxins in the Food Chain

One of the greatest long-term problems health-conscious individuals face is the pervasive contamination of America's food supply. For decades, the FDA (Food and Drug Administration) and other government agencies have allowed the multibillion-dollar food industry to grow and process its products with hundreds of questionably safe chemicals such as pesticides, industrial pollutants, dyes, stabilizers, and preservatives, as well as antibiotics, hormones, and other drugs given to animals. The long-term consequences of ingesting these chemicals is still not well understood. Many experts now believe that lifetime ingestion of these chemicals can play a major role in causing cancer, neurotoxicity (destruction of nerve tissue by toxic substances), birth defects, decreased immune function, food allergies, and chemical sensitivity.

In his book, *Diet for a Poisoned Planet*, David Steinman, former representative of the public interest at the National Academy of Sciences, makes an exhaustive study of how contaminated the food chain is with chemical residues. As a solution, he recommends the general principle of eating food as low on the food chain as possible. Animal products, high on the food chain, are laden with pesticides from the foods the animals consume, as well as antibiotics, sulfa drugs, and growth hormones. Plants, on the other hand, are relatively less contaminated, usually only by what's been freshly sprayed on them.

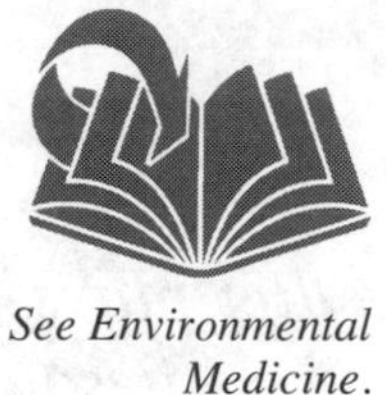

See Environmental Medicine.

"It seems like we've heard nothing but bad news about foods for the past few years," writes Steinman.[1] "Sometimes it seems that nothing is safe to eat, and that we live in a constant state of food anxiety . . . but you must not feel helpless. There is plenty of safe, delicious food to eat. And for your own well-being you need to find it."

Although many believe that the first step toward a healthy diet is knowing what to eat, it is more important to know what to avoid. Some areas of concern are:

Pesticides: Over four hundred pesticides are currently licensed for use on America's foods, and every year over 2.5 billion pounds are dumped on crop lands, forests, lawns, and fields. According to Steinman, a person gets several types of pesticides with a salad, different ones in meat or fish, still others in the vegetables on the side, and a separate dose with dessert. Wine has pesticides and, in many areas, water as well. In a single meal a person would easily consume residues of a dozen different neurotoxic or carcinogenic chemicals.

Yet, the Environmental Protection Agency's (EPA) Office of Pesticide Programs does not include the potential exposure to the same pesticide when calculating permitted residue levels of a given compound on a single crop. The agency sets these levels with "blinders" to the fact that people eat more than one product that has permitted residues of the same compound. EPA scientists have found that at times these residues, if totaled, exceeded 500 percent of the allowed daily intake.[2]

"Over four hundred pesticides are currently licensed for use on America's foods, and every year over 2.5 billion pounds are dumped on crop lands, forests, lawns, and fields."

Furthermore, many chemicals in food have not been adequately tested for human safety. And they have certainly not been tested with the "chemical cocktail syndrome" (multiple chemical exposure) in mind. The EPA does not have a scientifically acceptable method for determining the risk for multiple chemical exposure. Yet when scientists have done studies on multiple chemical exposure, it seems quite clear that the chemicals act synergistically. In one 1976 study, a scientific team used three chemicals on a group of rats. The chemicals were tested one at a time on the rats without ill-effect. When the scientists gave the rats two at a time, a decline in health was noted. When the rats were given all three chemicals at once, they all died within two weeks.[3]

Additives: Approximately two thousand food additives—artificial colors, artificial flavors, stabilizing agents, texturizers, sweeteners, antimicrobials, and antioxidants—are currently permitted in America's

TOP TEN FOOD ADDITIVES TO AVOID

Aspartame: *This chemical sweetener has the longest list of complaints the FDA (Food and Drug Administration) has ever received—over three thousand. Aspartame also goes under such brands as NutraSweet® and Equal®. Symptoms associated with aspartame sensitivity can range from rashes, mild depression, headaches, nausea, ringing ears, vertigo, and insomnia to loss of motor control, loss or change of taste, slurred speech, memory loss, blurred vision, blindness, suicidal depression, and seizures.[4] Many doctors now warn pregnant women to avoid any products containing aspartame.*

Brominated vegetable oil (BVO): *A potentially dangerous additive for some persons, BVO is used as an emulsifier in some foods and as a clouding agent in many popular soft drinks. Bromate, the main ingredient of BVO, is a poison. Just two to four ounces of a 2 percent solution of BVO can severely poison a child.[5]*

Butylated hydroxyanisole (BHA) and butylated hydroxytoluene (BHT): *Used to prevent fats, oils, and fat-containing foods from becoming rancid, BHA or BHT is often also added to food packaging materials. Researchers report that BHA in the diet of pregnant mice results in brain enzyme changes in their offspring including a 50 percent decreased activity in brain cholinesterase, which is responsible for the transmission of nerve impulses. BHA and BHT also affect the animals' sleep, levels of aggression, and weight. The authors of the study speculate that BHA and BHT can affect the normal sequence of neurological development in young animals too. Many consumers eat nearly twenty milligrams or more of BHA or BHT daily. Babies who are beginning to eat solid foods are estimated to ingest as much as eight milligrams per day.[6]*

Citrus Red Dye No. 2: *Used to color orange skins, Citrus Red Dye No. 2 is a probable carcinogen and may cause chromosomal damage. Some experts contend that this compound does not migrate from the organ skin into the pulp but the FDA has recommended a ban. Its continued use should be one more reason to seek organically grown foods.*

Monosodium glutamate: *Also known as MSG, monosodium glutamate is a flavor enhancer often found in fast food, processed food, and packaged food. Sensitivity symptoms include headaches, flushing of the skin, tightness of the chest, heart palpitations, and nausea.*

Nitrites: *Nitrites are used as preservatives in cured meats such as bacon, ham, and smoked fish to prevent spoilage. Nitrites form cancer-causing compounds known as nitrosamines in the gastrointestinal tract. They have been associated with human cancer and birth defects.[7]*

Saccharin: *Still widely used as an artificial sweetener, this additive is a possible human carcinogen. Every packet of Sweet 'n Low® has forty milligrams of saccharin. It is also used as a sweetener in soft drinks.*

Sulfur dioxide, sodium bisulfite, and sulfites: *These are used to preserve foods such as dried fruits to prevent them from drying and stiffening, and are also used on shrimp and frozen potatoes. The FDA has received hundreds of letters reporting adverse reactions in asthma sufferers who have consumed foods with sulfiting agents. At least four deaths caused by acute reactions to sulfites have been reported to the FDA.[8]*

Tertiary butyhydroquinone (TBHQ): *This chemical is often used along with BHA or BHT to spray the insides of cereal and cheese packages. TBHQ, which is toxic at extremely low doses, has been implicated in childhood behavioral problems. It is mainly found in candy bars, baking sprays, and fast foods.*

Yellow Dye No. 6: *Used in candy and carbonated beverages, Yellow Dye No. 6 increases the number of kidney and adrenal gland tumors in rats. It may also cause chromosomal damage as well as allergic reactions. It has been banned in Norway and Sweden.[9]*

food supply by the FDA. Yet studies show that some additives may be carcinogenic, such as Blue Dye No. 1, Blue Dye No. 2, and Green Dye No. 3, while others pose still different hazards. In 1981, researchers at the National Institutes of Health reported that Red Dye No. 3 may interfere with the neurotransmitters of the brain.[10] Meanwhile, aspirin-sensitive people have developed life-threatening asthmatic symptoms when ingesting Yellow Dye No. 5, which is found in breakfast cereal, bottled soft drinks, ice cream, sherbet, candy, bakery products, and pasta.[11]

Food additives can also have profound effects on behavior. Authorities at Tehama County Juvenile Hall in Red Bluff, California, had positive results in curbing antisocial behavior when they used honey in place of sugar and eliminated meats cured with nitrites and other foods with additives.[12] United States Naval Correction Center officials in Seattle, Washington, discovered that removing white bread and refined sugar from the diet of inmates reduced the incidence of violent behavior.[13]

In 1979, the New York City public schools ranked in the thirty-ninth percentile on standardized scholastic achievement test scores, meaning that 61 percent of the nation's public schools scored higher. That same year, the New York City Board of Education ordered a reduction of the sugar content of foods served in the schools and banned two synthetic food colorings. In 1980, New York's achievement test scores went up to the forty-seventh percentile. Next, the schools banned all synthetic colorings and flavorings. Test scores increased again, bringing New York City schools up to the fifty-first percentile. By 1983, when the additives BHA and BHT were removed from foods, New York City schools scored in the fifty-fifth percentile. Prior to the dietary changes, the academic performance of the students never varied more than 1 percent up or down in the course of a year.[14]

Irradiation: This process exposes food to radioactive materials like cesium-137 and cobalt-60 to kill insects, kill bacteria, kill molds, kill fungi, prevent sprouting, and extend shelf life. Irradiation may not be as dangerous as its harshest critics charge; however, this process leads to the formation of additional toxic substances in foods, including benzene and formaldehyde. Irradiation of foods may also have other hazardous consequences. For example, a study conducted by Ralston Scientific Services for the U.S. Army and the USDA (United States Department of Agriculture) found that mice fed a diet rich in irradiated chicken died earlier and had a higher incidence of tumors.[15]

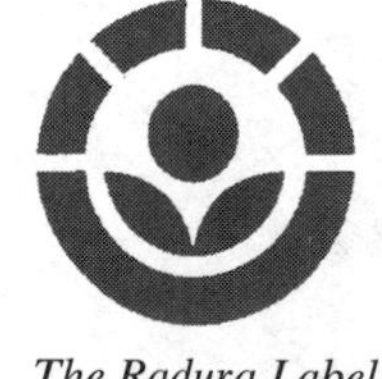

The Radura Label required on irradiated food by the U.S. FDA.

Furthermore, foods that have been irradiated lose much of their nutritional value. The vitamin C content of potatoes can be reduced by as much as 50 percent, according to a Japanese study.[16] In cooked pork, a dose of irradiation equal to one-third the level permitted by the FDA reduced thiamine levels by 17 percent.[17] Finally, irradiation plants pose hazards to workers as well as to the communities where they are located.

Unfortunately for consumers, while whole irradiated foods must be labeled with the flowerlike radura symbol, irradiated ingredients within foods are not identified. For example, commercially prepared spaghetti sauces may contain irradiated ingredients but not have to carry any warning.

Problems with Eating Red Meat

David Steinman reports that the combination of a high-fat diet and toxic overload may have a synergistic effect on human health. Fatty foods, he says, particularly red meat, can increase the toxicity of the chemicals that are lodged in them. In several animal studies, chemical carcinogens were more likely to produce tumors in the group that was fed fatty food than in the group fed low-fat foods.[18] Thus, a high-fat diet of animal foods can be especially troublesome because the most potent pesticides are concentrated in fat and the chemical properties of fat itself may actually increase their carcinogenicity.

Worldwide, a clear association consistently appears between the highest rates of breast, colon, and prostate cancers and nations that have the fattiest diets.[19] But the link between cancer and meat eaters' exposure to toxic chemicals goes even deeper. All fried and broiled foods contain mutagens, chemicals that can damage cellular reproductive material. But fried and broiled meats have far more mutagens than similarly prepared plant foods. One study indicates that some 20 percent of American meat eaters may have toxic mutagens in their digestive tracts that can be absorbed into the bloodstream where they can attack cells. The same study indicates that vegetarians are unlikely to have any mutagens in their digestive tracts.[20]

Fishing in Polluted Waters?

The industrial and agricultural pollution of the earth's rivers, lakes, and seas has led to widespread environmental contamination. Many of the most popular seafood dishes today are contaminated with pesticides and industrial chemicals that have been shown to cause cancer and birth defects. Industrial chemicals such as PCB's (polychlorinated biphenyls) and methyl mercury tend to accumulate in significant amounts in some fish and crustaceans.

Studies in Michigan indicate that PCB exposure during pregnancy causes a delay of the brain development in the infant, resulting in slower neuromuscular development, as well as causing decreased head

Safe Seafood

The shopping lists below and on the opposite page, compiled by David Steinman, author of Diet for a Poisoned Planet, *indicate the safest (i.e., green light) and the highest risk (i.e., red light) seafood choices.*

Green Light Seafood

Abalone
Arctic char
Crawfish
Dungeness crab
English Sole
Fish sticks
Flounder
Grouper
Haddock
Halibut
Mahimahi
Marlin
Octopus
Orange roughy
Pacific salmon (wild)
Red snapper
Scallops
Sea bass
Shrimp
Sole
Spiny lobster
Squid
Talapia
Tuna
Wahoo
Whiting
Yellowtail

HIGH RISK SEAFOOD

Red Light Seafood

Fish	Chemicals and Toxins Present
Bass (freshwater)	Dioxin, chlordane, DDT, dieldrin, PCB's
Black cod, also sold as California black cod, butterfish, and sablefish	DDT
Bluefish	PCB's, chlordane, DDT, dieldrin, HCB, nonachlor
Buffalo fish	Chlordane, DDT, dioxin, HCB, heptachlor, PCB's, mercury
Carp	PCB's, BHC, chlordane, DDT, dieldrin, dioxin, HCB, heptachlor
Catfish	BHC, chlordane, DDT, dieldrin, dioxin, heptachlor, PCB's, toxaphene
Caviar	Chlordane, DDT, PCB's
Chub	BHC, chlordane, DDT, dieldrin, dioxin,
Cod	DDT, PCB's
Coho salmon	BHC, chlordane, DDT, dieldrin, dioxin, HCB, heptachlor, PCB's
Croaker	Chlordane, DDT, dioxin, PCB's
Drum	DDT, dieldrin
Eel	BHC, chlordane, DDT, dieldrin, dioxin, HCB, heptachlor, PCB's
Great Lakes salmon	BHC, chlordane, DDT, dieldrin, dioxin, HCB, heptachlor, PCB's
Lake trout	Same as salmon
Maine lobster	PCB's
Mackerel	BHC, chlordane, DDT, HCB
Mullet	PCB's, DDT, dieldrin
Northern pike	Mercury
Norwegian salmon	BHC, lindane, PCB's
Ocean perchs	DDT, PCB's
Rock cod	DDT
Rockfish	DDT, PCB's
Sablefish	Same as black cod
Sea herring	BHC, chlordane, DDT, dieldrin, HCB, heptachlor, lindane, PCB's
Shark	DDT, PCB's, mercury
Sheepshead	BHC, chlordane, DDT, dieldrin, HCB, heptachlor, PCB's
Striped bass	PCB's, BHC, chlordane, DDT, dieldrin, HCB, nonachlor, mercury
Sturgeon	Same as striped bass, but no PCB's
Swordfish	Mercury, DDT, PCB's
Thresher shark	DDT, PCB's, mercury
Walleye	DDT, dioxin, PCB's, mercury
Weakfish	BHC, chlordane, DDT, dieldrin, HCB, nonachlor
White bass	BHC, see bass (freshwater)
White croaker	DDT, PCB's
Whitefish	Dioxin
White perch	DDT, dieldrin, dioxin, PCB's
Yellow perch	Dieldrin

BHC benzene hexachloride (hexachlorocyclohexane)
DDT chlorophenothane (dichlorodiphenyltrichloroethane)
PCB's polychlorinated biphenyls
HCB hexachlorobenzene

circumference, birth weight, and gestation period.[21] Such severe adverse birth defects were seen among infants whose mothers ate only two or three Great Lakes fish a month over several years, long before they ever considered the effects that such toxins could have on their pregnancies. Methyl mercury has also been shown to cause birth defects.

By rule, it is safest to avoid all freshwater fish, including farm-raised catfish, as well as swordfish and shark. Deep water fish such as red snapper, grouper, halibut, and flounder are generally safe.

Repetition versus Variety in the Diet

Nutritionist D. Lindsey Berkson, M.A., D.C., of Santa Fe, New Mexico, sees today's typical American diet as containing too few foods. "Unfortunately, most Americans tend to avoid variety and commit the dietary sin of monotony," she says, "eating the same foods meal after meal, only disguised by different names." They also consume food not according to what is best for them but according to what tastes best to them.

See Environmental Medicine.

According to Dr. Berkson, the American menu is actually made of various combinations of the same foods, usually wheat, beef, eggs, potatoes, and milk products. For example, she points out, a breakfast of eggs, sausage, white toast, and hash browns is the same as a lunch of a hamburger, white bun, and fries, which is the same as a dinner of steak and potatoes or white pasta. All of these meals, besides the fact that they are high-fat, high-calorie, low-fiber, and filled with toxins, are strikingly devoid of fruits and vegetables. They are also low in many of the essential nutrients. Such repetition can build deficiencies into the body.

The Dietary Guidelines for Americans (jointly issued by the Department of Agriculture and the Department of Health and Human Services) puts at the top of its dietary recommendations the suggestion that one "eat a variety of foods," in order to get the widest variety of nutrients.

Daily consumption of the same foods also tends to produce allergies and hypersensitivities to those foods, according to experts in environmental medicine. Instead of nourishing the body, these foods may start to act against it. Eating a varied diet minimizes these problems. The optimal diet should consist of more vegetables, fruits, and whole grains than any other foods.

The Whole Foods Diet

Both alternative and conventional medicine agree that Americans should consume far less fat, animal protein, and processed foods, and eat more complex carbohydrates, especially whole grains rich in fiber, and at least five servings daily of fruits and vegetables.

Buck Levin, Ph.D., R.D., Assistant Professor of Nutrition at Bastyr College in Seattle, Washington, offers a simple prescription for a healthy diet: one of natural, whole foods. "By whole foods we mean consuming a diet that is high in foods as whole as possible, with the least amount of processed, adulterated, fried, or sweetened additives," says Dr. Levin.

A whole foods diet is generously filled with a wide variety of different colored vegetables, fruits, and grains; raw seeds and nuts and their butters; beans; and fermented milk products such as yogurt and kefir; and fish, poultry, and bean products like tofu. It should also be lower in animal meats, fats, and cheeses as opposed to low-fat milk products.

A sense of balance is important in approaching one's diet. If the majority of meals are comprised of whole, fresh foods, then a little junk food, some alcoholic drinks, and a piece of candy here or there won't hurt. But when too few whole foods are consumed, as compared to "stressor" foods (those lacking in nutritional value), the body's physiology is damaged.

According to Buck Levin, Ph.D., "The average U.S. supermarket stocks over 24,000 items whose true 'natures' have often been drastically altered and ultimately devitalized."

Eating Lower on the Food Chain

While it is preferable that a whole foods diet be as plant-based as possible, it may not be necessary to become a complete vegetarian, eliminating meats and other animal foods from the diet totally. Today, many kinds of dairy products are completely fat-free, and many kinds of animal foods are low in fat. Even so, meats and other animal products should be eaten as a specialty rather than a staple, to add variety to one's diet once or twice a week. Always choose the leanest meats possible, as this will cut down effectively on calories, weight gain, and toxic exposure.

"Medical and scientific evidence points to the benefits of moving toward a vegetarian-based diet . . . In 1988, the American Dietetic Association published research showing a vegetarian lifestyle reduces the risk of heart disease, diabetes, colon cancer, hypertension, obesity, osteoporosis, and diverticular disease."

There are many reasons to stick to a more plant-based diet. First, important antioxidant nutrients including vitamin C, beta-carotene, vitamin E, and many cancer-fighting substances known as phytochemicals, are found in fruits, vegetables, and grains. These antioxidant nutrients are considered the best protection against age- and environmental-related diseases, from dandruff, bad breath, and wrinkling to cataracts, cancer, diabetes, and heart attacks. In many studies, vitamin A has been associated with increased immune response.[22]

Also, the high-fiber content of plant foods helps keep the digestive tract clean by absorbing and eliminating many potentially dangerous toxins. Plant foods also tend to have a lower toxicity than animal foods to begin with, because they are lower on the food chain, and as such have had less exposure to accumulating toxins.

Medical and scientific evidence also points to the benefits of moving toward a vegetarian-based diet. Dean Ornish, M.D., of the University of California at San Francisco, demonstrates that a diet free of animal protein, along with exercise and stress-reduction measures, can actually reverse heart disease.[23] James Anderson, M.D., has brought Type II diabetics off of insulin with a vegetarian diet. In 1988 the American Dietetic Association published research showing that a vegetarian lifestyle reduces the risk of heart disease, diabetes, colon cancer, hypertension, obesity, osteoporosis, and diverticular disease.[24]

Benefits of a Whole Foods Diet

According to Dr. Levin, a whole foods diet promotes health by decreasing fat and sugar intake and increasing fiber and nutrient intake. Ideally, it means more satisfaction and less overeating.

More Fiber: Most animal products, like meat, cheese, milk, eggs, and butter contain no fiber, compared to brown rice, broccoli, oatmeal, or almonds which have from six to fifteen grams per serving. Fiber is the transport system of the digestive tract, moving food wastes out of the body before they have a chance to form potentially cancer-causing and mutagenic chemicals. These toxic chemicals can cause colon cancer or pass through the gastrointestinal membrane into the bloodstream and damage other cells.

Less Fat: On a percentage-of-calories basis, most vegetables contain less than 10 percent fat, and most grains contain from 16 to 20 percent fat. By comparison, whole milk and

Stressor Foods

A whole foods diet is low in "stressor" foods. Stressor foods are those foods that rob the body rather than nourish it. Examples of stressor foods are refined sugars, commercial cola, refined grain flours and pastas, processed fats, hydrogenated fats, such as margarine, and deep fried foods. These foods can disturb the physiology of the body. For example, hydrogenated fats contain trans-fatty acids that inhibit normal essential fatty acid metabolism, and may negatively affect liver function and blood fat levels. Refined sugars, when consumed in excess, decrease immune functioning, increase risk of heart disease and obesity, promote dental decay, aggravate hyperactive behavior in some children, and provide no nutritional value at all. Commercial colas are high in phosphates that deplete the body of calcium and, when consumed daily, put women at risk of osteoporosis (excessive calcification of bones causing spontaneous fractures and marblelike appearance).

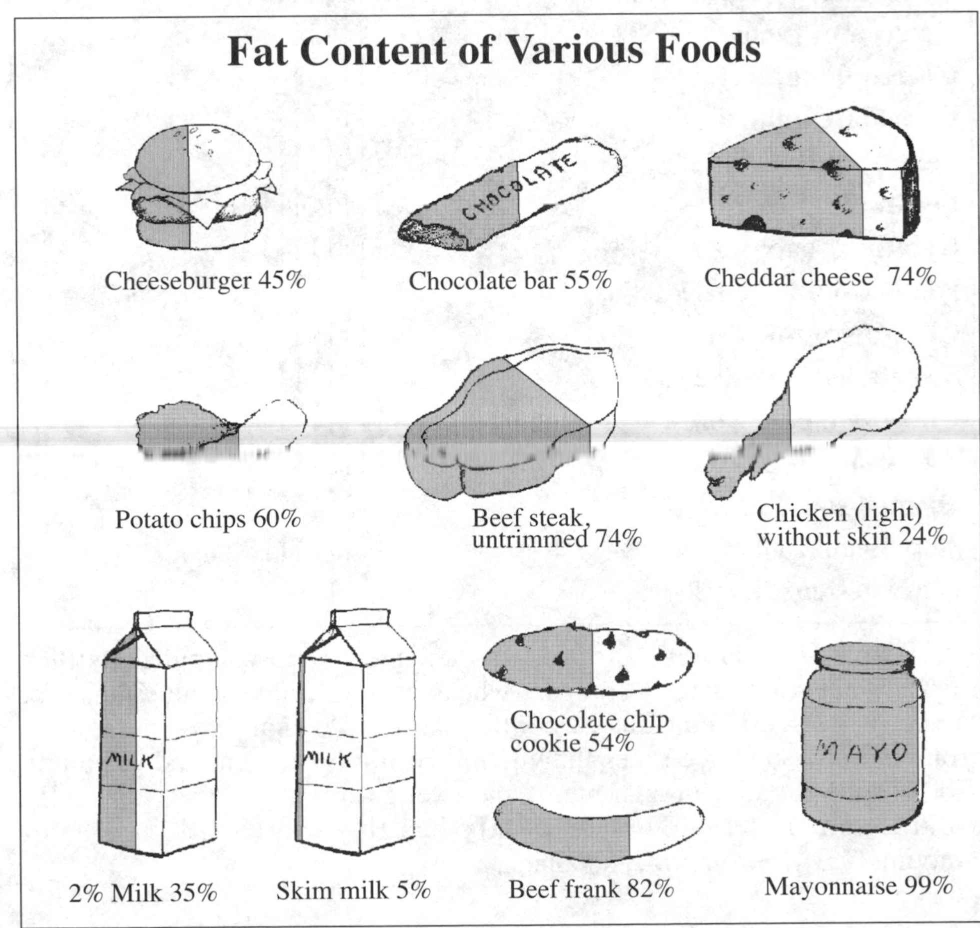

cheese contain 74 percent fat. A rib roast is 75 percent fat, and eggs are 64 percent fat. Low-fat milk or a skinned, baked chicken breast still has 38 percent fat. Not only do animal foods have more fat, but most of these fats are saturated fats, which research has shown to raise blood cholesterol levels. In addition, a lower fat, whole foods diet means fewer calories, since an ounce of fat contains twice as many calories as an ounce of complex carbohydrates. Studies have shown that a diet containing fewer calories can increase health and extend life.[25]

Labels can be very deceiving and misleading. The fat content of some of the foods on the previous page may be surprising.

Decreased Sugar Consumption: Eating a diet high in natural complex carbohydrates tends to be more filling, and decreases the desire to consume processed sugars. Lower sugar consumption also decreases overall food intake.

As with fat, sugar is a hidden and unwelcome ingredient in many processed foods. Here is a list of some of the culprits.

Sugar Content of Various Foods *(spoons of sugar per serving)*	
Pork and beans, 1 cup	5
Fruit yogurt, 8 oz.	8
Cola, 16 oz.	12
Chocolate cake, iced, 4 oz.	10
Ice cream, 1 cup	6
Glazed doughnut	6
Chocolate milk, 8 oz.	6
Peanut butter and jelly sandwich	7
Pecan pie, 5 oz.	12
Gelatin, 1 cup	8
Kool-Aid®, sweetened, 8 oz.	6
Chewing gum, 7 sticks	4
Sweetened cereal, 2 oz.	7
Chocolate bar, 2 oz.	7
Thick shake, 11 oz.	9
Orange soda, 12 oz.	12
Jelly beans, a handful	8
Liqueurs/cordials, 2 oz.	4

More Nutrients: Plant foods are richer sources of nutrients than their animal counterparts. Compare wheat germ to round steak. Ounce for ounce, wheat germ contains twice the vitamin B_2, vitamin K, potassium, iron, and copper; three times the vitamin B_6, molybdenum, and selenium; fifteen times as much magnesium; and over twenty times the vitamin B_1, folate, and inositol. The steak only has three nutrients in greater amounts—B_{12}, chromium, and zinc.

Increased Variation: A greater variety of vegetables also exposes the consumer to, literally, more colorful foods—red beets, chard, yellow squash, red peppers, cabbage. "This is more important than you may have imagined," says Dr. Berkson. "Variations in color are due to various minerals, vitamins, and other nutrients that perform important health-promoting functions in the human body."

More Food Satisfaction and Less Overeating: Foods such as vegetables, whole grains, and beans that are dense in nutrients and fiber require more eating (chewing) time and result in consumption of fewer calories. Eating whole foods makes a person satisfied more quickly which means he or she eats less. Eating less is associated with longevity and optimal health.[26]

MAKING THE TRANSITION TO A WHOLE FOODS DIET

Eating better means living better. The types of dietary changes that you make should not be threatening, limiting, or difficult to live with. Most Americans were raised eating meat and the transition to a vegetarian-oriented, whole foods diet may seem daunting. However, this change may be easier and more pleasurable than imagined and, considering the enormous health benefits, is worth it. Here are some tips:

***Eat more high protein plant foods** like grains, legumes, nuts, and seeds.*

***When dining out, try more exotic, foreign vegetarian foods.** Most ethnic restaurants—Indian, Chinese, Thai, Japanese, Mexican, Latin American, African, Middle Eastern—offer wonderful dishes with vegetables and grains. You can also prepare many of these at home.*

Experiment with spices and seasonings. For secrets to the exotic flavors found in vegetarian cooking, pick up several vegetarian or ethnic cookbooks. Get creative and invite friends to a buffet.

***Choose range-fed, hormone-free, additive-free meats** available at health food stores and quality markets.*

***Don't be rigid about your diet.** Allow yourself some meat and dairy. Move toward a whole foods diet gradually. "Don't become so worried about your diet that it becomes a burden," says D. Lindsey Berkson, M.A., D.C., of Santa Fe, New Mexico. "It is not what you eat once in a while that builds your optimal body but what you eat most of the time."*

***Achieve rhythm in your diet.** As important as what you eat is how and when you eat, adds Dr. Berkson. Eating regularly provides your body with a consistent intake of nutrients and avoids the stress associated with not knowing when your next meal will come or of going all day without food and then overeating in the evening.*

Exploring Your Biochemical Individuality

"Whether a food—even one that is whole and natural—acts to irritate or nourish your body depends largely," says Dr. Levin, "on your biological makeup." Each person is a unique product of genetics and environment. Roger Williams, Ph.D., a pioneering biochemist, referred to this concept as "biochemical individuality." One may have a genetic tendency to produce insufficient lactase—an enzyme required to break down the sugar (lactose) found in cow's milk. On the other hand, years of eating highly processed foods may render a person very chemically sensitive. For adults, stress and high-fat eating may cause an ulcer.

"Dietary needs are different for each of us, and in order to develop your ideal diet, you will need to explore your own biochemical individuality," says Dr. Levin. To do this he advises the following steps:

- **Take tests:** Many clinical tests are available to identify aspects of your biochemical nature:
  ELISA (Enzyme-Linked Immunosorbent Assay) is a commonly used test for determining food allergies that rates foods according to the intensity of the body's allergic reaction to them.
  A breath hydrogen test can help determine how effectively the body breaks down carbohydrates.
  A Heidelberg analysis can tell if the stomach acid level is within normal range.

See Detoxification Therapy, Fasting, Juice Therapy.

- **Have a nutritional assessment:** The assessment of nutritional deficiencies should be based on symptoms, physical manifestations, and genetic predispositions and performed by a qualified nutritional practitioner. The early stages of nutritional deficiencies are almost never detectable by conventional lab tests.

  Once you've reached initial conclusions about your own biochemical makeup, a nutritionist can help you develop a food plan to meet your specific needs. Most nutritionists use a computerized nutritional analysis to target your goals. Although the nutritionist you select need not be a registered dietitian, he or she should be licensed or certified by your state.
- **Monitor your food habits:** Keep a detailed record of what you eat, and pay close attention to the physiological results. When exploring food allergies, elimination and rotation diets can be extremely helpful.

Therapeutic Diets

When working with a qualified health professional and approaching specific health problems, diet takes on renewed importance that requires new understanding. During the therapeutic process, a dietary program can be divided into three parts, according to Dr. Berkson: the initial program is usually the most strict; the modified program is more lenient as health improves; and once optimal health is reached, the maintenance program is designed to maintain good habits and proper nutrition. After initiating a nutritional program, if a person gets worse, does not obtain results, or becomes nauseated, the most common cause is not the program itself, but due to the person's need for a bowel cleansing or rejuvenation program first, says Dr. Berkson.

The severity of the body's condition and health will influence how long one remains in each of the three dietary phases. It is important to recognize that healing occurs in stages and dietary practices differ at each stage.

Special Healing Foods

See Detoxification Therapy, Fasting, Juice Therapy.

All whole, natural foods have regenerative and restorative powers, says Dr. Levin. Indeed, meeting the health needs of the body is the aim of a balanced diet. Some foods, however, are unusually rich in nutrients and contain unique chemical components.

Garlic: This member of the lily family has well-documented health effects, including reduction of serum cholesterol and triglycerides, prevention of clot formation, reduction of blood pressure, and enhancement of immune capacity through stimulation of natural killer cell activity. Garlic has sulfur-rich compounds—allin and allicin, chromium, phosphorus, and sulfur-containing amino acids. Raw garlic swallowed in small pieces with water, like tablets, is a great flu remedy, or its cloves can be whole roasted and brushed lightly with oil. If you are worried about bad breath, chew a sprig of parsley.

Ginger: The roots of this reedlike plant contain compounds called *gingerols* and *shogaols* which relax the intestinal tract, prevent motion sickness, and relieve nausea and vomiting (especially during pregnancy). Ginger is an excellent source of minerals, especially manganese. Ginger ale can be a delicious bottled form of this food. Buy only natural brands at health food stores and avoid the overprocessed, sugar-sweetened, grocery store brands. A word of caution: ginger can aggravate problems associated with elevated estrogen levels in women.

Blackstrap Molasses: Drop for drop, it contains more calcium than milk, more iron than beef, and more potassium than bananas. It's easily used as a sugar substitute or eaten in place of jam and jelly.

Yeasts: These single-celled organisms contain high concentrations of B vitamins and many minerals including chromium, one of the key longevity nutrients. Yeasts can be purchased in dried form and sprinkled on top of many foods. Baker's, brewer's, and torula yeast are the three forms of "nutritional" yeasts most commonly available. Do not eat yeast or yeast products if you have candidiasis, the overgrowth of a naturally occuring fungus (*Candida albicans*) that may occur when the immune system is weakened. (This may contribute to other immune deficiency health conditions such as chronic fatigue syndrome).

Fermented Foods: Cheese, yogurt, buttermilk, sauerkraut, and beer are familiar examples of fermented foods. These foods are processed with enzymes from bacteria, yeasts, and molds that create gradual chemical changes in the structure of the foods. Fermented foods aid in digestion and balance bacterial populations in the gut. They also have a naturally long shelf life, and retain their vitamin content much longer than nonfermented foods.

See Candidiasis, Chronic Fatigue Syndrome, Herbal Medicine.

Raw Foods: While raw foods have a greater risk of contamination by microorganisms than cooked foods, this risk is minimal with high-quality foods, and is more than offset by the gain in nutrients and enzymes which would otherwise be lost in cooking. Also, high-fiber raw foods have water-absorbing properties which make them especially effective in absorbing digestive juices from the gastrointestinal tract, thus helping to regulate the digestive process. None of these benefits are possible though, unless the raw foods are well chewed.

Raw Juice: There is no better way to get the high-level nutrients from fresh, organic vegetables than to run them through a juicer. The bioflavonoids in the pulp of your peppers, for example, will be in the juice along with the vitamin C. Experiment with different combinations like parsley, spinach, and cucumber; or carrot, celery, and beet. Add fresh garlic and ginger for an immune boost.

Controversial Foods

While often touted by special interest groups, the safety of the following foods has been called into question.

Sucrose: The classic position on sugar is that its only harmful effects are obesity and dental cavities. But a substantial body of research suggests a correlation between high sugar intake and a variety of health problems such as colitis, mood swings, gallbladder disease, heart disease, childhood and adult hyperactivity, ulcers, immune responsiveness, effects on hunger mechanisms,[27] overeating, and even susceptibility to addictive behaviors such as excessive alcohol intake.

Milk: Milk has traditionally been viewed as just about the most perfect food—especially for children. However, more recently experts have begun to question the safety of milk—especially for children. Dr. Benjamin Spock, the world-famous child care expert, shocked the nation by appearing at a press conference in 1992 warning parents about the dangers of milk.[28]

According to the Physicians Committee for Responsible Medicine (PCRM), milk may cause diabetes, ovarian cancer, cataracts, iron deficiency, and allergies in both children and adults.[29] Additional medical research associates milk consumption with greater frequency of cancer of the lymph system.[30]

The statements of the PCRM may have some merit but much more research will be required for a final verdict. Until then, keep these safe eating guidelines in mind:[31]

- Breast milk is best for babies. Efficient breast pumps can be rented from hospitals to extract breast milk and make life easier for working mothers.
- Mothers who are breast-feeding infants whose siblings or parents had childhood diabetes should avoid drinking large amounts of cow's milk as some proteins from the cow's milk that can trigger this condition can be absorbed into their breast milk.
- Adults and children over the age of two should drink only skim or 1 percent low-fat milk.
- Those who suffer from recurring bouts of diarrhea, bronchitis, eczema, asthma, or runny nose, should be tested for a milk allergy.
- People who get gas, diarrhea, or cramps after drinking milk, should drink it in smaller quantities with meals, switch to a lactose-reduced milk, or try lactose pills (containing a key enzyme for digesting milk).

In addition, whole milk and whole dairy products like ice cream and cheese contain concentrated fat-soluble pesticides that have been shown to cause cancer in laboratory animals. They can also contain sulfa drugs and antibiotics as a result of mixing milk from healthy cows with the milk from ill or medicated cows. For protection against toxins in dairy products, rely on nonfat dairy products.

Another option is milk substitutes such as soy, almond, rice, or even goat's milk. Health food stores and many supermarkets sell these products, which are frequently made with organic (pesticide-free) ingredients.

Butter and Margarine: Many medical experts today are concerned about the safety of margarine because of its high content of hydrogenated oils. Hydrogenation is a process that turns liquid oils into semi-solid globules. This process artificially alters the chemical structure of the fatty acids in the product. Hydrogenated oils are also called trans-fatty acids. They are most often found in shortenings, cakes, crackers, cookies, french fries, and chips. They tend to act like saturated animal fats in the human body by raising cholesterol. Of margarines, the diet or whipped types have the fewest trans-fatty acids.

Butter, on the other hand, contains both saturated fat and, like other fatty dairy products, a whole host of carcinogenic pesticides and chemicals. Because neither butter nor margarine present a clear-cut option, it is best to use them in moderation, and find substitutes whenever possible.

The Whole Oil Story

There are three types of fats, or lipids, which are differentiated by their chemical makeup: saturated, monounsaturated, and polyunsaturated. The human body needs a certain amount of each of these lipids for its proper function. Common fats and oils have components of all of these lipids. For example, canola oil is made up of 62 percent monounsaturated fat, 32 percent polyunsaturated fat, and 6 percent saturated fat.

Saturated Fats: These are primarily found in animal foods and tropical oils such as coconut and palm oil. Due to their chemical structure, saturated fats tend to remain solid at room temperature. Though there is tremendous evidence that appears to support the relationship between high fat intake from animal sources and heart disease, some amount of saturated fat in the diet is necessary. Saturated fat is needed for the liver's production of cholesterol, an important component in the structure of cell membranes. In addition, stearic acid, one of the most common saturated animals fats, has been shown in some studies to be beneficial in fighting cardiovascular disease.[32]

Monounsaturated Fats: Monounsaturated fats are considered healthier than polyunsaturated fats because of their ability to lower LDL (commonly called bad) cholesterol while maintaining or raising HDL (or good) cholesterol. Canola oil and olive oil are naturally high in monounsaturated fats.

Although the evidence is not ironclad, a study published in the *Journal of the American Medical Association* surveyed 4,900 Italian men and women, whose ages ranged from twenty to fifty-nine, and found that those people who had a diet high in olive oil and low in butter and margarine also had lower overall levels of cholesterol and blood pressure than people whose diets included more butter and margarine.[33]

Polyunsaturated Fats: Plentiful in safflower, sunflower, and corn oil, polyunsaturated fats contain both omega-6 and omega-3 essential fatty acids (EFA's). Omega-6 is beneficial when a person is injured, causing blood to clot and blood vessels to constrict. In contrast, omega-3 inhibits harmful clotting, relaxes vascular smooth muscle, and has an anti-arrhythmic effect, reducing the risk of heart disease.

Humans evolved on a diet that contained small but roughly equal amounts of omega-6 and omega-3 fatty acids. Then, about one hundred years ago, the food supply began to change. The vegetable oil industry began to hydrogenate oil, which reduced the oil's omega-3 content. At the same time, the domestic livestock industry began to use feed grains, which happen to be rich in omega-6 fatty acid and low in omega-3's. As a result, the American diet now has an EFA ratio of 20-25:1 omega-6 to omega-3, rather than the 1:1 ratio with which humans evolved.[34] The modern diet is too high in omega-6's, which may contribute to heart disease.

There are many foods that can boost the intake of omega-3 essential fatty acids. Fish is a good source, as well as beans—especially Great

Northern, kidney, navy, and soy beans.[35] In oils, omega-3 is most abundant in flaxseed, but there is also canola oil with a 10 percent omega-3 content,[36] and soy, pumpkin seed, evening primrose, borage seed, walnut, and black currant oils.

Some of the symptoms of an omega-3 fatty acid deficiency include increased allergies, dry hair and skin, brittle nails, acne, eczema, rashes, or tiny lumps on the backs of your arms. To find out if any of these symptoms might be related to a lack of omega-3 in the diet, take a teaspoon or two daily of pure flaxseed (linseed) oil, the vegetable oil richest in omega-3 fatty acids, and see if symptoms diminish.

High temperature cooking, such as frying, destroys the EFA content of certain oils. Oils such as flaxseed and walnut should only be used for baking, and in soups and salads. When frying foods, use the more heat stable oils—canola, avocado, peanut, and olive.

Hydrogenated Oil: Many processed foods contain "partially hydrogenated oil" as an ingredient. Hydrogenated oils contain man-made molecules called trans-fatty acids, which may interfere with normal metabolic functions due to their unusual molecular shape. The natural form of fatty acids, called the *cis* form, has a molecular shape that is biochemically suited for human health. According to John R. Lee, M.D., of Sebastopol, California, "Trans-fatty acids enter our metabolic processes but are defective for our bodily uses. Our cell membranes, our hormone synthesis, our immune system, our ability to deal with inflammation and to heal, and many, many other vital systems all become defective when trans-fatty acids substitute for the health-giving cis fatty acids. Unknowingly, we are poisoning ourselves."

Many processed food products contain these hydrogenated oils. However, in the United states, the exact amount of trans-fatty acids in a product is not required to be listed on the label of the product. As Dr. Lee points out, "Other countries, such as Canada, are more enlightened; food labeling there now requires that the included fats be measured and identified in terms of cis or trans forms." For better nutrition, he advises, "Choose butter over margarine; olive oil and flaxseed oils over the many processed oils on the supermarket shelves; fresh vegetables over canned or otherwise processed ones; and learn to read labels."

Oxidized Oils: When oils are overheated and used for too long, as is the case with the cooking oils at fast food restaurants, they become oxidized. Oxidized oils are loaded with oxygen-damaging free radicals, according to Bernhard Hennig, Ph.D., R.D., of the Department of Nutrition and Food Science, College of Human Environmental Sciences, University of Kentucky.[37] To counteract the dangers of free radicals, Dr. Lee advises taking vitamin and mineral supplements. "Protect your metabolic processes and cell membranes with antioxidants such as vitamins C, A (or beta-carotene), and E, plus the mineral antioxidant, selenium," he says.

At the Market

Choosing the ingredients for an ideal diet in today's marketplace requires a healthy dose of skepticism, diligence, and a certain amount of fortitude to resist slipping into old convenience patterns. But all the improvements you make in your food choices will pay off in better health for you and your family.

Nutritionists recommend that you adopt a dual shopping strategy, buying some foods at major supermarkets and other foods at health food stores, obtaining the best from both. Consider these guidelines:

- **Read labels**. The cover of the package is the last place one is apt to find the truth about a product. Bold statements like "100% Natural" or "98% Fat-Free" might be legal, but deceiving. Go directly to the ingredient list and nutritional analysis. Fortunately, new labeling regulations will mean better and more accurate information for consumers.
- **Think starchy foods and complex carbohydrates.** The "main dish" approach centering on protein and a high-fat sauce is out. Replace those meat loafs and baby back pork ribs with whole grains and whole grain pastas, beans, and fresh vegetables.
- **Shop at your local health food store.** Here the emphasis is on quality and health. On the other hand, not all fresh fruits and vegetables sold in the health food store are organic. Look for labels that identify organically grown foods.
- **Buy organic foods.** Organic farming is a system of food cultivation that doesn't use artificial fertilizers, pesticides, herbicides, growth regulators, and livestock feed additives. Crop rotations, crop residues, animal manures, green manures, legumes, organic wastes, mineral-bearing rock, and biological pest controls are used by organic farmers to raise whole, natural foods. If you cannot buy all organic produce, buy the organic produce that substitutes for the most pesticide-contaminated crops such as apples, and buy the nonorganic fruits and vegetables that tend to be free from pesticides. For example, supermarket produce like bananas, pineapple, watermelon, and citrus foods, including oranges and tangerines, tends to be relatively pesticide free.
- **Buy seasonal foods.** By definition, foods grown out of season must be treated or manipulated to grow. Perhaps they were grown in greenhouse environments, with artificial lights, or induced to grow through chemical treatment. Often, the foods are imported from Third World nations where pesticides, banned in the United States, continue to be used, poisoning the food, the land, and farm workers. In-season foods are healthier, more abundant, and less expensive.
- **Eat colorfully.** Instead of being concerned with getting all the "right" vitamins and minerals in the most perfect ratios, Dr. Berkson suggests focusing on eating a colorful diet. By making an effort to get at least three different colored vegetables or fruits at both lunch and dinner, you will insure the best exposure to appropriate nutrients.

In the Kitchen

By its very nature, food has limitations. It needs to be stored and prepared with care. Overcooking vegetables can cut their vitamin B_1 content in half and destroy their enzyme content. Exposing milk to light can do the same thing to its B_2 content.

Cleaning and Storing Your Foods

Thoroughly wash produce in cold water, preferably filtered, says Dr. Levin. Use a vegetable brush with natural bristles to scrub the skins of sturdier vegetables to remove dirt and any residual surface toxins, but don't remove the skins as they contain vital nutrients.

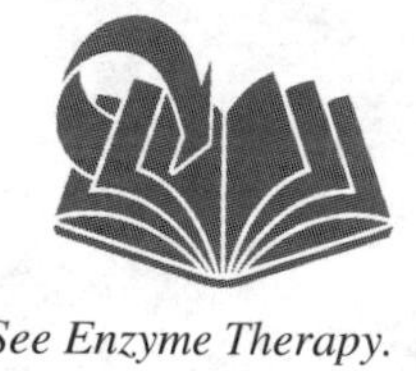

See Enzyme Therapy.

The main vitamin thieves in your kitchen are heat, air, and light. Vitamins A, B complex, C, and D are susceptible to damage by UV light. Vitamin E is damaged by oxygen. In general, the less exposure your food has to air, light, and heat, the better. Garlic, onions, potatoes, carrots, beets, and other root vegetables store well in cool, dark, dry places. Spices hold up well under refrigeration or even in the freezer, especially if purchased in large quantities and used over a period of months. Purchasing spices in whole seed form and then grinding with a mortar and pestle when ready for use is highly recommended. Better yet, grow your own. Parsley, basil, oregano, and thyme grow well on the windowsill in small pots and will provide fresh spices every night. Oils tend to store best under refrigeration, and dark glass containers are recommended to minimize exposure of fat-soluble vitamins to light.

Choosing Cookware

Glass (or Pyrex®), ceramics (including clay, terra-cotta, enamel, and porcelain), cast iron, and stainless steel should head your list for cookware materials. At the bottom of the list should be aluminum, plastic, and cookware featuring synthetic nonstick surfaces. According to Dr. Levin, here's why:

- Glass is your best choice. It does not interact with the food prepared in it and works well in the refrigerator, in the freezer, on the stove top, in the oven, and with the microwave.
- Ceramics are porcelain-covered metals, like cast iron, that combine the excellent heating capacities of metal with the friendly cooking surface of porcelain. Clay or "earthenware" pots are excellent for oven baking, but be careful about the glazes. Some contain lead or cadmium, both known to be hazardous.
- Cast iron is heavy, and requires the extra step of curing. (To cure cast iron, wash in hot, soapy water, rinse, towel dry, rub with refined oil, and place in an oven preheated to 300 degrees for three hours.) In exchange for the extra weight and care, your cast iron cookware may help prevent you from becoming anemic. One-half cup of spaghetti sauce prepared in a stainless steel skillet will provide you with less than one milligram of iron. Prepared in a cast iron skillet, the same sauce gives you six milligrams.
- Stainless steel adds neither the positive nutrient value to cooking

food that cast iron does, nor does it add any of the negative elements found in aluminum or plastic. However, stainless steel offers the chef an excellent and easy cooking surface along with hassle-free cleaning.

- Aluminum cookware can release traces of aluminum into the food which may make their way into the bone matrix, and may create changes in cognitive functioning.[38] Exactly how much aluminum is able to migrate from aluminum cookware into your food? Studies have shown that foods cooked in aluminum pans can pick up the element, but the quantity is disputable.[39] This debate is particularly fierce with respect to anodized aluminum. Anodized cookware is constructed of aluminum which has been placed in an electrolytic solution and subjected to an electrical current which changes its molecular structure. This process seals the pores of the aluminum and lessens—and some say eliminates—its interaction with food. In conclusion, there's at least a question mark associated with aluminum and its stability in cookware.
- Plastics for food preparation, particularly in the microwave, are controversial at best and they could be dangerous, as many of the resins used in plastics are cancer-causing substances. Molecules from polyvinyl chloride (PVC), polyethylene (PE), polyvinylidene chloride (PVDC), and plasticizers like di- (2-ethylhexyl) adipate (DEHA) in plastic wraps have been conclusively shown to migrate into foods at the high temperatures achieved in microwave ovens. The worst culprit in this regard is cyclic polyethylene terephthalate (PET) trimmer—the thin, mirrorlike, grey stripping which absorbs microwave energy and is often used to make microwave pizza crusts brown and microwave popcorn crunchy. You'll want to avoid microwave cookware containing these materials. Stick with glass and unleaded ceramics instead.

MICROWAVING FOODS

A microwave oven cooks by generating heat in the food itself. It contains a magnetron tube which converts electricity into electromagnetic radiation. The food is not irradiated nor does it become radioactive. Microwaves tend to diminish the formation of nitrosamine chemicals that can be formed in cured meats such as bacon and ham.[40] If you intend to eat these meats, cooking them in the microwave may be better than baking in a conventional oven or frying.

Microwave oven radiation is not very powerful. It drops off quickly as one moves away from the appliance. Yet, medical science has uncovered disturbing news about the effects of microwave radiation on health—including eye damage and carcinogenic effects.

There may be another more disturbing side to this modern convenience. Microwaving may cause chemical changes in foods beyond those associated with being exposed to heat.[41] Researchers reporting in the journal The Lancet *discovered that microwaving infant formula for ten minutes alters the structure of its component amino acids, possibly resulting in functional, structural, and immunological abnormalities.[42]*

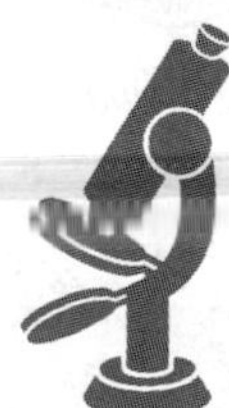

The results of studies that explore the immediate risks associated with food cooked in microwave ovens indicate the need for further research into the health risks of continuous microwave use.

Kitchen Cleansers

Many dishwashing liquids, bleaches, chlorinated scouring powders, all-purpose cleaners, and drain cleaners contain petrochemicals that do not belong in the kitchen. Nontoxic, environmentally safe alternatives are available in every category of cleanser and detergent. In general, look for products that are water-based, free of phosphates, biodegradable, and free of propellants. Baking soda makes an excellent scouring powder, and vinegar added to water can be used for cleaning windows.

Water and Water Filters

Drinking pure water is very important. It is also important to use pure water in the preparation and cleaning of food. Unfortunately, the public water supply is not always capable of providing optimally pure water. According to the Environmental Protection Agency, the tap water of 30 million people in the United States contains potentially hazardous levels of lead.[43] In addition, one out of every four public water systems has violated federal standards for tap water.[44]

America's water can contain many different contaminants, including pathogenic (disease-causing) bacteria, radioactive particles, heavy metals, industrial wastes, and chemical residues. Even chlorine and fluoride, intentionally added to public water supplies, are considered by many to pose a risk to health. While adding chlorine-type compounds to drinking water protects the public from several kinds of potentially deadly bacteria such as typhus, chlorine has been proven to form cancer-causing compounds in drinking water. Fluoride added to water to prevent tooth decay seems to also have negatives effects on the bones and even the teeth. Studies suggest that fluoride can cause mottling of the teeth[45] and can make bones more brittle in the elderly, leading to an increased rate of fracture.[46]

Drinking water containing lead can create health problems for both children and adults, including hypertension, mental deterioration, impotency, birth defects, and learning deficiencies. Unless a house has newer copper water lines, lead can leach out of the older water pipes and plumbing into the water.

In determining the quality of water in the home, ask the local water department for standards and analysis. It is also important to verify your home's water quality yourself. Easy-to-run tests usually cost about $100 and are worth every cent.

See sidebar on Fluoridation in Biological Dentistry chapter. See Osteoporosis.

Bottled water is also a viable alternative, but be careful about the source. Many waters are simply repackaged city supplies. Choose only those products that provide a full analysis of their contents upon request. Also, look for waters that have been purified through deionization. Many such brands are known as purified or distilled.

The best step is to buy a water filter. The cost can range from $150 for an under-the-sink model, combining carbon filtration with reverse osmosis, to $1,500 for a whole-house filter that will purify even the water for your shower. There are three basic types of filtration systems:

- **Solid block carbon filters** appear to be much more effective in removing organic chemicals such as solvents and trihalomethanes than do activated carbon filters, which use granulated or powdered carbon. If you prefer to leave dissolved minerals in your water, carbon block filters are a recommended choice since they do not remove these inorganic compounds.
- **Reverse osmosis systems** force water through a membrane under pressure. They are most effective against inorganic pollutants like nitrates, and against metals like lead. (Deionization resins are also used to accomplish this purpose.)
- **Distillation** purifies water by boiling and condensing it. Metals and inorganic compounds are effectively removed in this way because

they are heavier than the water, but all organic compounds are not heavier than water and they may not be removed from the supply.

The best systems combine several methods of filtration for optimal pollutant removal. Carbon block filtration combined with reverse osmosis units are effective against organic and inorganic pollutants, as are carbon block and distillation combinations.

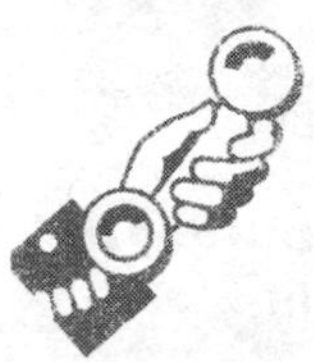

Where to Find Help

Educating yourself about healthier alternatives is the first step in the move toward an improved diet. The following list provides varied information, from where to find a naturopathic physician, to a list of organic food providers.

Locating a Nutritionist or Naturopathic Physician

American Association of Naturopathic Physicians
2366 Eastlake Avenue, Suite 322
Seattle, Washington 98102
(206) 323-7610

Contact them for the location of a licensed naturopathic physician in your area.

American College of Nutrition
722 Robert E. Lee Drive
Wilmington, North Carolina 28480
(919) 452-1222

A membership organization which produces a journal and newsletter. Annual meetings open to the general public. Provides lectures on nutrition research.

Food and Allergy Testing and Information

Doctor's Data, Inc.
P.O. Box 111
West Chicago, Illinois 60185
(800) 323-2784

Offers mineral and allergy testing.

Immuno Labs, Inc.
1620 West Oakland Park Boulevard
Fort Lauderdale, Florida 33311
(800) 231-9197

This laboratory specializes in allergy and immunological testing.

Meridian Valley Clinical Laboratory
24030 132nd Avenue S.E.
Kent, Washington 98042
(800) 234-6825

Offers a wide variety of specialized testing, including: micro-parasitology, allergies, food, essential fatty acid, and mineral and amino acid analysis.

MetaMatrix Medical Laboratory
5000 Peachtree Street Industrial Boulevard, Suite 110
Norcross, Georgia 30071
(800) 221-4640 (For doctors only)
(404) 446-5483

A full-service laboratory specializing in nutritional status, toxicology, and allergy testing.

Fighting Food Irradiation

Consumers United for Food Safety
P.O. Box 22928
Seattle, Washington 98122
(206) 747-2659

Contact them to find out more about the irradiation of food. The organization's newsletter, entitled The Food Activist, *provides updates on national developments in food irradiation.*

Learning More About Organics

International Federation of Organic Agriculture Movements
Okozentrum Imsbach
6695 Tholey-Theley, West Germany
011-49-6853-5190
011-49-6853-30110 (Fax)

This organization publishes a new journal, Ecology and Farming. *Write them for a subscription.*

The Organic Foods Production Association of North America
P.O. Box 1078
Greenfield, Massachusetts 01302
(413) 774-7511
(413) 774-6432 (Fax)

Publications and memberships are available.

Becoming Vegetarian and Cooking Vegetarian

Vegetarian Journal
Vegetarian Resource Group
P.O. Box 1463
Baltimore, Maryland 21203
(410) 366-8343

A nonprofit vegetarian resource group, whose main goal is to educate the public on health, nutrition, and environment.

Vegetarian Times
1140 Lake Street, Suite 500
Oak Park, Illinois 60301
(708) 848-8100

A glossy, color magazine that offers recipes as well as informative articles and the latest news in vegetarian lifestyles.

Exploring Nutrition and Politics

Community Nutrition Institute
2001 S Street N.W., Suite 530
Washington, D.C. 20009
(202) 462-4700

This organization focuses on consumer protection, food program development, and federal diet and health policies.

Food First/Institute for Food and Development Policy
145 9th Street
San Francisco, California 94103
(415) 864-8555

A nonprofit organization that investigates the root causes of hunger in a world of plenty. They survey and study social conditions and develop a profile of society through a "food window."

Physicians for Social Responsibility
1000 16th Street N.W., Suite 810
Washington, D.C. 20036
(202) 785-3777
(202) 785-3962 (Fax)

PSR is an organization of health professionals and concerned citizens committed to preventing nuclear war. They work to change public policy and to stop environmental degradation.

The Nutrition Action Health Letter
Center for Science in the Public Interest
1875 Connecticut Avenue Northwest, Suite 300
Washington D.C. 20009-5728
(202) 332-9111

A monthly newsletter published to educate the general public, covering all areas of dietary knowledge, studies, and statistics. Excellent reviews of books and recipes included.

Nutrition Week
2001 S Street Northwest
Washington, D.C. 20009
(202) 462-4700

This is an eight-page weekly covering legislation, regulations, and other developments regarding nutrition programs, food stamps, consumer issues, federal trade and environmental policies.

Food and Water Ecology

Natural Resources Defense Council
40 West 20th Street
New York, New York 10011
(212) 727-2700

An organization that attempts to steer America and Congress away from wasteful and destructive environmental policies. A nonprofit environmental law firm also concerned with public education.

Worldwatch Institute
1776 Massachusetts Avenue Northwest
Washington, D.C. 20036
(202) 452-1999

A nonprofit environmental research organization concerned with family planning, agriculture, national security, and the environment. They distribute a global publication on these issues.

Clean Water Action Project
1320 18th Street N.W., Suite 300
Washington, D.C. 20036
(202) 547-1196

A lobbying group that seeks to protect the environment. They are especially concerned with water, waste, sewage, pollution, and wildlife.

Earth Save
706 Frederick Street
Santa Cruz, California 95062
(408) 423-4069

A nonprofit organization that focuses on helping people realize how their diet affects the planet. Involved in several public education programs.

Greenpeace
1436 U Street Northwest
Washington, D.C. 20009
(202) 462-1177

An organization dedicated to monitoring and safeguarding the ecological soundness of the planet.

Pesticide Hotline
U.S. Environmental Protection Agency
NPTN Texas Tech University, Thompson Hall, Room S129
Lubbock, Texas 79430
(800) 858-7378

A telephone hotline open Monday-Friday, 8:00 A.M.-6:00 P.M. (EST) to answer questions on pesticides for the medical field, general public and veterinarians.

National Testing Laboratories
6555 Wilson Mills Road
Cleveland, Ohio 44143
(800) 458-3330
(216) 449-2525

A certified water testing facility, serving consumers, the beverage industry, and municipal customers. Call for laboratories in Michigan, Florida, and New Hampshire.

Watertest Corporation of America
28 Daniel Plummer Road
Gottstown, New Hampshire 03045
(800) 458-3330
(603) 623-1780

Socially Responsible Shopping

Seeds of Change
621 Old Santa Fe Trail, Suite 10
Santa Fe, New Mexico 87501
(505) 983-8956

An organic seed company that specializes in biodiversity. Their catalogue is available by mail or in certain health food stores.

Sources of Organically Grown, Hormone-Free, Nitrite-Free Meat and Poultry

Coleman Natural Beef. *Available at supermarkets throughout the United States including Grand Union stores in the New York City area as well as Purity Supreme in New England, A&P in New York and New Jersey, Bread & Circus in the Boston area, Big Y Foods in Massachusetts, and Farmer Jack stores in the Detroit, Michigan, area.*

Foster Farms *poultry is available in most supermarkets throughout the western U.S. Has a rigorous pesticide residue elimination program, screening all shipments of grain. Subtherapeutic doses of antibiotics and other drugs are not used.*

Holly Farms *poultry is available throughout the eastern and midwestern states. Has a rigorous residue elimination program. Subtherapeutic doses of antibiotics and other drugs are not used. Found in most supermarkets.*

Kohler Farms *of Wisconsin supplies hormone-free beef to supermarkets in Wisconsin and the Chicago area including Treasure Island. Look for the PURElean BEEF trademark.*

Larsen Beef, *produced without antibiotics or hormones, can be found in Kroger stores in Atlanta, Georgia, as well as King Kullen in Long Island, New York, Kash N Karry in the Tampa and Orlando, Florida areas and Dominicks in the Chicago area.*

Laura's Lean Beef, *produced without hormones, is available at Kroger stores in Kentucky and Southern Indiana.*

Maverick Ranch Lite Beef *is produced without hormones or antibiotics and is lab tested for pesticide residues. Available at King Super markets in Denver, Colorado, Schnucks in Saint Louis, Missouri, Kings Supermarkets in New Jersey, and Clemens in Philadelphia, Pennsylvania.*

Organic Cattle Co. *beef is certified organic and available at supermarkets in the New York City area.*

Quality Steaks *produces hormone-free beef that is available at Star Markets in Massachusetts, First National Supermarkets in New England, and ABCO in the Phoenix, Arizona, area.*

Center for Science in the Public Interest
Americans for Safe Food Project
1875 Connecticut Avenue N.W., Suite 300
Washington, D.C. 20009-5728
(202) 332-9110 Ext. 384

You can obtain a list of organic mail order suppliers or hormone-free beef suppliers, both supermarket chains and mail order home delivery, from this organization.

Eden Acres
Organic Network
12100 Lima Center Road
Clinton, Michigan 49236-9618
(517) 456-4288

Organic Network, a division of Eden Acres, offers a 150 page international directory or local statewide directories of suppliers of organic meats, poultry, fruits and vegetables.

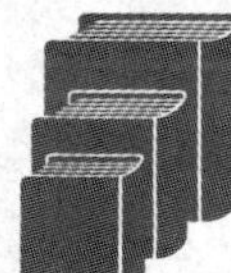

Recommended Reading

Cooking With Rachel. Albert, Rachel. Oroville, CA: George Ohsawa Macrobiotic Foundation, 1989.

Rachel Albert studied macrobiotics at the Kushi Institute of Great Britain, taught cooking classes, and owns a cafe. This book appeals to a wide range of tastes and food preferences.

Coping with Your Allergies. Golos, Natalie; and Golbita, Francis. Simon and Schuster, New York, 1986.

An excellent resource on food allergies.

Diet for a New America. Robbins, John. Walpole, NH: Stillpoint Publishing, 1987.

John Robbins provides a well-documented, factual account of the unhealthy and inhumane conditions animals are raised in to be eaten. He discusses the physical, emotional, and economic ramifications of these conditions.

Diet for a Poisoned Planet. Steinman, David. New York: Ballantine Books, 1990.

An in-depth guide for the consumer listing several foods and their contaminant levels.

***Diet for a Small Planet,* 10th ed.** Lappe, Frances Moore. New York: Ballantine, 1982.

An early classic in the field of diet, politics, and food supply. It explains how people can help change the impending situation of world hunger by changing their diets. Includes recipes, menus, and food combining charts.

Food Irradiation: Who Wants It? Webb, Tony; Lang, Tim; and Tuker, Kathleen. Rochester, VT: Thorsons Publishers, Inc., 1987.

The first authoritative study on food irradiation, the book provides maps locating irradiation facilities and charts of nutritional values, as well as discusses hazards faced by workers in these plants and how irradiation affects everyone.

The McDougall Plan. McDougall, John., M.D.; and McDougall, Mary. Piscataway, NJ: New Century Publishing, Inc., 1983.

This book encourages an adaptation of a specific vegetarian diet and lifestyle. This diet is centered on starchy plant foods such as rice, potatoes, pasta, and all fresh fruits and vegetables.

Perfect Health. Chopra, Deepak, M.D. New York: Harmony Books, 1990.

By determining your body type, Chopra seeks to restore inner balance to the body. He uses Ayurvedic techniques, diet, stress reduction, and exercise to strengthen the mind/body connection.

Shattering: Food, Politics, and the Loss of Genetic Diversity. Fowler, Carrie; and Mooney, Pat. Tucson, AZ: University of Arizona Press, 1990

An enlightening book for all, including politicians and plant lovers. A shocking account of the threat to the planet and world food security.

Staying Healthy with Nutrition. Haas, Elson, M.D. Berkeley, CA: Celestial Arts, 1992.

Combining Eastern philosophies with his knowledge of Western medicine, Dr. Haas seeks to rejuvenate and cure using a mind-body approach to overall health. A comprehensive guide to diet and nutrition.

Still Life with Menu. Katzen, Mollie. Berkeley, CA: Ten Speed Press, 1988.

Fifty original still lives accompanied by menus and recipes of meatless delicacies.

Transition to Vegetarianism. Ballantine, Rudolph. Honesdale, PA: Himalayan Publishers, 1987.

This book provides solid information on how to design an optimal vegetarian diet with advice on how to approach it gradually and wisely.

Vegan Nutrition—Pure and Simple. Klaper, Michael., M.D. Paui, HI: Gentle World, 1987.

An excellent sourcebook for those interested in the vegan vegetarian lifestyle. Provides daily menus, recipes, and books to refer to. A philosophical discourse on the question of eating animals.

"Let thy food be thy medicine and thy medicine be thy food."

—Hippocrates (460-377 BC)

Energy Medicine

Energy medicine uses diagnostic screening devices to measure the various electromagnetic frequencies emitted by the body in order to detect imbalances that may be causing present illness, or contributing to future disease. These disturbed energy flows can then be returned to their normal, healthy state through the input of electromagnetic signals that specifically counteract the affected frequencies to restore a normal energy balance within the body.

Imagine that you are sitting in the doctor's office. The doctor takes a small, hand-held probe connected to a meter and, with no further questions, gently presses certain points on your hands and feet while noting the figures displayed on the meter. From this he or she is able to tell you which parts of your body are functioning correctly and which organs are causing problems. Some small glass vials containing colorless liquids are placed into a container, which is also connected to the device, and the doctor remeasures some of the points. From this the doctor is able to tell you why there is a problem. Finally he or she gives you a few drops of a tasteless medicine. Before long you begin to feel better.

A description from a futuristic fantasy? No, this is precisely what is happening in some medical clinics around the world today with practitioners of energy medicine.

What Is Energy Medicine?

"For most of this century," says William Tiller, Ph.D., of Stanford University, "science and medicine have seen health as being dependent upon the balance of body chemistry and the functioning of physical structures. However, attempts to treat illnesses and imbalances chemically often lead to unwanted side effects or the body becoming insensitive to the chemicals."

This fact has led many physicians and health professionals to look beyond conventional drug-based therapies to the field of energy medicine. Many of the most sophisticated diagnostic systems used today in conventional medicine, such as the EKG (electrocardiogram), EEG (electroencephalogram), EMG (electromyelogram), and MRI (magnetic resonance imaging), employ the principles of energy medicine. Energy medicine, or bioenergetic medicine as it is sometimes called, refers to therapies that use an energy field—electrical, magnetic, sonic, acoustic, microwave, infrared—to screen for or treat health conditions by detecting imbalances in the body's energy fields and then correcting them.

The detection of energy level imbalances in the body is essential for providing an early warning system for potential disruptions in chemical balance that may lead to disease. Balance can then be restored using holistic therapies, or with treatment devices that rebalance the energy levels of the various fields before the chemical or structural disturbances can occur.

Types of Energy Medicine Devices

Most energy medicine devices are based on the acupuncture meridian system. Acupuncture works on the principle that there is a network of energy channels, called meridians, throughout the body. Different organs are associated with different energy meridians, and health problems in various organs show up as disturbances of energy in the associated meridians. Acupuncture points, or acupoints, are the points along these meridians where energy flow can be measured and manipulated.

Since the 1940s, research has established that acupuncture points possess electrical conductivity.[1] German doctors, led by Reinhold Voll, M.D., measured changes in electrical conductivity at each of the body's acupuncture points. They discovered that the electrical resistance of the skin decreases dramatically at the acupuncture points when compared to the surrounding skin. They also found that each point appeared to have a standard measurement for anyone who is in good health (when there is a steady flow of bioenergy, or *qi*, in the meridians). This measurement changes when health deteriorates.

“In the United States, electroacupuncture biofeedback devices have been approved on an experimental basis solely for screening purposes, despite the fact that it is estimated that there are between 85,000 to 100,000 practitioners in this field worldwide.”

These discoveries greatly simplified the task of locating acupoints rapidly and accurately. Based on the work of Dr. Voll and his colleagues, and later by researchers in Japan, a new field of energy medicine instruments have been developed both for assessment and treatment.

Assessment Instruments: Electroacupuncture Biofeedback

Dr. Voll developed a precise measuring instrument known as the Dermatron™ that allowed him to measure the electrical resistance at acupuncture points. He discovered that higher or lower readings than normal at a particular acupuncture point indicates a problem in the organ that corresponds to that acupoint; higher generally means there is irritation or inflammation in the organ and lower usually indicates fatigue or degeneration.

See Acupuncture.

The acupoints that correspond to specific organs and tissues are known as control measurement points (CMP) because they provide a general indication of the health of the organ or tissue as a whole. There are also specific points that indicate how the various parts of each organ are functioning. If the CMP for a particular organ gives a poor reading, the points for the various parts of that organ can then be checked. Whichever part of the organ shows an imbalance is the site of the dysfunction.

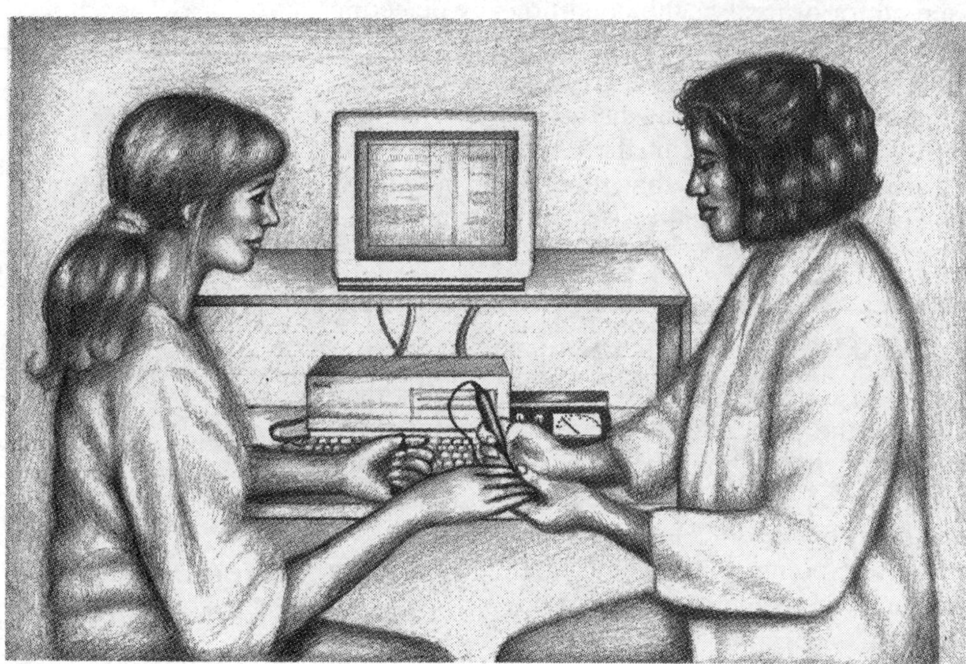

Electroacupuncture biofeedback testing.

To date there are over two thousand such points that have been established as having specific relationships with internal organs. A skilled physician can, in a relatively short time, discover not only which organs have problems, but which part of the organ is malfunctioning and what other organs, if any, it is affecting. Thus it becomes possible to find the root cause of any problem.

This assessment technique became known as "Electroacupuncture According to Voll" (EAV), and is the basis of all electroacupuncture biofeedback devices (also known as electrodermal screening devices) in use today.

Electroacupuncture biofeedback has been very successful in screening for a wide variety of conditions. However in screening for cancer it is advisable to also use traditional blood tests as well as blood analysis with a dark field microscope.

Dr. Voll later expanded his method not only to be able to learn what area of the body is being impacted, but to determine what the exact source of the problem is as well. He found that if a patient held sample homeopathic dilutions of known disease substances such as bacteria, viruses, or diseased tissue, when the patient came upon the one directly related to the cause of the problem, the EAV reading would return to normal. The reason for this is that homeopathic dilutions of a disease substance are actually remedies, following the homeopathic law of "like cures like." Therefore, the body is actually responding positively to what it perceives as "good medicine."

In this way, EAV can be used to detect almost every known disease, chemical toxin, food allergy, and disregulation in organ and glandular systems. EAV screening can be used to test various remedies to determine which medication will correct the problem, and if there are likely to be any side effects.

Electroacupuncture biofeedback devices are currently manufactured in Germany, France, Russia, Japan, Korea, England, and the United States. The Vega™ is another electroacupuncture biofeedback device similar to the original Voll device, but much faster. In recent years there have been several attempts to further speed up the testing procedure by using computers. Computerized versions of these instruments, such as the Computron, can quickly perform multiple screenings and can also allow the practitioner to build up a detailed data base of patient files useful for research purposes.

Today, these electroacupuncture biofeedback devices are widely used in Europe, and in Japan a system based on similar principles called *Ryo Do Raku* is used by an estimated 40,000 practitioners.[2] In the United States, however, electroacupuncture biofeedback devices have so far been approved on an experimental basis solely for screening purposes, despite the fact that it is conservatively estimated that there are between 85,000 to 100,000 practitioners in this field worldwide.[3]

Treatment Instruments

While electroacupuncture biofeedback devices can be a powerful tool for assessing health conditions within the body, treatment devices help complete the circle, allowing the energy medicine practitioner another viable therapy with which to combat disease and illness, oftentimes even before it can manifest, by successfully rebalancing the body's energy flow. The following are some of the more commonly used types of these instruments.

See Homeopathy.

The MORA: The MORA was created by Franz Morrel, M.D., a close colleague of Dr. Voll. He believed that all biological processes are essentially a matter of electromagnetic signals that can be described by a complex wave form. Health can be considered as a smooth wave, while disease is identified by unwanted variations on this wave, both higher and lower.

Dr. Morrel had the idea of taking the electromagnetic signals directly from the body and manipulating the aberrant wave forms by raising or lowering them to create normal waves. These corrected waves are then fed from the device back into the patient through the corresponding acupoints. The signals can be taken from any area of the body, modified, and then returned to that specific area.

Since the MORA uses only the electromagnetic signals coming directly from the patient, it can be characterized as a truly natural therapy. "The crucial point of the MORA is that disease is considered to be a question of 'wrong' electromagnetic information," says Anthony Scott-Morley, D.Sc., Ph.D., M.D. (alt. med.), of Dorset, England. "The MORA instrument 'reads' the wave information of the patient and corrects it. There is no artificial electrical signal introduced. In this sense it is an extremely pure form of treatment because it deals only with the wave information of the patient."

The MORA has been used successfully for treatment of skin disease, headaches, migraines, muscular aches and pains, and circulation problems, and can be used in combination with homeopathic prescriptions. Although used primarily for treatment, it can be used as a diagnostic instrument using Voll- and Vega-type measurements as well.

The MORA can also be used for color therapy, transforming individual colors into appropriate frequencies and transmitting them into the body. "The MORA color instrument reduces the frequency of each

See Light Therapy.

color to a lower harmonic, out of the spectrum of visible light to a lower electromagnetic range," states Dr. Scott-Morley. "This allows for deeper penetration of tissue and shorter treatment times than with the use of visible light color treatment."

The TENS Unit: A commonly used device for pain relief is the Transcutaneous Electrical Nerve Stimulator, or TENS. It is widely used in doctors' offices and physiotherapy clinics, and can be used at home. It works by simply applying an electrical current to the affected nerves, causing conduction to be blocked and pain to be relieved. TENS units are also believed to stimulate the productions of endorphins, the body's own natural painkillers.

Judy Zacharski, P.T., owner and Director of the Facial Pain and TMJ Clinic in Menomonee Falls, Wisconsin, uses TENS instruments to treat temporomandibular joint syndrome (TMJ), a painful condition of the jaw, usually caused by stress or injury.

A twenty-five-year-old patient of Zacharski's came to her with TMJ as a result of both an automobile accident in which her head struck the steering wheel, and a sports injury in which she was hit in the mouth with a baseball. The patient responded positively after the first two TENS treatments, and was given a unit to use at home. After ten days, the patient reported considerable reduction in discomfort.[4]

The Electro-Acuscope: Using a much lower electrical current than the TENS unit, the Electro-Acuscope™ reduces pain by stimulating tissue repair rather than by stimulating the nerves or causing muscle contractions. The current is continually adjusted to match the resistance from the damaged tissue in order to facilitate the repair process. The skill of the practitioner is of considerable importance for its effective use.

Because of its prolonged effects on tissue repair, the Electro-Acuscope can be applied to a broad range of clinical conditions such as muscle spasms, migraines, TMJ, bursitis, arthritis, surgical incisions, sprains and strains, neuralgia, herpes zoster infections (shingles), and bruises.

Steve Center, M.D., of San Diego, California, also uses the Electro-Acuscope to treat local skin infections, chronic fatigue syndrome, migraines, and carpal tunnel syndrome, though he says he predominantly uses it "for acute and chronic pain, mainly of musculoskeletal origin—automobile accidents, lumbosacral (lower back) sprains, shoulder strains, and sports injuries."[5]

George Godfrey, M.D., founding member of the American Trauma Society of the American College of Surgeons and Medical Director of Atlantic Industrial College of Surgeons in Atlantic City, New Jersey, finds that, "The most impressive results are found in the severe muscle contraction headaches associated with injuries to the muscles of the upper chest, upper thorax, and neck. At times the headache is gone within thirty seconds," he adds. He also uses the Electro-Acuscope treatment for chronic problems produced by strains and sprains, carpal tunnel syndrome, whiplash, trauma, skin ulcerations, arthritis, and the palliative care of ruptured disk patients who are either unable or unwilling to undergo surgery.[6]

Light Beam Generator (LBG): The Light Beam Generator™ radiates photons of light that help restore the cell's normal energy state, allowing the body to heal itself more readily. "The Light Beam Generator can be used anywhere on the body where there is a problem," says Robert Jacobs, N.M.D., D.Hom. (Med), of London, England, "and because of its deep penetration, it can help heal organs and structures deep within the body, as well as skin problems." Dr. Jacobs also points out that since healthy cells are in a stable energetic state, there are no adverse effects when the LBG is used in thirty- to forty-five-minute sessions.

Dr. Jacobs had a patient with a severe case of herpes zoster over his upper chest area. The condition was so painful that the man could not raise one of his arms and had difficulty sleeping. Medical treatments had not been able to help him. Dr. Jacobs gave him one forty-five-minute treatment with the LBG, after which the man was free of most of his pain. He could move his arm and the pustules were 60 percent reduced in size. After one additional treatment with the LBG he was fully healed. Another of Dr. Jacobs' patients had suffered from eczema for two years. After one treatment with the LBG his condition was fully improved.

According to Rena Davis, M.Sc., of St. Helens, Oregon, the effectiveness of the LBG is due to its stimulation of the lymphatic system. By opening sealed and calcified vessels, it stimulates blood circulation, reduces edema (swelling), and eliminates waste products stored in the tissues. Davis uses the LBG in conjunction with a dietary and nutritional program to treat a wide range of conditions, including tendonitis, bursitis, arthritis, bruises, sore throats, and allergies. One of Davis' patients was a sixty-year-old woman with severe rheumatoid arthritis in all of her joints. Davis treated her with the LBG for fourteen months, after which time she was completely healed.

Davis also finds the LBG is effective in draining varicose veins and for the fluid retention associated with premenstrual syndrome. Sports clinics use it to reduce swelling after sports injuries and it can also be used to remove the puffiness that gathers in the face and the abdomen with age, resulting in a more youthful appearance.

The Sound Probe: The Sound Probe emits a pulsed tone of three alternating frequencies that can destroy anything that is not in resonance with the body, such as bacteria, viruses, and fungi. The pad connected to the instrument is placed anywhere on the body where there is a problem or pain. The alternation of the frequencies ensures that the body does not adjust to the frequency, so that the treatment remains beneficial over time. It can also be used in sequence with the LBG. The Sound Probe is used first to kill off bacteria, viruses, etc., then the LBG is used to clear the debris from the system.

The Diapulse: The Diapulse™ uses radio waves to produce short, intense electromagnetic pulses that can penetrate deep into the tissues of the body. The heat energy produced reaches deep into tissues to improve blood flow, reduce pain, and promote healing. The Diapulse has been used successfully to reduce edema and inflammation following surgery and may be helpful in functional recovery from spinal cord injuries, according to Gary Emerson, D.C., of Santa Ana, California.

Cymatic Instruments: In addition to the electroacupuncture biofeedback devices discussed earlier, there are also therapeutic cymatic devices in which a sound transducer replaces the electrodes of the electroacupuncture biofeedback devices. This allows recording of the emitted sound patterns associated with different body parts.

The machines can be used for diagnosis as well as treatment. According to Sir Peter Guy Manners, M.D., D.O., Ph.D., of Bretforton, England, each organ, tissue, and molecule has its own harmonic signal. These signals are encoded into the cymatic device, which can be used to deliver to a particular body part a frequency pattern associated with its healthy state, restoring that particular body part to health.

See Qigong, Sound Therapy.

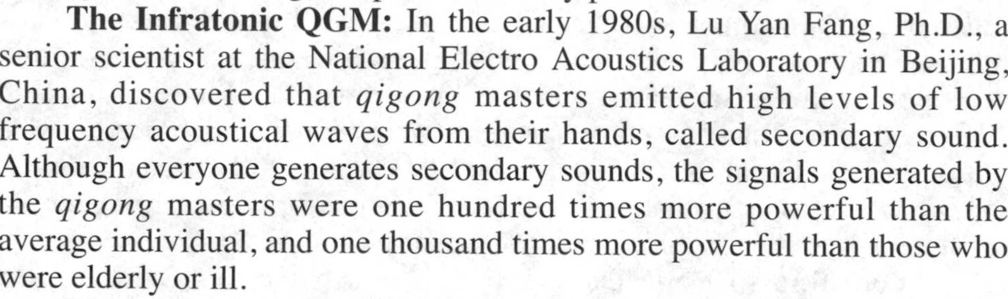

The Infratonic QGM: In the early 1980s, Lu Yan Fang, Ph.D., a senior scientist at the National Electro Acoustics Laboratory in Beijing, China, discovered that *qigong* masters emitted high levels of low frequency acoustical waves from their hands, called secondary sound. Although everyone generates secondary sounds, the signals generated by the *qigong* masters were one hundred times more powerful than the average individual, and one thousand times more powerful than those who were elderly or ill.

Using electroacoustical technology, Dr. Fang constructed an instrument that simulated this infratonic sound (eight to fourteen hertz, seventy decibels). When she directed these massage-like waves into hospitalized patients, she noted numerous improvements, particularly for the management of pain. Other benefits include increased circulatory functioning, migraine suppression, muscular relaxation, and the alleviation of depression. When used on the chest or back, the brain's production of alpha waves is also stimulated.

Today this machine is medically recognized as an effective pain management tool in China and is also used in Japan, Taiwan, Singapore, France, Spain, Mexico, and Argentina. In the United States, it is approved for sale by the FDA (Food and Drug Administration) as a therapeutic massage device.

The Teslar Watch: The Teslar Watch was developed as a device to minimize the harmful effects of electronic pollution, particularly those extremely low frequencies (ELF) which range from one to one hundred hertz. In-vitro research conducted by Glen Rein, Ph.D., of Stanford University Medical Center, demonstrated that the Teslar Watch enhanced immune response by 76 percent while simultaneously inhibiting the uptake of noradrenalin (an antidepressant) by 19.5 percent in the nerve cells.[7]

Dr. Scott-Morley also uses the Teslar Watch in his practice. One of his patients suffered from fatigue, headaches, and a case of eczema that she thought might be due to an allergic reaction. Within two days of wearing the watch, her headaches vanished, her skin cleared up, and her energy level significantly increased. "People who suffer from food allergies are invariably also sensitive to specific electromagnetic frequencies," Dr. Scott-Morley says. "When the Teslar is worn, their conditions very often improve, allowing easier subsequent treatment."

Applications of Energy Medicine

The level of accuracy of the electroacupuncture biofeedback devices is key to their future success and acceptance. Recently researchers at the University of Hawaii compared a diabetic population with a control group using electroacupuncture measurements on the spleen-pancreas meridian. The resulting data demonstrated a 95 to 97.5 percent correspondence between electroacupuncture biofeedback assessment and the conventionally confirmed diabetic group.[8]

Another study at the University of Hawaii compared electroacupuncture assessment of the allergy meridian with six other methods of assessing food allergies. The electroacupuncture biofeedback data gave the highest compatibility with the Food-Re-Challenge Test, the most sensitive of currently available diagnostic techniques for determination of food allergies.[9]

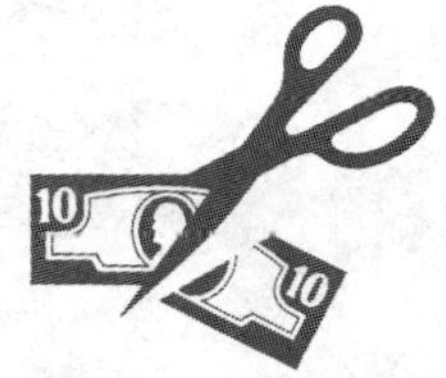

Electroacupuncture biofeedback testing provides a low-cost, highly effective way of screening for physiological and energetic imbalances before they develop into full-blown illnesses. It is an excellent tool for reducing the skyrocketing costs of medical care in this country.

Researchers at the University of California, Los Angeles, and the University of Southern California, were also able to demonstrate an 87 percent correlation between an electroacupuncture biofeedback diagnosis of lung cancer when compared with standard x-ray diagnosis.[10]

Electroacupuncture biofeedback devices can also be used to determine which bacteria, virus, or toxin is specifically responsible for an illness, infection, or disease, and which medications will help a particular health problem. Abram Ber, M.D., of Phoenix, Arizona, reports seeing a patient with Huntington chorea, a hereditary disease of the central nervous system. Characterized by progressive dementia and rapid, jerky motions, there is normally no treatment for this condition. He examined the patient with an electroacupuncture biofeedback device and found evidence of metal toxicity that he was able to treat with vitamin B_{12} injections and German homeopathic remedies. Within a year, the patient's symptoms abated and he is doing well at the present time.

Fuller Royal, M.D., of Las Vegas, Nevada, uses electroacupuncture biofeedback devices exclusively in his practice. He does not treat a specific disease, but rather treats the patient as a whole, looking for the underlying mechanisms that lead to disease. One patient came to him with angina, unable to walk across a room without pain. He had already undergone two bypass surgeries for sclerosis of the coronary artery and was facing a third. Using electroacupuncture biofeedback testing, Dr. Royal discovered the problem to be a wisdom tooth with a mercury amalgam filling. Once this filling was removed, the angina disappeared and the patient recovered completely.

In another case, Dr. Royal examined a six-month-old baby boy who was failing to thrive. The baby had been treated at the Mayo Clinic but still had not improved. Dr. Royal's electroacupuncture biofeedback device revealed the presence of a virus contracted from the mother when she had the flu. He treated the problem with homeopathic remedies, and now, a year later, the child is a normal eighteen-month-old, learning to walk and talk just like other children his age.

Robert D. Milne, M.D., of Las Vegas, uses electroacupuncture biofeedback devices to screen all his patients, many of whom come to him suffering from chronic fatigue syndrome (CFS). Using electroacupuncture biofeedback devices, he finds that virtually all female patients have digestive or pelvic problems predating the CFS. Once he treats these problems with diet, food supplements, Chinese herbs, enzymes, and homeopathic remedies, the condition abates.

Another of Dr. Milne's patients came to him with medically diagnosed intractable thyroiditis (Hashimoto's disease). Electro-acupuncture biofeedback testing, though, revealed that his body's energy system was congested. Using a combination of acupuncture, herbs, and homeopathic remedies to unblock the energy flow, Dr. Milne was able to resolve the problem to the extent that the patient's antimicrosomal antibody level, an indicator of thyroiditis, returned to normal.

Dr. Scott-Morley also employs energy devices in his practice. One of his patients was a thirty-six-year-old man who came to him with constant pain in the area of his liver. Two extensive medical investigations had found no evidence of anything wrong, and a third resulted in the suggestion that the man seek psychiatric treatment. Using an electroacupuncture biofeedback device, Dr. Scott-Morley measured the man's liver points and confirmed chronic inflammation and possible pathological damage. The test further revealed aflatoxin toxicity (frequently caused by a mold found on stale peanuts). Dr. Scott-Morley asked the man if stale peanuts had any significance for him and was told that the man had previously been a truck driver and had transported peanuts from Italy to England, eating several handfuls of them while en route. Upon arrival, shipment was found to be stale and condemned as unhealthy. Dr. Scott-Morley prescribed a homeopathic nosode of aflatoxin in conjunction with other remedies, and within a few weeks the man fully recovered. (A nosode is a potentized homeopathic remedy prepared from diseased tissue, such as bacteria, viruses, or pus, to treat the associated disease of the tissue material.)

Another woman came to Dr. Scott-Morley with pains in her abdomen and digestive disorders. Dr. Scott-Morley's test indicated liver malfunction along with an impaired right kidney. The toxic agent appeared to be Bilharzia, a parasite common in the Nile and irrigation canals of Egypt. But when Dr. Scott-Morley asked the woman when she had last been to Africa, she replied that she had never been outside of England. A second test again showed the presence of Bilharzia, leaving both Dr. Scott-Morley and the woman puzzled. Later that same evening, however, the woman phoned back to reveal that her mother had reminded her that she had been born in Egypt and had fallen into an irrigation ditch when she was eighteen months old. Dr. Scott-Morley was then able to use a Bilharzia nosode to resolve the woman's condition.

Dr. Scott-Morley also uses the MORA device to treat conditions. One of his patients had pain in both of his knees and required crutches in order to walk. After receiving treatment with the MORA in conjunction with MORA color for twenty minutes the patient was able to walk free of pain and without the need of crutches, and remains pain free three years later.

Another case history involved a thirty-two-year-old woman who had been unable to become pregnant for eight years, despite full medical examinations and treatment for infertility. Dr. Scott-Morley gave her five treatments with the MORA and she became pregnant after the fifth treatment.

Energy Medicine and Allergies

Professor Cyril Smith, of the University of Salford in England, has shown that extremely sensitive people can be affected by very small electrical signals of specific frequency. Working with highly allergic patients, he tuned an ordinary laboratory signal generator to specific frequencies causing the patients to experience symptoms of the allergy when exposed to them. He believes it is possible that these symptoms could be alleviated if a second, neutralizing frequency could be found.[11]

Dr. Royal uses electroacupuncture biofeedback devices in combination with homeopathy to determine the source of a patient's allergies and the proper neutralization dose. "We take an overview of the entire patient," explains Dr. Royal, "You can't afford to overlook anything." He tests the patient's diet; all the foods commonly eaten and the artificial dyes found in them; plus all the major chemicals in their environment, along with mold spores, house dust, and various pollens. They can all be tested within an hour with an electroacupuncture biofeedback device.

See Allergies, Environmental Medicine, Veterinary Medicine.

"For example, if someone is allergic to ragweed pollen, there will be an abnormal reading at the allergy control acupoint," he explains. "We then find a specific dilution of ragweed pollen that brings the reading back to zero when it is in the circuit. That solution, given by injection, will neutralize the patient's reaction to ragweed."

To further ensure accuracy, Dr. Royal performs intradermal skin tests as well. When all the tests are finished, separate serums are prepared for each group of allergens and injected for desensitization. Dr. Royal reports a high rate of success using this protocol.

Veterinary Energy Medicine

Bioenergetic veterinary medicine is identical to that used in humans. The only difference, according to H.C. Gurney, D.V.M., of Conifer, Colorado, is the fact that "animals do not have the power to reason whether a treatment is going to work or not; it either will or it won't." Due to an animal's basic impartiality to various treatment modalities, Dr. Gurney views veterinary energy medicine as blazing a trail in energy medicine by offering a workable model with the objective results to back it up.

Today, many veterinary professionals are moving into the field of energy medicine. Joanne Stefanatos, D.V.M., of Las Vegas, President of the American Holistic Veterinary Medicine Association, devotes her practice almost exclusively to energy medicine. She treats animals ranging from lions, tigers, snakes, and desert tortoises, to birds, domestic cats, and dogs. Using an electroacupuncture biofeedback device to screen for health problems, her treatment therapies include acupuncture, laser acupuncture, electroacupuncture, magnetic field therapy, and homeopathic remedies.

Dental Energy Medicine

As with acupuncture points, a relationship has been shown to exist between acupoints associated with specific teeth and organs. Using this fact, electroacupuncture biofeedback devices are now being used to screen for health problems in the body caused by the related teeth. It can also be used to determine a patient's compatibility with various dental materials and anesthetics before they are used. In this way, dental toxicity can be avoided. Electroacupuncture biofeedback devices can also be used to detect hidden infections below teeth, which cause no symptoms and often go undiagnosed for years, contributing to degenerative disease elsewhere in the body. Electroacupuncture biofeedback testing is sometimes the only way of detecting these infections.

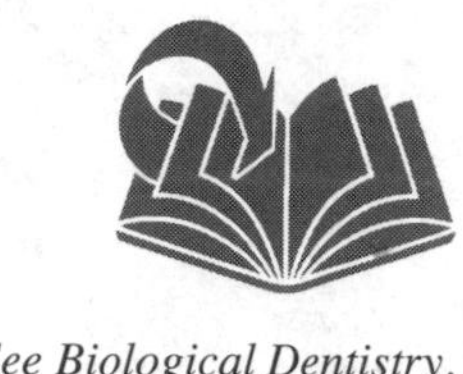

See Biological Dentistry.

Philip Jenkins, D.D.S., of Los Gatos, California, uses electroacupuncture biofeedback testing for this purpose. "For years I kept after patients to keep their teeth clean," he says, "but even some patients who followed all the instructions got worse." Now, using electroacupuncture biofeedback, Dr. Jenkins can find the infections, identify them, then determine the appropriate homeopathic remedies with which to treat them.

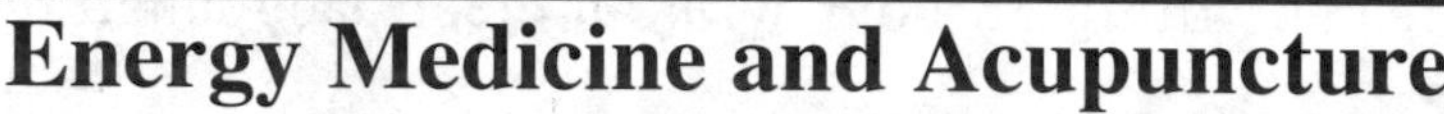

Energy Medicine and Acupuncture

Vaughn Cook, L.Ac., of the Utah Acupuncture Clinic in Salt Lake City, Utah, uses an electroacupuncture biofeedback device in his practice to record the energy flow in the patient's meridians and to feed this information directly back to him. Dr. Cook then uses acupuncture to rebalance the energy flow. He also uses TENS units and soft laser energy in his practice. The soft laser is used on the acupoints in much the same way as needles are in traditional acupuncture.

Dr. Cook uses these various methods to treat a broad range of patients with anything from headaches and back pains to postoperative problems, chronic fatigue syndrome, menstrual cramps, and allergies.

The Future of Energy Medicine

The main thrust of conventional chemical-based medicine is crisis intervention rather than prevention. Traditional drug therapies also pose a serious threat of side effects along with an alarming increase in iatrogenic (treatment-induced) diseases and problems. There also appears to be a dramatic rise in the number of chronic degenerative diseases in the Western world for which chemical medicine has no real answer. It is estimated that between 60 and 70 percent of the problems presented on a daily basis to primary care physicians defy diagnosis and are usually labeled as neurotic or psychosomatic in origin.[12]

"The medicine of the future will be energy medicine," says Dr. Jacobs, "and chemical medicine will be a subset of medicine as a whole. Probably 80 percent of medicine will be energy medicine, and 20 percent chemical medicine."

According to Dr. Jacobs, Russia is leading the world in the field of energy medicine today. "Russian physicians are using microwave energy at acupoints to treat many health problems successfully. At present, it is not known exactly how these different forms of energy work in the body, but there is substantial clinical evidence that they do work."

Dr. Jacobs is also carrying out new research of his own with world-renowned violinist Yehudi Menhuin. Menhuin is helping Jacobs design equipment which will analyze speech and hearing patterns to allow them to treat disease by aiming sound energy directly at the brain, where it will produce neurochemicals capable of restoring the body to health. "The body is controlled by the brain," says Dr. Jacobs, "and the brain has the capacity for self-healing. We hope to be able to activate this capacity using sound energy."

Just as significant as the treatment applications of energy medicine is electroacupuncture biofeedback testing, which can enable a practitioner to screen for the potential for illness before it happens. This makes energy medicine an excellent tool for reducing the skyrocketing costs of medical care in the United States. By catching diseases early, or preventing them from ever occurring, medical costs will be greatly minimized. Research is still needed to prove the value of electroacupuncture biofeedback testing, however. "The problem here is a very practical one," notes Dr. Scott-Morley. "Research costs money, and the skilled practitioners of these methods are busy working as doctors, not as researchers, and it would take two to three years to train researchers to a high enough level of competency in these methods for the research to be effective. Yet if some enterprising body were to give sympathetic and careful attention to our claims, then I feel we would discover that we have an undreamed of tool available to us which I'm sure can be further extended and refined."

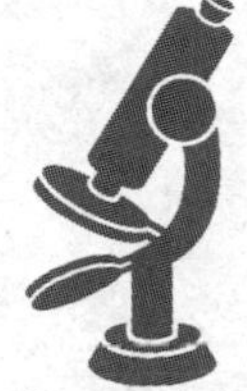

Research is needed to prove the value of electroacupuncture biofeedback testing. This can easily be verified by comparison of results of competent practitioners with traditional diagnostic methods.

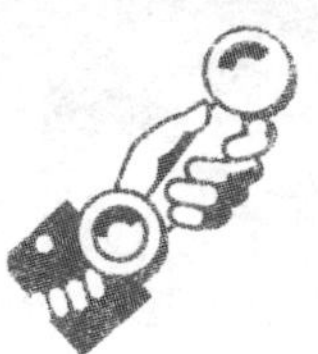

Where to Find Help

Due to various state laws and pending approval by the FDA, we cannot conscientiously offer referrals for electroacupuncture and biofeedback equipment or practitioners.

Electro Medical, Inc.
18433 Armistad
Fountain Valley, California 92708
(714) 964-6776
(800) 422-8726
(Outside California)

Marketing and education for the Electro-Acuscope™ and the Myopulse™. Referrals to doctors who use this equipment.

ELF Labs
1314 Burch Drive
Evansville, IN 47711
(812) 867-7942
(800) 540-4942

Makers of the Light Beam Generator, Sound Probe, and Teslar. Referrals to doctors who use this equipment.

Tools For Exploration
4460 Redwood Highway, Suite 2
San Rafael, California 94903
(800) 456-9887

Mail order catalog of nonmedical devices, machines, audiotapes, and books.

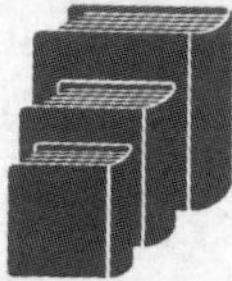

Recommended Reading

The Body Electric: Electromagnetism and the Foundation of Life. Becker, Robert O.; and Selden, Gary. New York: William Morrow and Company, Inc., 1987.

First-person account from one of the pioneers in the field of bioelectrics and regeneration, which details the relationship of electromagnetism and electricity to basic life processes, medical care, and environmental concerns, and the author's struggle against the politics of medicine and the resistance of the government.

Electromagnetic Man: Health and Hazard in the Electrical Environment. Smith, Cyril W.; and Best, Simon. New York: St. Martin's Press, 1989.

This book explains the connection between electromagnetism and living systems from large-scale phenomena in the solar system to the threat from man-made electromagnetic pollution. Provides new interpretations of the mechanisms underlying alternative medicine and shows what actions can be taken against the dangerous effects of electromagnetic fields as well as hot to make beneficial use of them.

Vibrational Medicine. Gerber, Richard, M.D. Santa Fe, NM: Bear & Company, 1988.

An examination of energy medicine, exploring alternative medical treatments such as flower essences, therapeutic touch, acupuncture, and herbal medicine. Includes thirty-four informative diagrams.

Environmental Medicine

Environmental medicine explores the role of dietary and environmental allergens in health and illness. Factors such as dust, molds, chemicals, and certain foods may cause allergic reactions that can dramatically influence diseases ranging from asthma and hay fever to headaches and depression. Virtually any chronic physical or mental illness may be improved by the care of a physician competent in this field.

In the past conventional medicine has been unwilling to attribute much importance to the complex relationship between individuals and their environment. This attitude has begun to change, however, due to extensive research by environmental specialists over the last thirty years. Today many physicians cite a link between their patients' illnesses and environmental factors such as diet, pollens, molds, and chemicals.[1]

The field of environmental medicine was pioneered by Theron G. Randolph, M.D., a prominent Chicago allergy specialist and professor at four medical schools. Since the late 1940s, Dr. Randolph has taught that sensitivity reactions to commonly eaten foods can cause a range of symptoms in susceptible individuals, including headaches, eczema, fatigue, arthritis, depression, and a variety of gastrointestinal disorders.

Further research by Dr. Randolph revealed that chemicals in the environment can also have profound negative effects throughout the body. His book, *Human Ecology and the Susceptibility to the Chemical Environment*, published in 1962, was the first textbook on the subject. Since then, many other physicians have followed in Dr. Randolph's footsteps attempting to educate the public that the widespread use of insecticides, herbicides, plastics, formaldehyde, food additives, petroleum products, gas, and other chemicals can lead to illness.

Symptoms of Environmental Sensitivity

Many common symptoms of illness can be caused by allergies or environmental sensitivity, according to William Crook, M.D., of Jackson, Tennessee.[2] Traditional allergists routinely treat patients with typical allergy complaints such as asthma, eczema, hives, sneezing, nasal congestion, a runny nose, and itching eyes or throat, as well as other symptoms frequently associated with hay fever. Doctors who specialize in environmental medicine do not limit themselves to these conditions, recognizing that other illnesses such as headaches, arthritis, fatigue, colitis, and lupus, can also be the result of, or aggravated by, allergies or chemical sensitivity.

AN UNUSUAL TREATMENT FOR MENTAL ILLNESS

In the late 1940s, Theron G. Randolph, M.D., agreed to evaluate Sally, a young woman who had been committed to a mental hospital due to an apparently untreatable psychosis. Dr. Randolph believed that nervous system reactions to certain foods might either be the cause of, or at least a contributing factor to, Sally's psychosis. He thought this could be proved by a test that eliminated those foods from her diet. However, if once the foods were removed, she remained as symptomatic as before, then probably they were not the cause.

Sally was hospitalized in an allergy-free environment and started on a spring water fast. Enemas were given to speed the complete evacuation of her intestinal tract. By the fourth day, her symptoms had cleared and she felt healthy and sane again. In order to ascertain which food or foods affected her physically or mentally and had triggered her psychosis, Dr. Randolph fed her single-food meals. As she reintroduced the foods one at a time into her diet, Sally was monitored for possible reactions.

Sally experienced no problems until she ate beet sugar. Within moments, her face began to contort, she lost contact with her surroundings, and she developed a blank, unknowing stare. She looked and acted as she had during her previous psychotic episodes. By subsequently eliminating beet sugar (fortunately her only food allergy) from her diet, Sally regained her mental health and no longer needed to be hospitalized.

Often an illness can be aggravated by environmental sensitivity. Marshall Mandell, M.D., of Norwalk, Connecticut, the father of bioecologic medicine, has discovered that even severe health conditions such as multiple sclerosis, cerebral palsy, and adult post-polio may be significantly complicated by superimposed allergic reactions, and likewise benefited when those allergies are treated.[3]

Richard S. Wilkinson, M.D., of Yakima, Washington, an expert in environmental medicine, points out that the following symptoms may be caused by environmental sensitivity or allergies. He groups these responses according to the different systems of the body and categories of illness:

- **Cardiovascular system:** migraine headaches, vasculitis (inflammation of a blood vessel), thrombophlebitis (inflammation of a vein combined with the formation of a blood clot), high blood pressure, angina, certain arrhythmias, edema (swelling), and fluid retention
- **Chronic pediatric disorders:** recurrent infections, recurrent ear infections, chronic headaches, stomachaches, muscle aches, bed wetting, and certain types of behavioral and learning disabilities
- **Endocrine system:** autoimmune thyroiditis (inflammation of the thyroid gland), hypoglycemia, and premenstrual syndrome (PMS)
- **Eye, ear, nose, and throat disorders:** hay fever, nasal congestion, sneezing, conjunctivitis, blurring of vision, itchy eyes, tearing, light sensitivity, swelling of the throat, recurrent ear infections, dizziness, loss of balance, ringing in the ears, and sinus headaches
- **Gastrointestinal system:** canker sores, irritable bowel syndrome, infant colic, gastroenteritis (inflammation of the stomach and intestines), diarrhea, constipation, gas, bloating, various abdominal pains, ulcerative colitis, and Crohn's disease (a chronic inflammatory condition affecting the colon and/or the small intestine)
- **Genitourinary system:** bed wetting, recurrent vaginitis, painful intercourse, and chronic cystitis

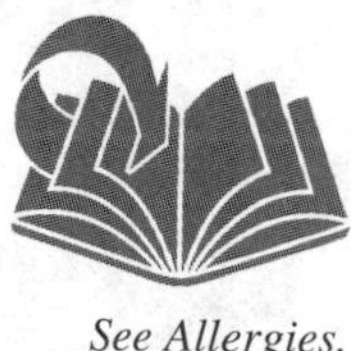

See Allergies.

- **Musculoskeletal system:** muscle spasm headaches, lupus erythematosus (a chronic inflammatory disease with symptoms including arthritis, fatigue, and skin lesions), rheumatoid arthritis, various muscle pains, and many forms of joint pain
- **Nervous system:** headaches, epilepsy, and sleep disorders
- **Neurobehavioral and psychiatric manifestations:** attention deficit disorder (hyperactivity), manic-depressive psychosis, sexual dysfunction, eating disorders, schizophrenia, irritability, anxiety, panic, and chronic fatigue syndrome
- **Respiratory system:** asthma and chronic bronchitis
- **Skin**: eczema, hives, and angioedema (a form of swelling)

Causes of Environmental Sensitivities

Dr. Wilkinson observes that it is not only the specific allergens (substances causing allergic reactions) that need to be identified and treated. Underlying genetic and nutritional factors, as well as exposure to toxic substances, often predispose the patient to develop sensitivities to foods, chemicals, airborne allergens, and other materials. Doctors of environmental medicine stress the importance of a thorough environmental- and nutritional-oriented history, as well as a careful physical examination, in order to uncover possible contributing factors to the patient's illness. According to Dr. Wilkinson, "In a thorough evaluation of the chronically ill, the history and physical exam might suggest nutritional problems, the presence of parasites or yeast, thyroid or adrenal disorders, the effect of dental work, psycho-spiritual issues, and other important considerations."

"An important question for the environmental physician to answer is: What are the underlying dietary and environmental causes of, and contributing factors to, my patient's physical and mental symptoms?"

An important question for the environmental physician to answer is: What are the underlying dietary and environmental causes of, and contributing factors to, my patient's physical and mental symptoms? According to the American Academy of Environmental Medicine (AAEM), a network of over six hundred physicians, some of the factors that may contribute to an individual's susceptibility include:

Heredity/Genetics: Sensitivity to dietary and environmental agents appears to be linked to one's heredity. AAEM members recognize that a genetic predisposition to the development of allergies can be passed down through successive generations of a person's bloodline. The number of family members in that chain who experienced severe allergies appears to increase the likelihood of their descendants experiencing allergies as well, and at an earlier age.

Poor Nutrition: A major cause of chemical sensitivity is poor or inadequate nutrition. A diet of refined, processed foods deficient in vitamins, minerals, enzymes, and other vital nutrients can severely impair the body's ability to function efficiently due to the increased levels of toxins such foods contain. Their ingestion can also result in an increase of free radicals (highly reactive destructive molecules), which can further predispose a person to allergic reactions.

Infection: Sensitivities to allergens can also be developed following severe infection, whether viral, bacterial, parasitic, or fungal (candida). Candidiasis or parasites can cause chronic inflammation or irritation of the lining of the intestinal tract. This inflammation can lead to "leaky gut syndrome," in which bacteria, bacterial toxins, and partially digested foods are able to travel from the intestine into the bloodstream, causing an allergic or immune reaction.

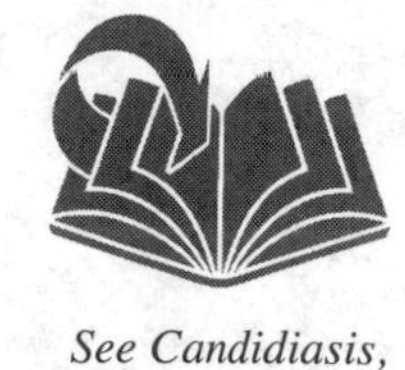

See Candidiasis, Gastrointestinal Disorders, Parasitic Infections.

Chemical Exposure: Current research has shown that due to their toxic effect on the body, exposure to pesticides, herbicides, petrochemicals, and other chemicals in the food and water supply, as well as in indoor and outdoor air, can lead to the development of allergic reactions.

Stress: Increased emotional or physical stress can also contribute to allergies in ways that are often both subtle and overlooked.

Other factors that can lead to allergies and sensitivity reactions include:

- Frequent use of antibiotics, steroids, and other medications
- Hormonal changes due to the menstrual cycle, aging, or surgery
- Glandular disorders such as low thyroid function, thyroiditis, and adrenal insufficiency
- Physical trauma such as accidents or surgery
- Electromagnetic disturbances of the environment
- Geopathic factors (harmful radiation from the earth)
- Dental amalgam fillings that contain large amounts of mercury and other dental involvements, such as infections under the teeth

Testing for Environmental Illness

The Occupational and Environmental Unit at Tri-Cities Hospital, in Dallas, Texas, is currently the only hospital in the United States where in-patient evaluations and treatments for environmental illness are performed. For most patients across the country the evaluation and treatment is performed on an out-patient basis. An environmental physician may use a number of options for evaluating illnesses to determine if they are caused or exacerbated by allergies.

Elimination Diet: Often a doctor will suggest an elimination diet to detect food allergies. This involves eliminating the suspected food or foods from one's diet for at least ten to fourteen days with the hope that the symptoms disappear. Though these vary from person to person, the foods that most frequently cause a reaction are milk and milk products, wheat, yeast, corn, eggs, coffee, soy, potatoes, tomatoes, beef, pork, chicken, peanuts, oranges, chocolate, and sugar.

Skin Testing: Skin testing is a commonly used and fairly accurate means to test for allergies to pollens, and it is about 35 percent accurate for molds. Unfortunately, it is not a satisfactory way to accurately identify a patient's food allergies.[4] The most commonly used form of skin testing is the scratch test, which is done on the surface of the skin. Many environmental physicians use intradermal testing (an injection into the outer layers of the skin) for dust, molds, and pollens, as well as foods and chemicals. The response to therapy based on the intradermal testing can be more rapid and the testing itself, in the hands of an experienced physician, is a safe procedure.[5]

Provocation/Neutralization: This form of testing is used by many environmental physicians for testing foods and determining what may be an effective neutralizing (symptom-relieving) dose. Control of symptoms can be achieved by injecting small amounts of allergenic material intradermally or subcutaneously (just beneath the skin), or by placing a few drops of the allergenic material under the tongue.

RAST (Radio Allergo Sorbent Test): This blood test is used by many doctors in diagnosing their patients' allergies. RAST testing can be a means of diagnosing allergies to pollens, molds, dust, bee venom, and other allergens. RAST testing, however, is not very accurate in testing foods, and it can be expensive.

Electroacupuncture Biofeedback: One potentially useful but much less frequently employed method of testing utilizes electroacupuncture equipment to measure minute changes in the electrical conductance of the skin. Some clinicians claim that this method correlates extremely well with skin testing, is much faster, and avoids the pain and slight risk of an allergic reaction associated with injecting allergens into the skin. "Investigational device" permits have been granted to some practitioners by the FDA (Food and Drug Administration) in order to review the usefulness of these devices as a diagnostic tool.

See Energy Medicine.

Thyroid Function: Another important factor in allergic diseases is the functioning of the thyroid gland. An overactive or underactive thyroid can result in increased allergies, skin problems, fatigue, nervousness, gastrointestinal problems, sleeping too much or too little, gaining or losing weight, swelling, and various types of pain. Thyroid function needs to be carefully evaluated.

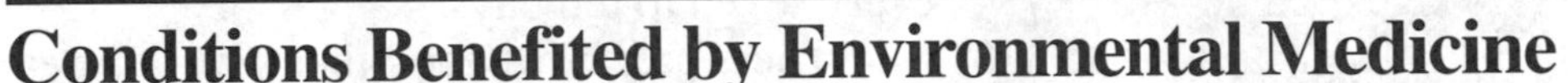

Conditions Benefited by Environmental Medicine

"Physicians who have been practicing environmental medicine for the past three or four decades point out that treating patients' illnesses has become more and more complicated over the years due to the increased use of chemicals and medications," says Dr. Wilkinson. Seldom is the solution to a problem as simple as finding one single food that causes all of the patient's symptoms. Effective treatment requires the full participation and cooperation of the patient, who may be asked to make changes in lifestyle, diet, and environment, and perhaps minimize the use of pharmaceutical medications.

Mold and Pollen Allergies

To treat mold and pollen allergies, a person's living environment needs to be as clean as possible. There are, as well, some medications that have minimal side effects and are effective for simple hay fever symptoms. These can often be prescribed for short-term, seasonal hay fever. In some cases it is necessary to test for allergies and then begin specific treatment to increase the body's resistance to those substances.

ALLERGIES AND CHILDREN

It has been clearly demonstrated that food intolerance is an important cause of hyperactivity in many children.[7] Dr. Joseph Egger, a pediatric neurologist in Germany, has demonstrated an effective treatment for hyperactive children who have their symptoms triggered by food sensitivity. The children avoided the foods to which they were allergic for several months and they were given a very low-dose injection therapy called enzyme potentiated desensitization—which is distinguished from conventional methods of desensitization by the fact that just prior to injection a minute amount of a naturally occurring enzyme in the body is added to the antigen solution. The injections were given three times at two-month intervals. Fifteen of seventeen patients were cured of their food sensitivities using this method.[8]

Marshall Mandell, M.D., of Norwalk, Connecticut, the father of bioecologic medicine and Doris Rapp, M.D., past President of the American Academy of Environmental Medicine, have documented on videotape the often serious effects that allergies have on the nervous systems of many children with emotional, behavioral, and learning problems, as well as autism and seizures. During feeding tests and tests with sublingual drops prepared from foods and other types of offenders (pollens, molds, food coloring, tobacco smoke), the children suddenly became angry, confused, and hyperactive. Rapid and dramatic improvement was seen in many of these children who avoided or decreased their exposure to the offending substances.

A few years ago, the New York City public school system decided to change the children's school diet. They decreased the amount of sugar, food colorings, synthetic flavorings, and two commonly used preservatives. Over the next four years, there was a dramatic 15.7 percent increase in academic performance by students in the city's schools. Prior to the dietary changes, the academic performance of the students never varied more than 1 percent up or down in the course of a year.[9]

This is best accomplished by giving the patient a customized mixture of treatment material prepared from the substances he or she is allergic to and administered in the form of drops taken under the tongue or shots.

According to Dr. Mandell, eating the wrong foods during a pollen season or peak mold season often makes the pollen and mold symptoms much worse, and greatly reduces the effectiveness of helpful medications and shots.

Food Allergies

Because frequently eaten foods remain constantly present in the system, allergic responses to them are responsible for many forms of chronic physical, mental, and emotional problems that are either misdiagnosed or inappropriately treated, according to Dr. Mandell. One effective and helpful method of treating food allergies is simply for the patient to avoid, or at least dramatically decrease, the intake of foods to which he or she is allergic. This is the most consistent and widely used method of treatment. According to Dr. Mandell, symptoms caused by eating a known food allergen daily or twice weekly may be reduced by eating the same food only once every seven to ten days.

There are, however, other ways to treat some types of food allergies, such as the provocation/neutralization technique. After skin testing for food allergies, treatments consisting of a mixture of very diluted symptom-relieving solutions of the offending foods can be administered to the patient by either injections or drops given under the tongue. A number of clinicians have found this technique to be an effective treatment for certain patients.[6]

One of Dr. Mandell's most interesting cases was an Italian woman with cerebral palsy who suffered for years from unpredictable attacks of fatigue, painful muscle spasms, and loss of balance. She had been told by her neurologist that these symptoms were from the cerebral palsy and she should learn to accept them because "That's the way cerebral palsy is."

Dr. Mandell was able to reproduce several episodes of these symptoms in his office by performing symptom-duplicating provocative tests with tomato extract. These office tests were confirmed by having the woman take several single-food test meals at home at seven-day intervals. The meals consisted of tomato juice and fresh tomatoes. If she ate tomato juice and tomatoes once every two weeks, there were no unpredictable flare-ups of her familiar cerebral palsy symptoms. However, the attacks could be brought on by eating tomatoes, in any form, less than twelve days apart.

“It has been clearly demonstrated that food intolerance is an important cause of hyperactivity in many children.”

Chemical Sensitivity and Allergy

Chemical susceptibility was first described by Dr. Randolph. Today it is commonly accepted that herbicides and pesticides in the earth's food supply and environment pose a hazard to human health. Even low-level exposure to a number of different chemicals can cause a wide variety of chronic diseases, according to Nicholas Ashford, Ph.D., J.D., of the Massachusetts Institute of Technology and Claudia Miller, M.D., M.S., M.A., of the University of Texas.[10]

In addition, Michael A. Evans, Ph.D., Associate Professor at the University of Illinois College of Medicine, believes 70 to 80 percent of human cancer is due to synthetic chemicals that are not themselves completely carcinogenic, but become carcinogenic when they interact with other environmental or genetic factors.[11]

The essential underlying causes of chemical sensitivity and allergies are still debated by medical researchers, even though in 1987 a National Academy of Sciences workshop estimated that approximately 15 percent of the United States population is chemically sensitive.[12] Many medical experts believe that at least part of this sensitivity is the result of the post-World War II petrochemical revolution.[13]

“Even low-level exposure to a number of different chemicals can cause a wide variety of chronic diseases.”

Today, people are exposed to chemical concentrations far greater than were previous generations. Also, ecological changes in the environment are occurring faster than the human body's capacity to adapt to them. There are currently about 55,000 chemical compounds in production.[14] 3,000 chemicals are added to food supplies, over 700 are added to drinking water,[15] and as many as 10,000 are used in the processing and storage of food.[16]

See Detoxification Therapy.

People are constantly exposed to products containing harmful substances that the body cannot properly break down: pesticides, gasoline, paints, industrial waste, household cleaners, smog, food preservatives, and dry cleaning chemicals. According to the EPA (Environmental Protection Agency), more than four hundred toxic chemicals have been identified in human tissue.[17] Certain pesticides like malathion, diazinon, and dursban accumulate in various parts of the nervous system and can cause brain disease, motor system dysfunction, and psychological disturbances. Studies have shown that environmental pollutants can cause cancer as well as neurotoxic diseases including depression, apathy, and a diminished capacity to think.[18]

Chemical sensitivities, like other forms of intolerance, vary in intensity. Some patients note mild irritation or headaches with exposure to certain perfumes, disinfectants, paints, tobacco smoke, or automobile exhaust. Others are so sensitive to virtually all man-made chemicals that, to minimize their reactions, they are forced to leave their troubling environment and move to clean housing in unpolluted, rural areas.

Frequently the milder forms of chemical sensitivity will improve with adequate intake of some of the antioxidant vitamins (vitamin C, vitamin E, zinc, and selenium), minerals, adjustments in diet, along with treatment for airborne allergens like pollens, molds, and dust mites. The more severe forms of allergies or sensitivity can be extremely complicated. Patients with severe cases of chemical sensitivity are the most difficult to treat. It takes persistence on the part of both the doctor and the patient to affect improvement.

Rheumatoid Arthritis

Rheumatoid arthritis has long confounded physicians. Conventional medicine essentially has nothing to offer the rheumatoid patient except various types of medication (which often cause serious side effects) or surgery to replace damaged joints. Environmental specialists know that adequate treatment of food, inhalant, and chemical allergies is an important factor in decreasing the lingering pain, disabling stiffness, and crippling effects associated with the disease. In a study of fifty-three patients with documented rheumatoid arthritis, the elimination of foods to which they were sensitive brought about a remarkable improvement in pain and flexibility.[19]

Dr. Mandell had a patient who was advised by an orthopedic surgeon to have both knees replaced because of very severe and painful arthritis. His symptoms were reproduced in Dr. Mandell's office by symptom-duplicating provocative testing that indicated certain foods were probably the culprits. These foods were definitely confirmed as major offenders by single-food test meals, taken every seven days for three weeks. The arthritis dramatically improved by elimination of these test-identified offenders. Today, Dr. Mandell's patient is walking comfortably, twelve years after the foods responsible for his severe arthritis were identified. The pain in his knees flares up only when these foods are eaten, or after exposure to certain chemical fumes.

See Arthritis.

Dr. Mandell emphasizes the fact that many people with arthritis may also have migraine headaches, asthma, and colitis that do not occur by coincidence. These symptoms represent bodywide allergies in predisposed individuals who have what Dr. Mandell has termed "biological weak spots." He also points out that the condition of the rheumatoid patient is further complicated by fatigue, which he considers a form of brain allergy. He has performed thousands of provocative sublingual tests on patients with arthritis and reports that while one food can cause joint pain and swelling, another can cause headache and fatigue, while a third might bring on all of the aforementioned symptoms. "Every patient is different," stresses Dr. Mandell. His findings point to the need for a more comprehensive approach to dealing with arthritis.

The Future of Environmental Medicine

A thorough understanding of physiology and the interaction of the body with the environment has equipped many specialists in environmental medicine to assist chronically ill patients in their quest for better physical and mental health. Due to the advancements in this field, conventional medicine is turning increased attention to the findings of environmental medicine.

"It's interesting to observe how conventional medicine is beginning to acknowledge that food and chemicals in the environment can cause a broad spectrum of physical ailments," says Dr. Wilkinson. "When I first became involved in environmental medicine twelve years ago, it was widely ridiculed by the mainstream of my profession. Now mainstream allergy conventions have lectures dealing with the possible links of food and environmental factors to allergy. Also, the American College of Allergy and Immunology has been sponsoring a conference on food allergy for the past few years."

Though conventional medicine is recognizing the demand of its own patients in the field of environmental medicine, Dr. Wilkinson points out that the realization of a problem does not rapidly translate into effective means of treatment. "Physicians who will continue to lead the way toward effective, physiologic therapy will be those who have spent years listening to their patients and exploring alternatives that offer the hope of helping them," he says.

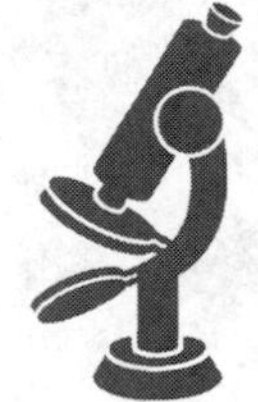

With the ever-growing threat of global pollution, more research is needed to fully understand the impact of environmental factors on health. To support the use of government funds for research in this field, write your elected representative.

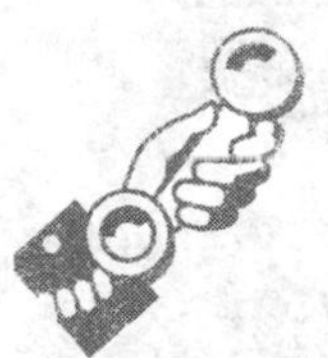

Where to Find Help

For more information about, and referrals for, environmental medicine, contact the following organizations:

American Academy of Environmental Medicine
P.O. Box 16106
Denver, Colorado 80216
(303) 622-9755
The academy offers extensive training for physicians interested in learning more about environmental medicine. For information on physicians practicing environmental medicine send three dollars and a self-addressed, stamped envelope stating your request.

Environmental Health Center
8345 Walnut Hill Lane, Suite 205
Dallas, Texas 75231
(214) 368-4132
This clinic handles severe cases of malnutrition and chemical exposure. Their therapy also treats heart problems, headaches, and joint pains.

Human Ecology Action League
P.O. Box 49126
Atlanta, Georgia 30359
(404) 248-1898
Contact HEAL for information on support groups located in many areas of the country that assist patients with environmental illness.

Natural Lifestyles Supplies
16 Lookout Drive
Asheville, North Carolina 28804
(704) 254-9606
For information on products and books especially prepared for patients suffering from environmental illnesses.

Occupational and Environmental Unit
Tri-Cities Hospital
7525 Scyene Road
Dallas, Texas 75227
(214) 275-1430
Detoxification clinic using dry heat, intravenous supplements, exercise, and massage.

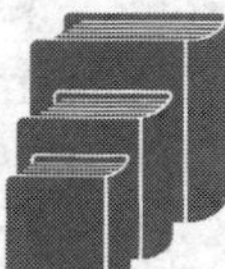

Recommended Reading

An Alternative Approach to Allergies. Randolph, Theron G., M.D.; and Moss, R. W., Ph.D. New York: Bantam Books, 1987.
This is an excellent overview of environmental medicine by the man generally regarded as the father of the field.

Brain Allergies: The Psychonutrient Connection. Philpott, William H., M.D.; and Kalita, D. K., Ph.D. New Canaan, CT: Keats Publishing, 1987.
Has excellent material on allergies and the benefits of "supernutrition."

Detecting Your Hidden Allergies. Crook, William G., M.D. Jackson, TN: Professional Books/Future Health, 1988.
Gives specific instructions on how to use an elimination diet to determine food allergies.

Dr. Mandell's 5-Day Allergy Relief System. Mandell, Marshall, M.D.; and Scanlon, L. New York: Harper & Row, 1988.
This is the first book on clinical ecology for the general public. Self-help and other information.

Dr. Mandell's Lifetime Arthritis Relief System. Mandell, Marshall, M.D. New York: Putnam/ Berkley Group, Inc., 1985.
Self-help and information on the role and importance of allergy in arthritis.

Help for the Hyperactive Child. Crook, William G., M.D. Jackson, TN: Professional Books, 1991.
An easy-to-use illustrated guide that provides exactly what the title suggests by a widely respected pediatrician.

Is This Your Child?: Discovering and Treating Unrecognized Allergies. Rapp, Doris, M.D. New York: William Morrow and Company, Inc., 1991.
This is an informative how-to book for parents or caregivers of "children who are complaining, cranky, slow learners, aggressive, hyperactive, unwell, or depressed."

Enzyme Therapy

Enzyme therapy can be an important first step in restoring health and well-being by helping to remedy digestive problems. Plant enzymes and pancreatic enzymes are used in complementary ways to improve digestion and absorption of essential nutrients. Treatment includes enzyme supplements, coupled with a healthy diet that features whole foods.

For every chemical reaction that occurs in the body, enzymes provide the stimulus. "Enzymes are substances that make life possible," stated Edward Howell, M.D., who pioneered enzyme therapy in the United States. "No mineral, vitamin, or hormone can do any work without enzymes. They are the manual workers that build the body from proteins, carbohydrates, and fats. The body may have the raw building materials, but without thc workers, it cannot begin."[1]

Both plant-derived and pancreatic enzymes are employed in enzyme therapy and they can be used independently or in combination. Plant enzymes are prescribed to enhance the body's vitality by strengthening the digestive system, while pancreatic enzymes are beneficial to both the digestive system and immune system. As proper digestive functioning is restored, many acute and chronic conditions may also be remedied.

Enzymes and Digestion

The human body makes approximately twenty-two different digestive enzymes, capable of digesting protein, carbohydrates, sugars, and fats. People digest food in stages: beginning in the mouth, moving to the stomach, and finally through the small intestine. At each step, specific enzymes break down different types of food. An enzyme designed to digest protein, for example, has no effect on starch, and an enzyme active in the mouth will not be active in the stomach. This process is balanced through acidity; each site along the digestive track has a different degree of acidity that allows certain enzymes to function while inhibiting others.

As enzymes begin digesting food in the mouth and continue their work in the stomach, plant enzymes (derived from food itself or taken as a supplement) also join in and become active. The food then enters the upper portion of the small intestine where the pancreas (a digestive organ that feeds enzymes into the gut) provides pancreatic enzymes to further break down the food. Final breakdown of remaining small molecules of food occurs in the lower small intestine. Ideally, these enzymes can work together, digesting food and delivering nutrients to cells to maintain their health. Protocols in enzyme therapy are based on this sequence of events.

Plant Enzyme Therapy

As plant enzymes are essential for the proper digestion of food, they can play an important role in promoting good health. This is the basis of treatment in plant enzyme therapy. According to Howard F. Loomis, Jr., D.C., of Forsyth, Missouri, "The ability to absorb the nutrients in the food we eat is at the foundation of good health. If we treat digestive disorders, other complaints often clear up as a result." In his own practice, Dr. Loomis tests his patients for enzyme deficiency and then replenishes this deficiency with enzyme supplements. Dr. Loomis adds, "Of course, if a patient is eating a diet of junk food, all the enzymes in the world won't improve his or her basic health. Enzyme therapy needs to be combined with good eating habits. Fresh fruits, vegetables, nuts, and seeds can provide plentiful plant enzymes, and plant enzyme supplements are only meant to supplement those that naturally occur in food."

"As plant enzymes are essential for the proper digestion of food, they can play an important role in promoting good health."

All four categories of plant enzymes have uses in plant enzyme therapy. Protease digests protein; amylase digests carbohydrates; lipase digests fat; and cellulase digests fiber. Plants are a person's only source of cellulase as the human body is unable to produce it. Numerous plant enzyme formulations on the market combine these enzymes.

Plant enzymes function in the stomach, predigesting the food, and plant enzyme therapy uses this to its advantage. This phenomenon was first proposed by Dr. Howell in the 1920s and the study of this process became his life's work.[2] He stated, "If the stomach is performing its proper role, and we are eating our foods uncooked, a large portion of the intake will be partially digested before reacting with the stronger digestive juices found there. Moreover, fewer of your body's internal digestive enzymes will be called upon to perform the digestive function." It is this easing of the body enzymes' workload that is thought to contribute substantially to the healing effects of enzyme therapy. When the body receives plentiful supplies of enzymes, according to Dr. Howell, "its internal enzyme supplies are preserved for the important work of maintaining metabolic harmony." As a result, many body systems are strengthened.[3]

This predigestion of food happens during an interim period, before enough hydrochloric acid (HCl) accumulates in the stomach to begin the next stage in digestion, but this is not commonly known. As Lita Lee, Ph.D., of Eugene, Oregon, states, "Many people don't believe this because they are told that gastric HCl excreted by the stomach destroys the enzymes." Actually, it takes thirty to sixty minutes before enough HCl accumulates in the stomach to initiate the digestion of food. Further, HCl does not destroy but merely deactivates these enzymes by making the environment more acidic. They are reactivated later in the duodenum (upper segment of the small intestine) if the optimum, more alkaline pH is achieved. Enzymes in the stomach can digest 30 percent to 40 percent of the starches we eat.[4] And Dr. Lee adds, "By eating raw foods and taking food enzymes, 30 percent of the protein and 10 percent of the fat can be digested in the stomach in less than one hour."

Cooking food can destroy these important plant enzymes. They are more heat-sensitive than vitamins and are the first to be destroyed during cooking. They are destroyed by being heated above 118 degrees Fahrenheit,[5] and, as Dr. Lee points out, "are deactivated or destroyed by pasteurizing, canning, and microwaving." However, while raw foods are recommended, a 100 percent raw foods diet is not necessary. Dr. Loomis points out that some people may have problems digesting uncooked food because of a lack of cellulase. "People who rarely eat raw food can have problems when they finally eat uncooked fruits and vegetables because they don't chew their food thoroughly," says Dr. Loomis. "Chewing liberates the cellulase out of the food, but when they eat the raw food and don't chew properly the cellulase is never released. Cellulase may also be lacking because of the way the food was handled by the suppliers. Some supermarket vegetables are missing cellulase because they have been sprayed with sulfites which can destroy these enzymes."

"Plant enzymes function in the stomach, predigesting the food."

Plant Enzyme Deficiency

In her practice, Dr. Lee has frequently seen the consequences of eating a predominantly cooked-foods diet—various inflammations, pancreatic hypertrophy (enlargement), a toxic colon, and allergies. Because of inflammation, conditions such as bronchitis, sinusitis, cystitis, rhinitis, and arthritis may occur, and may be accompanied by fever, redness, swelling, and pain. Pancreatic hypertrophy results when a diet lacking in enzymes puts an extra strain on the enzyme production of the pancreas. If the pancreas falls behind in its work, the organ will hypertrophy (enlarge) just as a thyroid grows a goiter when it cannot make enough hormones. This happens anytime an organ cannot produce enough secretions and enlarges in an attempt to make more secretion.

Low levels of enzymes can also lead to a toxic colon. Undigested food can remain in the intestine and not be excreted. Here, the molecules are converted into toxins that are transported by the blood to the liver for detoxification. If the liver is overworked, however, it will be unable to properly detoxify the blood. In his practice Dr. Loomis analyzes the urine and often finds toxins such as phenols (an organic molecule with a structure similar to alcohol) present. Presence of these phenols can lead to a wide range of problems, including allergies, acne, sciatica, and breast pathology.[6]

A meal of predominantly cooked foods can also lead to digestive leukocytosis (an increased white blood count). A rise in white blood cells is a sign that the immune system is being mobilized. It accompanies many pathological conditions, including infections and poisoning, but it can also immediately occur after eating breakfast, lunch, or dinner. Dr. Lee says, "Digestive leukocytosis occurs a mere thirty minutes after eating cooked food. This does not occur when a person eats raw food because of the presence of plant enzymes in this food." Such a response puts added stress on the immune system. "The concept of the immune system being stimulated every time you eat, was first reported in 1897 by Rudolph Virchow, the father of cellular pathology. In other words, your immune system is stimulated, as if you had an infection," confirms Dr. Loomis.

Benefits of Plant Enzyme Therapy

According to Dr. Lee, when a patient's plant enzyme deficiencies are addressed many other conditions can resolve, from digestive ailments and common sore throats to hay fever, ulcers, and candida. In one instance, Dr. Lee used plant enzymes to treat a case of chronic digestive disorders. A fifty-seven-year-old man had suffered from severe intestinal problems for most of his adult life. A number of medical specialists had provided him with varying diagnoses, including spastic colon, diverticulitis, yeast imbalance, and lactose intolerance, but none of them were able to discover the cause of the condition. He tried several changes of diet without success, and eventually was placed on Lomotil to treat his diarrhea. After meals, he continued to experience painful cramps, diarrhea, headaches, and an overall sense of weakness, and was finally told that there was no cure for this condition. Dr. Lee did a twenty-four-hour urinalysis and blood profile and diagnosed the patient's problem as a lipase enzyme deficiency, coupled with a fiber intolerance. After four months of enzyme supplements, the man's condition was completely improved with no recurrence of symptoms.

> *"People think that if they simply take vitamins and minerals they will be healthy, but every vitamin and mineral requires an enzyme. You can eat pounds and pounds of vitamins and minerals, but if you don't have the proper enzymes, they won't work."*
> —Lita Lee, Ph.D.

Plant enzyme therapy can also increase the absorption of nutrients. Dr. Lee recalls a case of myasthenia gravis (a disease characterized by extreme muscle weakness) which is associated with a deficiency in the B vitamins, vitamin E, and manganese. With enzymes, the patient was able to lower the vitamin and mineral dosage since these nutrients were now more easily absorbed. In another case a young child was diagnosed with severe iron anemia. Given a formulation of iron plus enzymes, the child's condition improved within three days. Dr. Lee points out, "People think that if they simply take vitamins and minerals they will be healthy, but every vitamin and mineral requires an enzyme. You can eat pounds and pounds of vitamins and minerals, but if you don't have the proper enzymes, they won't work."

Dr. Lee has also successfully treated patients who have had candidiasis for years. "They've tried all the popular yeast remedies, including nystatin, probiotics (substances such as acidophilus and bifidus that act to reestablish the intestinal flora), herbals, homeopathies, and fatty acids of many kinds," states Dr. Lee. "Many of them still had the yeast overgrowth plus liver damage due to the nystatin. I used a very potent remedy containing acidophilus, bifidus, and certain cellulase enzymes. This formula is taken to digest the yeast and reestablish friendly bowel bacteria. Along with this, a protease formula is used to remove the toxic debris. This treatment works very well with homeopathics and herbals and I do not hesitate to add these to the enzyme protocol when needed."

The FDA (Food and Drug Administration) has long approved the use of plant enzymes, but as dietary supplements only. As Dr. Loomis states, "All we are saying is that by clearing up digestive problems, we've found that many other problems seem to go away and new ailments may be prevented." And he is quick to add, "It cannot be said that a particular enzyme can help a particular illness. Any treatment is multifaceted, requiring various enzymes plus other modes of care, as well as adherence to a healthy diet with adequate raw foods."

"It cannot be said that a particular enzyme can help a particular illness. Any treatment is multifaceted, requiring various enzymes plus other modes of care, as well as adherence to a healthy diet with adequate raw foods."

—Howard Loomis, D.C.

Pancreatic Enzyme Therapy

The history of pancreatic enzyme therapy predates the work in plant enzyme therapy. In 1902, English embryologist John Beard injected pancreatic extracts directly into tumors of cancer patients with therapeutic success.[7] When others tried this method and failed, mainly due to the impurity of the extract preparations, the therapy fell into disrepute. Later in Germany, Max Wolf, M.D., and Karl Ransberger, Ph.D., used enzymes to successfully treat patients with multiple sclerosis, cancer, and viral infections. The two men provided some of the earliest research on enzymes and co-enzymes.[8]

Hector Solorzano del Rio, M.D., D.Sc., Coordinator of the Program for Studies of Alternative Medicine and Professor of Pharmacology of the University of Guadalajara in Mexico, is one of the many physicians who uses pancreatic enzyme therapy. He has treated a wide variety of diseases—inflammatory conditions such as rheumatic disorders, soft tissue trauma, viral infections, arthritis, multiple sclerosis, cancer, and autoimmune diseases, including AIDS. Dosages are given orally on an empty stomach or by injection, and may be combined with plant enzymes.

How Pancreatic Enzyme Therapy Works

Pancreatic enzymes are animal enzymes that include proteases, amylases, and lipases. Pancreatic enzymes function in the intestine and in the blood. Supplemental pancreatic enzymes can aid digestion in the intestine, sharing the workload of the body's own pancreatic enzymes that are active there. However, they do not digest food in the stomach, or contribute to the important step of predigestion. Dr. Loomis, who extensively trained in the use of both plant and pancreatic enzymes, recalls a case in point. A patient with chronic pancreatitis (inflammation of the pancreas) felt pain after every meal. He had been taking pancreatic enzymes but they had not helped. Since pancreatic enzymes are inactive in the stomach, they were not able to address the real problem. Dr. Loomis tried putting the man on plant enzymes instead, which predigest food in the stomach before it reaches the intestines. With the food first prepared for digestion, the condition was resolved. After taking plant enzymes, the patient's pain stopped at the very next meal.

By supplementing the body's own pancreatic enzymes, pancreatic enzyme therapy, like plant enzyme therapy, promotes health by lessening the demands on the body for supplying enzymes to convert food to usable nutrients and energy. Pancreatic enzymes also play a fascinating role in the immune system, directly assisting the defense mechanisms,[9] and this function has been shown to make a significant contribution to the therapeutic powers of these enzymes.

According to Dr. Loomis, "Protein molecules that are only partially digested in the small intestine are able to be absorbed into the bloodstream." The immune system now treats these as invaders. Antibodies couple with these antigens (foreign substances that provoke an immune reaction) and circulating immune complexes (CIC's) are formed. In a healthy person, these CIC's may be neutralized in the lymphatic system. But in a sick person, CIC's accumulate in the blood where they can initiate an "allergic" reaction. As too many CIC's accumulate, the kidneys cannot excrete enough and the CIC's begin to accumulate in soft tissues, causing inflammation. This brings unnecessary stress to the immune system. Dr. Loomis comments, "I always wonder why the diets for cancer and AIDS include such high amounts of protein when an excess of undigested protein can so obviously lead to demands on the immune system."

It is here that the pancreatic enzymes come into play. The pancreatic enzymes are able to break down CIC's so that they can pass through the kidneys for excretion. The enzymes are taken between meals so they will not be used for digesting food, but will make their way directly to the bloodstream. Because of their ability to digest foreign proteins, pancreatic enzymes are also able to clear out infecting organisms such as viruses, scar tissue, and the products of inflammation. For this reason, pancreatic enzymes are used in a variety of conditions, including lung infections, tooth infections, bone fractures, and are recommended prior to surgery.

VITAMINS, MINERALS, AND ENZYMES

"In enzyme therapy we recommend that patients eat whole, unprocessed foods with plenty of raw foods included," states Lita Lee, Ph.D. "This has many benefits, but not just because these foods provide enzymes. Whole foods also contain vitamins and minerals, embedded in the mother plant, that function as co-enzymes, molecules that also must be present for a chemical reaction to take place."

She continues, "One of the most important processes in the metabolism of food is the chain of reactions that convert glucose to energy. Several vitamin and mineral co-enzymes are necessary for these reactions. Co-enzymes are consumed in the process. Our bodies need a continuing supply. All the food we eat, that eventually becomes energy, passes through this same set of reactions, whether the food is a fast-food hamburger or a raw carrot. Co-enzymes are always needed, and when the food doesn't provide these, we use the vitamins and minerals stored in our body until these reserves are used up. Only when we eat whole and raw foods can we maintain a good supply of the parts that keep the metabolic machinery going."

Conditions Benefited by Pancreatic Enzyme Therapy

Pancreatic enzymes have been shown to be beneficial in a variety of disease conditions, including inflammation, viral disease, multiple sclerosis, and cancer.

Inflammation: Inflammation is a response to noxious stimuli, and is a way the body rids itself of harmful substances. The classical signs of inflammation are pain, redness, swelling, and heat. Once inflammation takes place, however, healing can begin. With sports injuries, enzymes are used to promote inflammation in order to accelerate healing, and taking them before performing athletics can promote faster healing if injury occurs.

Viral Diseases: Viruses have a protein coat, and enzymes are able to initiate reactions that can digest this protective layer so that the viruses can be destroyed. Enzymes also help in the removal of CIC's that are abundant in viral disease. Research also indicates that enzymes are beneficial in the treatment of herpes zoster (shingles), particularly in patients with immune deficiencies.[10] And enzymes can in part counteract the decreased immune function of HIV (human immunodeficiency virus) infection.[11]

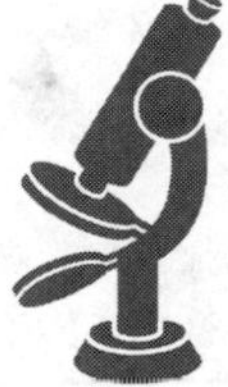

Further research into the benefits of pancreatic enzyme therapy is necessary as it has been clinically proven to alleviate a wide range of conditions.

Multiple Sclerosis: Although the cause of multiple sclerosis is unknown, it has been shown that demyelination (reduction of the fatty covering of the nerves) occurs. Dr. Solorzano tells of a wheelchair-bound patient diagnosed with multiple sclerosis for whom no traditional treatment had helped. Trying pancreatic enzyme therapy, the patient gained strength and could dress himself within one month. After three months, he could work with difficulty, and within six months his symptoms disappeared and he was able to resume a normal, productive life.

Cancer: Pancreatic enzymes can help in the treatment of cancer in several ways. Enzymes help expose antigens on the surface of cancer cells, so they can be recognized as foreign and destroyed by the immune system. They also help destroy CIC's produced when cancerous cells shed their antigens into the circulation to avoid detection by the immune system. Pancreatic enzymes can stimulate natural killer cells, T-cells, and tumor necrosis factor (anticancer agents), all toxic to cancer cells.[12]

According to Dr. Solorzano, by removing the "sticky" coating found on tumor cells, enzymes reduce the risk of tumors adhering to other areas of the body (i.e., preventing metastasis).[13] And pancreatic enzymes can enter cancer cells in their reproductive phase when they are not completely formed and more susceptible to destruction. Vitamin A increases these effects, as it releases enzymes contained in lysosomes (components of the intercellular digestive system), and is often given in combination with pancreatic enzymes. In Germany, pancreatic enzyme solutions have been injected directly into tumors, causing them to dissolve.[14]

The Future of Enzyme Therapy

The future of enzyme therapy seems assured. There are now over two thousand enzyme therapists in the United States and the field of enzyme therapy is rapidly expanding. "I think enzyme therapy is the wave of the future and will revolutionize the field of nutrition. All preventive therapies will include treatment of enzyme deficiencies and all food supplements will address our need for enzymes," states Dr. Lee.

The use of pancreatic enzyme therapy in the field of medicine has a head start because it already has been the subject of much research in Europe. And Dr. Loomis envisions, "If research funds were currently as available to study all types of enzyme therapy in the United States as they are in Europe, tremendous strides could be taken. The future could be particularly bright for plant enzyme therapy. Depletions of plant enzymes lead to a host of chronic diseases that could in part be avoided if we provided the body with the enzymes it needs. As it is, we are not aware of enzyme deficiencies because they take so long to manifest. When there are signs, the body is already in a state of exhaustion. It is here that the future of plant enzyme therapy lies, in its potentially enormous roll in nutrition and the prevention of chronic degenerative disease."

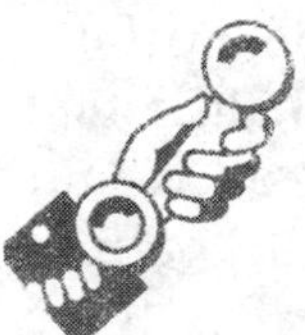

Where to Find Help

For more information on clinics and practitioners using enzyme therapy, contact:

Dr. Lita Lee
2852 Williamette Street,
Suite 397
Eugene, Oregon 97405
(503) 746-7621
For information on doctors using plant enzyme therapy. Dr. Lee also publishes a quarterly newsletter called Earthletter. *It covers current news and research of environmental medicine, enzyme therapy, and radiation.*

Dr. Howard Loomis
P.O. Box 883
North Highway 160
Forsyth, Missouri 65653
(417) 546-2411
For information on doctors using plant enzyme therapy.

NESS
P.O. Box 249 Highway 160
Forsyth, Missouri 65653
(417) 546-3121
For information on doctors using plant enzyme therapy.

Karl Ransberger
Medizinische
Enzymeforschungsgesellschaft
Alpenstrasse 29
D-8192 Geretstried 1
Germany
To contact Karl Ransberger, Ph.D., the father of pancreatic enzyme therapy.

Dr. Hector E. Solorzano de Rio
Universidad de Guadalajara
Apartado Postal No. 2-41
44280 Guadalajara, Jal.
Mexico
For further information on clinics and practitioners in Mexico.

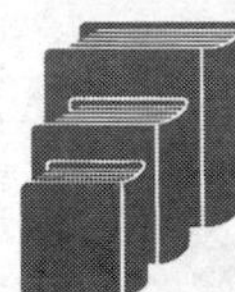

Recommended Reading

Enzyme Nutrition. Howell, Edward. Wayne, NJ: Avery Publishing Group, Inc., 1985.

In this excellent and accessible book, Dr. Howell emphasizes the importance of enzymes in diet as a prevention to degenerative disease and the key to longevity.

Enzyme Therapy. Wolf, Max, M.D., and Ransberger, Karl, Ph.D. New York: Biological Research Institute, 1972.

An in-depth study of pancreatic enzymes and their therapeutic qualities in treating aging, cancer, viral diseases, and more.

Food Enzymes. Santillo, Humbart, B.S., M.H. Prescott, AZ: Hohm Press, 1987.

A practical and concise guide that explains how food enzymes work and why they are so crucial and beneficial to all metabolic functions.

Radiation Protection Manual. Lee, Lita, Ph.D. Grassroots Network: Redwood City, CA, 1990.

Chemist and nutritionist Lita Lee discusses the sources and dangers of radiation in the environment, food, and appliances, and how to protect yourself through diet and nutritional supplements, including enzymes.

"The primary cause of our disease is in us, always in us."

—Antoine Beachamp. 1883

Fasting

Fasting is a low-cost, effective therapy for a wide range of conditions, including hypertension, headaches, allergies, and arthritis. By relieving the body of the task of digesting foods, fasting allows the system to rid itself of toxins while facilitating healing.

"One of the most overlooked and yet valuable modes of healing is the fast," says Evarts G. Loomis, M.D., co-founder of the American Holistic Medical Association (AHMA) and founder of the Meadowlark clinic in Hemet, California, America's first live-in health retreat. "In recent years, few physicians have seriously considered the fast as worthy of study, and most have used it in the treatment of obesity." Over a period of eighteen years at Meadowlark, Dr. Loomis successfully guided more than one thousand patients through a fast as part of their therapeutic regime.

For many people fasting can be used as an adjunct to the healing process, and is an invaluable aid for those seeking enhancement of their overall physical, mental, and spiritual health. Short fasts (two to five days) can be performed at home as part of a personal health maintenance program. Longer fasts, undertaken with medical supervision, can serve to strengthen the immune system, alleviate food allergies, and reduce or eliminate medications for certain health conditions.

How Fasting Works

A great deal of energy is needed to break down food into its nutritional components, convert food's carbohydrates and proteins into glycogen (a starch which can be converted into energy) for storage in the liver, and provide the body with the fuel necessary to perform its functions. When the intake of calories is restricted or eliminated, the body fuels itself through alternate means.

During the first two days of a fast, the liver converts stored sugars into glucose that the body can use for fuel, according to Steven Bailey, N.D., of the Northwest Naturopathic Clinic in Portland, Oregon. When these stores are depleted, fat is used as a source of energy. Fasting aids most health concerns because during a fast:

- The body continues its natural process of excreting stored toxins, while the intake of new toxins is decreased. In this way, total body toxicity is reduced.

- With the elimination of food and its allergens, the immune system's workload is also greatly reduced and the digestive tract is spared the constant inflammation due to allergic reactions.
- With the lowering of serum fats (after the fourth day of the fast), the thinner blood affords increased oxygenation of tissues and enhanced delivery of white blood cells throughout the body.
- Significantly less energy is directed at food digestion (which involves the use of blood, oxygen, and nutrients). This allows for greater reserves of energy and nutrients for use by the systems of self-regulation (immune function, cell growth, eliminatory processes).
- The metabolizing (burning) of fat and its conversion to energy-yielding molecules releases many fat-stored chemicals (pesticides, drugs) into the bloodstream at a time when the body has enhanced eliminatory capabilities.
- The innate ability of the body to recognize old, nonessential tissues and subsequently dissolve these, while recycling their important nutrients for new cell production, furthers elimination and leads to broadly enhanced physiological function.
- A person's awareness and sensitivity to diet and surroundings are elevated. Fasting has been used as a spiritual practice in many cultures to enhance health and well-being.

Conditions Benefited by Fasting

Some illnesses commonly benefited by fasting include heart disease, hypertension, arthritis, allergies, inflammatory diseases, psychological problems, and headaches.

Trevor Salloum, N.D., of Kelowna, British Columbia, Canada, has found that allergies, respiratory diseases, and acute illnesses are most responsive to a fast, while chronic degenerative diseases are the least responsive, often requiring several periods of fasting. He finds water fasts very beneficial for arthritis and tells of a woman from Australia confined to a wheelchair with rheumatoid arthritis who recovered her mobility after three separate thirty-day water fasts.

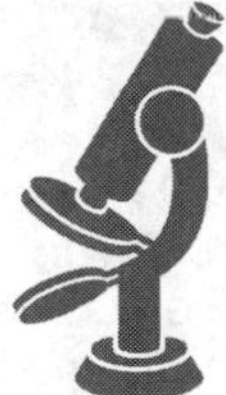

Further research into the benefits of fasting is necessary as it has been clinically proven to alleviate a wide range of conditions.

"As a general rule, patients with arthritis were likely to be off their medication with no increased discomfort within the space of a three- to four-day fast," says Dr. Loomis. "By the middle of the second week, they were generally 80 to 90 percent free of pain. The exception were those who had been on long-term use of cortisone derivatives. However, they were able to make a substantial reduction in their amount of medication. Patients with hypertension, for the most part, were able to reduce and then eliminate their medication, with a return to normal blood pressure within a period of two to three weeks."

Fasting can also help identify food allergies. A thirty-five-year-old woman, seen by Dr. Loomis, complained of depression, irritability, excruciating headaches, rapid heartbeat, a tremor of her hands, sinus congestion, and urinary problems. After a four-day water fast her symptoms were relieved. As various foods were reintroduced after the fast, Dr. Loomis found that following the ingestion of milk, her sinuses became congested; following a meal of corn, her tremor developed; a headache became evident subsequent to the ingestion of a meal of bananas; and her bladder symptoms followed both rice and strawberries. Two months later, after following a new dietary regimen, she reported no further headaches, bladder trouble, or depression. The subsequent month, she became lax with the dietary restrictions and practically all of her symptoms returned.

Dr. Bailey tells of a patient who called him stating that she was scheduled for a bilateral radical mastectomy (treatment of breast cancer in which the breast, involved skin, pectoral muscles, axillary lymph nodes, and subcutaneous fat are removed). In constant, severe pain and with only two weeks until surgery, she wondered if a naturopathic approach could help. Knowing that her problem had been a ten-year progressive condition recently biopsied as noncancerous, Dr. Bailey gave the woman no guarantees, but suggested she undertake a three-month intensive holistic approach while retaining surgery as an option. Hoping to avoid surgery and with pain as a great motivator, the woman began a three-week building diet to increase her nutritional intake prior to the fast. She ate whole grains and fresh vegetables, reduced nonessential fats, and eliminated caffeine. After two weeks she began a seven-day juice fast. By midfast her cysts had reduced in size and hardness and for the first time in many years she experienced a ceasing of pain. With this improvement as a springboard, she pursued a long-term program. Today, not only are her cysts almost completely inpalpable, but she is pain free and in control of her own health.

In the field of psychiatry, Professor Serge Nikoliav of the Moscow Psychiatric Institute, used fasting to treat six thousand patients for chronic refractory schizophrenia (a recurring mental disorder characterized by gross distortions of reality, which is resistant to treatment) who had not responded to the more usual types of psychiatric therapy. These patients were placed on water fasts, lasting from twenty-five to thirty days, and also engaged in aerobic exercise in the form of long periods of daily walking. Dr. Nikoliav's treatment of these cases shows a very high success rate.[1]

PREPARATION FOR FASTING

Short-term fasts (Dr. Chaitow's two-day weekend fast, or Dr. Bailey's five-day juice fast) may be carried out in a normal setting. They do not require extended rest periods and normal duties can be continued. There are no special preparations necessary for Dr. Chaitow's program. Dr. Bailey's clinical program includes a three-day bulking diet prior to beginning the juice fast. He also offers an initial individual consultation or group meetings to provide support and education prior to fasting. Dr. Loomis recommends a two-day transition diet of grains and steamed vegetables. If you are planning anything more than a two-day fast, a careful physical examination and history-taking are crucial to your safety, particularly if you are taking any kind of medication. In addition, blood tests measuring the levels of proteins, uric acid, sugar, creatinine, and cholesterol, along with liver function, should be performed. An EKG (electrocardiogram) may be an option.

A prolonged fast should not be carried out in the home or business environment. The setting should be a place of natural beauty removed from the everyday stressful distractions of newspapers, radio, television, telephone, and visitors (perhaps even including contact with immediate family).

Opinions concerning the use of enemas and colonics vary. Generally, vegetable juice fasts require regular enemas during the fasting period whereas water fasts often do not. Dr. Loomis recommends starting a fast with three nightly enemas, followed by a purge with a cathartic (laxative) such as sodium phosphate. A teaspoon (one gram) of vitamin C powder compounded with potassium, sodium, calcium, and magnesium is added to the enema solution. Dr. Loomis also suggests a nightly liver flush for an average of three days. Consult with a health professional to determine if internal cleansing, prior to or during the fast, is advisable.

Types of Fasts

There are differing ideas about what constitutes an ideal fast. In any case, it is essential to consult a health professional before undertaking a fast to ascertain your physical condition and to determine the length and type of fast (water or juice) that is most appropriate. During a prolonged fast (more than a couple of days), vitamin or mineral supplements may be necessary, as well as changes in dosage of any medication. Periodic blood tests are recommended during the fast to monitor one's physical condition.

Dr. Salloum favors a water fast and stresses the use of only pure water (distilled, spring or purified by reverse osmosis). He considers juice to be a food, since it supplies carbohydrates which inhibit the development of ketone metabolism (breakdown of fats), and maintains that a juice fast is, in effect, a restricted diet. Dr. Salloum believes that during a fast, water should be consumed according to thirst, with a minimum of three glasses a day.

Certain practitioners recommend a juice fast because of the withdrawal symptoms a water fast causes when nutrients and drugs (prescription and recreational) are released into the bloodstream for elimination. This detoxification process is much less severe on a juice fast.

For over ten years, Dr. Loomis exclusively used medically supervised water fasts with his patients. However, he noticed his patients often suffered from intense fatigue and other symptoms during the first few days of the fast. While visiting Zurich's Bircher-Benner Clinic and the Landhaus Nurpfli retreat, both in Switzerland, Dr. Loomis was introduced to the use of juice fasts. Not only did juice fasts prove to be as beneficial as water, but, unlike water fasters, juice fasters were far more likely to continue a healthy diet once they had broken the fast, as they had become accustomed to the taste of raw vegetables.

DR. CHAITOW'S TWO-DAY FAST[2]

Leon Chaitow, N.D., D.O., of London, England, recommends a two-day fast, as it can be conveniently followed over a weekend, and should not disrupt a work schedule. A two-day fast is also quite safe to perform at home with a doctor's approval, whereas longer fasts require continual professional supervision.[3] Dr. Chaitow explains the procedure:

Saturday: *Whether on a juice or a water fast, start the day with a slowly sipped glass of the fluid. Do stretching, relaxation, and breathing exercises, and spend the morning relaxing, reading, listening to music, or napping. Have a midmorning drink. After a lunchtime drink, nap for a while. Do more stretching exercises, have a massage, and, if possible, spend half an hour outside in the sun. Have another drink, relax, and meditate before going to bed early.*

Sunday: *Start the day like Saturday, and use an enema to cleanse the lower bowel. Rest outdoors. Drink midmorning, noon, and midafternoon, and have another massage if possible. Break the fast around 6:00 P.M. with a stewed apple or pear, live yogurt, or vegetable soup. You can have more of the same later if you are hungry.*

Monday: *Return to normal, but have a lighter breakfast than usual.*

Acceptable juice combinations include carrots (diluted with water 50:50) and green vegetables, according to Dr. Loomis. Fruit juices contain large amounts of sugar, and are not generally used in fasting. (For example, a glass of apple juice contains the equivalent of five apples—a considerable sugar load to ingest all at once.) Loomis's patients also take Bieler Broth (named after its inventor, Henry Bieler, M.D.), consisting of steamed green beans, zucchini, celery, and parsley, that are pureed and eaten with a spoon. Herbal teas are also permitted on this type of fast.

If Dr. Loomis feels a patient requires a more intense detoxification, a detoxifying cocktail is taken at bedtime, consisting of a blend of one garlic clove, the juice of one-half of a lemon, the juice of two grapefruits (which can be replaced by apple juice if preferred), and two tablespoons of olive oil. Also known as a "liver flush," this works to detoxify the liver, a main organ of elimination most active between the hours of 11:00 P.M. and 1:00 A.M.

See Juice Therapy.

Dr. Bailey believes that two five-day juice fasts a year are ideal for maintaining health. However, some of his patients with chronic health problems have gone on juice fasts in excess of thirty days. He prefers to use vegetable juices, since they provide adequate supplies of vitamins and minerals. Dr. Bailey recommends a beet/carrot/celery blend (equal parts of each), but the beet can be omitted if sugar is a health concern. This combination supplies excellent energy, vitamins, and minerals, live enzymes, and other nutrients needed to maintain health during the fast. By providing much of the body's daily caloric needs with easily absorbed juices, the release of toxins from fat cells is much more gradual and gentle. Dr. Bailey also advocates water fasts but believes that the further one's diet is from a nonprocessed, whole foods regimen, the greater the need for gradual detoxification, as provided by juice fasts.

A person's nutritional status and degree of toxicity prior to the fast will determine the type of fast undertaken and its length. Also important to consider is whether the fast is being undertaken for detoxification purposes or to counteract a specific disease.

STAGES OF A PROLONGED FAST (ONE TO THREE WEEKS)

Evarts G. Loomis, M.D., divides a fast into four stages:

***Stage 1** is a period of general excitation of the involuntary nervous system and major detoxification, manifested through the increased electrical activity observed with the EEG (electroencephalogram). At this time, the blood picture reveals an increased number of white blood cells. This stage lasts about three days.*

***Stage 2** is heralded by increasing evidence of acidosis, the presence of hypoglycemia (low blood sugar), and a psychomotor depression. Stage two is marked by a loss of appetite. The length of the second stage depends on the toxicity of a person prior to fasting and the number of medications he or she is taking. This stage may begin after three or four days of fasting, or not until the second week of the fast.*

***Stage 3** is a normalization period accompanied by a feeling of increased well-being that surpasses any preexisting the fast. This state is usually reached in the second week of the fast, but can occur earlier in less toxic people.*

***Stage 4** is usually accompanied by a vast improvement in energy, clarity of mind, and a heightened sense of well-being. Again, the time frame depends on the individual, and can occur anywhere from four days into the fast to the second week of the fast.*

What to Do During a Fast

Many bodily changes can occur during a fast, especially due to the release of toxins. Patients should be aware of these symptoms so there is no cause for alarm.

Physical Effects: A coated tongue and unpleasant taste in the mouth usually accompany a fast. These can be remedied by frequent rinsing of the mouth (with lemon juice). Headaches and a general feeling of "unwellness" may occur. Fatigue is likely, body odor will increase, and the skin may appear blotchy, dry, and scaly. The patient may experience dizziness, nausea, insomnia, aching limbs, and visual and hearing disturbances. None of these are serious or permanent conditions.

Cardiac arrhythmia (irregular beating of the heart) is a possibility during a fast. The irregular beating does not usually persist, and is probably due to the realignments going on within the human frame.[4] Blood pressure and pulse rate can drop, particularly during a longer fast. When detoxification occurs, hallucinogenic flashbacks and return of previous illness symptoms may occur temporarily.

Weight loss during the early days of the fast can be dramatic, especially in women who have a water retention problem, often the case with obese people. Sometimes the loss can be as much as four to seven pounds in a single day, and ten to twenty pounds in a week is not unusual, according to Dr. Loomis. By the end of the first week, however, the weight loss will have leveled off to an average of three-fourths of a pound a day, and there will be days of no loss, and perhaps even days of gain. If diuresis (water loss) seems to be incomplete, diuretic herb teas such as goldenrod, chamomile, watercress, parsley, or rosehips are frequently recommended.

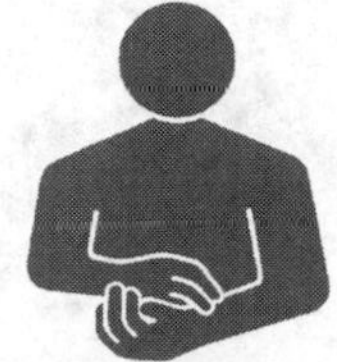

Fasting is ideally suited to self-care and can become an important part of one's personal health maintenance program.

Personal Hygiene: There is likely to be considerable body odor due to the elimination of toxins. A morning shower is suggested, but water temperatures should not be extreme as a long hot shower can be physically taxing. Cosmetics and deodorants should be avoided during the fast, as they tend to drive impurities back into the system. A coated tongue can be brushed, and the mouth rinsed. Also, it is important that dentures remain in the mouth during the fast to avoid any shrinkage of the gums.

Exercise: Opinions on exercise vary from those who advise bed rest to those who believe in long daily periods of walking, cycling, or swimming. Variations of exercise to suit the particular faster are recommended, but strenuous exercise is not advised.

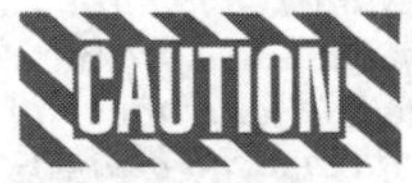

Certain conditions contraindicate fasting. These include: diabetes, eating disorders, epilepsy, hypochondria, kidney disease, malnutrition, pregnancy, lactation, severe bronchial asthma, terminal illness, tuberculosis, ulcerative colitis. Long-term fasts should be done under professional supervision.

Sunlight: Sunlight is important for general health during fasting, and ten to thirty minutes of sunbathing a day is recommended.

Rest: Rest is very important during a fast. Napping during the day is beneficial.

Coming off the Fast

The time suggested to come off a fast varies. One may follow a set time schedule or wait for traditional indicators of detoxification (improved breath, clear tongue, removal of original symptoms, return of appetite). Always, when the hunger-free stage of fasting has passed and a strong hunger returns, it is time to return to juices and broths.

The reason for ending a fast when a strong hunger returns is that continued fasting may cause the body to enter a starvation stage in which it begins to burn vital protein mass. As a rule, approximately the same length of time should be given to the withdrawal phase as was spent on the fast. At the end of the fast, the amount of digestive juices available is limited and the stomach may have shrunk considerably, so the initial meals should be in small amounts at frequent intervals. Gorging after a fast, as some occasionally do, or eating highly refined or spiced foods, can have serious consequences, such as severe abdominal pain, diarrhea, and vomiting.

The longer the fast, the more care is needed in its method of termination. The usual procedure to break a water fast is with fruit or vegetable juices. Meadowlark's routine is one glass of fruit juice for breakfast and two to three glasses of vegetable juices during the remainder of the day. In the case of water fasts that have continued longer than a week, the juices should at first be diluted. These are sipped at intervals throughout the day and not gulped down as a substitute for a meal. Water intake should also be continued. Follow a one-week water fast with two to three days of juice fasting; for a two-week fast, double this amount. In cases of obesity, one can remain considerably longer on the juice, if so desired.

The longer the fast, the more care needed in its method of termination.

After the juice portion of a water fast (or at the end of a juice fast) solid foods may be introduced. A good beginning is a breakfast of fruits or of freshly prepared muesli, made by soaking oatmeal in pineapple juice overnight and, the next morning, adding fresh fruit and a scattering of ground nuts. The other two meals should be of vegetables, raw or very lightly steamed. Dr. Loomis notes that many people lose their appetite for meat as well as junk foods on completion of the fast.

Fasting and the New Medicine

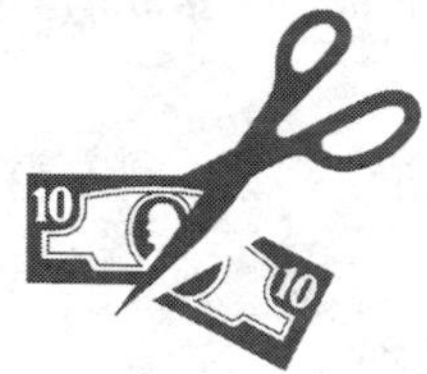

Fasting is a natural and inexpensive preventive method for maintaining health and can be a cost-effective therapy for numerous health conditions.

Fasting can play an integral role in any health maintenance program. It can aid in detoxification and strengthen the immune system. Fasting often allows a patient to reduce or eliminate medications for certain conditions. As medical costs soar, an alternative to high-cost medical procedures will be sought. "Fasting is now coming under much scientific study, particularly in Scandinavia, where medical professionals find it very beneficial in rheumatoid arthritis," says Dr. Salloum. "Results suggest that it will become the therapy of choice for many people in the future. All it requires is water [or juice] and a practitioner to supervise."

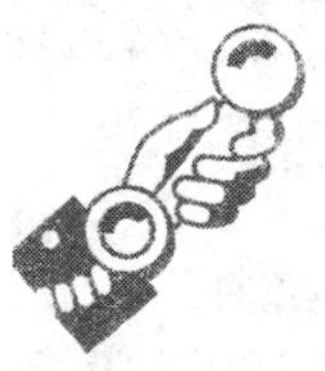

Where to Find Help

Fasting remains a simple and effective therapy for a wide range of health problems and is an important tool of alternative medicine. For more information on fasting, contact one of the following organizations or practitioners:

American Association of Naturopathic Physicians
2366 Eastlake Avenue, Suite 322
Seattle, Washington 98102
(206) 323-7610
(800) 206-7610
Provides referrals to a nationwide network of accredited or licensed naturopathic physicians for health professionals and the general public; supported by members and corporate sponsors. It hosts an annual convention, and works to move legislature and licensure in various states.

International Association of Professional Natural Hygienists
Regency Health Resort and Spa
2000 South Ocean Drive
Hallandale, Florida 33009
(305) 454-2220
A professional organization of doctors who specialize in therapeutic fasting. All follow the same protocol for fasting. Represents doctors in the United States, Canada, Australia, England, Greece, Israel, Japan, and Poland.

National College of Naturopathic Medicine
11231 Southeast Market Street
Portland, Oregon 97216
(503) 255-4860
For referrals to naturopathic doctors in your area.

Northwest Naturopathic Clinic
2606 Northwest Vaughn
Portland, Oregon 97210
(503) 224-8083
For information and guidance on juice fasting.

Trevor Salloum, N.D.
557 Bernard Avenue
Kelowna, British Columbia V1Y 6N9
(604)763-5445
For information and guidance on water fasts.

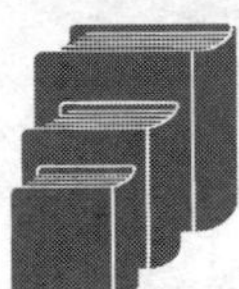

Recommended Reading

Body/Mind Purification Program. Chaitow, Leon. New York: Simon and Schuster, 1990.
A holistic approach to enhance your physical, spiritual, and emotional well-being in a toxic world. Dr. Chaitow guides you through detoxification and introduces a clean nutritious diet, as well as exercises, stretches, massage, and other therapies. This book is currently available only from Educating Hands Bookstore, 261 Southwest 8th Street, Miami, Florida 33139, (305) 285-6991, (305) 857-0298 (Fax).

Fasting Signs and Symptoms—A Clinical Guide. Salloum, Trevor K. East Palestine, OH: Buckeye Naturopathic Press, 1992.
Most extensive work on the subject of therapeutic fasting. The author focuses on specific diseases and his tested method of treatment through water and juice fasts.

Healing for Everyone. Loomis, Evarts. Marina del Rey, CA: DeVorss & Co., 1975.
Loomis writes on nutrition, exercise, yoga, and self-realization as the root to health and wholeness. His extensive research and studies on fasting are very informative.

The Hygienic System, Volume III. Shelton, Herbert M. Chicago: Natural Hygiene Press, 1971.
The most extensive work on the subject of therapeutic fasting. Shelton gives a thorough history of fasting plus explains its physiology, acute chronic diseases, and the symptomology of fasting.

Flower Remedies

The emotions play a crucial role in the health of the physical body. Flower remedies directly address a person's emotional state in order to help facilitate both psychological and physiological well-being. By balancing negative feelings and stress, flower remedies can effectively remove the emotional barriers to health and recovery.

"Behind all disease lies our fears, our anxieties, our greed, our likes and dislikes," wrote English physician Edward Bach, M.B., B.S., D.P.H., in the early 1930s.[1] Dr. Bach based his revolutionary belief upon his personal observations of patients whose physical illnesses seemed to be predisposed by negative psychological or emotional states such as fear, anxiety, insecurity, jealousy, shyness, poor self-image, anger, and resentment. Today, numerous studies conducted at major universities and medical centers have verified Dr. Bach's early conviction, revealing a definite connection between negative emotional states and a reduction of the body's natural resistance to disease.

"True healing involves treating the very base of the cause of the suffering. Therefore no effort directed to the body alone can do more than superficially repair damage. Treat people for their emotional unhappiness, allow them to be happy, and they will become well."
—Dr. Edward Bach

"True healing involves treating the very base of the cause of the suffering," said Dr. Bach. "Therefore no effort directed to the body alone can do more than superficially repair damage. Treat people for their emotional unhappiness, allow them to be happy, and they will become well." [1]

In Dr. Bach's day, conventional medicine had no real methodology to address the link between emotional and physical illness, relying instead upon the use of drugs which often did more harm than good. In an attempt to fill this void, he began to investigate the healing potential of the wildflowers native to the English countryside. After several years of extensive research and testing, he was able to identify thirty-eight flowering plants and trees, which, when prepared according to a specific homeopathic process he developed, had a profound effect on the underlying psychological and emotional states that influence physical illness. These special preparations became known as the Bach flower remedies.

Since the late 1970s, companies have researched and produced additional flower essences derived from flowers native to America, Hawaii, and Australia, but the original thirty-eight remedies discovered by Dr. Bach still remain the core of all flower remedies today.

How Flower Remedies Work

"Think of the patient, not the disease," was Dr. Bach's motto concerning health and the use of his flower remedies. He felt that the physical condition of the patient should not be the primary focus of concern. "The main reason for the failure of modern medical science is that it is dealing with results and not causes," said Dr. Bach.[2]

Flower remedies, on the other hand, set out to affect physical problems of the body by addressing their emotional and psychological causes, according to Dr. Bach. "As the emotions stabilize and general health—especially emotional outlook—improves, the illness begins to dissipate. This seems to be accomplished by the triggering of mechanisms that stimulate the internal healing processes."[3]

These "mechanisms" that represent the link between the mind and the body have received intense scrutiny from the scientific community over the last two decades, leading to the emergence of a new field called psychoneuroimmunology. Clinical studies have confirmed that the psychological and emotional state of a person influences a myriad of bodily processes, for better or for worse, by stimulating or suppressing immune cell activity, adrenal gland hormones, and neurotransmitters.[4]

"Unlike most pharmacological drugs, flower remedies have a subtle effect, gently resolving underlying emotional stress by triggering mechanisms which serve to mobilize the body's own internal healing processes," says Leslie Kaslof, researcher, writer, educator, and authority on the Bach remedies. Most often, as the remedies take effect, one will not even have a sense of having had an emotional problem. Only in retrospect will a person be able to determine where attitudes have changed or resolved themselves.[5]

HOW FLOWER REMEDIES ARE PREPARED AND ADMINISTERED

Flowers are picked in the morning, when heavy with dew, and at their fullest bloom. After being placed in a bowl of spring water and exposed to full sunlight for three hours, the flowers are removed with a twig from the same plant. A sterile bottle is filled half with the flower water from the bowl and half with brandy. This is the "Mother Essence," which is then diluted to make the remedy.

An alternative method is used for certain other flowers—the flowers, leaves, and twigs are placed in a saucepan then covered with two pints of spring water and brought to a boil. After cooling, the liquid is decanted then filtered through three layers of blotting paper and again mixed with brandy 1:1 to make the Mother Essence, before diluting to make the concentrate.

The remedy concentrates can then be administered in a variety of ways, as well as in varying strengths, depending on the patient's specific need. Generally, though, for immediate or acute situations, two to four drops of the concentrate can be placed directly under the tongue. For alcohol-sensitive persons, the concentrate can be diluted and sipped in a quarter of a glass of juice or water, or can be rubbed on the temples, behind the ears, wrists, crook of the elbows, or knees. The remedies can also be sprayed from an atomizer onto or around the patient.[6]

For long-term use, two to four drops of the concentrate should be added to a one-ounce bottle of spring water (avoid distilled). A teaspoon of brandy or other rectified spirits may be added as a preservative (if alcohol-sensitive, use apple cider vinegar). Four drops are placed under the tongue upon rising, between meals, and at bedtime.[7]

To maximize shelf life, the remedies should always be kept tightly stoppered and away from sunlight and heat.

See Mind/Body Medicine.

Usually flower remedies prove effective in removing the emotional blocks to recovery within one to twelve weeks. However, in some instances of deeply rooted psychological patterns or beliefs, it may take longer. Once a patient's emotional state has improved, though, the remedy, or remedies, no longer need to be taken. Furthermore, flower remedies will not create any physical dependencies, as chemical drugs often can, because the remedies have a self-diminishing effect.[8] This means that both the need for and the effectiveness of the remedies diminish as the patient moves toward a more balanced and healthy emotional level.

Conditions Benefited by Flower Remedies

"Flower remedies are different from other forms of medicine and complementary therapies insofar as they do not directly treat a physical condition," states Julian Barnard of Hereford, England, an authority on flower remedies. "There is not a specific remedy for heart disease and then another for eye problems. Practitioners who use flower remedies take little account of the named illness or disease. Rather, they focus on the emotional state by asking, 'How do you feel?' In this way the individual personality is treated rather than the nature of a particular disease."

In practice this means that flower remedies, rather than relating to any specific physical manifestations or symptoms, relate only to specific psychological and emotional states. As there is no universal corresponding psychological equivalent for every physical condition, each patient must be diagnosed individually. "You rarely use the same remedy, or combination of remedies, with any two people," says Abram Ber, M.D., of Phoenix, Arizona, "even if they display similar physical conditions." For example, two patients can suffer from chronic headaches, yet for one, fear may be the overriding emotional cause, while for the other, it may be loneliness.[9]

DR. BACH'S EMERGENCY STRESS FORMULA

One of the best-known combination remedies is Dr. Bach's emergency stress formula, alternatively called Rescue Remedy, Nature's Rescue, and Five Flower Remedy Combination. It contains five of the thirty-eight flower remedies and has been in use for over fifty years. The formula has a positive, calming effect in acute emergency situations including bereavement, anxiety, hysteria, and physical trauma or accidents. (The use of this formula should not take the place of emergency medical treatment, though, but should be used as an adjunct therapy only.) This emergency formula is also available as a cream that can be applied to bruises, bumps, sprains, insect bites, cuts, and burns. It can also be used for tension headaches and muscle stiffness.

In his book, *The Twelve Healers and Other Remedies*, Dr. Bach carefully outlines and describes the various emotional and psychological states and personality traits for which the remedies are used. These descriptions, though stated in simple terms, coincide with and reveal a more complex assessment of underlying discordant patterns.

Alec Forbes, M.D., Medical Director of the Cancer Help Center in Bristol, England, and a former member of the World Health Organization's Expert Advisory Panel on Traditional Medicine, has used flower remedies for over twenty years. Dr. Forbes states, in addition to personally using flower remedies to help him through many family crises, he has used them in his practice to take hundreds of patients off antidepressants, sedatives, and tranquilizers. "I use flower remedies regularly at the Cancer Help Center and find them to be most helpful in alleviating the emotional and psychological stress many of the cancer patients experience," he says.[10]

J. Herbert Fill, M.D., a psychiatrist and former New York City Commissioner of Mental Health, uses flower remedies almost exclusively over tranquilizers and psychotropic drugs. He has found flower remedies to have a more profound and long-lasting effect on his patients, free from any side effects. "I deal with emotional problems as well as physical ones," says Dr. Fill. "In my observations, these remedies appear to work on a much deeper level, apparently assisting the individual in resolving deep-rooted conflict, as opposed to simply relieving the symptoms."

"I deal with emotional problems as well as physical ones. In my observations, these remedies appear to work on a much deeper level, apparently assisting the individual in resolving deep-rooted conflict, as opposed to simply relieving the symptoms."

—J. Herbert Fill, M.D., former New York City Commissioner of Mental Health

John Bolling, a specialist in behavioral and drug abuse problems and former Assistant Professor and Chief Resident in Psychiatry at New York University's Bellevue Medical Center, found significant health improvements in 80 percent of the patients he treated with flower remedies during a recent clinical study. Although other types of treatment were simultaneously used, such as meditation and hypnosis, Dr. Bolling found the most impressive part of the study "was the dramatic improvement shown in the overcoming of blocked emotional patterns by 20 percent of this group, who prior to the study had been deemed resistant to any form of treatment."

States Dr. Bolling, "Clearly Dr. Bach's remedies were the primary factor here. In addition to the marked improvement in their emotional state, these patients are now more open and receptive to other treatment modalities which had not been effective before."[11]

Along with medical doctors, many other health professionals have found that flower remedies combine well with their specific treatment therapies. Chiropractic physicians who use flower remedies along with standard chiropractic techniques report that using both methods in conjunction has a greater and more permanent health-enhancing effect than using either alone. George Goodheart, D.C., of Detroit, Michigan, the founder of applied kinesiology states, "I have used the thirty-eight traditional flower remedies over the past number of years with remarkable success. I have found them to alleviate a wide range of emotional problems and emotionally based physical problems. I have seen them dispel worry, anxiety, and negative attitudes, very often in a surprisingly short period of time, instilling a more positive attitude toward recovery."[12]

See Energy Medicine.

Harold Whitcomb, M.D., of Aspen, Colorado, uses electroacupuncture biofeedback testing (a method of testing based on measurement of the electrical properties of acupuncture points) to determine appropriate flower remedies, especially in his treatment program for chronic fatigue syndrome. He finds that deep-seated, buried emotions are common in people with chronic fatigue syndrome and that the flower remedies help to bring these emotions to the surface and allow them to heal.

Flower remedies can also be used as an adjunct to acupuncture and Traditional Chinese Medicine. As acupuncture treatments open blocked energy channels, stored emotional energy is released. As flower remedies work to balance any negative emotional energy, the two therapies work well together, according to Susan Lange, O.M.D., of the Meridian Health Center in Santa Monica, California.

A forty-year-old man suffering from chronic asthma since age three came to see Dr. Lange. The man's long treatment history included prednisone (a steroid hormone with the same effects as cortisone), and inhalants. Dr. Lange learned that the initial outbreak of asthma coincided with the onset of his parent's marital difficulties. His parents fought openly in the home, and his mother eventually committed suicide.

Dr. Lange performed acupuncture to open blockages in the man's chest and treated him adjunctively with fuchsia, a flower essence native to America that addresses the repression of deep-seated emotions such as anger and grief. Because the man masked his suffering behind a cheerful facade, Dr. Lange incorporated Bach's traditional flower remedies elm and agrimony.

As the energy held in the man's chest released, Dr. Lange treated him for blockage in the solar plexus and administered the flower essence sunflower for issues of self-worth. Finally, he was treated for repressed kidney energy and was given basil and sticky monkey flower essence, and the flower remedy rock rose. These remedies addressed his repressed sexual feelings and his fear of intimacy. Within three months the man was able to discontinue all previous medication and was free of asthma, reports Dr. Lange.

When treating children, Dr. Lange also likes to treat the parents simultaneously. She finds that their problems often interconnect. In one case, a mother was experiencing postnatal depression and couldn't relate to her child. Mariposa lily, a flower essence native to America, was given to both the mother and the child to help them with parent/child bonding. The child was also given pink yarrow essence which is used to treat those who overidentify with the emotions of others. The health of both mother and child improved as did their relationship.

Julian Barnard reports seeing a nine-year-old girl suffering from repeated migraines who was tense, anxious, and depressed. She was given a treatment bottle containing the flower remedies gentian, water violet, walnut, and Bach's emergency stress formula. Within days her mother reported marked improvements, noting that her daughter had been transformed back to her happy, outgoing self.

In another instance, a three-year-old child stung on the throat by a bee became frightened and hysterical, screaming in pain. He was given Bach's emergency stress formula directly into his mouth by Barnard, and immediately became calm and quiet. With the stinger removed, Bach's emergency formula cream applied to the skin helped to alleviate inflammation. The entire episode was over in two minutes.

"Flower remedies are particularly beneficial in helping to relieve acute trauma associated with accidents, bruises, and injuries, as well as grief that would occur following the loss of a loved one," adds Dr. Ber. He also believes that using flower remedies can be a tremendous preventative therapy, and that by correcting underlying emotional problems, one can ensure that many physical problems will never recur.

Selecting Flower Remedies

To assist in the selection of Bach remedies, a self-help questionnaire follows. Read and answer each question carefully. After completing the questionnaire, count only the yes answers in each section. If there are two or more, that remedy is indicated.

Up to six remedies may be combined and taken at one time. The fewer remedies taken the better; the ideal being the single remedy. This will allow for an easier integration and adjustment of internal processes.

Check only those questions which evoke a yes answer. If your answer is no or sometimes, leave the box blank.

Caution: *The following questionnaire has been developed from the original writings of Dr. Edward Bach, and has been provided for your interest and self-assessment. Both the author and publisher make no claims as to the efficacy of the traditional flower remedies in the conditions described in the questionnaire or elsewhere in the text. As previously stated, persistent conditions, and those conditions requiring medical attention, should be referred to a physician of one's choosing, immediately.*

Aspen

__Do you have vague fears that you cannot explain?
__Do you often find yourself distressed and anxious, but are unable to put your finger on the problem?
__Do you wake with a sense of apprehension and foreboding, feeling that something bad may happen, but don't know what it may be?

Mimulus

__Do you have specific fears you can identify and would like to overcome?
__Are you shy and easily frightened by particular circumstances and things?
__When faced with situations or things that frighten you, do you become nervous and too paralyzed to act?

Cherry Plum

__Do you fear losing control of your mind or body?
__Are you compulsive, or have impulses to do things you know are wrong but have difficulty controlling your actions?
__Do you fear losing control and hurting yourself or others?

Red Chestnut

__Do you worry over the health and safety of your friends and family?
__Do you fear that something may happen to those close to you?
__Does your overconcern and worry for others cause you considerable distress?

Rock Rose

__Do you suffer from extreme terror?
__Do you tend to panic and become hysterical?
__Are you troubled by nightmares?

Cerato

__Do you lack confidence in your ability to judge things on your own and make decisions?
__Do you find yourself asking other people's advice, even when you know what you want?
__After taking advice from others, do you find yourself confused by the choices, constantly changing your direction according to the latest recommendation?

Scleranthus

__Do you suffer from indecision, uncertainty, or hesitancy?

__Do you have difficulty choosing between one thing and another?

__Do you experience extreme mood swings, or have difficulty in keeping your balance?

Wild Oat

__Are you dissatisfied with your current position in life, feeling that life is passing you by?

__Have you tried many different jobs but nothing seems to bring satisfaction?

__Would you like to find a new career or change your old one, but have difficulty deciding what you should be doing?

Larch

__Do you lack confidence?

__Do you not try things for fear of failing?

__Do you feel inferior, and that others are more capable and qualified than you?

Hornbeam

__On rising in the morning, do you find yourself tired, not wanting to work?

__Do you feel some part of you needs to be strengthened before you can tackle your job?

__Do you find once you've started working, your tiredness is forgotten, and you're able to complete your task?

Clematis

__Are you absentminded, or does your attention easily wander, making it difficult to concentrate?

__Do you find you have little interest in present circumstances, often daydreaming, wishing you were somewhere else?

__Do you find yourself dozing off frequently, regardless of where you are?

Honeysuckle

__Do you find you are caught between living in the present and dwelling in memories of the past?

__Are there things you would like to have done with your life but never had the opportunity to do?

__Do you find yourself reminiscing about the good old days, wishing you were able to live your life over again?

Wild Rose

__Do you find you are indifferent and apathetic toward life?

__Are you resigned to your current circumstances, making little effort to improve things or find joy?

__Do you feel you've given up and don't care one way or another what happens?

White Chestnut

__Are you troubled by persistent unwanted thoughts?

__Do you worry or have mental arguments which circle around in your mind?

__Do you have difficulty sleeping due to mental chatter and worries?

Chestnut Bud

__Do you find you don't learn from past experiences, repeating the same mistakes or patterns of behavior?

__Due to lack of observation, do you find it necessary to go over things already done?

__Is there a particular situation or condition continually recurring in your life which you would like to overcome?

Olive

__Are you now going through, or have you recently gone through, an illness or personal ordeal which left you physically and mentally drained?

__Do you tire easily with no reserve energy to complete your tasks or enjoy the day?

__Do you feel sapped of strength and vitality, where even the least effort exhausts you?

Water Violet
__Do others find you aloof, prideful, and at times condescending?
__Do you keep to yourself, not wishing to be interfered with or to interfere in other people's affairs?
__Are you self-reliant and do you prefer spending your time alone?

Impatiens
__Do you find yourself losing patience, becoming tense and irritable with people and things that move too slowly for you?
__Do you do things in a rush, racing from one place or situation to another?
__Do you find you need to work alone, because others can't keep up your pace?

Heather
__Do you find others avoiding conversation with you because you tend to talk a great deal?
__Do you dislike being alone and seek the company of anyone willing to listen to your troubles?
Do you feel the need to steer conversations back to your special interests or problems, and are you reluctant to discontinue them even when the listener has to leave?

Agrimony
__When worried or in pain, do you tend to conceal it from others, making light of even the most trying of circumstances?
__Do you go out of your way to avoid burdening others with your problems, giving in to the wishes of others in order to avoid an argument or quarrel?
__When troubled, do you find yourself drinking alcohol or using stimulants or other drugs to assist in keeping up a happy disposition?

Centaury
__Are you easily imposed on because of your willingness to help others?
__Is it difficult for you to say no when you're asked for help, becoming more a servant than a willing helper?
__Do you neglect your own needs, because you are too busy taking care of other people's needs?

Walnut
__Are you involved in a relationship or situation you would like to be free of, but cannot break away from?
__Are you currently in a state of transition or change?
__In the midst of this change, do you find that you're having difficulty in letting go of past attachments or in starting new beginnings?

Holly
__Are you suspicious and mistrusting of other people's motives and intentions?
__Do others find you spiteful, envious, jealous, or vengeful?
__Do you find yourself lacking compassion or warmth toward others?

Pine
__Are you rarely content with your accomplishments, feeling that you could always do a better job?
__Do you blame yourself for other people's mistakes, feeling that their shortcomings are in some way your fault or responsibility?
__Are you hard on yourself, when you fail to live up to the standards or expectations you've set for yourself?

Elm
__Do you tend to overextend your work commitments?
__Do you find yourself overwhelmed by your work, and despite being capable feel you have taken on more than you can do?
__Do you become despondent when faced with the magnitude of your responsibilities?

Star of Bethlehem

__Have there been past traumas, or shocks in your life, which you may not have completely recovered from?

__Do you feel a past surgery or accident is responsible for your present condition?

__Have you recently, or in the past, suffered a personal loss which you haven't quite gotten over?

Sweet Chestnut

__Do you feel you've reached the limits of your endurance, and there's nothing but annihilation left to face?

__Do you suffer from mental anguish and deep despair?

__Do you feel that the burden of life is more than you can bear?

Gorse

__Have you lost hope that you will recover from or be helped in overcoming an illness or difficulty?

__Do you feel it is useless to seek further help for your problems?

__Have you given up hope that things will change for the better in some circumstance or situation in your life?

Mustard

__Do you ever become gloomy and depressed for no known reason?

__Does this depression envelop you like a dark cloud, hiding the joy of life?

__Do you find this gloom and depression, for no apparent reason, lifts as suddenly as it comes?

Gentian

__Are you easily discouraged when things don't go your way?

__When setting out to accomplish a task, do you become oversensitive to small delays and hindrances which may lead to self-doubt, and at times to depression?

__Is it hard for you to start over again once you've encountered difficulties?

Oak

__Are you one who tirelessly struggles on despite oppositions and delays?

__Can you always be depended on to complete what you set out to do, regardless of the challenge?

__Do you tend to throw yourself into your work, neglecting your own needs, as well as the needs of those close to you?

Willow

__Through no fault of your own, do you feel that life has been unfair or unjust to you?

__Have you become resentful and bitter toward those who may have treated you poorly?

__Despite all you have done, do you feel your best efforts have largely gone unrewarded, while others not as deserving as yourself have gained?

Crab Apple

__Do you feel unclean or ashamed over an act you should not have committed; or over someone or something having violated you personally?

__Do you find yourself preoccupied with small physical problems such as pimples, small blemishes or rashes, while overlooking more serious conditions?

__Do you feel there is something wrong with, or some things you would like changed, in your physical appearance?

__Are you compulsive about cleanliness, even at times to the extreme?

__Are you afraid of becoming, or feel you have already become, contaminated and need to be cleansed?

Chicory
__Are you possessive of those close to you and feel you know what's best for them, often directing and correcting even small details of their lives?
__Do you feel you are not appreciated by those you care for?
__Do you find yourself needing the attention and devotion of those you love, feeling it's their duty to stay in close contact with you?

Beech
__When assessing people and situations, do you look for what you can find wrong?
__Do the small habits and idiosyncracies of others bother you?
__Are you critical and intolerant of those who don't measure up to your standards or expectations?

Vervain
__Do you have strong opinions which you attempt to convince others are right?
__Are you easily incensed by injustices, arguing for and defending principles that you believe in?
__Are you high-strung and at times tense and overenthusiastic, always teaching and philosophizing?

Rock Water
__Do you feel you have a mission in life to conform with or live up to?
__Are you strict in your adherence to a religious or social discipline, or in a particular way of living?
__Do you feel it's important to make an example of yourself by living up to your ideals, so that others may follow?

Vine
__Do you tend to take charge in circumstances and situations you're involved with?
__Are you strong-willed and expect complete obedience (without question) from those around you?
__When taken to an extreme, can you become tyrannical and domineering?

Used with permission by Ellon USA, Inc.

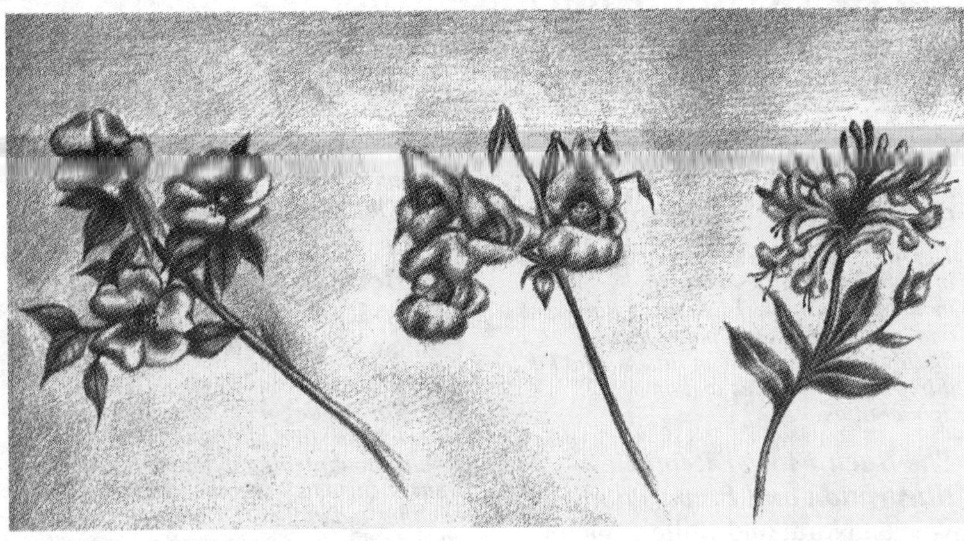

Wild Rose *Impatiens* *Honeysuckle*

Where to Find Help

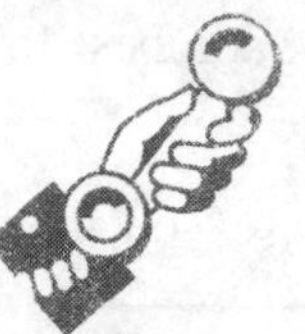

To receive information regarding remedies and to obtain flower essences contact:

Ellon USA, Inc.
644 Merrick Road
Lynbrook, New York 11563
(516) 593-2206

Ellon USA (formerly Ellon Bach USA) was responsible for introducing, on a large commercial scale, Dr. Bach's thirty-eight flower remedies into North America, and was the first and only official distributor of these remedies in North America for nearly fifteen years. Today, Ellon USA manufactures and distributes worldwide its own complete line of Dr. Bach's thirty-eight flower remedies under the trade name of "Traditional Flower Remedies from Ellon" and Dr. Bach's emergency stress formula under the trade name of "Nature's Rescue.™" These preparations are subject to strict FDA and homeopathic labeling and quality control laws.

Flower Essence Society
P.O. Box 459
Nevada City, California 95959
(916) 263-9162

FES distributes California flower essences, and imports Healing Herbs, made in the United Kingdom, a full line of the thirty-eight flowers as discovered by Dr. Bach.

Pegasus Products, Inc.
P.O. Box 228
Boulder, Colorado 80306
(800) 527-6104 Outside Colorado
(303) 667-3019 In Colorado

Pegasus manufactures and distributes various flower essences.

Perelandra, Ltd.
P.O. Box 3603
Warrenton, Virginia 22186
(703) 937-2153

Perelandra sells their own line of flower essences as well as books. Call for a catalog.

Recommended Reading

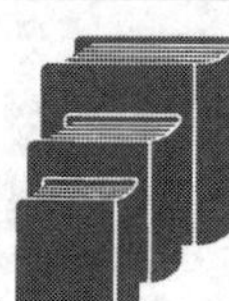

The Bach Flower Remedies. Bach, Edward; and Wheeler, F. J. New Caanan, CT: Keats, 1979.

The first book of Bach's writings published in the United States. This single volume includes two books by Edward Bach and one by F. J. Wheeler, including Bach's findings on the nature of illness, and his thirty-eight remedies and their applications.

The Bach Flower Remedies: Illustration and Preparation. Weeks, Nora; and Bullen, Victor. Saffron Walden, England: CW Daniel, 1990.

A conscientious list of Bach flowers with color photos of each, an emphasis on proper preparation, and warnings about common misuse and misunderstanding.

The Bach Remedies: A Self-Help Guide. Kaslof, Leslie J. New Canaan, CT: Keats, 1988.

A clear and concisely written self-help guide for the beginner, as well as the professional. In addition to outlining details on clinical and double blind studies, this easy-to-understand reference contains a detailed self-help questionnaire specifically designed to assist one in choosing the appropriate flower remedy or remedies for one's needs.

Bach Flower Therapy. Scheffer, Mechthild. Rochester, VT: Inner Traditions, 1987.

Each of the thirty-eight remedies are described in depth, with an emphasis on their spiritual and psychological implications. This book also includes lists of symptoms and a section of questions that frequently arise.

Guide to the Bach Flower Remedies. Barnard, Julian. Saffron Walden, England: CW Daniel, 1979.

A straightforward guide to the Bach flower remedies and how to use them.

Handbook on the Bach Flower Remedies. Chancellor, Phillip M. New Caanan, CT: Keats, 1971.

A complete sourcebook for laypeople and practitioners on Bach flowers with detailed descriptions of each remedy. Provides useful case histories for each.

Healing Herbs of Edward Bach. Barnard, Julian and Martine. Hereford, England: Flower Remedy Programme, 1988.

This book contains color photographs and botanically correct illustrations. Edward Bach's remedies are explained with instructions on which plants are used, where and when they can be found, and how to prepare them.

The Medical Discoveries of Edward Bach, Physician. Weeks, Nora. New Caanan, CT: Keats, 1979.

A biography of Bach's life, work, discoveries, the controversy they aroused, and his remedies continued success, written by the woman who was his assistant and carried on his work.

"When health is absent
Wisdom cannot reveal itself,
Art cannot become manifest,
Strength cannot be exerted,
Wealth is useless and
Reason is powerless."

—Herophilies, 300 B.C.

Guided Imagery

Using the power of the mind to evoke a positive physical response, guided imagery can reduce stress and slow heart rate, stimulate the immune system, and reduce pain. As part of the rapidly emerging field of mind/body medicine, guided imagery is being used in various medical settings, and, when properly taught, can also serve as a highly effective form of self-care.

"The imagination is probably a person's least utilized health resource," says Martin L. Rossman, M.D., co-founder of the Academy for Guided Imagery. "It can be used to remember and recreate the past, develop insight into the present, influence physical health, enhance creativity and inspiration, and anticipate possible futures."

All of us have to some extent experienced the effects of the imagination on the body. Getting goose bumps while listening to a frightening story, breaking out in chills at the thought of fingernails scratching a chalkboard, or becoming physically aroused from a sexual fantasy, are all examples of the body reacting to a sole stimulus—the imagination.

What Is Imagery?

Imagery is simply a flow of thoughts that one can see, hear, feel, smell, or taste in one's imagination. As an inner representation of experience, as well as fantasy, imagery is a rich, symbolic, and highly personal language. "An image may or may not represent external reality, but it always represents internal reality," says Dr. Rossman. "It is the language of the emotions and the interface between mind and body."

"An image may or may not represent external reality, but it always represents internal reality."
—Martin L. Rossman, M.D.

Perhaps the most common human experience of imagery is worrying. Most people worry sometimes and some people worry constantly, even to the point where they experience butterflies in the stomach, or tightening in the shoulders. Whatever the case, the body is not reacting to external events, but to thoughts or images about these events, even though the worrier may not be consciously aware of them. Other thoughts may be verbal, but what all thoughts have in common is that they exist in the mind, and the body reacts to them.

"If you are a good worrier," says Dr. Rossman, "and especially if you ever worry yourself sick, you may be an especially good candidate for learning how to positively affect your health with imagery, as the internal process involved in worrying yourself sick and imagining yourself well are quite similar."

David Bresler, Ph.D., L.Ac., Co-director of the Academy for Guided Imagery, and former Director of the UCLA Pain Center, defines imagery as one of the two "higher order" languages of the human nervous system—the other one being the more familiar, more educated faculty of thinking in words. Imagery is a natural way the nervous system stores, accesses, and processes information. This makes it especially effective for maintaining the dialogue between mind and body, which is the source of its power in the healing process.

"If you are a good worrier and especially if you ever worry yourself sick, you may be an especially good candidate for learning how to positively affect your health with imagery, as the internal process involved in worrying yourself sick and imagining yourself well are quite similar."

—Martin L. Rossman, M.D.

The Healing Power of Imagery

Imagery has three main characteristics that lend it great value in medicine and healing:

- It directly affects physiology.
- Through the mental processes of association and synthesis, it provides insight and perspective into health.
- It has an intimate relationship with emotions, which are often at the root of many common health conditions.

The Physiological Effects of Imagery

Relax for a moment and imagine holding a juicy, yellow lemon. Feel its coolness, its texture, its weight in your hand. Imagine cutting it in half. Notice the cut surfaces—the pale yellow of the pulp, the whiteness of the inner peel, perhaps a seed or two. Carefully cut one of the halves in two and pick up one of the freshly cut lemon quarters. Imagine lifting this lemon wedge to your mouth. Smell its lemony scent. Now imagine biting into the lemon and sucking its sour juice into your mouth. What happened as you imagined doing that? Did you salivate or grimace? Did you have any other kind of physical reaction? Most people do—much more than if you simply asked them to salivate.

This is a simple illustration of the type of physiological response that imagery can induce. If thinking of a lemon makes you salivate, what other more important effects on physiology might certain types of imagery have? For instance, can thinking of pain relief cause endorphins to be secreted?

Research using biofeedback, hypnosis, and meditative states has demonstrated that people possess a remarkable range of self-regulatory capacities. Focused imagery in a relaxed state of mind is a common and central factor in most of these techniques.

Imagery of various types has been shown to affect heart rate, blood pressure, respiratory patterns, oxygen consumption, carbon dioxide elimination, brain wave rhythms, electrical characteristics of the skin, local blood flow and temperature of tissues, gastrointestinal motility and secretions, sexual arousal, levels of hormones and neurotransmitters in the blood, and immune system function.[1]

The healing potentials of imagery go far beyond its remarkable ability to directly affect physiology, however.

IMAGERY AND THE BRAIN

According to Martin L. Rossman, M.D., co-founder of the Academy for Guided Imagery, imagery seems to arise from unconscious processes, body processes, and memories and perceptions from the part of the brain known as the cerebral cortex. Some imagery, however, having to do with smell or feelings, may arise from older, more primitive brain centers. Wherever its origin, imagery is believed to have its effect by sending messages from the higher centers of the brain through to the lower centers that regulate most of a person's physiologic functions, such as breathing, heart rate, blood flow and pressure, digestion, immunity, and temperature, as well as waking and sleeping rhythms, hunger, thirst, and sexual function.

Recent research utilizing PET scans (a test involving radioactive material that is used to examine brain tissue) indicates what parts of the brain are active when a person is performing certain tasks. The PET scans seem to show that the optic cortex, the same part of the brain activated when a person is seeing, is activated when a person visualizes.

Similarly, when people imagine hearing things, the auditory cortex is active, and when they imagine feeling sensations, the sensory cortex is active. Therefore, it appears that the cortex can create these imaginary realities and, in the absence of conflicting information, the lower centers of the nervous system respond to this information.

This is one reason why health care professionals use sensory recruitment, an approach that utilizes as many senses in the imagery process as possible. Sensory recruitment increases the subjective reality of the image and probably increases the amount of information sent through the lower brain centers and autonomic nervous system, making it more likely to elicit the desired response.

Associations and "Getting the Big Picture"

"Recovering from or coping with a serious or chronic illness may well demand more than simply imagining getting well," says Dr. Rossman. "It may also require changes in your lifestyle, your attitudes, your relationships, or your emotional state." Imagery can help to develop the insight and self-awareness that it takes to deal with a chronic or life-threatening illness in more positive and constructive ways. This is due to the mental processes of association and synthesis that are central to imagery. "Imagery tends to give us the 'big picture' of a situation and can help us recognize how things are related in ways we might not expect," Dr. Rossman explains. "Becoming aware of these relationships may facilitate a shift in attitude or behavior that can be helpful in relieving, altering, or coping with illness or symptoms."

For example, Dr. Rossman tells of a woman whose chronic arm pain had not responded to medical treatment for two years. She kept seeing an image of her pain as pieces of iron. This made little sense to her until she was asked to describe the qualities of the iron. She described it as hard, cold, and rigid, and then immediately associated these qualities with her grandfather, whom she had been caring for during the past two years, as he displayed these same qualities. This association allowed her to deal with repressed feelings about her role as a caregiver and led to a rapid resolution of her arm pain as well as a great deal of personal growth.

Emotional Connections

Emotions are powerful events in the body. They are physiologically distinct from one another and each affects human physiology in different ways. In fact, Dr. Rossman points out, many physical ailments are direct manifestations of emotions that are locked within the unconscious. "Through imagery you can access those emotions and consciously alter their effect on your health," he says.

Emotions themselves are a normal, healthy response to life. Failure to acknowledge and express important emotions, however, can be an important factor in illness, and is unfortunately all too common. People often suppress those emotions they find to be the most distressing, such as fear, grief, and anger.

The natural expression of emotion is often suppressed by family, friends, and society, as well. "Yet strong emotion has a way of finding routes of expression," says Dr. Bresler, "and if it is not recognized and dealt with it can manifest itself indirectly in the form of physical pain and illness, or destructive behaviors like smoking, heavy drinking, and overworking, all of which can in turn lead to serious health problems." In fact, studies in England and the United States have found that 50 to 75 percent of all problems presented to a primary care clinic are emotional, social, or familial in origin, though they are being expressed by pain or illness.[2]

"Studies in England and the United States have found that 50 to 75 percent of all problems presented to a primary care clinic are emotional, social, or familial in origin, though they are being expressed by pain or illness."

By directly accessing emotions, imagery can help the individual understand the needs that may be represented by an illness and can help develop ways to meet those needs. Imagery is also one of the quickest and most direct ways of becoming aware of emotions and their effects on health, both positive and negative. For instance, one of Dr. Rossman's patients with inflammatory bowel disease reported that she imagined her bowels being "red, inflamed, and irritated." As this image was explored, she became aware of how her bowels responded to the irritation, frustration, and anger she frequently felt. By learning to recognize what triggered her frustration, and by developing more effective means to express herself when angry, she had progressively less trouble with her bowels. She also learned to use simple relaxation and imagery to imagine her own hands gently soothing her bowels with a cooling, calming balm whenever they became upset. A few minutes of doing this would relieve her abdominal pain and leave her feeling relaxed and at ease.

Imagery in Medicine and Healing

Imagery can be a key factor in dealing with either a simple tension headache or a life-threatening disease. It is a proven method for pain relief, for helping people tolerate medical procedures and treatments and reducing side effects, and for stimulating healing responses in the body. Imagery can assist in clarifying attitudes, emotions, behaviors, and lifestyle patterns that may be involved in producing illness. It can also facilitate recovery, and be used to help people find meaning in their illnesses, cope more effectively with their health problems, and come to grips with life's limitations.

Learning to relax is fundamental to self-healing, and imagery is a part of almost all relaxation and stress-reduction techniques. For many people, imagery is the easiest way to learn to relax, and its active nature makes it more comfortable than other methods of relaxation.

Treating People Rather Than Symptoms

Beyond simple relaxation, imagery can have specific effects in relieving numerous common symptoms. Dr. Bresler states that because imagery is a way of treating people rather than symptoms or diseases, it can be applied to almost any health care concern. The following areas of application are some examples of where imagery can be useful, but this list is by no means complete.

Imagery is often used for relief of chronic pain, and other symptoms, including headaches, neck and back pain, allergies (including hay fever and asthma), high blood pressure, benign arrhythmias (heartbeat irregularities), stress-related gastrointestinal symptoms (including chronic abdominal pain and spastic colon), functional urinary complaints, and reproductive irregularities including premenstrual syndrome, irregular menstruation, dysmenorrhea (painful menstruation), and even excessive uterine bleeding. It can also accelerate healing and minimize discomfort from all kinds of acute injuries, including sprains, strains, and broken bones, as well as from the symptoms of the common cold, flus, and infections. Because imagery can affect immune system function, within limits, there is a great deal of interest among researchers of mind/body medicine for applying it to a broad spectrum of autoimmune diseases, including rheumatoid arthritis, ulcerative colitis, and systemic lupus erythematosus (a chronic inflammatory disease with symptoms including arthritis, fatigue, and skin lesions).

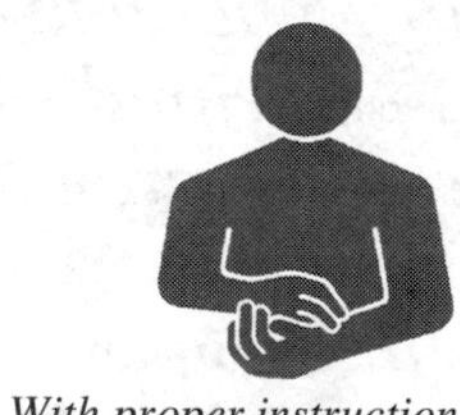

With proper instruction imagery can be uniquely suited to self-care.

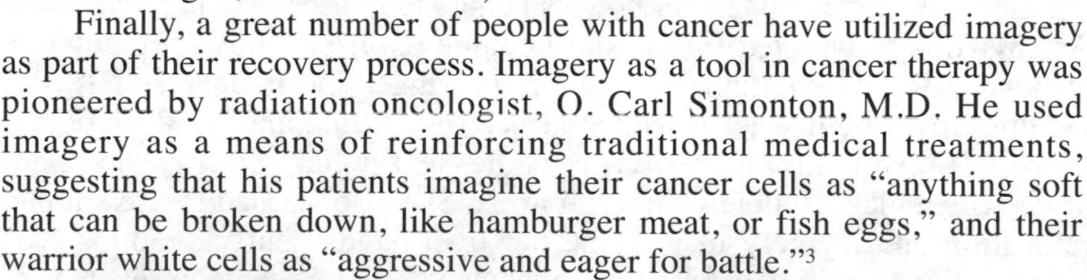

Finally, a great number of people with cancer have utilized imagery as part of their recovery process. Imagery as a tool in cancer therapy was pioneered by radiation oncologist, O. Carl Simonton, M.D. He used imagery as a means of reinforcing traditional medical treatments, suggesting that his patients imagine their cancer cells as "anything soft that can be broken down, like hamburger meat, or fish eggs," and their warrior white cells as "aggressive and eager for battle."[3]

Dr. Simonton first employed this technique in 1971 with a throat cancer patient whose condition has been diagnosed as "hopeless." The man was sixty-one years old. He was extremely weak, his weight had dropped to ninety-eight pounds, and he was having trouble breathing and swallowing his own saliva. Although he was scheduled to receive radiation treatment, his doctors were concerned that treating him would further deteriorate his condition.

Dr. Simonton outlined a program of relaxation and imagery for the man, instructing him to devote five to fifteen minutes three times a day. The imagery exercise consisted of imagining the radiation treatment as "bullets of energy" striking his cells, healthy and cancerous alike, with the healthy cells remaining healthy and the cancer cells dying off. The man would then visualize his cancer shrinking in size and his health returning to normal. As a result of this program, the man was able to receive radiation treatment with minimum discomfort. Halfway through his treatment, he began eating again, and regaining weight and strength. Within two months, his cancer completely disappeared.[4]

Patricia Norris, Ph.D., a pioneer in the field of imagery and author of *Why Me?*, works with people with serious illnesses. Dr. Norris likes to distinguish between two types of imagery: That which uses images preconceived by the therapist as a means of suggesting healing; and imagery created by the patient as a way to better understand the meaning of symptoms or to access inner resources. Dr. Norris's most well-known case using the latter type of imagery was that of nine-year-old Garrett Porter, who was diagnosed with an inoperable, terminal brain tumor. By creating an imagery scenario with Garrett (based on his favorite TV show, "Star Trek"), used in combination with biofeedback, Dr. Norris was able to guide Garrett through a year of intensive therapy, after which the boy's tumor completely disappeared.[5]

Even when cancer patients are not cured through imagery, they report benefits from its use, including relief from anxiety and pain, increased self-esteem, and an increased sense of control over their bodies. They also report an increased ability to tolerate chemotherapy or radiation therapy. In addition, by coming to grips with the illness, they are often able to resolve personal and family issues.

In addition to being used to explore diseases and symptoms, imagery can be helpful for enhancing tolerance to medical procedures such as MRI's (magnetic resonance imaging), bone marrow biopsies, cancer chemotherapy, and radiation. Imagery can also help prepare people for surgery and postsurgical recovery.

In fact, imagery can be applied to almost any medical situation where problem solving, decision making, relaxation, or symptom relief is useful. Imagery can be considered as an adjunct treatment to health care no matter how minor the condition. According to Jeanne Achterberg, Ph.D., President of the

AN IMAGERY RELAXATION EXERCISE

This simple technique can be used as a stress reducer either for a few minutes, or half an hour. It's best when learning it to have another person read and guide you through the steps until they are familiar. You can also tape the exercise yourself and listen to it before going to bed at night.

Get comfortable, either lying down or sitting up. Take a few deep breaths and begin to imagine that with each in-breath, you take in calmness and peacefulness—with each out-breath you release tension, discomfort, and worry. Let your breath find its own natural rate and rhythm and continue to imagine breathing in calmness and peacefulness, and breathing out tension and worry.

Invite your body to relax. Imagine breathing calmness into your feet and legs—release any tension on the out-breath. Breathe into your pelvis, hips, and low back, and release on the out-breath—don't struggle or make an effort—just imagine this happening in your own way. Breathe calmness into your abdomen and release tension on the out-breath, breathe into your chest and release tension as you exhale, breathe peacefulness into your neck and shoulders, and release tension as you exhale. Breathe calmness into your arms and hands all the way to the fingertips, and relax as you let go of the breath, breathe into your face and jaws, into your scalp and forehead, into your eyes and release all tension. Allow your whole body to sink into a peaceful, relaxed state.

Now imagine yourself in a place that is particularly peaceful and beautiful, perhaps a place you've actually visited, or a place imagined—a special place you'd really like to be. Imagine yourself there now—notice the details—what you see, the colors, shapes, living things. Notice what you hear in this special place, smell any aromas or odors you associate with this place, pay special attention to any feelings of peacefulness and relaxation that you feel and allow yourself to experience them as fully as possible.

Whenever you are ready, simply allow the images to fade and, taking all the time you need, bring yourself back to the outer world, gently opening your eyes and stretching as you return.

Association for Transpersonal Psychology, establishing healing patterns is far easier when the individual is relatively healthy than when faced with a serious disease. Once someone is diagnosed as being seriously ill, the person often lacks the emotional resources and belief system to employ imagery to its best advantage.[6]

Interactive Imagery

Beyond these relatively direct applications, "receptive" uses of imagery can have profound effects on health and medical care. These typically involve imaginary dialogues with images representing symptoms or illness, or with an inner store of wisdom or healing that can provide insights into the meaning of body sensations and symptoms. This can lead to better understanding of how lifestyle choices and behavior are affecting health. The following stories demonstrate how imagery can be used to help identify thoughts and fears at the root of physical pain.

Natural ability, skills, motivation, practice, and the availability of good instruction are all factors in how effectively you can work with imagery. Some conditions respond better than others, but no matter what the condition, imagery can help you better cope and minimize your suffering.

Alice was a forty-year-old woman who had recently undergone cancer surgery and radiation. However, she continued to have persistent pain in her upper back. Because doctors could not identify the problem, she decided to try guided imagery with Dr. Rossman. First, he asked her to relax and imagine herself at some beautiful place. Alice saw herself on a beach surrounded by cliffs. Next, she was invited to have a dialogue with an imaginary "inner advisor." Alice asked for an image to appear and saw a wise old man tending a fire. He looked like Merlin the Magician. When Alice asked him about her pain, he told her that she needed to "ask for help." Alice immediately broke into tears, for throughout her ordeal she had never asked for help from her husband or family. She suddenly realized that she had been afraid to ask for help, thinking she would be too much of a burden on them. Her "inner advisor" then told her how much better her family members would feel if they were included in her healing process. Finally, she imagined asking her husband for help and having him agree to provide it. At the end of her session, her pain had substantially decreased and she found the courage to turn to her family for assistance. "In my experience," says Dr. Rossman, "this receptive use of imagery as an interface language between what we call 'mind' and what we call 'body' often yields the most profound healing response."

In a similar case, Dr. Bresler worked with a fifty-two-year-old cardiologist who suffered from excruciating pain in the lower back after receiving successful treatment for rectal cancer. Further surgery was ruled out because the area had been so heavily irradiated, and because the man had developed tolerance to his pain medications.

Reviewing the man's medical records, Dr. Bresler read that in a psychiatric workup the man had described his pain as "a dog chewing on my spine." Dr. Bresler suggested guided imagery as a way to make contact with the dog, and invited the man to imagine what the dog looked like. The patient described "a nasty little terrier" named Skippy. During the following sessions, Skippy began revealing critically important information about the patient, including the fact that he had never wanted to be a doctor but had been pressured into medical school by his mother. As a consequence, the man resented not only his mother, but also his patients and colleagues. Skippy told him that this hostility had contributed to both his cancer and to his subsequent back pain. Finally, Skippy said, "You're a damn good doctor. It may not be the career you wanted, but it's time you recognized how good you are at what you do. When you stop being so resentful and start accepting yourself, I'll stop chewing your spine." Following these insights, the man experienced an immediate alleviation of his pain, and within a few more weeks it progressively subsided to the point where he felt like a new person.

Imagery is an adjunctive treatment for illness. Make sure you are well aware of all of the medical options for your condition, and seek proper medical care.

The Future of Imagery

"One of the most appealing aspects of guided imagery," Dr. Bresler says, "is that it lends itself so readily to the process of patient education and self-care. It also provides a formal methodology for increasing personal empowerment and self-control. While research studies of its cost-effectiveness are still underway, it appears to offer significant and effective therapeutic benefits after only a few weeks or months of therapy."

Dr. Bresler and Dr. Rossman both predict that in the very near future training in guided imagery will be an integral part of all psychotherapeutic approaches and that its benefits will become more widely available for medical and psychological problems and as a means of achieving greater personal insight, creativity, and self-actualization.

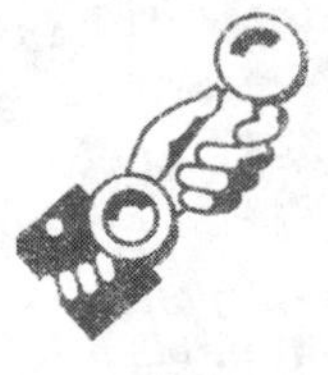

Where to Find Help

Mastering guided imagery comes with time and training. There are groups and classes that teach imagery around the country. Check local hospitals for wellness programs, patient support groups, or behavioral medical units for referrals. You can also inquire with mental health practitioners, especially those with an interest in health psychology, or with alternative medicine practitioners in your area. For further information contact:

The Academy for Guided Imagery
P.O. Box 2070
Mill Valley, California 94942
(800) 726-2070

The Academy trains health professionals to use Interactive Guided Imagery™, offering a 150-hour certification program. They publish a directory of imagery practitioners and also carry books and tapes for professionals and lay people, specifically relating to imagery in medicine and healing. Send for free catalog.

American Holistic Medical Association and
American Holistic Nurses Association
4101 Lake Boone Trail, Suite 201
Raleigh, North Carolina 27607
(919) 787-5146

Both of these organizations have members who favor holistic approaches to treatment and will be familiar with and supportive of the use of imagery in healing.

Center for Applied Psychophysiology
Menninger Clinic
P.O. Box 829
Topeka, Kansas 66601-08829
(913) 273-7500 Ext. 5375

This organization conducts research and provides treatment and workshops in all areas of mind/body medicine, including extensive work with imagery.

Exceptional Cancer Patients
1302 Chapel Street
New Haven, Connecticut 06511
(203) 865-8392

This organization, founded by Dr. Bernie Siegel, has a referral list of professionals who work with imagery and cancer patients. They also have an extensive catalogue of books and tapes related to healing, with special emphasis on cancer and catastrophic illness.

Health Associates, Inc.
P.O. Box 220
Big Sur, California 93920
(408) 667-0248 (Fax)

Co-directed by Jeanne Achterberg, Ph.D., and Frank Lawlis, Ph.D., Health Associates provides imagery workshops and offers training in transpersonal uses of imagery, including its applications in healing.

Simonton Cancer Center
P.O. Box 890
Pacific Palisades, California 90272
(310) 459-4434

0. Carl Simonton, M.D., pioneered the use of imagery in people recovering from cancer. His organization has trained professionals around the country in his methods and may be able to refer you to someone in your area.

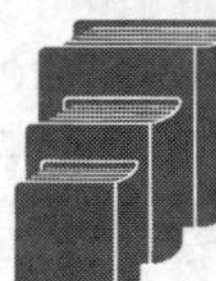

Recommended Reading

Free Yourself from Pain. Bresler, David, Ph.D. Topanga, CA: The Bresler Center, 1992.

This self-help book for managing chronic pain and depression includes several chapters illustrating the use of imagery for pain control. (Available from The Bresler Center, 115 South Topanga Canyon Boulevard, Suite 158, Topanga, California 90290. (310) 455-3634.)

Getting Well Again. Simonton, Carl, M.D. and Stephanie; and Creighton, J. Los Angeles: Jeremy P. Tarcher, 1978.

A self-help book combining deep relaxation with mental imagery to reinforce the goals of medical treatment.

Healing from Within. Jaffe, Dennis T. New York: (Fireside) Simon and Schuster, 1988.

In simple language, Jaffe explores the meaning of growth, freedom, and personal responsibility, while showing how to develop one's inner resources and creative energy.

Healing Yourself: A Step-by-Step Program for Better Health through Imagery. Rossman, Martin L. New York: Pocket Books, 1989.

A simple how-to on unleashing the body's natural healing powers.

Imagery in Healing: Shamanism and Modern Medicine. Achterberg, Jeanne. Boston, MA: New Science Library/Shambala, 1985.

The author explains how the systematic use of imagery can help patients through painful events ranging from childbirth to burn treatment, as well as acting as a positive influence on disease states such as cancer.

Minding the Body, Mending the Mind. Borysenko, Joan. Reading, MA: Bantam, 1988.

Learn to control conditions from allergies to cancer, as well as your emotional well-being, using imagery.

Why Me? Harnessing the Healing Power of the Human Spirit. Porter, Garrett; and Norris, Patricia. Walpole, NH: Stillpoint International, 1985.

An uplifting account of a nine-year-old's successful struggle against cancer using imagery and biofeedback.

Herbal Medicine

Herbal medicine is the most ancient form of health care known to humankind. Herbs have been used in all cultures throughout history. Extensive scientific documentation now exists concerning their use for health conditions, including premenstrual syndrome, indigestion, insomnia, heart disease, cancer, and HIV.

Herbs have always been integral to the practice of medicine. The word drug comes from the old Dutch word *drogge* meaning "to dry," as pharmacists, physicians, and ancient healers often dried plants for use as medicines. Today approximately 25 percent of all prescription drugs are still derived from trees, shrubs, or herbs.[1] Some are made from plant extracts; others are synthesized to mimic a natural plant compound.

The World Health Organization notes that of 119 plant-derived pharmaceutical medicines, about 74 percent are used in modern medicine in ways that correlated directly with their traditional uses as plant medicines by native cultures.[2]

Yet, for the most part, modern medicine has veered from the use of pure herbs in its treatment of disease and other health disorders. One of the reasons for this is economic. Herbs, by their very nature, cannot be patented. Since herbs cannot be patented and drug companies cannot hold the exclusive right to sell a particular herb, they are not motivated to invest any money in that herb's testing or promotion. The collection and preparation of herbal medicine cannot be as easily controlled as the manufacture of synthetic drugs, making its profits less dependable. In addition, many of these medicinal plants grow only in the Amazonian rain forest or other politically and economically unstable places, which also affects the supply of the herb. Most importantly, the demand for herbal medicine has decreased in the United States because Americans have been conditioned to rely on synthetic, commercial drugs to provide quick relief, regardless of side effects.

"The World Health Organization notes that of 119 plant-derived pharmaceutical medicines, about 74 percent were used in modern medicine in ways that correlated directly with their traditional uses as plant medicines by native cultures."

Yet, the current viewpoint seems to be changing. "The revival of interest in herbal medicine is a worldwide phenomenon," says Mark Blumenthal, Executive Director of the American Botanical Council. This renaissance is due to the growing concern of the general public about the side effects of pharmaceutical drugs, the impersonal and often demeaning experience of modern health care practices, as well as a renewed recognition of the unique medicinal value of herbal medicine.

"The scope of herbal medicine ranges from mild-acting plant medicines such as chamomile and peppermint, to very potent ones such as foxglove (from which the drug digitalis is derived). In between these two poles lies a wide spectrum of plant medicine with significant medical applications," says Donald Brown, N.D., of Bastyr College, in Seattle, Washington, and an educator in herbal medicine. "One need only go to the *United States Pharmacopoeia* to see the central role that plant medicine has played in American medicine."

What Is an Herb?

The word herb as used in herbal medicine (also known as botanical medicine or, in Europe, as phytotherapy or phytomedicine), means a plant or plant part that is used to make medicine, food flavors (spices), or aromatic oils for soaps and fragrances. An herb can be a leaf, a flower, a stem, a seed, a root, a fruit, bark, or any other plant part used for its medicinal, food flavoring, or fragrant property.[3]

"There are an estimated 250,000 to 500,000 plants on the earth today (the number varies depending on whether subspecies are included). Only about 5,000 of these have been extensively studied for their medicinal applications."

Herbs have provided humankind with medicine from the earliest beginnings of civilization. Throughout history, various cultures have handed down their accumulated knowledge of the medicinal use of herbs to successive generations. This vast body of information serves as the basis for much of traditional medicine today.

There are an estimated 250,000 to 500,000 plants on the earth today (the number varies depending on whether subspecies are included). Only about 5,000 of these have been extensively studied for their medicinal applications. "This illustrates the need for modern medicine and science to turn its attention to the plant world once again to find new medicine that might cure cancer, AIDS, diabetes, and many other diseases and conditions," says Norman R. Farnsworth, Ph.D., Professor of Pharmacology at the University of Illinois at Chicago. "Considering that 121 prescription drugs come from only ninety species of plants, and that 74 percent of these were discovered following up native folklore claims," says Dr. Farnsworth, "a logical person would have to say that there may still be more jackpots out there."[4]

How Herbal Medicine Works

In general, herbal medicines work in much the same way as do conventional pharmaceutical drugs, i.e., via their chemical makeup. Herbs contain a large number of naturally occurring chemicals that have biological activity. In the past 150 years, chemists and pharmacists have been isolating and purifying the "active" compounds from plants in an attempt to produce reliable pharmaceutical drugs. Examples include such drugs like digoxin (from foxglove [*Digitalis purpurea*]), reserpine (from Indian snakeroot [*Rauwolfia serpentina*]), colchicine (from autumn crocus [*Colchicum autumnale*]), morphine (from the opium poppy [*Papaver somniafera*]), and many more.

According to Andrew Weil, M.D., of Tucson, Arizona, because herbs and plants use an indirect route to the bloodstream and target organs, their effects are usually slower in onset and less dramatic than those of purified drugs administered by more direct routes. "Doctors and patients accustomed to the rapid, intense effects of synthetic medicines may become impatient with botanicals for this reason," Dr. Weil states.[5]

Herbal medicine has most to offer when used to facilitate healing in chronic ongoing problems. By skillful selection of herbs for the patient, a profound transformation in health can be effected with less danger of the side effects inherent in drug-based medicine. However, the common assumption that herbs act slowly and mildly is not necessarily true. Adverse effects can occur if an inadequate dose, a low-quality herb, or the wrong herb is prescribed for the patient.

The Action of Herbs

A great deal of pharmaceutical research has gone into analyzing the active ingredients of herbs to find out how and why they work. This effect is referred to as the herb's action. Herbal actions describe the ways in which the remedy affects human physiology. In some cases the action is due to a specific chemical present in the herb (as in the antiasthmatic effects of ma-huang) or it may be due to a complex synergistic interaction between various constituents of the plant (the sedative valerian is an example). A much older, and far more relevant approach is to categorize herbs by looking at what kinds of problems can be treated with their help. Plants have a direct impact on physiological activity and by knowing what body process one wants to help or heal, the appropriate action can be selected. The qualities of herbs which make them beneficial in treating the human body, include:

- **Adaptogenic:** Adaptogenic herbs increase resistance and resilience to stress, enabling the body to adapt around the problem and avoid reaching collapse. Adaptogens work by supporting the adrenal glands.
- **Alterative:** Herbs that gradually restore proper functioning of the body, increasing health and vitality.
- **Anthelminitic:** Herbs that destroy or expel intestinal worms.
- **Anti-inflammatory:** Herbs that soothe inflammations or reduce the inflammatory response of the tissue directly. They work in a number of different ways, but rarely inhibit the natural inflammatory reaction as such.
- **Antimicrobial:** Antimicrobials help the body destroy or resist pathogenic (disease-causing) microorganisms. Herbs help the body strengthen its own resistance to infective organisms and throw off illness. While some contain chemicals that are antiseptic or poisonous to certain organisms, in general they aid the body's natural immunity.

- **Antispasmodic:** Antispasmodics ease cramps in smooth and skeletal muscles. They alleviate muscular tension and can ease psychological tension as well.
- **Astringent:** Astringents have a binding action on mucous membranes, skin, and other tissue. They have the effect of reducing irritation and inflammation, and creating a barrier against infection that is helpful to wounds and burns.
- **Bitter:** Herbs with a bitter taste have a special role in preventative medicine. The taste triggers a sensory response in the central nervous system leading to a range of responses, including: stimulating appetite and the flow of digestive juices; aiding the liver's detoxification work; increasing bile flow, and motivating gut self-repair mechanisms.
- **Carminative:** Plants that are rich in aromatic volatile oils stimulate the digestive system to work properly and with ease. They soothe the gut wall; reduce any inflammation that might be present; and ease griping pains and help with the removal of gas from the digestive tract.
- **Demulcent:** Demulcent herbs are rich in mucilage and soothe and protect irritated or inflamed tissue. They reduce irritation down the whole length of the bowel, reduce sensitivity to potentially corrosive gastric acids, help prevent diarrhea, and reduce the muscle spasms that cause colic.
- **Diuretic:** Diuretics increase the production and elimination of urine. They help the body eliminate waste and support the whole process of inner cleansing.
- **Emmenagogue:** Emmenagogues stimulate menstrual flow and activity. With most herbs, however, the term is used in the wider sense for a remedy that affects the female reproductive system.
- **Expectorant:** Herbs that stimulate removal of mucous from the lungs. Stimulating expectorants "irritate" the bronchioles (a subdivision of the bronchial tubes) causing expulsion of material. Relaxing expectorants soothe bronchial spasm and loosen mucous secretions, helping in dry, irritating coughs.
- **Hepatic:** Hepatics aid the liver. They tone and strengthen the liver and in some cases increase the flow of bile. In a broad holistic approach to health they are of great importance because of the fundamental role of the liver in maintaining health by not only facilitating digestion but by removing toxins from the body.
- **Hypotensive:** Hypotensives are plant remedies that lower abnormally elevated blood pressure.
- **Laxative:** These are plants that promote bowel movements. They are divided into those that work by providing bulk, those that stimulate the production of bile in the liver and its release from the gallbladder, and those that directly trigger peristalsis (wavelike contractions of the smooth muscles of the digestive tract).
- **Nervine:** Nervines help the nervous system and can be subdivided into three groups. Nervine tonics strengthen and restore the nervous system. Nervine relaxants ease anxiety and tension by

soothing both body and mind. Nervine stimulants directly stimulate nerve activity.

- **Stimulating:** Stimulants quicken and invigorate the physiological and metabolic activity of the body.
- **Tonic:** Tonics nurture and enliven. They are used frequently in Traditional Chinese Medicine and Ayurvedic medicine, often as a preventative measure. Tonic herbs like ginseng build vital energy, or *qi*.

THE POLITICS OF HERBS

The World Health Organization (WHO) recognizes that nearly 80 percent of the world population is dependent on traditional medicine for primary health care.[6] Herbal medicine constitutes a large part of what is practiced as traditional medicine around the world. WHO has published guidelines for the assessment of herbal medicines in an attempt to help the ministries of health of all governments develop regulations that ensure medicines are labeled properly, and that consumers and practitioners are given proper directions for their use.[7]

However, expert FDA (Food and Drug Administration) panels that stringently review over-the-counter drug ingredients for safety and efficacy have eliminated many herbal ingredients from sanctioned use in nonprescription medicine.[8]

At the same time, the FDA is banning formerly used herbal ingredients from use in over-the-counter drugs, an increasingly large segment of the population is requesting and using natural medicines.

Herbal medicine is more readily accepted in Europe than in the United States. The British Herbal Pharmacopoeia, *though not officially recognized by Parliament, is nevertheless the accepted publication in the field.[9] In Germany, the Ministry of Health has a separate commission that deals exclusively with herbal medicine. German doctors study herbal medicine in medical school, and since 1993, all physicians in Germany must pass a section on these medicines in their board exams before becoming licensed.[10]*

As part of the unifying efforts going on among members of the European community, European physicians, health professionals, and researchers have formed ESCOP, the European Scientific Cooperative for Phytotherapy. This organization is publishing monographs on individual herbs used in clinical medicine as well as those used for self-medication. These monographs, representing the culmination of all the scientific information known on each herb, are intended to be published in the next edition of the European Pharmacopoeia *and will become the guiding information for regulations of each herb in all of Europe.[11]*

There is no licensing body for the practice of herbal medicine in the United States. The result is that many herbal practitioners are outside of the "system." However, there are numerous qualified practitioners of herbal medicine who utilize approaches based on either the Western bio-medical model, or on Oriental approaches, such as Traditional Chinese Medicine and Ayurveda. Within the Western medical community, naturopathic physicians have a solid foundation in botanical medicine and phytochemistry.

Herbs in Many Forms

Herbs and herbal products come in many forms, and are now available not only in natural food stores, but also grocery stores, drugstores, and gourmet food stores. Also, a number of multilevel marketing organizations sell a variety of herbal products, as do mail order purveyors.

HOW TO MAKE AN HERB TEA

Loose teas are usually steeped in hot water: three to five minutes for leaves and flowers (this method is called infusion), or fifteen to twenty minutes in a rolling boil for denser materials like root and bark (called a decoction).

Infusions: *Infusions are the simplest method of preparing an herb tea and both fresh or dried herbs may be used, such as peppermint, chamomile, and rosehips. Due to the higher water content of the fresh herb, three parts fresh herb replace one part of the dried herb. To make an infusion:*

- *Put about one teaspoonful of the dried herb or herb mixture for each cup into a teapot.*
- *Add boiling water and cover. Leave to steep for five to ten minutes. Infusions may be taken hot, cold, or iced. They may also be sweetened.*
- *Infusions are most appropriate for plant parts such as leaves, flowers, or green stems where the medicinal properties are easily accessible. To infuse bark, root, seeds, or resin, it is best to powder them first to break down some of their cell walls before adding them to the water. Seeds like fennel and aniseed should be slightly bruised to release the volatile oils from the cells. Any aromatic herb should be infused in a pot that has a well-sealing lid, to reduce loss of the volatile oil through evaporation.*

Decoctions: *For hard and woody herbs, ginger root and cinnamon bark for example, it is best to make a decoction rather than an infusion, to ensure that the soluble contents of the herb actually reach the water. Roots, wood, bark, nuts, and certain seeds are hard and their cell walls are very strong, requiring more heat to release them than in an infusion. These herbs need to be boiled in the water. To make a decoction:*

- *Put one teaspoonful of dried herb or three teaspoonfuls of fresh material for each cup of water into a pot or saucepan. Dried herbs should be powdered or broken into small pieces, while fresh material should be cut into small pieces.*
- *Add the appropriate amount of water to the herbs.*
- *Bring to a boil and simmer for ten to fifteen minutes.*

When using a woody herb that contains a lot of volatile oil, it is best to make sure that it is powdered as finely as possible and then used in an infusion, to ensure that the oils do not boil away. Decoctions can be used in the same way as an infusion.

Whole Herbs: Whole herbs are plants or plant parts that are dried and then either cut or powdered. They can be used as teas or for a variety of products at home.

Teas: Teas come in either loose or teabag form. Because of the obvious convenience, most Americans today prefer to purchase their herbal teas in teabags, which include one or a variety of finely cut herbs. When steeped in boiled water for a few minutes, the fragrant, aromatic flavor and the herbs' medicinal properties are released. As a general rule, most teas are consumed for three reasons: 1) as alternatives to caffeinated tea or coffee (although some herbal teas do contain caffeine, e.g., maté); 2) as a component to a meal strictly for the flavor (peppermint, spearmint, rosehips, lemon grass, anise); and 3) for their mild medicinal effects (peppermint and chamomile for upset stomach or to improve digestion, chamomile or hops as a nighttime sleep aid or insomnia remedy, cinnamon tea as a home remedy for diarrhea).

Capsules and Tablets: One of the fastest growing markets in herbal medicine in the past fifteen to twenty years has been capsules and tablets. These offer consumers convenience and, in some cases, the bonus of not having to taste the herbs, many of which have undesirable flavor profiles, from intensely bitter due to the presence of certain alkaloids (goldenseal root) to highly astringent due to the presence of tannins (oak bark).

Extracts and Tinctures: These offer the advantage of high concentration in low weight and space. They are also quickly assimilated compared to tablets, which take more time to disintegrate and ingest. Extracts and tinctures almost always contain alcohol. The alcohol is used for two reasons: as a solvent to extract the various non–water-soluble compounds from an herb, and as a preservative to maintain shelf life. Properly made extracts and tinctures have virtually an indefinite shelf life. Tinctures usually contain more alcohol than extracts (sometimes up to 70 to 80 percent alcohol, depending on the particular herb and manufacturer).

Essential Oils: Essential oils are usually distilled from various parts of medicinal and aromatic plants. Some oils, however, like those from lemon, orange, and other citrus fruits, are actually expressed directly from the peels. Essential oils are concentrated, with one or two drops often constituting adequate dosage. Thus, they are to be used carefully and sparingly when employed internally. Because some oils may irritate the skin, they should be diluted in fatty oils or water before topical application. There are a few exceptions, most notably eucalyptus and tea tree oils, which can be applied directly to the skin without concern of irritation.

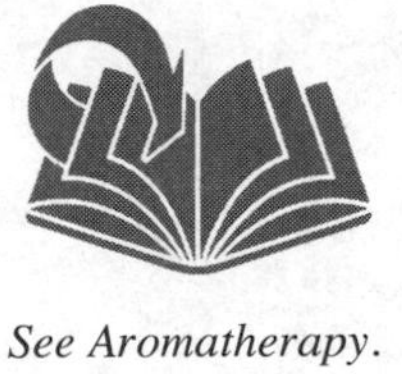

See Aromatherapy.

Salves, Balms, and Ointments: For thousands of years, humans have used plants to treat skin irritations, wounds, and insect and snake bites. In prehistoric times, herbs were cooked in a vat of goose or bear fat, lard, or some vegetable oils and then cooled in order to make salves, balms, and ointments. Today, a number of such products, made with vegetable oil or petroleum jelly, are sold in the United States and Europe to treat a variety of conditions. These products often contain the following herbs: aloe, marigold, chamomile, St. John's Wort, comfrey, and gotu kola.

Conditions Benefited by Herbal Medicine

Herbal remedies can be used for a wide range of minor ailments that are amenable to self-medication, including stomach upset, the common cold, flus, minor aches and pains, constipation and diarrhea, coughs, headaches, menstrual cramps, digestive disturbances, sore muscles, skin rashes, sunburn, dandruff, and insomnia. A growing number of American health consumers use herbal remedies for these conditions, which have been traditionally the domain of the nonprescription or over-the-counter drugs.

Other conditions that respond well to herbal medicine include: digestive disorders such as peptic ulcers, colitis and irritable bowel syndrome; rheumatic and arthritic conditions; chronic skin problems such as eczema and psoriasis; problems of the menstrual cycle and especially premenstrual syndrome; anxiety and tension-related stress; bronchitis and other respiratory conditions; hypertension; and allergies.

Herbal medicines can also be used for a number of conditions normally treated by prescription only. One example is milk thistle seed extract for use in cirrhosis and hepatitis.[12] Another example is the use of hawthorn as a heart tonic.[13] This herb is highly recommended for cardiac patients by physicians in Germany (see The Herbal Medicine Chest section in this chapter).

"When treating chronic illness with herbal medicine it is extremely important to treat the entire body, as the illness may be simultaneously affecting many systems of the body at various levels," says Mary Bove, N.D., L.M., head of the Department of Botanical Medicine at Bastyr College of Natural Health Sciences, in Seattle, Washington. "The course of the treatment must include nutritional, tonic, and restorative plants in conjunction with herbs that support the body's elimination functions. We find the alterative and adaptogenic plants to be very effective. Digestive function is also an important consideration in most chronic diseases. The duration of treatment is often longer, with a constant dose of the remedy being given over a longer period of time."

Dr. Bove reports, "I had a thirty-eight-year-old female patient who came in with a ten-year-old case of colitis. She had been seen by several M.D.'s and N.D.'s over the past decade with some improvement. After discussing her long history, I chose to treat her from a different perspective. Primarily I gave her digestive nervines and tonic herbs like catnip, lemon balm, and tilia flowers. Within three days, she went from eleven stools per day to two per day. I continued with these herbs, adding some others for gut healing. We had excellent results which were supported by diagnostic imaging."

Herbal medicine has also had great results with arthritic conditions. Consider the case of a forty-two-year-old woman with rheumatoid arthritis, confined to a wheelchair due to extreme and almost constant pain and swelling. She consulted with David Hoffmann, B.Sc., M.N.I.M.H., past President of the American Herbalists Guild, whose treatment involved herbal medicine and a reevaluation of her diet and lifestyle. Herbs were selected initially to ease the digestive problems caused by medications she was taking and to help her sleep. Once such side effects were alleviated, a program was started that enabled her to completely abandon the wheelchair after six months. Though she still had some arthritic pain, she was able to live with it comfortably.

The uniqueness of each individual is important in evaluating any holistic therapy, whether it be homeopathic, herbal, or nutritional. In order to prescribe effectively, it is critical that a physician be knowledgeable and adaptable to each patient's individual situation. John Sherman, N.D., of the Portland Naturopathic Clinic in Oregon tells of a woman he treated who came to his clinic complaining of heart palpitations. She was also concerned about the drugs she'd been prescribed for her heart arrhythmia. She told Dr. Sherman that the drugs had been "sapping" her energy and only partially helping her heart problem. Dr. Sherman prescribed a combination herbal tincture of cactus, hawthorn, valerian, and lily of the valley, which is a standard combination naturopathic physicians use to combat arrhythmia and a "feeble" heart. He also analyzed her diet to determine her intake of specific minerals which affect the heart, including calcium, potassium, and sodium.

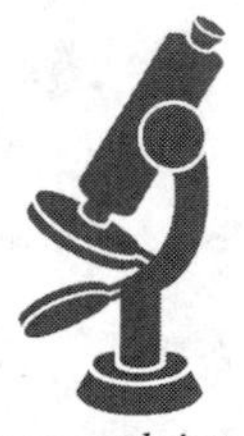

Additional research into the medicinal benefits of herbs will speed the integration of herbal medicine into the American health care system.

She returned to Dr. Sherman's clinic two weeks later, still complaining of heart palpitations and feeling even more frustrated. Dr. Sherman decided to change the herbal formula slightly by adding scotch broom. Within a few days, she happily reported the absence of any heart symptoms and was subsequently able to wean herself off the prescription drugs.

DIFFERENT SYSTEMS OF HERBOLOGY

There is a great diversity and richness in the various herbal traditions of the world, most of which still thrive today. Native American cultures contain a cornucopia of healing wisdom as do European traditions, from the Welsh to the Sicilian. There are a number of highly developed medical systems around the world that utilize medicinal plants in their healing work. These include ancient systems such as Ayurveda from India and Traditional Chinese Medicine. The essential differences between these various systems of medicine are their cultural contexts rather than their goals or effects.

Traditional Chinese Medicine: *The restoration of harmony is integral to Chinese herbal medicine. Harmonious balance is expressed in terms of the two complementary forces—*yin *and* yang*; and the five elements—fire, earth, metal, water, and wood. The five elements are of particular importance to the Chinese herbalist; they give rise to the five tastes by which all medicinal plants are evaluated. Fire gives rise to bitterness, earth to sweetness, metal to acridity, water to saltiness, and wood to sourness. Each taste is said to have a particular medicinal action: bitter-tasting herbs drain and dry; sweet herbs tonify and may reduce pain; acrid herbs disperse; salty herbs nourish the kidneys; sour herbs nourish the* yin *and astringe, preventing unwanted loss of body fluids or* qi*. Herbs that have none of these tastes are described as bland—a quality that indicates that the plant may have a diuretic effect. The taste of a plant can also indicate the organ to which it has a natural affinity. Besides defining particular herbal tastes, the Chinese ascribe different temperatures to herbs—hot, warm, neutral, cool, and cold.*

Ayurveda: *Ayurvedic medicine has ancient roots in the Indian subcontinent. It also recognizes five elements: ether, fire, water, air, and earth. These five elements manifest themselves in the body to form the* tridosha *or three basic humors:* vata *(the principle of air or movement);* pitta *(the principle of fire); and* kapha *(the principle of water). Ayurvedic medicine sees all universal energies as having their counterparts within the human being. The healing process seeks to achieve in individuals a balance between the elements of air or wind (*vata*), fire or bile (*pitta*), and water or phlegm (*kapha*).*

Ayurvedic medicine holds that the taste of an herb is indicative of its properties. The Sanskrit word for taste, rasa*, means "essence." There are six essences: sweet, sour, salty, pungent, bitter, and astringent. For example, pungent, sour, and salty-tasting herbs cause heat and so increase* pitta *(fire); sweet, bitter, and astringent herbs have precisely the opposite effect, cooling and decreasing* pitta*. As in Chinese herbal medicine, Ayurvedic texts categorize all plants according to this system, so that their herbalists can prescribe herbs more easily.*

Western medicine: *The use of medicinal plants is also fundamental to Western society's pharmacologically based approach to medicine. The majority of medicinal drug groups were discovered or developed from the plant kingdom, even if they are now manufactured synthetically. However, most modern health professionals view medicines as biochemical "magic bullets," which should be expected to provide instant results. This approach has been very successful in certain areas, such as the treatment of acute illness, but has major limitations when it comes to chronic or degenerative disease.*

See Ayurvedic Medicine, Traditional Chinese Medicine.

The Herbal Medicine Chest

Each of the following twenty-five herbal medicines has a long history of use.

Aloe Vera (*Aloe vera)*: Aloe is such a widely used ingredient in cosmetics (hand lotions, shaving creams, etc.), it is considered a mainstream cosmetic product and many people do not realize that it is a medicinal herb. Aloe gel is used externally on the skin primarily for its emollient (skin softening) property.

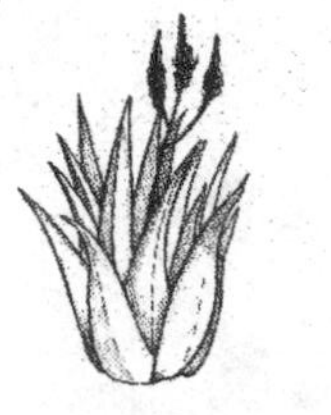

Aloe Vera

Another use for aloe comes from the latex of the leaf. Aloe latex is recognized as a safe and effective laxative ingredient by the FDA (Food and Drug Administration) as well as a number of European countries. For example, in Germany, aloe latex is employed as a stimulant laxative. Normal precautions regarding stimulant laxatives apply to aloe. Like other stimulant laxatives, anthraquinone-containing (a plant-based, organic compound) purgatives like aloe need to be used for the short-term only and not during pregnancy or lactation. Long-term use or misuse may also cause an electrolyte imbalance, resulting in depletion of potassium salts and thus may adversely effect heart function.[14] Keep in mind that these warnings are for aloe *latex* used as a laxative, not the aloe *gel* or *juice* commonly consumed by health enthusiasts for "inner cleansing."

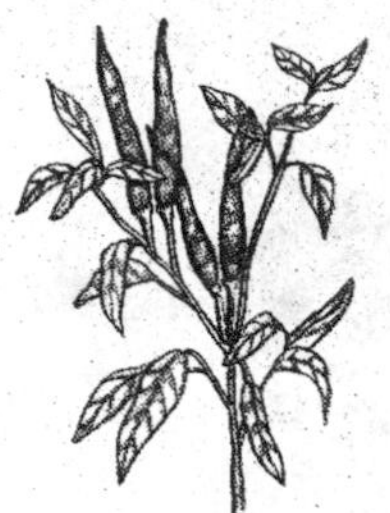

Cayenne

Cayenne *(Capsicum annuum)*: Cayenne or red pepper is the most useful of the systemic stimulants. It stimulates blood flow, strengthening the heartbeat and metabolic rate.[15] A general tonic, it is helpful specifically for the circulatory and digestive systems. It may be used in flatulent dyspepsia (imperfect or painful digestion) and colic.[16] If there is insufficient peripheral circulation, leading to cold hands and feet and possibly chilblains (a form of cold injury characterized by redness and blistering), cayenne may be used. It is also useful for debility as well as for warding off colds.[17] Externally it is used in problems like lumbago (a dull, aching pain in the lumbar region of the back) and rheumatic pains.[18]

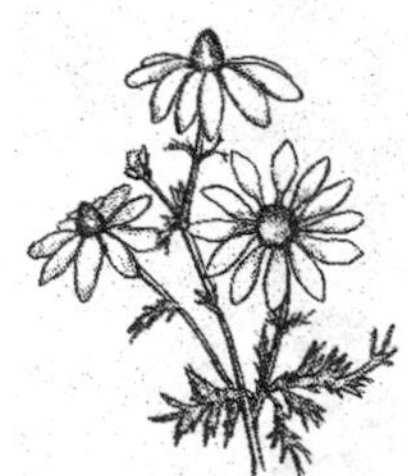

Chamomile

Chamomile *(Matricaria recutita)*: Chamomile flower is used in many cultures for its pleasant-tasting tea, consumed as an after-dinner beverage to help digestion. In Europe, chamomile is noted as a digestive aid, as a mild sedative, and for its anti-inflammatory property, especially in over-the-counter preparations for oral hygiene and skin creams.[19] In Germany, chamomile is licensed as an over-the-counter drug for internal use against gastrointestinal spasms and inflammatory diseases of the gastrointestinal tract. Externally, the extract is approved for skin and mucous membrane inflammations, for bacterial skin diseases of the mouth and gums, for inflammation of the mucous membranes of the throat and airways, and as an external bath and rinse for inflamed conditions of anal and genital regions.[20]

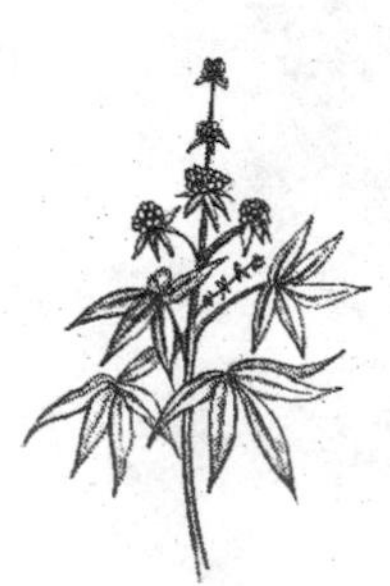

Chasteberry

Chasteberry *(Vitex agnus-castus):* Chasteberry is becoming widely used as an herb that addresses various hormonal imbalances in women. The clinical results are thought to be due to some regulatory effect upon the pituitary gland.[21] Recent findings confirm that chasteberry helps restore a normal estrogen-to-progesterone balance.[22] It is indicated for irregular or painful menstruation,[23] premenstrual syndrome,[24] and other disorders related to hormone function. It is especially beneficial during menopausal changes, relieving symptoms such as hot flashes. It may be used to aid the body in regaining a natural balance after the use of birth control pills. Other ailments treatable with chasteberry include fibroid cysts that occur in smooth muscle tissue or body cavities. It may also be of value in treating endometriosis. Several studies indicate chasteberry can help control acne in teenagers, both among young women and men.[25]

Echinacea *(Echinacea angustifolia)*: Often called purple coneflower, the term echinacea refers to several species of plants that are generally found in the Great Plains region of North America. It was the most widely used medicinal plant of the Native Americans of this area. Native Americans often exploited echinacea for its external wound-healing and anti-inflammatory properties. Ironically, it was a German researcher, Dr. Gerhard Madaus, who imported echinacea seeds to Europe and initiated the first modern scientific research on the immunostimulating properties of this plant. Due to his work, echinacea has become one of the most important over-the-counter remedies in Germany, where it is employed for relieving the common cold and flus.

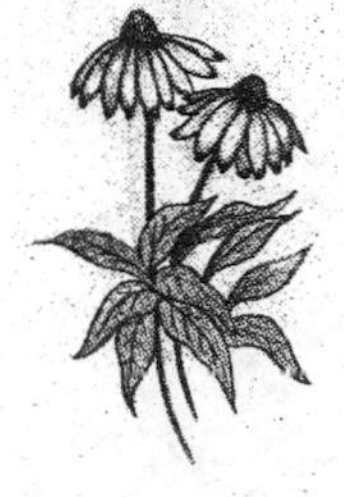

Echinacea

Over 180 products are marketed in Germany, including extracts and fresh-squeezed juices from both the roots and leaves of echinacea.[26] The German government has approved oral dosage of echinacea for use in recurrent infections of the respiratory and urinary tracts, progressive systemic disorders such as tuberculosis, leukosis (abnormal growth of white blood cells), connective tissue disease, multiple sclerosis, and, when applied topically, for surface wounds with a poor tendency to heal. Liquid echinacea preparations have been shown to have immune-stimulating activity when administered both orally and parenterally (denoting any medication route other than the intestine, e.g., intravenously): they increase the number of leukocytes (white blood cells) and splenocytes (white blood cells of the spleen) and enhance the activity of granulocytes (granular white blood cells) and phagocytes (cells that have the ability to ingest and destroy substances, such as bacteria, protozoa, and cell debris).[27]

Ephedra or Ma-huang *(Ephedra sineca):* Ephedra is a medicinal plant that has been cultivated for over five thousand years in China, where it was used for asthma and hay fever-like conditions. Also known as ma-huang, the stems contain two primary alkaloids, ephedrine and pseudoephedrine, which are now approved for use in over-the-counter decongestant and bronchial drugs. Ephedrine has a marked peripheral vasoconstricting (causing constriction of the blood vessels) action. Pseudoephedrine is a bronchodilator (able to dilate the windpipe), approved for use in asthma and certain allergy medicines. Ma-huang and its extracts are found in a number of herbal formulas that are designed to increase energy and reduce appetite. Both ephedrine and pseudoephedrine have central nervous system (CNS)-stimulating properties, ephedrine being more active. The CNS activity of these alkaloids has been characterized as being stronger than caffeine and weaker than methamphetamine (a central nervous system stimulant). Hence, as is the case with caffeine, this herb should be used with caution or avoided by those with high blood pressure, diabetes, glaucoma, and related conditions where hypertensives are contraindicated.[28]

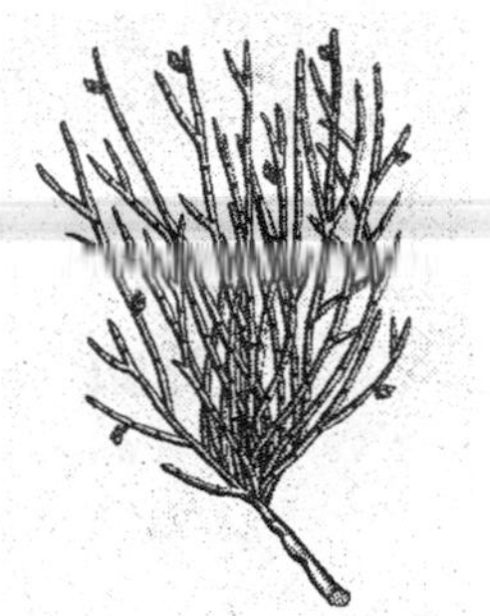

Ephedra or Ma-huang

Feverfew *(Tanacetum parthenium):* Feverfew is an herbal remedy that dates back to Greco-Roman times. It was formerly employed as a remedy for difficulties associated with young women's menstrual cycles (the word parthenium is derived from the Greek word *parthenos,* meaning "virgin") and was later used in European herbalism to reduce fevers (the common name feverfew being a corruption of the Latin word *febrifuga,* an agent that lowers fevers).[29] Interest in this herb has been generated in the past ten years because of several clinical studies that have been published in British medical journals. Research shows that feverfew leaves not only bring relief in a significant number of migraine patients who have not responded positively to conventional medications, but also helps to prevent the onset of additional episodes.[30] Recently, the Canadian government's Health Protection Branch (equivalent to the United States' FDA) has approved feverfew leaf extract for migraine prevention, as long as the products contain a minimum of 0.2 percent parthenolide, a substance in the feverfew leaf that has been identified as being the primary active component.[31] Early herbal literature also attributes anti-rheumatic properties to feverfew, but this has not been confirmed by twentieth century research.[32]

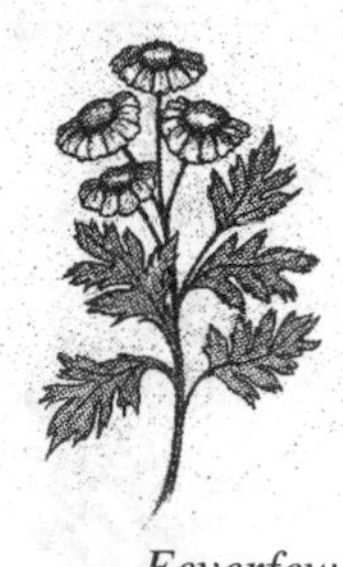

Feverfew

Garlic *(Allium sativum):* Garlic is probably the most well-recognized medicinal herb. It is used by traditional medicines all over the world and its applications are as varied as its geographical distribution. The chemistry and pharmacology of garlic is well studied; over one thousand research papers have been published in the past twenty to twenty-five years. Garlic and its preparations are known for their antibiotic, antifungal, and antiviral activity; for use in helping clear congested lungs; for coughs and bronchitis; as a preventive measure for the common cold and flus; and for intestinal worms, dysentery, sinus congestion, certain ulcers, gout, and rheumatism.[33] Garlic even has chemopreventive properties—helping to prevent certain cancers. Recent reports by the National Cancer Institute on a large population of subjects in China indicate that the consumption of garlic and other members of the *allium* genus (onions, leeks, shallots) can help lower the incidence of stomach cancer.[34]

Western countries have shown interest in the herb's ability to provide important cardiovascular benefits, including slightly lowering blood pressure, aiding in the thinning of the blood, and reducing platelet aggregation (the clustering of disks found in human blood that facilitates blood coagulation). The chemical basis of garlic's anti-thrombotic effect (the ability to prevent harmful blood clotting) has been studied.[35] It has shown an ability to aid certain immune functions, particularly increasing natural killer cells' activity.[36]

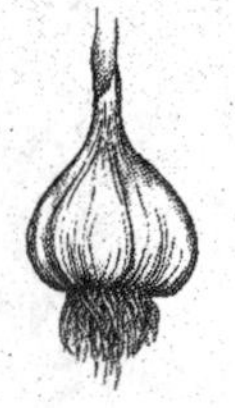

Garlic

Studies indicate general benefits from almost any type of garlic, be it raw garlic, dried garlic, garlic oil, or a prepared commercial product.[37] However, odorless or odor-controlled garlic preparations have a high degree of activity and are appropriate for those who do not wish to suffer the problems associated with garlic's characteristic odor, such as bad breath. In Germany, garlic extracts are approved over-the-counter drugs to supplement dietary measures in patients with elevated blood lipid (liquid fat) levels and to avert age-associated vascular changes."[38] A scientific panel of the European community has also endorsed garlic for its cardiovascular benefits.[39]

Ginger *(Zingiber officinalis):* In addition to its very popular food flavoring qualities, ginger is widely used as a medicinal herb in Chinese and Ayurvedic medicine, often added to herbal formulas to increase digestion and the activity of other herbs. In the past ten years, ginger has become best known for its anti-nausea and anti-motion sickness activity. A number of clinical studies have confirmed ginger's ability to act on the gastrointestinal system and allay nausea.[40] Unlike the leading over-the-counter drug, Dramamine, ginger does not relieve nausea by suppressing central nervous system activity. Rather, the effect is explained by the antiemetic (preventing or relieving nausea and vomiting) effects of this herb, which are well documented,[41] though more research is needed. Ginger is also known to have cardiotonic properties.[42] The herb has been used in traditional medicine for migraine relief,[43] and fresh ginger juice has been applied topically in Traditional Chinese Medicine as a burn remedy.[44]

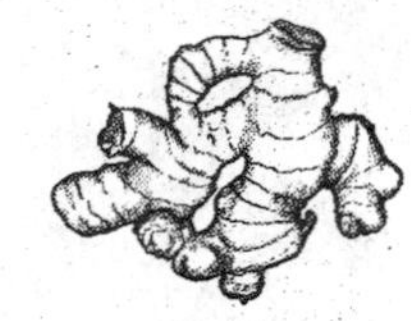

Ginger

Ginkgo *(Ginkgo biloba):* Ginkgo is an excellent example of why protecting plants and animals from extinction can help create new medicine. Ginkgos are the oldest living trees on earth. They first appeared about 200 million years ago and, except for a small population in northern China, were almost completely destroyed in the last Ice Age. Ginkgo leaves contain several compounds called ginkgolides that have unique chemical structures. The leaves were mentioned in a major Chinese herbal text of the Ming dynasty in 1436 and another in 1505. A standardized extract was developed in the past twenty years in Germany to treat a number of conditions associated with peripheral circulation.[45] It is currently licensed in Germany for the treatment of cerebral dysfunction, with the following symptoms: difficulty in memory, dizziness, tinnitus, headaches, and emotional instability coupled with anxiety. It is also licensed as a supportive treatment for hearing loss due to cervical syndrome and for peripheral arterial circulatory disturbances, such as intermittent claudication (a severe pain in the calf muscles resulting from inadequate blood supply).[46] Ginkgo leaf extracts are also used for heart and eye diseases, and accidents involving brain trauma. At least three volumes of technical papers on the chemistry, pharmacology, and clinical studies on *Ginkgo biloba* extract have been published.[47]

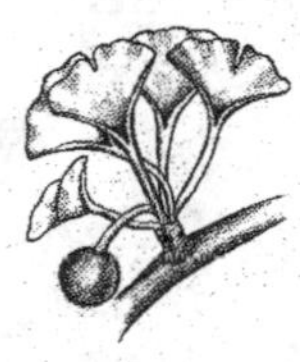

Ginkgo

Ginseng (*Panax ginseng*, Oriental ginseng; *Panax quinquefolius*, American ginseng): Ginseng has an ancient history and as such has accumulated much folklore about its actions and uses. The genus name *Panax* is derived from the Latin word *panacea* meaning "cure all." Many of the claims that surround ginseng are exaggerated but it is clearly an important remedy, receiving attention by researchers around the world.[48] It is a powerful adaptogen,[49] aiding the body to cope with stress, primarily through effects upon the functioning of the adrenal gland.[50] Ginseng has antioxidant,[51] antihepatotoxic (liver-protecting),[52] and hypoglycemic[53] effects. Thus there is a wide range of possible therapeutic uses. The main application is with weak, debilitated, stressed, or elderly people, where

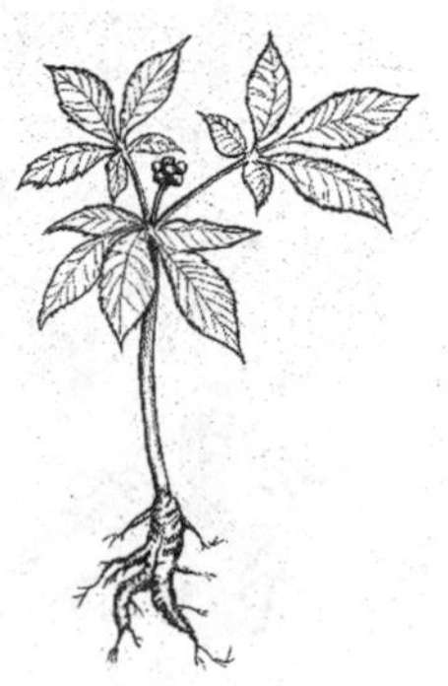

Ginseng

these properties can be especially useful.[54] In addition, ginseng may lower blood cholesterol[55] and stimulate a range of immune system[56] and endocrine responses.[57] If ginseng is abused, however, serious side effects can occur, including headaches, skin problems, and other reactions. For this reason, the proper dosage for the individual should be determined and respected.

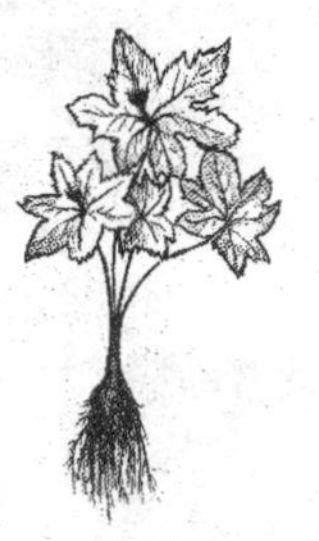

Goldenseal

Goldenseal *(Hydrastis canadensis)*: One of the most widely used American herbs, goldenseal is considered to be a tonic remedy that stimulates the immune response, and is directly antimicrobial itself. In addition, because of its bitter effects it can help in many digestive problems, from peptic ulcers to colitis.[58] Its bitter stimulation helps in loss of appetite, and the alkaloids it contains stimulate production and secretion of digestive juices. The antimicrobial properties are due to alkaloids, such as berberine.[59] Berberine, found in a number of other herbs as well, has marked antimicrobial activity. Not as powerful as an antibiotic, it nonetheless has a broad spectrum of activity. Effects have been demonstrated against bacteria, protozoa, and fungi, including *Staphylococcus sp., Streptococcus sp., Candida albicans*, and *Gardia lanbia*.[60] Berberine's action in inhibiting candida prevents the overgrowth of yeast that is a common side effect of antibiotic use. This alkaloid has also been shown to activate macrophages (cells that digest cell debris and other waste matter in the blood) in a number of ways.[61] Traditionally, goldenseal has been used during labor to help contractions, and for this reason it should be avoided during pregnancy. Applied externally it can be helpful in eczema, ringworm, itching, earache, and conjunctivitis.[62]

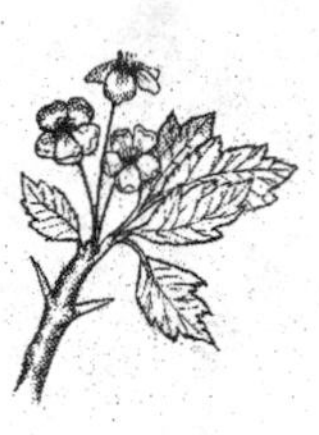

Hawthorn

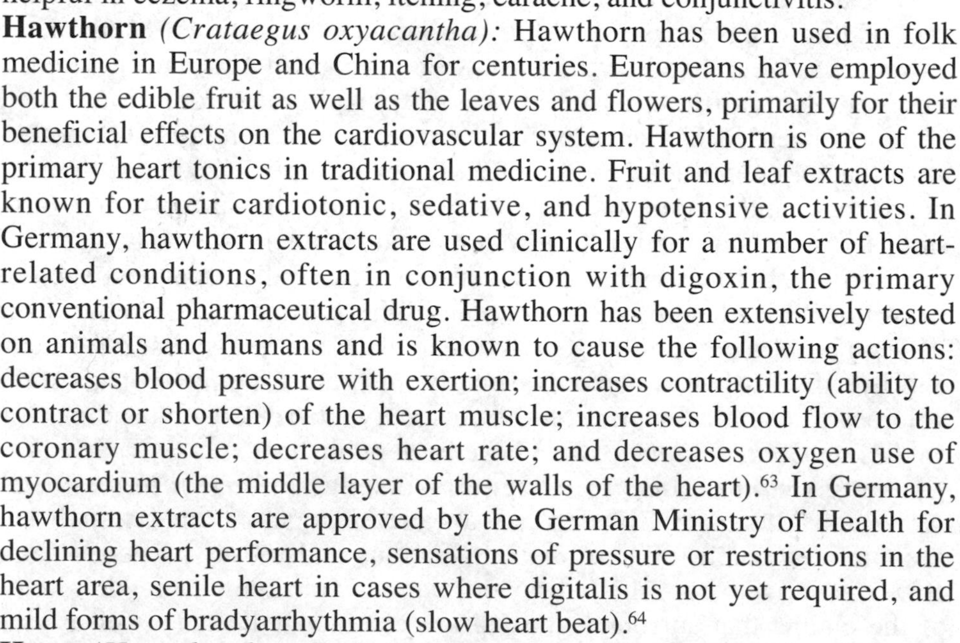

Hawthorn *(Crataegus oxyacantha):* Hawthorn has been used in folk medicine in Europe and China for centuries. Europeans have employed both the edible fruit as well as the leaves and flowers, primarily for their beneficial effects on the cardiovascular system. Hawthorn is one of the primary heart tonics in traditional medicine. Fruit and leaf extracts are known for their cardiotonic, sedative, and hypotensive activities. In Germany, hawthorn extracts are used clinically for a number of heart-related conditions, often in conjunction with digoxin, the primary conventional pharmaceutical drug. Hawthorn has been extensively tested on animals and humans and is known to cause the following actions: decreases blood pressure with exertion; increases contractility (ability to contract or shorten) of the heart muscle; increases blood flow to the coronary muscle; decreases heart rate; and decreases oxygen use of myocardium (the middle layer of the walls of the heart).[63] In Germany, hawthorn extracts are approved by the German Ministry of Health for declining heart performance, sensations of pressure or restrictions in the heart area, senile heart in cases where digitalis is not yet required, and mild forms of bradyarrhythmia (slow heart beat).[64]

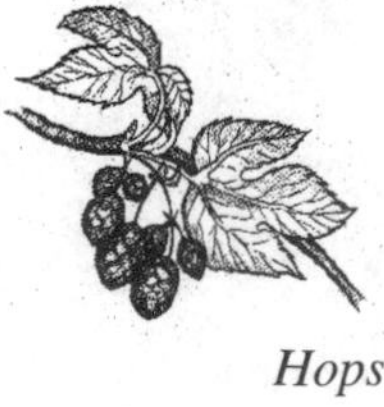

Hops

Hops *(Humulus lupulus):* Hops has been used as a bittering and preservative agent in brewing for centuries. In Germany, hops is licensed for use in states of unrest and anxiety as well as sleep disorders, due to its calming and sleep-inducing properties. European medicinal plant researchers have approved the use of hops for such conditions as nervous tension, excitability, restlessness, and sleep disturbances, and as an aid to stimulate appetite. Unlike other types of sedatives, there are neither dependence nor withdrawal symptoms reported with the use of hops, nor are there any reports of adverse side effects.[65]

Licorice *(Glycyrrhiza glabra):* Licorice is a traditional herbal remedy with an ancient history. Modern research has shown it to have effects upon the endocrine system and liver and other organs. Constituents of this herb, called triterpenes, are metabolized in the body into molecules that have a similar structure to the adrenal cortex hormones, which is possibly the basis for licorice's anti-inflammatory action.[66] Glycyrrhizin, a triterpene, inhibits liver cell injury caused by many chemicals and is used in the treatment of chronic hepatitis and cirrhosis, especially in Japan.[67] Glycyrrhizin inhibits the growth of several DNA (deoxyribonucleic acid) and RNA (ribonucleic acid) viruses, inactivating herpes simplex virus particles irreversibly.[68] Licorice is used as a treatment for peptic ulceration and gastritis, and can be used in the relief of abdominal colic. It is also used for bronchial problems such as bronchitis and coughs. There is a small possibility of affecting electrolyte balance with extended use of large doses of licorice. It can cause retention of sodium, thus raising blood pressure. The whole herb has constituents that counter this but it is best to avoid licorice in cases of hypertension or kidney disease, or during pregnancy.

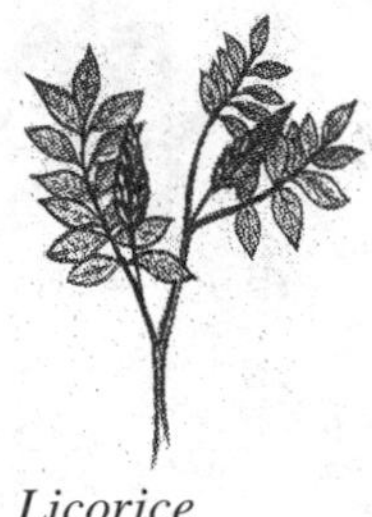
Licorice

Milk Thistle *(Silybum marianum):* Historically this herb has been used in Europe as a liver tonic and current phytotherapy indicates its use in a whole range of liver and gall bladder conditions, including hepatitis and cirrhosis. A wealth of laboratory and clinical research on this herb is revealing exciting data about reversal of toxic liver damage as well as protection from potential hepatotoxic agents.[69] These clinical findings highlight a role for milk thistle in the treatment of toxic/metabolic liver disease (including both alcohol- and drug-induced forms), some forms of hepatitis, cirrhosis of the liver, and fatty degeneration of the liver.[70] The best results are found in toxic metabolic hepatitis and cirrhosis. Milk thistle shortens the course of viral hepatitis, minimizes post-hepatitis complications, and protects the liver against problems resulting from liver surgery. It is an excellent remedy for use in the prevention and treatment of many liver disorders. A recent article in a European journal stated that the leading milk thistle extract product "is undoubtedly the best documented pharmaceutical agent for the treatment of liver diseases."[71]

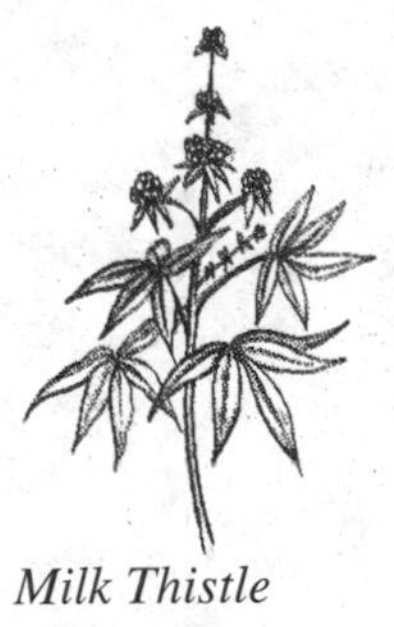
Milk Thistle

Nettle *(Urtica dioica):* Nettle is one of the most widely used herbs in the Western world. However, this common plant has received little attention from the medical community. Throughout Europe nettle is used as a spring tonic and detoxifying remedy. If used regularly over the long-term it can be remarkably successful in cases of rheumatism and arthritis.[72] Based upon its traditional uses, it might be inferred that nettle is a safe immunomodulating tonic. A lectin (plant protein) found in a nettle's leaf stimulates the proliferation of human lymphocytes.[73] Traditional use of nettle in the treatment of allergic rhinitis (hayfever) is gaining research support.[74] It is especially indicated for cases of childhood eczema and beneficial in all the varieties of this condition. Fresh nettle has been used as a safe diuretic.[75]

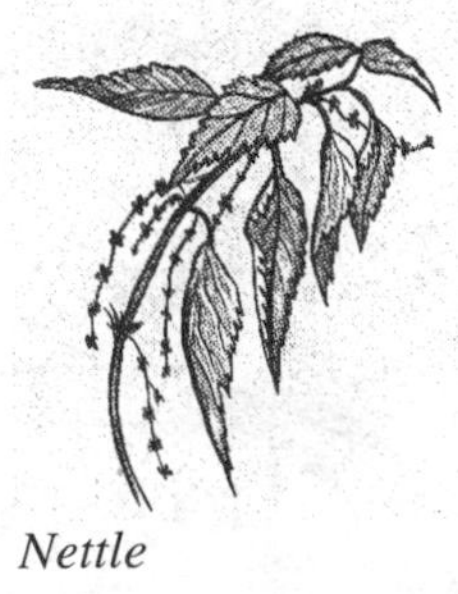
Nettle

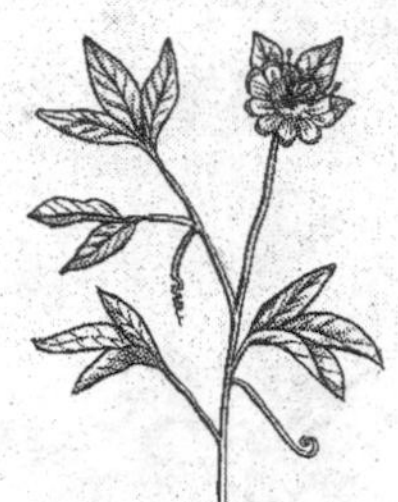
Passion flower

Passion Flower *(Passiflora incarnata):* Passion flower has enjoyed a tradition of use for its mildly sedative properties. In Germany, passion flower is approved as an over-the-counter drug for states of "nervous unrest."[76] In Europe, passion flower is often added to other calming herbs, usually valerian and hawthorn. Passion flower and hawthorn are often used together as antispasmodics for digestive spasms in cases of gastritis and colitis. Pharmacological studies indicate antispasmodic, sedative, anxiolytic (anxiety-allaying), and hypotensive activity of passion flower extracts.[77]

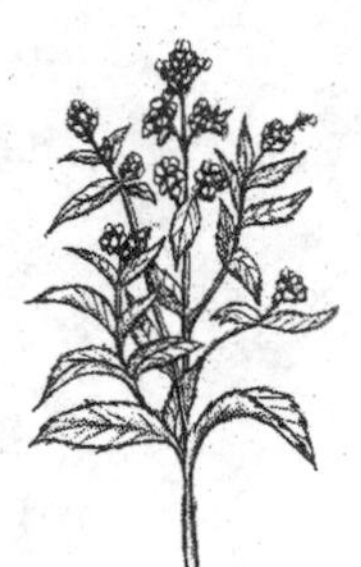
Peppermint

Peppermint *(Mentha piperita):* Peppermint has been a popular folk remedy for digestive disorders for over two hundred years and is currently one of the most economically significant aromatic food/medicine crops produced in the United States.[78]

In some countries in Europe, peppermint leaf is recognized as a digestive aid due to the carminative (gas-preventing) and cholagogue (bile increasing) action of the aromatic oil. In Germany, peppermint oil is approved as an over-the-counter drug for upper gastrointestinal cramps and spastic conditions of bile ducts, catarrh (inflammation of mucous membranes) of upper respiratory area, and inflammation of oral mucosa.[79] It is also approved (in enteric, coated capsules) for irritable bowel syndrome, as the oil exerts a relaxing effect on the smooth muscles of the bowel. Peppermint oil also has antibacterial properties, as do many essential oils. Peppermint oil and menthol are common ingredients in over-the-counter external analgesic products like balms and liniments. In Germany, this combination is approved for external use for muscle and nerve pain.[80] In addition to the above conditions, peppermint oil is approved by ESCOP (the European Scientific Cooperative in Phytotherapy) for gallbladder inflammation and gallstones, and skin conditions such as pruritis (severe itching) and urticaria (eruption of wheals with intense itching).[81]

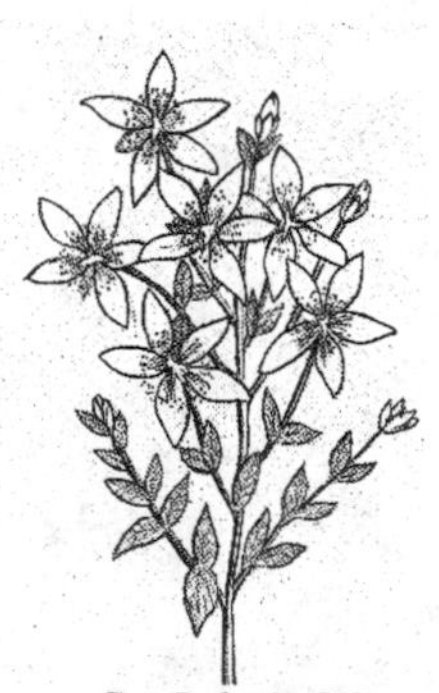
St. John's Wort

St. John's Wort *(Hypericum perforatum):* A remedy long used as an anti-inflammatory, wound-healing nervine, valued for its mild sedative and pain-reducing properties, St. John's Wort has recently regained medical attention. Taken internally, it has traditionally been used to treat neuralgia, anxiety, tension, and similar problems. In addition to neuralgic pain, it will ease fibrositis, sciatica, and rheumatic pain.[82] It is especially regarded as an herb to use in the case of menopausal changes triggering irritability and anxiety. It is increasingly recommended in the treatment of depression.[83] Recent research has suggested a role for this herb in the treatment of virus infections, from influenza to HIV,[84] and thus it is currently the focus of intense investigation. Used externally, it is a valuable healing and anti-inflammatory remedy.[85] As a lotion it will speed the healing of wounds and bruises, varicose veins, and mild burns. The oil is especially useful for healing sunburn.[86]

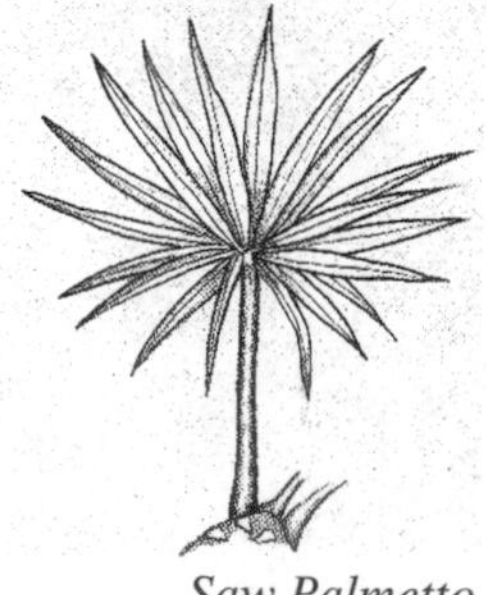
Saw Palmetto

Saw Palmetto *(Serenoa repens):* Saw palmetto is an herb that acts to tone and strengthen the male reproductive system. It may be used with safety where a boost to the male sex hormones is required. It is most effective in cases of benign prostatic hypertrophy (enlargement of the prostate gland).[87] The treatment of this condition with plant-based medicines is attracting the attention of the medical community.[88] It can help in cases of prostatitis (inflamed prostate gland) if combined with echinacea and bearberry.

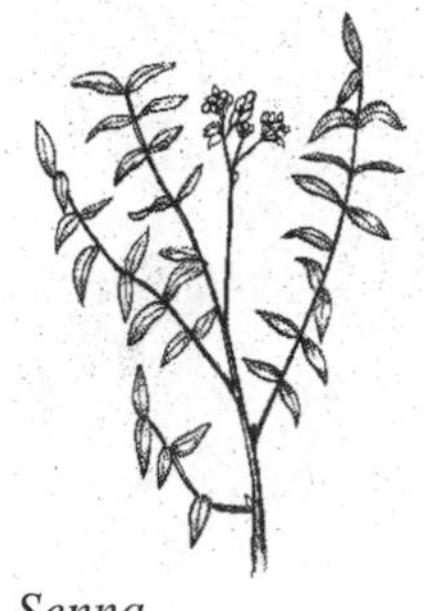
Senna

Senna *(Cassia angustifolia):* Senna is a laxative from the leaves and pods of the senna plant, a member of the pea family that is derived from ancient Arabic medicine. In Europe and in the United States, extracts from senna are approved in over-the-counter stimulant laxative products. The German government has approved senna for all conditions in which constipation and the need for soft stools is indicated. There are no known adverse side effects connected with the use of senna, other than those normally associated with the use of stimulant laxatives, in which case, long-term use or misuse can result in dependency and electrolyte loss.[89] Like other stimulant laxatives, senna should not be used during pregnancy or lactation unless professionally supervised.[90]

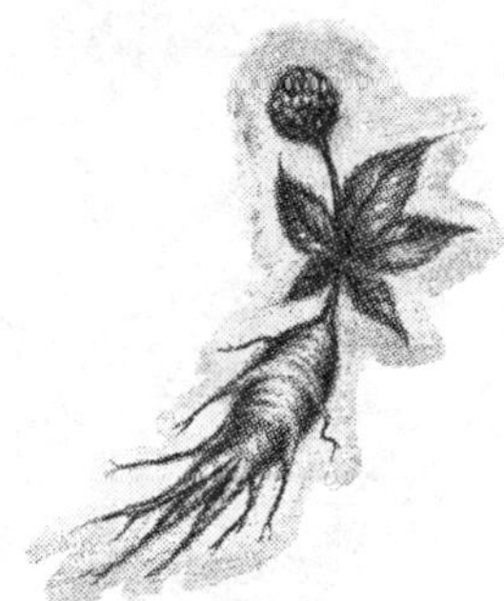
Siberian Ginseng

Siberian Ginseng or Eleuthero *(Eleutherococcus senticosus):* Siberian ginseng is one of the best adaptogen herbs, increasing the body's ability to resist and endure stress. This herb has a very low toxicity. A wealth of clinical and laboratory research has been conducted on Siberian ginseng in the former Soviet Union. Initial findings from controlled experiments indicate a dramatic reduction of total disease occurrence, especially in diseases related to environmental stress.[91] There is a long list of illnesses that improve with the use of this herb, including chronic gastritis, diabetes, and atherosclerosis (hardening of the arteries). Results from surgical studies show that Siberian ginseng speeds postoperative recovery and is being used in this way in the treatment of cancer patients, easing the stress response that can aggravate metastasis (the spreading of a tumor from its site of origin to distant sites).[92] Siberian ginseng reduces the cytotoxicity (cell-attacking nature) of antineoplastic (cancer-fighting) drugs, and the narcotic effects of sedatives.[93]

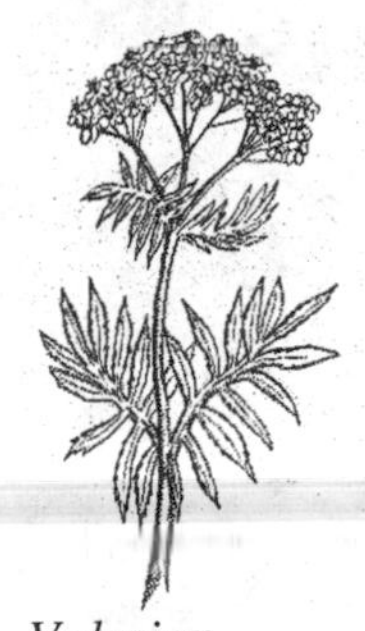
Valerian

Valerian *(Valeriana officinalis):* The odorous root of valerian has been used in European traditional medicine as a stimulant for centuries. In Germany, valerian root and its teas and extracts are approved as over-the-counter medicines for "states of excitation" and "difficulty in falling asleep owing to nervousness."[94] A scientific team representing the European community has reviewed the scientific research on valerian and concluded that it is a safe nighttime sleep aid. These scientists also found that there are no major adverse reactions associated with the use of valerian and, unlike barbiturates and other conventional drugs used for insomnia, valerian does not have a synergy with alcohol.[95] Christopher Hobbs, founder of the American School of Herbalism, notes that other uses include nervous heart conditions, children's anorexia caused by excitement, trembling, and stomach complaints. He recommends a valerian-hops preparation as a good daytime sedative as it will not interfere with or slow one's reflexive responses.[96]

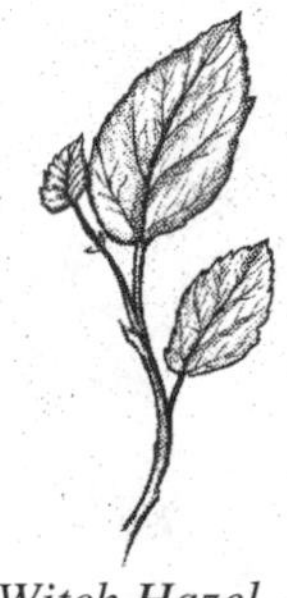
Witch Hazel

Witch Hazel *(Hamamelis virginiana):* Witch hazel is found in most households in the form of a distilled liquid. As such, it is a safe astringent for common usage. As with all astringents, this herb may be used wherever there has been bleeding, both internally or externally. It is especially useful in the easing of hemorrhoids.[97] Topically it has a well-deserved reputation in the treatment of bruises and inflamed swellings, and also with varicose veins.[98] Witch hazel will stop diarrhea and aid in the treatment of dysentery.

The Future of Herbal Medicine

According to James Duke, Ph.D., a scientist and USDA (United States Department of Agriculture) specialist in the area of herbal medicine, one of the reasons that research into the field of herbal medicine has been lacking is the enormous financial cost of the testing required to prove a new "drug" safe. Dr. Duke has seen that price tag rise from 91 million dollars over ten years ago to the present figure of 231 million dollars. Dr. Duke asks, "What commercial drug dealer is going to want to prove that saw palmetto is better than his multimillion dollar drug, when you and I can go to Florida and harvest our own saw palmetto?"

Yet the future looks bright for those who want to explore the benefits of herbal medicine. The demand for an alternative to synthetic and pharmaceutical drugs is growing, and herbal medicine is working to meet it. "I feel very optimistic about the future of herbal medicine," says David Hoffmann, past President of the American Herbalist Guild. "It has an abundance of gifts to offer both individuals in search of health and a society in search of compassionate and affordable health care. With the growing recognition of the value of herbs, it is surely time to examine the professional therapeutic use of these herbs. There are profound changes happening in the American culture and herbal medicine, 'green medicine,' is playing an ever-increasing role in people's experience of this transformation."

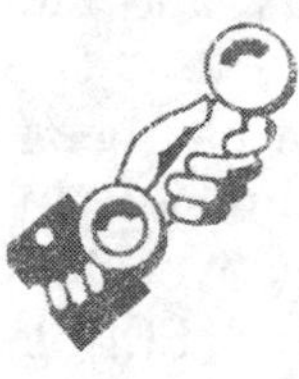

Where to Find Help

As part of a resurgence in environmental awareness, herbs and herbal remedies are receiving increased attention as a natural, cost-effective alternative to pharmaceutical products. For more information on herbalism, or to find a physician who uses herbal remedies, contact:

American Association of Acupuncture and Oriental Medicine
4101 Lake Boone Trail, Suite 201
Raleigh, North Carolina 27607
(919) 787-5181

The AAAOM is a national professional trade organization of acupuncturists who meet acceptable standards of competency. They also can provide you with the names and locations of local members.

American Association of Naturopathic Physicians
2366 Eastlake Avenue, Suite 322
Seattle, Washington 98102
(206) 323-7610

Provides referrals to a nationwide network of accredited or licensed practitioners. Publishes a quarterly newsletter for both professionals and the general public. Also offers a series of brochures and pamphlets on a variety of subjects.

American Botanical Council
P.O. Box 201660
Austin, Texas 78720
(512) 331-8868

Nonprofit research and education organization. Publishes HerbalGram *magazine, booklets on herbs, and reprints of scientific articles.*

The American Herbalists Guild
P.O. Box 1683
Sequel, California 95073

The Guild, with members ranging from clinical practitioners to ethnobotinists has become an important influence in the reemergence of medical herbalism in the United States. A directory of schools and teachers is available.

Herb Research Foundation
1007 Pearl Street, Suite 200
Boulder, Colorado 80302
(303) 449-2265

Co-publishes HerbalGram *with ABC. Provides research materials for consumers, pharmacists, physicians, scientists, and industry.*

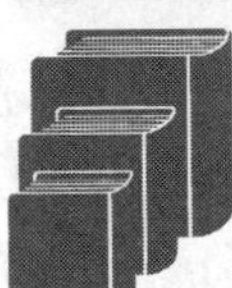

Recommended Reading

The American Herb Association Newsletter. P.O. Box 353, Rescue, California 96672

This publication, one of the oldest in the field, covers a wide range of herbal topics: media coverage, internal developments, research, regulatory issues, quality control, and more.

Foster's Botanical & Herb Reviews. B & H Reviews, P.O. Box 106, Eureka Springs, Arkansas 72632
(501) 253-7442 (Fax)

An excellent quarterly publication by noted botanist/author Steven Foster. Reviews recent books, publications, articles, videos. Botanical subjects, including herbs and herbal medicine.

The Healing Herbs. Castleman, Michael. Emmaus, PA: Rodale Press, 1991.

An A to Z guide on herbs and their medicinal qualities along with a history and description of each herb. Castleman includes a paragraph or two on the safety factor and dosage as well as on how to grow the herbs.

HerbalGram. American Botanical Council, P.O. Box 201660, Austin, Texas 78720
(512) 331-8868
(800) 373-7105 (Phone orders)
(512) 331-1924 (Fax)

The quarterly magazine of the American Botanical Council and the Herb Research Foundation. Loaded with information on the medical and scientific updates on herbs; feature articles; reviews on medicinal plants; reviews of media coverage; updates on legal and regulatory matters, conferences, book reviews, networking, and more.

The Herbs of Life. Tierra, Lesley. Freedom, CA: Crossing Press, 1992.

A concise, well-organized book of both Western and Chinese herbs and their uses.

Medical Herbalism. Bergner Communications, P.O. Box 33080, Portland, Oregon 97233
(503) 242-9815

Written primarily for practitioners, this newsletter deals with the appropriate use of herbs in a clinical setting, case histories, dosages, contraindications, and toxicity issues of both Western and Asian herbs. Published six times a year.

The New Holistic Herbal. Hoffmann, David. Rockport, MA: Element Books, 1992.

A revised and updated version of the best-selling comprehensive guide to the use of herbs in healing. The New Holistic Herbal *is an indispensable reference work for all those who want to find out more about the healing properties of plants.*

Weiner's Herbal. Weiner, Michael, Ph.D. Mill Valley, CA: Quantum Books, 1990.

An A to Z compendium of herbs with illustrations, therapeutic index, and excellent descriptions and recommendations.

Homeopathy

Homeopathy is a low-cost, nontoxic system of medicine used by hundreds of millions of people worldwide. It is particularly effective in treating chronic illnesses that fail to respond to conventional treatment, and is also a superb method of self-care for minor conditions such as the common cold and flu.

The word homeopathy derives from the Greek word *homoios*, meaning "similar," and *pathos*, meaning "suffering." Homeopathic remedies are generally dilutions of natural substances from plants, minerals, and animals. Based on the principle of "like cures like," these remedies specifically match different symptom patterns or "profiles" of illness, and act to stimulate the body's natural healing response.

Throughout its 180-year history, homeopathy has proven effective in treating diseases for which conventional medicine has little to offer. However, due to its low cost, which threatens pharmaceutical profits, as well as its divergence from conventional medical theory, homeopathy has been continually attacked by the medical establishment.

"The World Health Organization has cited homeopathy as one of the systems of traditional medicine that should be integrated worldwide with conventional medicine in order to provide adequate global health care by the year 2000."

Nonetheless, homeopathy is practiced around the world, with an estimated 500 million people receiving homeopathic treatment. The World Health Organization has cited homeopathy as one of the systems of traditional medicine that should be integrated worldwide with conventional medicine in order to provide adequate global health care by the year 2000.[1]

In the United States, an estimated three thousand medical doctors and licensed health care providers practice homeopathy, and the number continues to rise annually. The FDA (Food and Drug Administration) recognizes homeopathic remedies as official drugs and regulates their manufacturing, labeling, and dispensing. Homeopathic remedies also have their own official compendium, the *Homeopathic Pharmacopoeia of the United States* first published in 1897.

In Europe, the birthplace of homeopathy, there are approximately six thousand practitioners in Germany and five thousand in France. All French pharmacies are required to carry homeopathic remedies along with conventional drugs. In fact, the homeopathic remedy Oscillococcinum™ is the largest selling cold and flu remedy in France. In Britain, homeopathic hospitals and out-patient clinics are part of the national health system, and homeopathy is recognized as a postgraduate medical specialty by virtue of an act of Parliament. Homeopathy has also enjoyed the patronage of the British royal family for the past four generations.[2] It is also widely practiced in India (where over twenty-five thousand doctors practice homeopathy), Mexico, Argentina, and Brazil.

How Homeopathy Works

Homeopathy was founded in the late eighteenth century by the celebrated German physician Samuel Hahnemann, known for his work in pharmacology, hygiene, public health, industrial toxicology, and psychiatry. Reacting to the barbarous practices of his day, such as bloodletting (the use of leeches), and toxic mercury-based laxatives, Dr. Hahnemann set out to find a more rational and humane approach to medicine.

“In Britain, homeopathic hospitals and out-patient clinics are part of the national health system, and homeopathy is recognized as a postgraduate medical specialty by virtue of an act of Parliament. Homeopathy has also enjoyed the patronage of the British royal family for the past four generations.”

Dr. Hahnemann's breakthrough came during an experiment in which he twice daily ingested cinchona, a Peruvian bark well known as a cure for malaria. Soon after Dr. Hahnemann began his experiment he developed periodic fevers common to malaria. As soon as he stopped taking the cinchona, his symptoms disappeared. Dr. Hahnemann theorized that, if taking a large dose of cinchona created symptoms of malaria in a healthy person, this same substance, taken in a smaller dose by a person suffering from malaria, might stimulate the body to fight the disease. His theory was borne out by years of experiments with hundreds of substances that produced similar results. Based on his work, Dr. Hahnemann formulated the principles of homeopathy:

- Like cures like (Law of Similars).
- The more a remedy is diluted, the greater its potency (Law of the Infinitesimal Dose).
- An illness is specific to the individual (a holistic medical model).

Like Cures Like

According to Dr. Hahnemann, “Each individual case of disease is most surely, radically, rapidly, and permanently annihilated and removed only by a medicine capable of producing (in the human system) the most similar and complete manner of the totality of the symptoms.”[3] In other words, the same substance that in large doses produces the symptoms of an illness, in very minute doses cures it.

Dr. Hahnemann referred to this phenomenon as the Law of Similars, a principle first recognized in the fourth century B.C., by Hippocrates, who was studying the effects of herbs upon disease. This Law of Similars was also the theoretical basis for the vaccines of physicians Edward Jenner, Jonas Salk, and Louis Pasteur. They would “immunize” the body with trace amounts of a disease component, often a virus, to strengthen its immune response to the actual disease. Allergies are treated in a similar fashion by introducing minute quantities of the suspected allergen into the body to bolster natural tolerance levels.

The More Dilute the Remedy, the Greater Its Potency

Most people believe that the higher the dose of a medicine, the greater the effect. But the opposite holds true in homeopathy where the more a substance is diluted, the higher its potency. Dr. Hahnemann discovered this Law of the Infinitesimal Dose by experimenting with higher and higher dilutions of substances to avoid toxic side effects.

Today, homeopathic remedies are usually prepared through a process of diluting with pure water or alcohol and succussing (vigorous shaking). Homeopathic solutions can be diluted to such an extent that literally no molecules of the original substance remain in the remedy. Yet, the more dilute it gets the more potent it becomes. This phenomenon has been the source of great fascination among practitioners and researchers in the field of homeopathic medicine, as from the point of view of conventional chemistry, diluted homeopathic remedies may contain no trace of the original substance. In fact, any homeopathic remedy over 24X potency (twenty-four successive dilutions and succussions) will have no chemical trace of the original substance remaining.

A "special" report on homeopathy that aired in the United States on NBC's "DateLine" in December, 1992, which offered a one-sided argument against homeopathy, contended that a homeopathic remedy received from a prominent homeopathic physician was chemically tested in a laboratory and the results showed that it was "only" water and alcohol. According to homeopathic experts, however, this is exactly the case. After successive dilutions, no molecules of the original substance remain in the remedy.

According to Trevor Cook, Ph.D., DI Hom., President of the United Kingdom Homeopathic Medical Association, the explanation of the therapeutic action of the highly dilute homeopathic remedies appears to lie in the domain of quantum physics and the emerging field of energy medicine. A study using nuclear magnetic resonance (NMR) imaging demonstrated distinctive readings of subatomic activity in twenty-three different homeopathic remedies. This potency was not demonstrated in placebos (substances having no pharmacological effect).[4]

See Energy Medicine.

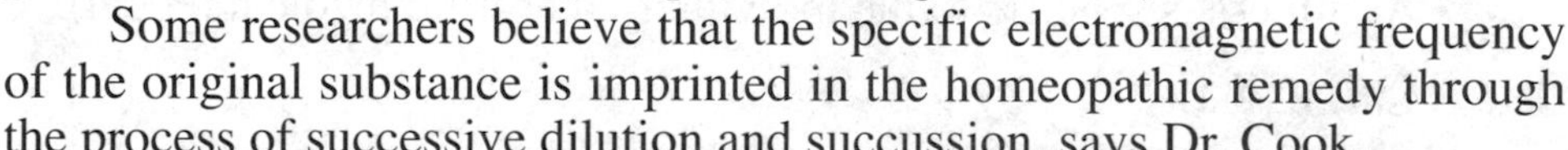

Some researchers believe that the specific electromagnetic frequency of the original substance is imprinted in the homeopathic remedy through the process of successive dilution and succussion, says Dr. Cook.

The distinguished Italian physicist Emilio del Giudici has set forth a theory that helps explain homeopathy's mode of therapeutic action. Del Giudici proposes that water molecules form structures capable of storing minute electromagnetic signals.[5] This proposition is given added weight by the findings of Dr. Wolfgang Ludwig, a German biophysicist, who has demonstrated in preliminary research that homeopathic substances give off measurable electromagnetic signals. These signals show that specific frequencies are dominant in each homeopathic substance.[6]

If del Giudici's model is accurate, a homeopathic remedy may convey an electromagnetic "message" to the body that matches the specific electromagnetic frequency or pattern of an illness in order to stimulate the body's natural healing response. What Dr. Hahnemann may have been doing in his empirical research was unwittingly "matching the frequencies of the plant extract with the frequency of the [patient's] illness."[7]

Illness Is Specific to the Individual

A session with a homeopathic practitioner is a unique experience for someone accustomed to conventional medicine. For instance, you may suffer from chronic headaches, perhaps migraines. While the conventional medical treatment for this condition is the same for most everyone (some form of analgesics or anti-inflammatories), homeopathy recognizes over two hundred symptom patterns associated with headaches, and has corresponding remedies for each.

Your headache may be in the front of your head. It may get worse with a cold sensation and improve with heat. It may be better while you are laying down, or while you are sitting up. You may be a person who is thin, and easily excited, or the docile, sedentary sort. The first task of the homeopathic practitioner is a process called "profiling," or recording all of the qualities—physical, mental, and emotional—that will determine the patient's remedy or combination of remedies.

Practitioners of classical homeopathy consult vast compendiums called repertories and *materia medicas* to determine the remedy that most closely matches the total picture of the patient's symptomology. These compendiums are compilations of the findings of thousands of tests, for over two hundred years, that record how healthy individuals react to different substances. The very detailed reactions of the subjects are catalogued in these compendiums and the homeopathic practitioner's task is to match them exactly to the patient's profile.

The Healing Crisis and Hering's Laws of Cure

In homeopathy, the process of healing begins by eliminating the immediate symptoms, then progressing to the "older," underlying symptoms. Many of these "layers" are residues of fevers, trauma, or chronic disease that were unsuccessfully treated or suppressed by conventional medicine. As the stages of homeopathic healing progress, the patient may get worse before getting better. This is often referred to as the "healing crisis."

In the mid-nineteenth century, Dr. Constantine Hering, the father of American homeopathy, stated that healing progresses from the deepest part of the body to the extremities; from the emotional and mental aspects to the physical; and from the upper part of the body (head, neck, ears, throat) to the lower parts of the body (fingers, abdomen, legs, feet). Hering's Laws of Cure also state that healing progresses in reverse chronological order, from the most recent maladies to the oldest. By Hering's laws, homeopaths are able to track the progress of their treatment and restore a patient's health, layer by layer.

> *"The long-term benefit of homeopathy to the patient is that it not only alleviates the presenting symptoms but it reestablishes internal order at the deepest levels and thereby provides a lasting cure."*
>
> —George Vithoulkas, Director, Athenian School of Homeopathic Medicine

An excellent example of homeopathic treatment is the case of a woman who suffered from lupus, a disease where the body's immune system attacks its own tissue. After years of unsuccessful conventional treatment, she was told that she could only expect a life of continued pain and drug dependency. In desperation, she turned to a homeopathic physician.

First she was treated for drug dependency and the condition it was to relieve, pericarditis, an intensely painful inflammation of the outer lining of the heart. She was prescribed the remedy *Cactus grandiflorus*, a substance that, in healthy people, produces heart palpitations and depression. The homeopathic dose of *Cactus grandiflorus* reduced the inflammation, and a new set of symptoms emerged—anger, bitterness, and stress—powerful emotions she'd experienced prior to the emergence of her pericarditis.

"The highest ideal of cure is the speedy, gentle, and enduring restoration of health by the most trustworthy and least harmful way."
—Samuel Hahnemann, founder of Homeopathy

Nux vomica (poison nut) was then administered. A substance that produces hyperirritability and nervous cramping in healthy individuals helped her to overcome her emotional problems and progress to the next layer of healing. A recurrence of an old back pain and her phobia of cars emerged, the result of a serious accident and injury. As these conditions were treated, the woman was able to return fully to her life, healthy and free of pain.[8]

Conditions Benefited by Homeopathy

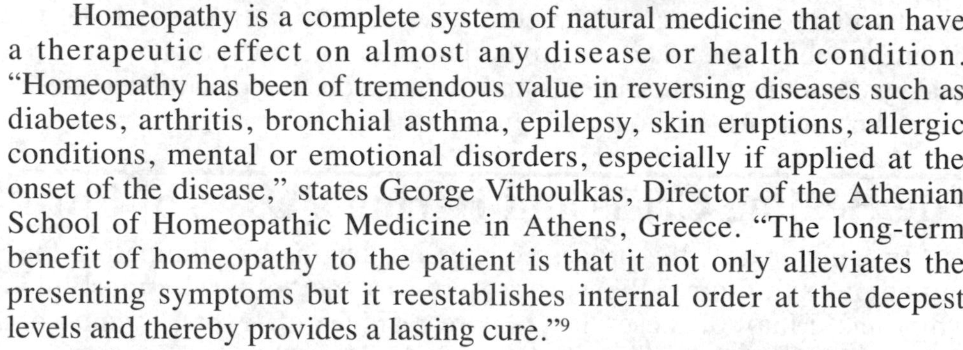

Homeopathy is a complete system of natural medicine that can have a therapeutic effect on almost any disease or health condition. "Homeopathy has been of tremendous value in reversing diseases such as diabetes, arthritis, bronchial asthma, epilepsy, skin eruptions, allergic conditions, mental or emotional disorders, especially if applied at the onset of the disease," states George Vithoulkas, Director of the Athenian School of Homeopathic Medicine in Athens, Greece. "The long-term benefit of homeopathy to the patient is that it not only alleviates the presenting symptoms but it reestablishes internal order at the deepest levels and thereby provides a lasting cure."[9]

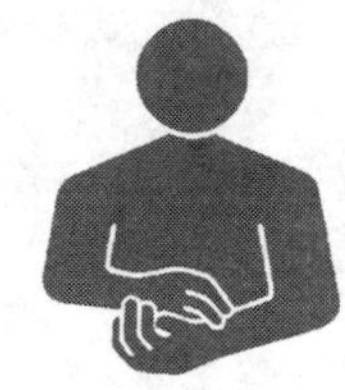

Homeopathy is well suited to self-care and can become an integral part of your and your family's health maintenance program.

Robert D. Milne, M.D., of Las Vegas, Nevada, reports excellent results in the prevention and treatment of acute cold and flu-like symptoms using homeopathic remedies. "The quick use of remedies, such as *Aconite*, *Bryonia*, and/or *Belladonna*, have been a great help in alleviating the acute symptoms of colds," says Dr. Milne. He also has had success treating conditions such as headaches and female health problems, including symptoms such as fatigue, irritability, premenstrual symptoms, neck stiffness, low back pain, and bloating with homeopathic remedies.

Official acceptance of homeopathy and its integration into the American health care system could prove to have an enormous impact on lowering the cost of national health care due to the low cost, safety, and effectiveness of homeopathic remedies.

Increasingly, clinical studies are supporting the effectiveness of homeopathic remedies. In a recent article published in the *British Medical Journal*, 107 controlled clinical studies (performed between 1966 and 1990) were reviewed. Eighty-one of these studies showed that homeopathic medicines were beneficial in treating headaches, respiratory infections, diseases of the digestive system, ankle sprains, postoperative infections and symptoms, and other health-related disorders.[10]

Studies attesting to the effectiveness of homeopathic treatment for rheumatoid arthritis have appeared in both *The Lancet* and the *British Journal of Clinical Pharmacology*.[11] In a double-blind study on the effects of homeopathic remedies on influenza, it was found that twice as many of the patients who took the homeopathic remedy were cured in forty-eight hours, as opposed to those who took a placebo, as reported in the *British Journal of Clinical Pharmacology*.[12]

Another clinical study shows the efficacy of treating hay fever with homeopathic remedies.[13] A double-blind trial indicates that homeopathic remedies are extremely effective in dealing with dental neuralgic pain following tooth extraction.[14] German research reports successful homeopathic treatment of Parkinson's disease, bronchitis, sinusitis, migraines,[15] influenza, and motion sickness with homeopathic remedies.[16]

See Part III for complete listings of homeopathic remedies for specific health conditions.

HOMEOPATHY IN THE UNITED STATES

Homeopathy has a long and distinguished history in the United States, and was popular from the mid-nineteenth to early twentieth centuries. Dr. Constantine Hering, a student of German physician Samuel Hahnemann, and father of homeopathy in the United States, established the first homeopathic medical school in the U.S. in 1835 in Allentown, Pennsylvania. By 1844, there were so many physicians claiming to be homeopathic practitioners that the homeopathic medical profession formed the American Institute of Homeopathy, the first national medical association in the United States. The American Medical Association (AMA) was formed three years later and denounced homeopathy as a delusion. AMA members were forbidden to associate with homeopathic physicians either professionally or socially, and physicians practicing homeopathy were expelled or blocked from becoming members.[17]

Still, homeopathy continued to gain attention in America due in part to its great success in treating acute and epidemic diseases, notably cholera and yellow fever. During an 1849 cholera epidemic in Cincinnati, Ohio, only 3 percent of those patients treated homeopathically died, as compared to the 40 to 70 percent death rate among those treated with conventional medicine.[18]

In the 1879 epidemic of yellow fever, homeopaths in New Orleans treated 1,945 cases with a mortality rate of 5.6 percent, while the mortality rate with standard medical treatment was 16 percent.[19] At this time some of homeopathy's more illustrious supporters included John D. Rockefeller, Thomas Edison, and Mark Twain.

By 1900, there were twenty-two homeopathic medical schools and nearly one hundred homeopathic hospitals in the United States. In fact, 15 percent of all American physicians practiced homeopathy at the turn of the century, according to Trevor Cook, Ph.D., DI Hom., President of the British Homeopathic Medical Society.[20] However, by the same time, the bond between the AMA and the pharmaceutical companies was firmly established. Paid advertisements from pharmaceutical companies in the AMA journal were the AMA's main source of revenue (as it is today), prominent physicians were paid to endorse proprietary drugs, and doctors were deluged with free samples of pharmaceutical drugs. Through a series of maneuvers including a new rating system for medical schools aimed at eliminating homeopathic colleges, the practice of homeopathy had nearly disappeared as a force in American medicine by 1930.[21]

However, homeopathy is again becoming recognized as a viable alternative medicine, and statistics now show that the American public is returning to this form of treatment in dramatic numbers, with annual sales of homeopathic medicines in the United States now reaching $150 million.[22]

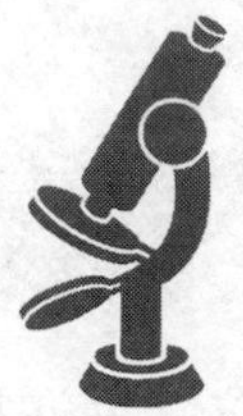

The government should provide funds for research into homeopathy due to its 180 years of clinical success. The results of recent European research also indicate that it deserves to become an integral part of America's health care system. Write your congressional representatives and demand that research be carried out in this important field of health care.

Combination Remedies

Today, many homeopathic practitioners use "combination" formulas that contain several remedies to cover a broad range of symptoms for an acute condition. For example, people with colds experience runny noses, watery eyes, sneezing, fever, and headaches. A combination cold remedy contains remedies for each of these symptoms. The appropriate remedies in a formula will have a therapeutic effect, while the unnecessary remedies will be shed off and have no effect at all. Combination homeopathic remedies have a unique effect on the body—the body assimilates what it needs, and throws off what it doesn't, making it a completely safe, nontoxic form of medicine.

The Future of Homeopathy

The official acceptance of homeopathy and its integration into the American health care system could prove to have an enormous impact on lowering the cost of national health care, due to its low cost and tremendous health benefits. Although controlled clinical studies might prove costly, homeopathy's history of clinical success and the results of studies being carried out in Europe indicate that this is an area where the United States government should provide funds for research. Because homeopathic remedies are derived from natural substances, and as such, are unpatentable, no pharmaceutical company will provide the necessary funds for research to gain FDA approval. The low cost of homeopathic remedies also guarantee that it would be impossible for a company to recoup its research investment. Clearly, homeopathy, like other forms of natural medicine including herbal medicine and nutritional supplementation, is caught in an economic catch-22. But as part of the growing tide of national awareness of alternative medicine, homeopathy should soon receive the attention it deserves from the United States government and become part of the solution to America's national health care crisis.

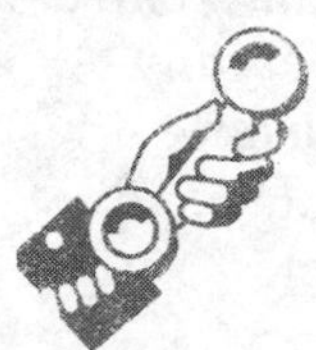

Where to Find Help

For more information on homeopathy contact:

British Institute of Homeopathy and College of Homeopathy
520 Washington Boulevard
Suite 423
Marina Del Rey, California 90292
(310) 306-5408
Offers a two-hundred-hour course in classical modern homeopathy for health care professionals and lay people and a home study course.

Homeopathic Educational Services
2124 Kittredge Street
Berkeley, California 94704
(510) 649-0294
(800) 359-9051
Offers access to homeopathic books, tapes, and software.

International Foundation for Homeopathy
2366 Eastlake Avenue, East
Suite 301
Seattle, Washington 98102
(206) 324-8230
Provides educational courses for professionals and the general public. Offers referrals to homeopathic health professionals.

National Center for Homeopathy
801 North Fairfax, Suite 306
Alexandria, Virginia 22314
(703) 548-7790
Provides a referral list of practicing homeopaths and information. Gives courses for lay people and professionals, and organizes study groups around the country.

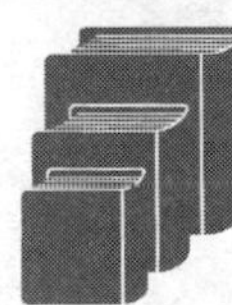

Recommended Reading

Discovering Homeopathy: Your Introduction to the Science and Art of Homeopathic Medicine. Ullman, Dana. Berkeley, CA: North Atlantic Books, 1991.
A wonderful introductory book to natural medicine. Ullman notes the conventional approach and explains why it often fails and under what circumstances homeopathic treatments succeed. Includes well-cited studies and clinical experiments.

Divided Legacy: A History of the Schism in Medical Thought, Vol. 3: Science and Ethics in American Medicine, 1800-1914. Coulter, Harris, L. Berkeley, CA: North Atlantic Books, 1973.
Coulter thoroughly explains the history of natural medicine and the battle between its supporters and the American Medical Association and pharmaceutical companies.

Everybody's Guide to Homeopathic Medicines. Cummings, Stephen, M.D., and Ullman, Dana, M.P.H. Los Angeles: Jeremy P. Tarcher, Inc., 1991.
This book details common health conditions and discusses treatments using natural alternative homeopathic methods and medicines. Offers advice on when to seek professional care.

The Family Guide to Homeopathy: Symptoms and Natural Solutions. Lockie, Andrew. New York: Prentice Hall Press, 1993.

A comprehensive book, cataloging areas of the body, ailments, pain, conditions, and homeopathic treatments. An A-Z list of nutritional supplements and special diets. Useful sources included at the end of the book as well.

Homeopathic Medicine for Children and Infants. Ullman, Dana. Los Angeles: Jeremy P. Tarcher, 1992.

A guide of natural remedies geared toward the family, babies, and children.

Homeopathic Medicine Today: A Study. Cook, Trevor. New Canaan, CT: Keats Publishing, 1989.

Cook describes the early history of homeopathy, its development nationally and internationally, its decline and recent revival. A detailed examination of remedies, principals, and techniques, prescribing methods of treatment, current research, and future trends.

Homeopathic Medicines at Home: Natural Remedies for Everyday Ailments and Minor Injuries. Panos, Maesimund B., M.D., and Heimlich, Jane. Los Angeles: Jeremy P. Tarcher, 1981.

An informative guide to cure everyday common ailments and injuries.

"Health is the proper relationship between the microcosm, which is man, and the macrocosm, which is the universe. Disease is a disruption of this relationship."

—Dr. Yeshe Donden, physician to the Dalai Lama

Hydrotherapy

Hydrotherapy is the use of water, ice, steam, and hot and cold temperatures to maintain and restore health. Treatments include full body immersion, steam baths, saunas, sitz baths, colonic irrigation, and the application of hot, and/or cold compresses. Hydrotherapy is effective for treating a wide range of conditions and can easily be used in the home as part of a self-care program.

The therapeutic use of water in all of its forms dates back to the beginning of civilization. Hydrotherapy has been used to treat disease and injury by many different cultures, including the Egyptians, Assyrians, Babylonians, Persians, Greeks, Hebrews, Hindus, Chinese, and Native Americans. Today, many alternative practitioners prescribe baths, jacuzzis, steam, saunas, mineral tubs, wraps, rubs, flushes, fasts, enemas, colonic irrigations, douches, sitz baths, and compresses to remedy a great variety of health conditions. Hot or cold water administered externally or internally can be effective in treating conditions ranging from stress and pain to the many toxins, bacteria, and viruses that can cause disease.

How Hydrotherapy Works

The external hydrotherapies fall into three categories—hot water, cold water, or contrast. "Heat relaxes while cold stimulates," says Douglas Lewis, N.D., Chairperson of Physical Medicine at the Bastyr College Natural Health Clinic in Seattle, Washington. "Hot water produces a response that stimulates the immune system and causes white cells to migrate out of the blood vessels and into the tissue where they clean up toxins and assist the body in eliminating wastes." Therapeutically, hot water soothes and relaxes the body, and through the reflex action of the nerves, it can affect nearly every organ and system of the body.

"Cold water," says Dr. Lewis, "discourages inflammation by means of vasoconstriction (constricting blood vessels), and by reducing the inflammatory agents by making the blood vessels less permeable. Cold water also tones muscular weakness and may be useful in cases of incontinence." Dr. Lewis cautions that, contrary to the popular belief, short cold water treatment may actually increase fever and only long cold water treatment pulls heat from the body for fever reduction.

Contrast therapies are those that alternate between hot and cold water in the same treatment. They can stimulate the adrenal and endocrine glands, reduce congestion, alleviate inflammation, and activate organ

See AIDS, Chronic Fatigue Syndrome, Detoxification Therapy, Hyperthermia.

function. According to Leon Chaitow, N.D., D.O., of London, England, certain contrast therapies are designed to improve circulation in the digestive areas and the pelvis and to improve the detoxifying capability of the liver.[1]

Clinical Application of Hydrotherapy

Many forms of hydrotherapy are used by naturopathic physicians, alternative practitioners, and physical therapists at clinics, hospitals, and health spas to treat a wide range of conditions. Most therapies can also be performed at home, however the following—hyperthermia, whirlpool baths, and neutral baths—are only available in a clinical setting.

Hyperthermia (fever-induction therapy) is a form of hydrotherapy that deliberately induces fever in the patient who is unable to mount a natural fever response to pathogens (disease-causing organisms and toxins). Fever is often regarded as an undesirable symptom of illness, but holistic practitioners see it as the body's defense against invading organisms. Fever stimulates the immune system by increasing the production of antibodies and interferon (a group of proteins released by white blood cells that combat a virus).[2]

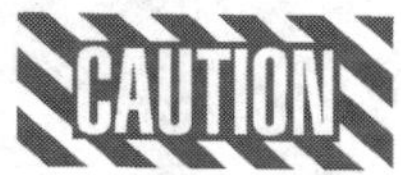

Hyperthermia can be hazardous for certain people and conditions, and should only be performed under the supervision of a qualified doctor.

Laboratory research has proven that HIV (human immunodeficiency virus) is temperature sensitive and suffers greater inactivation per unit time at progressively higher temperatures above the normal body temperature of 37 degrees centigrade (98.6 degrees Fahrenheit).[3] Dr. Lewis believes that a hot immersion bath, if done without raising body temperature and heart rate too quickly, can be used as an adjunctive treatment for "a diverse number of diseases; from upper respiratory infections to sexually transmitted diseases, from cancer to AIDS."

In the treatment of chronic fatigue syndrome, Bruce Milliman, N.D., an Associate Professor at Bastyr College in Seattle, Washington, reports a 70 percent success rate using hyperthermia.

Hyperthermia can also be used to remove fat-stored chemicals such as pesticides, PCB's, and drug residue from the body. Zane Gard, M.D., of Beaverton, Oregon, has developed a successful heat stress detoxification program for this purpose. Dr. Gard's BioToxic Reduction Program™ (BTR) is a medically-managed detoxification program designed to reduce the body's internal "toxic load" of chemicals, heavy metals, medical or street drugs, and alcohol.

Whirlpool Baths can rehabilitate injured muscles and joints, and alleviate the stresses and strains of everyday life. Whirlpools are also effective in healing skin sores, infected wounds, edema (swelling), and minor frostbite pain. Physical therapists use it to soothe burn patients and improve the circulation of paraplegic and polio victims.

Neutral Baths are a full immersion therapy that submerges the body up to the neck in water from 92 to 98 degrees Fahrenheit. The soothing nature of the neutral bath calms the nervous system and is

NATURAL HEALING WATERS

There are many natural healing waters that spring from the earth. The balance of minerals in seawater is similar to that of human blood. The water from natural springs carries concentrated levels of sodium, calcium, magnesium, bicarbonate, and sulphur. Bicarbonate spring water can aid cuts, burns, hardening of the skin, digestive problems, and allergies. Sulphur has been known to help arthritis, rheumatism, chronic poisoning, diabetes, skin disease, and urinary disease.

effective for treating emotional and mental disturbances, and insomnia. According to Dr. Chaitow, clinical studies reveal that two hours in a neutral bath is effective in reducing excessive fluid retention in patients suffering from mild heart conditions and cirrhosis of the liver.[4] It is also beneficial to the swollen joints of rheumatoid patients. Neutral baths help promote detoxification from alcohol and drug abuse as the neutral bath helps the body rid itself of large amounts of toxin-laden fluids.

CAUTION

Those who suffer from eczema and other skin conditions, or acute heart disease, should avoid neutral bathing.

Hydrotherapy at Home

Many of the hydrotherapy techniques used in spas and therapy centers around the world can be performed in the comfort and privacy of your own home. The following section describes these methods. Experiment to find which ones work best for you. Dr. Chaitow suggests that you vary the treatments from day to day, or week to week, to increase "the efficiency of your body's response."

The following methods are recommended for people who are in good health. If you have any health-related problems or illnesses, consult your doctor before beginning a hydrotherapy program.

Ice and Contrast are effective therapies for trauma relief. Any injury, like sprains and strains, or acute inflammation, like tendinitis, calls for an immediate application of cold. Apply ice as often as twenty minutes every hour for the first twenty-four to thirty-six hours post-trauma.

Trauma or chronic conditions also respond well to contrast therapy. Alternating hot and cold increases circulation to bring vital nutrients to the area and move waste products out. Simply apply alternating hot and cold packs to the effected area beginning with hot for three minutes, then cold for thirty to sixty seconds. Repeat three times in one sitting, always finishing with cold, one to three times per day, depending upon the severity of the condition.

Baths and Showers are soothing, both mentally and physically. Not only do they relieve general aches and pains, they can also ease internal congestion and digestive ills.

Again, water temperature varies according to your needs. Hot baths and showers are relaxing and stimulating to the immune system. By inducing perspiration, they facilitate the detoxification process. Cold baths and showers can tonify muscles, reduce inflammation, and act as a bracer against fatigue. Long cold baths are useful for reducing fevers but are not recommended for home use and should only be used under the direction of your physician.

Cold showers also can increase the nerve force, stimulate the glandular system, and have a positive effect on the central nervous system.[5] Alternating hot and cold showers can be an excellent way to increase circulation and stimulate organ function. Remember, though, always start with hot and end with cold.

SALT RUBS

A salt rub, or "salt glow," is excellent for stimulating circulation. Take a small handful of slightly damp sea salts or Epsom salts and vigorously massage them into your already wet skin until it turns slightly pink. One to two pounds of salt is needed for the whole body. Follow the "salt glow," with a warm—not hot—shower or bath. Again, vigorously rub your skin while rinsing and drying. The salt glow may make you perspire and help you sleep more soundly. Do it at least once a month, or weekly as part of your detoxification program. It is not for people with skin rashes or lesions.

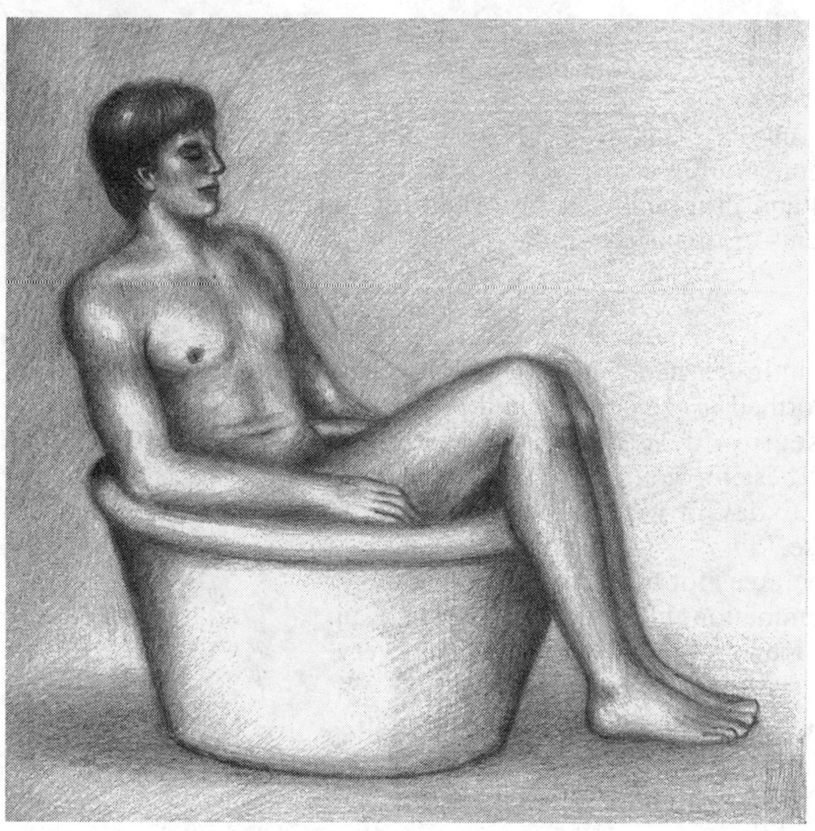

A sitz bath.

Sitz Baths are a traditional European folk remedy in which the pelvis is immersed in hot or cold water. A hot sitz bath is particularly helpful for problems involving the pelvic region, including uterine cramps, painful ovaries or testicles, and hemorrhoids. A cold sitz bath, taken for two minutes or less, can be used for inflammation, constipation, vaginal discharge, and impotence, but should not be used for urinary tract infections. (For instructions on how to prepare sitz baths, see "Hydrotherapy Procedures.")

Foot and Hand Baths are excellent for drawing blood away from inflamed parts of the body, or drawing congestion away from an organ. They can help relieve insomnia, sore throats, colds, menstrual cramps, feet and leg cramps, and pain from gout, neuralgia, and headaches.

According to Agatha Thrash, M.D., and Calvin Thrash, M.D., of Seale, Alabama, a hot foot bath is the ideal remedy for shivering, cold hands or feet, nausea, dizziness, or faintness.[6] To relieve a sore throat or avert a cold, add a tablespoon of mustard powder per quart of hot water to a foot bath container.

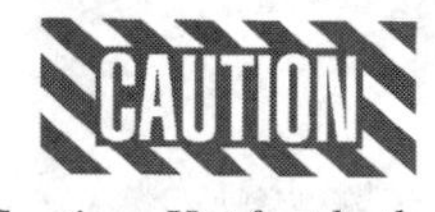

Caution: Hot foot baths are not good for those with arteriosclerosis, Buerger's disease, or diabetes mellitus.

Alternating hot and cold foot baths has a profound effect on the nerve and reflex points of the feet. These baths also help relieve toothaches, neuralgia, headaches (when used in conjunction with a cold compress on the head), ankle swelling, foot infections, blood poisoning, and abdominal congestion.

Fill two tubs—one with hot water, the other with cold water. Place your feet and ankles in the hot water for three minutes, then plunge your feet into the cold water for twenty to thirty seconds. Repeat three times, ending with cold water, then thoroughly dry your feet. You may do this several times per day, as needed.

Hands also contain many reflex points that affect the entire body. A cold hand bath can stop a nosebleed and relieve sunstroke. A hot hand bath can relieve cramps in the hands from overuse in athletics, writing, or sewing, and even alleviate asthma attacks.

Cold Water Treading is one of the "most important preventive water treatments," says Dian Dincin Buchman, Ph.D.[7] After a shower or bath, immerse your feet in cold water and march in place for five seconds to five minutes. (For safety, you may need the support of a wall or handle.) Afterward, rub your feet vigorously with a towel, especially the soles. Dr. Buchman believes that by building tolerance to cold it is possible to develop resistance to infectious disease, and she recommends this practice be a part of the daily self-care routine for everyone, young and old.

HEALING BATHS: HERBS, ESSENTIAL OILS, AND HOME REMEDIES

A number of herbs, oils, and minerals may be added to a bath to enhance its therapeutic effects. Here are a few of the more common herbs used in hydrotherapy, available at most natural food stores:

Chamomile: Soothes skin, opens pores, eliminates blackheads, aids digestive problems, and promotes sleep.

Ginger: Relaxes sore muscles, improves circulation, and tones the skin.

Oat straw: Relieves sore feet, ingrown toenails, and blisters.

Sage: Stimulates the sweat glands.

A few drops of various essential oils may also be added to the bath or rubbed directly onto the skin after a shower. According to Dr. Chaitow, they influence blood pressure, stimulate nerve function, and aid digestive functioning. These are a few of the dozens of essential oils available at health stores and body shops:

Cedarwood: Promotes elimination through mucous membranes and acts as an antiseptic and sedative.

Lemon: Increases urine flow and acts as an antiseptic.

Rose: Stimulates liver and stomach functions, and acts as an antidepressant.

Tea tree: Enhances skin function, and can be used as an antifungal and antibiotic.[8]

Also, try adding the following common household ingredients to your bath:

Apple cider vinegar: Detoxifies, combats fatigue, relieves poison ivy, and restores the skin's natural acid covering. Add one cup to your bath.

Baking soda: Relieves skin irritation and itching, and acts as a mild antiseptic. Add up to one pound to your bath.

Epsom salts: Induces perspiration, aborts illness, relaxes muscles, relieves swollen and irritated joints. Dissolve one half to one pound in hot bath.

Cornstarch: Helps reduce itchiness from poison ivy, poison oak, and eczema. Add one cup to one pound of cornstarch to the bath (can be added in conjunction with other substances such as oatmeal). Cornstarch can also be an effective cooling agent.

Oatmeal: Coats, soothes, and restores the skin, and is especially good for itchiness, hives, sunburn, and chafing. Put one cup of uncooked oatmeal in a blender, finely blend it, and add it to a warm or mild bath. (This is also good for soothing diaper rashes.)

Steam is an excellent cleanser and deep moisture treatment for the skin. It also helps break up congestion from the common cold and flus. To create a simple home vaporizer boil water in a clean kettle or pot. Add a few drops of eucalyptus or wintergreen oil, or one to two tablespoons of mint leaves to the water. Lean over the steaming pot, holding a towel or sheet over your head like a tent. Be careful not to get too close to the boiling water. Breathe slowly and deeply, inhaling the vapors to warm and soothe the respiratory tract.

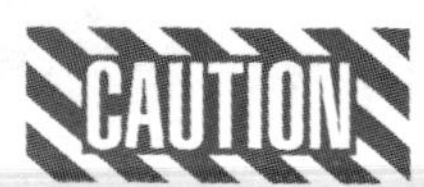

Caution: Cold treading should not be used if you have rheumatism of the toes or ankles, sciatica, pelvic inflammation, or problems with the bladder or digestive tract.

Compresses and Packs are particularly effective for applying heat or cold to specific parts of the body. According to Tori Hudson, N.D., Clinical Director of the National College of Naturopathic Medicine, in Portland, Oregon, they stimulate the immune system and increase the body's white blood cell count.

One can treat sciatica, for example, by applying hot compresses to the lower back and legs for thirty minutes or longer. For gallstones, intestinal colic, or painful menstrual periods, hot, moist compresses can be applied every half hour around the torso, between the shoulders and the navel. (For instructions on how to prepare compresses and packs, see "Hydrotherapy Procedures.")

Hydrotherapy Procedures

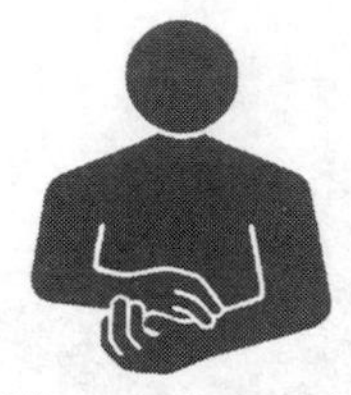

Many varieties of hydrotherapy are well suited to home treatment and can become effective and inexpensive additions to your personal health maintenance program.

The following hydrotherapy procedures described by Dr. Lewis are intended to be general and applicable in a variety of situations. According to Dr. Lewis, most of these are best used in conjunction with other treatments to enhance recovery, while some may be used alone. The procedures described in this section correspond to suggestions for hydrotherapy procedures in Part III, Health Conditions. Please use discretion and consult your physician if you have questions about your condition or the appropriateness of these treatments for you.

Cold Compresses (See also Ice Packs and Sitz Baths sections of this chapter.)

Description: An application that is applied cold and restored as it warms. It is generally applied as a cold cloth wrung from ice water (not usually as cold as an ice pack).

Purpose: Cold compresses are commonly used where it is beneficial to force blood from an area or to prevent its accumulation. (Such an accumulation might cause congestion which might then cause pain or discomfort.) They may also be applied to relieve heat in an affected part.

Uses: To reduce a minor inflammatory reaction, to relieve or prevent headache accompanying fever, following a hot application to stimulate blood flow.

Materials: A cloth of appropriate size to cover the area to be treated (terry cloth face, hand, or bath towel) and a basin of ice water.

Procedure: Wring a cloth of appropriate size from ice water and apply to the area to be treated. Restore as necessary to keep the cloth cold or for the comfort of the person treated.

Cold Friction Rub

Description: A cold application with friction.

Purpose: The cold friction rub is very stimulating and increases the function of the various organs.

Uses: Immune stimulation (very useful in chronic fatigue syndrome, upper respiratory infections, pneumonia, etc.); to stimulate blood flow into an area to enhance healing.

Materials: Ice water bath; terry cloth towel or mitten.

Procedure: The patient is prepared with a heating process (see also Hot Packs, Immersion Baths, Steam/Sauna, Hot Blanket Packs, and Sprays/Showers sections of this chapter). Briskly rub the area to be treated with the cold, wet cloth until the skin turns pink. Wrap up and stay warm.

Variations: This treatment may be applied to the trunk (front and back) when treating general conditions or it may be applied to a small area or extremity when treating specific conditions.

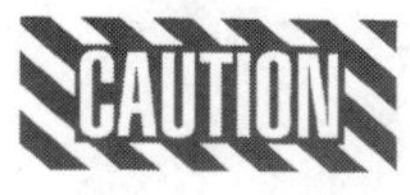

Precautions/Special Considerations: *Adequate preheating will produce a better reaction in most people.*

Constitutional Hydrotherapy

Description: An application of first hot then cold to the trunk, front and back.

Purpose: The treatment is useful to balance body functions, strengthen the immune system, and promote healing.

Uses: Constitutional hydrotherapy is useful in the treatment of, or as an adjunct to, the treatment of any condition. It is perhaps most useful in the treatment of acute conditions such as upper respiratory infections, bronchitis, asthma, the stomach flu, and in chronic conditions such as irritable bowel, ulcerative colitis, premenstrual syndrome, and arthritis. (When in doubt, try constitutional hydrotherapy.)

Materials: A bed or treatment table, one double sheet folded end to end (or two twin sheets), two wool blankets (or acrylic), three bath towels (a small bath towel is best, one that when folded in half reaches side to side across the patient and from shoulders to hips), one hand towel, and a source of hot and cold water.

Procedure: This is a version of the constitutional hydrotherapy treatment used by naturopathic physicians. It has been simplified for use at home.

- Have the patient undress to the waist and lie face up between the sheets, under one blanket.
- Place two hot, folded bath towels (four layers) on the patient's trunk, shoulders to hips, side to side.
- Cover with sheet and one blanket, and leave on five minutes.
- Return with one hot bath towel and one cold hand towel.
- Place the new hot towel on top of two old towels and flip all three towels. Remove the two old hot towels leaving the new hot towel in place. Place the cold towel on top of the new hot towel and flip again. Remove the hot towel leaving the cold in place.
- Cover the patient and add an extra layer of blanket. Leave ten minutes or until the cold towel is well warmed.
- Remove the towel.
- Have the patient roll over, face down.
- Repeat steps applying the towels to the patient's back.

Variations: The contrast may be narrowed (not as hot or cold) for the very ill or weak patient or may be pushed to the hot for sedation or to cold to tonify and strengthen.

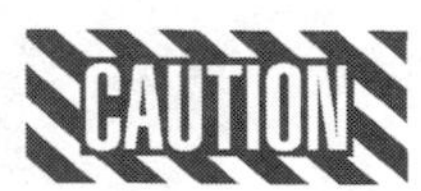

Precautions/Special Considerations: *A person should take the following precautions when using constitutional hydrotherapy.*

- *If using the patient's bed, take care not to get it wet.*
- *Hot water from the tap is usually hot enough. The hot towel should be hot enough that it's just possible to wring it out.*
- *The cold towel should be quite cold (use ice water), but wring it out thoroughly and use only one layer.*
- *If the patient has trouble warming the cold towel, massage the back (through the blankets and towel) and feet.*
- *Patients with asthma often react negatively to cold applications on the chest. For these persons, begin with a smaller cold towel applied to the abdomen only. With later treatments, gradually increase the size of the cold towel until you're able to cover the entire chest and abdomen without any negative reaction.*

Contrast Applications (See also Immersion Baths, Sitz Baths, and Sprays/Showers sections of this chapter.)

Description: An application of alternating hot and cold generally applied as three to four minutes hot followed by thirty to sixty seconds cold, repeated three to five times. It may be applied with hot and cold compresses or with immersion.

Purpose: Contrast applications are the most effective for increasing blood flow through an area. This aids in removing wastes that accumulate in areas of inflammation and helps bring nutrients and oxygen into those areas. It is also known to increase the functional activity of the organs that are in reflex relationship to the areas of skin being treated (e.g., contrast applied to the skin over the liver will increase the functional activity of the liver itself). Whole body contrast treatments have been shown to be effective in stimulating immune function.

Uses: Contrast hydrotherapy is the appropriate treatment to follow ice in acute injuries. Once the acute phase is over (usually twenty-four to thirty-six hours), ice should be discontinued and contrast begun. Contrast is useful in postacute, subacute, and chronic cases of tendinitis, bursitis, arthritis, as well as local infections such as otitis, mastitis, urethritis, or even many infected wounds.

Materials: Hot and cold compresses (terry cloth hand, face, or bath towel), or basin of hot and cold water for immersion.

Procedure: Apply hot compress to, or immerse the affected part in hot water (approximately 110 degrees Fahrenheit) for three to four minutes. Follow with cold (ice water) for thirty to sixty seconds (not longer, the effects of short cold are desirable here). Repeat three to five times; always end with cold.

Variations: Chemical hot packs and gel cold packs may be used if desired, but wet hot and cold applications are more effective and more readily available. Hand towels and face cloths are readily available and may be adequately heated from hot tap water and cooled from a basin of ice water.

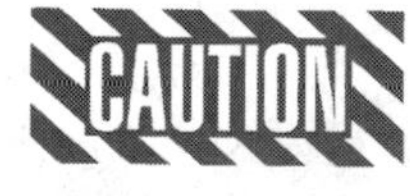

Precautions/Special Considerations: *The same precautions apply as with hot and cold applications alone.*

Enema/Colon Irrigation

Description: An irrigation of the large bowel using a small amount of water or solution.

Purpose: To aid in, and encourage, elimination from the bowel.

Uses: Used in detoxification from chemical exposure or abuse, to relieve constipation.

Materials: Enema bag (fountain syringe) available at most pharmacies, sea salt, baking soda, and lubricant (hand lotion, surgical lubricant, vegetable oil).

Procedure: Prepare enema solution of one tablespoonful of sea salt and one tablespoonful of baking soda per quart of water, at about 98 degrees Fahrenheit. Place solution in enema bag and place bag about three feet above the patient. Lubricate the anus and the enema tubing. Insert the tubing just past the inner sphincter (about one and a half to two inches), and hold in place. Release the valve to allow the solution to enter the colon. Introduce the solution slowly and don't try to take too much (about one pint is usually adequate at one time). Hold the solution for a few minutes before releasing into the toilet. Repeat the procedure several times during each enema.

Variations: It is possible to take the enema while lying on the floor or sitting on the toilet. Choose which is most comfortable for you.

- Often it is useful to stand and walk or massage the abdomen after taking a small amount of solution and before releasing into the toilet.
- If there is spasm and tension in the bowel, warmer water (about 102 degrees Fahrenheit) will often help relax the bowel.
- If the bowel is weak and flaccid, colder water may help to strengthen it. (Use water at about 75 to 80 degrees Fahrenheit.)
- The use of large amounts of solution introduced at once into the bowel during frequent enemas may cause the bowel to become stretched. To avoid this, remember to introduce the smallest amount of solution necessary to produce results.
- It is possible to use water without salt and baking soda. It is also possible to use other solutions for other effects.

Precautions/Special Considerations: *Do not use hot water or very cold water. Do not give enema if there is bleeding from the rectum. Consult your physician before giving enemas to children, the elderly, the very ill, persons with hypertension, persons with bowel disease, or pregnant women. If constipation persists after giving an enema, check with your physician.*

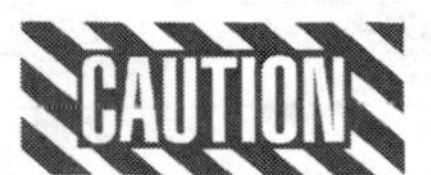

Heating Compresses (See also Wet Sheet Pack section of this chapter.)

Description: A heating compress is a cold application that is left in place for a long period of time. It is heated by the body and so becomes a hot application.

Purpose: The heating compress requires an active response from the body and therefore stimulates increased metabolic and healing activity in its vicinity.

Uses: Because it encourages blood flow into an area, it can be used to reduce congestion in another area. (Wet socks may be used to reduce congestion headaches, sinus congestion, and lung congestion.) Its tendency to bring blood into an area makes it useful for chronic joint pain or chronic bronchitis. It may be used in acute and chronic sore throats, tonsillitis, and ear infections. A whole body treatment may be achieved by the use of the wet sheet pack.

Materials: One pair light cotton socks, one pair heavy wool or acrylic socks, or a light-weight cotton fabric cut in width and length to wrap around the area to be treated (joint, neck). You will also need a wool cloth, cotton tee shirt, or wool sweater to cover the body.

Procedure: The wet sock treatment is especially useful in treating children with upper respiratory infections. Before bedtime, wring a pair of cotton socks in ice water, pull over feet, and cover with wool socks; leave in place overnight. By morning the socks should be warm and dry.

Variations: Knees, ankles, elbows, and wrists may easily be treated by wrapping the area with a cotton cloth wrung from cold water. (One or two layers are adequate.) Then cover with wool and leave several hours until quite warm (overnight is easiest). Throat conditions may be treated the same way. Shoulders and hips may also be treated this way but will require more creative wrapping techniques.

You can also use a chest pack. By far the easiest way to make one is to use a cotton tee shirt. Wring the shirt in ice water, pull it on, and cover yourself with a wool sweater. Leave in place overnight.

Hot Blanket Packs

Description: A hot blanket pack with a hot water bottle or electric heating pad.

Purpose: To produce a mild increase in body temperature.

Uses: The hot blanket pack may be used to produce hyperthermia for immune stimulation or detox. It may also be used to prepare for cold applications (see also Wet Sheet Packs, Cold Friction Rub, and Sprays/Showers sections of this chapter).

Materials: A dry sheet, two wool or acrylic blankets, two hot water bottles (or an electric heating pad), and a cold compress.

Procedure: Lay out two blankets with a dry sheet covering them. Have the patient undress and wrap in the sheet. Place one hot water bottle on the abdomen and one at the feet. (Or place the electric heating pad on the abdomen.) Mop the face with the cold compress as needed. Leave the patient in the pack for twenty to sixty minutes depending on the amount of heating desired.

Variations: A hot half-pack may be used where it is desirable to heat only the lower half of the body. In this case wrap only from the waist to the feet with a hot water bottle or heating pad between the legs. This treatment is milder than the hot foot bath and may be used with people who have peripheral vascular diseases or loss of peripheral sensations. Consult your physician.

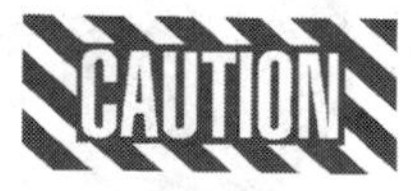

Precautions/Special Considerations: *Take care not to overheat the patient with the hot water bottles or heating pad. Always follow the hot blanket pack with a cool rinse.*

Hot Packs (See also Immersion Baths, and Hyperthermia sections of this chapter.)

Description: A hot application used to warm a local area.

Purpose: To relieve muscle spasms, produce local hyperthermia, encourage local blood flow, or relieve pain.

Uses: To relieve muscle spasms from various causes, to bring out local infections, or to prepare for cold applications.

Materials: Commercially available chemical hot packs or towels soaked in hot water from the tap (or heated in the microwave).

Procedure: Prepare hot packs to about 120 degrees Fahrenheit. Place two to three layers of toweling over the area to be treated. Place the hot pack on the toweling and cover. If the pack gets too hot for comfort, add additional layers of toweling as needed. Leave the pack in place five to twenty minutes depending on the time needed to obtain the desired effect. Packs may need to be restored if they cool too much. Follow with a short cold application when done (thirty seconds). Local redness and perspiration will occur.

Variations: Towels may be wrung from tap water at a temperature that will allow them to be placed directly on the skin. If the desired effect requires that they stay in place for more than five minutes, they should be renewed frequently so that they stay warm.

Precautions/Special Considerations: *Hot packs should be used with caution when treating children or persons with decreased sensation. Burns are possible if care is not taken to protect the skin from hot packs.*

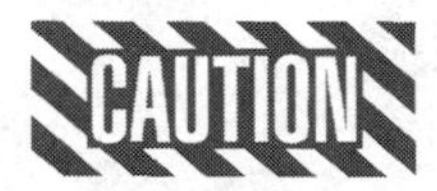

Never apply toweling that has been heated in a microwave directly to the skin. Microwave heating often creates hot and cold spots, so you may not be aware of an area that is too hot. In general, hot packs wrung from hot tap water are the safest. If you can wring them out with your hands, they're not likely to be hot enough to cause burns.

Hyperthermia (See also Immersion Baths, Steam/Sauna, and Hot Blanket Packs sections of this chapter.)

Description: A local or whole body treatment intended to raise the temperature of the tissues (also called artificial fever).

Purpose: To destroy heat sensitive organisms (viruses, bacteria, etc. that are sensitive to increases in body temperature), to enhance immune function and to encourage elimination of toxic material from the body.

Uses: Hyperthermia may be very useful in the adjunct treatment of various infectious diseases ranging from upper respiratory infections to pneumonia, from influenza to AIDS. It is also very useful in helping to eliminate toxic material from the body by encouraging sweating. In addition, it has been used in the treatment of many different types of cancer.

Materials: A hot tub or deep hot bath at 103 to 104 degrees Fahrenheit, or a hot blanket pack, or steam/sauna bath; a basin of ice water and terry cloth towel; and drinking water.

Procedure: Hyperthermia treatments may safely be done by immersing the body in hot water (103 to 104 degrees Fahrenheit) for up to sixty minutes at a time. Maintain the bath temperature for the entire time. To prevent a headache, apply cold to the head during treatment. Liberal use of cold water is advised. Begin early in the treatment and a headache can be prevented. (It is much more difficult to get rid of a headache than to prevent one.) Check the oral temperature every ten to fifteen minutes. If the oral temperature exceeds 104 degrees Fahrenheit, cool the bath and apply more cold to the head. Following the treatment, rinse in a cool shower. Then wrap up and stay warm.

Variations: If a bath or hot tub is not available, it is possible to heat the body in a steam or sauna bath. The hot blanket pack may also be used to raise body temperature. Local hyperthermia may be achieved by the use of hot packs or through the inhalation of steam. When inhaling steam for upper respiratory illness, avoid inhaling the steam deeply into the lungs.

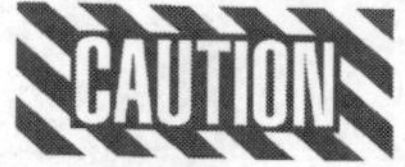

Precautions/Special Considerations: *A person should take the following precautions when using hyperthermia treatment.*

- *Hotter water can generally be tolerated for short periods, but it may cause an increase in body temperature that occurs too quickly. This may cause the treatment to be ended soon and leave the patient feeling uncomfortable.*
- *Consult your physician before doing this treatment if you have any of the following: high or low blood pressure, serious illness, diabetes mellitus, multiple or muscular sclerosis.*
- *Do not use this treatment if you are or may be pregnant.*
- *Watch for signs of hyperventilation. These include numbness and tingling in the lips, hands, or feet. If hyperventilation occurs, reduce the bath temperature; breathe from the abdomen, not the chest; or breathe into a paper bag until the tingling passes.*
- *Stand slowly after finishing the treatment and be careful in the shower for the cool rinse.*
- *Having an attendant near or at hand may be a good idea for the first few times the treatment is done.*

Ice Packs (See also Immersion Baths section of this chapter.)

Description: A very cold application using ice or gel packs.

Purpose: To reduce swelling, inflammation, pain, or reduce congestion.

Uses: To relieve swelling and inflammation from acute injuries and conditions such as sprained ankles, blows, crushing injuries, tendinitis, and bursitis. To reduce congestion from vasodilation.

Materials: Commercially available cold pack, crushed ice in bag, bag of frozen vegetables, ice cubes, frozen paper cup of water, or ice water bath.

Procedure: Apply a cold pack to the affected part twenty minutes out of every hour for the first twenty-four to thirty-six hours after acute injury, depending on the severity.

Variations: An immersion bath may be used if more convenient (e.g., an ankle sprain). Add ice to a basin of water and immerse the affected part as in one above. (The disadvantage with immersion is that it is difficult to elevate a part that is immersed in a water bath.)

In the case of an acute tendinitis or muscle spasm, it may be useful to rub the area with an ice cube or frozen cup. Rub vigorously over the painful area until a feeling of burning occurs and the area begins to feel numb (usually about ten to twelve minutes). This may be repeated hourly in acute cases.

CAUTION

Precautions/Special Considerations: *Do not apply cold to suspected frost bite or to areas where there is loss of sensation. For this reason it may be inappropriate to apply cold to the extremities of persons with diabetes or other peripheral neuropathy.*

Immersion Baths (See also Sitz Baths section of this chapter.)

Description: A bath in which all or part of the body is immersed in water. It may be used for contrast or for the effects of hot or cold alone.

Purpose: Immersion may be the easiest way to apply hydrotherapy to the body either because of the irregularity of a part like a hand or foot or if a large area is to be covered. It may be useful in cases of edema to provide pressure to force fluid back into circulation. Water is also a powerful solvent and may dissolve and remove "toxic" materials from the body through the skin.

Uses: Extremities may be treated in the immersion bath for any of the various effects of hot, cold, or contrast. Chemicals may be added for various effects such as Epsom salt for its anti-inflammatory and "drawing" effects. Full immersion baths may be given to produce a hyperthermia response (artificial fever), for the relaxing and sedative effects of a neutral bath, to relieve sore muscles, to "detoxify," or for the stimulation of a cold plunge.

Materials: A basin (or two for contrast) large enough to accommodate the part to be immersed, filled with hot or cold water (or one of each), plastic wastebaskets are often the best for a foot, leg, or arm. A double-bowl kitchen sink may also serve. A hot tub, whirlpool bath, or bathtub may serve for full immersion when needed.

Procedure: For a local application, cover the part entirely. The hot bath may be approximately 110 degrees Fahrenheit. The cold should be ice water. Most conditions respond best to contrast unless within the first twenty-four to thirty-six hours of an acute inflammatory condition (see also Contrast Applications section of this chapter). Epsom salt may be added to the hot bath if desired, generally one-quarter to one-half pound per gallon, for its anti-inflammatory action.

Variations: A full immersion bath may be useful in promoting a fever (see also Hyperthermia section of this chapter), for the relief of sore, aching muscles, or to aid in "detoxification." For the latter two, soak in a tub (102 to 104 degrees Fahrenheit) fifteen to twenty minutes and follow with short cold plunge or shower. (Epsom salt may be added, one-quarter to one-half pound per gallon.)

In cases of insomnia, anxiety, or nervousness, a neutral bath (97 degrees Fahrenheit) may be taken for anywhere from thirty minutes to several hours. Do not follow with cold.

A cold plunge may be useful after exercise or after any whole body hot application.

Precautions/Special Considerations: *The same precautions apply as with any hot or cold application. Both the hot bath and cold plunge may be contraindicated for persons with cardiovascular disease or during pregnancy. It is also contraindicated for persons with peripheral vascular diseases or who have loss of sensation in the hands or feet. Consult your physician.*

Sitz Baths

Description: A bath in which the pelvis is immersed in hot and/or cold water.

Purpose: To provide the benefits of hot, cold, or contrast to the pelvic organs.

Uses: May be used in infections of the bladder, prostate, or vagina; hemorrhoids; menstrual problems; or bowel problems such as anal fissures, colitis, diverticulitis, or other inflammatory bowel diseases. Cold sitz alone may be used to tonify the pelvic musculature in cases of bladder or bowel incontinence or prolapse.

Materials: One (or two) basins adequate to sit in such that water will cover up to the level of the navel, or bathtub of water filled to reach the level of the navel and a basin of ice water and bath towel if needed for contrast treatment.

Procedure: Warm soaks alone may be useful for the treatment of local anal or vaginal irritation. Hemorrhoids and anal fissures may be treated by soaking in a warm bath for ten to fifteen minutes. Other conditions will respond better to contrast. Use one tub of hot water (about 110 degrees Fahrenheit) and one tub of ice water. Follow directions as for contrast applications; three to four minutes hot, thirty to sixty seconds cold, repeated three to five times. Always end with cold.

Variations: If two tubs are not available, the following is very effective. Sit three to four minutes in a hot half-bath (water up to the level of the navel in a bath tub), then stand in the hot water and pull a cold towel between the legs and over the pelvis in the front and back. Hold in place thirty to sixty seconds, then sit back into the hot bath. Repeat as with contrast three to five times. End with cold.

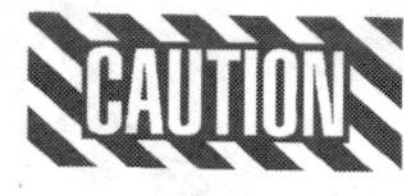

Precautions/Special Considerations: *When sitting and standing around water be careful that your footing is secure so you don't slip and fall. Also, when sitting in hot water it is possible that you may become light-headed and dizzy when standing up. It is best to have an assistant present when doing any type of contrast sitz.*

Sprays/Showers

Description: A hot or cold spray of water from a hose or shower.

Purpose: Hot—to prepare for cold; cold—to stimulate and increase function.

Uses: Contrast showers—to improve immune function; cold sprays—to increase organ function or stimulate the nervous system.

Materials: A household shower, and a hose attached to a faucet or bathtub filler spout.

Procedure: For general immune stimulation follow a hot cleansing shower with a two-minute cold rinse.

Variations: Following a hot shower (or other heating application), a cold spray on each side of the spine is very stimulating and invigorating. A gentle cold spray over mild varicose veins (without preheating) may help to tone the veins.

Precautions/Special Considerations: *Don't use a strong spray over varicose veins. Cold showers and sprays may be approached gradually, starting with cool and working gradually to all cold.*

Steam/Sauna

Description: A full-body application of heat in a humid environment.

Purpose: To increase body temperature and/or promote sweating.

Uses: May be used to prepare for cold applications (see also Contrast Applications, Wet Sheet Packs, and Sprays/Showers sections of this chapter), to produce an artificial fever, or to encourage the breakdown and elimination of "toxic" material.

Materials: Steam room, steam cabinet, sauna.

Procedure: No more than fifteen to twenty minutes should be spent in a steam room or sauna where it is necessary to breathe hot air or steam. This is due to the fact that hot air, moist or dry, reduces the ability of the lungs to exchange oxygen and carbon dioxide. It may be preferable to work your way up to the longer times. Begin with three to four minutes in the hot environment then exit and do a cool rinse. Gradually increase your time in the heat and increase the degree of cold water for the rinse. It may be useful to take a basin of ice water and a cloth into the steam room to apply cold to the head and face. This may reduce the tendency to headache that can occur with whole-body heating.

Variations: Where available, a Russian steam room or steam cabinet is preferable. This is a room or cabinet that allows the head to be outside the hot environment. This allows the patient to breathe room temperature air and an attendant may easily apply cold compresses to the face and head. It is possible for a person to remain in this environment for a much longer period of time. Treatment times of up to sixty minutes may be achieved depending on the tolerance and response of the patient.

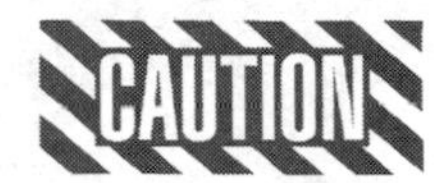

Precautions/Special Considerations: *Women who are or may be pregnant should limit applications of heat to ten minutes or less. Persons with cardiovascular disease should consult their physician before doing any treatment involving very hot or very cold temperatures. Persons with multiple sclerosis may not tolerate hot applications well.*

Prolonged applications of heat may encourage hyperventilation. If there is any evidence of tingling in the lips, fingers, or toes treatment should be discontinued and a cold rinse applied.

A headache is a common side effect to prolonged heating that may occur immediately or some time following the treatment. Most headaches can be avoided by applying cold to the head and face during treatment. It is probably not possible to overdo the use of cold in this way.

Wet Sheet Packs

Description: A full-body wrap in a cold wet sheet. The treatment progresses in three phases: cold or cooling, neutral, and heating.

Purpose: To stimulate, relax, or detoxify depending on phase.

Uses: The treatment is stimulating and tonifying if it is stopped before the sheet is warmed (first phase). There are easier ways to achieve this stimulation and therefore it is rarely used this way. However, the cold application is useful to control a fever that is rising too rapidly or is too high.

The neutral phase is useful to relax and sedate.

The final phase of heating is commonly used to aid in cleansing through the skin. It promotes sweating and elimination and is therefore useful in detoxifying from environmental or chemical exposure or from drug, alcohol, or tobacco use.

Materials: A bed or treatment table, wool blankets (one to three may be needed), pillows (two—one for the head, one for under the knees), a cotton (poly/cotton) sheet soaked in ice water, a terry cloth bath towel, and a terry cloth hand towel.

Procedure: Lay out one blanket with a pillow for the head and one to support the knees. The blanket should be high enough to fold over the shoulders of the patient.

- Thoroughly wring the sheet from ice water and lay it out over the blanket.
- Have the patient undress and lie down on the center of the wet sheet and pull the far half over themselves.
- Return and arrange the sheet by pulling the far half under the arms and around the far leg. Have the patient place the arms in a comfortable position across the abdomen. (If the patient is claustrophobic, one arm may be left out.) Wrap the near half of the sheet over the shoulders, arms, and around the near leg. Next, bring the blanket across the patient, draping it over the shoulders. Any extra length of wet sheet should be folded up over the blanket.
- Add extra layers of blanket to hold in heat produced by the patient to warm the sheet. (If the treatment is used to reduce fever, extra blankets are not needed.)
- If general detoxification is desired, leave the patient in the wet sheet until profuse sweating has occurred and as long as he or she tolerates. This may require two to four hours or more. The heating/detoxifying stage will be reached sooner if the patient has undergone some sort of heating before getting into the wet sheet pack (exercise, hot shower, hot tub, etc.).

Variations: If the relaxing effects of the neutral phase are desired, the patient should be removed from the pack before he or she begins to perspire. A warm (not hot) shower following is acceptable.

If the tonifying, fever-reducing effects are sought, remove the patient as soon as he or she begins to heat the sheet. It may be appropriate and necessary to restore the cold wet sheet one or more times to reach the desired effect of the cold.

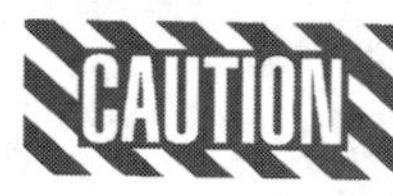

Precautions/Special Considerations: *A person should take the following precautions when using wet sheet packs:*

- *Hot drinks such as hot ginger tea will promote sweating. However, don't burn the patient (test the temperature of the drinks first) and don't give too much fluid. The need to urinate could end the treatment too soon if too much fluid is given.*
- *Water to drink may be necessary during the elimination phase.*
- *The bath towel may be used to cover the patient's head and eyes to enhance the heating phase and shade the eyes.*
- *The hand towel may be used as a cold compress and to mop the patient's face once perspiration begins in the elimination phase.*

The Future of Hydrotherapy

"In Europe," says Dr. Lewis, "hydrotherapy is commonly found in health clinics, both as a primary and an adjunctive treatment modality. In the United States, there is also a definite resurgence of interest in hydrotherapy, which I feel is due to the growing dissatisfaction people have with the overuse of medications. People are looking for other alternatives." Dr. Lewis points out that hydrotherapy has numerous clinical applications and provides a number of safe, natural, and effective adjunct treatments for conditions that include digestive problems, female health conditions, chronic fatigue syndrome, cancer, and AIDS. The most important application of hydrotherapy, however, may be in the home, where it can be used as a simple and inexpensive means of both preventing and treating the common cold, flus, and many common health conditions. Because of this, hydrotherapy has great potential to play an important role in medicine in the coming years.

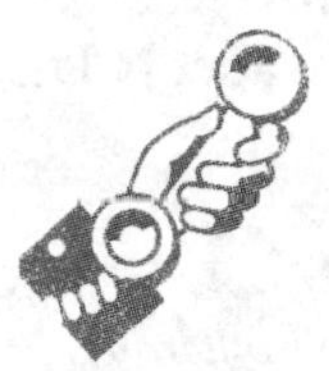

Where to Find Help

To find a hydrotherapy facility in your area look under "Physical Therapy," or "Health Spas" in your phone book, or make inquiries at your local hospital. To find a referral to a naturopathic physician in your area who practices hydrotherapy, contact:

American Association of Naturopathic Physicians
2366 Eastlake Avenue, Suite 322
Seattle, Washington 98102
(206) 323-7610

Provides referrals to a nationwide network of accredited or licensed naturopathic physicians for health professionals and the general public; supported by members and corporate sponsors. It hosts an annual convention, and works to move legislature and licensure in various states.

Bastyr University
Natural Health Clinic
1307 North 45th Street, Suite 200
Seattle, Washington 98103
(206) 632-0354

Both National and Bastyr Colleges offer postgraduate training in naturopathic medicine and support teaching clinics. The Physical Medicine Department of the Natural Health Clinic of Bastyr College and the teaching clinic of National College of Naturopathic Medicine use hydrotherapy treatment, including hyperthermia, for detox and for conditions ranging from upper respiratory infection and chronic fatigue syndrome to HIV.

National College of Naturopathic Medicine
11231 Southeast Market Street
Portland, Oregon 97216
(503) 255-4860

For referrals to naturopathic doctors in your area.

Uchee Pines Institute
30 Uchee Pines Road, Suite 75
Seale, Alabama 36875
(205) 855-4764

Uchee Pines Institute is a healing center that provides many health care alternatives including hyperthermia treatment.

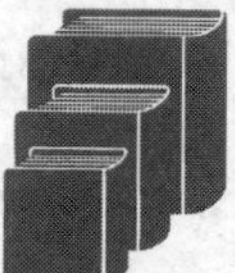

Recommended Reading

Back to Eden: A Herbal Guide. Kloss, Jethro. Loma Linda, CA: Gordon Press, 1991.

A classic guide to home remedies, herbal medicine, and natural foods. Contains a major section on various forms of hydrotherapy.

Home Remedies. Thrash, Agatha, M.D., and Calvin, M.D. Seale, AL: New Lifestyle Books, 1981.

A helpful book for anyone interested in hydrotherapy and home remedies with useful information on hyperthermia treatment.

How to Get Well. Airola, Paavo. Sherwood, OR: Health Plus Publishers, 1974.

A handbook of natural healing. Contains a chapter on therapeutic baths.

Lectures in Naturopathic Hydrotherapy. Boyle, Wade, N.D., and Saine, Andre, N.D. East Palestine, OH: Buckeye Naturopathic Press, 1988.

A useful book on general hydrotherapy topics, not specific to hyperthermia.

"The greatest danger of pollution may well be that we shall tolerate levels of it so low as to have no acute nuisance value, but sufficiently high, nevertheless, to have delayed pathological effects and spoil the quality of life."

—Rene Du Bois, Scientist, Environmentalist

Hyperthermia

Fever is one of the body's most powerful defenses against disease. Hyperthermia artificially induces fever in the patient who is unable to mount a natural fever response to infection, inflammation, or other health challenges. It is used locally or over the entire body to treat diseases ranging from viral infections to cancer, and is an effective self-help treatment for the common cold and flu.

The body protects itself from viruses, bacteria, and other harmful substances through the use of numerous defense systems. One of these is fever. Fever raises the body's temperature above normal in an attempt to destroy invading organisms and sweat impurities out of the system. Fever is a highly effective and natural process of curing disease and restoring health, and has been recognized as such for thousands of years. Hyperthermia deliberately creates fever in the patient in order to utilize this natural healing response.

How Hyperthermia Works

A state of hyperthermia exists when body temperature rises above its normal level of 98.6 degrees Fahrenheit. An increase in body temperature causes many physiological responses to occur in the body. Hyperthermia takes advantage of the fact that many invading organisms tolerate a narrower temperature range than body tissues and are therefore more susceptible to increases in temperature (they may die from overheating before harm is done to human tissue). Examples are viruses such as rhinovirus[1] (responsible for one-half of all respiratory infections), HIV (human immunodeficiency virus),[2] and the microorganisms and bacteria that cause syphilis and gonorrhea.[3]

“Hyperthermia takes advantage of the fact that many invading organisms tolerate a narrower temperature range than body tissues and are therefore more susceptible to increases in temperature.”

Hyperthermia treatments may not be able to kill every invading organism, but they can reduce their numbers to a level the immune system can handle. Hyperthermia stimulates the immune system by increasing the production of antibodies and interferon (a protein substance produced by virus-invaded cells that prevents reproduction of the virus). Hyperthermia is also a useful technique in detoxification therapy because it releases toxins stored in fat cells.

Methods of Inducing Hyperthermia

Body temperature can be swiftly increased by the external application of heat. This approach causes blood vessels to swell and the body to perspire in an attempt to prevent an increase in temperature. An increase in body temperature may be accomplished by such low-tech methods as immersing the body in hot water, sitting in a sauna or steam bath, or wrapping oneself in blankets with a hot water bottle.

Other, high-tech approaches, more commonly found in hospital and medical centers rather than in alternative medical settings, include the use of shortwave or microwave diathermy, ultrasound, radiant heating, and extracorporeal heating.

- **Diathermy** is the application of radio frequency electromagnetic energy to the body to cause a temperature rise.
- **Ultrasound** is the application of high energy sound waves to cause an increase in body temperature as a result of friction produced at the molecular level that is created as the sound waves strike different body tissues. For whole body or large area treatments, multiple ultrasound applicators may be used.
- **Radiant heating** devices produce infrared heat that is applied to the body.
- **Extracorporeal heating** is accomplished by removing blood from the body, heating it, and returning it to the body at a higher temperature.

Hyperthermia can be produced either locally or over the whole body. Locally-applied hyperthermia is most often employed to treat infections such as upper respiratory infections (with inhalation of steam or a local application of diathermy), or for infected wounds in a hand or foot (generally produced with immersion in a hot water bath). Whole-body hyperthermia, on the other hand, is used when there is a general infection, when a local application is impractical, or when a general whole-body response is desirable.

For whole-body hyperthermia, practitioners normally utilize the methods of full-immersion baths, saunas, steam, and blanket packs. For a localized application, immersion baths, steam, or, occasionally, diathermy are used. In conventional medical settings, whole-body treatment usually involves the more high-tech approaches of diathermy, ultrasound, radiant and extracorporeal heating; for localized treatments, diathermy and ultrasound are used.

Hyperthermia in all of its forms is often employed in the treatment of bronchitis, pneumonia, sinusitis, and other conditions of the lungs and body cavities, and is used as a modality for physical therapy.

History of Hyperthermia

The beneficial effects of hyperthermia in the form of hot packs, baths, and saunas have been recognized for thousands of years. In 500 B.C., the Greek physician Parmenides stated that if only he had the means to create fever, he could cure all illness. The early Romans built elaborate baths which included saunas, cold plunge baths, and swimming areas. The sauna has long been a part of Finnish tradition, and the Russians use steam baths regularly. Native American cultures use sweat lodges in cleansing practices. Over the last few centuries, physicians have observed that people suffering from certain illnesses, such as cancer, gonorrhea, and syphilis, often become free of these illnesses following a high fever from another infection. This has led to research into the production of fever by various methods (injection of foreign substances, hot packs, hot baths) to treat a wide variety of health problems from the common cold to AIDS and cancer.

Conditions Benefited by Hyperthermia

Hyperthermia can be used in the treatment of upper and lower respiratory tract infections, bladder problems, and urinary tract infections such as cystitis. For these problems, hot baths are the most common method used to induce hyperthermia.

Viral Diseases

Douglas Lewis, N.D., Chair of Physical Medicine at the Bastyr College Natural Health Clinic in Seattle, Washington, states that a hot immersion bath, if done without raising body temperature and heart rate too quickly or too high, can be used as an adjunctive treatment for a "diverse number of diseases—from upper respiratory infections and sexually transmitted diseases to cancer and AIDS." Hyperthermia in the form of hot baths has also proved useful in the treatment of herpes simplex and herpes zoster (shingles). At first the treatment aggravates the situation, but conditions improve considerably after a short time. It is also useful in treating the common cold and flu, as well as chronic fatigue syndrome. Bruce Milliman, N.D., of Seattle, Washington, reports a 70 percent success rate using hyperthermia to treat chronic fatigue syndrome.

"Over the last few centuries, physicians have observed that people suffering from certain illnesses such as cancer, gonorrhea, and syphilis often become free of these illnesses following a high fever from another infection. This has led to research into the production of fever to treat a wide variety of health problems from common colds to AIDS and cancer."

Dr. Lewis has also had good results treating chronic fatigue syndrome with hyperthermia. For certain cases, Dr. Lewis prescribes hyperthermia as a form of self-care. In one instance, he suggested a patient take hot tub treatments at home three to four times weekly. "During the following year," Dr. Lewis reports, "her condition improved wonderfully. While not fully recovered, her energy level is substantially higher, and she credits this to her hot tub routine."

Acute viral infection is another condition Dr. Lewis treats with hyperthermia. In one case, a patient came to him suffering from a combination of pneumonia and bronchitis. His infection had initially been treated with natural remedies, and then antibiotics, both of which produced only minor results. Dr. Lewis prescribed two treatments of hyperthermia forty-eight hours apart, with an additional treatment given at home one week later. The patient began to improve with the first treatment and was significantly better by the time of the final treatment. "In treating acute conditions," Dr. Lewis says, "sometimes the patient will have more difficulty tolerating higher temperatures than those who are suffering from chronic conditions. As the fever response is stimulated, however, usually a higher tolerance follows."

HIV Infection

At the Natural Health Clinic of Bastyr College, hyperthermia is commonly used in the treatment of HIV and other chronic and acute viral infections. In 1988 and 1989, the Natural Health Clinic conducted a "Healing Aids Research Project" (HARP). Hyperthermia treatment was included in the treatment protocol developed for the study because of its immune-stimulating, detoxifying, and disinfecting properties.

According to Leanna Standish, N.D., Ph.D., Director of HARP, participants reported that hyperthermia was the facet of their treatment that had the greatest impact. They found a decrease in night sweats and in the frequency of secondary infection. Also, many participants reported having a greater sense of well-being after hyperthermia treatments.[4]

Laboratory research has proven that HIV is temperature sensitive and suffers greater inactivation at progressively higher temperatures above 98.6 degrees Fahrenheit. For example, after thirty minutes heating in a water bath at 107.6 degrees Fahrenheit, 40 percent inactivation of HIV has been reported, and at 132.8 degrees Fahrenheit, 100 percent inactivation.[5] "I don't believe that hyperthermia is the answer for all HIV patients," says Dr. Lewis, "but I do think it is an appropriate adjunct treatment for all but a few very sick patients."

Cancer

Current medical literature is filled with references to the use of hyperthermia in conventional medical settings as an adjunct cancer treatment. Studies have shown that hyperthermia treatment modifies cell membranes in such a way as to protect healthy cells and make tumor cells more susceptible to chemotherapy and radiation.[6] This makes hyperthermia a useful adjunct in cancer therapy, as its application enables the use of lower doses of chemotherapy and radiation.

Other studies have shown that hyperthermia treatments play a role in stimulating the immune system. White cell counts appear to drop immediately following treatment, but rise within a few hours. Not only do the number of white cells increase, but their ability to destroy target cells appears to increase as well.[7] A recent study has shown an increase in the production of interleukin-1 (a compound produced by the body in response to infection, inflammation, or other immunologic challenges) with whole-body hyperthermia.[8] These studies indicate that increased body temperature plays a positive role in the healing process of the body. According to A.C. Guyton, M.D., an authority in the field of medical physiology, the metabolic rate would be increased 100 percent for every 10 degrees centigrade rise in temperature.[10] This increased metabolic rate no doubt accounts for some of the increased immune activity.

Hyperthermia at Home

Hot baths are the simplest method of inducing a fever at home and can be used to treat upper respiratory tract infections (colds, flu) and even lower respiratory tract conditions, such as bronchitis and pneumonia. To treat viral infections, hot baths can be combined with hot drinks and blanket-wrapping to stimulate the immune system. After the bath, wrap yourself in dry blankets. You may also want to put a hot water bottle over your abdomen. Allow yourself to perspire heavily for as long as you can tolerate. This may take several hours. Follow with a cool shower.

It is also possible to produce a mild fever at home by simply wrapping up in a dry blanket pack. Again, you can allow yourself to perspire heavily for several hours and follow with a cool shower.

Also, a wet sheet pack may be used to produce a therapeutic fever. Wrap yourself in a very cold wet sheet and several blankets. Like the dry pack, you will need several hours to produce a fever. The cold sheet produces reactions in the body that encourage the production of heat. It is often useful to precede the wet sheet with some kind of heating such as exercise or a hot bath or shower.

Local hyperthermia can also be useful at times. One study shows that the inhalation of steam is useful in the treatment of head colds.[9] Hot soaks or hot packs may also be used to treat local conditions. An infection in a hand or foot might benefit from immersion in hot water. If immersion would be uncomfortable, as in the case of an infected wound, hot packs may be applied to the area instead.

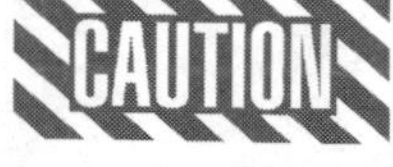

If you practice hyperthermia at home, you should consult your physician. Douglas Lewis, N.D., cautions patients to be careful to monitor their temperature and not let it go above 102 degrees Fahrenheit, measured orally.

Detoxification

Zane Gard, M.D., and Erma Brown, B.S.N., P.H.N., incorporate hyperthermia as part of their detoxification program known as the BioToxic Reduction (BTR) Program™.[11] "The human body stores a mix of toxins in the fat found in cells and cell walls, as well as in actual fat cells," says Dr. Gard. "These toxins include pesticides, herbicides, and solvents, as well as prescription and recreational drugs." According to Dr. Gard, hyperthermia is an excellent way to stimulate the release of toxins from the cells and allow their elimination, first through the skin, and later through the bowels and kidneys.[12]

See Detoxification Therapy, Hydrotherapy.

The program developed by Dr. Gard is comprehensive and requires careful medical supervision. The treatment consists of a daily schedule of exercise and sauna sessions, supplementation of vitamins, minerals, niacin, trace elements, oil, and amino acids, pre- and post-program blood chemistry analysis, and personality and perception testing. The daily treatments must last for at least two weeks to be effective.

Patients are monitored closely after exiting the sauna. Large amounts of toxins are sometimes released into the blood by the hyperthermia treatment and may cause a medical emergency (difficulty breathing, heart problems, and, in the case of recreational drug toxins, flashbacks and hallucinations).

Dr. Lewis describes a patient who was being treated at the Natural Health Clinic using hyperthermia produced with a steam cabinet. The patient had a long history of oral and intravenous drug abuse. After a short period of heating, the old accumulation of drug residues was released and he got "high" from the drugs rushing through the bloodstream. Several times during his first few treatments he became incoherent and babbled away about nothing in particular. Gradually, over several sessions this reaction diminished to almost nothing.

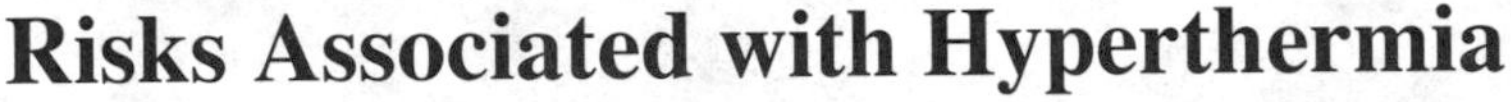

Risks Associated with Hyperthermia

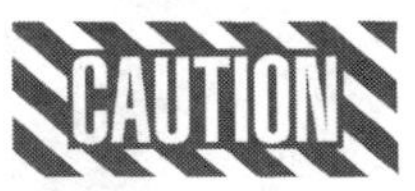

When used knowledgeably and with care, hyperthermia is a safe and effective treatment for many conditions. However, many people are sensitive to the effects of heat, such as those with anemia, heart disease, diabetes, seizure disorders, and tuberculosis, as well as women who are or may be pregnant. People with these conditions should take great care.

When used knowledgeably and with care, hyperthermia is a safe and effective treatment for many conditions. Ill-effects of hyperthermia usually appear only when body temperatures exceed 106 degrees Fahrenheit. However, certain individuals are sensitive to the effects of heat, such as those with anemia, heart disease, diabetes, seizure disorders, tuberculosis, and women who are or may be pregnant.[13] People with these conditions should take great care.

Other reported risks of hyperthermia include herpes outbreaks[14] (including herpes zoster), liver toxicity,[15] and nervous system injury. Some substances used to induce hyperthermia are not recommended. These include blood products, vaccines, pollens, and benign forms of malaria,[16] as secondary infection from the injection of blood products and these other substances is extremely dangerous. Hyperthermia for detoxification should only be performed under medical supervision for the reasons described in the previous section.

Additional notes of caution:

- Patients with temperature regulatory problems, especially the old and the very young, should not use hyperthermia.

- Microwave diathermy can burn the tissue around the eyes, and should never be used by people with pacemakers.
- People with peripheral vascular disease or loss of sensation should not use hyperthermia due to the risk of burns.
- Caution is advised with patients who have cardiovascular disease, in particular arrhythmia (irregularity or loss of rhythm, especially of the heartbeat) and tachycardia (abnormally rapid heart rate), and severe hypertension or hypotension.

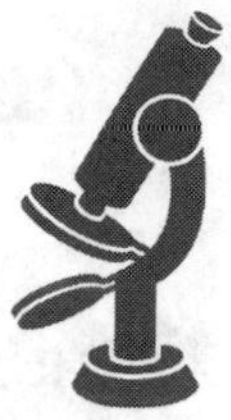

In a time when medical treatment consists primarily of high-tech drugs and surgical intervention, it would be very useful for some of America's tax dollars to be spent researching low-cost alternative therapies such as hyperthermia.

The Future of Hyperthermia

As is true with many treatments that offer little or no potential profit from their development, hyperthermia has seen limited research. Also, to be effective, it is labor intensive, and requires the supervision of a qualified medical professional who is able to deal with a crisis situation that can arise as the body throws off toxins. Because of these factors, Dr. Lewis realizes that many health professionals do not use hyperthermia as a means of treatment.

However, Dr. Lewis foresees the situation changing. "As we really begin to recognize the degree to which we have poisoned our environment and ourselves, we will begin to look for effective ways to detox," Dr. Lewis says. "And hyperthermia is certainly an important way of doing so, both as a primary method and adjunctly. Likewise, as it becomes evident that our immune functions are suffering, we will begin to explore ways to support immune function, and hyperthermia can be a useful tool in that quest." In a time when medical treatment consists primarily of high-tech drugs and surgical intervention, it would be very useful for some of America's tax dollars to be spent researching low-cost alternatives such as hyperthermia.

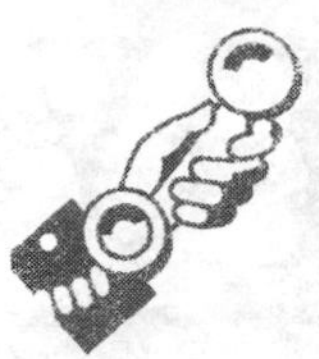

Where to Find Help

For additional help and information concerning hyperthermia contact:

Bastyr University
Natural Health Clinic
1307 North 45th Street, Suite 200
Seattle, Washington 98103
(206) 632-0354

Offer, postgraduate training in naturopathic medicine and support teaching clinics. The physical medicine department of the Natural Health Clinic of Bastyr College uses hyperthermia treatment for detox and in conditions ranging from upper respiratory infection to chronic fatigue syndrome and HIV.

National College of Naturopathic Medicine
11231 Southeast Market Street
Portland, Oregon 97216
(503) 255-4860

Offers postgraduate training in naturopathic medicine and support teaching clinics. The teaching clinic uses hyperthermia for a wide variety of conditions.

Uchee Pines Institute
30 Uchee Pines Road, Suite 75
Seale, Alabama 36875
(205) 855-4764

Uchee Pines Institute is a healing center that provides many health care alternatives including hyperthermia treatment.

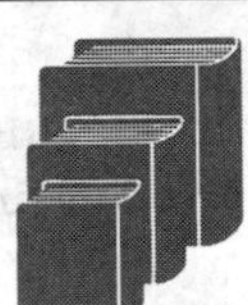

Recommended Reading

Home Remedies. Thrash, Agatha, M.D., and Calvin, M.D. Seale, AL: New Lifestyle Books, 1981.

A helpful book for anyone interested in hydrotherapy and home remedies with useful information on hyperthermia treatment.

Lectures in Naturopathic Hydrotherapy. Boyle, Wade, N.D., and Saine, Andre, N.D. East Palestine, OH: Buckeye Naturopathic Press, 1991.

A useful book on general hydrotherapy topics, including, but not specific to, hyperthermia.

Hypnotherapy

Hypnotherapy is used to manage numerous medical and psychological problems. Hypnotic techniques can help a person stop smoking, overcome alcohol and substance abuse, and reduce overeating. Hypnotherapy is also effective in treating stress, sleep disorders, and mental health problems such as anxiety, fear, phobias, and depression.

For thousands of years the power of suggestion has played a major role in healing in cultures as varied as ancient Greece, Persia, and India. Hypnotherapy uses both the power of suggestion and trancelike states to access the deepest levels of the mind to effect positive changes in a person's behavior, and to treat a range of health conditions, including migraines, ulcers, respiratory conditions, tension headaches, and even warts.

In 1955, the British Medical Association approved the use of hypnotherapy as a valid medical treatment. The American Medical Association (AMA) followed suit in 1958, and its Council on Scientific Affairs continues to encourage more research on the subject of hypnotherapy. At the same time, the American Society of Clinical Hypnosis, a professional association of physicians, psychologists, and dentists, has grown from twenty members in 1957 to over 4,300, and attendance at hypnotism courses by physicians and other medical specialists is steadily increasing. Approximately fifteen thousand doctors now combine hypnotherapy with traditional treatments, and recent studies show that 94 percent of patients benefit from hypnotherapy, even if the only benefit is relaxation.[1]

Therapeutic Applications of Hypnotherapy

Hypnotherapy has therapeutic applications for both psychological and physical disorders. A skilled hypnotherapist can facilitate profound changes in respiration and relaxation on the part of the client to create positive shifts in behavior and an enhanced well-being. A physiological shift can be observed in a hypnotic state, as can greater control of autonomic nervous system functions normally considered to be beyond one's ability to control. Stress reduction is a common occurrence, as is a lowering of blood pressure rate.

Recently, hypnotherapy has become more widely used as a method for treating a variety of medical conditions. "Because hypnotherapy induces a deep, multilevel relaxation, increases tolerance to adverse stimuli, eases anxiety, and enhances affirmative imagery, it can be adapted to maximize the mind's contribution to healing, both in and out of the hospital," says Gerard V. Sunnen, M.D., Associate Clinical Professor of Psychiatry at the New York University-Bellevue Hospital Medical Center.

Maurice Tinterow, M.D., Ph.D., an anesthesiologist at the Center for the Improvement of Human Functioning in Wichita, Kansas, has employed hypnotherapy to control pain for conditions that include headaches, facial neuralgia, sciatica, osteoarthritis, rheumatoid arthritis, whiplash, menstrual pain, and tennis elbow.[2] Dr. Tinterow has also used hypnotherapy in place of anesthesia in a variety of surgical operations, including hysterectomies, hernias, breast biopsies, hemorrhoidectomies, cesarian sections, and for the treatment of second and third degree burns.[3]

One of Dr. Tinterow's earliest and most dramatic cases involved a fifteen-year-old girl who required open heart surgery. Because the girl proved allergic to all anesthetic agents, Dr. Tinterow used hypnosis over a period of eight weeks, and by the final session before surgery the girl was able to relax quite easily. She was hypnotized before the operation and remained conscious throughout the four-hour procedure. The operation was a success, and today, thirty years later, the woman is healthy and living a full life.

Gary Lalonde, C.Ht., of Wales, Michigan, also uses hypnotherapy to treat a variety of health conditions. One of his clients suffered from reflex sympathetic dystrophy (RSD), a chronic condition where pain does not subside and muscle function begins to deteriorate. "This man had pierced one of his feet with a three-and-a-half-inch nail after stepping on a piece of wood at a construction site," Lalonde relates. "He was treated for the injury, but the pain persisted and grew so bad that he could not return to work. For two years, his condition grew worse. Finally, a thermograph showed that the foot's temperature was eleven degrees colder than the rest of his body. When his doctors told him it might have to be amputated, he came to see me."

Lalonde worked with this client for seven months using hypnotherapy not only for pain relief, but also to explore any link between

History of Hypnosis

Franz Anton Mesmer, a German physician, introduced hypnosis to the medical community in the late eighteenth century under the name Mesmerism. Mesmer theorized that a universal fluid present in all objects produced disease when it was out of balance in the human body. But Mesmer soon fell out of favor and was banned from France after a committee headed by American statesman Benjamin Franklin and Joseph de Guillotin, a French physician, could not verify his findings. James Braid, an English ophthalmologist, later changed the name to hypnosis based on "hypnos," the Greek word for sleep. Although hypnosis is not sleep, the word became entrenched in the English vocabulary.

In the mid-1800s, James Esdaile, an English surgeon stationed in India, performed a variety of operations using only hypnotic anesthesia. Some of the surgical procedures he performed while administering hypnosis included amputations of the arm, breast, and penis, as well as the removal of tumors.

One of the more well-known proponents of hypnosis was Sigmund Freud, the nineteenth century father of modern psychiatry. Freud delivered two papers on the subject, and included it in his own practice. "There was something positively seductive in working with hypnosis," he wrote. "For the first time there was a sense of having overcome one's helplessness; and it was highly flattering to enjoy the reputation of being a miracle worker."

By the early 1890s, however, Freud rejected hypnosis in favor of his own theories of analysis and, shortly afterward, the practice became the focus of dispute, disagreement, and argument. It wasn't until the middle of this century that the British and American Medical Societies recognized its use as an adjunct to treating pain.

the man's condition and his unconscious beliefs. It was discovered that within his unconscious he doubted his ability to provide for his family and that his condition took care of that need by enabling him to collect worker's compensation pay. Lalonde worked with the man to change his belief. As he gained confidence in himself, his pain began to diminish. At the end of twelve sessions, the man was free of all pain and the temperature of his foot returned to normal, something his doctors had told him would not be possible.

Dentistry is another field where hypnotherapy has been used with excellent results. Kay Thompson, D.D.S., of Pittsburgh, Pennsylvania, regularly uses hypnotherapy in her practice. She describes how hypnotherapy was used to extract a molar in a patient who was allergic to all novocaine-type drugs.

To prepare the patient for the extraction, Dr. Thompson taught her how to go into a trance using hypnotic induction techniques. After one session with the patient, Dr. Thompson was able to perform the extraction using only hypnosis. Because the molar was so badly decayed, the operation lasted forty-five minutes, yet the patient had no swelling or discomfort afterward, and even ate dinner that night. Meanwhile, a co-worker who underwent a similar procedure without hypnosis needed two days off from work because of a swollen jaw, according to Dr. Thompson.

"Most people are not aware that they can control their own healing and even influence their circulation," says Dr. Thompson, who believes that her patient's ability to control her circulatory system through hypnosis enhanced the healing process. Dr. Thompson and her colleagues have also used hypnotherapy to help treat hemophiliacs, and have been able to perform surgery on these patients without them having any postoperative bleeding.

The long-term benefits of hypnotherapy are beginning to be borne out. One comprehensive study of 178 patients suffering from chronic pain between 1981 and 1983 reported that 78 percent remained pain-free after six months; 47 percent after one year; 44 percent after two years; and 36.5 percent after three years.[4] Another study showed the efficacy of hypnotherapy as compared to psychoanalysis and behavior therapy. After 600 sessions of psychoanalysis, 38 percent of the patients reported recovery from their conditions; those receiving behavior therapy improved in 72 percent of all cases after twenty-two sessions; while hypnotherapy produced a 93 percent success rate after only six sessions.[5]

How Hypnotherapy Works

"All hypnosis is self-hypnosis," states A. M. Krasner, Ph.D., founder and Director of the American Institute of Hypnotherapy in Santa Ana, California. "The hypnotherapist is a facilitator. The fact is that there can be no hypnosis unless the client is willing to participate in the process. The client always enters hypnosis in a natural way, of his or her own accord, simply by following the suggestions of the hypnotherapist."

Generally speaking, hypnosis is an artificially induced state characterized by a heightened receptivity to suggestion. The state is attained by first relaxing the body, then shifting attention away from the external environment toward a narrow range of objects or ideas as suggested by the hypnotherapist or by oneself (self-hypnosis).

In the *superficial* hypnotic state, the patient accepts suggestions but does not necessarily carry them out. Patients who reach the deep, or *somnambulistic*, state benefit most from hypnotherapy. It is in this state that posthypnotic suggestions (suggestions that take effect after the patient awakens from the trance) to relieve pain are most successful. According to the World Health Organization (WHO), 90 percent of the general population can be hypnotized, with 20 to 30 percent having a high enough susceptibility to enter the somnambulistic state, making them highly receptive to treatment.[6]

Research has demonstrated that a person's body chemistry actually changes during a hypnotic trance. In one experiment, a young girl was unable to hold her hand in a bucket of ice water for more than thirty seconds. Testing showed that the blood levels of cortisol in her body were high, indicating she was undergoing severe stress. Under hypnosis, she was able to keep the same hand in ice water for thirty minutes while there was no rise in blood cortisol levels.[7]

See Mind/Body Medicine.

There are many ways of inducing hypnosis. Regardless of what procedure is used, the main concern during hypnosis is to quiet the patient's conscious mind and to make the unconscious mind more accessible. Because the unconscious mind is basically noncritical, suggestions have a better chance of being effective than they would if given during a normal waking state.

Three conditions are essential to successful hypnotherapy: 1) rapport between hypnotist and subject; 2) a comfortable environment, free of distraction; and 3) a willingness and desire by the subject to be hypnotized. People who benefit most from hypnotherapy are those who understand that hypnosis is not a surrender of control; it is only an advanced form of relaxation.

"Research has demonstrated that a person's body chemistry actually changes during a hypnotic trance."

"The client must be led to accept his or her physician-hypnotist's words as valid descriptions of reality," says Dr. Tinterow. "The physician-hypnotist must manipulate his or her words and the situations in such a way as to lead the subject to believe that the suggestions are literally true statements. These suggestions should be accepted without criticism or analysis."

Dr. Tinterow had the fifteen-year-old girl on whom he performed open heart surgery concentrate on her favorite sport—water skiing. "It was just a matter of having her take deep breaths, close her eyes, and feel herself relaxing from the top of her head to the tips of her toes," he recalls. "You start with the feet and legs and then just have it go all the way to the top of the head."

Eventually Dr. Tinterow distracted the girl from the surgical procedure by shifting her attention to what she liked to do best. "I told her to picture herself going to the lake and getting on the skis and waterskiing. She was listening to music with her headset on, and we just kept talking to her." Dr. Tinterow even had the girl perform simple arithmetic problems during the surgery to make sure her mind was functioning properly. Dr. Tinterow adds that after the operation the girl didn't even take an aspirin.

What to Expect During a Hypnotherapy Session

During an initial visit to a hypnotherapist it's common for the therapist to address any concerns that you may have and then perhaps illustrate how suggestion works in everyday life, as well as point out what you can expect while in a trance state. Possible effects, according to Dr. Krasner, include physical relaxation, distraction of the conscious mind, a narrowed focus of attention, increased sensory awareness, reduced awareness of physical surroundings, and increased awareness of internal sensations. Following this, you might then be tested for suggestibility based on a variety of methods at the hypnotherapist's disposal.

You may also be asked about your specific condition. The value of this, according to Anne H. Spencer, Ph.D., C.Ht., founder of the International Medical and Dental Hypnotherapy Association, is that it provides the hypnotherapist with insights into any pattern associated with the condition, as well as an idea of what the client's goals are in terms of wellness. "What I look for in this discussion," says Dr. Spencer, "are clues as to how my client deals with life, as well as indications of any beliefs which may be contributing to his or her condition. These clues very often can then provide me with the most effective approach to use in the actual hypnotherapy session."

A hypnotherapy session will usually last from one hour to ninety minutes. The number of sessions required to produce results varies according to each individual. According to Dr. Spencer, six to twelve sessions, once a week, is about the average.

Although hypnosis is a very safe practice in the hands of a qualified practitioner, it is a very powerful tool that should be used only with utmost caution. WHO cautions that hypnosis should not be performed on patients with psychosis, organic psychiatric conditions, or antisocial personality disorders.

Is Hypnotherapy Safe for Everyone?

Although hypnosis is a very safe practice in the hands of a qualified practitioner, it is a very powerful tool that should be used only with utmost caution. WHO cautions that hypnosis should not be performed on patients with psychosis, organic psychiatric conditions, or antisocial personality disorders.

Hypnotherapy is not a cure-all and few doctors are willing to invest the time to master its techniques. Many patients, because of the severity of their conditions, do not make good subjects and are unable to reach the proper depth for posthypnotic suggestions to be effective.

The Future of Hypnotherapy

Since its formal sanction by the AMA in 1958, more and more physicians have come to accept hypnotherapy's value and are making fuller use of its techniques. While hypnosis is still far from being fully understood, it is scientifically respected and has achieved almost unanimous professional acceptance. Experiments to determine how hypnosis works and to quantify its effects are ongoing. And new breakthroughs on how hypnotherapy may be applied to medical and psychological problems are constantly being reported.

In hospitals today, it is not at all uncommon to find on staff an anesthesiologist, surgeon, nurse, or therapist who is also a trained hypnotherapist. As George Pratt, Ph.D., a clinical psychologist and hypnotherapist in La Jolla, California, notes, "With its focus on the whole person, hypnosis holds the great promise of becoming a humanizing force for the field of medicine as a whole . . . Realizing that even unconscious patients hear and remember information that pertains to them, physicians, surgeons, nurses, and anesthesiologists will communicate more effectively with comatose, critically ill, and anesthetized patients, thus replacing fear and isolation with encouragement and positive expectations."[8]

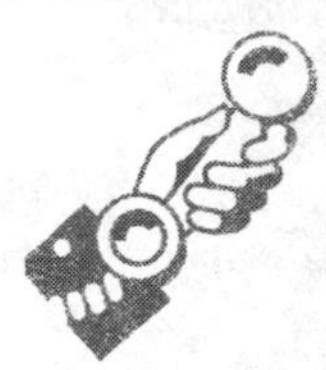

Where to Find Help

In choosing a hypnotherapist to treat your condition, it is important that you be assured that he or she has been competently trained and certified. The following organizations can refer you to legitimate practitioners in your area:

The American Institute of Hypnotherapy
1805 East Garry Avenue
Suite 100
Santa Ana, California 92705
(714) 261-6400

Trains and certifies hypnotherapists in a wide range of hypnotherapy applications. Also the only institution of its kind to be authorized to grant a doctorate degree in hypnosis. Provides a comprehensive range of books and tapes on all aspects of hypnotherapy.

The American Society of Clinical Hypnosis
2200 East Devon Avenue
Suite 291
Des Plaines, Illinois 60018
(708) 297-3317

Membership is comprised of M.D.'s and dentists trained in the use of hypnosis for treating health conditions. Send a stamped, self-addressed envelope for referrals to practitioners in your area.

International Medical and Dental Hypnotherapy Association
4110 Edgeland, Suite 800
Royal Oak, Michigan 48073
(313) 549-5594
(800) 257-5467 Outside Michigan

Trains and certifies M.D.'s, dentists, and hypnotherapists in the therapeutic use of hypnotherapy for treating health challenges. Has members throughout the United States, Canada, Europe, Japan, Mexico, and the Virgin Islands. Provides a referral list of certified practitioners throughout the United States and Canada, available by sending a stamped, self-addressed envelope.

The National Guild of Hypnotists
P.O. Box 308
Merrimack, New Hampshire 03054
(603) 429-9438

The oldest certifying guild in the United States. Offers basic certification programs and trainer programs, and supplies a complete range of books and tapes on hypnotherapy.

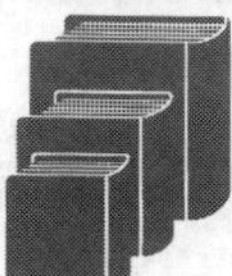

Recommended Reading

Hypnosis, Acupuncture and Pain. Tinterow, Maurice M., M.D. Wichita, KA: Bio-Communication Press, 1989.

Tinterow's techniques combine hypnosis and acupuncture to relieve pain and physical suffering.

Hypnotherapy. Elman, Dave. Glendale, CA: Westwood Publishing Company, 1984.

This classic text provides a comprehensive look at the many therapeutic applications of hypnosis, including actual transcripts of sessions treating a variety of physical conditions. Originally written for doctors, this book nonetheless provides a fascinating overview of hypnotherapy for the lay reader.

The Wizard Within: The Krasner Method of Clinical Hypnotherapy. Krasner, A. M., Ph.D. Santa Ana, CA: American Board of Hypnotherapy Press, 1990.

A straightforward explanation of hypnotherapy, including its history, applications, and a broad sampling of induction techniques. Also includes a comprehensive chapter on self-hypnosis applications.

"The art of medicine consists of amusing the patient while Nature cures the disease."

—Voltaire

Juice Therapy

Juice therapy uses the fresh, raw juice of vegetables and fruits to nourish and replenish the body. Used as nutritional support during periods of stress and illness, juice therapy can also be used as part of a comprehensive health maintenance plan.

For centuries, plant juices and extracts have been used for their healing and medicinal properties. The word chemical comes from the Greek word *chemia*, meaning "the juice of a plant."

Juice therapy offers a balanced way to supplement the diet, according to Steven Bailey, N.D., of the Northwestern Naturopathic Clinic in Portland, Oregon. "One of the most convenient therapies available is the use of raw fruit and vegetable juices to augment the typical diet. Juice can also aid in a patient's treatment program by stimulating the immune system, reducing blood pressure, aiding in detoxification, and protecting the body from harmful environmental factors. It is also used to help diagnose and treat food allergies, and is the ideal nutritional remedy for individuals suffering from nausea or digestive problems."

The Healing Properties of Juice

Juice therapy follows a system of cleansing and restoration, and uses fresh juices to provide a nutritional foundation for the body's curative processes. Fresh juices play an important role with virtually any regime to cleanse the body and restore vitality. With juice therapy, nutrients are supplied in a concentrated, raw, and unprocessed form that is easy to consume and digest, making juice an ideal companion to fasting and health maintenance regimens.

Juicing is the easiest and most efficient method for extracting the high level of nutrients stored within the individual cells of fruits and vegetables. When a fruit or vegetable is juiced, the fibrous plant cell wall is cut open and the juice of the cell, which contains the cell sap, sugars, starches, proteins, enzymes, and other nutrients, is released.

Nutritional Qualities

Fresh fruit and vegetable juices are a concentrated source of energy, and are rich in carbohydrates, vitamins, and minerals. "By separating the juice from the pulp, you end up with a liquid that contains most of the nutrients with a much reduced mass," says Dr. Bailey. "For example, it takes approximately five pounds of carrots to make one quart of carrot juice. Although eating five pounds of vegetables two to three times a day is nearly impossible, most people can easily drink two to three quarts of juice a day."

Juices with a high content of vitamin C, such as citrus fruits or cabbage, help the body absorb iron when added to a meal.[1] This is particularly beneficial for the health of children, who often get inadequate amounts of iron from their diets.

Nutrient-rich juices, such as collard and kale, may also be added to soups and stews or used as a substitute for other liquids in cooking recipes. Ideally, the juices are added last to minimize heat destruction of vitamins and enzymes.

Since fruit juices have a high sugar content and ferment rapidly in the stomach, they should be diluted with water 1:1. People with diabetes or hypoglycemia should be sure to only drink fruit juices with food. Tomato and orange juices are not recommended as they are highly acidic and tend to upset the body's natural pH (acid-base) balance.

Nutrients Found in Juices

Nutrient	Juice
Beta-carotene	Carrot, cantaloupe, papaya
Folic acid	Orange, kale, broccoli
Vitamin B_6	Kale, spinach, turnip greens
Vitamin C	Peppers, citrus fruit, cabbage
Vitamin E	Asparagus, spinach
Vitamin K	Broccoli, collard, kale
Calcium	Kale, collard greens, bok choy
Chromium	Apple, cabbage, sweet peppers
Manganese	Brussels sprouts, cabbage, turnip greens
Potassium	Celery, cantaloupe, tomato
Selenium	Apple, turnip, garlic
Zinc	Carrot, ginger, green peas

Vegetable juices are used extensively in fasting and as nutritional supplements because of their high vitamin and mineral content. Fruit juices, however, provide a quicker pick-me-up as they are immediately absorbed.

Fruit juices also remain stable for a longer period of time and "travel" better than vegetable juices, which oxidize quickly, breaking down the protective enzymes and vitamins. It is always preferable to juice fresh, organic fruits and vegetables oneself just prior to drinking in order to maximize nutritional value. If this isn't possible, juices should be purchased from a health food store the same day that they are made.

Medicinal Qualities

Many fruits and vegetables have scientifically proven medicinal qualities. So far, scientific studies have documented only the medicinal effects of fruit juices, with very little research applied to vegetable juices. Cherie Calbom, M.S., C.N., a nutritionist from Seattle, Washington, and co-author of *Juicing For Life*, recommends the following juice remedies:

- **Apple:** Apples are rich in sorbitol, a form of sugar and a gentle laxative.
- **Apple, grape, and blueberry:** These fruits are a source of polyphenols (an antioxidant). In laboratory tests, polyphenols have been shown to kill viruses.[2]
- **Beet:** Beet greens are rich in magnesium, beta-carotene, vitamin C, and vitamin E. Beetroot is rich in potassium, folic acid, and the antioxidant glutathione. Beet juice is valued for its vitamin, mineral, and nutrient content. Due to its strong taste, it should be mixed with other juices.

- **Blueberry and cranberry:** When consumed on a regular basis, these juices can help prevent recurrent urinary tract infections.[3]
- **Cabbage:** Cabbage juice is famous for its ulcer-healing capabilities,[4] but should be used only in conjunction with a doctor's prescribed therapy for ulcer treatment.
- **Cantaloupe:** Cantaloupe has a blood-thinning effect that can help prevent heart attacks and strokes.[5]
- **Carrot:** Carrot juice is an excellent source of beta-carotene, potassium, trace minerals, and anticancer nutrients including phthalide and glutathione (antioxidants). Yellowish coloration of the skin may occur when large amounts are consumed. This coloration is harmless, and will fade when consumption is reduced.
- **Celery:** Celery juice contains the anticancer nutrients phthalide and polyacetylene (antioxidants). It is rich in potassium and sodium and helps lower blood pressure. Celery juice can be diluted with water and used as a sports drink to replace fluid and mineral loss due to sweating. It contains the same ulcer-healing factors found in cabbage juice.
- **Cherry:** A traditional remedy for the pain of gout.
- Garlic: This herb is a treasure house of healing compounds. It acts as a natural antibiotic and blood thinner and can reduce cholesterol levels.[6] Juice a clove and add it to your favorite vegetable mix.
- **Ginger:** The root of the ginger plant has anti-inflammatory properties and will also protect the stomach from irritation caused by nonsteroidal anti-inflammatory drugs.[7] Migraines and motion sickness can also be relieved by ginger juice.[8] A small amount goes a long way; use only one-quarter- to one-half-inch slice per drink.
- **Lemon:** Lemon juice is a traditional appetite stimulant. Place one or two tablespoons of fresh, unsweetened lemon juice in a glass of water and drink half an hour before meals. This remedy stimulates the flow of saliva and digestive juices.
- **Pineapple:** The raw juice of this plant contains the enzyme bromelain. Bromelain has been shown to have gentle anti-inflammatory properties.[9] Swish the raw juice around the site of a tooth extraction to reduce swelling or eat a frozen pineapple juice pop to soothe a sore throat.
- **Fruit juice:** A glass of fruit juice (lemon juice excepted) one hour before dinner will act as a natural appetite suppressant due to the sugar in the juice.

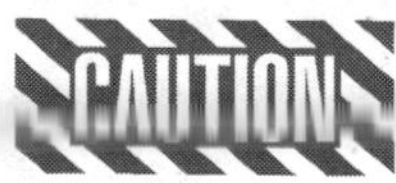

The information on the nutritional qualities of juices is intended to supplement, not replace, the advice of a trained health professional. If you know or suspect that you have a health problem, consult your doctor.

Juices as Preventive Agents

The qualities listed below are found in specific juices and can be useful when dealing with cancer and other degenerative diseases.

Anticarcinogenic: Certain substances found in fruits and vegetables can prevent carcinogens from reaching and reacting with the body's tissues.[10] These substances, dubbed "anutrients," are found in cabbage, kale, broccoli, cauliflower, garlic, onions, leeks, shallots, oranges, grapefruit, and lemons. Anutrients act as blocking agents to prevent carcinogens from reaching or reacting with tissues, and work by creating a barrier between the carcinogen and its target.[11]

Suppressive: Certain nutrients act as agents to suppress the development of cancer in a cell already exposed to a carcinogen. These include D-limonene (an antioxidant), found in oranges; vitamin A, found in carotene-rich fruits and vegetables; calcium, found in leafy greens; and antioxidant nutrients (beta-carotene, vitamin C, vitamin E, and selenium), found in orange and green fruits and vegetables.[12]

"Certain substances found in fruits and vegetables can prevent carcinogens from reaching and reacting with the body's tissues."

Growth Retarding: Cells that exhibit a marked increase in their rate of division after exposure to certain chemicals are more susceptible to cancer-causing agents. Phthalides and polyacetylenes, compounds found in carrots, celery, and parsley, act indirectly to decrease cell duplication rates by regulating prostaglandin E-2 (hormone-like fatty acids) production. Other compounds found in garlic and onions also modulate prostaglandin synthesis, which regulates white blood cells in the body's immune system.[13]

See Detoxification Therapy, Environmental Medicine, Fasting.

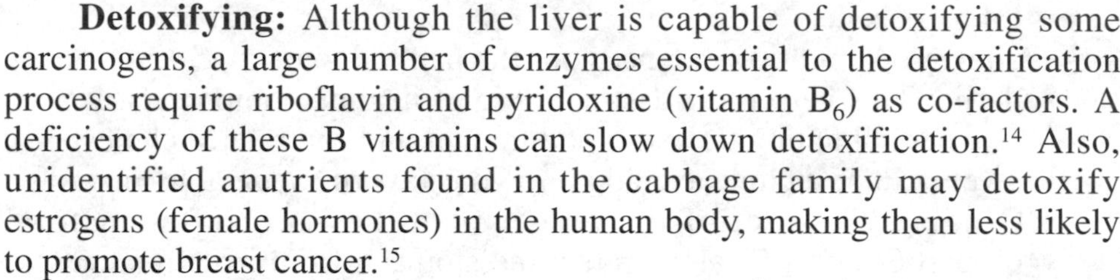

Detoxifying: Although the liver is capable of detoxifying some carcinogens, a large number of enzymes essential to the detoxification process require riboflavin and pyridoxine (vitamin B_6) as co-factors. A deficiency of these B vitamins can slow down detoxification.[14] Also, unidentified anutrients found in the cabbage family may detoxify estrogens (female hormones) in the human body, making them less likely to promote breast cancer.[15]

Conditions Benefited by Juice Therapy

Dr. Bailey utilizes juice therapy in the form of fasts and nutritional supplementation for a variety of conditions, including allergies and arthritis, and as an adjunct therapy with cancer and AIDS patients.

Another benefit of juicing is derived from the rich supply of enzymes contained in the fruits and vegetables. "When fruits or vegetables are juiced, their enzymes are released and immediately go to work when they are consumed," says Dr. Bailey. "This aids the body in its constant work of dissolving and eliminating wastes, as well as speeding delivery of the vital nutrients contained in the juice."

Also, juice therapy in the form of juice fasts can help identify food sensitivities, according to Dr. Bailey. "A hypo-allergenic (lowered potential for causing an allergic reaction) juice fast of five or more days will frequently result in either significant improvement or complete elimination of chronic symptoms caused by undetected food allergies and sensitivities," he observes. "The recurrence of old symptoms following a return to the normal diet allows the patient to identify and remove the allergic food."

One of Dr. Bailey's patients, a woman diagnosed with rheumatoid arthritis, had been on prescription medicines for twenty-five years with only minimal relief. A juice fast supervised by Dr. Bailey indicated an allergy to potatoes. Since their removal from her diet, she has remained symptom and drug free.

Many of Dr. Bailey's patients have been alleviated of symptoms related to allergies such as rashes, digestive problems, chronic urinary or prostate problems, emotional swings, muscle and joint pain, and respiratory problems, while on a prescribed juice program. Dr. Bailey maintains that conventional allergy tests can often be inconclusive for food sensitivities. He has found juice fasting to be one of the least expensive, most accurate methods available.

A thirty-year-old man with a three-plus-year condition of chronic prostatis came to Dr. Bailey as an alternative to conventional medicine which had yet to have any success with long term antibiotic therapy. The patient's symptoms improved with diet changes, increased fluid intake, and herbal medicines, but it was only after a two week juice fast with accompanying herbal therapy that he became symptom free. His prostate has remained stable and uninfected for seven years.

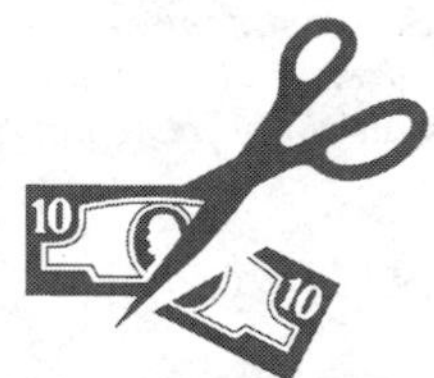

Juice therapy is a cost-effective means to help maintain health and deal with some common health problems.

Dr. Bailey believes that juice therapy can help provide cancer patients with an excellent nutritional foundation and can strengthen the body's curative processes. The addition of juices to the diet can help supply the required nutrients in a form that is easy to assimilate.

Dr. Bailey also uses juice therapy as an adjunct in the treatment of AIDS patients. At advanced stages these patients are often weak and nauseated, making normal eating difficult. Using vegetable juices allows them to maintain a higher nutritional state, and helps to retain strength and muscle mass.

For maintaining optimum health, Dr. Bailey recommends at least two five-day juice fasts per year, one in the spring and one in the fall. Juice fasts should not be undertaken during the cold months, as the body creates heat through the metabolic processes needed to digest a regular solid diet. Dr. Bailey recommends a beet/carrot/celery blend and excludes citrus and tomatoes, as he considers them common allergens, and too acidic.

"I did my first ten-day juice cleanse in 1975, and the experience changed my life and health."

—Elson Haas, M.D.

Elson Haas, M.D., of San Rafael, California, also uses juice fasts as a form of medical therapy. According to Dr. Haas, he has used juice fasting regularly himself, as have thousands of his patients over the course of nearly twenty years. "I did my first ten-day juice cleanse in 1975, and the experience changed my life and health. I realized the importance of diet and fasting in preventing disease and maintaining health. I cleared my allergies and back pains, normalized my weight, and felt a new level of vitality and creativity." Dr. Haas finds juice therapy very helpful with congestion of colds and flus, recurrent infections, allergies, skin disorders, and gastrointestinal problems, as well as other congestive or chronic disorders.

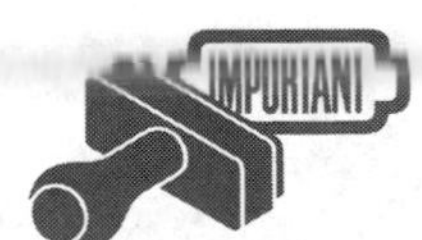

Due to the high amount of pesticides and residual chemicals found in today's foods, it is important to select organically grown fruits and vegetables, as these often contain a more complete vitamin and mineral base. If possible, avoid irradiated fruits and vegetables.

Juice therapy can also benefit athletic training, because fresh juices take a fraction of the energy needed to digest solid foods. Portland marathon winner Debra Myra set her collegiate personal records for one thousand, five thousand, and ten thousand meters while on a supervised juice fast with Dr. Bailey.

Juice therapy can be used to maintain an increased nutrient need, and can be combined with other dietary regimens. Because juicing removes

Consult a health professional before any fast. Infants, young children, and the elderly should not practice juice fasting.

the fiber from the fruit or vegetable, juices are not a whole food and should not be considered a dietary substitute for whole fruits and vegetables. However, juices in their raw and unprocessed form are an excellent supplement to a whole foods, low-fat diet. It is also important to use organically grown fruits and vegetables that are free of pesticides, as these often contain a more complete vitamin and mineral base.

There are very few contraindications to juice therapy. Never drink juices from fruits or vegetables that you are allergic or sensitive to. If you react to sugars (are hypo- or hyperglycemic), dilute high sugar content juices such as carrot and beet with other low sugar juices such as celery. Always dilute fruit juices with water 1:1. Consider stabilizing blood sugar with juices of Jerusalem artichokes and green beans. If yeast is a concern, add two cloves of garlic per quart of juice. Avoid juice fasts if you are pregnant or lactating. For diabetics, close supervision is required.

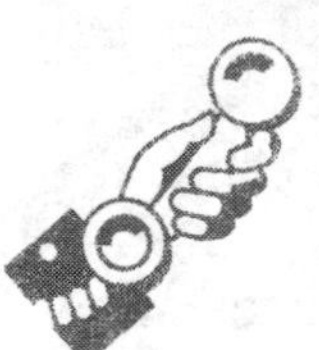

Where to Find Help

There is much helpful, published information on the use of juice. Below are some sources to contact.

American Association of Naturopathic Physicians
2366 Eastlake Avenue, Suite 322
Seattle, Washington 98102
(206) 323-7610

Contact this association to locate a naturopathic physician who practices juice therapy anywhere in the United States.

Choices Magazine
Trillium Health Products
655 South Orcas, Suite 220
Seattle, Washington 98108
(206) 762-8403

A monthly magazine devoted to juicing and natural living. It prints articles on nutrition and diet, juicing techniques, and fresh juice recipes, as well as fitness and exercise.

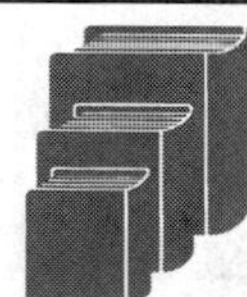

Recommended Reading

The Complete Book of Juicing. Murray, Michael. Rocklin, CA: Prima Publishing, 1992.

The author of this book is a licensed naturopathic physician. He includes juice drink recipes as well as information on the nutritional content of various fruits and vegetables. This book stresses disease prevention and includes recommendations for juicing programs for all age levels. Also includes a buying guide as well as a glossary of the nutrient and anutrient content of various fruits and vegetables.

Juicing for Good Health. Keane, Maureen B. New York: Pocket Books, 1992.

Juicing for Life. Calbom, Cherie, and Keane, Maureen B. New York: Avery Publishing Group, 1992.

Written in easy-to-understand language, this book provides complete nutritional programs for dealing with over fifty health problems.

Light Therapy

Light and color have been valued throughout history as sources of healing. Today, the therapeutic applications of light and color are being investigated in major hospitals and research centers worldwide. Results indicate that full-spectrum, ultraviolet, colored, and laser light can have therapeutic value for a range of conditions from chronic pain and depression to immune disorders and cancer.

Many health disorders can be traced to problems with the circadian rhythm, the body's inner clock, and how it governs the timing of sleep, hormone production, body temperature, and other biological functions. Disturbances in this rhythm can lead to health problems such as depression and sleep disorders. Natural sunlight and various forms of light therapy can help reestablish the body's natural rhythm and are becoming an integral treatment for many related health conditions.

More recently, the ability of light to activate certain chemicals has become the basis of treatment for skin disorders such as psoriasis and for certain forms of cancer. Exposure to ultraviolet light under controlled conditions has also proved beneficial for certain conditions, particularly when combined with light-sensitive medications.

How Light Therapy Works

When light enters the eye, millions of light- and color-sensitive cells called photoreceptors convert the light into electrical impulses. These impulses travel along the optic nerve to the brain where they trigger the hypothalamus gland to send chemical messengers called neurotransmitters to regulate the autonomic (automatic) functions of the body.

The hypothalamus is part of the endocrine system whose secretions govern most bodily functions—blood pressure, body temperature, breathing, digestion, sexual function, moods, the immune system, the aging process, and the circadian rhythm. Full-spectrum light (containing all wavelengths) sparks the delicate impulses that regulate these functions and maintain health.

After twenty years of clinical research, John Downing, O.D., Ph.D., Director of the Light Therapy Department at the Preventive Medical

Center of Marin in San Rafael, California, has expanded the theory regarding the action of visually perceived light to encompass its effects on other areas of the brain, including the cerebral cortex, where it stimulates motivation, learning, thinking, creativity, memory, and even motor cortex body movements; the limbic system, where visually perceived light brings in the emotional impressions of the world; and the brain stem, where light helps to provide coordination and balance.

The Importance of Natural Sunlight

Poor light poses a serious threat to health, according to the numerous published studies of photobiologist John Nash Ott, D.Sc. (Hon.).[1] He firmly believes that the kind of light adequate for maintaining health must contain the full wavelength spectrum found in natural sunlight.

Most artificial lighting, both incandescent and fluorescent, lacks the complete balanced spectrum of sunlight and, as Dr. Ott discovered, interferes with the body's optimal absorption of nutrients, a condition he calls "malillumination." Windows, windshields, eyeglasses, smog, and suntan lotions all filter out parts of the light spectrum and contribute to this problem. Research reveals that if certain wavelengths aren't present in light, the body can't fully absorb certain nutrients.[2] Malillumination contributes to fatigue, tooth decay, depression, hostility, suppressed immune function, strokes, hair loss, skin damage, alcoholism, drug abuse, Alzheimer's disease, and cancer.[3] It has also been linked, in a recent study at the Clinical Pathology Department of the National Institutes of Health, to a loss of muscle tone and strength.[4]

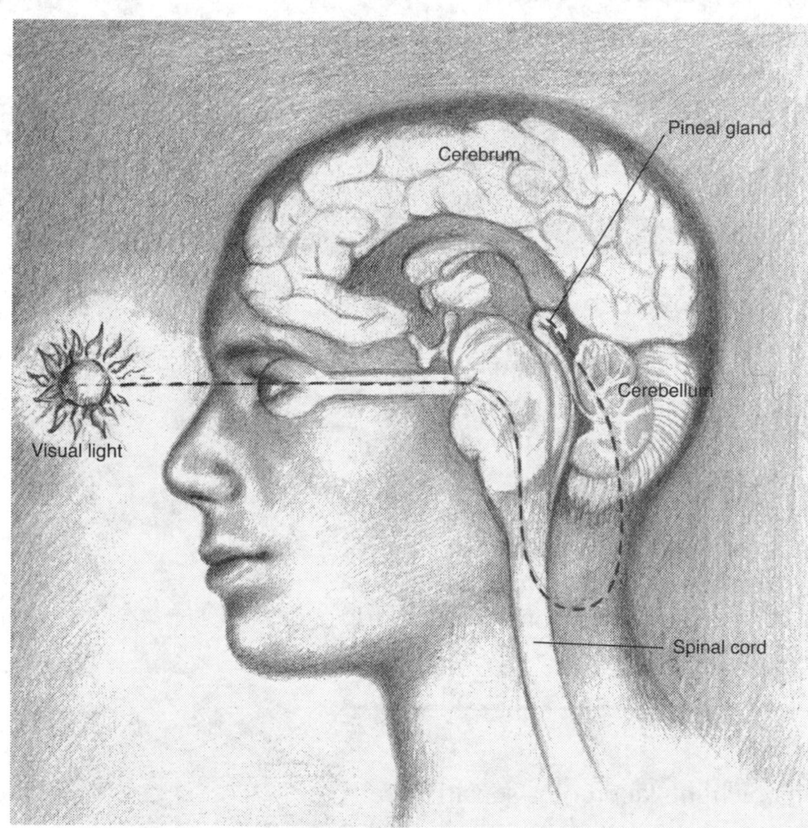

The interactions of light with the brain.

According to John Zimmerman, Ph.D, founder and President of Bio-Electro-Magnetics Institute in Reno, Nevada, most offices, even those with uncovered windows and the lights on, have a light level of only 500 lux (the international unit of illumination, one lumen per square meter), as compared to outdoor light, which has about 50,000 lux, or approximately 100 times more. Night shift workers are usually exposed to a light level of only 50 lux.

According to Dr. Downing, "By spending 90 percent of our lives indoors, under inadequate lighting conditions, we cause or worsen a wide range of health problems, including depression, heart disease, hyperactivity in children, osteoporosis in the elderly, and lowered resistance to infection."[5] In order to maintain health it is important to be exposed to light containing the full wavelength spectrum found in natural sunlight.

See Energy Medicine.

A recent study carried out by the U.S. Navy compared the risk of melanoma (a malignant, dark pigmented skin mole or tumor) for different naval occupations. It was discovered that personnel holding indoor occupations had the highest incidence rate of melanoma while workers in occupations that required spending time both indoors and outdoors had the lowest rate. In addition, a higher rate of melanoma occurred on the trunk of the body as opposed to the head and arms which are commonly exposed to sunlight. The authors of the study theorized that the anatomical site of melanoma suggests a "protective role for brief, regular exposure to sunlight."[6]

This is in keeping with recent laboratory studies that show vitamin D (whose production is stimulated by ultraviolet light) suppresses the growth of malignant melanoma cells. These new findings also call into question the belief that indoor occupations can provide safety for fair-skinned, freckled individuals who are at high risk for skin cancers. This and other studies indicate that an occupational deprivation of sunlight can lead to a vitamin D deficiency, which in turn could favor the development of melanoma.[7]

Light and the Internal Clock

The body's internal clock, known as the circadian system, is regulated by the pineal gland. This gland is controlled by the presence or absence of external light, and serves to synchronize and coordinate the biological events of the body.

Melatonin, the chief hormone of the pineal gland, is produced only during darkness. Its production is actually inhibited by light. Melatonin has sedative qualities and helps reduce anxiety, panic disorders, and migraines as well as inducing sleep. It is also thought to be a primary regulator of the immune system.

Researchers have found that when a person ignores the twenty-four-hour dark-light cycle and keeps irregular hours of work and rest, the body's internal rhythms go awry. The number of hours one sleeps is less important than when one sleeps in respect to daylight.

People who work in rotating shifts or at night have been shown to experience a higher incidence of heart disease, back pain, respiratory problems, ulcers, and sleep disorders. These people also have a higher rate of error and accidents and often experience a significant loss of alertness and ability to make decisions. However, researchers are using carefully timed, high-intensity bright lighting (five to ten times brighter than ordinary room level), as well as the administration of melatonin to help shift workers adjust to their schedules.[12]

Travel between time zones often results in jet lag, a less serious, but often debilitating and disorienting condition caused by the upset of the body's internal clock. Melatonin, full-spectrum, and bright light therapies are being explored as useful antidotes. Some airports are now considering the installation of full-spectrum lights in their first class lounges to help passengers adjust to their destination time zones.

Forms of Light Therapy

The oldest form of light therapy is natural sunlight. The sun is the ultimate source of full-spectrum light, which means it contains all possible wavelengths of light, from infrared to ultraviolet (UV). Numerous forms of light therapy are now also available, including full-spectrum light therapy, bright light therapy, various forms of UV light therapy, syntonic optometry, cold laser therapy, and colored light therapy. Electromagnetic devices such as the Light Beam Generator and the MORA™ also use specific light frequencies in treatment.

Full-Spectrum Light Therapy

Sunlight and full-spectrum light can be applied to the skin in order to relieve hypertension, depression, insomnia, premenstrual syndrome, migraines, and carbohydrate cravings associated with metabolic imbalances.[8] A ten-year epidemiological study conducted at Johns Hopkins University Medical School in Baltimore, Maryland, showed that exposure to full-spectrum light (including the ultraviolet frequency) is positively related to the prevention of breast, colon, and rectal cancers.[9]

“Most artificial lighting, both incandescent and fluorescent, lacks the complete balanced spectrum of sunlight and interferes with the body’s optimal absorption of nutrients, a condition known as ‘malillumination’. In order to maintain health it is important to be exposed to light containing the full wavelength spectrum found in natural sunlight.”

In Russia, a full-spectrum lighting system was installed in factories where colds and sore throats had become commonplace among workers. This lowered the bacterial contamination of the air by 40 to 70 percent. Workers who did not receive the full-spectrum light were absent twice as many days as those who did.[10]

In a recent study undertaken by Dr. Ott and his associates, Lewis Mayron, Ph.D., Rick Nations, Ph.D., and Ellen L. Mayron, M.S., the effect of full-spectrum lighting in the classroom was tested on first grade students in Sarasota, Florida. Using four classrooms, two as a control with standard fluorescent lighting, and two outfitted with full-spectrum lights, the researchers tracked the students behavior levels for a full semester, using a hidden camera. Their results demonstrated conclusively that the students exposed to the full-spectrum lighting had a marked diminishment of hyperactivity, whereas those in the control classrooms actually became more hyperactive.

A similar study in Wetaskiwin, Alberta, Canada, clearly showed that students in classrooms with full-spectrum light also had less absenteeism and a higher academic achievement record when compared with classes conducted under ordinary fluorescent lighting.[11]

SAD: Full-spectrum light and bright white light (often preferred because the additional UV light found in full-spectrum light is not necessary to achieve the antidepressant effect of the therapy, and can be harmful with protracted direct exposure to the eyes) are effective treatments for seasonal affective disorder (SAD), also known as the “winter blues.” The symptoms of SAD are depression, excess sleeping and eating, a withdrawn feeling, and lowered sex drive. It is currently being investigated by Charmane Eastman, Ph.D., Director of the Biological Rhythms Research Laboratory at Rush Presbyterian St. Luke’s Medical Center in Chicago.

Melatonin levels are found to be very high in patients with SAD. Daily exposure to sunlight or to full-spectrum light has been known to eliminate SAD symptoms.[13] In one study, SAD patients who took morning walks and received a minimum one hour of sunlight showed positive results.[14]

Light boxes are used in the majority of SAD cases. They measure two feet by two feet and enclose a full-spectrum light or bright white light that is angled toward the face. The patient sits about eighteen inches from the box, and without looking directly at the light, keeps the head and eyes toward the light while reading or doing other tasks. Most studies find that early morning sessions ranging from thirty minutes to two hours using varying intensities of light bring improvement within a week. [15]

Jaundice: Light therapy is used to treat jaundice in newborn babies. In 1956 Sister Ward of Rochford General Hospital in England discovered the treatment by accident. On warm summer days she would wheel the premature infants into the courtyard. One day a doctor came into the ward and noticed that an unclothed infant was pale yellow except for a bright yellow (heavily jaundiced) triangle across the abdomen. A few days later, laboratory tests on a blood specimen left on a windowsill showed a lower bilirubin (the pigment responsible for jaundice) level than when previously tested. These two events led to the discovery that sunlight was an effective therapy against jaundice. Today, newborns with jaundice are placed near a brightly lit window or, in extreme cases, under intense lights to correct the condition. Often an intense blue light is used since it has a higher luminosity than full-spectrum light.

Bright Light Therapy

"Bright light therapy involves the use of bright white light ranging in intensity from 2,000 to 5,000 lux," says Dr. Zimmerman. While the intensity of this light therapy isn't near that of sunlight (50,000 lux), it is significantly higher than that of the average office and workspace (50 to 500 lux). "Brighter lights in the workplace have been shown to reduce mistakes on the job, and drowsiness, especially among night shift workers," adds Dr. Zimmerman. Bright light therapy is also used to treat SAD and the following conditions:

Bulimia: Because of serotonin's involvement in appetite regulation, bright light therapy has proven helpful in cases of bulimia (bingeing on large amounts of food, followed by self-induced purging). "During two weeks of bright light therapy, seventeen women, twenty to forty-five years old, experienced a 50 percent reduction in the number of binges and purges, as well as in their feelings of depression," says Raymond W. Lam, M.D., assistant professor of psychiatry at the University of British Columbia, Vancouver.

Delayed Sleep Phase Syndrome: Delayed sleep phase syndrome [falling asleep late (2:30-3:00 A.M.)] may also be treated with bright light. "People who have delayed sleep phase syndrome have seen it disappear for the first time in their lives using light therapy," says Michael Terman, Ph.D., of the New York State Psychiatric Institute at Columbia Presbyterian Medical Center, New York. By getting a dose of bright light in the morning, the day starts earlier and patients fall asleep earlier at night. Bright light early in the night works similarly for those who fall asleep early and wake early, allowing them to sleep later.

See Female Health, Sleep Disorders.

Menstrual Cycles: Researchers two decades ago reported that a one-hundred-watt bedside light could shorten and regulate the menstrual cycles among women with long and irregular cycles. According to Daniel F. Kripke, M.D., a professor of psychiatry at the University of California, San Diego, "More recently, we repeated this experiment and achieved the same result. This needs more research, but it offers intriguing implications for treating infertility and improving upon contraception."

Ultraviolet Light Therapy

In the 1890s, Danish physician Niels Finsen observed that tubercular lesions occurred commonly during the winter but were very rare in the summer. He suspected a lack of sunlight to be the cause of the lesions and successfully treated skin tuberculosis with ultraviolet light. Known as the "father of photobiology," Dr. Finsen won the Nobel Prize in 1903 for his work. Today, ultraviolet light therapies are used to treat diseases ranging from high cholesterol to premenstrual syndrome and cancer.

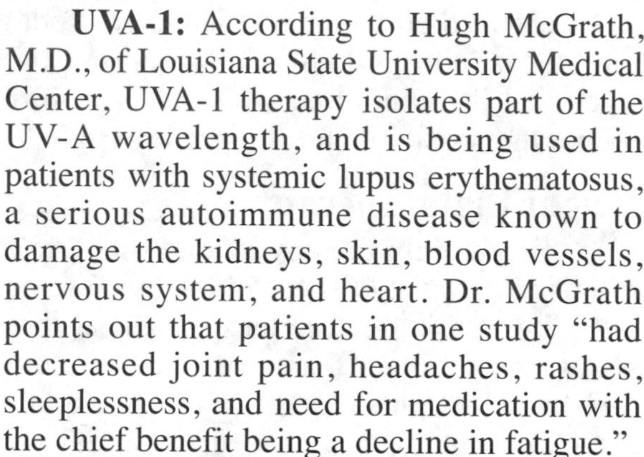

ULTRAVIOLET LIGHT AND THE SUN

Ultraviolet light from the sun can be divided into three types of rays: UV-A, UV-B, and UV-C, depending upon the wavelength.

Although there is some difference of opinion concerning the three types, generally UV-C is thought of as the most harmful, but because very little of it penetrates the ozone layer, it is not considered dangerous. UV-A penetrates the skin (responsible for slow tanning), but because it has the longest wavelength, it is considered the least harmful.

According to most sources, it is UV-B that poses the greatest danger to humans. UV-B easily penetrates the skin, is responsible for sunburn, and can damage the eyes. Similarly, UV-B reflected from snow can burn the cornea, causing snow blindness. UV-B reflected from the sand and water is responsible for burning the skin more than the direct UV-B rays from the sun. Too much exposure of the eyes to UV-B can result in cataracts, a clouding of the lens of the eye, so the eyes should always be protected in strong sunlight. Chronic exposure of the eyes to UV-B is also responsible for retinal damage, pterygium (abnormal growths on the cornea), and activation of ocular herpes.[17]

UVA-1: According to Hugh McGrath, M.D., of Louisiana State University Medical Center, UVA-1 therapy isolates part of the UV-A wavelength, and is being used in patients with systemic lupus erythematosus, a serious autoimmune disease known to damage the kidneys, skin, blood vessels, nervous system, and heart. Dr. McGrath points out that patients in one study "had decreased joint pain, headaches, rashes, sleeplessness, and need for medication with the chief benefit being a decline in fatigue."

Hemoirradiation: Also known as photophoresis, this therapy involves the removal of up to a pint of blood from the body, irradiating it with ultraviolet light, and reinjecting it. The absorbed light energy activates oxidation of the blood. (The process of hemooxidation therapy involves hemoirradiation of blood to which oxygen has been added.)

In his practice, William Campbell Douglass, M.D., of Clayton, Georgia, uses an instrument called the Photolume to irradiate blood with ultraviolet light. According to Dr. Douglass, ultraviolet light can have the following physiological effects: calcium metabolism improves; body toxins become inert; bacteria are killed either directly or indirectly (by increased systemic resistance); chemical balances are restored; and oxygen absorption is increased. He has successfully used ultraviolet light therapy to treat infections, cancer, rheumatoid arthritis, bronchial asthma, and symptoms of AIDS. His method has also been used to improve peripheral blood circulation in the treatment of blood poisoning.[16]

See Oxygen Therapy.

PUVA Light Therapy: In PUVA (psoralen UV-A) light therapy, patients are first given the light sensitive drug psoralen, and one to two hours later are exposed to full-body UV light. This approach is used to treat vitiligo, a depigmentation problem, and works by stimulating pigment-producing cells to come to the skin surface.

Psoriasis, a chronic skin disease, also responds to PUVA light therapy. The ultraviolet light used in treatment helps stop the disease cells

Colored Light Therapy

There is mounting evidence that different colors of light have different effects on the body. In 1942, the Russian scientist S. V. Krakov demonstrated that red light stimulates the sympathetic nervous system, while white and blue light stimulate the parasympathetic nervous system. Earlier experiments revealed that certain colors stimulate hormone production, while other colors inhibit it.[18] Specific colors can also have an effect on specific diseases. In the late nineteenth and early twentieth centuries, it was noted that symptoms of acute eruptive diseases such as smallpox and measles were relieved when patients were put in a room with red windows. Melancholiacs also recovered after a few hours in such rooms.

Norman Shealy, M.D., Ph.D., of Springfield, Missouri, uses flashing bright lights and colored lights to treat pain and depression. According to Dr. Shealy, these treatments have been shown to alter neurochemical production in the brain and this may account for their positive effects. Dr. Shealy believes the brain has specific responses to different frequencies of flashing light and the different frequencies of various colors. "Sleep problems can often be cured in one day by this method," he says, "but mood alteration usually takes one to two weeks of treatments." Dr. Shealy believes that it is the relaxation induced by these methods that is responsible for the effects seen in patients suffering from pain. "I believe tension is a primary factor in 100 percent of pain," he says, "and once you relax the tension, the pain eases."

Dr. Shealy has found that photostimulation with flashing opaque white or violet lights induces relaxation, reducing stress and chronic pain. "Photostimulation, or brain wave synchronization, has been used as a tool to assist relaxation and the induction of hypnosis since 1948," he says. "It has been used with the EEG (electroencephalogram) as an adjunct to the diagnosis of epilepsy."

Another method of colored light therapy known as monochromatic red light therapy is used to treat a range of problems, including shoulder pain, endocrine problems, dysmenorrhea, diabetes, gastrointestinal problems, depression, impotence, and frigidity. Gerald Hall, D.C., of El Paso, Texas, uses monochromatic red light therapy to treat the acupoints of the ear as well as points elsewhere on the body.

Ray Fisch, Ph.D., C.H., of Los Angeles, uses monochromatic red light therapy for headaches (applying the light across the brow), arthritis, allergies, sore throats, sinus problems, stress reduction, and wound healing. The red light is also applied to acupressure points or to sites of localized pain. For localized pain such as tendinitis, two five-minute applications directly to the painful area are followed by ten to fifteen seconds to the surrounding area. This is followed by a gentle massage of the area. Treatment is repeated two to three times a day for a week, then twice a day for a week followed by once a day for another week. "There are virtually no side effects to this treatment, and it can be done at home," says Dr. Fisch.

from dividing, according to Meyrick Peak, Ph.D., Senior Scientist at the Center of Mechanistic Biology and Biotechnology at Argonne National Laboratory in Argonne, Illinois, and can often result in dramatic cures.

"In study settings, 90 to 95 percent of [psoriasis] patients respond favorably," adds Warwick L. Morrison, M.D., Associate Professor of Dermatology at Johns Hopkins University, "with the treatment usually involving thirty PUVA sessions spanning ten weeks."

Photodynamic Therapy and Cancer

"The very thing that can lead to skin cancer can also be used to cure it," says Dr. Peak. In photodynamic therapy, dyes that absorb light are absorbed by tumors then exposed to specific types of light. "Light photons are absorbed by the pigment of the dye, which becomes chemically reactive and causes the cancer cells to die," says Dr. Peak. "This therapy has been used in China for over twenty years and has been very successful in eliminating some types of tumors," he adds.

Nicholas J. Lowe, M.D., Clinical Professor of Dermatology at the UCLA School of Medicine, and Director of the Skin Research Foundation of California, mentions that, "Photodynamic therapy is currently being tested for basal and squamous cell cancers (skin cancers). However, the concern with some of these treatments is unwanted phytotoxicity—some treatments are likely to make the patient sensitive to sunlight for long periods of time."

Warren Grundfest, M.D., of Cedars-Sinai Medical Center in Los Angeles, is using a type of photodynamic therapy called light-activated chemotherapy to treat patients with lung and bladder cancer.

"What we're doing," says Dr. Grundfest, "is using light to cause a chemical change in the drug. Because it is located only in the cancer tissue, or predominantly in the cancer tissue, it causes only the cancer cells to die." Dr. Grundfest reports that after eighteen months of treatment bladder tumors showed an 85 percent successful response.

Syntonic Optometry

Syntonic therapy applies colored light directly into the eyes to augment the control centers of the brain that regulate various functions of the body. For example, in the 1930s it was shown by Harry Riley Spitler, M.D., D.O.S., M.S., Ph.D., founder of the College of Syntonic Optometry, in Fall River, Massachusetts, that focusing blue light into the eyes reduces inflammation and pain.

Solomon Slobin, O.D., Director of the College of Syntonic Optometry, uses an instrument called the Lumatron Light Stimulator® for visual evaluation, increasing the visual fields (peripheral vision), relieving headaches, and treating traumatic brain injuries.

Developed by Dr. Downing, the Lumatron emits eleven pure wave bands of biologically active light, ranging through the spectrum from ruby to violet. This light is focused into the eyes where it travels to the brain and activates the autonomic nervous system to regulate disruptions in the system, thereby triggering the healing process. Patients sit in a darkened room in front of the Lumatron for approximately twenty-five minutes while it bathes their eyes with the appropriate colored light, emitted at a rate of two to sixteen flashes per second. This exposure is normally found to be immediately soothing, with a lessening of symptoms within a few days.

Cold Laser Therapy

According to Marvin Prescott, D.M.D., of Los Angeles, cold laser therapy, sometimes referred to as soft or low-level laser therapy, utilizes a beam of low-intensity laser light to initiate a series of enzymatic reactions and bioelectric events that stimulate the natural healing process at the cellular level. "Cold laser therapy has been successfully applied to pain control, orthopedic myofascial syndrome (inflammation of the muscles and their surrounding membranes), neurology, trauma, dermatology, and dentistry," says Dr. Prescott, who adds that, "The effects on microcirculation, increased synthesis of collagen in the skin, production of neurotransmitters, and pain relief have all been documented."

Cold laser therapy is often used in patients who do not like the needles used in traditional acupuncture. John Diamond, M.D., of Reno, Nevada, uses cold laser therapy to treat pain, particularly in children, who are often afraid of acupuncture. He finds it very useful for back pain, bursitis, and tendinitis, and uses it to treat chronic problems, in conjunction with homeopathy, herbs, and nutrients.

WHOLE-BRAIN LIGHT THERAPY

When light rays strike the retina of the eye, they are converted into nerve currents, sometimes termed photocurrents. By measuring the amount of light-generated photocurrents traveling from the retina to the higher brain centers and then comparing them to symptoms of patients, John Downing, O.D., Ph.D., Director of the Light Therapy Department at the Preventive Medical Center of Marin in San Rafael, California, has found many people to have a decreased level of photocurrent transmission. This condition, termed photocurrent deficit, can cause diminished brain function, and can lead to numerous symptoms. Among these are:

- *Learning disabilities*
- *Poor concentration*
- *Poor memory*
- *Mental fogginess*
- *Poor physical coordination and performance*
- *Sleeping problems*
- *Poor self-esteem*
- *Mood swings*
- *Seasonal affective disorder*
- *Depression*
- *Fear and anxiety*
- *Hyperactivity*
- *Fatigue*
- *Headaches*
- *Light sensitivity*
- *Poor peripheral vision*
- *Night blindness*

Dr. Downing has found that stimulation by way of the eyes with the appropriate colored light can increase the ability of the neurovisual pathways to transmit photocurrents to the higher brain centers and thus significantly reduce or eliminate this photocurrent deficiency.

To administer this therapy, Dr. Downing developed the Lumatron Light Stimulator®, a device that focuses light of various colors into the eye to trigger the healing process.

A thirty-five-year-old woman who was involved in an auto accident suffered pains in the face and head, was mentally sluggish, confused, and severely fatigued. Dr. Downing treated her with forty sessions of indigo and violet light. The pains disappeared, the mental sluggishness and confusion cleared, and her energy returned to the point where she needed only five hours sleep a night instead of ten, reports Dr. Downing.

Dennis Tucker, Ph.D., L.Ac., of Nevada City, California, uses cold laser therapy to stimulate acupuncture points as an aid to healing wounds, and to reduce inflammation and balance the energy flow in the acupuncture meridians. Dr. Tucker also finds cold laser therapy very effective in treating infections under teeth. Cold laser therapy is applicable with little prior knowledge, either by a health provider or by self-application, with no demonstrable side effects when used properly. With the development of microelectronics, pen-sized, low-level laser instruments are now available.

See Biological Dentistry.

The Future of Light Therapy

"Light is the medicine of the future," says Jacob Liberman, O.D., Ph.D., Director of the Aspen Center for Energy Medicine, adding that those working in the field today are discovering new applications all the time for not only improving one's physical health, but also one's psychological and spiritual well-being. Additionally, many of the new light therapies can be used at home, providing a pain-free and inexpensive alternative to surgery and drugs.[19]

"I remember when people didn't know that smoking was dangerous," adds Dr. Eastman, "and people didn't pay much attention to their diets. One of the next steps will be for people to realize that the amount of natural light they receive, as well as when they receive it, is another important component to health. People will watch when they get light just as they now watch their diets and the amount of exercise they get. In the future it will become commonplace for people to take natural light exposure into account."

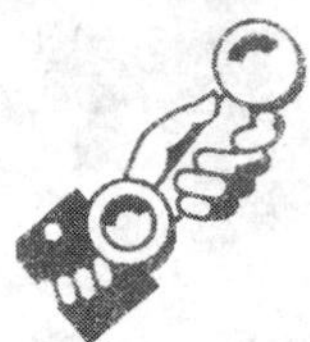

Where to Find Help

Though light therapy is a growing field, information may be difficult to find. Below are some organizations that can answer questions and provide you with further information.

College of Syntonic Optometry
1200 Robeson Street
Fall River, Massachusetts
02720-5508
(508) 673-1251

An organization of optometrists who incorporate optometric phototherapy into their treatments. The college will refer you to one of their members who practices in your area.

Dinshaw Health Society
100 Dinshaw Drive
Malaga, New Jersey 08328
(609) 692-4686

The Dinshaw Health Society, in existence since 1975, advocates the value of color therapy. Through publishing books like Let There Be Light, *they seek to help people treat themselves with color therapies. Not a referral service.*

Environmental Health & Light Research Institute
16057 Tampa Palms Boulevard
Suite 227
Tampa, Florida 33647
(800) 544-4878

The Institute continues the work of light pioneer, Dr. John Ott, and can provide information on full-spectrum lighting.

Society for Light Treatment and Biological Rhythms
P.O. Box 478
Wilsonville, Oregon 97070
(503) 694-2404

For information on treatment of seasonal affective disorder.

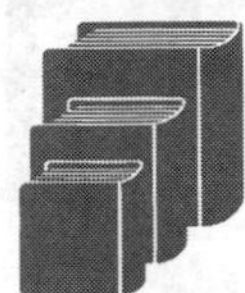

Recommended Reading

Color Therapy. Amber, Reuben, B. Santa Fe, NM: Aurora Press, 1983.

A two-part book on the theory and philosophy of chromotherapy and a specific-applications guide for daily use.

Health & Light. Ott, John D.Sc. Old Greenwich, CT: The Devin-Adair Co., 1988.

As an outgrowth of his work with time-lapse photography, Ott explores the influence natural and artificial light have on the human endocrine system.

Let There Be Light. Dinshaw, Darius. Malaga, NJ: Dinshaw Health Society, 1985.

An in-depth study of color therapy and how and why it works as a treatment. This book also contains a list of diagnosed disorders with specific treatments for each.

Light: Medicine of the Future. Liberman, Jacob. Santa Fe, NM: Bear & Co. Publishing, 1993.

The book discusses the use of light in the treatment of various cancers, depression, stress, visual problems, premenstrual syndrome, sexual dysfunction, learning disabilities, and the human immune system.

Magnetic Field Therapy

Electromagnetic energy and the human body have a valid and important interrelationship. Magnetic field therapy can be used in both diagnosing and treating physical and emotional disorders. This process has been recognized to relieve symptoms and may, in some cases, retard the cycle of new disease. Magnets and electromagnetic therapy devices are now being used to eliminate pain, facilitate the healing of broken bones, and counter the effects of stress.

The world is surrounded by magnetic fields: some are generated by the earth's magnetism, while others are generated by solar storms and changes in the weather. Magnetic fields are also created by everyday electrical devices: motors, televisions, office equipment, computers, microwave ovens, the electrical wiring in homes, and the power lines that supply them. Even the human body produces subtle magnetic fields that are generated by the chemical reactions within the cells and the ionic currents of the nervous system.[1]

"The use of magnets and electrical devices to generate controlled magnetic fields has many medical applications, and has proven to be one of the most effective means for diagnosing human illness and disease."

Recently, scientists have discovered that external magnetic fields can affect the body's functioning in both positive and negative ways, and this observation has led to the development of magnetic field therapy.

What Is Magnetic Field Therapy?

The use of magnets and electrical devices to generate controlled magnetic fields has many medical applications, and has proven to be one of the most effective means for diagnosing human illness and disease. For example, MRI (magnetic resonance imaging) is replacing x-ray diagnosis because it is safer and more accurate, and magnetoencephalography is now replacing electroencephalography as the preferred technique for recording the brain's electrical activity.

In 1974, researcher Albert Roy Davis, Ph.D., noted that positive and negative magnetic polarities have different effects upon the biological systems of animals and humans. He found that magnets could be used to arrest and kill cancer cells in animals, and could also be used in the treatment of arthritis, glaucoma, infertility, and diseases related to aging.[2] He concluded that negative magnetic fields have a beneficial effect on living organisms, whereas positive magnetic fields have a stressful effect.

"Scientifically designed, double-blind, placebo-controlled studies, however, have not been done to substantiate the claims of there being different effects between positive and negative magnetic poles," says John Zimmerman, Ph.D., President of the Bio-Electro-Magnetics Institute. "But numerous anecdotal, clinical observations suggest that such differences are real and do exist. Clearly, scientific research is needed to substantiate these claims."

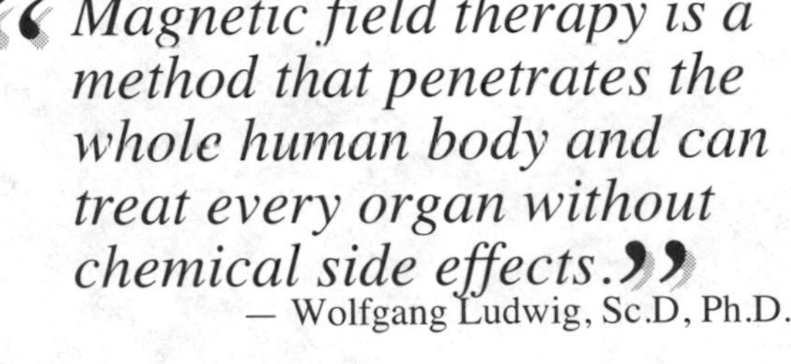

"Magnetic field therapy is a method that penetrates the whole human body and can treat every organ without chemical side effects."
— Wolfgang Ludwig, Sc.D, Ph.D.

Robert Becker, M.D., an orthopedic surgeon and author of numerous scientific articles and books, found that weak electric currents promote the healing of broken bones. Dr. Becker also brought national attention to the fact that electromagnetic interference from power lines and home appliances can pose a serious hazard to human health. "The scientific evidence," writes Dr. Becker, "leads only to one conclusion: the exposure of living organisms to abnormal electromagnetic fields results in significant abnormalities in physiology and function."[3]

According to Wolfgang Ludwig, Sc.D., Ph.D., Director of the Institute for Biophysics in Horb, Germany, "Magnetic field therapy is a method that penetrates the whole human body and can treat every organ without chemical side effects." Magnetic field therapy has been used effectively in the treatment of:

- Cancer
- Rheumatoid disease
- Infections and inflammations
- Headaches and migraines
- Insomnia and sleep disorders
- Circulatory problems
- Fractures and pain
- Environmental stress

Dr. Ludwig adds that magnetic changes in the environment can affect the electromagnetic balance of the human organism and contribute to disease. Kyoichi Nakagawa, M.D., Director of the Isuzu Hospital in Tokyo, Japan, believes that the time people spend in buildings and cars reduces their exposure to the natural geomagnetic fields of the earth, and may also interfere with health. He calls this condition magnetic field deficiency syndrome, which can cause headaches, dizziness, muscle stiffness, chest pain, insomnia, constipation, and general fatigue.[4] Researchers suggest that magnetic therapy can be used to counter the effects caused by the electromagnetic pollution in the environment.

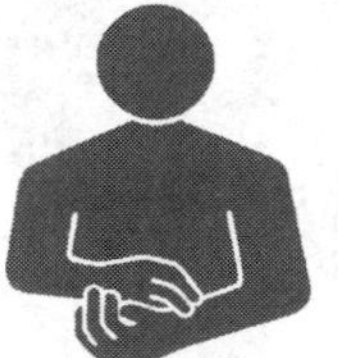

Magnetic field therapy can be safely used in a self-care program to alleviate symptoms from pain, or to encourage sleep. To better understand the therapeutic uses of magnets, consult a practitioner for guidance.

Electromagnetic Fields Can Pose a Serious Health Hazard

According to Robert Becker, M.D., John Zimmerman, Ph.D., and many other scientists and researchers, we live in an environment that is filled with stress-producing, electromagnetic fields generated by the electrical wiring in homes and offices, as well as from televisions, computers and video terminals, microwave ovens, overhead lights, electrical poles, and the hundreds of motors that can generate higher than naturally occurring gauss strengths.

The frequency at which a magnetic field is pulsed determines whether or not it is harmful. For example, the voltage of the electrical current used in homes in the United States is sixty cycles per second. In contrast, normal frequencies of the human brain during waking hours range from eight to twenty cycles per second, while in sleep the frequencies may drop to as low as two cycles per second. The higher frequencies present in artificial electrical currents may disturb the brain's natural resonant frequencies and in time lead to cellular fatigue, according to Dr. Zimmerman.

In 1979, Nancy Wertheimer, Ph.D., an epidemiologist at the University of Colorado, found that there was a statistically significant increase in childhood cancers among those who were exposed to the AC (alternating current) electromagnetic fields that emanate from the electrical power lines that run along many of the nation's city streets.[5] Ten years later, in 1987, a large-scale study conducted by the New York State Department of Health confirmed Dr. Wertheimer's findings and added that it also affected the neuro-hormones of the brain.[6] In 1988, Marjorie Speers, Ph.D., at the University of Texas Medical Branch, found that workers exposed to electromagnetic fields showed a thirteenfold increase in brain tumors compared to the unexposed group.[7] Other studies have shown increases in suicides,[8] depression,[9] chromosomal abnormalities,[10] and learning difficulties.[11]

In another study by Dr. Wertheimer, it was observed that users of electric blankets had a higher incidence of miscarriages.[12] Add to this the possible perils from fluorescent lighting, microwave ovens, hair dryers, electric shavers, and heaters, and one can see why more research is urgently needed. "Only a few farsighted individuals, such as Dr. Robert O. Becker, have given much thought to the fact that the new electromagnetic environment created by twentieth century technology may be exerting subtle, yet very important effects upon biology," states Dr. Zimmerman. "This may include alterations in gene expression, immune function, viral pathogenesis, and future genetic tendencies."

How Magnetic Field Therapy Works

"The healing potential of magnets is possible because the body's nervous system is governed, in part, by varying patterns of ionic currents and electromagnetic fields," reports Dr. Zimmerman. There are numerous forms of magnetic field therapy, including static magnetic fields produced by natural or artificial magnets, and pulsating magnetic fields generated by electrical devices. The magnetic fields produced by magnets or electromagnetic generating devices are able to penetrate the human body and can affect the functioning of the nervous system, organs, and cells. According to William H. Philpott, M.D., of Choctaw, Oklahoma, an author and biomagnetic researcher, magnetic fields can stimulate metabolism and increase the amount of oxygen available to cells. When used properly magnetic field therapy has no known harmful side effects.

All magnets have two poles: one is called positive, and the other negative. However, as there are conflicting methods of naming the poles of a magnet, a magnetometer should be used as a standard method of determination (if one is using a compass to locate the poles, the arrowhead of the needle marked "N" or "North" will point to the magnet's negative pole). Dr. Philpott and other researchers claim that the negative pole generally has a calming effect and helps to normalize metabolic functioning. In contrast, the positive pole has a stress effect, and with prolonged exposure interferes with metabolic functioning, produces acidity, reduces cellular oxygen supply, and encourages the replication of latent microorganisms.

Industrial magnets often have different positive and negative pole identifications than the magnets used in medicine and therapy. Use a magnetometer or compass to confirm proper identification.

The strength of a magnet is measured in units of gauss (a unit of measuring the intensity of magnetic flux), or Tesla (1 tesla=10,000 gauss), and every magnetic device has a manufacturer's gauss rating. However, the actual strength of the magnet at the skin surface is often much less than this number. For example, a 4,000 gauss magnet transmits about 1,200 gauss to the patient. Magnets placed in pillows or bed pads will render even lower amounts of field strength at the skin surface, because a magnet's strength quickly decreases with the distance from the subject.

How Magnets Are Used Therapeutically

Magnetic therapy can be applied in many ways, and devices range from small, simple magnets to large machines capable of generating high magnitudes of field strength (used for treating fractures and pseudoarthrosis, a joint affliction caused by nerve breakdown). Magnetic blankets and beds have also been manufactured for the purposes of promoting sleep and reducing stress. Specially designed ceramic, plastiform, and neodymium (a rare earth chemical element) magnets can be placed either individually or in clusters above the various organs of the body, on lymph nodes, or on various points of the head. In Japan, small *tai-ki* magnets have been designed to stimulate acupuncture points, but no clinical studies have yet explored this procedure.

Magnetic devices are quite popular in Germany, where the use of certain devices is covered by medical insurance. After simple instruction is given to the patient, these devices can be used at home.

Conditions Benefited by Magnetic Field Therapy

Research into the therapeutic benefits of magnetic field therapy is needed. This type of therapy could provide a safe and effective way to curb rising health care costs.

Treatments can last from just a few minutes to overnight and, depending upon the situation and severity, may be applied several times a day, or for days or weeks at a time. Sometimes, though, the results of magnetic therapy can be quite dramatic, as in a case cited by Dr. Ludwig. A forty-six-year-old man had suffered for years from severe heart flutter, diarrhea, and nausea. No treatment seemed to help, but when a magnetic applicator with less than one gauss of energy was placed upon his solar plexus for only three minutes, his symptoms immediately ceased. Two years later, he had experienced no relapse.

In a case described by Dr. Philpott, a seventy-year-old man who had undergone coronary bypass surgery continued to suffer from heart pain.

His walk was reduced to a shuffle, his speech was slurred, and he lived in a state of chronic depression. He decided to try magnetic therapy and a plastiform magnet was placed over his heart. Within ten minutes, the pain disappeared. Magnets were applied to the crown of his head while he slept, and within a month, his depression was gone, his speech was clear, and his walking returned to normal.

In other cases cited by Dr. Philpott, magnets have helped to eliminate toothaches, eliminate periodontal disease, and eradicate fungal infections like candidiasis. Kidney stones and calcium deposits in inflamed tissues have also been known to dissolve. Magnetic therapy has been shown to be particularly effective in reducing swelling and edema. According to Dr. Philpott, "Symptoms of cardiac atherosclerosis and brain atherosclerosis have been observed to disappear after six to eight weeks of nightly exposure to a negative static magnetic field."

See Chronic Pain, Stress.

Stress

A negative magnetic field applied to the top of the head has a calming and sleep-inducing effect on brain and body functions, due to the stimulation of the production of the hormone melatonin, according to Dr. Philpott. Melatonin has been shown to be antistressful, antiaging, anti-infectious, anticancerous, and to have control over respiration and the production of free radicals.[13]

A free radical is a highly destructive molecule that is missing an electron, and readily reacts with other molecules. This can lead to the aging of cells, the hardening of muscle tissue, the wrinkling of skin, and, in general, a decreased efficiency of protein synthesis. As there are literally hundreds of diseases that are related to stress, infections, and aging, magnetic field therapy could be considered an important adjunct in their treatment and researchers are currently studying its contributions.

Bacterial, Fungal, and Viral Infections

"A negative magnetic field can function like an antibiotic in helping to destroy bacterial, fungal, and viral infections," says Dr. Philpott, "by promoting oxygenation and lowering the body's acidity." Both these factors are beneficial to normal bodily functions but harmful to pathogenic (disease-causing) microorganisms, which do not survive in a well-oxygenated, alkaline environment. Dr. Philpott theorizes that the biological value of oxygen is increased by the influence of a negative electromagnetic field, and that the field causes negatively charged DNA (deoxyribonucleic acid) to "pull" oxygen out of the bloodstream and into the cell. The negative electromagnetic field keeps the cellular buffer system (pH or acid-base balance) intact so that the cells remain alkaline. The low acid balance also helps maintain the presence of oxygen in the body.

Pain Relief

A negative magnetic field normalizes the disturbed metabolic functions that cause painful conditions such as cellular edema (swelling of the cells), cellular acidosis (excessive acidity of the cells), lack of oxygen to the cells, and infection.

Dr. Philpott cites the case of a woman in her seventies who had experienced pain and weakness in her left leg for thirty-three years stemming from a blood clot in the groin area, and could not climb stairs without stopping several times due to pain. After twelve months of sleeping on a negative magneto-electric pad, the woman found that she could walk a long flight of stairs without any pain or weakness in her leg.

A negative magnetic field cannot take the place of local anesthetics and analgesics, however. A positive magnetic field, on the other hand, can increase pain due to its interference with normal metabolic function.

THE PHYSIOLOGICAL EFFECTS OF POSITIVE AND NEGATIVE MAGNETIC FIELDS

According to many researchers, negative magnetic fields seem to affect all the metabolic processes involved in growth, healing, immune defense, nonimmune microorganism defense, and detoxification. The following chart was prepared by Dr. Philpott and is based on his clinical observations of the effects that positive and negative magnetic fields have upon living organisms.

BIOLOGICAL RESPONSE TO ANTISTRESSFUL NEGATIVE STATIC MAGNETIC FIELDS	**BIOLOGICAL RESPONSE TO STRESSFUL POSITIVE STATIC MAGNETIC FIELDS** (Stress starts at 100 gauss and is strongly developed by 200 gauss)
pH normalizing	*Acid producing*
Oxygenating	*Oxygen deficit producing*
Resolves cellular edema	*Evokes cellular edema*
Usually reduces symptoms	*Often evokes or exacerbates the existing symptoms*
Can relieve addictive withdrawal symptoms	*Stress evokes endorphin production and can therefore be addicting*
Inhibits microorganism replication	*Accelerates microorganism replication*
Biologically normalizing	*Biologically disorganizing*
Governs rest, relaxation, and sleep	*Governs wakefulness and action*
Evokes anabolic hormone production—melatonin and growth hormone	*Evokes catabolic hormone production and inhibits anabolic hormone production*
Counters and processes metabolically-produced toxins out of the body	*Produces toxic end products of metabolism and does not counter or process these toxins out of the body*
	Produces free radicals
Cancels out free radicals	

Central Nervous System Disorders

"When a negative magnetic field is placed directly over an area of electrical activity in the brain, the electrical excitement can be reduced," says Dr. Philpott. It can stop such symptoms as hallucinations, delusions, seizures, or panic without disrupting the patient's mental alertness and orientation. Small disc magnets (made from ceramic neodymium or iron oxide) can be placed around the head to alleviate these kinds of symptoms. Dr. Philpott has pioneered the use of magnetic therapy for numerous psychiatric disorders, and he believes that in the future subtle uses of magnets will be used to control a variety of symptoms and central nervous system disturbances.

A woman who had a benign tumor removed from her spine could not walk without dragging her feet. When Dr. Philpott placed a positive magnetic pole over the area where the tumor had been removed, she could walk perfectly. With practice, and with the help of both a positive and negative magnetic field, the neuronal function returned. The positive field stimulated the nonfunctioning neurons and produced (as a reaction to stress) endorphins (natural opiates produced in the brain), while the negative field prevented the neurons from becoming overly excited. Because of the potential dangers relating to positive magnetic fields, the period of exposure was quite brief.

Caution: *The body's subtle electromagnetic fields can be affected by even the weakest of magnets. Since even minor alterations in the field can cause mild to serious symptoms, magnetic therapy should only be practiced under the supervision of a qualified professional. For some patients, magnetic field therapy can cause pain, while others may have symptomatic reactions to various medications they are taking. Toxins may also be released into the body, causing severe reactions. Dr. Philpott adds the following precautions:*

- *Don't use magnets on the abdomen during pregnancy.*
- *Don't use a magnetic bed for more than eight to ten hours.*
- *Wait sixty to ninety minutes after meals before applying magnetic therapy to the abdomen, to prevent interference with peristalsis (wavelike contractions of the smooth muscles of the digestive tract).*
- *Do not apply the positive magnetic pole unless under medical supervision. It can produce seizures, hallucinations, insomnia, hyperactivity, stimulate the growth of tumors and microorganisms, and promote addictive behavior.*[14]

The Future of Magnetic Field Therapy

With the rising popularity of magnetic field diagnostic techniques such as MRI (magnetic resonance imaging), magnets and electrical devices are beginning to gain mainstream medical acceptance as human diagnostic and treatment tools.

According to Dr. Philpott, the application of magnets provides the most predictable results of any treatment he has observed. "It is not only valuable as a medically supervised technique, but for many self-help problems such as insomnia, chronic pain, and tension."

Because magnets do not introduce any foreign substance to the body, this will, Dr. Philpott believes, make them safer over the long-term than aspirin or other over-the-counter medications.

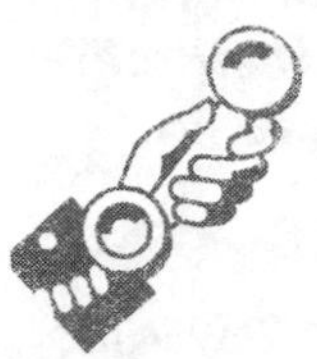

Where to Find Help

The following organizations offer referrals and information on professional and self-care treatment of magnetic field therapy.

Bio-Electro-Magnetics Institute
2490 West Moana Lane
Reno, Nevada 89509-3936
(702) 827-9099

A private, nonprofit organization established to provide research, education, support, and technical assistance in matters relating to bioelectromagnetics. A national clearinghouse for information relating to both health risks from power line magnetic fields and the health benefits from magnetic therapy.

Enviro-Tech Products
17171 Southeast 29th Street
Choctaw, Oklahoma 73020
(405) 390-3499

This service includes self-help information, information for physicians, and information and guidance for research projects under the Institutional Review Board of the Bio-Electro-Magnetic Institute of Reno, Nevada.

Dr. Wolfgang Ludwig
Silcherstrasse 21
Horb A.N.1
Germany
011-49-7451-8648 (Fax)

For information regarding German instruments utilizing magnetic energy and pulsing frequencies such as Endomet and Magnetron.

MagnetiCo, Inc.
4562 14th Street, N.E.
Calgary, Alberta, Canada
T1Y 6C1
(403) 291-0085

Manufactures and markets a SleepPad™, engineered to produce a negative magnetic field, designed to restore energy while you sleep, as well as other magnetic products.

Prometheus Italia SrL
Centro Commerciale, VR-EST,
Viale del Lavoro 45
I-36037, S. Martino B.A. (VR),
Italy

This company produces magnetic blankets according to Dr. Ludwig's design.

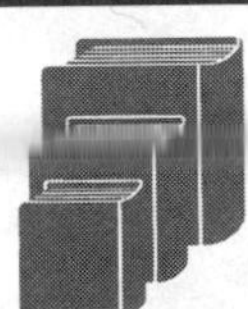

Recommended Reading

Biomagnetic Handbook. Philpott, William; and Taplin, Sharon. Choctaw, OK: Enviro-Tech Products, 1990.

This handbook details what Dr. Philpott observed in over three thousand patients from 1985 to 1990. It's a self-help, informative guidebook in the area of magnetics.

Cross Currents. Becker, Robert O., M.D. Los Angeles: Jeremy P. Tarcher, Inc., 1990.

This book describes two opposing trends: the rise in the use of electromedicine and the parallel rise of electropollution. Becker teaches how to engage the healing energies of electromagnetism and offers practical ways people can protect themselves from the dangers of electromagnetic fields in the environment.

Magnetism and Its Effects on the Living System. Davis, Albert; and Rawls, Walter. Kansas City, MO: Acres U.S.A., 1993.
To order: P.O. Box 9457, Kansas City, MO 64133
(816) 737-0064

A scientific, but generally accessible, text on the "natural science" of biomagnetics, which explains the effects of magnetism on living systems. Contains detailed illustrations and diagrams.

BEMI Currents—Journal of the Bio-Electro-Magnetics Institute, 2490 West Moana Lane, Reno, Nevada, 89509-3936
(702) 827-9099.

Published since the Spring of 1989 with twelve issues to date, BEMI Currents *is a journal for those interested in electromagnetics, with articles, published studies, and a recommended reading list. A list of the table of contents is available upon request.*

"The natural force within each one of us is the greatest healer of disease."

—Hippocrates

Meditation

Meditation is a safe and simple way to balance a person's physical, emotional, and mental states. It is easily learned and has been used as an aid in treating stress and pain management. It has also been employed as part of an overall treatment for other conditions, including hypertension and heart disease.

Meditation has been practiced for several thousand years. It is only during the past three decades that scientific study has focused on its clinical effects on health. During the 1960s, reports reached the West of yogis and meditation masters in India who could perform extraordinary feats of bodily control and altered states of consciousness. These reports captured the interest of Western researchers studying self-regulation and the possibility of voluntary control over the autonomic nervous system.[1] At the same time, new refinements in scientific instrumentation made it possible to duplicate and substantiate some of these reports at medical research institutes. Health care professionals who were often dissatisfied with the side effects of drug treatments for stress-related disorders embraced meditation as a valuable tool for stress reduction, and today both patients and physicians enjoy the health benefits of regular meditation practice.

What Is Meditation?

According to Joan Borysenko, Ph.D., a pioneer in the field of mind/body medicine, meditation can be broadly defined as any activity that keeps the attention pleasantly anchored in the present moment. When the mind is calm and focused in the present, it is neither reacting to memories from the past nor being preoccupied with plans for the future, two major sources of chronic stress known to impact health. "Meditation," says Dr. Borysenko, "helps to keep us from identifying with the 'movies of the mind.'"

> *"Meditation helps to keep us from identifying with the 'movies of the mind."*
>
> —Joan Borysenko, Ph.D.

Although there are numerous approaches to meditation, most techniques can be grouped into two basic approaches: concentrative meditation and mindfulness meditation. Concentrative meditation focuses the attention on the breath, an image, or a sound (*mantra*), in order to still the mind and allow a greater awareness and clarity to emerge. This form of meditation can be compared to the zoom lens of a camera that narrows its focus to a selected field.

A SIMPLE MEDITATION EXERCISE

The first step to practicing meditation is learning to breathe in a manner that facilitates a state of calmness and awareness. The following exercise is recommended as an effective method for achieving calmness by Jon Kabat-Zinn, Ph.D., founder and Director of the Stress Reduction Clinic at the University of Massachusetts Medical Center. Find a quiet place where you will not be disturbed and practice the following for several minutes each day:

Assume a comfortable posture lying on your back or sitting. If you are sitting, keep the spine straight and let your shoulders drop.

Close your eyes if it feels comfortable.

Bring your attention to your belly, feeling it rise or expand gently on the in-breath and fall or recede on the out-breath.

Keep the focus on your breathing, "being with" each in-breath.

Every time you notice that your mind has wandered off the breath, notice what it was that took you away and then gently bring your attention back to your belly and the feeling of the breath coming in and out.

If your mind wanders away from the breath, then your "job" is simply to bring it back to the breath every time, no matter what it has become preoccupied with.

Practice this exercise for fifteen minutes at a convenient time every day, whether you feel like it or not, for one week and see how it feels to incorporate a disciplined meditation practice into your life. Be aware of how it feels to spend time each day just being with your breath without having to do anything.

The simplest form of concentrative meditation is to sit quietly and focus the attention on the breath. The connection between the breath and one's state of mind is a basic principle of the practice of yoga and meditation. When a person is anxious, frightened, agitated, or distracted, the breath will tend to be shallow, rapid, and uneven. On the other hand, when the mind is calm, focused, and composed, the breath will tend to be slow, deep, and regular. Focusing the mind on the continuous rhythm of inhalation and exhalation provides a natural object of meditation. As the meditator focuses his or her awareness on the breath, the mind becomes absorbed in the rhythm of inhalation and exhalation, breathing slows and becomes deeper, and the mind becomes more tranquil and aware.

Mindfulness meditation, according to Dr. Borysenko, "involves opening the attention to become aware of the continuously passing parade of sensations and feelings, images, thoughts, sounds, smells, and so forth without becoming involved in thinking about them." The meditator sits quietly and simply witnesses whatever goes through the mind, not reacting or becoming involved with thoughts, memories, worries, or images. This helps the meditator gain a more calm, clear, and nonreactive state of mind. Mindfulness meditation can be likened to a wide-angle lens—a broad, sweeping awareness that takes in the entire field of perception.

How Meditation Works

Hans Selye, a pioneering Canadian stress researcher, describes two types of stress—negative stress and positive stress. The difference between the two depends upon whether or not the individual feels in control of the stress.[2] By allowing one to become more aware of one's reactions to stress, meditation can assist in providing the individual with an increased internal sense of control.

See Mind/Body Medicine.

Studies have also shown that meditation [in particular research on Transcendental Meditation™ (TM), a popular form of meditation practiced in the West for the past thirty years], can bring about a healthy state of relaxation by causing a generalized reduction in multiple physiological and biochemical markers, such as decreased heart rate, decreased respiration rate, decreased plasma cortisol (a major stress hormone), decreased pulse rate, and increased EEG (electroencephalogram) alpha, a brain wave associated with relaxation.[3] The first research on the physiology of meditation was conducted by R. Keith Wallace at U.C.L.A. Studying Transcendental Meditation, Wallace found that whereas the body gains a state of profound rest, the brain and mind become more alert, indicating a state of "restful alertness." Studies show that after TM, reactions are faster, creativity greater, and comprehension broader.

"Through meditation we can learn to access the relaxation response (the physiological response elicted by meditation) and to be aware of the mind and the way our attitudes produce stress," says Dr. Borysenko, former Co-director of Harvard's Mind/Body Clinic. "In addition, by quieting the mind, meditation can also put one in touch with the inner physician, allowing the body's own inner wisdom to be heard."

Transcendental Meditation

Transcendental Meditation™ is a simple mental technique introduced by Maharishi Mahesh Yogi from the Vedic tradition of India. TM is easily learned, can be practiced for fifteen to twenty minutes, twice daily, and requires no change in lifestyle or belief. Since 1958, 4 million people have learned TM and over five hundred scientific studies have been conducted on it at over two hundred universities worldwide.[5]

Physiological research shows that during TM, the body gains a deeper state of relaxation than during ordinary rest.[6] EEG (electroencephelogram) changes indicate a state of heightened awareness and coherence.[7] Regular practice of TM has been found to produce a state of increased stability, adaptability, and integration during all phases of activity. Also, TM has been found to increase intelligence, creativity, and perceptual ability[8] and to reduce high blood pressure and illness rates by more than 50 percent.[9] Meta-analysis (research comparing large numbers of studies) have found that TM is one of the most effective techniques known for reducing drug and alcohol abuse,[10] decreasing anxiety and increasing self-actualization.[11]

Conditions Benefited by Meditation

Patricia Norris, Ph.D., Director of the Biofeedback and Psychophysiology Clinic at the Menninger Foundation, reports: "In our practice at Menninger we use meditative techniques to enhance immune functioning in cancer, AIDS, and autoimmune patients. We also use meditation in conjunction with neuro-feedback to normalize brain rhythms and chemistry in alcohol and drug addiction, as well as other addictive conditions. Almost all of our patients use meditative techniques in learning self-regulation for disorders such as anxiety and hypertension, and for stress management. We consider meditation a recommended practice for anyone seeking high-level wellness."

In addition to the growing body of research literature on meditation, physicians, psychotherapists, and other professionals are increasingly adding meditative techniques to their practice. According to David Orme-Johnson, Ph.D., Dean of Research for Maharishi International University in Fairfield, Iowa, over six thousand physicians have begun the practice of Transcendental Meditation and regularly recommend the TM technique to their patients. Other physicians who advocate meditation include Dean Ornish, M.D., who recently demonstrated that heart disease can be reversed with a comprehensive program that includes meditation.[4] Ron Hunninghake, M.D., has made meditation a key element in the integrated health program at the Center for the Improvement of Human Functioning International in Wichita, Kansas. Jon Kabat-Zinn, Ph.D., founder and Director of the Stress Reduction Clinic at the University of

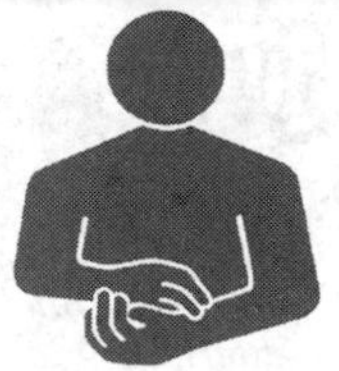

Meditation is well-suited to self-care, and can become part of your personal health maintenance program.

Massachusetts Medical Center, has taught Buddhist meditation and yoga to thousands of patients, most of whom were referred by their physicians. "Many well-known physicians," adds Dr. Norris, "such as Larry Dossey, M.D., Deepak Chopra, M.D., Bernie Siegel, M.D., and Norman Shealy, M.D., also use and advocate meditation for total well-being."

WALKING MEDITATION

According to Jon Kabat-Zinn, Ph.D., founder and Director of the Stress Reduction Clinic at the University of Massachusetts Medical Center, one simple way to bring awareness into your life is through walking meditation. "This brings your attention to the actual experience of walking as you are doing it, focusing on the sensations in your feet and legs, feeling your whole body moving," Dr. Kabat-Zinn explains. "You can also integrate awareness of your breathing with the experience."

To do this exercise, focus the attention on each foot as it contacts the ground. When the mind wanders away from the feet or legs, or the feeling of the body walking, refocus your attention. To deepen your concentration, don't look around, but keep your gaze in front of you.

"One thing that you find out when you have been practicing mindfulness for a while is that nothing is quite as simple as it appears," says Dr. Kabat-Zinn. "This is as true for walking as it is for anything else. For one thing, we carry our mind around with us when we walk, so we are usually absorbed in our own thoughts to one extent or another. We are hardly ever just walking, even when we are 'just going out for a walk'. Walking meditation involves intentionally attending to the experience of walking itself."

The benefits of an ongoing meditation practice can be classified into three categories: physiological, psychological, and spiritual.

Physiological Benefits

The Transcendental Meditation technique has proven to be a successful coping strategy in helping to deal with drug addiction,[12] a useful tool in psycho-neuro-immunology by helping to control the immune system,[13] and an effective manager of stress and pain.

A strong link has also been established between the practice of TM and longevity.[14] Only two factors have been scientifically determined to actually extend life: caloric restriction and lowering of the body's core temperature. Meditation has been shown to lower core body temperature.[15]

Stress Control: The term stress was first popularized in the 1950s, based on Dr. Selye's physiological studies of animals injured or placed under extreme conditions. People now use the term to refer to any or all the various pressures experienced in life. These stressors can stem from work, family, illness, or environment and can contribute to such conditions as anxiety, hypertension, and heart disease. According to Dr. Kabat-Zinn, "How an individual sees things and how he or she handles them makes all the difference in terms of how much stress he or she experiences."

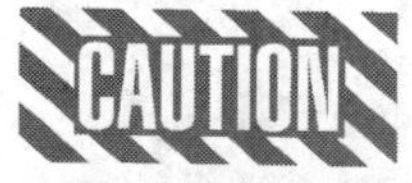

Although meditation can be an important part of your health care program it is not an alternative to medical treatment. If you have a stress-related disorder, consult your physician. If you decide to learn meditation, it is advised that you find an experienced instructor.

In one research project conducted by Dean Shapiro, Ph.D., of the University of California at Irvine, individuals reported self-regulation effects that long-term meditators (average four plus years) could identify as positive attributes from meditation. Those studied agreed that learning to control stress was an enormous benefit. Becoming more relaxed, learning to control negative thinking, and being able to handle situations with calmness and equanimity were other noted benefits.[16]

Pain Management: "Chronic pain can systematically erode the quality of life," says Dr. Kabat-Zinn. Although great strides are being made in traditional medicine to treat recurring pain, treatment is rarely as simple as prescribing medication or surgery.

In one study overseen by Dr. Kabat-Zinn, 72 percent of the patients with chronic pain conditions achieved at least a 33 percent reduction after participating in an eight-week period of mindful meditation, while 61 percent of the pain patients achieved at least a 50 percent reduction. Additionally, these people perceived their bodies as being 30 percent less problematic, suggesting an overall improvement in self-esteem and positive views regarding their bodies.[17]

See Hypertension, Stress.

Chronic Illness: Dr. Ainslie Meares, an Australian psychiatrist who uses meditation with cancer patients, studied seventy-three patients who had attended at least twenty sessions of intensive meditation, and wrote: "Nearly all such patients can expect significant reduction of anxiety and depression, together with much less discomfort and pain. There is reason to expect a 10 percent chance of quite remarkable slowing of the rate of growth of the tumor, and a 50 percent chance of greatly improved quality of life."[18]

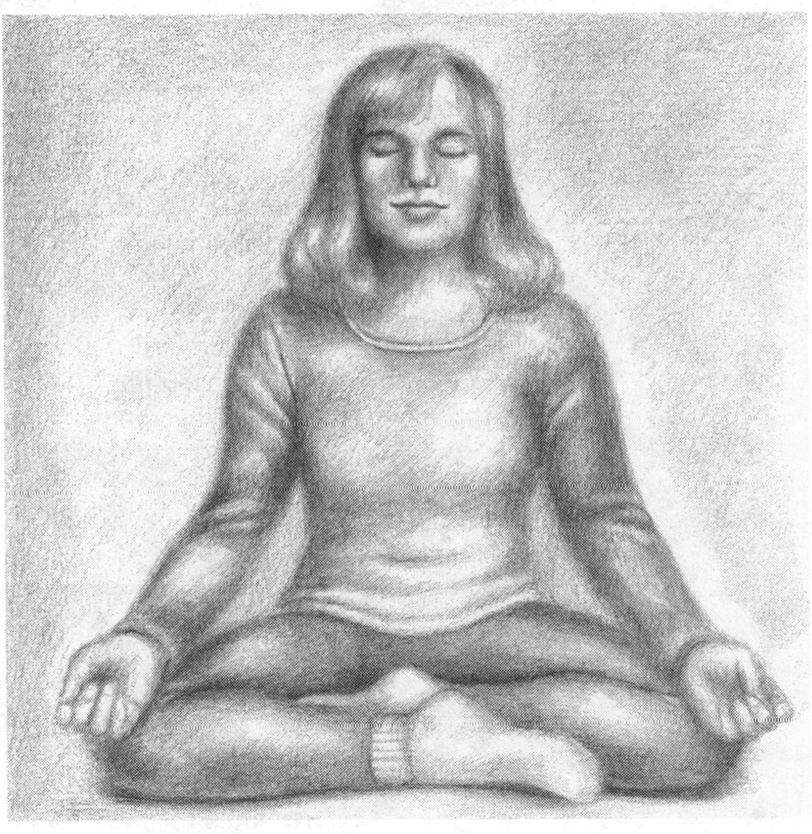

The practice of meditation.

Psychological Benefits

Meditation can help most people feel less anxious and more in control. The awareness that meditation brings can also be a source of personal insight and self-understanding. Drs. Benson and Borysenko note that even among patients with little psychological orientation, "approximately 20 percent [of these patients] with a wide range of psychophysiological disorders who joined stress reduction and relaxation programs involving mindfulness meditation became interested in psychotherapy for further expansion of self-understanding."[19]

Dr. Borysenko notes that "meditation may also lead to a breakdown of screen memories so that early childhood abuse episodes and other traumas suddenly flood the mind, making the patient temporarily more anxious until these traumas are healed. Many so-called meditation exercises are actually forms of imagery and visualization that are extraordinarily useful in healing old traumas, confronting death anxieties, finishing 'old business', learning to forgive, and enhancing self-esteem."

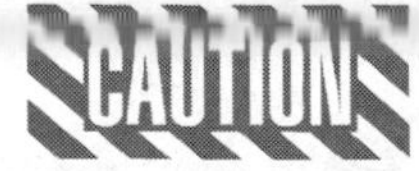

Although meditation can be an important part of your health care program it is not an alternative to medical treatment. If you have a stress-related disorder, consult your physician. If you decide to learn meditation, it is advised that you consult an experienced instructor.

Spiritual Benefits

The longer an individual practices meditation, the greater the likelihood that his or her goals and efforts will shift toward personal and spiritual growth.[20] One practitioner in Dr. Shapiro's study noted, "I began meditating to decrease my stress and fear of public speaking. But as my practice deepens, not only do I have decreased heart rate, but I also am developing a more open heart—more sensitivity, greater compassion, and less negative judgment toward others." Many individuals who initially learn meditation for its self-regulatory aspects find that as their practice deepens they are drawn more and more into the realm of the "spiritual."

In her work with many cancer and AIDS patients, Dr. Borysenko has observed that many are most interested in meditation as a way of becoming more attuned to the spiritual dimension of life. She reports that many die "healed," in a state of compassionate self-awareness and self-acceptance.

The Future of Meditation

Because meditation can be practiced in a hospital, home, office, or hospice environment, it is well suited for many individuals as a means of contributing to overall health.

With the increasing amount of negative emotional, work, and environmental, influences that people have little control over, it is important to set aside times to rejuvenate the body and the mind. According to Dr. Kabat-Zinn, "The more complicated the world gets and the more intrusive it becomes on our personal psychological space and privacy, the more important it will be to practice non-doing."

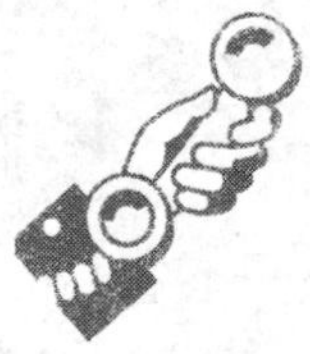

Where to Find Help

Meditation instruction has been added to the curriculum of universities, continuing education services, recreational organizations, alternative health clinics, and some religious programs. Specific organizations that may be a helpful resource for meditation are:

Institute of Noetic Sciences
P.O. Box 909
Sausalito, California 94966
(415) 331-5650

A resource of meditation researchers and teachers. Excellent support organization for those interested in consciousness.

Institute of Transpersonal Psychology
P.O. Box 4437
Stanford, California 94305
(415) 327-2066

A source of information about meditation research, activities, and teachers.

Maharishi International University
1000 North 4th Street
Fairfield, Iowa 52556
(515) 472-5031

A Transcendental Meditation organization-sponsored school, and research facility. They will provide information about where to learn Transcendental Meditation.

Mind-Body Clinic
New Deaconess Hospital,
Harvard Medical School
185 Pilgrim Road
Cambridge, Massachusetts 02215
(617) 632-9530

A treatment program at a medical center where the relaxation response can be learned.

Mind/Body Health Sciences, Inc.
393 Dixon Road
Boulder, Colorado 80302
(303) 440-8460

This organization helps groups organize workshops and provides expert speakers on meditation and mind/body medicine. They also have a mail order selection of books on meditation and music on tape.

Stress Reduction Clinic
University of Massachusetts Medical Center
55 Lake Avenue, North
Worcester, Massachusetts 01655
(508) 856-2656

An actual training program at a medical center to teach meditative-type awareness.

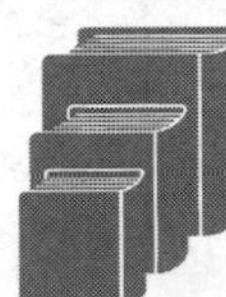

Recommended Reading

Beyond the Relaxation Response. Benson, Herbert; and Procter, William. New York: Putnam/Berkley, Inc., 1984.

Herbert Benson continues his studies in the field of meditation. In this book he discusses how everyone has the ability within to heal him-or herself. An excellent follow-up to his previous book, The Relaxation Response.

Full Catastrophe Living. Kabat-Zinn, Jon. New York: Delacorte Press, 1990.

An excellent description of the stress reduction and relaxation program at the University of Massachusetts Medical Center, a pioneering center using mindfulness training for addressing stress and pain. The technique is based on Buddhist mindfulness meditation, but is taught in a secular manner.

The Meditative Mind. Goleman, Daniel. Los Angeles: Jeremy P. Tarcher, Inc., 1988.

A very helpful book surveying the way in which meditation has been used in different religious traditions, both East and West.

Minding the Body, Mending the Mind. Borysenko, Joan. New York: Bantam Books, 1988.

A clear, lucid, thoughtful, and compassionate book discussing the author's work while director of the Mind/Body Clinic at Harvard Medical School.

The Neurophysiology of Enlightenment. Wallace, Robert Keith. Fairfield, IA: Maharishi International University Neuroscene Press, 1986.

Provides a good understanding of the mechanics of Transcendental Meditation, as well as scientific research carried out on Transcendental Meditation.

The Relaxation Response. Benson, Herbert. New York: Outlet Books, Inc., 1993.

Still a classic in the field, this book explains the relaxation response, a meditative technique derived from Transcendental Meditation, and its ability to relieve stress, anxiety, and stress-related illness.

Transcendental Meditation. Roth, Robert. New York: Donald I. Fine, Inc., 1988.

A simple, readable introduction to Transcendental Meditation.

Mind/Body Medicine

Mind/body medicine may soon revolutionize modern health care. Recognizing the profound interconnection of mind and body, the body's innate healing capabilities, and the role of self-responsibility in the healing process, mind/body medicine utilizes a wide range of modalities, including biofeedback, imagery, hypnotherapy, meditation, and yoga.

For the last three hundred years Western civilization has been shaped by a rational, scientific, mechanistic world view that has helped to bring about enormous technological and material advances. The practice of Western medicine reflects this mind-set and relies upon the technology it has produced, according to James S. Gordon, M.D., Director of the Center for Mind/Body Studies, and Clinical Professor in the Departments of Psychiatry and Community and Family Medicine at the Georgetown University School of Medicine. "Since the philosopher Descartes separated a transcendent and nonmaterial mind from the material and mechanical operations of the body, science has been concerned with ever more accurately resolving the body into its component parts," says Dr. Gordon. "This approach has produced extraordinary achievements—in the treatment of infectious diseases, in the synthesis of such desperately needed substances as insulin, and in the creation of exquisitely sophisticated and life-saving surgical procedures."

Unfortunately, the power and real achievements of this biomedical model have tended to narrow human perspective over time. People have come to view all illness as primarily a malfunction of mechanical parts and to regard physicians as technicians responsible for their repair. People have lost sight of the importance of the psychological, social, economic, and environmental influences on health and illness and of the extraordinary power of the mind to affect the body.

The Mind/Body Connection

In the last thirty years, scientists have begun to explore the complex interconnections between mind and body. "Psychological, sociological, and anthropological studies have confirmed what was clinically obvious—that people who are beset with poverty, job dissatisfaction, prejudice, cultural dislocation, long-term loneliness, or the sudden loss of a loved one are far more vulnerable to illness and death than those who are fulfilled in their social and interpersonal world," states Dr. Gordon.

Mood, attitude, and belief can affect virtually every chronic illness: fear, cynicism, as well as a sense of hopelessness and helplessness, can have a detrimental effect on health; whereas courage, good humor, a sense of control, and hopefulness can all be beneficial. Optimistic people are less likely to become ill and, when they do become ill, tend to live longer and suffer less. Studies at Yale and Rutgers Universities by Ellen Idler, Ph.D., Professor of Sociology at Rutgers, and Stanislav Kasl Ph.D., Professor of Epidemiology at Yale, indicate that the opinion of one's health status—how well one thinks one is—may be the best predictor of well-being and future health.[1]

See Biofeedback Training, Guided Imagery, Hypnotherapy, Meditation, Neuro-Linguistic Programming.

The scientific underpinnings for these clinical studies and anecdotal reports may be found in the new and rapidly expanding field of psychoneuroimmunology (PNI). The fruits of this approach are already being harvested in comprehensive programs of mind/body medicine at Harvard University, the University of Massachusetts, Stanford University, the University of Miami, and the University of California at San Francisco. Here people with such life-threatening and debilitating illnesses as cancer, AIDS, coronary heart disease, and chronic pain are learning to change their habits and attitude, what they eat, when they exercise, and how they think. A number of landmark studies have shown that these men and women are functioning far more effectively, feeling better, and in some particularly striking instances, living longer.[2]

Psychoneuroimmunology

In the 1970s, great advances in the study of the immune system helped to clarify the relationship between body and mind, which gave rise to the field of psychoneuroimmunology. Researchers found that naturally occurring substances known as peptides or neuropeptides (messenger molecules made up of amino acids), could cause alterations of mood, pain, and pleasure.[3] Among the first of these substances identified were endorphins, which is shorthand for endogenous morphines, meaning "the brain's own morphine." When endorphins are released they produce pleasurable responses, similar to those associated with opiates.

"We have come to theorize that these neuropeptides and their receptors are the biochemical correlates of emotions," says Candace Pert, Ph.D., visiting Professor at the Center for Molecular and Behavioral Neuroscience, Rutgers University, and former Chief of the Section on Brain Biochemistry of the Clinical Neuroscience Branch at the National Institute of Mental Health. "It took us fifteen years of research before we dared make that connection," adds Dr. Pert, "but we know that these neuropeptides are released during different emotional states.

"But the astounding revelation is that these endorphins and other chemicals like them are found not just in the brain, but in the immune system, the endocrine system, and throughout the body. When people discovered that there were endorphins in the brain that caused euphoria and pain relief, everyone could handle that. However, when they discovered they were in the immune system, as well, it just didn't fit, so these findings were denied for years. The original scientists had to repeat their studies many, many times to be believed."

Emotions, previously thought to be purely psychological, could now be linked to specific chemical processes taking place throughout the body, not just in the brain. Likewise, these peptides were seen to affect the functioning of all the systems of the body, including the immune system. "Viruses use the same receptors [as a neuropeptide] to enter into a cell," explains Dr. Pert, "and depending on how much of the natural peptide for that receptor is around, the virus will have an easier or harder time getting into the cell. So our emotional state will affect whether we'll get sick from the same loading dose of a virus."

"The immune system, like the central nervous system, has a memory and the capacity to learn. Thus, it could be said that intelligence is located in literally every cell of the body, and that the traditional separation of mind and body no longer applies."

Statistics have always borne out this relationship between the emotional state of an individual and his or her health, adds Dr. Pert. "You know the data about how people have more heart attacks on Monday mornings, and how death peaks in Christians the day after Christmas and in Chinese people the day after the Chinese New Year," but now science has been able to confirm that "emotional fluctuations and emotional status directly influence the probability that the [human] organism will get sick or be well."

Researchers also discovered that the immune system, like the central nervous system, has a memory and the capacity to learn. Thus, it could be said that intelligence is located in literally every cell of the body, and that the traditional separation of mind and body no longer applies.

Robert Ader, Ph.D, Director of the Division of Behavior and Psychosocial Medicine at the University of Rochester School of Medicine in New York, considered by many to be the father of psycho-neuroimmunology, conducted several studies that confirmed this belief. In one study, rats were given an immune-suppressing drug flavored with saccharin. Eventually, they were conditioned to suppress their immune systems in response to the taste of saccharin alone.[4] Another study showed that their immune systems could be similarly enhanced through conditioning. Since the immune systems of the rats are comparable to those of human beings, Dr. Adler suggests that people "can learn to influence the balance that maintains health in relation to the outside world."[5]

See Stress.

"Conditioning is a powerful bridge between mind and body," states Joan Borysenko, Ph.D., for "the body cannot tell the difference between events that are actual threats to survival and events that are present in thought alone."[6]

The implications of this work for human learning are vast, for they strongly suggest that internal and external stimuli (memories, thoughts, emotions, body movements, sounds, smells, tastes, situations, settings) can affect a variety of previously conditioned immune responses.

The Effect of Consciousness on the Body

The extent by which consciousness can affect control over the body is remarkable. Biofeedback research, for example, has shown that individuals can learn to control brainwave activity, affect cardiovascular and respiratory functioning, reduce skin temperature, and voluntarily modify many other autonomic processes of the body. John Basmajian, M.D., Professor Emeritus, Department of Medicine, McMaster University, Canada, who is a pioneer in biofeedback research, demonstrated that people could learn to consciously control individual neurons and muscle cells.[7] Single cell control through consciousness offers the possibility that one can affect any part of one's body, knowing how this process works.

Numerous other studies have demonstrated that consciousness can be used to relieve tension headaches, hypertension, urinary and fecal incontinence, temporomandibular joint syndrome, involuntary muscle spasms, muscle paralysis caused by cerebrovascular accidents, and dyskinesia. Consciousness can also be directed toward lowering blood pressure, reducing certain malfunctions of the heart, and modifying gastrointestinal secretions that cause ulcers, stomach acidity, and irritable bowel syndrome.[8]

"This extension of conscious control over involuntary systems has far-reaching implications for psychology and medicine," add pioneering researchers Elmer Green, Ph.D., and Alyce Green, founders of the Voluntary Controls Program at the Menninger Clinic in Topeka, Kansas. "It suggests that human beings are not biological robots, controlled entirely by genes and the conditioning of life experiences."[9]

Steven Fahrion, Ph.D., Director of the Center for Applied Psychophysiology at the Menninger Clinic, recalls one patient, a forty-three-year-old middle management executive, who came to him for treatment of hypertension and elevated blood pressure. Dr. Fahrion noted that the man talked rapidly, was

Fight or Flight Response

Virtually everyone has experienced the "fight or flight" response to some degree in his or her life. This response is the body's natural, unconscious reaction to threats, either real or imagined. It is often characterized by an adrenalin rush, dilated pupils, and a racing heart, all conditions that better equip the body to deal with whatever danger is perceived, be it from an animal, another person, a vehicle, or an imaginary threat, such as a noise in the middle of the night or a bad dream. The body's physiological processes adapt to their emotional reaction to danger. According to Joan Borysenko, Ph.D.,"It's what allows a small woman whose child has been run over to lift a two-ton truck off of that child."

Originally it was thought that the immune system played no part in the fight or flight mechanism, but recently new evidence has pointed to a different conclusion. In one study done immediately after the 1987 Los Angeles earthquake, blood was taken from nineteen people two to four hours after the trembler, and then again several times over the next year. What the study found was an increase in killer cells (such as antibodies) in the bloodstream just after the earthquake. The distress the individuals were experiencing, coupled with the fear that the "big one" might be coming next, correlated directly with the increase in killer cells.[10]

While the alarm response mobilizes the body's ability to fight or get away from a threat, the immune system activation may be seen as the body preparing itself to deal with the results of such a response, i.e., cuts and bruises sustained while fleeing, or any injuries from a hostile encounter.

This response is healthy and normal in situations of extreme stress or danger. However, when fight or flight manifests itself too often as a reaction to everyday stresses, the cumulative result can strain the various systems of the body, including the immune system. The body can become conditioned to react in this way, sometimes with little or no impetus, particularly among people who tend to internalize their emotions. This suggests a link between the body's emotional state and its overall health. Relaxation and the "venting" of pent-up emotions, negative or otherwise, have shown positive results counteracting this overactive fight or flight response.[11]

overscheduled, and felt he never had enough time. The patient was given biofeedback exercises so that he could learn to relax by consciously controlling the temperature of his hands and feet. He also learned to meditate and use visualization techniques in order to slow down his racing mind. As the man was able to sit quietly, he also began to have insights into his feelings and the way he managed his life, which he discussed with Dr. Fahrion. After three and a half months, the man's blood pressure had returned to normal.

"This extension of conscious control over involuntary systems has far-reaching implications for psychology and medicine. It suggests that human beings are not biological robots, controlled entirely by genes and the conditioning of life experiences."
—Elmer Green, Ph.D., and Alyce Green, founders of the Voluntary Controls Program at the Menninger Clinic

Principles of Mind/Body Medicine

The new mind/body medicine extends beyond the parameters of psychoneuroimmunology to include the fields of psychology and physics in a new "science of consciousness," a view which sees energy as the underlying pattern of the universe. This view bears similarities to many Asian philosophies that see human beings as part of an interconnected, universal energy field. These Eastern traditions (Ayurveda, *qigong,* yoga) have for centuries believed that consciousness plays an essential role in governing physical and psychological health.[12]

Mind/body medicine encompasses the following basic principles, which are often ignored or unrecognized by contemporary Western medicine:

Each Person Is Unique

No two people are alike, so even if they have the same disease, the paths to recovery may be different. Conversely, the same disease can be the result of different factors with different people. Although these principles have been long recognized in Traditional Chinese Medicine and Ayurvedic Medicine, it is a relatively new concept in Western medicine. One person, for example, may contract pneumonia as a result of a serious infection or cold, while someone else may come down with the same disease as a result of psychological stress. Yet a third person could become susceptible due to a nutritional or biochemical imbalance. Roger Williams, Ph.D., a pioneer in biochemistry, called this phenomenon "biochemical individuality," for he recognized that each of us is genetically unique, requiring slight variations in nutrient intake in order to function optimally.[13]

See Acupuncture, Ayurvedic Medicine, Qigong, Traditional Chinese Medicine, Yoga.

Chronic Stress

A basic premise in mind/body medicine is that chronic stress and lack of balance contribute to illness. Likewise, relaxation, positive methods of coping with stress, and restoration of balance lead to health. More important than the stressors themselves is the person's ability to cope. When stressors are met as a challenge and the individual feels competent to cope effectively, health may be enhanced. On the other hand, stress can also cause people to turn to desperate measures to try to cope, as in the case of substance abuse.

In the general adaptation syndrome model, developed by Hans Selye, a pioneering stress researcher, chronic activation of the fight or flight response leads to strain on an organ system over time, and interferes with its ability to adapt. Ultimately, the system breaks down and illness can set in.[14]

British cardiologist Peter Nixon explains that increased stress and arousal causes numerous changes in body functioning that eventually interfere with immune function, protein synthesis, and cardiac functioning. Repetitive stress also uses up the body's reserves, leading to increased stress on other physiological functions. This, in turn, can result in heart disease, cancer, or depression.[15]

If stress contributes to illness, then stress reduction should promote healing. This is the basis of numerous healing modalities such as progressive relaxation, guided imagery, and biofeedback. One such stress reduction method, the relaxation response technique, developed by Herbert Benson, M.D., of Harvard University, is a distillation of basic meditative practice, and has been shown to decrease heart rate and blood pressure, enhance health, and reduce the incidence of illness.[16] These basic stress reduction practices can be learned and practiced by anyone.

Multiple Personalities

The phenomenon of the multiple personality patient may offer evidence of how mental states directly affect physiology. Often a multiple will switch medical conditions when another personality takes over. By changing personalities, a multiple can switch physiological states, going from drunk to sober, sedated to alert, or left to right handed.[20]

John Sward, Ph.D., of the Center for the Improvement of Human Functioning International in Wichita, Kansas, experienced this several years ago when a female patient he was working with manifested allergies while in a different personality state. Working along with an allergist who would first test the woman for a certain allergy, Dr. Sward would then hypnotize her into a different personality state and the reaction would cease. Additionally, Dr. Sward found that the allergist could send the person into a different personality merely by placing different antigens on her skin.

The ability for a multiple personality patient to substitute personalities when in pain is an example of how mind/body medicine can accelerate the healing process.

Taking Self-Responsibility for Healing

Mind/body medicine supports the view that the patient is an active partner in all stages of treatment, rather than a passive recipient of medical intervention. Lawrence LeShan, Ph.D., a pioneer in mind/body medicine for the treatment of cancer, has documented that cancer patients who took charge of their life directions were more likely to recover than those who passively accepted their diagnosis.[17]

Taking action also decreases the fear and depression that so often accompanies life-threatening illness. By becoming actively involved in self-healing, one shifts from the feelings of helplessness and hopelessness that have been shown to increase depression and the risk of death to a sense of control.[18]

“By becoming actively involved in self-healing, one shifts from the feelings of helplessness and hopelessness that have been shown to increase depression and the risk of death to a sense of control.”

Immune functions are also affected by the experiences of helplessness or control. In one study, rats that were conditioned to experience helplessness were more likely to develop cancer from injected tumor cells and die than other rats. Rats that were trained to have a sense of control were best able to reject the tumor cells.[19]

The Body's Innate Healing Capabilities

The body has a natural, biological tendency to move toward health and balance, a phenomenon that can be observed in the simple healing of a cut in which the body automatically closes the wound and repairs the damage.

The well-known "placebo effect" (in which a neutral substance is found to effectively cure an ailment or disease) also demonstrates the body's capacity to heal itself. Erik Peper, Ph.D., Associate Director of the Institute for Holistic Healing Studies at San Francisco State University, suggests that "the placebo effect can decrease or remove the constraints that are interfering with the body's intrinsic drive toward wholeness." These constraints can include feelings of helplessness and hopelessness, negative beliefs about the illness, and negative self-images.

Jeanne Achterberg, Ph.D., President of the Association for Transpersonal Psychology, adds that the effectiveness of the placebo varies "depending upon how much the patient expects to benefit." In other words, those who think they will get better have a significantly greater recovery rate than those who think they will not get better, or think they will get worse.[21]

The Importance of the Client-Provider Relationship

The relationship between the client and the physician can strongly influence the healing process. For example, when a physician is perceived as powerful and trustworthy, the client gets better faster, and one study has even shown that physician reassurance and support raises the threshold of pain tolerance in hospital patients.[22]

Mind/body medicine recognizes that the practitioner is constantly communicating (consciously and unconsciously) with the client. Just as the placebo is seen as a way of promoting healing through the patient's belief system, the positive attitude of the doctor can influence the outcome of a given treatment, while discouraging statements or prejudices can evoke what some call a "nocebo" effect by undermining the patient's confidence and hindering the healing process.

Unfortunately, this dimension of the healing process is rarely noticed or addressed. Thus, a doctor who thinks of a patient as hopeless will convey this to the patient even if the thought is unspoken. In the ideal client/provider relationship, the healing process is viewed as a working partnership in which both parties respect the knowledge and intuition of the other. In this respect, the health care provider seeks to convey the potential for wholeness in each client.

A Systems Approach

Mind/body medicine is based upon a systems perspective that recognizes that human lives are influenced by many interrelated factors, including genetics, family and socioeconomic background, diet, exercise, social support, risk-taking behaviors, attitudes, and spiritual practices. An illness may be only a manifestation of imbalance on the physical level, but the imbalance may also originate in other aspects of the self, such as the mental or emotional state.

Any movement toward health mobilizes the other healing potentials of the body. As a person makes a change in one area, other areas tend to change as well. For example, if a person begins to exercise, the person may feel more socially confident and might spontaneously change his or her eating habits, thus improving overall physical and emotional health. While any disease may be a problem in but a small part of the total person, the factors that influence its manifestation and subsequent healing can be extraordinarily complex.

The Energy Field Perspective

Each of us has various fields of energy that can be measured instrumentally with an EKG (electrocardiograph), an EEG, (electroencephalograph), or electroacupuncture biofeedback testing, a method of testing based on measurement of the electrical properties of acupuncture points. These energy fields are continuously affected by changes in physical or psychological health, and can even be influenced by the energy fields of others.

Robert Becker, M.D., a pioneer in the study of the effects of electromagnetism on health, found that small electric currents can stimulate cells to regenerate, fractures to heal faster, and tissue to repair itself.[23] Research in neuropsychiatry over the past few decades has also shown that small electric currents between specific points in the brain give rise to the same behavioral changes that are observed with the injection of certain brain-stimulating chemicals.[24]

The energy field perspective can even be applied to hospital settings. Dolores Krieger, Ph.D., R.N., a former Professor of Nursing at New York University, has developed a technique known as Therapeutic Touch, which has been proven to be effective in treating a variety of medical conditions. According to Dr. Krieger, Therapeutic Touch "is a contemporary interpretation of several ancient healing practices in which the practioner consciously directs or sensitively modulates human energies."[25]

The proper use of Therapeutic Touch can increase hemoglobin and decrease anxiety,[26] reduce pain, accelerate the healing of surgical wounds, and help correct dysfunctions of the autonomic nervous system.[27] This technique has been taught to more than 37,000 nurses, doctors, and health practitioners.[28]

See Bodywork, Energy Medicine.

The importance of human touch is greatly emphasized in mind/body medicine, especially for children. "In a child, absence of touch can cause the pituitary gland not to secrete enough growth hormone," says Dr. Borysenko. "The child will dwarf, developing what is called 'failure to thrive' syndrome. The child can't assimilate nutrients and may actually sicken and die."

Handling and physical affection have been shown to increase the survival rate of infants, improve psychological skills and functioning, promote physical growth and immune function, and, most importantly, enable a person to respond effectively to stress.[29] Also, autopsies on rats that were given extra handling and care showed much less damage to their cardiovascular and intestinal systems than those who were not handled.[30]

Illness as Message, Not Enemy

In many ways, contemporary medicine conveys the notion of all-out war against disease, in which illness is seen as an enemy and death as a failure. From a mind/body perspective, illness is seen as a communication from the body, a warning signal that something needs attention. People can use this "message" to review the entire mind/body system and see how it is functioning as a whole. If a person experiences back pain, he or she might ask, "Am I carrying too much emotional weight? Am I under too much stress? Am I using my body properly or exercising it well?"

"In mind/body medicine, one looks beyond the immediate problem to include a larger dimension of one's life. For example, a heart attack may be a signal for a person to become less defensive and hostile, to become less competitive at work, and to give more attention to relaxation, hobbies, family, and the enjoyment of life."

In mind/body medicine, one looks beyond the immediate problem to include a larger dimension of one's life. For example, a heart attack may be a signal for a person to become less defensive and hostile, to become less competitive at work, and to give more attention to relaxation, hobbies, family, and the enjoyment of life. In this process a person's heart will heal both literally and symbolically. The highly successful program for healing heart disease conducted by Dean Ornish, M.D., Assistant Clinical Professor of Medicine at the University of California at San Francisco, utilizes these components.[31]

How Does Healing Occur from a Mind/Body Perspective?

Ultimately people do not know how healing occurs. The best people can do is to support and encourage the body's intrinsic healing mechanisms. Mind/body medicine often begins by promoting physical and mental relaxation, and developing better ways of coping with stress. Various techniques include meditation, biofeedback, hypnotherapy, guided imagery, hypnosis, neuro-linguistic programming, *qigong*, massage, bodywork, exercise, yoga, breathwork, and progressive relaxation techniques. Even herbal remedies and acupuncture may be used to promote relaxation. Lifestyle changes may also be required in this holistic approach to health.

By taking time to relax, one becomes more mindful of one's condition, grows more aware of the body's subtle signals, and responds to stress long before its destructive effects can take hold. By incorporating many short relaxation practices throughout the day and conditioning oneself to relax instead of tensing when encountering a source of stress, the depleted energy reserves can be rebuilt.

How a person frames or perceives experiences may also have a direct impact on the immune system. Symbolic threats produce real physiological consequences, as every good worrier knows. Perception of meaning, and the language used, may also be an essential element of healing.

Health Requires Emotional Balance

Grief, bereavement, depression, fear, and panic have been shown to suppress the immune response, while laughter, play, love, faith, hope, and self-acceptance help to stimulate and balance immune function. Part of healing, then, involves the recognition and release of negative emotions such as resentment, guilt, anger, and self-hatred, and the fostering of feelings of well-being, adequacy, and self-control. Studies have shown that having a sense of control, commitment, and connectedness—along with viewing change as a challenge rather than a threat—promotes the maintenance of good health even when under stress.[32]

Sharing and Support

Satisfaction in relationships and work are also essential to one's happiness and health. Healthy relationships are characterized by a mutual flow of giving and receiving, mutual support and respect, and the ability to work out conflicts and difficulties.

To be able to share feelings and pain with one another is an essential component to healing, for it shows us that people are not alone and that they have something to offer. This can be accomplished in therapy, in social groups, and through the development of friends or close family relationships. David Spiegel, a psychiatrist at Stanford University, demonstrated that women with breast cancer who participated in a weekly support group lived twice as long as than those who did not.[33]

"There is overwhelming evidence that people who have few social contacts are more likely to get sick and less likely to recover from an illness," says Dr. Peper. One long-term study found that people with the lowest amount of social ties were two to three times more likely to die of all causes than those with the most social connectedness.[34] "Isolation and loneliness have also been shown to result in immune problems in bereaved individuals who have recently lost their loved ones," adds Dr. Fahrion.

PSYCHOLOGICAL FACTORS ENHANCE HEALTH AND HEALING

In a recent issue of the journal Science, *sixty-two studies were cited showing that supportive social relationships—friends, extended family, marital ties, and group membership—had a positive effect upon surgical recovery, recovery from chronic and infectious disease, and improvements of cardiovascular activity and immune function. A lack of these supportive relationships significantly increased the incidence of death.[37]*

Jeanne Achterberg, Ph.D., President of the Association for Transpersonal Psychology, cites numerous additional studies demonstrating that:

- *Feelings of helplessness and hopelessness increase cancer growth and digestive problems.*
- *Anxiety and stress increase the production of adrenal corticosteroids which interfere with healing, compromise the immune system, and encourage cardiovascular disease.*
- *Fear and anxiety inhibit the cell's repair mechanisms.*
- *Feelings of security, coupled with the ability to cope, counter the deleterious effects of negative emotions.*
- *Joy and relaxation increase circulation to painful or wounded areas and improve tissue repair.[38]*

Guided Imagery in Healing

Guided imagery is an important tool for healing. Dr. Achterberg suggests that every image a person has in the mind can affect immune function, blood flow, and heart rate.[35] Other studies have shown that guided imagery can decrease chronic nightmares,[36] reduce substance abuse, and alleviate many other psychological and physiological problems.

Breath

Regulation of breathing plays an important role in mind/body medicine, because it is capable of bringing about a state of relaxation. Shallow chest breathing and hyperventilation, for example, are part of the body's response to stress. These dysfunctional breathing patterns can cause increased heart rate, blood vessel constriction, and muscle tension, as well as chains of negative thoughts.

A person who suppresses unpleasant feelings and thoughts may also unknowingly restrict his or her breathing. Thus, it is important to express and release these emotions in order to maintain proper breathing. Likewise, proper breathing can help facilitate an emotional release. Many psycho-oriented therapies such as Reichian therapy emphasize emotional release through deliberate alteration of breathing patterns.

Slow, conscious, diaphragmatic breathing is a powerful tool for promoting relaxation and awareness. It is an essential component of many therapeutic approaches to the body and the mind, and is utilized in most forms of meditation as well as in the practice of yoga and *qigong*. When cardiac patients, who are usually shallow chest breathers, learn slow diaphragmatic breathing, there is a 50 percent drop in recurrence of coronary events.[39] It can also be used to reduce panic attacks, headache, chest pain, and other symptoms.

In a study at San Francisco State University, Dr. Peper, along with his student Vicci Tibbets, worked with a group of asthmatics to help them learn self-regulation approaches. Participants met in a group for sixteen weeks, utilizing the power of group support. They were given slow diaphragmatic breathing and biofeedback training for calming the upper body muscles. Once breathing techniques were mastered, the participants learned to use them in increasingly stressful situations. As they began to feel in control, their fears decreased, and a sense of hope emerged. Those participants who took charge of their lives and continued with their training were found to be in better shape at the fifteen-month follow-up, showing that self-responsibility contributed to the enhancement of their health.[40]

The Future of Mind/Body Medicine

Mind/body practitioners believe that the present Western medical model will become a subset of the holistic mind/body medicine of the future. As patients recover from surgery or illness, they can be taught skills to speed up the body's healing processes, reduce pain, and reflect upon those changes necessary to improve the quality of their lives. The goal will be not to simply remove the symptom but to help the person attain a greater state of wholeness. It is a process that should continue throughout life.

Since this new healing philosophy places so much power and responsibility in the hands of the patient, an educational approach is needed. Relaxation, stress reduction, guided imagery, and behavioral change can and should be taught at all levels, from elementary school to college.

There is already a program in holistic healing studies at San Francisco State University that includes Traditional Chinese Medicine, Western and Eastern perspectives on holistic health, relaxation training, peak performance training for athletes, meditation, and biofeedback. In addition to cognitive study, students practice daily relaxation, imagery, and other healing techniques. They report decreases in chronic headaches, improved sleep, enhanced self-awareness and self-esteem, and much greater ability to cope with stress. Many have adopted improved diet and exercise patterns or quit smoking. Some have even been able to eliminate long-standing health problems.

Throughout the United States, major hospitals and university medical centers are also beginning to incorporate the principles of mind/body medicine. At Parkland Hospital in Dallas, Texas, mind/body medicine has been implemented throughout the organizational system, focusing on what practioners call "patient-centered" care, which includes personalized attention, education, self-health improvement at home, and prevention. Parkland's seven community center clinics have been able to cut their average hospital expenses in half by implementing these types of programs.

At Case Western Reserve University in Cleveland, Ohio, and at the Menninger Clinic, biofeedback, guided imagery, and other stress reduction techniques are being used to treat conditions ranging from migraines to cancer and heart disease. At the University of Massachusetts Medical Center, Jon Kabat-Zinn, Ph.D., established the Stress Reduction Clinic where patients suffering from chronic pain are taught meditation and a new philosophy of health and well-being.

"We need to take what's most valuable from all the various consciousness traditions, integrate them into Western behavioral science and mainstream medicine, and study them as best we can in terms of the most sophisticated and stringent scientific methodologies," adds Dr. Kabat-Zinn. "We need to ask, 'What is it about these ancient traditions that tells us something valuable about healing and the mind?'"

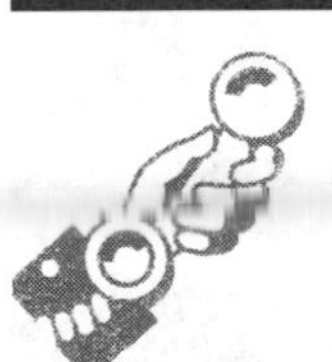

Where to Find Help

A growing field, mind/body medicine is currently practiced at many locations throughout the country. The following programs are among the most renowned:

The Center for Applied Psychophysiology
Menninger Clinic
P.O. Box 829
Topeka, Kansas 66601-0829
(913) 273-7500 Ext. 5375

The Center for Applied Psychophysiology has research and treatment in all phases of mind/body medicine. They work with disorders of the cardiovascular, gastrointestinal, immune, and respiratory systems. They also work with programs on peak performance for athletes, as well as drug and alcohol abuse.

The Center for the Improvement of Human Functioning
3100 North Hillside Avenue
Wichita, Kansas 67219-3904
(316) 682-3100

A medical research educational organization, the center offers clinical services, diagnostic testing, educational classes, conferences and seminars. The center publishes books, has a large library and performs clinical and basic research.

The Center for Mind/Body Studies
5225 Connecticut Avenue, Northwest, Suite 414
Washington, D.C. 20015
(202) 966-7338
(202) 966-2589 (Fax)

The Center for Mind-Body Studies is an educational program for health and mental health professionals and those who are interested in exploring their own capacities for self-knowledge and self-care. Directed by James S. Gordon, M.D., its work is grounded in an appreciation of the interpenetration of life's biological, psychological, spiritual, and social dimensions. The Center's projects include: 1) the development of a comprehensive model program of mind/body studies for medical students and residents; 2) a community health services program to bring the mind/body approach to nonprofit groups that serve the working poor and indigent; 3) a mind/body education program for teenagers; 4) educational and support groups for people with chronic illness; 5) stress management groups; 6) a supervision group for psychotherapists and community workers; 7) a training program in mind/body health care for professionals; 8) a program of public workshops in mind/body health care.

Mind-Body Clinic
New Deaconess Hospital
Harvard Medical School
185 Pilgrim Road
Cambridge, Massachusetts 02215
(617) 632-9530

Provides treatment program at a medical center where the relaxation response can be learned. The Mind-Body Clinic uses yoga, meditation, and stress reduction as part of its program.

Stress Reduction and Relaxation Program
University of Massachusetts Medical Center
55 Lake Avenue, North
Worcester, Massachusetts 01655
(508) 856-2656

The Stress Reduction and Relaxation Program is a training program to teach meditative-type awareness.

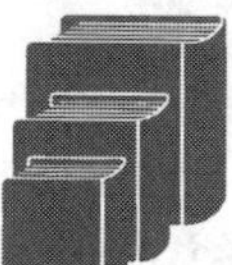

Recommended Reading

Creating Wholeness: A Self-Healing Workbook Using Dynamic Relaxation, Images and Thoughts. Peper, Erik; and Holt, Catherine. New York: Plenum, 1993.

A simple and accessible self-help program that teaches physical, cognitive, and imagery-based techniques to reduce stress and promote health.

Full Catastrophe Living: Using the Wisdom of Your Body and Mind to Face Stress, Pain, and Illness. Kabat-Zinn, Jon. New York: Delta, 1990.

A comprehensive look at how meditation can be applied to modern life. Provides a variety of self-help exercises, along with actual case histories which illustrate how the mind can be used to create wellness in daily life.

Head First: The Biology of Hope. Cousins, Norman. New York: Thorndike Press, 1991

Based on hundreds of interviews with doctors, patients, medical students, and research scientists, this book chronicles how an optimistic outlook, faith, hope, laughter, the will to live, and a strong relationship with the doctor can make illness less painful and increase a person's chances of survival.

Healing and the Mind. Moyers, Bill. New York: Doubleday, 1993.

The transcripts of fifteen interviews with different doctors who are investigating the power of the mind. An investigation by Moyers of a new approach to illness.

The Healer Within. Locke, Steven; and Colligan, Douglas. New York: Mentor, 1986.

An accessible, authoritative, and complete study of how emotions and attitudes can affect health and the treatment of diseases from the common cold to cancer.

Healing Yourself: A Step-by-Step Program for Better Health through Imagery. Rossman, Martin L. New York: Pocket Books, 1989.

A simple how-to book on unleashing the body's natural healing powers.

Imagery in Healing Shamanism and Modern Medicine. Achterberg, Jeanne. Boston: Shambala Publications, Inc. 1985.

The author explains how the systematic use of imagery can help patients through painful events ranging from childbirth to burn treatment, as well as act as a positive influence on disease states such as cancer.

Mind/Body Medicine: How to Use Your Mind for Better Health. Goleman, D.; and Gurin, Joel. New York: Consumer Reports Books, 1993.

A comprehensive, informative book on the power of the mind. A well-researched collection of essays and case histories by more than twenty-four different researchers and doctors.

Minding the Body, Mending the Mind. Borysenko, Joan. New York: Bantam Books, 1988.

Based on ground-breaking work at the Mind/Body Clinic at New England Deaconess Hospital, this book tells of dramatic success with conditions ranging from allergies to cancer. A unique blend of physical and mental exercises are explained, which show how to elicit the mind's relaxation response, boost the immune system, overcome chronic pain, and alleviate stress-related illnesses.

Quantum Healing. Chopra, Deepak. New York, Bantam Books, 1989.

Draws from Western medicine, neuroscience, physics, Ayurvedic medicine, ancient wisdom, and case histories, including recoveries from severe illnesses, to explain mind/body medicine in a thought-provoking and personal way.

The Relaxation Response. Benson, Herbert. New York: Outlet Books, Inc. 1993.

Still a classic in the field and an excellent introduction to learning meditations.

"A cheerful heart is good medicine,
But a downcast spirit dries up the bones."

—Proverbs 17:22

Naturopathic Medicine

Naturopathic medicine treats health conditions by utilizing the body's inherent ability to heal. Naturopathic physicians aid the healing process by incorporating a variety of alternative methods based on the patient's individual needs. Diet, lifestyle, work, and personal history are all considered when determining a treatment regimen.

The spirit of naturopathic medicine is reflected in the definition of health advocated by the World Health Organization (WHO)—"a state of complete physical, mental, and social well-being, not merely the absence of infirmity."[1] In fact, WHO, in a report on traditional medicine, has recommended the integration of naturopathic medicine into conventional health care systems.[2]

Naturopathic medicine is not a single modality of healing, but an array of healing practices, including diet and clinical nutrition; homeopathy; acupuncture; herbal medicine; hydrotherapy; therapeutic exercise; spinal and soft-tissue manipulation; physical therapies involving electric currents, ultrasound, and light therapy; therapeutic counseling; and pharmacology.

Principles of Naturopathic Medicine

Although the term naturopathy or naturopathic medicine was not used until the late nineteenth century, its philosophical roots date back thousands of years. Drawing from the healing wisdom of many cultures including Indian (Ayurveda), Chinese (Traditional Chinese Medicine), Native American, and Greek (Hippocratic), naturopathic medicine is a system of medicine based on six time-tested principles:

- **The healing power of nature:** The body has considerable power to heal itself, and the role of the naturopathic physician is to facilitate this natural process with the aid of natural, nontoxic therapies.
- **Treat the cause rather than the effect:** Naturopathic physicians seek the underlying cause of a disease rather than simply suppressing the symptoms. They avoid suppression of the natural healing wisdom of the body, such as fever and inflammation. Symptoms are viewed as expressions of the body's natural attempt to heal while the causes can spring from the physical, mental/emotional, and spiritual levels.

- **First, do no harm:** By employing safe and effective natural therapies, naturopathic physicians are committed to the principle of causing no harm to the patient.
- **Treat the whole person:** The individual is viewed as a whole, composed of a complex interaction of physical, mental/emotional, spiritual, social, and other factors. This multifactorial approach results in a therapeutic approach in which no disease is automatically seen as incurable.
- **The physician is a teacher:** Naturopathic physicians are first and foremost teachers who educate, empower, and motivate the patient to assume more personal responsibility for his or her health by adopting a healthy attitude, lifestyle, and diet.
- **Prevention is the best cure:** Naturopathic physicians are preventive medicine specialists. Prevention of disease is accomplished through education and a lifestyle that supports health.

“In the naturopathic system of medicine, disease is seen as the manifestation of the causes by which the body naturally heals itself.”

How Does Naturopathic Medicine Work?

In the naturopathic system of medicine, disease is seen as a manifestation of the natural causes by which the body heals itself. For example, fever and inflammation are viewed as the body's way of dealing with an imbalance that is undermining the healthy functioning of the body. However, if the cause of the imbalance is not removed, the inflammatory responses will continue, either at a lower level of intensity or intermittently. This can be the origin of chronic disease. Healing a chronic disease requires removal of the underlying cause. This usually culminates in a return of an acute episode, called a “healing crisis” or “reaction,” a keynote of naturopathic medical theory. Following this the condition improves.

Although naturopathic physicians emphasize therapeutic choices based on individual interest and experience, as well as the legal parameters of the state in which he or she practices, they maintain a consistent philosophy. All have been trained in the basic tools of natural therapeutics, and most work with diet and nutrition while specializing in one or more other therapeutic methods.

“After identifying which conditions in the patient manifest in disease, the naturopathic physician advises the patient on building better conditions for the return to health.”

After identifying which conditions in the patient manifest in illness, the naturopathic physician advises the patient on the methods most appropriate for creating a return to health. In order to become free of illness, it is often necessary for the patient to make both dietary and lifestyle changes. Homeopathy or acupuncture are often used to stimulate recovery. Herbal medicines may be used as tonics and nutritive agents to support and strengthen weakened systems, while specific nutritional agents such as vitamin and mineral supplements and glandular tissue extracts might also be utilized. Hydrotherapy and various types of physical therapy may be required. Additionally, it is important that major emotional stresses be eased to allow the digestive system to function in the relaxed environment required for proper digestion.

Finally, underlying many illnesses is a spiritual disharmony. This may be experienced as a feeling of deep unease or insufficient strength of will necessary to sustain the healing process. For lasting good health to be established, this disharmony must be overcome. Naturopathic physicians can play an important role in guiding patients to discover the course of action most appropriate.

Conditions Benefited by Naturopathic Medicine

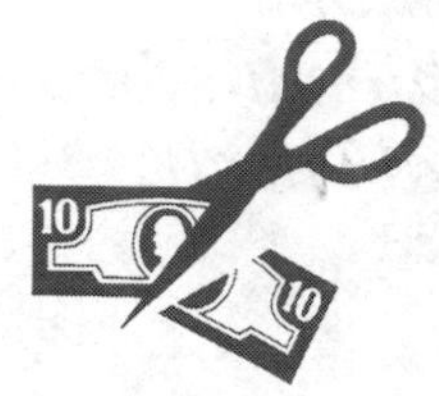

With its emphasis on prevention and natural care, naturopathic medicine may offer long-term savings to the consumer.

Naturopathic medicine can be applied in any health care situation, but its strongest area is in the treatment of chronic and degenerative disease. Naturopaths are, for the most part, licensed primary care/general practice family physicians. For severe, acute traumas such as a serious automobile accident, emergencies of childbirth, or orthopedic problems requiring corrective surgery, naturopathic medicine is not recommended, although it can contribute to such cases, especially in the recovery phase.

In other acute cases, such as ear infections and common illnesses with fever, the naturopathic physician addresses the associated pain, infection, and fever of the condition, as well as any related concerns of the patient. How this acute condition might relate to underlying causes, such as diet, life stresses, and occupational hazards, is also addressed. The physician will then usually prescribe a variety of means to deal with the immediate problem.

In chronic cases, the procedure is different. Typically, a thorough case exploration will detail the history and nature of the patient's symptoms and complaints, his or her complete health history, and the patient's lifestyle. Finally, a physical examination and appropriate laboratory tests are performed. For naturopathic physicians, understanding the patient as an individual is essential when searching for causative factors, particularly in the areas of the physical, mental/emotional, and spiritual.

See Acupuncture, Diet, Herbal Medicine, Homeopathy, Hydrotherapy, Nutritional Supplements.

After determining causative factors, the physician will discuss his or her findings with the patient, and an attempt will be made to tie together and interpret the symptoms. Symptoms usually relate to a central problem that has many manifestations. As an example, many symptoms can be tied to the effects of toxemia on the different systems of the body such as the immune system, nervous system or circulatory system. Others may be due to emotional factors, such as a chronic urinary tract infection when there is a history of sexual abuse.

Finally, dietary factors are determined and appropriate changes are recommended. Any other perceived causes are addressed with either counseling, exercise, or other methods of treatment.

Healing the Person, Not the Disease

Naturopathic medicine does not focus on disease symptoms, but, rather, the underlying causes. For example, the body has four major organs that assist in elimination: the lungs, kidneys, bowels, and skin. Most skin diseases are viewed by naturopathic physicians to be the result of excessive metabolic toxicity in the body, forcing the skin to be used as an extra route of elimination. The skin excretes both water-soluble and oil-soluble wastes through the sweat and oil glands. Because the elimination of toxins is irritating to the skin, the result is often various forms of skin-related disorders such as dermatitis and acne.

"Naturopathic medicine does not focus on disease, but rather the underlying causes."

A woman suffering from dermatitis, an itchy and often inflamed skin rash, sought the help of Jared Zeff, N.D., L.Ac., of Portland, Oregon. She was also partially blind from an incurable condition known as retinitis pigmentosa, a progressive form of retinal degeneration which results in blindness. After assessing her condition, Dr. Zeff viewed the dermatitis as a result of the elimination of toxins through the skin generated by maldigestion. He prescribed a specific diet to help improve her digestion, and recommended a series of hydrotherapy treatments, also to improve digestion and to stimulate other mechanisms of elimination. Dr. Zeff also prescribed a botanical digestive tonic, and later a homeopathic remedy.

As a result of Dr. Zeff's diagnosis and subsequent treatment, not only did the woman's dermatitis begin to clear, but she reported to Dr. Zeff that instead of seeing him as a blurry shape, she was able to make out the specific features of his face. Her eyesight improved to the point where she could read large print books. Dr. Zeff had not specifically sought to improve her retinal degeneration, assuming it was not possible for her destroyed tissue to be regenerated. Her story is just one example of the body's amazing capacity to recuperate.

Another patient of Dr. Zeff was an older gentleman afflicted with bladder cancer. Although this form of cancer has a high rate of success from conventional treatment, his had not responded to chemotherapy. When Dr. Zeff applied pressure to specific reflex points of the patient's body, he was told they did not hurt, even though he could see pain expressed in the man's face. When questioned more deeply, it was discovered that the patient's only child had committed suicide five years previously. The man had been unable to grieve, and had apparently shut off his feelings, which resulted in a physical manifestation of feeling cut-off from his body.

WHAT TO EXPECT WHEN YOU VISIT A NATUROPATHIC PHYSICIAN

A typical office visit with a naturopathic doctor takes one hour. Your naturopathic physician considers teaching you how to live healthfully one of his or her primary goals, so the time devoted to discussing and explaining principles of health maintenance, as well as your medical condition, is one of the factors that sets naturopaths apart from conventional physicians, who often seem to be rushing from patient to patient.

The relationship begins with a thorough medical history and interview process designed to view all aspects of your lifestyle. If needed, the physician will perform standard diagnostic procedures including a physical exam and blood and urine analysis. Once a good understanding of your health and disease status is established (diagnosing an illness is only one part of this process), you and your doctor work together to establish a treatment and health-promoting program.

Dr. Zeff prescribed a diet and a series of hydrotherapy treatments. He also instructed the patient's wife on how to treat her husband at home. She assisted with the hydrotherapy sessions and administered a therapeutic touch technique taught by Dr. Zeff that involved placing her hands over

ORIGINS AND DEVELOPMENT OF NATUROPATHIC MEDICINE

Naturopathic medicine grew out of the alternative healing movement of the eighteenth and nineteenth centuries. The European tradition of "taking the cure" at natural springs and spas had gained a foothold in America by the middle of the nineteenth century, and this atmosphere helped make the United States especially receptive to the principles of naturopathy.

The early naturopaths attached great importance to a natural, healthy diet, as did many of their contemporaries. John Kellogg, a physician and vegetarian, ran the Battle Creek Sanitarium in Battle Creek, Michigan, which utilized natural therapies such as hydrotherapy, while his brother Will built and ran a factory in Battle Creek to produce health foods like shredded wheat and granola biscuits. The Kellogg brothers, along with a former employee, C. W. Post, helped popularize naturopathic ideas about food, and at the same time founded the cereal companies which today bear their names.

Naturopathic medicine flourished in the United States until the mid-1930s, at which point the medical profession started to conglomerate into the single-view, omnipotent establishment it is today. Naturopathic medicine, and nearly every other natural healing modality, was effectively wiped out.

Yet, naturopathic medicine has experienced a tremendous resurgence in the last two decades. This is largely due to increased public awareness of the role of diet and lifestyle in the cause of chronic disease, as well as the failure of modern medicine to deal effectively with these disorders.

and under her husband's bladder and sacrum for ten minutes each session. Because she was also not well, suffering from chronic bronchitis, Dr. Zeff outlined for her a specific diet, as well as a dose of *Ignatia*, a homeopathic remedy to relieve the effects of suppressed grief. Dr. Zeff also instructed the couple to walk together for half an hour each day.

In both husband and wife, the cause of their illnesses—the grief and the inability to release it—was the same, yet on the physical level the unexpressed grief manifested differently. Their illnesses were addressed by informal discussion, a referral to a counselor, and a homeopathic remedy, as well as mutual treatments between husband and wife. In ten weeks the patient was rechecked for cancer. Not only had it disappeared, but his wife's chronic bronchitis had also cleared up.

What Is a Naturopathic Physician Trained to Do?

Modern naturopathic doctors provide complete diagnostic and therapeutic services. As family doctors, many practice natural childbirth (usually in the home setting), pediatrics, gynecology, and geriatrics. Naturopathic physicians make recommendations on lifestyle, diet, and exercise, and utilize a variety of natural and noninvasive healing techniques.

The current scope of treatments naturopathic physicians are trained in include: clinical nutrition; botanical or herbal medicine; homeopathy; acupuncture; hydrotherapy; physical medicine including massage and therapeutic manipulation; counseling and other psychotherapies; and minor surgery.

- **Clinical nutrition:** The use of diet as a therapy serves as the foundation of naturopathic medicine. There is an ever-increasing body of knowledge that supports the use of whole foods and nutritional supplements in the maintenance of health and treatment of disease.
- **Herbal medicine:** Plants have been used as medicines since antiquity. Naturopathic physicians are professionally trained herbalists and know both the historical and medicinal uses of plants.

- **Homeopathy:** The term homeopathy is derived from the Greek word *homoios*, meaning "similar," and *pathos*, meaning "suffering." Homeopathy is a system of medicine that treats a disease with dilute, potentized remedies that will produce the same symptoms as the disease when given to a healthy individual. The fundamental principle operating here is that like cures like. Homeopathic medicines are derived from a variety of plant, mineral, and chemical substances.
- **Acupuncture:** Acupuncture is an ancient Chinese system of medicine involving the stimulation of certain specific points on the body to enhance the flow of vital life energy *qi* along pathways called meridians. Acupuncture points are stimulated by the insertion and withdrawal of needles, the application of heat (moxibustion), acupressure (deep finger pressure), lasers, electrical means, or a combination of these methods.
- **Hydrotherapy:** Hydrotherapy uses water in all its temperatures (hot, cold), forms (ice, steam), and methods of application (sitz baths, douches, spas, whirlpools, saunas, showers, immersion baths, packs, poultices, foot baths, fomentations, wraps, colonic irrigations), in the maintenance of health or treatment of disease. It is one of the most ancient methods of treatment. Hydrotherapy has been used to treat disease and injury by many different cultures, including the Egyptians, Assyrians, Persians, Greeks, Hebrews, Hindus, Chinese, and Native Americans.
- **Physical medicine:** Physical medicine refers to the use of physical measures in the treatment of disease. These include: therapeutic exercise, massage, joint mobilization (manipulation) and immobilization techniques, and hydrotherapy. Physical medicine also includes physiotherapy equipment such as ultrasound (high frequency sound waves that act as a micro-massage to tissues, stimulating or restoring function or blood circulation), diathermy (high frequency currents used to generate heat within the body), electric currents used in the body to stimulate function or relieve pain, and light therapy (applications of light that are used to stimulate heating responses in the body, such as endocrine function or increased circulation).
- **Counseling and lifestyle modification:** Counseling and lifestyle modification techniques are essential to naturopathic medicine. A naturopathic physician is formally trained in the following counseling areas: 1) Interviewing and responding skills, active listening, body language assessment, and other contact skills necessary for the therapeutic relationship; 2) Recognition and understanding of prevalent psychological issues including developmental problems, sexual dysfunction, abnormal behavior, addictions, and stress; 3) Various treatment measures including hypnosis and guided imagery, counseling techniques, correction of underlying organic factors, and family therapy.
- **Minor surgery:** Some naturopathic physicians are trained in a variety of minor surgical techniques. These include laceration

repair (sutures), skin biopsies, skin lesion removal, sclerosing therapy for spider veins and varicose veins, noninvasive hemorrhoid surgery, abscess incising and draining, circumcision, and the setting of fractures.

Licensing is currently available for naturopathic physicians in only seven states. It is important to encourage your state government to license naturopathic medicine in your state.

The Future of Naturopathic Medicine

"To the uninformed, naturopathic medicine, as well as the entire concept of natural medicine, appears to be a fad that will soon pass away," says Michael Murray, N.D., of Seattle, Washington. "To the informed, however, it is quite clear that naturopathic medicine is at the forefront of the future."

One of the great fallacies promoted by the United States medical establishment is that there is not firm scientific evidence for the use of many natural therapies. "This assumption is simply not true," according to Dr. Murray. "In fact, during the last ten or twenty years there has been a literal explosion of information in the scientific literature supporting the use of natural medicine."

"To the uninformed, naturopathic medicine, as well as the entire concept of natural medicine, appears to be a fad that will soon pass away. To the informed, however, it is quite clear that naturopathic medicine is at the forefront of the future."
—Michael Murray, N.D.

Today, science and medicine have the technology and understanding necessary to appreciate many aspects of natural medicine. It is becoming increasingly common for medical organizations which in the past have spoken out strongly against naturopathic medicine to embrace it, endorsing naturopathic techniques such as lifestyle modification, stress reduction, exercise, and a high-fiber diet.

"This illustrates the paradigm shift that is occurring in medicine," says Dr. Murray. "What was once scoffed at is now becoming generally accepted as an effective alternative. In fact, in most instances the naturopathic alternative offers significant benefit over standard medical practices. Undoubtedly in the future many of the concepts, philosophies, and practices of naturopathy will be vindicated. Certainly the future looks very bright for naturopathic medicine."

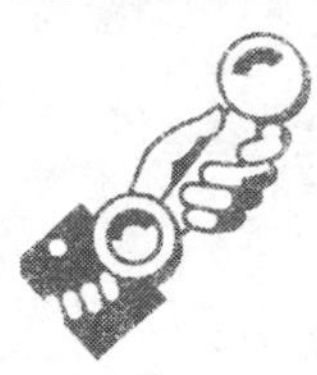

Where to Find Help

Licensing for naturopathic physicians in the United States is currently available in seven states (Alaska, Arizona, Connecticut, Hawaii, Montana, Oregon, and Washington), as well as in five Canadian provinces (Alberta, British Columbia, Manitoba, Ontario, and Saskatchewan). However, the profession is expanding, and additional licensing efforts are underway in eight other jurisdictions. There are currently two accredited colleges in the United States, and one in Canada. A third, the Southwest College of Naturopathic Medicine, has recently opened in Scottsdale, Arizona. These colleges offer degrees in naturopathic medicine and in other health-related sciences.

American Association of Naturopathic Physicians
2366 Eastlake Avenue, Suite 322
Seattle, Washington 98102
(206) 323-7610

Provides a directory of naturopathic physicians and offers referrals to a nationwide network of accredited or licensed practitioners. Publishes a quarterly newsletter for both professionals and the general public. Also offers a series of brochures and pamphlets on a variety of subjects.

Bastyr University
144 NE 54th
Seattle, Washington 98105
(206) 523-9585

Bastyr University is an accredited educational institution that offers degree programs in the natural health sciences. These include programs in naturopathic medicine; homeopathy; midwifery; acupuncture; nutrition; Chinese herbal medicine; marriage and family counseling; and applied behavioral science. Bastyr also offers a limited number of Distance Learning courses in these areas for students unable to attend classes at its Seattle, Washington facility.

The Institute for Naturopathic Medicine
66 1/2 North State Street
Concord, NH 03301-4330
(603) 225-8844

A non-profit, charitable organization dedicated to increasing public awareness of the options and solutions provided by natural medicine in solving the underlying causes of our health care crisis. The Institute's mission is to change the emphasis of the health care system from strictly disease management to health promotion and disease prevention. It serves the needs of consumers, the media, policy makers, medical educators, and others for accurate and reliable information about health care alternatives. In addition, the Institute promotes research into the clinical outcomes and cost effectiveness of natural therapeutics.

National College of Naturopathic Medicine
11231 SE Market Street
Portland, Oregon 97216
(503) 255-4860

Provides a listing of naturopathic doctors in the United States and offers a degree program in naturopathic medicine.

Southwest College
6535 E. Osborn Road
Scottsdale, Arizona 85251
(602) 990-7424

A degree program in naturopathic medicine is offered.

Canadian College of Naturopathic Medicine
60 Berl Avenue
Etobicoke, Ontario M8Y 3C7
Canada
(416) 251-5261

This school offers a diploma in naturopathic medicine. This is the Canadian equivalent of a degree in the United States.

Recommended Reading

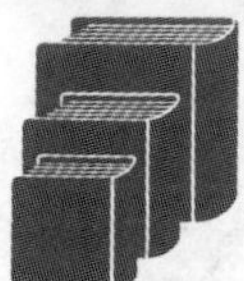

Divided Legacy, A History of the Schism in Medical Thought, Vol. 3. Coulter, Harris L. Washington, D.C.: Wehawken Book Company, 1973.

Coulter thoroughly explains the history of natural medicine and the battle between its supporters and the American Medical Association and pharmaceutical companies.

Encyclopedia of Natural Medicine. Murray, Michael, N.D.; and Pizzorno, Joseph, N.D. Rocklin, CA: Prima Publishing, 1991.

A definitive guide for the layperson on naturopathic medicine.

Lectures in Naturopathic Hydrotherapy. Boyle, Wade, N.D., and Saine, Andre, N.D. East Palestine, OH: Buckeye Naturopathic Press, 1988.

A useful book on general hydrotherapy topics.

Textbook of Natural Medicine, **Vols. 1 - 2**. Murray, Michael, N.D., and Pizzorno, Joseph, N.D. Seattle: John Bastyr College Publications, 1989.

A comprehensive two-volume textbook for the health professional interested in natural medicine. Chapters on the therapeutic modalities used in naturopathic medicine, and descriptions and treatments of certain diseases.

"The ultimate cause of human disease is the consequence of our transgression of the universal laws of life."

—Paracelsus

Neural Therapy

Neural therapy uses injections of anesthetics to remove short circuits in the body's electrical network. This process frees up the body's flow of energy and normalizes cellular function, making neural therapy an effective treatment for a variety of health conditions, especially chronic pain.

"Neural therapy treats pain and illness and resolves trauma in the body by working to reverse the cumulative effects of injury," says William Faber, D.O., of Milwaukee, Wisconsin. "The structural integrity of the body can be disturbed by injury, causing the energy flow to be blocked."

Neural therapy corrects these blockages in the body through the use of anesthetics injected into the nerve sites of the autonomic (independent) nervous system, acupuncture points, scars, glands, and other tissues. The most commonly used anesthetics are procaine and lidocaine. "These are very easily metabolized by the body," explains Marvin Penwell, D.O., of Linden, Michigan, "meaning that the body is able to break down their molecules into other chemical forms that can be readily eliminated. This safeguards against side effects."

By using the pathways of the autonomic nervous system, neural therapy delivers energy to cells short-circuited by disease or injury, and helps to regulate biological energy. Although a series of injections is usually required, a single injection can relieve pain instantly and, in many cases, restore complete health, even if the disease has lingered for years.

How Neural Therapy Works

To grasp how neural therapy works, it is necessary to understand a basic premise of biological energy. Everything alive is charged with electricity and every living cell has its own specific frequency range. As long as energy flow throughout the body is within its normal frequency range, the tissues will remain healthy.

Most chronic illnesses are caused by changes in the electrical conductivity of autonomic nerves and cells. These changes disrupt the flow of biological energy. Illness begins when energy flow is disrupted, creating what is known as an interference field in the "ground system" of the body. The ground system lies between the cell membranes, arteries, veins, lymph vessels, and nerve endings, and is composed of connective tissue—fibroblasts (cells that are the precursors of bone, collagen, and other connective tissue cells), collagen (the protein of the connective tissue), elastin (extracellular protein that makes the tissue elastic), water, and glycoproteins (proteins combined with sugars). When normal electrical impulses travel unimpeded, there is communication among the various systems of the body, fostering vibrant health. If this delicate balance breaks down, however, disruptions in the normal function of cells occur, and eventually chronic disorders develop.[1]

“Illness begins when energy flow is disrupted, creating what is known as an interference field in the ‘ground system’ of the body.”

Any part of the body that has been traumatized can create an interference field and can cause disturbances not only at a specific trauma site, but elsewhere in the body. For instance, extracting a wisdom tooth produces an interference field that can frequently cause heart problems.[2] Scars are another form of trauma that can create an interference field.

The task of the neural therapist is to locate the source of the abnormal activity and eliminate the disturbance. Once the cells regain their normal electrical activity, they can eliminate toxic wastes that have built up as a result of this disturbance, and begin to function normally again.

Congestion in the lymph system can be especially debilitating. Lymphatic vessels in a chronic state of imbalance can severely disrupt the flow of lymph fluid. Neural therapy can increase the flow of lymph, and help clear the tissues of wastes and restore them to normal function.[3]

Interference fields often lie dormant until activated by further trauma or by general illness such as malnutrition, emotional stress, or food sensitivity. Interference fields can also be activated by weight gain, as excess weight can stretch scar tissue.

Indicators of an underlying interference field include failure to respond to other therapies; a condition that worsens after other therapies; a situation where all symptoms are located on only one side of the body; or where one illness after another continually develops. To effect a longstanding cure, it is necessary to identify and clear interference fields from the body.

Conditions Benefited by Neural Therapy

German research claims that 40 percent of all illness and chronic pain may be due to interference fields in the body. Neural therapy has become one of the most widely used treatments for chronic pain in Germany.[4] One study compiled in Germany in the 1970s collected statistics from twenty-five doctors who used neural therapy with procaine to treat 639 cases of trigeminal neuralgia. The results were:

See Chronic Pain.

- 34% cures
- 37% substantial improvements
- 14% improvements
- 15% no improvements

In 267 of these cases, or 42 percent, an interference field was held to be either the cause or a mitigating factor of the disease. This report also stated that those who experienced the least result from neural therapy were those who had previously undergone surgery.[5]

There are hundreds of conditions that respond to neural therapy. "About the only conditions that do not respond to neural therapy are metabolic disorders and cancer," says pain specialist Dietrich Klinghardt, M.D., Ph.D., of Santa Fe, New Mexico, President of the American Academy of Neural Therapy. "Interestingly enough," he adds, "the people who are the hardest to treat with any other modality are the easiest to treat with neural therapy. Those who come to us haven't responded to conventional medicine, chiropractic, acupuncture, nerve blocks, physical therapy, or surgery. This is the very group that is most likely to respond rapidly to neural therapy."

Conditions that normally respond to neural therapy include:

- Allergies
- Arthritis
- Asthma
- Arteriosclerosis
- Back pain
- Bladder dysfunction
- Chronic pain
- Circulatory disorders
- Colitis
- Depression
- Dizziness
- Ear problems
- Emphysema
- Gallbladder disease
- Glaucoma
- Hayfever
- Headache
- Heart disease
- Hemorrhoids
- Hormonal imbalance
- Inflammatory eye disease
- Kidney disease
- Liver disease
- Menstrual cramps
- Migraine
- Muscle injuries
- Postoperative recovery
- Prostate disorders
- Sinusitis
- Skin diseases
- Sports injuries
- Thyroid disease
- Ulcers
- Whiplash

See Applied Kinesiology.

"In my experience, between one and six treatments, given twice weekly, are all that's needed," adds Dr. Klinghardt. "Often, we can get a person well with one treatment, although it sometimes takes a bit of sleuthing and listening for the body's response to target the source of the problem."

"German research claims that 40 percent of all illness and chronic pain is due to interference fields in the body."

Sally suffered from chronic fatigue syndrome for the better part of a decade. At first, Dr. Klinghardt suspected an appendectomy scar was causing the interference in her body's electrical field, so he injected it with procaine. When this did not bring about the expected result, he used applied kinesiology and found weakness in a strong indicator muscle when she touched her pelvic area. Immediately after injecting the Frankenhåuser ganglion (autonomic nerve centers in the pelvis), Sally started coughing. The cough indicated the presence of an interference field in the chest. When Dr. Klinghardt injected her chest, the chronic fatigue syndrome cleared within hours.

In retrospect, Sally remembered coming down with the flu and developing a cough immediately before the chronic fatigue syndrome had set in. Her body's attempt to fight the virus created chest congestion, and this affected the autonomic nerve endings in her lungs and created an obstruction of electrical impulses within her body's ground system. The injection of procaine into her chest reestablished the normal electrical potential of the cells and eliminated the interference field in her lungs so that her energy could circulate freely.

Dr. Penwell uses neural therapy as a large part of his practice. He recounts one particular case, an eighty-year-old woman who came to him with degenerative arthritis in her knee. She was experiencing a great deal of pain, which extended down her leg and up through her hip joint. This condition had crippled her to such an extent she was forced to depend on a walker and posed a very poor surgical risk. Following his examination, Dr. Penwell gave her several injections in her leg, including her knee joint. When the patient very reluctantly got up off the table to bear weight on the knee joint, she was amazed. Asked to move around, the patient took several steps and smiled broadly. In answer to the doctor's question about how she felt, the woman reached for her walker, folded it up, put it under her arm, and walked out the door and down the hallway. She was given follow-up injections at weekly intervals for four weeks and as the pain did not return, she concluded the therapy.

Eduardo Guerrero, M.D., P.A., a neural therapist from Houston, Texas, reports that his best results occur when he combines homeopathic remedies with anesthetics to clear interference fields. Dr Guerrero once treated a man whose two operations failed to relieve his back pain. "He was getting so bad, he couldn't function as a foreman anymore, so he changed to a janitorial job," Dr. Guerrero relates. "One day, while sweeping, the man reinjured his back and couldn't walk. When I administered nerve blocks to the sacral area, he felt pain in the lumbar area. Since the lumbar area corresponds to the urogenital system, I asked him if he'd ever had problems there. 'Oh, yes!,' he said. 'When I was in the army, I had gonorrhea.' Within a week of treating him for that complaint, his back pain disappeared.

"I believe the most important contribution neural therapy has brought to modern medicine is the understanding of interference fields," concludes Dr. Guerrero. "As long as you have a short circuit in the body's electrical network, you cannot recharge your biological energy."

HISTORY OF NEURAL THERAPY

Neural therapy was developed in Germany by two brothers, Ferdinand and Walter Huneke, both medical doctors. The idea first took shape in 1925, when they published a paper showing how the injection of a local anesthetic affected other places in the body. Years later, Ferdinand found, to his amazement, that injecting a woman in her leg for pain caused her chronic shoulder pain to immediately disappear. This gave rise to the concept of ster-felder, *or fields of interference.*

In Germany and South America, neural therapy is the most commonly used treatment for chronic pain. Today the "ground system theory," the foundation of neural therapy, is widely accepted in Europe. This theory states that it is actually the connective tissues between cells that control health, and that disease results from disturbances in this tissue.

In the United States, Dietrich Klinghardt, M.D., Ph.D., of Santa Fe, New Mexico, has trained nearly two hundred practitioners through his American Academy of Neural Therapy, and there are other practicing neural therapists who have trained outside the United States.

According to James A. Carlson, D.O., past President of the National Association of Orthopedic Medicine and a sports medicine specialist who practices neural therapy in Knoxville, Tennessee, there are cases where poor results are achieved with neural therapy due to a counter magnetic field surrounding the patient. "This can be caused by dental metal fillings and metal bridges, total joint replacements, external watches, rings, even metal eyeglass frames," Dr. Carlson says. "Many times, once these factors are eliminated from the patient's field, he or she will readily begin to respond to neural therapy with lasting, positive results."

See Acupuncture, Biological Dentistry.

Neural Therapy in Dentistry

Reinhold Voll, M.D., discovered in the 1950s that each tooth in the mouth relates to a specific acupuncture meridian. He observed that if the organ related to that meridian is not functioning normally, the tooth related to the same meridian may be symptomatic (i.e., painful, decayed). When the meridian is under stress, the acupuncture points are sensitive to local pressure, and this phenomenon can be used for diagnosis and treatment. For example, if the patient suffers a gallbladder attack (intense abdominal pain), the acupuncture point close to his or her right canine will be tender when probed. If neural therapy is used to inject this acupuncture point with a local anesthetic, the abdominal pain will subside. Toothaches, tooth sensitivity, jaw pain, gingivitis, and other local problems respond well when the corresponding oral acupuncture point is treated with neural therapy.

Dental acupoints and corresponding organs.

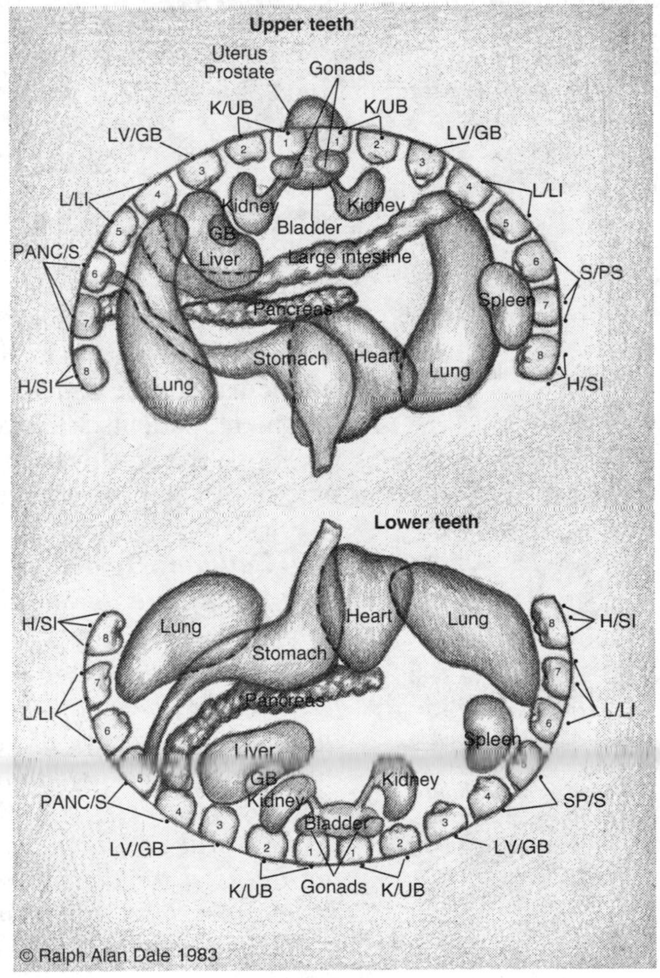

The acupuncture points in the retromolar area (the space behind the last molar of the lower jaw) are indispensable for treating neck pain, low back pain, and temporomandibular joint-related pain with neural therapy. Acupuncture points in the upper jaw are sensitive to pressure in cases of sinus infections, tension headaches, and indigestion. Sensitivity adjacent to the wisdom teeth indicates heart problems, intestinal disorder, arm/elbow/shoulder problems, vertigo, migraines, and lymphatic problems.

Sensitivity in the lower jaw is associated with lumbago, spinal problems, sciatica, indigestion, and hormonal malfunctions. Lingual sensitivities accompany vertigo, cervical syndrome, migraines, hearing difficulties, and kidney/bladder disorders.

How Interference Fields Are Diagnosed.

Locating interference fields begins with a study of patient history of past illness, surgery, or trauma. There are certain empirical relationships between interference fields and illness. Some of these are: Tonsils—knee joints; abdominal scars—large joints and low back; leg scars—sciatica; tonsils and teeth—migraine headaches; prostate, stomach, and sinuses—neck; gallbladder scar—shoulder; pelvic scars—premenstrual syndrome; and depression—arthritis, according to Peter Dosch, M.D.,[6] of Austria. A scar that crosses an acupuncture meridian is likely to cause disturbances in the corresponding body part. Scars may also be responsible for problems in nearby joints. According to Dr. Faber, scars that do not fade within two years or seem excessively hard or tight across the skin can signal an interference field. Also, the relationship between specific teeth and organs, such as the upper and lower front four teeth to the urogenital system, can be responsible for pelvic pain, chronic kidney disease, and even pelvic malignancies.

TYPES OF NEURAL THERAPY

Direct techniques: *The direct or "local" technique in neural therapy treats pain or illness with an injection of anesthetics specifically at the site of the interference field causing the problem. The injections can be made by infiltrating scar tissue, into nerve junctions, or into the area surrounding the spinal cord.*

Indirect technique: *If the neural therapist cannot pinpoint the exact location of the interference field, the source of pain can be tracked down by injecting related interference fields until the original blockage is found. In other cases, an indirect approach is needed when the problem area is too delicate to receive a direct injection.*

Neural therapists listen to the patient to pick up clues to past problems that the patient may believe to be insignificant. After the initial treatment, patients are asked to keep a record of any changes that occur in the body over the next forty-eight hours, as these can guide the practitioner in further treatments.

CAUTION

Neural therapy is contraindicated for certain conditions—cancer, diabetes, coagulation disorders (such as hemophilia), renal failure, myasthenia gravis—and for those people treated with morphine or antiarrhythmics.

Caution: *By definition, neural therapy can influence disturbances only if they are due to autonomic (independent) causes or if neural or humoral (body fluid) factors are part of the original cause.[7] Neural therapy cannot reverse any major structural changes and therefore does not take the place of orthodox diagnostic or therapeutic measures. Neural therapy is ineffective in genetic disease and nutritional deficiencies, and not beneficial in psychiatric disorders (except depression) or end-stage chronic diseases.*

Several conditions are contraindicated for neural therapy. It should not be used for cancer patients, since the stimulation of the lymphatic system may lead to the spread of cancer cells throughout the body. It is contraindicated in diabetes mellitus because it may cause instability of the disease.

Patients allergic to local anesthetics should definitely not receive neural therapy. It should not be used for patients with renal failure or myasthenia gravis (a disease characterized by extreme muscle weakness), or for patients treated with morphine or antiarrhythmics similar in chemical structure to local anesthetics. It is also contraindicated for patients with coagulation disorders (such as hemophilia) or for those receiving anticoagulant therapy.

The Future of Neural Therapy

Currently, chronic pain is the single largest cause of disability in the United States. Employers and insurance companies have begun researching the far-reaching benefits of neural therapy in efforts to reduce the high cost of health care. According to Dr. Faber, individuals treated with neural therapy for chronic pain are able to resume their productivity earlier and with no side effects.

Because neural therapy can remedy a broad range of pain and illness by improving the patients range of motion, it is gaining respect by health care professionals who are moving away from drug-based treatments for pain. "These results will hopefully move practitioners into employing neural therapy, realizing that the body has the ability to heal itself, rather than viewing the body as being deficient in some pharmaccutical," says Dr. Faber.

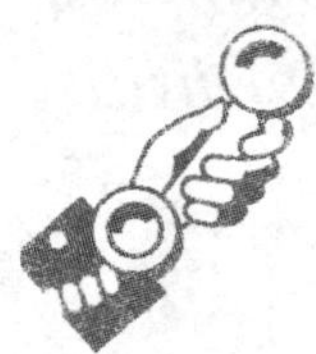

Where to Find Help

Locating a neural therapist may be difficult. For information about neural therapy and referral contact:

The American Academy of Neural Therapy
1468 South Saint Francis Drive
Santa Fe, New Mexico 87501
(505) 988-3086

Offers introductory and advanced courses in neural therapy and pain management techniques to doctors, and provides referrals for neural therapists nationwide.

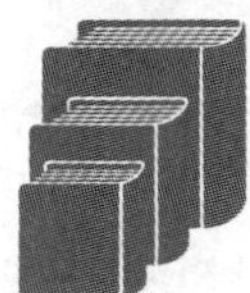

Recommended Reading

Books available through: Medicina Biologica, 2937 N.E. Flanders, Portland, Oregon 97232, or phone (503) 287-6775.

Facts About Neural Therapy According to Huneke. A Brief Summary for Patients. Dosch, Peter, M.D. Heidelberg, Germany: Karl Haug Publishers, 1985.

An introductory guide that is not only excellent for the patient, but for physicians unfamiliar with neural therapy.

Manual of Neural Therapy According to Huneke. Dosch, Peter, M.D. Heidelberg, Germany: Karl Haug Publishers, 1985.

A main textbook on neural therapy and a comprehensive teaching and reference manual. Enables any interested practitioner to learn and apply these methods effectively.

Matrix and Matrix Regulation Basis for an Holistic Theory in Medicine. Pischinger, Alfred, M.D. Heidelberg, Germany: Karl Haug International, 1991.

This fundamental work on Pischinger's basic or ground regulation system provides a new basis for a total biological theory of medicine.

Neuro-Linguistic Programming

Neuro-Linguistic Programming (NLP) helps people detect and reprogram unconscious patterns of thought and behavior in order to alter psychological responses and enhance the healing process. NLP has provided positive results for people suffering from various conditions, including AIDS, cancer, allergies, arthritis, Parkinson's disease, and migraine headaches.

Neuro-Linguistic Programming focuses on how people learn, communicate, change, grow, and heal. "Neuro" refers to the way the brain works and how human thinking demonstrates consistent and detectable patterns. "Linguistic" refers to the verbal and nonverbal expressions of the brain's thinking patterns. "Programming" refers to how these patterns are recognized and understood by the mind and how they can be altered, allowing a person to make better choices in behavior and health.

How NLP Works

People who have difficulty recovering from physical illness have often adopted negative beliefs about their recovery. They perceive themselves as helpless, hopeless, worthless, and express statements like "I can't get healthy," "There is no hope," and "I am not worth the effort." The primary goal of the NLP practitioner is to move a person from his or her present state of discomfort to a desired state of health and well-being by helping to reprogram beliefs about healing.

> *"The primary goal of the NLP practitioner is to move a person from his or her present state of discomfort to a desired state of health and well-being by helping to reprogram beliefs about healing."*

NLP practitioners ask questions to discover how a client relates to issues of identity, personal beliefs, and life goals. By reading autonomic body changes—skin color changes, moisture changes on the lips or eyes—as well as other physiological responses, NLP practitioners show people how to tap into their way of healing, as individuals, based on how they process information and how they view their health conditions.

According to Janet Konefal, Ph.D., of Miami, Florida, identity can be a major component of the way a person deals with his or her health condition, particularly someone suffering from chronic disease. Dr. Konefal states, "Too often people tend to identify directly with their illnesses. A person doesn't usually say, 'I'm John, who has this condition of diabetes,' he says, 'I'm a diabetic.' A person doesn't usually say, 'I'm Mary, a carrier of this virus,' she says, 'I'm an AIDS patient.' The disease moves in and actually shifts a person's identity."

One of the first priorities of an NLP practitioner is to separate a person's negative or false identifications and then to have that person recapture or regain his or her identity.

NLP practitioners are trained to ensure that any changes will ultimately benefit all the various aspects of the individual, not just the particular problem that is being addressed. Special care is taken to keep not only a client's family, social, and work relationships in balance, but also his or her internal systems: thoughts, strategies, behaviors, capabilities, values, and beliefs. This is known as an ecology check, and is used to ascertain if NLP will be compatible with a person's specific needs. It is accomplished through the careful questioning of the individual client both before and after a session.

As a next step, the practitioner will ask a client to see him- or herself in a state of health. By doing so, an outcome is set that will facilitate the healing process. The brain's natural response is to duplicate whatever images or beliefs are created about getting better.[1] The brain then triggers the necessary immunological responses to guide the body toward its goal of health and well-being.

THE HISTORY OF NLP

In the early 1970s, John Grinder, a professor of linguistics at the University of California at Santa Cruz, and Richard Bandler, a student of psychology and mathematics at Santa Cruz, collaborated in an effort to define the qualities of excellence in several accomplished individuals. They studied the thinking processes, language patterns, and behavioral patterns of Fritz Perls, father of Gestalt therapy; Virginia Satir, an exceptional family psychotherapist; Milton Erickson, M.D., an innovative hypnotherapist; and Gregory Bateson, a well-known British anthropologist and writer on communication theories. As a result, they discovered that many of the behavioral and psychological elements that allowed these individuals to achieve excellence were unconscious and intuitive and that the participants could not describe their own exceptional qualities.

By analyzing speaking patterns, voice tones, and the selection of words, as well as the gesticulations, postures, and eye movements of these individuals, Grinder and Bandler were able to make strong connections between body language and speaking patterns. They then related this information to the internal thinking process of each participant. Based on their findings, Grinder and Bandler then trained themselves to assist people experiencing emotional difficulties. Clients were asked questions about their problems and their body cues were observed as they responded.

According to Grinder and Bandler, eye movements, posture, voice tone, and breathing patterns reveal unconscious patterns affecting a person's emotional state. Once these unconscious patterns are distinguished, the client can be assisted in adopting new patterns. From their work they devised a method to teach others how to analyze a person's language, thoughts, and behavior.

When a client is asked questions about life and his or her condition, the NLP practitioner observes the language patterns, eye movements, postures, muscle tension, and gestures. These relay information and report internal sensations about how the client relates to his or her present condition in both conscious and unconscious ways, revealing what limiting beliefs may exist. These belief structures can then be altered using NLP.

See Mind/Body Medicine.

Yet changing a person's belief structures is not the only issue for NLP practitioners, warns Dr. Konefal. "I think what people need to achieve in order to become healthy—to actually make some changes in their health state—is not only a shift in their beliefs, but a shift in their behavior," she says. "They need to have alignment or congruency at all levels, not just a shift in beliefs. If they change their beliefs, but in fact don't change any of their behavior, then there's an incongruency. It's much more impactful if people tell themselves that they need to eat better than if a doctor or health counselor tells them. They're much more likely to listen to themselves."

Engaging the Body's Natural Ability to Heal

From childhood, Sarah had been severely allergic to dairy products. Whenever they were ingested, she would almost immediately experience sinus blockage, a sore throat, and stomach pain, followed a day or two later by an outbreak of boils. As an adult, Sarah had learned to carefully avoid all dairy products.

NLP practitioner Tim Hallbom asked Sarah to think of something similar to a dairy product, yet something to which she was not allergic. She chose tofu, a soybean product she ate as a substitute for cheese. As Sarah thought of tofu, Hallbom carefully observed her eye movements, skin color, muscle tones, and breathing.

> *"I think what people need to achieve in order to become healthy—to actually make some changes in their health state—is not only a shift in their beliefs, but a shift in their behavior."*
> —Janet Konefal, Ph.D.

Sarah was then asked to think of a food that would cause an allergic reaction. As she thought of cheese, Hallbom observed the changes: her skin color became mottled, her muscle tension changed, her eyes looked down and to the left (compared to looking up and to the right when she thought about tofu). Hallbom explains, "When she thinks of cheese her immune system reacts as though the cheese is a foreign invader such as a virus. The killer cells are called out, but as there is nothing to fight, they attack healthy cells. If this occurs on a large scale, problems such as those Sarah experienced may occur. Essentially what is happening, however, is a mistake—an overreaction of the immune system. On the other hand, when Sarah thinks of tofu, her body enters a different (healthy) state, responds appropriately, and she feels fine."

Hallbom uses touch to create a positive association to that healthy state. NLP practitioners call this an anchor because it holds the positive state stable through a client's nervous system. (Anchors can also be created using visual and auditory methods, depending on the client's needs.) As Hallbom anchored Sarah's positive state (associated with eating tofu), he asked her to imagine herself in an audience watching a movie of herself eating tofu, enjoying it, and seeing herself fully healthy.

Hallbom then asked Sarah to imagine that the "Sarah" on the movie screen was eating cheese. In order for her to have the full experience, he had her feel its texture, taste, and smell. By using the anchor of touch to hold the tofu state constant, it sent a message to Sarah: when she visualizes herself eating the cheese, it's pleasing to her. In order to create a bridge from this point into some future real-life experience, Hallbom then had Sarah imagine a future time when she will eat cheese.

When Sarah was able to hold the healthy state while imagining seeing herself eating cheese on the movie screen, the path was clear for the real change to occur. The "Sarah" in the movie and the "Sarah" in the room were reassociated. In other words, Sarah no longer imagined watching herself eating the cheese, but rather imagined herself actually doing it. When Sarah was able to hold the healthy "tofu" state while imagining that she was actually eating the cheese, Hallbom knew the change had occurred. Sarah has since been able to eat at least one dairy product every day with no allergic response.

Conditions Benefited by NLP

By identifying and removing an individual's limiting belief about his or her condition, NLP has been shown to benefit a variety of health conditions and illnesses. Once these beliefs are redirected, the body is better able to utilize the immune system.

David Paul, M.D., Medical Director of Vail Valley Medical Center in Vail, Colorado, uses NLP frequently in his medical practice. One specific application is as a drugless technique for placing dislocated shoulders back into their sockets. Standard medical practice involves a significant amount of medication to induce pain relief and muscle relaxation, followed by manipulation of the shoulder to put it back in place.

Dr. Paul and his group have developed a technique that uses language patterns based on NLP to help the patient achieve relaxation and not pay any attention to the discomfort involved in the actual physical manipulation. "We use phrases like 'allow your arm to relax,'" explains Dr. Paul, "'and allow your muscles to relax; notice as your arm goes up the discomfort becomes more bearable'—all positive, no negative commands, and also very specific. Ninety-five percent of the time the shoulder can be put back in its socket in one minute or less without the use of morphine, valium, or similar products." According to Dr. Paul, prior to using this technique, his average success rate was between 40 and 50 percent.

Over the past five years Dr. Paul and his group have used this technique to treat more than one thousand patients, and feels that NLP is an essential adjunct to his physical practice. Dr. Paul has also found NLP techniques helpful in the treatment of traumatic injury cases such as car accidents.

"A lot of times a person involved in a car accident feels much worse after four or five days," says Dr. Paul. "He or she replays the accident over and over in his or her head, sometimes even going through it in slow-motion. However, this causes the muscles to tense, and this creates a lot of discomfort. If the practitioner can get involved quickly enough—in the emergency room, for instance—and change the internal representations of that experience, the accident victim will be less prone to a lot of the 'whiplash,' muscle spasms, or prolonged pain usually associated with major trauma. NLP techniques help to remove blocks that stand in the way of the body's natural healing process."

NLP has also been found to be helpful in cases of chronic disease. NLP trainer Robert Dilts recalls how his mother, after having earlier undergone chemotherapy, experienced a recurrence of breast cancer that metastasized to her skull, spine, ribs, and pelvis. He worked with his mother to uncover her conscious and unconscious beliefs about herself and her illness. Her cancer had reappeared during a transition period in her life. Numerous changes in her family life had caused her to feel frustrated, upset, to question her place in the family system, and to question her whole identity. She also worked long hours as a nurse, commenting that she was literally "dying" to take a vacation. When her cancer recurred in the midst of these changes, her prognosis was poor, with her doctor saying all he could do was "make her comfortable." Dilts assisted his mother in changing her limiting beliefs and unconscious conflicts. She also made lifestyle changes that included diet and exercise. As a result, her health improved dramatically and she elected not to receive any further chemotherapy or radiation treatments. Eventually she fully recovered and resumed a normal lifestyle.[2]

Submodalities

According to NLP, information in the brain is coded by the five senses of sight, hearing, touch, taste, and smell. Each of these senses, also called modalities in NLP, has a subset of qualities called submodalities, which are similar to the controls on a television set. As information is retrieved from the brain through memory, the submodalities determine the memory's shape in terms of contrast, color, and volume. For example, when remembering a person from the past, the submodalities would determine whether in your mind's eye the person appeared near or far to you, if you saw him or her distinctly and in color or black and white, and so forth. The way that the submodalities arrange the memory plays a significant role in how the memory itself affects people. NLP can be used to adjust internal memories and feelings by adjusting the submodalities of the experience. Pleasant memories can be reinforced by increasing their proximity to you in your inner vision, while upsetting memories can be diminished by making them dimmer and placing them further away from you.

NLP trainers Steve and Connierae Andreas studied how the mind codes healing and discovered a technique to engage the body's natural ability to heal. Their discovery was prompted by a personal experience. Shortly after the birth of her first child, Connierae developed a sore lump in her breast. A bright red patch of skin and a high fever soon followed. She was diagnosed with a breast infection, put on antibiotics, and within twenty-four hours the fever was gone and eventually the lump vanished.

When the symptoms returned after the birth of her second child, Connierae incorporated her NLP experience and began to experiment. She thought of influenza as something her body was capable of healing. Connierae explains, "When I saw myself healing from influenza I was lying in bed and the image started out in grayish tones. In a split second I went from that position, like a fast action clip, to standing up—healthy, well, in full color." But when she compared the submodalities of this image to the submodalities of the image she had of herself trying to heal the breast infection, she noticed a difference. "The image I had for the breast infection was a grayish, still image of myself lying in bed. There was no movement to it."

NLP AND AIDS

Dr. Janet Konefal, Ph.D., of Miami, Florida, has utilized NLP for the past ten years in the treatment of HIV (human immunodeficiency virus) and AIDS patients. Dr. Konefal has worked with patients in all phases of the disease, from those just recently diagnosed to cases of full-blown AIDS. One of her clients has been HIV positive for eleven years, another for nine years, and many have been HIV positive for six and seven years. Dr. Konefal explains, "Part of what I'm examining with NLP is: What is the quality of life and what can be done to enhance that, and what is the client's goal? Some goals are longevity; how long a person wants to live. With AIDS it might be, 'Let's make a career out of becoming healthy for a while and then you can get on with your life.'

"One of the things that happens, though, is that when a person is out there and surviving five, six years, they begin to think they are on borrowed time. They start to think, 'Oh my gosh! I've beaten this thing for this long, now for sure something will happen.' "

When this happens, Dr. Konefal has her clients come back and go through another kind of NLP process that lets them extend the possibility that they're not on borrowed time. "I tell them, 'Yes, you can survive and have the virus. Some people put cancer in remission. There isn't any reason why we cannot put the AIDS virus into remission, but just keep it a secret,' she says. "I warn them not to go around telling everybody because what happens is that someone will say to them it's not possible, and then they have to expend a lot of energy and create a lot of stress for themselves defending their position. They can also join a network of people who can support each other in the healing process."

Dr. Konefal has had success by combining NLP with other alternative therapies such as acupuncture, chinese herbs, homeopathy, and nutrition. "One of the things I like to do is not depend solely on any one method. If this is what you want to do, I say, good for you."

Another issue that AIDS has raised is the question of false hope. Research shows that when a person feels hopeless the immune system compromises itself. Because AIDS has been labeled a fatal disease, the immune system of someone suffering with AIDS can be compromised inadvertently and unknowingly. When it is perceived that there is no hope for their AIDS patients, most medical doctors are under the impression that it is their ethical duty to inform their patients that they are going to die.

"I think this process is detrimental," says Dr. Konefal, who always asks the people she works with to envision building a future. "I'll ask a patient, 'If you could survive this, if you could be one of the people who figures out how you're going to live with this virus, what would your life be like?' Then immediately the patient has a future instead of a black hole or a coffin, and the whole way he or she approaches daily activity or the rest of his or her life changes."

Connierae identified how her brain coded healing influenza in terms of the submodalities of her healing pictures, sounds, and feelings. She analyzed this pattern and then coded her image of healing her breast infection with the same submodalities. At first her image of healing from the breast infection was grayish, inactive, and distant. To adjust the image she changed the location, color, and size of herself in the picture by imagining herself moving up off the bed and seeing the image become colorful as she became larger, until she was standing healthy and well. This encoded her brain with the new imprint for healing and her brain then triggered the necessary immunological responses to heal the breast infection.[3]

AN EXERCISE USING NLP SUBMODALITIES

By becoming familiar with your submodalities and how they operate, you can learn to adjust your internal memories and feelings. The following exercise illustrates how this process can work for you.

Close your eyes and allow yourself to recall an unpleasant memory. Depending on how you code and process your experiences, the memory will appear to you primarily as an image, a sound, or a feeling. Whichever way it happens will be the way that is most appropriate for you.

As the memory arises, become aware of the emotions you are experiencing because of it. Now notice the memory itself. If it is visual, notice its size, its proximity to you, and whether or not you are seeing it in color. If your experience is primarily auditory, notice the qualities of the sounds. Are they loud, grating, or harsh? If your memory evokes a kinesthetic sensation, notice how it feels. These qualities comprise the submodalities of your experience. By adjusting them, you can literally change the experience itself.

You can adjust the submodalities in the same way that you can use the controls on a TV set. If you are seeing an image, allow it to become blurry and indistinct. If it is in color, allow it to become black and white. Now allow it to recede from you, becoming smaller and smaller, until it is so small that you can hardly see it anymore. You can do the same thing with sounds and sensations, changing them until they are comfortable for you. Once you accomplish this, notice how your emotions with regard to the memory have also changed. You may be surprised to discover how relaxed and in control you feel, and how the memory is no longer able to provoke an unpleasant reaction in you.

This same exercise can also be used to reinforce positive memories, thereby creating more powerful resourceful states for yourself.

As you focus on a pleasant memory, allow it to become clearer, closer, and brighter for you, then add whatever other appealing qualities you wish to create your desired state.

By regularly experimenting with this exercise, you will find yourself gaining greater control over your emotions and the memories that trigger them. This, in turn, will enhance your sense of well-being.

Memory Imprints

Another way of changing a limiting belief is by a technique called reimprinting. An imprint is a memory formed at an earlier age. Whereas positive imprints are empowering, negative imprints often result from trauma or confusion that is forgotten, but which can serve as a root for limiting beliefs. Tim Hallbom says, "A negative imprint laced with unhealthy beliefs can create serious problems when the brain duplicates these messages and sends them out to the immune system where they can serve as a catalyst for undesirable health conditions. Many unhealthy immunological responses result from limiting beliefs created through trauma or confusion." The NLP practitioner can help to identify a limiting belief formed during the imprinting event, and assist in its reimprinting or replacement.

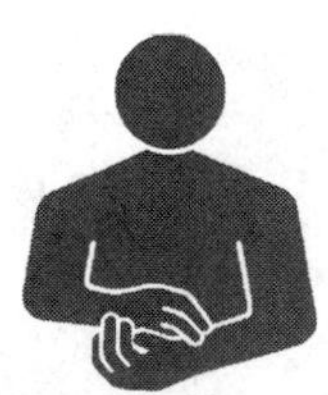

By helping individuals become aware of the interrelationship between mind and body, NLP can be a safe, cost-effective form of self-care.

The Future of NLP

"According to standard medical literature, 50 percent of all medical complaints are recognized today as having a strong psychological component," states to Dr. Paul. "If a practitioner has the tools and technology to deal with this psychological component, patients will receive better care, be in better health, and utilize fewer health-related services. The organizations that consistently apply these principles and integrate them into the practice of medicine are going to be the successful medical models for how we take care of people in a cost-efficient and caring manner. I think it's going to become an economic necessity."

John Sward, Ph.D., of the Center for the Improvement of Human Functioning International, in Wichita, Kansas, notes that these economic necessities, along with greater medical openness, have moved NLP out of the "fad" phenomena and into acceptability and respectability. "NLP is starting to be accepted in academically credible ways, bringing it into the awareness of business people, and people who strongly influence the economy.

"Economics drives a lot of things in our culture, including our health care system," admits Dr. Sward, "and NLP is certainly efficient. So I think one of the good things that will come out of this trend is that NLP will become increasingly more acceptable and understood as an adjunctive modality, and as a separate methodology all its own."

"The organizations that consistently apply these principles and integrate them into the practice of medicine are going to be the successful medical models for how we take care of people in a cost-efficient and caring manner."

—David Paul, M.D.

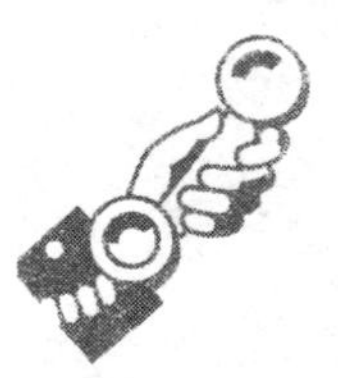

Where to Find Help

NLP can be effective in assisting the healing process of many physical conditions. Some NLP practitioners, however, have not been trained in the aspects of physical healing. When selecting an NLP practitioner, ask if he or she has been trained in the area of NLP you are seeking.

Dynamic Learning Center
P.O. Box 1112
Ben Lomond, California 95005
(408) 336-3457
(408) 336-5854 (Fax)

The Center provides NLP certification training, as well as NLP classes open to the general public. Dynamic Learning Publications provides books, audio tapes, and educational materials.

NLP Comprehensive
2897 Valmont Road
Boulder, Colorado 80301
(303) 442-1102

Connierae and Steve Andreas are internationally known trainers and authors in the field of NLP. Through NLP Comprehensive they conduct a variety of training seminars and NLP certification programs.

Western States Training Associates
2290 East 4500 South, Suite 120
Salt Lake City, Utah 84117
(801) 278-1022
(801) 278-1088 (Fax)

WSTA provides NLP training to individuals, businesses, and government organizations. Founders Tim Hallbom and Suzi Smith can be contacted for further information about their training seminars and NLP certification programs. References are provided for people with health-related issues.

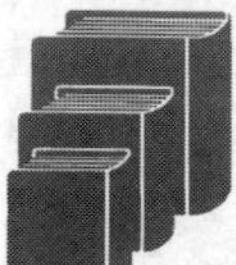

Recommended Reading

Applications of NLP. Dilts, Robert. Cupertino, CA: Meta Publications, 1983.

A comprehensive text detailing the history, principals, and applications of NLP.

Beliefs: Pathways to Health and Well Being. Dilts, Robert; Hallbom, Tim; and Smith Suzi, Portland, OR: Metamorphous Press, 1990.

The first book of its kind to demonstrate how the advanced technology of neuro-linguistic programming can be used to identify limiting or destructive beliefs, and how to rapidly and effectively alter these ideas and promote positive change.

Heart of the Mind. Andreas, Connierae, and Steve; Moab, UT: Real People Press, 1989.

An accessible introductory book that provides examples of common NLP patterns, including easy-to-apply techniques, to deal with weight loss, stage fright, phobias, abuse, grief, as well as tools for becoming more independent, creating motivation, and promoting self-healing.

Introducing Neuro-Linguistic Programming: The New Psychology of Personal Excellence. O'Connor, J.; and Seymour, J. London, England: Mandala, an imprint of HarperCollins Publishers, 1990.

This working handbook offers easy-to-understand descriptions and practical skills to be used as tools for improving the quality and effectiveness of one's communication and for achieving personal excellence in all areas of one's life.

Magic of NLP Demystified. Lewis, B.; and Pucelik, F. Portland, OR: Metamorphous Press, 1990.

Written in an informal and entertaining style, this book introduces the reader to the NLP approach to the study of human communication and therapeutic exchange.

Nutritional Supplements

Recent research has demonstrated that diet alone may not be sufficient to supply the nutrients necessary for overall good health. While most experts agree that nutritional supplements are vital for a variety of illnesses, injuries, and age-related problems, vitamin and mineral supplements can also help to maintain optimal physical and psychological health, and promote longevity and chronic disease prevention.

Ever since the term "vitamins" was coined almost one hundred years ago to describe the discovery of the essential life substances in foods, scientists have debated the issue of nutritional adequacy. Medical science has long held that healthy adults do not need supplementation if they consume a healthful, varied diet. Until recently, it was widely believed that supplements were only considered necessary if a person had an outright, or "severe", nutrient deficiency, usually manifested by overt illness.

Today, research indicates that people can have "mild" or "moderate" nutrient deficiencies, and that nutritional supplements are necessary to maintain health, according to nutritionist D. Lindsey Berkson, M.A., D.C., of Santa Fe, New Mexico. These mild disorders may not cause tangible health disorders, making them difficult to diagnose, but can result in a variety of symptoms along with a general decrease in wellness. Unaddressed, these deficiencies can often put the body at risk for future health problems. Therefore, it is important for individuals to be sure they are receiving the proper amounts of nutrients for overall emotional and physical well-being.

The Modern Diet and a New Understanding of Nutrition

"Nutrient density is the hallmark of good food," says Paul McTaggart, a nutrition researcher from Ventura, California. Defined as the relative ratio of nutrients to calories, foods low in nutrient density are often termed "empty-calorie" or "junk" foods.

The leading nutritional problem in the United States today is "overconsumptive undernutrition," or the eating of too many of these empty-calorie foods, says Jeffrey Bland, Ph.D., a biochemist and nutrition expert from Gig Harbor, Washington. Although people in the United States consume plenty of food, it is not the right kind of food. Statistically, studies have concluded that almost two-thirds of an average American's diet is made up of fats and refined sugars having low to no nutrient density. This contributes to nutrient deficiencies that can rob the body of its natural resistance to disease and premature aging, while weakening its overall physiological and psychological performance. Consequently, the remaining one-third of the average diet is counted on for the essential nutrients needed to maintain health, which may or may not be from high-nutrient-density food.

The United States Department of Agriculture (USDA) has found that a significant percentage of the United States population receives well under 70 percent of the U.S. Recommended Daily Allowance (U.S. RDA) for vitamin A, vitamin C, B-complex vitamins, and the essential minerals calcium, magnesium, and iron.[1] A separate study found that most typical diets contained less than 80 percent of the RDA for calcium, magnesium, iron, zinc, copper, and manganese, and that the people most at risk were young children and women, adolescent to elderly.[2] The chart on pages 389-392 indicates the adult RDA requirements for vitamins and minerals, as well as adult maintenance and therapeutic ranges recommended by many nutritional experts.

See Diet, Orthomolecular Medicine.

The standard American diet has been continually cited by numerous studies conducted since the 1960s as a contributing, causative factor in a variety of "killer" diseases, including coronary heart disease, atherosclerosis, strokes, high blood pressure, diabetes, arthritis, and colitis. According to Dr. Berkson, there may also be increased risk of female disorders associated with diets high in processed fats (trans-fatty acids) and increased consumption of refined sugar and caffeine.

Additionally, other contributing factors such as environmental pollution and stressful life patterns are creating even greater nutrient requirements. As the typical American diet is resulting in dangerous deficiencies people are constantly requiring more nutrients to maintain good health, even though they may appear to be adequately fed.

Symptoms of Nutritional Deficiency

Historically, doctors and nutritional scientists only recognized nutritional deficiencies if they actually manifested as diseases such as beriberi, pellagra, or rickets. If a patient had no overt symptoms or disease, he or she was regarded as healthy and adequately nourished. Today, doctors and scientists are beginning to recognize mild and moderate nutritional deficiencies, the symptoms of which may often be subtle, overlapping, and varied, according to Dr. Berkson. Many times these symptoms are taken for granted as being part of the aging process. Nutritional doctors and scientists are learning, however, that these symptoms are actually subtle deficiency signs that can be responsive to nutrient supplementation and dietary improvement. Greater understanding and better testing methods are leading to the diagnosis of more and more subtle nutrient imbalances.

For example, the first signs of B vitamin deficiency may include subtle changes in behavior: insomnia, mood swings, and an inability to concentrate. These early warning signs, according to Myron Brin, Ph.D., demonstrate that social function may be adversely affected by chronic vitamin deficiency.[3]

Other symptoms of nutritional deficiencies can include fatigue, nervousness, mental exhaustion, confusion, anemia, and muscle weakness. It has been reported that marginal deficiencies of vitamins A, C, E, and B_6 may also reduce immunocompetence, impairing the body's ability to ward off disease and repair tissues.[4]

While these can all be signs of deficiencies, they can also have a root in other, separate health problems. Therefore, one needs to always have any deficiencies properly assessed by a qualified health care provider trained in this field.

Biochemical Individuality

Scientists have increasingly begun to examine whether the standardized U.S. RDA guidelines are sufficient for individual nutritional needs. One of the first to question the guidelines was Roger Williams, Ph.D., a pioneering biochemist who discovered vitamin B_5 (pantothenic acid) in the 1930s. In his book, *Nutrition Against Disease*, Dr. Williams expresses his belief that each person is genetically unique, and therefore requires slight variations in nutrient intake to function optimally. He calls this principle biochemical individuality. Dr. Williams also believes that all living creatures are greatly affected by the overall quality, balance, and quantity of food ingested.

The concept of biochemical individuality has brought about many changes, including the emergence of new preventive diagnostic procedures, such as nutrition assessment and risk factor analysis. These utilize physiological data, personal and family health history, dietary intake analysis, and scientifically advanced biochemical screenings to help nutritional practitioners determine individual biochemistry and nutritional status.

Recommended Daily Allowances

The generally accepted reference standard for nutritional adequacy in the United States is the U.S. Recommended Daily Allowance (U.S. RDA). Developed by a group of government-sponsored scientists, its function is to provide levels of essential nutrients that prevent classic deficiency diseases, and set marginal daily guidelines for average population groups. As it was difficult for the scientists to agree upon the RDA's, they built within the guidelines instructions to keep reviewing and changing the RDA's every four years as new information is discovered. Today, in the wake of overwhelming clinical evidence that shows a wide variance in each person's individual nutritional needs, a growing number of scientists have begun to dispute the validity of RDA standards.

While a diet adequate in RDA's may be appropriate to avoid severe nutritional deficiency diseases such as rickets, scurvy, or beriberi, it may not be appropriate to avoid more mild deficiency reactions such as nervousness, insomnia, mental exhaustion, improper immune function, or proneness to injury.

Emmanuel Cheraskin M.D., D.M.D., suggests that IDA's—Ideal Daily Allowances—should replace RDA's, to make up for the limiting nature inherent in the current method. In line with the growing body of research regarding nutrients, the FDA (Food and Drug Administration) in 1994 will introduce a new nutritional label reference known as the Reference Daily Intake (RDI), to ensure that food labeling be more consistent with the latest data on nutrient allowances.

Essential Nutrients

"Essential nutrients are those nutrients derived from food that the body is unable to manufacture on its own," says Dr. Bland. These are absolutely necessary for human life and include eight amino acids, at least thirteen vitamins, and at least fifteen minerals, plus certain fatty acids, water, and carbohydrates.

Amino acids are the building blocks of protein. The essential amino acids are L-isoleucine, L-leucine, L-valine, L-methionine, L-threonine, L-phenylalanine, and L-tryptophan.

Essential vitamins are broken up in two groups: fat-soluble and water-soluble. The essential vitamins classified as fat-soluble include vitamin A, vitamin D, vitamin E and vitamin K. The water-soluble essential vitamins are vitamin C (ascorbic acid), vitamin B_1 (thiamine), vitamin B_2 (riboflavin), vitamin B_3 (niacin), vitamin B_5 (pantothenic acid), vitamin B_6 (pyridoxine), vitamin B_{12}, folic acid, and biotin.

The essential minerals include calcium, magnesium, phosphorus, iron, zinc, copper, manganese, iodine, chromium, potassium, sodium, and a number of trace elements. They make up part of the necessary elements of body tissues, fluids, and other nutrients and play an active role in the body's regulatory functions. Low levels of these nutrients have been linked to such conditions as heart disease, high blood pressure, cancer, osteoporosis, depression, schizophrenia, and problems relating to menopause.

Essential fatty acids required for proper metabolism include linoleic and linolenic acid, found in seafood and unrefined vegetable oils, plus oleic and arachidonic acids, found in most organic fats and oils and peanuts. These also play an important role in reducing heart disease and in the treating of conditions such as eczema[5] and premenstrual stress.[6]

Accessory Nutrients

There are also many nonessential nutrients, called accessory nutrients or co-factors, that work in harmony with the essential nutrients to aid in the breakdown and conversion of food into cellular energy, and also help support all of the body's physical and mental functions.

According to Dr. Bland, some of the accessory nutrients that help support metabolism include vitamin B-complex co-factors choline and inositol, as well as coenzyme Q10 (a close relative of the B-vitamins), and lipoic acid.

Other accessory nutrients which have demonstrated preventative functions include B-complex co-factor PABA (para-aminobenzoic acid), and substance P or bioflavonoids which work with vitamin C. Certain amino acids found in protein are also considered nonessential because they can be synthesized by the body from the essential amino acids.

Vitamin and Mineral Supplement Ranges

U.S. RDA Adult	Adult Daily Supplement Range

FAT-SOLUBLE VITAMINS

Beta-carotene pro-vitamin A: Converted by the body to vitamin A as needed. Primary antioxidant which helps protect the lungs and other tissues.

Not established	**10,000 - 50,000 IU**

Possible side effects: Prolonged ingestion of relatively high doses may cause a nonharmful yellowing of the skin, especially palms and soles. Avoid beta-carotene supplement while taking the prescription drug Accutane, especially during pregnancy.

Vitamin A (preformed retinol): Essential for growth and development, maintenance of healthy skin, hair, and eyes. Involved in wound healing.

4000 - 5000 IU	**5,000 - 10,000 IU**

Possible side effects: Prolonged ingestion of excess vitamin A (50,000 IU+/day) may be toxic. Avoid vitamin A supplement while taking the prescription drug Accutane, especially during pregnancy.

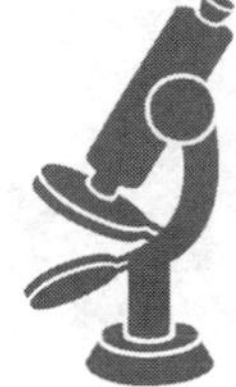

Because the current U.S. RDA's are an inadequate guide to the therapeutic benefits of nutritional supplements, research should be made to develop an accurate guide to the ranges of supplementation.

Vitamin D cholecalferol: Essential for calcium and phosphorus metabolism, required for strong bones and teeth.

400 IU	**200-400 IU**

Possible side effects: Prolonged ingestion of excess vitamin D (1,000 IU+/day) may be toxic and cause hypercalcemia (excess of calcium in blood).

Vitamin E (alpha tocopherol): Primary antioxidant which protects red blood cells and is essential in cellular respiration.

12 -15 IU	**200 - 800 IU**

Possible side effects: Prolonged ingestion of vitamin E may produce adverse skin reactions and upset stomach.

Vitamin K (phylloquinone): Integrally involved in the blood clotting mechanism.

65 mcg.	**50-500 mcg.**

Possible side effects: Unlike the other fat-soluble vitamins, vitamin K is not stored in significant quantity in the liver. Synthetic vitamin K (menadione) is toxic in excess dosages.

WATER-SOLUBLE VITAMINS

Vitamin C (ascorbic acid): Primary antioxidant, essential for tissue growth, wound healing, absorption of calcium and iron and utilization of the B vitamin folic acid. Involved in neurotransmitter biosynthesis, cholesterol regulation, and formation of collagen.

60 mg.	**300-3,000 mg.**

Possible side effects: Essentially nontoxic in oral doses. However, excessive ingestion may cause abdominal bloating, gas, flatulence, and diarrhea. Acid-sensitive individuals should take buffered ascorbate form of vitamin C supplement.

US RDA - Adult	Adult Daily Supplement Range

Vitamin B_1 (thiamine): Essential for food metabolism and release of energy for cellular function.

1.2-1.5 mg.	5-100 mg.

Possible side effects: Essentially nontoxic in oral doses.

Vitamin B_2 (riboflavin): Essential for food metabolism and release of energy for cellular function. Important in the formation of red blood cells and activation of other B vitamins.

1.4-1.8 mg.	5-100 mg.

Possible side effects: Essentially nontoxic in oral doses. Moderate to high doses of vitamin B_2 may cause nonharmful bright yellow coloration of urine.

Vitamin B_3 (niacin): Essential for food metabolism and release of energy for cellular function. Vital for oxygen transport in the blood, and fatty acid and nucleic acid formation. A major constituent of several important coenzymes.

16-20 mg.	20-100 mg.

Possible side effects: Essentially nontoxic in normal oral doses. High doses (100 mg+) may cause transient flushing and tingling in the upper body area, as well as stomach upset. Prolonged ingestion of excess vitamin B_3 (1,000 mg-2,000 mg+/day) may elevate liver enzymes and cause liver damage.

Vitamin B_5 (pantothenic acid): Involved in food metabolism and release of energy for cellular function. Vital for biosynthesis of hormones and support of the adrenal glands.

4-7 mg.	10-1,000 mg.

Possible side effects: Essentially nontoxic in oral doses. Extremely high doses (10,000 mg+) will produce diarrhea.

Vitamin B_6 (pyroxidine): Involved in food metabolism and release of energy. Essential for amino acid metabolism, and formation of blood proteins and antibodies. Helps regulate electrolytic balance.

2.0-2.5 mg.	5-200 mg.

Possible side effects: Prolonged high doses (500 mg+/day) may be toxic and cause neurological damage. Prescription oral contraceptives may cause deficiency of vitamin B_6.

Vitamin B_{12} (cobalamin): Essential for normal formation of red blood cells. Involved in food metabolism, release of energy and maintenance of epithelial cells (cells that form the skin's outer layer and the surface layer of mucous membranes) and the nervous system.

3.0-4.0 mcg.	10-500 mcg.

Possible side effects: Essentially nontoxic in oral doses.

Folate (folic acid, folacin): Essential for blood formation, especially red blood cells and white blood cells. Involved in the biosynthesis of nucleic acids including RNA/DNA.

400 mcg.	200-800 mcg.

Possible side effects: Essentially nontoxic in oral doses. An excess intake of folate can mask a vitamin B_{12} deficiency.

US RDA - Adult	Adult Daily Supplement Range

Biotin: Essential for food metabolism and release of energy. Assists in the biosynthesis of amino acids, nucleic acid, and fatty acids. Utilization of other B vitamins.

150-300 mcg.	**300-600 mcg.**

Possible side effects: Essentially nontoxic in oral doses.

B vitamins should also be taken in a B-complex form because of their close interrelationship in metabolic processes.

MINERALS

The functions of minerals are highly interrelated to each other and to vitamins, hormones, and enzymes. No mineral can function in the body without affecting others.

Calcium (Ca++): Essential for strong bones and teeth. Serves as a vital cofactor in cellular energy production, and nerve and heart function.

800-1,200 mg.	**200-1,200 mg.**

Possible side effects: Prolonged ingestion of excess calcium, along with excess vitamin D may cause hypercalcemia of bone and soft tissue (such as joints and kidneys) and may also cause a mineral imbalance.

Magnesium (Mg++): Essential catalyst for food metabolism and release of energy. A cofactor in the formation of RNA/DNA, enzyme activation, and nerve function.

300-350 mg.	**150-600 mg.**

Possible side effects: Extremely high doses (30,000 mg+) may be toxic in certain individuals with kidney problems. Doses of 400 mg+ may produce a laxative effect, causing diarrhea.

Potassium (K+): A primary electrolyte, important in regulating pH (acid/base) balance and water balance. Plays a role in nerve function and cellular integrity.

Not established	**1,875-5,625 mg.***

* (A typical healthy diet contains adequate potassium. Very active individuals may require additional electrolytes).
Possible side effects: Extremely high doses (25,000 mg+/day) of K chloride may be toxic in instances of kidney failure.

Sodium (Na+): A primary electrolyte, important in regulating pH (acid/base) balance and water balance. Plays a role in nerve function and cellular integrity.

Not established	**Limit your daily intake to 1,500 mg.**

Possible side effects: Prolonged ingestion of excess sodium has been linked to high blood pressure and increased incidence of migraine headaches. Extremely high intakes of sodium can result in swelling of tissues called edema.

Phosphorus (P): Constituent of the molecule phosphate, which plays a major role in energy production and activation of B vitamins. Component of RNA/DNA, bones, and teeth.

900-1,200 mg.	**300-600 mg.**

Possible side effects: Although essentially nontoxic, a disproportionately large amount of phosphorus relative to calcium intake may cause a deficiency in calcium and mineral imbalance.

US RDA - Adult	Adult Daily Supplement Range
Zinc (Zn++): Cofactor in numerous enzymatic processes and reactions. Structural constituent of nucleic acids and insulin. Involved in taste, wound healing, and digestion.	
15 mg.	**15-30 mg.**
Possible side effects: Extremely high doses (2,000 mg+/day) can be toxic. Excess zinc intake (50 mg+/day) may cause copper deficiency and mineral imbalance.	
Iron (FE++ or FE+++): Combines with other nutrients to produce vital blood proteins. Involved in food metabolism.	
10-18 mg.	**10-30 mg.**
Possible side effects: Prolonged ingestion of excess iron can be toxic, affecting the liver, pancreas, heart, and nucleus and increasing susceptibility to infection. Poorly utilized forms of iron (Fe sulfate or Fe gluconate) may cause constipation and/or stomach upset. Iron supplements should be taken with food and supplemental vitamin C.	
Manganese (Mn++): Important catalyst and cofactor in many enzymatic processes and reactions. Helps maintain skeletal and connective structural tissue, as well as cellular integrity.	
2.5-5.0 mg.	**2-10 mg.**
Possible side effects: Prolonged ingestion of excess manganese may result in nonharmful elevated concentrations in the liver and may cause a mineral imbalance.	
Copper (Cu++): Essential for production of red blood cells. Involved in the maintenance of skeletal and cardiovascular systems. Works with vitamin C in the biosynthesis of collagen and elastin.	
2-3 mg.	**2-3 mg.**
Possible side effects; Prolonged ingestion of excess copper may be toxic, especially with Wilson's disease, a rare metabolic disorder resulting in an excess accumulation of copper in the liver, red blood cells, and the brain.	
Iodine (I-): Essential component of thyroid hormones which regulate growth and rate of metabolism.	
150 mcg.	**50-300 mcg.**
Possible side effects: Prolonged ingestion of excess iodine may cause "iodine goiter," an enlargement of the thyroid gland. May also induce acne-like skin lesions or aggravate preexisting acne conditions.	
Chromium (Cr+++): Vital as cofactor of GTF (glucose tolerance factor), which regulates the function of insulin. Involved in food metabolism, enzyme activation, and regulation of cholesterol.	
50-200 mcg.	**200-500 mcg.**
Possible side effects: Essentially nontoxic in oral doses.	
Selenium (Se): Important constituent of the antioxident enzyme gluathione peroxidase which is contained in white blood cells and blood platelets. Synergistic nutritional partner of vitamin E.	
55-200 mcg.	**100-200 mcg.**
Possible side effects: Prolonged ingestion of excess selenium may be toxic.	

How Nutrients Work Together

Vitamins and minerals help regulate the conversion of food to energy in the body, according to Dr. Bland, and can be separated into two general categories: energy nutrients, which are principally involved in the conversion of food to energy, and protector nutrients, which help defend against damaging toxins derived from drugs, alcohol, radiation, environmental pollutants, or the body's own enzyme processes.

"The B-complex vitamins and magnesium are examples of energy nutrients," says Dr. Bland, "for they activate specific metabolic facilitators called enzymes, which control digestion and the absorption and use of proteins, fats, and carbohydrates. These nutrients often work as a team, their mutual presence enhancing the other's function."

In the process of converting food to energy, oxygen-free radicals are produced that can damage the body and set the stage for degenerative diseases, including arthritis, heart disease, certain forms of cancer, and premature aging. Protector nutrients such as vitamin E, beta-carotene (a close relative of vitamin A), vitamin C, and the minerals zinc, copper, manganese, and selenium, play a critical role in preventing or delaying these degenerative processes. Vitamins E, A, and C work together as a team, protecting against breakdown and helping each other maintain adequate tissue levels.

Dr. Berkson notes that vitamins and minerals are what make the chemical and electrical circuitry of the body work, and that the body's functioning is therefore profoundly affected by how nutrients either work together or against each other. Nutrients can help each other or inhibit each other when taken simultaneously. For example, iron is best absorbed when taken separately from pancreatic enzymes and should also not be taken with vitamin E, says Dr. Berkson. There are also certain nutrients that can help "potentiate" the other nutrients. For example, vitamin C taken with iron provides the maximum absorption of the iron.

Benefits of Nutritional Supplementation

Many studies support the use of nutritional supplements to achieve adequate levels of nutrients. Research by Raymond Shamberger, Ph.D., and Derrick Lonsdale, M.D., from the Cleveland Clinic in Ohio, found that while consumption of empty-calorie diets can lead to such problems as lassitude, fatigue, mood swings, insomnia, and a variety of health complaints that had no other related medical diagnosis, when patients were given supplementary nutrients over a period of six to twelve weeks, many of their symptoms improved.

A study conducted by Ruth Harrell, Ph.D., David Benton, Ph.D., and Guilyn Roberts, Ph.D., at the University of Wales, found that the administration of multivitamin supplements to children suffering from marginal nutrient insufficiency brought about significant improvement in their academic performances.[7] A similar observation was made in studying the mental capacity of elderly individuals.[8]

Current studies lend strong support to the importance of vitamin C in slowing the development of cataracts, heart disease, and cancer. A recent study, conducted by James E. Enstrom, M.D., an epidemiologist at the University of California at Los Angeles, suggests that men who consume vitamin C every day, at levels 500 to 666 percent of the U.S. RDA, live about six years longer than men who don't.[9]

Robert Cathcart, M.D., of Los Altos, California, has also documented the effective use of vitamin C in treating various infectious diseases, including the common cold, flu, pneumonia, hepatitis, mononucleosis, and several childhood diseases.[10]

Other clinical studies have also shown a relationship between low intakes of beta-carotene (pro-vitamin A), vitamin E, and vitamin C and higher incidences of cancer.[11] Research done at Johns Hopkins University found that there were approximately 50 percent fewer heart disease cases in a group of people with the highest levels of beta-carotene, compared to the group with the lowest levels.[12] A similar study at Harvard University found that of two groups with prior evidence of heart disease, the group given a beta-carotene supplement had 40 percent fewer heart attacks than the group given a placebo.[13]

Due to current FDA labeling regulations, health-food stores and/or pharmacies are not allowed to present information regarding dosage or treatment of nutritional supplements and herbs, regardless of scientific support.

Research has also found that vitamin B_3 (niacin) can help combat heart disease, while vitamin B_6 can help prevent atherosclerosis.[14] Other studies have shown similar results with vitamin E and heart disease.[15] Large doses of vitamin E have also been found to strengthen immune functioning and reduce the severity of age-related diseases such as Parkinson's disease.[16]

According to Eric Braverman, M.D., of New Jersey, amino acid supplementation has been used to treat heart disease, as well as herpes, alcoholism, and a variety of psychiatric disorders.[17] Zinc supplementation has also been found to improve progressive hearing loss and other related ear problems.[18]

Accessory nutrients can also be taken as supplements for specific purposes. For example, bioflavonoids, which are present in various foods like citrus rind and buckwheat, can help to increase vitamin C's antiviral activity in treating herpes simplex.[19] Coenzyme Q10 helps to improve heart function.[20] Evidence suggests that gamma-linolenic acid may help to regulate the cardiovascular, nervous, and immune systems of the body.[21]

In addition to disease control, nutritional supplements can also help people cope with specific lifestyle, environmental, and emotional/psychological factors. For example, smokers require more vitamin E, vitamin C, and beta-carotene than nonsmokers, and persons who consume a significant amount of alcohol require more vitamin B_1 and magnesium than the average person.[22]

Individuals engaged in heavy exercise programs need to make sure they are getting adequate nutrients to meet their increased caloric demands. Weight-loss dieters also need supplemental vitamins and minerals to make up for deficiencies that result from reduced calorie intake, according to Dr. Berkson.

Women taking oral contraceptives may need to increase their zinc, folic acid, and vitamin B_6 intakes, while pregnant women may require more folic acid for proper fetal development. Lactating women also need additional magnesium and protein, and postmenopausal women require increased calcium and vitamin D to maintain strong bones.

When recovering from surgery, a person may need higher levels of zinc,[23] and individuals who are exposed to smog or other pollutants require higher levels of the protector nutrients such as selenium, vitamin E, and vitamin C.[24] Also, anyone who is under heavy emotional or physical stress will need higher intakes of all the B vitamins.[25]

Using Nutritional Supplements

Today, an estimated 46 percent of adult Americans take nutritional supplements, many on a daily basis.[26] It is no longer just a fad, but part of a growing trend as more and more people take a proactive approach to their own health care.

Although researchers are learning more and more every day about the connection between nutrients and health, there is still no definitive scientific "how-to guide" for this very complex issue, especially since each individual's needs are different.

How to Take Nutritional Supplements

Before taking any nutritional supplement you should ask what scientific data supports its safety and what are the safe intake levels for the nutrients you are considering taking. Jeffrey Bland, Ph.D., of Gig Harbor, Washington and D. Lindsey Berkson, M.A., D.C., of Santa Fe, New Mexico, make the following recommendations:

- *Nutritional supplements should be taken with meals to promote increased absorption. Fat-soluble vitamins (such as vitamin A, beta-carotene, vitamin E, and the essential fatty acids linoleic and alpha linolenic acid) should be taken with the meal which contains the most fat during the day.*
- *Amino acid supplements should be taken on an empty stomach at least an hour before or after a meal, and taken with fruit juice to help promote absorption. Whenever taking an increased dosage of an isolated amino acid be sure to supplement with an amino acid blend.*
- *If you become nauseated when you take tablet supplements, consider taking a liquid form, diluted in a beverage.*
- *If you become nauseated or ill within an hour after taking nutritional supplements, consider the need for a bowel cleanse or rejuvenation program prior to beginning a course of nutritional supplementation.*
- *If you are taking high doses, do not take the supplements all at one time, but divide them into smaller doses taken throughout the day.*
- *Take digestive enzymes with meals to assist digestion. If you are taking pancreatic enzymes for other therapeutic reasons, be sure to take them on an empty stomach between meals.*
- *Take mineral supplements away from the highest fiber meals of the day as fiber can decrease mineral absorption.*
- *Whenever taking an increased dosage of an isolated B vitamin, be sure to supplement with a B-complex.*
- *When taking nutrients be sure to take adequate amounts of liquid to mix with digestive juices and prevent side effects.*

While it is always recommended that a person try to obtain as many nutrients as possible through the consumption of a variety of high-nutrient-density foods, this can be unrealistic for many, due to reduced calorie intake; the dislike of certain foods; loss of nutrients in cooking;

the variable quality of food supply; lack of knowledge, motivation, or time to plan and prepare balanced meals; and nutrient depletion caused by stress, lifestyle, and certain medications. This is where nutritional supplements can play an important role in filling any nutrient gaps.

Nutritional supplements are not a panacea, however, and it is important to be aware of some potential risks. Prolonged intake of excessive doses of vitamin A, vitamin D, and vitamin B_6, for example, may produce toxic effects. Other vitamins, minerals, and accessory nutrients can also sometimes cause side effects when they interact with medications, or due to health conditions or simply a person's biochemical individuality. However, alternative practitioners may sometimes recommend dosages higher than those currently considered safe by conventional medicine. The scientific literature and numerous clinical trials support these elevated dosages for short periods of time and only under medical supervision. "For example," says Dr. Berkson, "many alternative practitioners use extremely elevated levels of vitamin A for several days to a week to act as a natural antibiotic for acute infection."

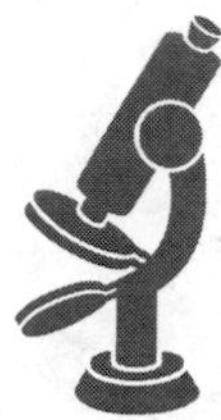

Since nutritional supplements cannot be patented, there is little financial incentive for pharmaceutical companies to invest the millions of dollars needed to meet the government's stringent research requirements in order to receive FDA approval for treatment of specific conditions. Alternative sources of funding must be found in order to make nutritional supplements an accepted part of mainstream medicine.

Nutritional supplements should also never take the place of proper dietary habits or appropriate medical care when warranted. If someone is currently under medical care, is taking any medications, or has a history of specific problems, it is important for him or her to always consult with a physician before making any changes in diet or lifestyle, including the use of supplements.

It can take years of personal research and experimentation to put together a good dietary and supplement program. To eliminate a lot of guesswork and frustration, a person should consult a qualified health professional trained in the intricacies of nutritional biochemistry, to help the person assess his or her personal needs and to help develop an effective dietary and nutritional supplement program tailored to biochemical individuality.

High-quality nutritional supplements can often be obtained through these professionals, or from a source recommended by them. When making a decision to purchase nutritional supplements without the advice of an expert, do so as an informed consumer. It is worthwhile to read some of the many books and magazines published about good dietary habits and nutritional supplements. Reputable health food stores are a good source of quality supplements and are also usually staffed by people who have a knowledgeable understanding of nutrition and supplementation. Some pharmacies specialize in nutritional and natural remedies as well; there are also several good mail order and direct outlets.

The current challenge for medicine and nutritional science is to look beyond statistical guidelines in order to gain a greater understanding of the role and proper level of nutrients that will help every individual achieve and maintain a high level of wellness. Through education and involvement, a person can develop an understanding of the proper diet and nutritional needs specifically suited to the body, and should make this knowledge an integral part of living well.

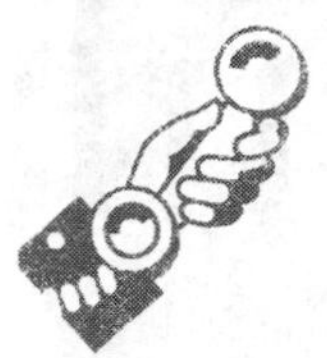

Where to Find Help

To obtain referrals to physicians trained in nutritional medicine, contact:

American College of Advancement in Medicine
P.O. Box 3427
Laguna Hills, CA 92654
(714) 583-7666

ACAM provides a directory listing of physicians worldwide who have been trained in nutritional and preventative medicine. The directory also provides an extensive list of books and articles on nutritional supplementation.

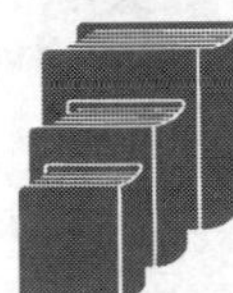

Recommended Reading

Dr. Wright's Guide to Healing with Nutrition. Wright, Jonathan V., M.D. New Canaan, CT: Keats Publishing, Inc., 1990.

A very readable and informative book, it contains many case histories describing how Dr. Wright approaches patients' problems. He describes the patients' exams, tests, and treatments that solved long-standing disorders.

The Healing Nutrients Within. Braverman, Eric R., M.D.; and Pfeiffer, Carl C., M.D., Ph.D. New Canaan, CT: Keats Publishing, Inc., 1987.

This book focuses on protein and amino acids and their function in the treatment of depression and insomnia, addiction, detoxification, and nutritional support for surgery. The authors have found amino acid therapy effective in cases of cancer, arthritis, allergy, physical and emotional health problems, and other disorders. This book is useful to health care professionals and understandable to lay readers.

The Nutrition Desk Reference. Garrison, Robert, H. Jr., M.A.R., Ph.D.; and Somer, Elizabeth, M.A., R.D. New Canaan, CT: Keats Publishing, Inc., 1990.

Reference for personal health and professional research. Basic nutritional information. Research findings on vitamins and minerals and their role in disease treatment and prevention.

Nutritional Influences on Illness. 2nd Edition. Werbach, Melvyn A., M.D. Tarzana, CA: Third Line Press, 1992.

This is a sourcebook that abstracts and organizes many studies dealing with the way nutrition affects illness.

Prescription for Nutritional Healing; A Practical A-Z Reference to Drug-Free Remedies Using Vitamins, Minerals, Herbs, and Food Supplements. Balch, James, M.D.; and Balch, Phyllis, R.N., Garden City Park, NY: Avery Publishing, 1990.

A complete guide to dealing with health disorders through nutritional, herbal, and supplemental therapies written by a medical doctor and a nutritionist. It provides all the information needed for the average person to design his or her own nutrition program.

Staying Healthy with Nutrition. Haas, Elson M., M.D. Berkeley, CA: Celestial Arts Publishing, 1992.

A comprehensive guide to diet and nutritional medicine. Includes an analysis of the building blocks of nutrition and their uses in medicine; an evaluation of diets around the world; the environmental aspects of nutrition; nutritional therapies; and help in creating individualized diets.

Orthomolecular Medicine

Employing vitamins, minerals, and amino acids to create optimum nutritional content and balance in the body, orthomolecular medicine targets a wide range of conditions, including depression, hypertension, schizophrenia, cancer, and other mental and physiological disorders.

In 1968, Nobel Prize-winner Linus Pauling, Ph.D., originated the term "orthomolecular" to describe an approach to medicine that uses naturally occurring substances normally present in the body. "Ortho" means correct or normal, and orthomolecular physicians recognize that in many cases of physiological and psychological disorders health can be reestablished by properly correcting, or normalizing, the balance of vitamins, minerals, amino acids, and other similar substances within the body.

"Our physical bodies are made up of water, fat, protein, carbohydrates, and similar substances," says Jonathan Wright, M.D., of Kent, Washington, explaining a basic principle of orthomolecular medicine. "Therefore, it's logical to expect that if something is wrong with our bodies, proper manipulation of the elements of which they are made will be a major factor in reestablishing health."

"Our physical bodies are made up of water, fat, protein, carbohydrates, and similar substances. Therefore, it's logical to expect that if something is wrong with our bodies, proper manipulation of the elements of which they are made will be a major factor in reestablishing health."
—Jonathan Wright, M.D.

The premise behind orthomolecular medicine extends back to the 1920s, when vitamins and minerals were first used to treat illnesses unrelated to nutrient deficiency. During that time, it was discovered that vitamin A could prevent childhood deaths from infectious illness, and that heart arrhythmia (irregular heartbeat) could be stopped by dosages of magnesium. Scientific evidence supporting nutritional therapy did not fully emerge, however, until the 1950s, when Abram Hoffer, M.D., and Humphrey Osmond, M.D., began treating schizophrenics with high doses of vitamin B_3 (niacin). Their studies showed that niacin, in combination with standard medical therapy, doubled the number of recoveries in a one-year period.[1]

As research continued it was found that malnutrition and improper nutrition could place a person at risk, directly causing or contributing to the development of disease and psychiatric disorders. Furthermore, it was noted that health can be impaired, due, in part, to the consumption of refined, empty-calorie foods such as white bread and pastries and the overconsumption of sugar. Decreased intake of dietary fiber, bran, minerals, and complex carbohydrates were also found in patients with certain forms of mental illness, along with a loss of vitamins and an increase in dietary fat. At the time, the notion that diet could contribute to disease was a new and controversial idea.

Basic Principles of Orthomolecular Medicine

Even today many physicians disregard the value of proper nutrition in relation to health. The prevalent notion is that a balanced diet will provide all the nutrition one needs. What is overlooked, however, is the fact that the majority of the United States food supply is processed and grown in nutritionally depleted soil. Orthomolecular physicians recognize these factors, as well as the fact that biochemical individuality can also play a crucial role in health.

The concept of biochemical individuality is based on the work of Roger J. Williams, Ph.D. In treating his patients, Dr. Williams realized that each individual is unique. Although the government minimum, or recommended daily allowances (RDA), for nutrients may prevent severe deficiency disease, orthomolecular physicians say that these levels do not provide for optimal health, and people may need many more times the RDA levels. For example, studies of guinea pigs show a twentyfold variation in their requirement for vitamin C. Similar studies have been done with humans: children have been shown to have varying needs for vitamin B_6, and Canadian soldiers and Japanese prisoners of war who suffered from starvation were shown to require a much greater intake of vitamins than usual.

In 1987, Richard Kunin, M.D., of San Francisco, California, summarized the principles of orthomolecular medicine:[2]

- Nutrition comes first in medical diagnosis and treatment, and nutrient-related disorders are usually curable once nutritional balance is achieved.
- Biochemical individuality is the norm in medical practice; therefore universal RDA values are unreliable nutrient guides. Many people require an intake of certain nutrients far beyond the RDA suggested range (often called a megadose), due to their genetic disposition and/or the environment in which they live.
- Drug treatment is used only for specific indications and always mindful of the potential dangers and adverse effects.
- Environmental pollution and food adulteration are an inescapable fact of modern life and are a medical priority.
- Blood tests do not necessarily reflect tissue levels of nutrients.
- Hope is the indispensable ally of the physician and the absolute right of the patient.

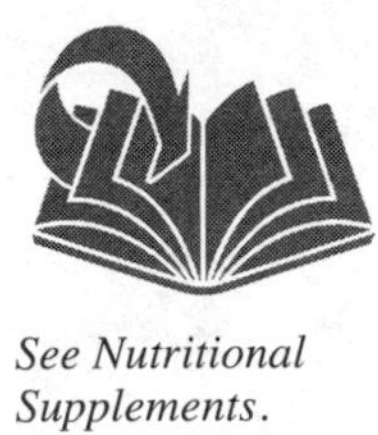

See Nutritional Supplements.

"Megavitamin Therapy"—How Does it Work?

The basis of orthomolecular medicine lies in creating a healthier diet. Junk foods, refined sugar, and food additives are eliminated. Every effort is made to eat nutritious, whole foods, high in fiber and low in fat. Depending on the condition to be treated, various vitamins, minerals, and other nutrients are supplemented. The types and amounts of the nutrients are determined by blood tests, urine analysis, and tests for nutrient levels. Frequently, supplementation is based not only on a patient's symptoms, but on results reported in medical journals, and, quite commonly, the clinical experience of the doctor. Prescribed doses of vitamins are sometimes injected to speed the initial response, and follow-up treatment usually consists of vitamin pills several times a day until adequate dosage is achieved. This dosage has often been called a megadose because amounts of nutrients taken are often far greater than the levels needed to prevent deficiency. As a result, orthomolecular medicine has also been called megavitamin therapy.

"The total number of fatalities from overdoses of major pharmaceutical drugs for the eight-year reporting period from 1983 to 1990 equals 2,556, whereas the total number of fatalities resulting from high doses of vitamin supplements during the same period is zero."

One of the arguments against megavitamin treatment is that high doses of certain vitamins are toxic and may cause certain reactions. A major study, however, indicates that the total number of fatalities from overdoses of major pharmaceutical drugs for the eight-year reporting period from 1983 to 1990 equals 2,556, whereas the total number of fatalities resulting from high doses of vitamin supplements during the same period is zero.[3]

Nevertheless, orthomolecular physicians are aware of the problems associated with megavitamin therapy, and if symptoms arise, the dosage of the offending vitamin is reduced. In some cases these reactions are carefully observed as an indication that the body has been saturated with the vitamin. When this occurs, the dose is lowered until the symptoms disappear and the body is supplied with optimal levels of the nutrient. An example is the method of administering vitamin C to bowel tolerance for the common cold, flus, and other conditions pioneered by Robert Cathcart III, M.D., of Los Altos, California.[4]

See Diet.

Conditions Benefited by Orthomolecular Medicine

Since the mid-1950s, niacin has been used as a treatment for schizophrenia. Other orthomolecular discoveries include:

- Studies have shown over the years that higher levels of beta-carotene (a precursor of vitamin A) are associated with lower rates of certain cancers.[5]
- Folic acid (a B vitamin) has been used by a number of mainstream physicians to prevent neural tube defects,[6] a condition that causes improper brain and spinal cord development in newborns. It is now a recommended preventive measure for pregnant women. Folic acid is also used in the treatment of cervical dysplasia, a precancerous condition of the uterus, and, for this reason, is also given to women who take birth control pills[7] or who are pregnant.[8]

- Intravenous magnesium sulphate (a mineral compound) is given in some hospitals to heart attack victims to speed recovery time.[9] Injections of vitamin C, magnesium sulphate, vitamin B_6, and zinc sulphate are also used by some orthomolecular physicians to help prevent high blood pressure during surgery and help prevent postsurgical complications.
- Chromium (a trace mineral) is now given to help regulate the body's response to sugar and insulin. It may help those with diabetes[10] and hypoglycemia.[11] It can also aid in lowering cholesterol.
- Essential fatty acids (unsaturated fats that the body cannot make for itself and must obtain from food sources), including omega-3 and omega-6, are now linked to a decrease in risk factors for heart disease[12] and a lessening of symptoms of other afflictions, including psoriasis[13] and rheumatoid arthritis.[14]

In many of these examples, the doses of nutrients are far greater than those suggested by the RDA, but there is general agreement among orthomolecular physicians concerning dosage and usage.

Numerous case histories illustrate the effectiveness of orthomolecular medicine, in many cases, even after other approaches to healing had failed. A dramatic example concerns a patient of Alan R. Gaby, M.D., of Baltimore, Maryland.

The patient, a thirty-six-year-old woman, had a six-year history of progressively diffuse muscle pain and spasm, which began after an auto accident. The condition had caused severe and incapacitating symptoms, which had resulted in eleven hospitalizations for persistent pain. She had spent an estimated one hundred thousand dollars on various treatments over the six years. Numerous prescription medications had been tried with only mild to moderate relief. At the time of her initial visit, she was taking five medications for muscle pain, spasm, and fatigue. Physical examination revealed severe tenderness to light touch at numerous areas of her body.

Dr. Gaby began her treatment with a therapeutic trial of intravenous nutrients consisting of magnesium chloride hexahydrate, calcium glycerophosphate, ascorbic acid (vitamin C), vitamin B_6, vitamin B_5, vitamin B_1, vitamin B_{12}, and B complex. There was no change after the first two injections. After the third injection, however, she reported a 90 percent improvement in fatigue and muscle complaints. After three days, she discontinued all five medications. During the ensuing two months, she received one injection approximately every two weeks. She has reported continued improvement, but the effects of the vitamins begin to wear off after two weeks if she does not maintain her injection schedule.

Dr. Wright reports success in cases of childhood asthma treated with orthomolecular medicine. One of his patients was a four-year-old boy described by his parents as "being allergic since birth." The boy suffered from chronic nasal congestion. He was admitted to emergency rooms numerous times for acute wheezing. When the boy was first brought to Dr. Wright he was on long-term antihistamine medication.

Dr. Wright's examination revealed that the boy had "allergic shiners" under his eyes and showed a maldigestion/malabsorption pattern. Dr. Wright taught the boy's parents how to inject the boy intramuscularly with vitamin B_{12} shots. His parents reported that their son stopped wheezing within the first week of treatment and has slowly been able to come off medication without ill effects. With additional supplementation of glutamic acid hydrochloride capsules as a digestive aid, a low-dose multimineral complex, and 50 milligrams twice daily of magnesium, combined with B_{12} shots given once every two weeks, he has experienced no further wheezing episodes. When Dr. Wright saw him two years later, the boy was still healthy and his digestive and absorption abilities had also improved significantly. [15]

Dr. Wright has also successfully treated numerous other conditions using orthomolecular medicine. Among them: acne, chronic anemia, angina, high blood pressure, cholesterol imbalance, cystic mastitis, headache, herpes simplex, infertility, and prostate enlargement.[16]

Mood and behavior are other factors that can be improved by orthomolecular medicine. According to Phyllis J. Bronson, a nutritional-

HOW TO DETERMINE THE PROPER DOSE OF VITAMIN C FOR THE TREATMENT OF ILLNESS

In his twenty-three years of clinical experience, Robert Cathcart III, M.D., has found that taking vitamin C to bowel tolerance (bowel tolerance refers to the amount of vitamin C that can be tolerated by the body before diarrhea occurs) can effectively treat diseases which may involve free radical damage. These include: the common cold, infections, allergies, autoimmune diseases, burns, and viral pneumonia. Free radicals are atoms within the body that contain an unpaired electron. As free radicals seek to replace their missing electrons they wreck havoc on body tissue, thus depleting the body. Free radicals are neutralized by electrons called reducing equivalents that are carried by high doses of vitamin C.

Powdered ascorbic acid (vitamin C) is mixed with water and taken several times in a twenty-four-hour period. The amount taken is increased until diarrhea develops and is slightly adjusted until the diarrhetic condition stops. The more severe the problem, the more vitamin C that can be taken before diarrhea occurs. Dr Cathcart suggests the following amounts of vitamin C be taken for certain problems

In many conditions, symptoms are greatly reduced but will return rapidly if the dose levels are not maintained. In serious problems, doses may have to be taken every half hour, and delays may prolong the illness.

	Grams per 24 hours	Number of Doses Per 24 hours
Hay fever, asthma	**5-20**	**4-8**
Mild cold	**30-60**	**6-10**
Influenza	**100-150**	**8-15**
Viral pneumonia	**50-200+**	**12-18**

CAUTION

***Caution**: Before beginning this type of program, it is advisable to seek out the guidance of your physician. People suffering from hypertension or kidney problems should also ascertain that the form of vitamin C they use does not contain sodium ascorbate, a form of salt that can result in heart and kidney complications.*

biochemical consultant in Aspen, Colorado, amino acid levels in the brain play a significant role. "Chemical impulses in the brain are relayed via nerve transmitters, some of which affect emotions, others which affect muscle function," Bronson states. "Almost all of these neurotransmitters are composed of amino acids. By using supplements of the amino acids which make up specific neurotransmitters, you can actually change the nature and intensity of the brain messages they carry."

Bronson focuses the large part of her practice on treating people for depression and anxiety disorders. "The traditional treatment for most types of anxiety disorders is the use of Xanex and Valium, which seem to work by stimulating the production of GABA (gammaaminobutyric acid) in the brain," she says. Such drugs have a myriad of side effects, Bronson points out, and they can also have toxic effects on kidney and liver function. Bronson prefers to use GABA itself. "GABA is the brain's natural opiate, and is related to the endorphins which are the brain's natural painkillers. It can quiet anxiety, reduce muscle tensions, and induce sleep." Bronson notes that for many people suffering from depression or anxiety disorders there is a long history of deficient GABA reserves. "Once they begin taking GABA supplements, their improvement can be quite dramatic," she says. But she cautions against using GABA without the supervision of a competent physician or nutritionist. An individually prescribed supplementation program takes into account the Krebs cycle, which is the final step in the metabolism of fats, carbohydrates, and proteins. Therefore, says Bronson, "To attempt supplementation on one's own is not advisable."

The Future of Orthomolecular Medicine

Unfortunately, there is still some prejudice against nutritional therapy. Most medical schools have limited programs in nutrition education. As a result, most graduating doctors have little knowledge of the power of nutrition against disease. Also, since conventional medicine has a history of rejecting nutritional intervention, most doctors are not trained to think along these lines and consequently do not use nutrition in their practices.

Abram Hoffer, M.D., Ph.D., one of the pioneers in orthomolecular medicine, foresees a change. "It takes approximately forty years for innovative thought to be incorporated into mainstream thought," he says. "I expect and hope that orthomolecular medicine, within the next five to ten years, will cease to be a specialty in medicine and that all physicians will be using nutrition as an essential tool in treating disease."

Richard P. Huemer, M.D., of Vancouver, Washington, a colleague of Dr. Linus Pauling, and himself a pioneer in the field of orthomolecular medicine, agrees. "We need a paradigm shift, and I think it's beginning to occur," he says. "Nutrition needs to be looked at, not as a means of preventing specific deficiency diseases, but as a means of contributing to the overall health of the person

"I expect and hope that orthomolecular medicine, within the next five to ten years, will cease to be a specialty in medicine and that all physicians will be using nutrition as an essential tool in treating disease."

—Abram Hoffer, M.D., Ph.D.

and his or her resistance to chronic diseases. We have to start looking for the optimum levels of nutrients necessary for optimum health instead of the minimum amount needed to prevent diseases. This is going to produce a big upsurge in human health in the next twenty years."

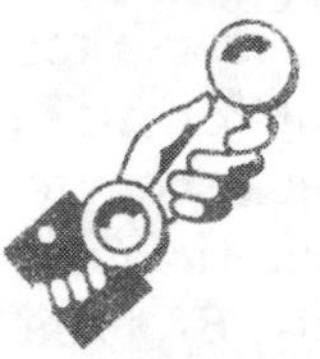

Where to Find Help

For more information about nutritional therapy, or to locate an orthomolecular physician, contact:

International Academy of Nutrition & Preventive Medicine
P.O. Box 18433
Asheville, NC 28814
(704) 258-3243

This resource serves as a clearinghouse of information and as a referral service for physicians practicing orthomolecular medicine.

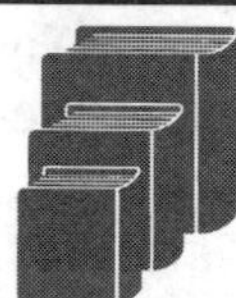

Recommended Reading

Dr. Wright's Guide to Healing with Nutrition. Wright, Jonathan, M.D. New Canaan, CT: Keats Publishing, Inc., 1990.

Dr. Wright's book contains case histories describing his approach to patients' problems. Details about the patients' exams, tests, and treatments that solved long-standing disorders are provided.

Nutritional Influences on Illness. 2nd ed. Werbach, Melvyn, M.D. Tarzana, CA:Third Line Press, 1992.

This sourcebook abstracts and organizes many studies dealing with the way nutrition affects illnesses.

Orthomolecular Nutrition, Rev. ed. Hoffer, Abram, M.D.; and Walker, Morton. New Canaan, CT: Keats Publishing, Inc., 1978.

Description of the development of orthomolecular medicine from early psychiatric studies to the present. Authors discuss individual nutrients; the relationship between food and health; and benefits to be gained from optimal nutrition.

The Real Vitamin and Mineral Book. Lieberman, Shari; and Bruning, Nancy P. Garden City Park, NY: Avery Publishing Group, Inc., 1990.

All of the major nutrients are discussed in this helpful book and research supporting their therapeutic value is cited. Amounts of vitamin treatment are suggested for certain conditions. Optimal amounts of each nutrient for daily supplementation are suggested.

The Roots of Molecular Medicine: A Tribute to Linus Pauling. Huemer, Richard, P., M.D., Ed. New York: W.H. Freeman and Company, 1986.

This is a tribute to Nobel laureate Dr. Linus Pauling and a comprehensive overview of orthomolecular medicine applications. Chapters include: discussions on the biochemistry of disease, the role of nutrition and health, immunology, vitamin C, orthomolecular psychiatry, and free radical reactions.

Osteopathy

Osteopathy is a form of physical medicine that helps restore the structural balance of the musculoskeletal system. Combining joint manipulation, physical therapy, and postural reeducation, osteopathy is effective in treating spinal and joint difficulties, arthritis, digestive disorders, menstrual problems, and chronic pain.

Osteopathy considers and treats the patient as a whole rather than narrowly focusing on a specific ailment. According to Leon Chaitow, N.D., D.O., of London, England, diagnosis of structural problems within the musculoskeletal system and corresponding manipulative treatment are the most fundamental aspects of osteopathy. Doctors of osteopathy believe that the structure of the body is intimately related to its function, and that both structure and function are subject to a wide range of disorders. In treating patients, osteopaths utilize various forms of physical manipulation which allow the body's innate self-healing mechanism to operate more efficiently.

Although osteopathy is very effective in treating pain and chronic illness, it typically looks for the deeper causes underlying serious health conditions. One example is coronary heart disease. Osteopathy views this disease as having a musculoskeletal component, and with the appropriate manipulation substantial benefits can result.

How Osteopathy Works

"At its simplest we can say that when the mechanical structure of the body is normalized or improved it will improve in function," says Dr. Chaitow.

To illustrate, Dr. Chaitow points out the implications of one structural problem, a restriction of movement in the upper spinal or rib area that also involves the muscles of that region. The causes of this problem are numerous, and can include occupational or sport-related injuries (including overuse through repetitive activities), emotional tensions, and internal diseases. "A person with these restrictions may have a breathing problem, such as asthma, bronchitis, emphysema, or problems relating to a heart condition. Osteopathic treatment can bring more suppleness and mobility to this area, which will ultimately benefit breathing function and help prevent future problems."

Any mechanical restriction in the physical body can influence entire systems and organs. Restriction of any area of the spine can directly affect the organs and systems related to that area. "This is why" says Dr. Chaitow, "osteopathic care has been able to, if not cure, allow the patient mobility enough to move in the direction of a cure, especially concerning digestive ailments (including liver and pancreatic dysfunction), bowel disorders, bladder and menstrual problems, prostate congestion, and a multitude of joint and muscle-related problems."

Effects of Musculoskeletal Restriction

The musculoskeletal system is the body's largest energy user. Tension or restriction in this system wastes energy and can cause any number of health problems.

"With chronic fatigue syndrome, for instance," says Dr. Chaitow, "it has been found that the person affected has a tendency toward hyperventilation (overbreathing) which is always associated with shortened muscles in the upper chest/neck area and with some restriction of mobility of ribs and the spinal joints.

"The musculoskeletal system is the body's largest energy user. Tension or restriction in this system wastes energy and can cause any number of health problems."

"Osteopathic attention to the ribs and spine combined with physical therapy to retrain the area is probably the most effective method for normalizing a problem like hyperventilation, with all of its devastating consequences (phobias, panic attacks, anxiety, fatigue). This has clearly been demonstrated in London's Charing Cross Hospital's cardiovascular unit, where hundreds of people have been dramatically helped in this way."

Also, observes psychiatrist Michael Lesser, M.D., "Chronic muscular tensions in the upper spine are a prime cause of hypoglycemia (low blood sugar) since these tissues are burning fuel at an amazing rate, creating a constant requirement for glucose which the person may try to meet through sugar-rich snacks and stimulants."[1]

Conditions Benefited by Osteopathy

Research has confirmed what has already been observed through practical application, that there are few health concerns that cannot benefit from osteopathic care. "Osteopathy can help or resolve many problems that previously have failed to respond to medicine and surgery," states William Faber, D.O., of Milwaukee, Wisconsin, head of the Milwaukee Pain Clinic.

"Osteopathy can help or resolve many problems that previously have failed to respond to medicine and surgery."
—William Faber, D.O.

More specifically, osteopathy has provided aid for patients with spinal and joint conditions, arthritis, allergies, cardiac diseases, breathing dysfunctions, chronic fatigue syndrome, hiatal hernias, high blood pressure, headaches, sciatica, and various other neuritis (inflammation of nerves) disorders.[2]

Research into the effects of osteopathy on children has produced marked benefits in terms of quicker recovery rates and fewer negative effects from measles[3] and respiratory infections.[4] For these conditions manipulation is used to improve blood circulation, to boost immune function, and to maintain nerve supply to affected organs and tissues at optimum levels. According to Dr. Chaitow, without a good supply of blood, nutrients cannot be used normally and the defenses of the body are retarded.

The effectiveness of osteopathic treatment depends on a number of factors:

- The level of organic disease
- The level of musculoskeletal involvement
- The patient's nutritional status
- The effectiveness of the body's healing mechanisms

Dr. Faber reports the story of how his plumber suffered from locking in his left knee due to a cartilage tear. An MRI (magnetic resonance imaging) scan confirmed the tear and Dr. Faber referred the man to an orthopedic specialist who treated the condition with physical therapy and a cortisone injection. Two months of treatment failed to correct the problem and the plumber returned to Dr. Faber for help. "I did a myofascial release (a manipulative treatment) of the muscles and connective tissue around the knee," Dr. Faber says. "The results were immediate, with the locking and pain relieved. After a second treatment, the problem was completely resolved."

"It is not uncommon for patients with internal organ disease to cite musculoskeletal pain as their primary complaint."

"Just before the 1980 Moscow Olympics, the then world record holder for the 1,500 meters, Sebastian Coe, consulted Terry Moule, D.O., a British osteopath, for a recurrent low back and hip problem that posed a threat to his career," relates Dr. Chaitow. "He had been through the entire medical process without success, including conventional orthopedic treatment. Within weeks of commencing osteopathic care from Dr. Moule, Coe was pain free and running faster than ever. He went on a few weeks later to win two gold medals in Moscow. The treatment primarily utilized the 'neuromuscular technique', an osteopathic soft tissue treatment now widely taught in the United States."

It is not uncommon for patients with internal organ disease to cite musculoskeletal pain as their primary complaint. For example, an osteopathic physician who treats a patient for pain in the right shoulder would, because of the relationship between the internal organs and the musculoskeletal system, look for reflex pain patterns in the upper thoracic (pertaining to the chest or thorax), lower cervical, and rib regions. In doing so, the physician may find a pain pattern relative to gallbladder disease that would lead to palpating the abdomen and discovering a tender and swollen gallbladder. The osteopathic physician would then treat both the musculoskeletal component of the pain and the gallbladder disease.

What to Expect During an Osteopathic Examination

Osteopathic treatment addresses the cause of mechanical problems within the body. Diagnostic methods include screening and evaluation of:

- Posture and gait—how a person holds him- or herself while standing and sitting, and during activities such as walking.
- Motion—testing evaluates all moving parts for restrictions. For example, a patient may be asked to complete various body movements such as bending, side-bending, extension, or rotation for both specific and general areas of the body.
- Symmetry—to notice one-sided use of any part of the body and subsequent stress. Physicians also look for increased or decreased curve to the normal spinal pattern.
- The soft tissues—by inspection and palpation for skin changes, hardening of muscles, temperature changes, tenderness, reflex activity, excessive fluid retention.

In conjunction with evaluation, x-ray, blood test, and MRI are used if there is a suspicion of deeper pathology.[5]

Types of Therapy Used

Different manipulative approaches are available to the osteopathic physician. These include:

- **Gentle mobilization:** Moving a joint slowly through its range of motion, gradually increasing the motion to free the joint from restrictions.
- **Articulation:** When motion is severely limited, a quick thrust (similar to chiropractic) may be used.
- **Functional and positional release methods:** Placing the patient in a specific position to allow the body to relax and release muscular spasms that may have been caused by strain or injury.
- **Muscle energy technique:** Gently tensing and releasing specific muscles to produce relaxation.
- **Other soft tissue techniques:** Techniques to relax and release restrictions in the soft tissues of the body.
- **Cranial manipulation:** Very gentle and subtle cranial techniques used to treat conditions such as headaches, strokes, spinal cord injury, and temporomandibular joint syndrome dysfunction. Cranial osteopathy can also be of particular benefit for young children who suffer from hyperactivity, mood disorders, dizziness, or dyslexia.

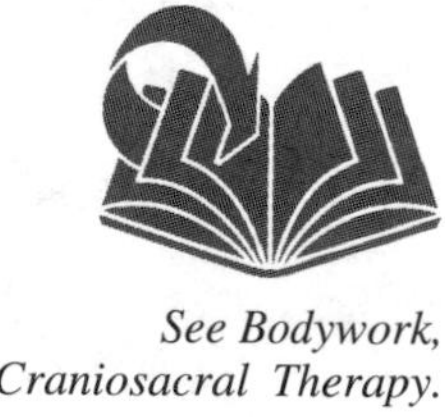

See Bodywork, Craniosacral Therapy.

Patient Reeducation: Keeping Your Body Healthy

Reeducation is the important final step of osteopathic treatment. Patients who learn how to keep their bodies functioning in a relaxed and healthy state have less anxiety and tension, and are better able to cope with stress.

- Relaxation techniques may be used to reduce the levels of excessive tension often present in the muscles of people with joint and back problems. These methods, combined with specifically designed exercises and stretches, help the patient to restore functional integrity, restore balance, coordinate muscular activity, and reduce stress on the joints, making any manipulative treatment easier and more effective.
- Improved breathing methods may be taught where necessary in order to cut down on the excessive stress endured by certain muscles in the back and neck when breathing patterns are dysfunctional. This helps restore normal diaphragmatic breathing, allowing for improved lung capacity while lessening the wear and tear on joints which were previously restricted by the excessive contraction of muscles inappropriately overworking.
- Postural correction teaches patients how to use their bodies in less stressful, more efficient and economical ways (in terms of energy output), reducing damage and tension affecting the joints and soft tissues, as well as decreasing levels of fatigue. These methods draw on systems such as Feldenkrais, Trager, and Alexander, along with osteopathic innovations, and are particularly useful in relation to patterns of overuse and misuse found commonly in work and sports related activities.
- Individualized nutritional guidance taking into account the particular requirements of the patient, may be used, as well as the known links between specific nutrients and the tissues of the system.

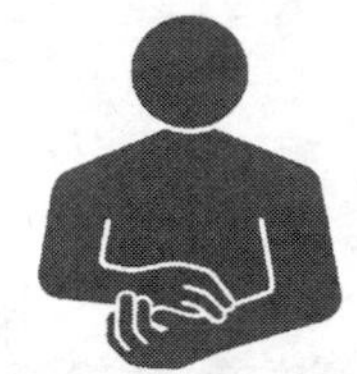

Patient reeducation is an integral part of osteopathic treatment and provides important tools for self-care.

ORIGINS OF OSTEOPATHY

Osteopathy originated in the United States in the last quarter of the nineteenth century as a result of the work of Andrew Taylor Still, a registered physician who founded the first school of osteopathy in Kirksville, Missouri, in 1892. Dr. Still continually sought better methods of medical treatment for his patients, especially for those faced with the epidemic diseases of the time, and the terrible side effects of the drugs used for their problems.[6]

By the time of Still's death there were over five thousand licensed osteopaths in the United States, and the first school had been established in the United Kingdom. Today, there are over fifteen osteopathic medical colleges in the United States, many associated with major universities.

Osteopathic training in the United States blends conventional medical, surgical, and obstetrical practices with osteopathic manipulative treatments, providing a comprehensive system of health care. American D.O.'s (Doctors of Osteopathy, of which there are over 33,500) carry the same license and scope of practice as M.D.'s.[7] However, some osteopaths focus on the conventional medical approach while others give priority to the manipulative therapies. (To make sure you find what you are looking for from an osteopathic physician, contact the American Osteopathic Association, listed in the Where to Find Help section of this chapter.)

There are also many thousands of registered osteopaths in Europe, with schools in France and Belgium. Practitioners trained in the United Kingdom and other English-speaking countries, such as Australia, New Zealand, and Canada, where osteopathy focuses on manipulative treatment, are considered an integral part of alternative and complementary health care.

Health concerns, from heart and breathing dysfunction to fatigue and hyperventilation, can be helped by therapeutic correction of the underlying mechanical disorder. A complete osteopathic treatment to normalize the musculoskeletal system will keep the body working smoothly and efficiently, a fact that is synonymous with health.

The Future of Osteopathy

When seeking an osteopath, ask whether he or she practices manipulative therapies since many D.O.'s focus on conventional medicine.

Osteopathic medicine is a uniquely American system which has spread worldwide, helping to pioneer the creation of a bridge between conventional and alternative health care. On July 1, 1993, Queen Elizabeth signed into law the Osteopath's Bill, making osteopathy the first alternative health care system to achieve legal statutory recognition in Europe, clearing the way for others to follow.

A truly holistic system, osteopathy takes into account all of a patient's needs, with a particular emphasis on a person's structural and functional integrity. "If you consider that the musculoskeletal system makes up the largest body system, using far and away the greatest amount of energy," says Dr. Chaitow, "and if you reflect on the fact that it is through the musculoskeletal system that you live your life, you will begin to appreciate osteopathy's importance."

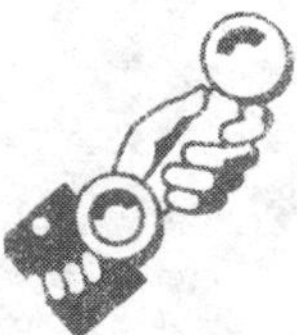

Where to Find Help

For further information on the use of osteopathic techniques in the treatment of health problems, or to locate a doctor of osteopathy, contact:

American Academy of Osteopathy
3500 DePauw Boulevard
Suite 1080
Indianapolis, Indiana 46268
(317) 879-1881
(317) 879-0563 (Fax)

The American Academy of Osteopathy (a practice affiliate of the American Osteopathic Association) represents D.O.'s who provide skilled osteopathic manipulative treatments as part of their practices.

The Cranial Academy, a component society of the American Academy of Osteopathy represents osteopathic physicians who practice cranial osteopathy.

American Osteopathic Association
142 East Ontario Street
Chicago, Illinois 60611
(312) 280-5800

All D.O.'s are trained in the use of osteopathic manipulative treatments. Some specialize in osteopathic manipulative treatments while others focus less on manipulation and more on other medical specialties. There are many superbly skilled osteopaths in the United States. The American Osteopathic Association is the national organization which represents all D.O.'s.

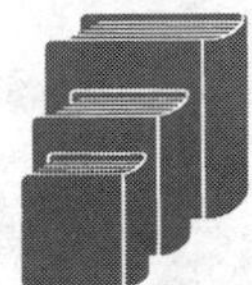

Recommended Reading

The American Academy of Osteopathy publishes and offers for sale a variety of books on osteopathy. Contact the Academy for a current catalog of titles.

Andrew Taylor Still—1828-1917. Trowbridge, Carol. Kirksville, MO: Thomas Jefferson University Press, 1991.

The author has carefully researched Still's life by scrutinizing hundreds of letters and other materials in Still's handwriting plus hundreds of documents of that time. Firmly planted in the dynamic intellectual and medical developments of the late nineteenth and early twentieth centuries, Still emerges as a physician who not only was on the cutting edge of medicine but was a medical pioneer in the founding of osteopathy.

Osteopathic Medicine: An American Reformation. Northup, George, D.O. Chicago: American Osteopathic Association, 1987.

Provides an overview of the history and development of osteopathy in the United States with a good background to its basic beliefs and methods of treatment. To order, call: (312) 280-5827

Osteopathic Self-Treatment. Chaitow, Leon, D.O. San Francisco, CA: Thorsons, 1990.

This book provides information on some of the safe "soft-tissue" methods used in osteopathic treatment, many of which are ideal for first aid use or to accompany treatment from a professional (osteopath, chiropractor, massage therapist, physical therapist).

"The greatest discovery of any generation is that human beings can alter their lives by altering the attitudes of their minds."

—Albert Schweitzer

Oxygen Therapy

Oxygen therapies alter the body's chemistry to help overcome disease, promote repair, and improve overall function. These therapies have been found to be effective in treating a wide variety of conditions, including infections (viral, fungal, parasitic, bacterial), circulatory problems, chronic fatigue syndrome, arthritis, allergies, cancer, and multiple sclerosis.

Oxygen therapy refers to a wide range of therapies utilizing oxygen in various forms to promote healing and destroy pathogens (disease-producing microorganisms and toxins) in the body. These therapies are grouped according to the type of chemical process involved: the addition of oxygen to the blood or tissues is called "oxygenation," and "oxidation" is the reaction of splitting off electrons (electrically charged particles) from any chemical molecule. Oxidation may or may not involve oxygen (oxidation refers to the chemical reaction and not to oxygen itself). One therapy that utilizes the process of oxygenation is hyperbaric oxygen therapy, which introduces oxygen to the body in a pressurized chamber. Hydrogen peroxide therapy, on the other hand, uses the process of oxidation. Ozone therapy utilizes both of these chemical processes. Although various oxygen therapies have been utilized in Europe for many years for a wide range of conditions, in the United States, most remain controversial and are currently unapproved by the FDA (Food and Drug Administration). Legality of oxygen therapies varies from state to state.

How Oxygenation Therapy Works

All human cells, tissues, and organs need oxygen to function. Oxygenation saturates the body with oxygen through the use of gas, sometimes at high-pressure (hyperbaric), increasing the total amount of available oxygen in the body. Insufficient oxygenation may promote the growth of pathogens, whereas excessive oxygenation may damage normal tissues. However, oxygenation employed under strictly controlled conditions can have very positive therapeutic effects.

Otto Warburg, Director of the Max Planck Institute for Cell Physiology in Germany and a two-time Nobel laureate, proposed that a lack of oxygen at the cellular level may be the prime cause of cancer, and that oxygen therapy could be an effective treatment for it.[1] He showed that normal cells in tissue culture, when deprived of oxygen, become cancer cells, and that oxygen can kill cancer cells in tissue cultures.

Oxygen therapy may be professionally administered in many ways: orally, rectally, vaginally, intravenously (into a vein), intra-arterially (into an artery), through inhalation, or by absorption through the skin. High concentrations of oxygen gas can also be given orally through masks or tubes, via oxygen tents, or within pressurized hyperbaric chambers. Oxygen may also be injected subcutaneously (beneath the skin). Ionized oxygen, both positively and negatively charged, is administered by inhalation or dissolved in drinking or bath water.

Hyperbaric Oxygen Therapy

Hyperbaric oxygen therapy (HBOT) dates back to the beginning of this century, although its modern use in the United States dates only to the formation of the Undersea Medical Society in the United States in 1967. HBOT may be administered in individual oxygen chambers that consist of acrylic tubes about seven feet long and twenty-five inches in diameter. The patient lies on a stretcher which slides into the tube. The entry is sealed and the tube pressurized at up to two and a half Atmospheres Absolute (two and a half times the pressure of the atmosphere at sea level) with pure oxygen for 30 to 120 minutes. The increased pressure makes it possible to breathe oxygen at a concentration higher than that allowed by any other means. After treatment, the chamber is depressurized slowly with the patient resting inside. Most of the hyperbaric facilities in the United States are either part of, or affiliated with, American hospitals or the military.

Multiplace chambers which accommodate many patients at once, and in which oxygen is delivered by mask, are now used at the University of Maryland, Duke University, the University of Texas, Scripps Institute, and the Hyperbaric Oxygen Institute in San Bernardino, California. These chambers allow nurses and technical personnel to attend to patients during the treatment. An added advantage of multiplace chambers is that a patient can be removed immediately if problems arise, whereas in individual chambers, the patient cannot be removed until the entire chamber is depressurized.

EARLY HISTORY OF OXYGEN THERAPIES

The scientific community has been aware of oxygen and its characteristics for over two hundred years. Oxygen was discovered by Englishman Joseph Priestly in 1771. Hydrogen peroxide was discovered by French chemist Louis Jacques Thenard in 1818, and ozone was discovered by Christian Friedrich Schonbein in 1840. The first hyperbaric operating room was created as early as 1879 by a French physician, Dr. J. A. Fontaine.

Doctors and scientists began treating diseases and conditions with oxygen over one hundred years ago. Skin conditions were first treated with ultraviolet light (which activates oxidation when absorbed by the blood) in the late nineteenth century by Niels Finsen, and the use of peroxide appears in the health literature as early as 1884. A. L. Cortelyou of Marietta, Georgia, successfully treated diphtheria with a peroxide nasal spray in 1898. In a 1919 influenza epidemic, Drs. T. H. Oliver and D. U. Murphy administered intravenous hydrogen peroxide which significantly reduced mortality rates.

Ozone application was used successfully in World War I to combat battlefield infections, and as early as 1924, Frederick Koch, M.D., advocated oral hydrogen peroxide for cancer patients in the United States .

Conditions Benefited by Hyperbaric Oxygen Therapy

Today in the United States, HBOT is primarily used for traumas such as crash injuries, burns, wounds, gangrene (death of tissue, usually due to deficient or absent blood supply), carbon monoxide poisoning, decubitus ulcers (bed sores), stasis (the stagnation of the normal flow of fluids), radiation necrosis (death of an area of tissue or bone surrounded by healthy parts), and recalcitrant skin grafting (skin grafting that doesn't take). Some microsurgical procedures for the repair and restoration of severed limbs are made possible only by the use of HBOT during the surgery.

According to David Hughes, D.Sc., of the Hyperbaric Oxygen Institute, HBOT postsurgery improves early healing in about 60 percent of time in most cases, and guarantees there will be no surgical edema (retention of excessive amounts of fluid by body tissues).

"In West Germany, HBOT has been used extensively to treat stroke victims, and government sponsorship of HBOT has reduced aftercare costs for stroke victims by 71 percent," says Dr. Hughes. "In France, it is employed for peripheral vascular and arterial problems, and in Russia, it is used in drug and alcohol detoxification. In Japan, the medical establishment boasts that no citizen is ever more than half an hour away from a hyperbaric chamber." In Great Britain, more than twenty-five thousand multiple sclerosis patients have benefited from HBOT.[2]

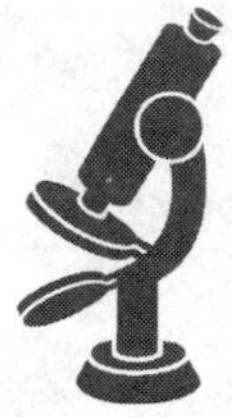

Reaserch is needed on the effects of hyperbaric oxygen therapy for the treatment of early complications of stroke. This type of therapy could prove revolutionary by preventing permanent damage to stroke patients and could be a great money saver.

Pulmonary crises such as carbon monoxide poisoning, low blood volume anemia, and cyanosis (a bluish discoloration of the skin due to abnormal amounts of oxygenated hemoglobin in the blood), have also been treated with HBOT, according to Dr. Hughes. Much work has been done with HBOT as an adjunct to radiation therapy for cancer and to minimize the side effects of some chemotherapy protocols. "Non-cancerous cells are much less sensitive to radiation when the oxygen concentration in their vicinity is increased," explains Dr. Hughes. "HBOT prior to radiation treatment enhances its effectiveness."

According to Dr. Hughes, HBOT has also demonstrated its value as an adjunct to antibiotics in the treatment of anaerobic (able to live without oxygen) infections. HBOT has begun to be used experimentally to treat the symptoms of HIV (human immunodeficiency virus) infection and its accompanying fatigue. "HBOT is a valuable adjunct in treating opportunistic infections which threaten the immunosuppressed patient," Dr. Hughes says.

He cites the case of an eighteen-year-old boy involved in a near drowning incident, who was brought to an HBOT clinic after being in a vegetative coma for nine days. After seventy treatment sessions, the boy was able to return to school. He continued with the treatment and made good progress toward a full recovery.

HBOT also aided a seventy-year-old woman who had been bedridden from multiple sclerosis. After eighteen HBOT sessions with Dr. Hughes, she had recovered enough of her motor skills to drive a car and walk without assistance, and within six months she was able to resume her original duties at work.

In another case, Dr. Hughes was brought a twenty-eight-year-old woman suffering from viral encephalitis (inflammation of the brain), leaving her unable to speak and with right side hemiplegia (paralysis of only one side of the body). She couldn't walk and had acute optic neuralgia (severe, sharp pain along the optic nerves). After thirty sessions, she had improved enough to walk and talk normally, the optic neuralgia had resolved, and the only persistent symptom was right arm and hand weakness.

Hyperbaric oxygen therapy may cause problems for those with a history of middle ear infection, emphysema, or spontaneous pneumonthorax due to the pressure it requires, according to Dr. Hughes. The use of HBOT for illnesses including AIDS, heart disease, and detoxification from recreational drug addiction and alcoholism, is in debate. Yet HBOT is gaining acceptance and is used by both alternative and conventional physicians. Its broad spectrum of applications gives it enormous potential to be used as an adjunct therapy in the future.

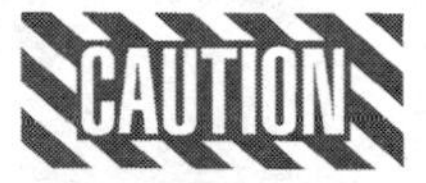

Hyperbaric oxygen therapy may cause problems for those with a history of middle ear infection, emphysema, or spontaneous pneumonia due to the pressure it requires.

How Oxidation Therapy Works

The word oxidation refers to a chemical reaction whereby electrons are transferred from one molecule to another. Oxygen molecules are frequently, but not always, involved in these reactions. The molecules that "donate" electrons are said to be oxidized, whereas the molecules that accept electrons are called oxidants.

A healthy state of oxidative balance is necessary for optimal function of the body, but when the body is exposed to repeated environmental stresses, its oxidative function is weakened. When oxidation is partially blocked by toxicity in the body or pathological (disease-causing) organisms, oxidation therapy may help by "jump-starting"[3] the body's oxidative processes and returning them to normal, according to Charles Farr, M.D., Ph.D., of Oklahoma City, Oklahoma.

When properly administered, oxidation therapy selectively destroys pathogenic (disease-producing) bacteria, viruses, and other invading microbial organisms, and deactivates toxic substances without injury to healthy tissues or cells.[4] For example, if diluted hydrogen peroxide is placed on a wound, the normal cells thrive while the pathogens die.

"When properly administered, oxidation therapy selectively destroys pathogenic (disease-producing) bacteria, viruses, and other invading microbial organisms, and deactivates toxic substances without injury to healthy tissues or cells."

Oxidation therapy must be administered under clinical supervision, since uncontrolled oxidation may be destructive to the body. Oxidation therapy may be given intravenously, orally, rectally by enema, vaginally, or transcutaneously (absorbed through the skin).

Hydrogen Peroxide Therapy

Hydrogen peroxide is a liquid the molecular structure of which is made up of two atoms of hydrogen and two atoms of oxygen (H_2O_2). Because it is less stable than water (H_20), hydrogen peroxide readily enters into oxidative reactions, ultimately becoming oxygen in water.

It was Dr. Farr who first characterized the oxidative effects of hydrogen peroxide in humans in 1984.[5] Today, the use of hydrogen peroxide for its oxidative effects has spread to over thirty-eight countries, and remains one of the least expensive, yet effective oxidation therapies.

Oxidation administered through hydrogen peroxide therapy regulates tissue repair, cellular respiration, growth, immune functions, the energy system, most hormone systems, and the production of cytokines (chemical messengers that are involved in the regulation of almost every system in the body). Oxidation therapy can also work as a defense system, directly destroying invading bacteria, viruses, yeast, and parasites, according to Dr. Farr.

Conditions Benefited by Hydrogen Peroxide Therapy

Dr. Farr uses hydrogen peroxide for a variety of health problems, including AIDS, arthritis, cancer, candidiasis, chronic fatigue syndrome, depression, lupus erythematosus (a chronic inflammatory disease with symptoms including arthritis, fatigue, and skin lesions), emphysema, multiple sclerosis, varicose veins, and fractures.

According to Dr. Farr, other conditions that may benefit from hydrogen peroxide therapy include arteriosclerosis, vascular headaches (migraines, cluster headaches) gangrene, strokes, allergies, asthma, lung infections, diabetes mellitus, herpes simplex, herpes zoster (shingles), fungal, bacterial, viral and parasitic infections, acne, and wounds.[6] Hydrogen peroxide injections have been used for inflamed, damaged, and injured tissues, inflamed nerves such as in herpes, or trigger points causing pain and muscle spasms.[7]

Dr. Farr has demonstrated rapid recovery from Type A/Shanghai influenza with intravenous hydrogen peroxide treatments. Two-thirds of his patients recovered after only a single injection. One-third returned for a second injection and only 10 percent required a third. Recovery time was half that of a control group treated with conventional methods: antibiotics, decongestants, and analgesics.[8]

Robert Haskell, M.D., of San Rafael, California, treated a forty-four-year-old man with multiple sclerosis who was confined to a wheelchair. After six treatments of intravenous hydrogen peroxide he began taking a few steps and by the eighteenth treatment, he was able to walk for four hours without resting.[9]

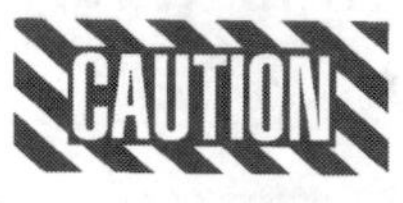

Oxidation therapy needs to be administered under clinical supervision, since uncontrolled oxidation may be destructive to the body.

There are few side effects with hydrogen peroxide therapy. In rare cases, a problem involving inflammation of veins at the site of injection will occur. Hydrogen peroxide should not be taken orally as it causes nausea and vomiting, and rectal administration can lead to inflammation of the lower intestinal tract. Other side effects observed include temporary faintness, fatigue, headaches, and chest pain.

Most problems stem from the use of either an inappropriate administration route, administration above patient tolerance, the mixing of oxidative chemicals with other substances, or using oxidative chemicals in too great a concentration, reports Dr. Farr.

Ozone Therapy

Ozone therapy relies on the process of oxidation as well as oxygenation. Approximately one-fifth of the air humans breathe is comprised of two atoms of oxygen (O_2). Ozone (O_3) contains three oxygen atoms and is a less stable form of molecular oxygen. Because of this added molecule, ozone is more reactive than oxygen and readily enters into reactions to oxidize other chemicals. During oxidation in the body, the extra oxygen molecule in ozone breaks away, leaving a normal O_2 molecule. This increases the oxygen content of the blood or tissues. For this reason, ozone therapy is a combination of both oxygenation therapy and oxidation therapy.

See Light Therapy.

Ozone is a common substance in nature, but can also be a source of air pollution when produced by man-made combustion. Medical grade ozone is made from pure oxygen. Used medically, ozone increases local oxygen supply to lesions, improves and accelerates wound healing, deactivates viruses and bacteria and increases local tissue temperature, thus enhancing local metabolic processes, according to Gerard Sunnen, M.D., of New York City.

"A healthy state of oxidative balance is necessary for optimal function of the body, but when the body is exposed to repeated environmental stresses, its oxidative function is weakened."

Ozone can be administered intravenously, intra-arterially, intramuscularly (within the muscle), intra-articularly (into the joint), and subcutaneously. In the case of an intravenous or intramuscular injection, up to a quart of blood is removed from a vein and mixed with ozone gas, then reinjected into the body. Ozone may also be applied topically as a gas or dissolved in water or olive oil. As a gas it may be insufflated (blown in) vaginally or rectally. It may also be taken orally, rectally, or vaginally in the form of ozonated water.

Laboratory studies have shown that ozone is capable of inactivating HIV in solution.[10] It has also been shown to inhibit the growth of human lung, breast, and uterine cancer cells in tissue culture.[11]

Conditions Benefited by Ozone Therapy

Jonathan Wright, M.D., of Kent, Washington, finds ozone therapy very effective against any sort of chronic infection, particularly viruses and candidiasis. He also treats hepatitis B with ozonation of the blood along with an herbal remedy—*Phyllanthus*—and high doses of intravenous ascorbate (a salt of the ascorbic acid vitamin C). "You can't just use ozone alone," says Dr. Wright. "You need to combine it with a proper diet, [nutritional] supplements, herbs, botanicals, acupuncture, and chiropractic." He adds that antioxidants (chemicals or substances that can donate, or give up, electrons) such as vitamin C should be given along with any oxidative therapy since they prevent uncontrolled oxidation which is detrimental to the body.

Due to its wide application for a number of conditions, oxygen therapy can save money in long-term health costs.

Dr. Wright has successfully treated a cancer patient with ozone therapy. The patient had a goose egg-sized tumor on her right ear. Her doctor said it could not be treated and gave her six months to live. Dr. Wright treated the tumor with topical ozone (applied externally to the site

THERAPEUTIC USES OF OZONE THERAPY

The administration of ozone therapy is as varied as the many conditions it can treat. Below are the most typical methods of treatment:

- *Intra-arterial (injected into an artery): For arterial circulatory disturbances and to dissolve arteriosclerotic plaque*
- *Intestinal insufflation (blown into the intestines from a gas tank using a catheter): For mucous colitis (fungal infection in the intestine) and fistulae (abnormal openings)*
- *Intramuscular (injected into the muscle): To treat inflammatory infections, allergic diseases, and cancer (with autohemotherapy)*
- *Autohemotherapy (ozonation of blood): To address arthritis, hepatitis, allergies, and herpes infections*
- *Ozonized water (ozonation of water that is taken orally, rectally, or vaginally): Disinfection during surgery and dentistry*
- *Intra-articular (injected into a joint): During surgery and with diseased joints*
- *External application (by covering the area with a tent and infusing ozone): For treating fungal infections, leg ulcers, infected or poorly healing wounds, and burns.*

of the tumor) and injected ozone directly into the tumor. The tumor regressed in size, and although a small lump remained, the patient recovered.

Jeff Harris, N.D., of Seattle, Washington, successfully treated a patient suffering from multiple sclerosis (MS) with ozone therapy administered by rectal insufflation. When the patient came to see Dr. Harris, she had been unable to work effectively for seven years due to the deteriorating effects of MS, which included numbness in her right leg as well as incontinence, and had spent the last three months on unemployment. Dr. Harris also used vitamin and mineral supplementation, vegetarian diet, amalgam removal, counseling, and craniosacral therapy as part of the treatment protocol. She received vitamin B_{12} and folic acid injections daily for two to three weeks and then ozone therapy was started. After the first ozone treatment, she said she felt full of energy. Dr. Harris taught her how to do the treatments herself, which she does daily, and she has now returned to work and states that she is feeling well and full of energy.

Adverse effects associated with intravenous ozone have been reported to include phlebitis (inflammation of a vein), circulatory depression, chest pain, shortness of breath, fainting, coughing, flushing, cardiac arrhythmias, and gas embolus (bubbles). Rectal administration of ozone can lead to inflammation of the lower intestinal tract. Although it is easily tolerated in other tissues, in high concentrations ozone causes inflammation of the lung tissues.

Ozone Therapy and AIDS

The late German physician, Alexander Preuss, of Stuttgart, used ozone as part of a regimen including vitamins, minerals, and other treatments to enhance the immune system. He achieved remission in a number of patients with AIDS-associated infections.[12] In a similar study, French researchers Bertrand Vallancien and Jean-Marie Winkler reported on a group of patients with HIV, herpes, and hepatitis.[13] After nine weeks of transfused ozone, T4 and T8 cells (cells of the immune system) moved toward normal levels in all cases. The ozone treatments caused no further health problems.

John Pittman, M.D., of Raleigh, North Carolina, initiated a study with nine HIV positive patients whom he treated with a regimen of ozone one day, hydrogen peroxide the next, and chelation therapy on the third day for twenty-three days (the study was then stopped for legal reasons).

In patients whose T-cell count was greater than 100 initially, a 20 to 30% rise was seen. There was no effect on those with T-cell counts below 100 to start with. He believes ozone is helpful in AIDS because it is known to damage viruses which have a lot of fat in their membranes (HIV membranes have a high fat content). Healthy cells have antioxidant enzymes to break down ozone and prevent damage; viruses do not. He believes ozone may also stimulate the immune system.

Since the FDA has not approved the practice of ozone therapy in the United States, it is difficult to get data on its use. Many physicians also have been forced to use ozone therapy without calling attention to themselves, for fear of FDA reprisals. However, numerous patient anecdotes are available. One doctor, for instance, reports of good results with HIV positive patients. He gave these patients three ozone treatments a week for seven weeks. For each treatment, 250 to 300 cc's of blood were removed, treated with ozone, and injected back into the patient. This helped reduce opportunistic infections. Other treatments were also employed to help strengthen the immune system.[14] Patients who have difficulty tolerating AZT (an AIDS medication) treatments may also benefit from ozone therapy.

OZONE THERAPY IN VETERINARY MEDICINE

The value of ozone therapy in veterinary medicine was discovered by accident while animal tests were being conducted to substantiate the hazards of ozone to humans. However, the results proved the positive effects of ozone/oxygen mixtures on the survival rate of animals, and researchers concluded that the results from the experiments constituted "a critical item worthy of serious consideration."[15]

Ozone therapy can be used on animals to treat intestinal disorders, arthritis, canine paralysis, skin problems, acute and chronic cystitis, oncological disorders, and helminthiasis (intestinal parasites or worms). Ozone is a disinfectant to bacteria and germs, and causes inactivation of viruses and fungi. It is used by colonic insufflation for colitis and improves wound healing.

Dr. Wright also uses ozone therapy with AIDS patients by ozonating the blood and returning it to the patient, or by rectal insufflation. In 1985, he treated an HIV positive patient who was feverish and had swollen glands. The patient was given ozone twice a week for six months, along with vitamin and mineral supplements and botanicals. The patient's symptoms were greatly relieved, and he continues doing well, returning for ozone treatment whenever he has a fever or other symptoms.

Like many oxygen therapies, ozone therapy is widely used and practiced in Europe, but still not readily available in the United States. According to Dr. Sunnen, prospective patients and doctors in America must await two further animal studies before the FDA sanctions a phase-one clinical trial with humans, and ultimately approves the therapeutic use of ozone.

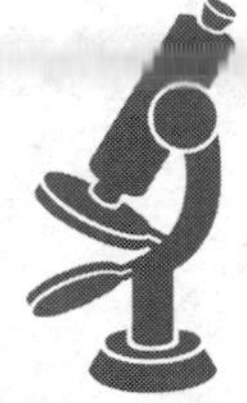

Reaseach is needed into the many conditions oxygen therapy can benefit. Because oxygen therapy can help the body repair itself, it is an ideal treatment to integrate into a comprehensive health care system.

The Future of Oxygen Therapy

The main stumbling blocks for all oxygen therapies, according to Dr. Hughes, are the FDA, the insurance companies, and the entrenched medical establishment. "I'm a bottom liner, I believe all forms of oxygen therapy ought to be considered and ought to be used if they can help a patient or a certain condition," he says. "The problem is that most of the areas of conventional medicine in this country are driven by the pharmaceutical companies. The incentive is always to sell pills, and you can't sell oxygen pills. This tends to hold it back, especially since a very large percentage of the research that's done at universities is funded by pharmaceutical companies."

Despite this fact, as Dr. Farr points out, oxygen therapies are widely used in other countries, particularly Germany and Russia. In the United States, indications are that the medical profession is becoming more receptive to oxygen therapy's potential benefits. For example, ten to twelve years ago there were only eight indications in America for the use of hyperbaric oxygen. Now, according to Dr. Hughes, there are twenty-eight, and it's expanding all the time. "More and more people are becoming familiar with HBOT, and we're getting more and more requests from the medical profession about what other conditions it can help."

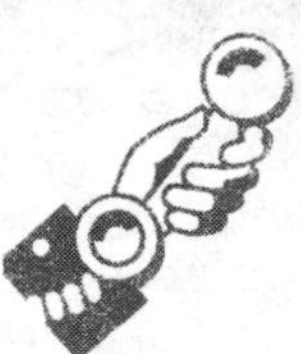

Where to Find Help

The following organizations can provide information and answer questions about the various oxygen therapies:

The American College of Hyperbaric Medicine
Ocean Medical Center
4001 Ocean Drive, Suite 105
Lauderdale-by-the-Sea, Florida 33308
(305) 771-4000

A group of physicians dedicated to the clinical aspects of hyperbaric medicine. Their purpose is to foster ethical growth and development of the science and practice of hyperbaric oxygen therapy. Promotes research and education.

ECH_2O_2 Newsletter
9845 NE 2nd Avenue
Miami, FL 33138
(305) 758-8710

A public forum for those interested in the oral use of hydrogen peroxide and ozone. Publishes a quarterly newsletter for the public and professionals addressing thousands of uses for hydrogen peroxide and ozone in areas including farming and agriculture, waste and water treatment, industry, bathing, and dentistry.

International Bio-oxidative Medicine Foundation
P.O. Box 13205
Oklahoma City, Oklahoma 73113-1205
(405) 478-IBOM Ext. 4266

The foundation publishes and distributes a newsletter, as well as scientific research data. Supports educational programs that highlight current research and the therapeutic use of oxidative therapies. Encourages basic and clinical research. Membership available.

International Ozone Association
31 Strawberry Hill Avenue
Stamford, Connecticut 06902
(203) 348-3542

A professional scientific organization disseminating information on use and production of ozone through meetings, synopsis, and world congresses. Publishes books and journals on ozone.

Medical Society for Ozone Therapy
Klagen Furtestrasse 4
D. 7000 Stuttgart 30, Germany

An excellent informational resource for the public and professionals. Addresses the differences between free ozone and medical ozone. The Society can explain how medical ozone is used to treat diseases, give treatment applications, and explain where and why medical ozone is used.

Medizone International, Inc.
123 East 54th Street
New York NY 10022
(212) 421-0303

Developers of ozone-based blood purification systems and treatment for diseases caused by lipid-enveloped viruses, including AIDS, hepatitis B, and herpes.

North Carolina Bio-Oxidative Health Center
4505 Fair Meadow Lane, Suite 111
Raleigh, North Carolina 27607
(800) 473-9812 (U.S. and Canada)
(407) 967-6466 (Outside North America)

Outpatient facility which focuses on metabolic and intestinal detoxification. Comprehensive and synergistic treatment regimens for each patient are developed utilizing therapies such as colon hydrotherapy, intravenous therapies (including ozone), and external ozone hydrotherapy. Supportive elements such as acupuncture and lymphatic massage, as well as techniques to address the psychological/emotional components of health and illness are also part of the program.

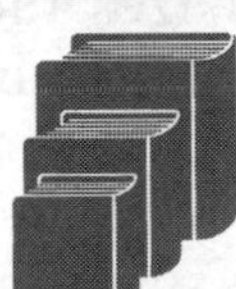

Recommended Reading

Hydrogen Peroxide Medical Miracle. Douglass, William Campbell. Atlanta, GA: Second Opinion Publishing, 1992.
To order, call (800) 728-2288

This book explores the importance of H_2O_2 in the proper function of the immune system, and in its ability to rid the body of disease and metabolize protein, carbohydrates, fats, vitamins, and minerals.

Oxygen Therapies. McCabe, Ed. Morrisville, NY: Energy Publications, 1988.

Discusses the effects of a low-oxygen environment resulting from sedentary lifestyles, poor food, lack of exercise, and the breathing of polluted air. This book explores how cells in this condition can become breeding grounds for harmful viruses and microbes. Included are methods of increasing cellular oxygenation, medical studies, case histories of former AIDS and other degenerative disease victims, as well as contacts.

Underwater Medicine and Related Sciences: A Guide to the Literature. Shilling, Charles. New York: Plenum Publications, Volume 1, 1973; Volume 2, 1975.

An invaluable book for researching hyperbaric medicine.

***The Use of Ozone in Medicine*, First English Edition.** Rilling, Siegfried; and Viebahn, Renate. Heidelberg, Germany: Haug Publishers, 1987.

A history of ozone/oxygen therapy treatments of lesions, burns, virus infections such as herpes and hepatitis, circulatory disturbances, and rheumatic/arthritic complaints. Includes a listing of indications and applications with exact treatment guide. This book is available through Medicina Biologica, 2937 N.E. Flanders, Portland, Oregon 97232, or phone (503) 287-6775.

Qigong

Qigong combines movement, meditation, and breath regulation to enhance the flow of vital energy in the body, improve blood circulation, and enhance immune function. Because qigong can be used by the healthy as well as the severely ill, it is one of the most broadly applicable systems of self-care in the world. In China, it is estimated that 200 million people practice qigong everyday.

Qigong (also referred to as *chi-kung*) is an ancient Chinese exercise that stimulates and balances the flow of *qi*, or vital life energy, along the acupuncture meridians (energy pathways). Like acupuncture and Traditional Chinese Medicine, the *qigong* tradition emphasizes the importance of teaching the patient how to remain well. In China, the various methods of *qigong* form the nucleus of a national self-care system of health maintenance and personal development. *Qigong* cultivates inner strength, calms the mind, and restores the body to its natural state of health by maintaining the optimum functioning of the body's self-regulating systems.

> "*In China, the various methods of* qigong *form the nucleus of a national self-care system of health maintenance and personal development.*"

Recent medical studies in both China and the United States show that *qigong* can reduce stress, increase circulation, and provide resistance to disease. Today, most hospitals in China include *qigong* as part of their health care programs, with certain hospitals devoted solely to its study and practice. Thousands of *qigong* institutes also provide *qigong* instruction, while major centers in Beijing, Shanghai, and Guangzho train *qigong* teachers and carry out government-supported research.

See Acupuncture, Traditional Chinese Medicine.

How *Qigong* Works

Qigong practice can range from simple calisthenic-type movements with breath coordination, to complex exercises where brain wave frequency, heart rate, and other organ functions are altered intentionally by the practitioner. When practiced regularly, *qigong*'s combination of movement, deep relaxation, and breathing can improve strength and flexibility, reverse damage caused by prior injuries and disease, and promote relaxation, awareness, and healing.

Traditional Chinese Medicine holds that *qigong* stimulates and nourishes the body's internal organs by circulating *qi*. *Qigong* can break down energy blocks and facilitate the free flow of energy throughout the body, promoting blood and lymph flow and the even flow of nerve impulses necessary for proper health maintenance. "The overall benefit of *qigong* is to mobilize and harmonize the body's naturally occuring healing resource (known as *qi* in China)," according to Roger Jahnke, O.M.D., of Santa Barbara, California.

Like acupuncture, *qigong* activates the electrical currents that flow along the meridian pathways of the body. According to Dr. Jahnke, *qigong* stimulates human bioelectrical conductibility. Dr. Jahnke explains, "The human body has the ability to conduct an electrical charge." This affects the entire body, and it is responsible for maintaining the function of the organs and tissues. For example, one *qigong* exercise involves breathing regulation and deep relaxation while lifting the arms and rising upward on the toes. According to Dr. Jahnke, this exercise can help prevent tension headaches, constipation, insomnia, and other disorders by improving circulation of the cardiovascular and lymphatic systems, as well as modulating brain chemistry.

"In the United States, qigong *is now being taught by qualified instructors at innovative hospital programs, at adult education centers, and in community fitness programs."*

In the United States, *qigong* is now being taught by qualified instructors at innovative hospital programs, at adult education centers, and in community fitness programs. Applicable to young and old alike, and for people in any state of health, *qigong* is unique among fitness programs as it can be performed standing, walking, sitting, or lying down. *Qigong* exercises can even be performed by those confined to bed or a wheelchair.

In a comprehensive overview of applied physiology and *qigong* research, Dr. Jahnke cites a number of current studies in which the following physiological mechanisms are enhanced by regular *qigong* practice:

- Initiates the "relaxation response" which decreases the sympathetic function of the autonomic nervous system (triggered by any form of mental focus that frees the mind from its many distractions). This decreases heart rate and blood pressure, dilates the blood capillaries, and optimizes the delivery of oxygen to the tissues.
- Alters the neurochemistry profile (neurotransmitters, also called information molecules, bond with receptor sites on tissue, enzyme, immune, and other cells to excite or inhibit their function) moderating pain, depression, and addictive cravings, as well as optimizing immune capability.
- Enhances the efficiency of the immune system through increased rate and flow of the lymphatic fluid.
- Improves resistance to disease and infection by accelerating the elimination of toxic metabolites (metabolic by-products) from the interstitial spaces in the tissues, organs, and glands through the lymphatic system.
- Increases the efficiency of cell metabolism and tissue regeneration through increased circulation of oxygen and nutrient rich blood to the brain, organs, and tissues.

"Today in China, many hospital practitioners combine qigong *with conventional medicine in order to treat cancer, bone marrow disease, and diseases of old age."*

- Coordinates right/left brain hemisphere dominance promoting deeper sleep, reduced anxiety, and mental clarity.
- Induces alpha and, in some cases, theta brain waves which reduce heart rate and blood pressure, facilitating relaxation, mental focus, and even paranormal skills; this optimizes the body's self-regulative mechanisms by decreasing the activity of the sympathetic nervous system.
- Moderates the function of the hypothalamus, pituitary, and pineal glands, as well as the cerebrospinal fluid system of the brain and spinal cord, which mediates pain and mood and potentiates immune function.

Conditions Benefited by *Qigong*

Qigong has been shown to be effective in helping resolve digestive problems, asthma, arthritis, insomnia, pain, depression, and anxiety, as well as helping cancer, coronary heart disease, and cases of HIV/AIDS. According to Wong Chong-xing, M.D., Director of Research at the Rei Jin Hospital in Shanghai, China, several thousand hypertensive patients experienced dramatic improvement after they had been instructed in basic *qigong* exercises. His studies suggest that daily *qigong* practice lowers blood pressure, pulse rates, metabolic rates, and oxygen demand. David Eisenberg, M.D., a clinical research fellow at Harvard Medical School, says these studies also indicate that *qigong* triggers the body's relaxation response by reducing the level of dopamine, an enzyme that controls neurological activity.[1]

Stephen Chang, M.D., a doctor of Traditional Chinese Medicine, cites numerous scientific studies documenting the effects of *qigong*. In one study, 2,873 terminal cancer patients practiced *qigong* for six months: 12 percent of the patients were cured, while 47 percent showed significant improvement. In another study, *qigong* eye exercises significantly reduced farsightedness and nearsightedness in a group of Chinese school children. Sinus allergies, hemorrhoids, and prostrate problems have also been effectively treated.[2]

Today in China, many hospital practitioners combine *qigong* with conventional medicine in order to treat cancer, bone

TYPES OF QIGONG

Over its long history, qigong *has developed into a number of branches. Personal self-healing and health maintenance practice is called* internal qigong. *Internal* qigong *can be performed with little or no movement. In this form, it is known as* quiescent qigong. *When internal practice includes movement, it is called* dynamic qigong. *According to Roger Jahnke, O.M.D., internal, self-applied* qigong *practice may include laying down, sitting, standing, or walking forms. Meditation is an example of quiescent* qigong *while* tai chi *is an example of a mildly dynamic* qigong.

One of the most provocative aspects of qigong *is known as* external qigong. *In external* qigong, *a* qigong *master or* qigong *doctor projects or emits his or her own* qi *to serve or heal another. When patients are severely ill and their own level of* qi *is very low or stagnant, receiving* qi *from a* qigong *master can prove to be a powerful stimulant toward healing. Generally, however, people who receive external* qigong *from a* qigong *master, simultaneously do their own internal practice.*

"External projection," states Dr. Jahnke, "while seeming to be a fantastic aspect of qigong, *is not unlike what Western cultures call magnetic healing or psychic healing, both which operate through the same natural laws of physics as the phenomena of* qi *emission."*

In a study conducted by Fong Li-da, M.D., from the Beijing Institute of Traditional Chinese Medicine, a qigong *master practicing external* qigong *was able to project her* qi *to either kill or promote the growth of bacteria in test tubes.*[5]

marrow disease, and diseases of old age. At the Kuangan Men's Hospital in Beijing, China, ninety-three cases of advanced malignant cancer were treated with a combination of drugs and *qigong* exercises, while a control group of thirty patients were treated by drugs alone. Eighty-one percent of the *qigong* group gained strength, 63 percent improved appetite, and 33 percent were free from diarrhea compared to control group improvements of 10 percent, 10 percent, and 6 percent, respectively.[3]

Qigong is often found to be more effective than chemotherapy, surgery, and even acupuncture for the prevention and treatment of disease. According to Liu Guo Long, M.D., Ph.D., of the Beijing College of Traditional Chinese Medicine, *qi* energy directed to the site of an injury "facilitates the signals to the brain stem." As a result of increased blood and lymph flow, and a greater supply of nutrients regenerating the cells, the area of injury can heal more effectively.[4]

As Director of the Health Action Clinic and Chairperson of the Qigong Department of the Santa Barbara College of Oriental Medicine, Dr. Jahnke draws from a broad experience with *qigong*. "In regular classes at Health Action, and at a regional hospital, we have seen constant testimonials of the health benefits of *qigong*. After only two weeks of practice, six people out of a group of thirty had specific improvement—(three cases experienced increased breath volume and relief of constricted breathing, one person found relief from constipation, one person improved sleep, and one had a lessening of headaches). Twenty-five of the thirty participants reported a heightened sense of well-being in this very brief period of practice. One of our patients had set an appointment for glaucoma surgery before joining a weekly *qigong* class. After six weeks in the class she went to the laboratory for preoperative testing. The results of the tests showed that the glaucoma problem had resolved itself and surgery was no longer necessary."

Dr. Jahnke also cites a group of arthritis patients who have been regular participants in *qigong* classes. "After approximately six months, several patients remarked that the stiffness and pain in their hands had

THE INFRATONIC QGM—A MACHINE THAT PRODUCES QI ENERGY

In the early 1980s, Lu Yan Fang, Ph.D., a senior scientist at the National Electro Acoustics Laboratory in Beijing, China, discovered that the hands of qigong *masters emitted high levels of low frequency acoustical waves called secondary sound. Although everyone generates secondary sounds, the signals generated by the* qigong *masters were one hundred times more powerful than the average individual, and one thousand times more powerful than those who were elderly or ill. Using electroacoustical technology, Dr. Fang constructed an instrument that simulated this infratonic sound (eight to fourteen hertz, seventy decibels). By directing these massage-like, secondary sounds into hospitalized patients, Dr. Fang noted numerous improvements, particularly for the management of pain.*

Over 1,100 human patients were studied and treated. When used on the chest or back, the brain's production of alpha waves is stimulated. Therapeutic benefits include pain reduction (including migraines), increased circulatory functioning, muscular relaxation, and the alleviation of depression.[5]

Dr Fang's device, the Infratonic QGM, has received awards of recognition from the China Ministry of Health, the China Central Technological Committee, and the National Committee for Traditional Chinese Medicine. It is used as an effective pain management tool in China as well as in Japan, Taiwan, Singapore, France, Spain, Mexico, and Argentina. In the United States, it is approved for sale by the FDA (Food and Drug Administration) as a therapeutic massage device. Dr. Jahnke cautions, however, "These machines mimic the human qi. Please remember, it is always preferable to develop one's personal practice instead of just relying on a machine."

“With qigong, *individuals learn to heal themselves and maintain their health—a profoundly cost-effective feature.”*
—Roger Jahnke, O.M.D.

diminished and the deformed knuckles characteristic of arthritis had begun to return to normal. The most incredible thing about *qigong* practice is that people actually can feel the operation of the physiological mechanisms of healing in their body. The increase of blood and lymph flow, and a shift in neurotransmitters creates an actual sensation that is clearly perceptible to the individual. The Chinese call this ‘*qi* sensation.’ ”

Qigong Practices

Following is a series of *qigong* practices compiled by Dr. Jahnke. They are designed for maximum result along with maximum ease and can be done by almost anyone regardless of health, age, or physical condition.

To make the practice of *qigong* more beneficial and accessible to the person just starting out, Dr. Jahnke suggests:

- Take it easy and don’t rush. Excess effort and trying too hard go against the natural benefits of *qigong*. Remember, *qigong* is intended to help you heal.
- Although *qigong* may seem simplistic, a dedication to these practices can mobilize one’s inherent healing forces.
- Results come over time, so don’t overdo it or expect too much too soon.
- If performed correctly, *qigong* is safe to practice as often as you like.
- Feel free to make up your own routine and to change the practices to suit your needs, likes, and limitations.
- Always approach each practice with an intention to relax; direct the mind toward quiet indifference.
- Regulate the breath so that both the inhalation and exhalation are slow and deep, but not urgent or exaggerated.

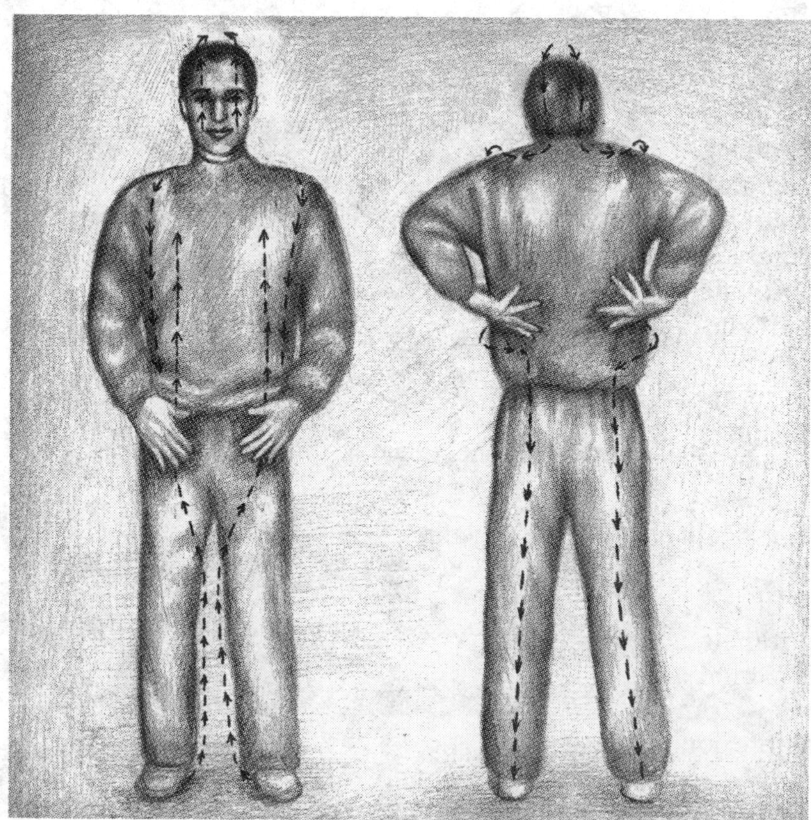

Practice 1.

The Practices

1. Tracing acupuncture meridians to circulate the vital life energy: The goal of this practice is to move the *qi* along the meridians. Rub your hands together to build up heat. The Chinese say this increases *qi*. They will become warmer if you are relaxed and the environment is comfortable. As if washing your face, stroke the palms upward across the cheeks, eyes, and forehead. Continue over the top and side of the head, down the back of the neck, and along the shoulders to the shoulder joint.

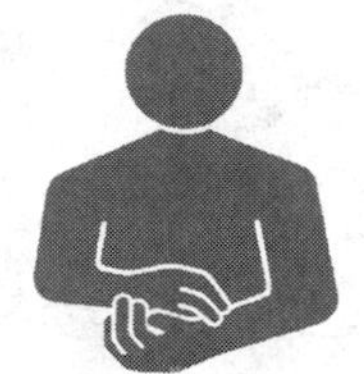

Qigong *can easily become a part of your self-care health maintenance program.*

Continue under the arm and down the sides to the rib cage. At the lower edge of the rib cage, move the palms around to the back, across the buttocks, down the back and sides of the legs, and out the sides of the feet. Trace up inside the feet and the inner surface of the legs, up the front side of the torso and onto the face again, beginning the second round. You may rub the palms together before each round.

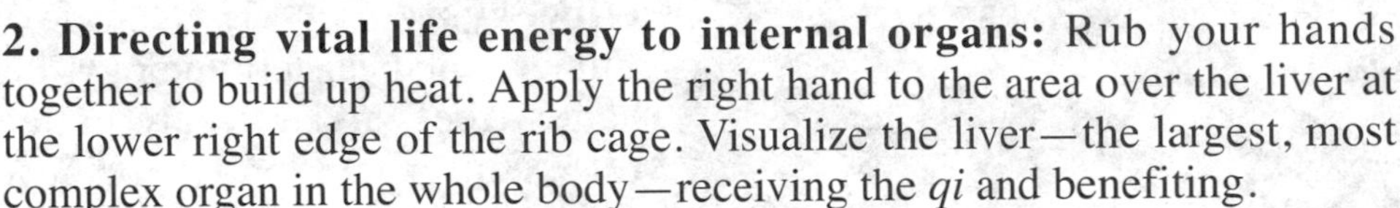

2. Directing vital life energy to internal organs: Rub your hands together to build up heat. Apply the right hand to the area over the liver at the lower right edge of the rib cage. Visualize the liver—the largest, most complex organ in the whole body—receiving the *qi* and benefiting.

Apply the left hand to the area over the spleen and pancreas at the lower left side of the ribs. The spleen—an immense lymph organ—is the producer of white blood cells, and the pancreas is a critical link in energy metabolism and digestion. Move the hands circularly continuing to create heat, breathing full breaths, and relax. Feel the heat, or *qi*, passing in through the surface of the skin and penetrating to the organs as the entire metabolic process becomes more efficient.

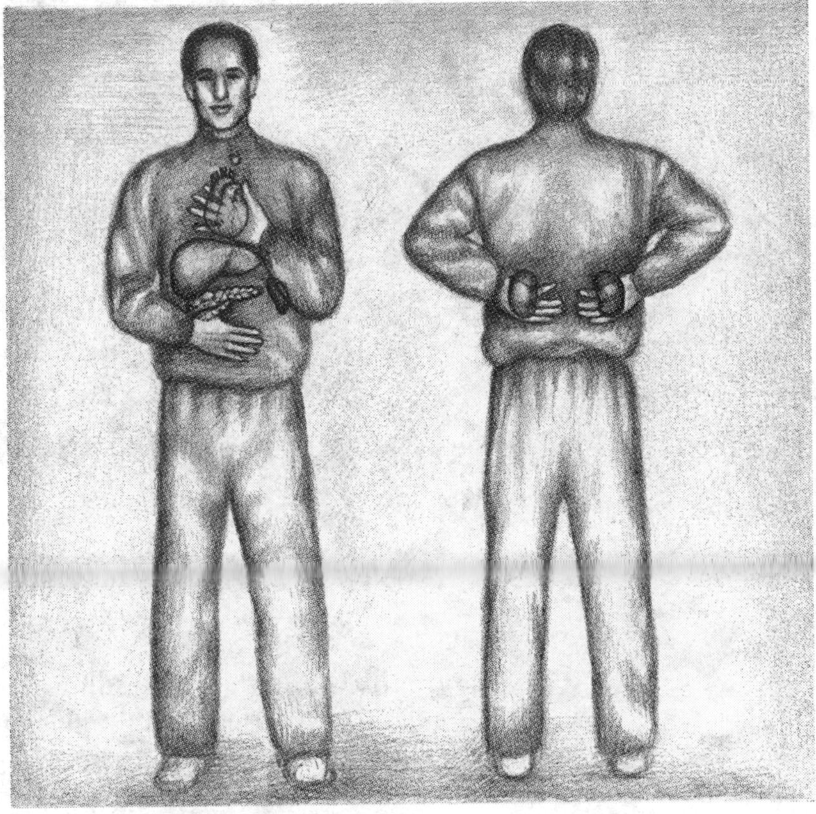

Practice 2.

Holding the hands still over the organs, continue to feel the heat penetrate. On exhalation, visualize the *qi* circulating from the center of the body out the arms, into the hands, and penetrating from the hands into the organs.

Now, move the palms to cover the navel and breastbone. The navel is the human original connection to life and nourishment, and the Chinese feel that in adulthood it still connects to the whole body. The breastbone protects several vital organs, the heart, and the thymus. The heart pumps the blood, of course, but the Chinese believe it is the resting place of one's emotional and spiritual self. The thymus is the source of T-cells, some of the most powerful immune agents. Visualize them benefiting from the warmth, the *qi*, pouring into the navel, heart, and thymus, being more able to do their essential functions.

Move the palms around to cover the lower back. In Traditional Chinese Medicine, this area is thought to be directly connected to the kidneys, which not only remove toxins from the blood but also is the storehouse of vital life energies. The adrenal glands rest on top of the kidneys and control much of what the Chinese associate with the regulation of those energies. Rub these areas, penetrating the *qi* deep into the body to improve the ability of the kidneys and adrenals to do their work. Visualize the kidneys and adrenals receiving the *qi* and being empowered to more efficiently help eliminate waste products, produce energy, and activate healing throughout the whole body.

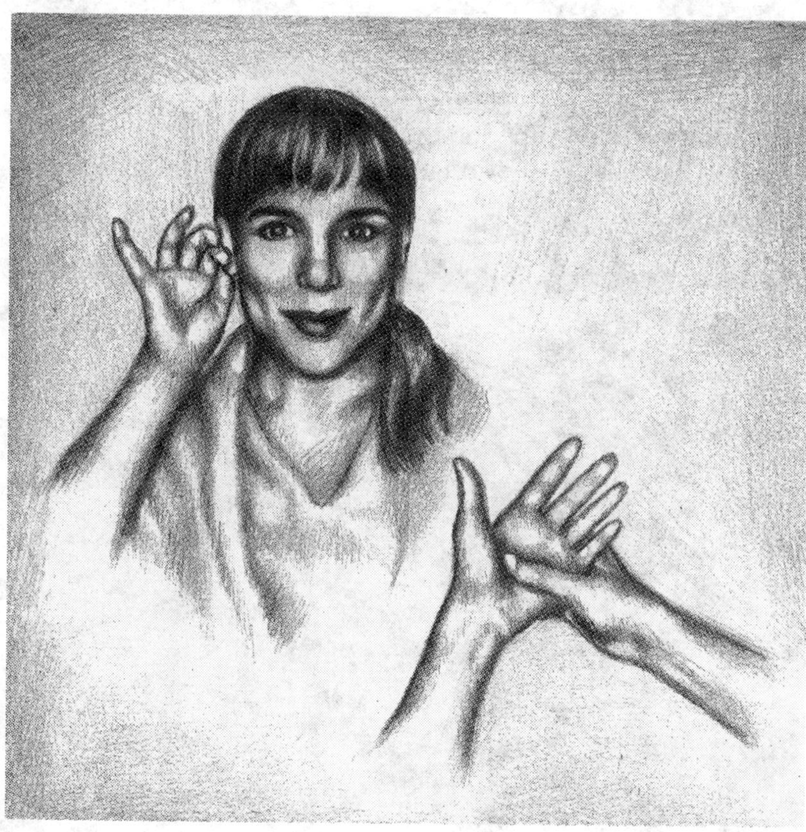

Practice 3.

3. Massaging the acupuncture microsystems: In modern Chinese medical terminology, the hands, feet, and ears are called reflex microsystems. Pressure applied to these areas, usually with the thumbs, stimulates *qi* throughout the body.

With your thumbs, vigorously press all areas of the palms and the soles of the feet. Find sore points and concentrate pressure on them several times.

Press out along each segment of the fingers and toes. At the tips of the fingers and toes press on the lateral sides of the base of the finger- or toenails (feel for an indentation). Continuing to press, roll the receiving finger or toe under the pressure of the thumb and forefinger of the working hand. Return to give additional pressure to those hand or foot points that were particularly tender.

Now using the thumbs and forefingers, massage the ears simultaneously. Begin with moderate pressure and work over the entire ear on both sides, until the ears begin to feel hot. Notice any areas of discomfort and rub the uncomfortable areas vigorously.

4. Building up vital life energy with breathing: Sit or stand, keeping your eyes lightly closed or just slightly open; attention focused inward. Shoulders are relaxed and the head rests directly on top of the shoulders and spine. Hands are held palm facing upward, fingertips pointing toward each other two inches below the navel.

Slowly inhaling, bring the hands upward to the lower edge of the breastbone. Then, take in three additional short puffs of breath to maximally fill the lungs, raising the hands a bit with each puff to the level of the arm pits. Hold for a moment. Slowly turn the palms face down and exhale slowly, lowering the hands slowly to the navel. Exhale three additional puffs of breath, to maximally empty the lungs. Lower the hands a bit to the beginning level. Hold for a moment. Repeat.

On the exhalations you may feel a warm or tingling sensation spreading outward from the center of your body toward your hands. On inhaling, visualize the *qi* accumulating deep inside the pelvic and abdominal cavities (known as "the sea of energy"). Continue visualizing with exhalation.

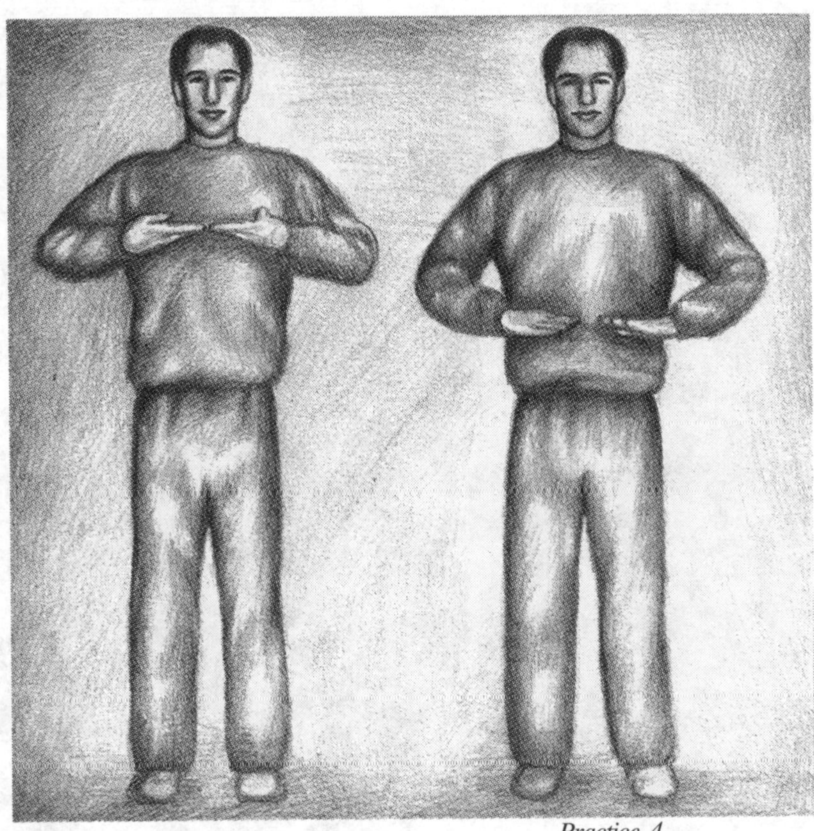

Practice 4.

5. Contracting and relaxing with breathing: In this exercise, the whole body musculature contracts on exhalation and deeply relaxes on each inhalation. The breath and the contraction together help to cleanse the tissues of the body.

While sitting or standing, bring the hands in front of the heart/breastbone, inhale, and relax. Begin to exhale, pressing the hands forward as if pushing something heavy. Contract as many of the body's muscles as possible. Grip the floor or ground with the toes and, while the hands slowly push forward, contract the perineal muscles (located on the pelvic floor between the genital and anal area).

Practice 5.

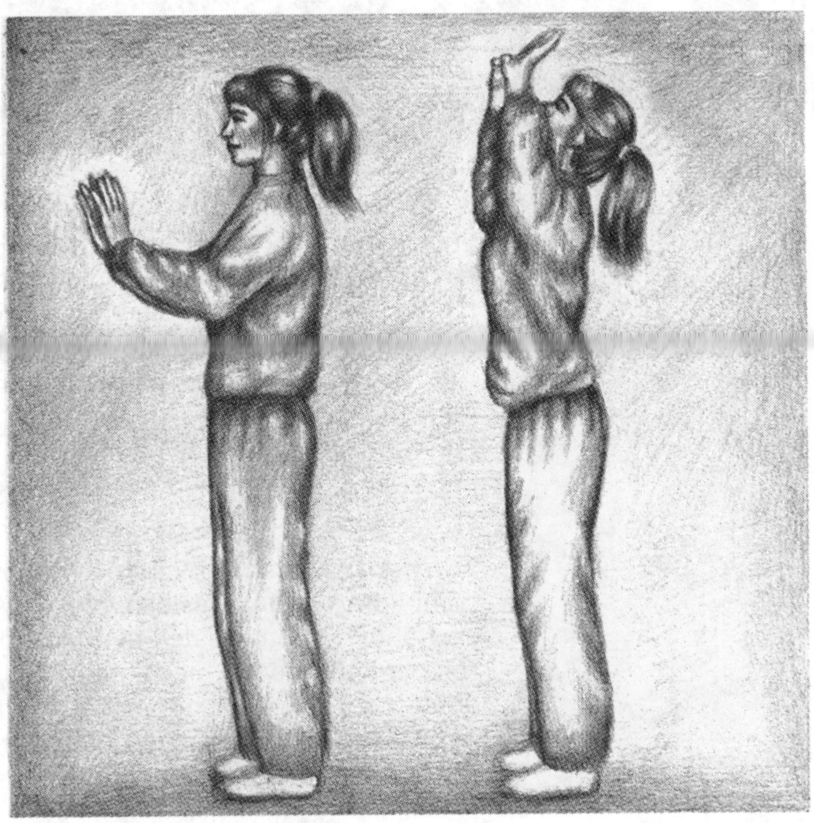

When the hands are extended, all muscles contracted, breath is completely exhaled; relax. Release tension from all muscles and float the hands back toward the heart with a deep inhalation. Release the toes, the perineum, and the abdomen.

Repeat the same cycle, pressing the hands upward as high as possible, as if lifting a great weight off of yourself, exhaling and contracting. Then relax completely, inhale slowly, and return the hands to the position before the heart.

Next, repeat pushing out to the sides, then pressing downward. Continue forward, then up, then to the sides and finally downward. Contraction and release of muscles pump large volumes of lymphatic fluid away from the tissues, carrying away metabolic by-products and pollutants through the bloodstream.

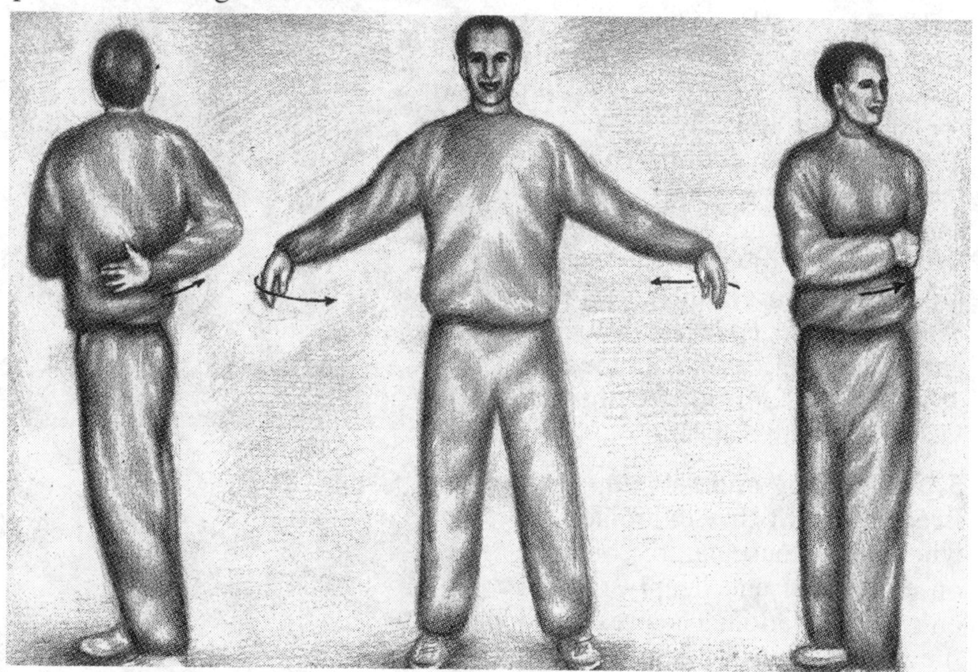

Practice 6.

6. Twisting the waist: Standing, with your feet at shoulder width, rotate your torso. This can be done seated. Upper body movement should come from moving the waist. Shoulders follow the waist and the arms follow the shoulders, they just dangle and swing. Turn the head completely, as far as it will comfortably go, to look behind you.

Breathe fully and note a dynamic relationship between action and relaxation. Bring as much relaxation to the movement as possible. Notice that the arms and hands hit the body. This hitting or thumping can become purposeful when aimed at the reflexes of the kidneys, spleen, and liver around the lower torso.

7. Spontaneous movement: Spontaneous movement *qigong* is very common in China. Instead of following a prescribed set of instructions each individual is guided to move about or not move at all by an internal sense of the body's needs, a sense of the *qi*. Some people seem to be doing nothing or almost nothing, others may be sitting and moving their arms about in coordination with the breath. Still others may be dancing about in a deeply energized state.

Standing with feet at shoulder width or sitting in an armless chair, begin to wiggle the fingers and shake or rock the body; deepen the breath. Increase the body's activity and allow hands and arms to shake. Add shaking of the head and shoulders. Relax the jaw, allowing some sound to be generated on the exhalation, like a giant sigh of relief. This is one of the best exercises to bring about an immediate sensation of the energy or *qi*. Exaggerate the movement, prolong it; shift weight from foot to foot; make sounds; find your own best way to use this exercise.

8. *Qigong* meditation: This practice can be done standing, sitting, or lying down. In the severely ill, it can mobilize important healing resources. If the person is healthy, it can help maintain health and coordinate body, mind, and spirit.

In this practice, natural forces accelerate through breath, relaxation, intention, and visualization. On inhalation, visualize a concentration of *qi* in the abdominal area. On exhalation, visualize these resources circulating out from the center to all the parts of the body: extremities, organs, tissues, and glands. Continue, through thought and visualization, to circulate healing energy with deep breathing and deep relaxation.

With its proven ability to enhance health and prevent disease, qigong *can serve as an effective system of self-care, saving thousands of dollars in long-term health costs.*

Qigong in America

Although *qigong* exercises are widely practiced in the United States, the conventional medical community has been resistant to its use in a medical context. "Yet," says Dr. Jahnke, "one factor makes *qigong* an inevitable innovation in Western culture: the staggering cost of postsymptomatic medical intervention. With *qigong*, individuals learn to heal themselves and maintain their health—a profoundly cost-effective feature." Dr. Jahnke adds that ancient, low-impact, self-healing traditions like *qigong, tai chi,* yoga, and *pranayama* are being referred to as "self applied health enhancement methods" (SAHEM) in the international medical literature. This name allows Western culture to embrace *qigong* and its benefits in terms that are familiar. SAHEM combines gentle body movement, self-massage, relaxation exercises, breathing, meditation, and visualization, and is now being implemented in hospitals, schools, YMCAs, corporate wellness programs, and communities at large throughout the country.[6]

Where to Find Help

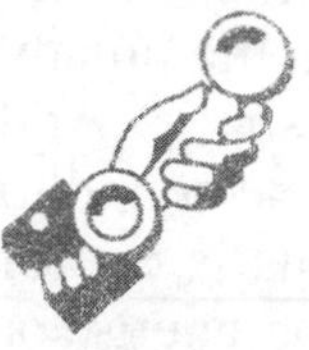

Though there are many books on *qigong*, classes should be taken from a qualified teacher. Consult your telephone book for a *qigong* center, or ask an acupuncturist or doctor of Traditional Chinese Medicine for a referral.

American Foundation of Traditional Chinese Medicine
505 Beach Street
San Francisco, California 94133
(415) 776-0502

This foundation has a national referral bank and an international listing of classes, sponsors continuing education programs, and publishes Gateways, *a quarterly newsletter.*

The Healing Tao Center
P.O. Box 1194
Huntington, New York 11743
(516) 367-2701

The Center offers classes in the United States, Europe, Australia, India, and South America. Videotaped demonstrations of qigong *exercises are also available.*

Health Action
243 Pebble Beach
Santa Barbara, California 93117
(805) 682-3230

This organization offers a comprehensive and clinical program of alternative therapies including Traditional Chinese Medicine, publishes various books, and presents qigong *training throughout the United States, Europe and China.*

Qigong Institute/East-West Academy of the Healing Arts
450 Sutter Street, Suite 916
San Francisco, California 94108
(415) 788-2227

The Institute offers monthly lectures and demonstrations and promotes education, research, and clinical work. The Institute sponsors a qigong *science program and provides an index listing of six hundred related abstracts on* qigong.

Qigong Universal
2828 Beverly Boulevard
Los Angeles, California 90057
(213) 487-2672

The company presents qigong *trainings in Southern California.*

Recommended Reading

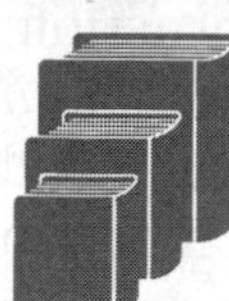

Chi Kung, The Ancient Chinese Way to Health. Dong, Paul; and Esser, Aristide H., M.D. New York: Paragon House, 1990.

This book approaches qigong *as a therapeutic system, combining mental concentration and breathing exercises and shows exercises and relationships between* qigong *and the Western world.*

Chi Self-Massage: The Taoist Way of Rejuvenation. Chia, Mantak. Huntington, NY: Healing Tao Books, 1986.

This practice of qi *massage is broken down into a logical, easy-to-follow, sequence.*

The Complete System of Self-Healing: Internal Exercises. Chang, Stephen T. San Francisco, CA: Tao Publishing, 1986.

A philosophy "workbook" for those devoted to inner healing.

Iron Shirt Chi Kung I. Chia, Mantak. Huntington, NY: Healing Tao Books, 1986.

Iron Shirt Chi Kung I *teaches ways to direct the internal power and increase* qi.

The Most Profound Medicine. Jahnke, Roger. Santa Barbara, CA: Health Action Books, 1990.

Part I describes the history and tradition of qigong. *Part II is an in-depth exploration of* qigong *practice. [To order, call (805) 682-3230.]*

Qigong for Health: Chinese Traditional Exercise for Cure and Prevention. Takahashi, Masaru; and Brown, Stephen. Tokyo, New York: Japan Publications, 1986.

An examination of qigong *and its applications through lifestyle and exercise.*

Qigong Magazine
Pacific Rim Publishers, Inc.
P.O. Box 31578
San Francisco, California 94131
(800) 824-2433

A quarterly magazine for professionals and the general public.

QI: The Journal of Traditional Eastern Health and Fitness
P.O. Box 221343
Chantilly, Virginia 22022
(800) 787-2600

A quarterly magazine geared to educating the public about the benefits of Asian traditions of healing.

The Self-Applied Health Enhancement Methods. Jahnke, Roger. Santa Barbara, CA: Health Action Books, 1989.

A how-to manual for beginning a personal qigong *practice. [To order, call (805) 682-3230.]*

Taoist Ways to Transform Stress into Vitality. Chia, Mantak. Huntington, NY: Healing Tao Books. 1985.

This book teaches techniques to help to cool down the system, eliminate trapped energy, and clean toxins out of the organs.

"The next major advance in the health of the American people will be determined by what the individual is willing to do for himself."

—John Knowles, Former President of the Rockefeller Foundation

Reconstructive Therapy

Reconstructive therapy uses injections of natural substances to stimulate the growth of connective tissue in order to strengthen weak or damaged tendons or ligaments. As a simple, cost-effective alternative to drug and surgical treatments, reconstructive therapy is an effective treatment for degenerative arthritis, low back pain, carpal tunnel syndrome, migraine headaches, and torn ligaments and cartilage.

Joint, tendon, ligament, cartilage, and arthritic problems are among the most common afflictions Americans suffer from today. Many remedies are used to treat these problems, such as rest, medication, traction, exercise, cortisone injections, physical therapy, and surgery, but for many patients, these fail to provide lasting relief. In many cases, however, reconstructive therapy (also known as sclerotherapy, prolotherapy, or proliferative therapy), a nonsurgical method that stimulates the body's natural healing abilities to repair injured tissues and joints, can provide an answer.

"Ligaments, tendons, cartilage, and bones have poor healing abilities due to the lack of blood supply to these tissues," says William Faber, D.O., Director of the Milwaukee Pain Clinic and a leading authority in the field of reconstructive therapy. "This is why injuries to these areas are so long lasting. When these tissues become damaged, the joint becomes unstable, and in order to compensate, the body forms bony, arthritic spurs. This causes increased friction, increased pain and weakness, and a loss in joint mobility. Further injury often results."

Reconstructive therapy can facilitate the healing process for specific injuries. In the case of injured joints, a local anesthetic and a natural irritant (sodium morrhuate, a purified derivative of cod liver oil), dextrose, phenol, minerals, or other natural substances are injected into areas where ligaments, tendons, and cartilage are torn or weak. "The injection stimulates the body to produce more connective tissue, which helps to strengthen the weak or damaged areas," says Dr. Faber. "As a result, the patient will often experience less pain and greater strength and endurance."

How Reconstructive Therapy Works

According to Dr. Faber, "Mild, irritating reconstructive solutions cause dilation of blood vessels and a migration of fibroblasts [healing cells] to the injured areas. These healing cells lay down collagen [a structural protein] to repair the area." This regrowth has been substantiated by research studies dating back almost forty years.

In a study conducted in the 1950s by surgeon George Hackett, M.D., 1,600 patients with severe sacroiliac sprain were treated with reconstructive injections. When the patients were examined by independent physicians two to twelve years later, 82 percent had remained free of pain or recurrences.[1] Dr. Hackett's experiments were repeated in 1983 and 1985 by the University of Iowa's Department of Orthopedic Research. Both studies found that the patients' tendons became more firmly attached to the bone and increased in strength and structure by 30 to 40 percent above normal.[2]

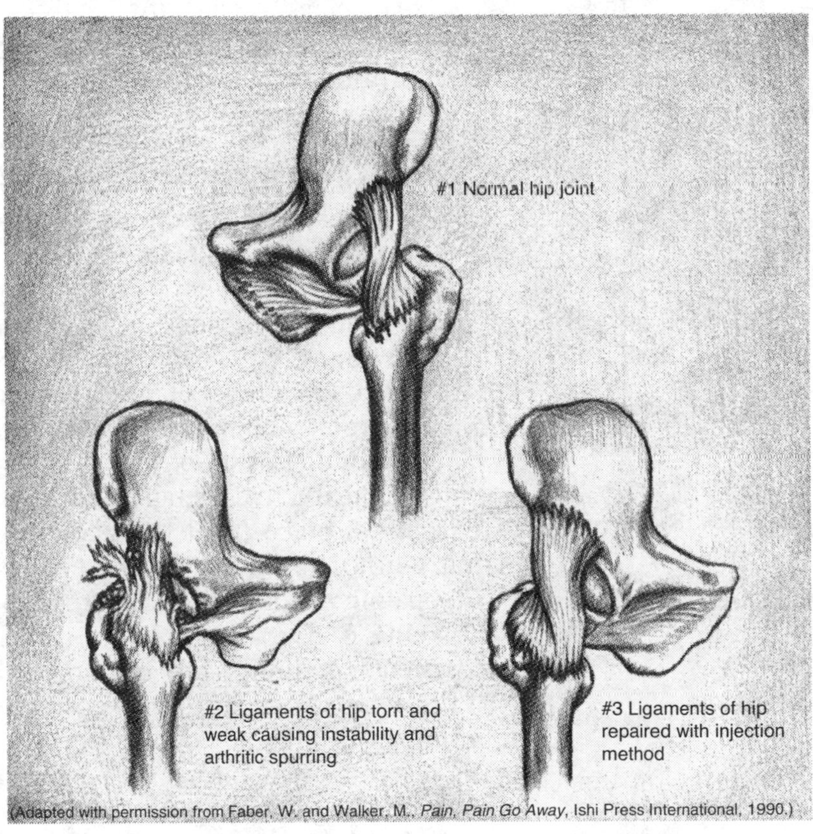
#1 Normal hip joint
#2 Ligaments of hip torn and weak causing instability and arthritic spurring
#3 Ligaments of hip repaired with injection method
(Adapted with permission from Faber, W. and Walker, M., *Pain, Pain Go Away*, Ishi Press International, 1990.)

Damaged joint regenerated by reconstructive therapy.

In 1987, at the Sansum Medical Clinic of Santa Barbara, California, rheumatologist Robert Klein, M.D., and internist Thomas Dorman, M.D., conducted a double-blind study of eighty-one patients who suffered from continuous low back pain for more than ten years. They found that 88 percent of the patients injected with a reconstructive solution of dextrose, glycerine, and phenol demonstrated moderate to marked improvement.[3] A similar study, reported in the *Journal of Spinal Disorders*, showed an 80 percent improvement.[4] Both studies support Dr. Hackett's findings.

Studies conducted by Harold Walmer, D.O., of Elizabeth, Pennsylvania, have also shown that reconstructive therapy increases mechanical strength in ligaments and joints.[5] This may explain why so many patients with advanced degeneration of bones and soft tissues, or those who suffer from a wide range of musculoskeletal problems, have improved so dramatically when given reconstructive injections.

Conditions Benefited by Reconstructive Therapy

Reconstructive therapy has been practiced in the United States for over sixty years as a treatment for America's most common afflictions: tendon, ligament, and arthritic problems. To date, over six hundred thousand patients have been successfully treated with reconstructive therapy. Common symptoms and conditions that respond well to reconstructive therapy include:

- Degenerative arthritis
- Back and neck pain
- Torn ligaments and cartilage
- Degenerated discs
- Migraines
- Bursitis
- Carpal tunnel syndrome
- Achilles tendon tears
- Tennis elbow
- Rotator cuff tears
- Bunions
- A wide range of musculoskeletal problems caused by failed surgery, compression fractures, degenerated disks, polio, and muscular dystrophy

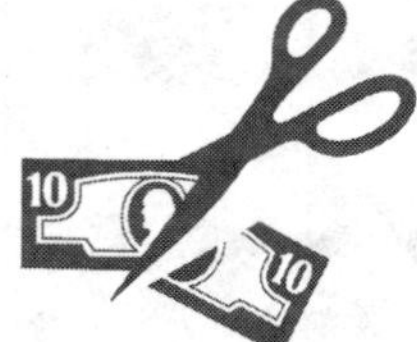

Reconstructive therapy can provide a more cost-effective solution to musculoskeletal and joint problems than traditional surgery.

Reconstructive therapy is also recommended for weak joints; joints requiring a brace; joints that continually pop, snap, and grind; or joints that cannot maintain alignment (particularly when chiropractic or osteopathic manipulations fail to help).

One of Dr. Faber's cases involved a physician who had been experiencing chronic low back pain since the age of fourteen. At the age of thirty he had sprained his neck, worsening his condition, and a cervical laminectomy (removal of a cervical disk) was surgically performed. However, his back problems persisted, and ten years later, he injured his back once again. Diagnosis showed a herniated lumbar disk. Another operation followed, but his back pain persisted, and when it became so severe that he could barely move without pain, he sought reconstructive therapy. The pain was relieved immediately, Dr. Faber reports, with his neck and back steadily strengthening during the days after his first treatment. Further treatments provided more relief. "He told me that reconstructive therapy was the most valuable of any of the treatments he had received, and it only cost a fraction of the $120,000 he had spent on surgery, medications, and other physical therapies," says Dr. Faber.

Another case reported by Dr. Faber involved a college football player who had suffered repeated injuries to his left shoulder. He relied upon various medications and therapies until the pain became too great, and then underwent orthopedic surgery, but his condition worsened. Chiropractic treatments afforded him only temporary relief, and his chiropractor suggested reconstructive therapy. After receiving reconstructive injections his condition improved dramatically. In fact, in a metered punching test, it was found that he wound up with more strength in the left shoulder than in the right.

Degenerative muscle and joint complaints seem to particularly benefit from reconstructive therapy. James Carlson, D.O., an orthopedic and sports medicine specialist in Knoxville, Tennessee, and past President of the American Association of Orthopedic Medicine, believes that reconstructive therapy is the most effective treatment for Osgood-Schlatter disease, a muscle ailment that strikes adolescents between the ages of eleven and sixteen. "These kids have such severe pain in the knees, they can't participate in exercise, sports, or dance, and traditional medicine just dictates 'don't do anything athletic,'" says Dr. Carlson. "Reconstructive therapy is the best thing I've ever seen." His own son, an aspiring baseball catcher, couldn't squat down or kneel. After therapy, he made the team as a catcher, and later, became a top school athlete.

"Reconstructive therapy is estimated to be three to ten times more cost-effective than surgery or joint replacement."

Another patient of Dr. Faber suffered from lumbar spondylolisthesis (a forward slipping of one vertebrae on the one below it) for more than two years. He experienced constant pain caused by a break in a vertebra. After receiving reconstructive therapy from Dr. Faber he was pain free. Eight years later he reported no recurrences. Today he does landscaping, hunts, and even waterskis.

What to Expect from Reconstructive Therapy

Reconstructive therapy is estimated to be three to ten times more cost-effective than surgery or joint replacement. Dr. Carlson notes that any pain or discomfort associated with receiving multiple injections is compensated for by the benefits received from reconstructive therapy. According to Kent Pomeroy, M.D., an Arizona physical medicine and rehabilitation specialist, and co-founder and past President of the American Association of Orthopedic Medicine, "Dramatic results should be noted by the patient within the first week of treatment. But if swelling occurs, improvement may not be noticed until the swelling subsides. If marked improvement is not obtained after the first six treatments, then further examination is recommended to find out why the patient's body is failing to reconstruct tissue."

Generally, a patient improves dramatically after the first six injections. Most patients will need twelve to thirty treatments to bring the joint back to full strength and function. The benefits of reconstructive therapy over other methods of treatment include

- Eliminating the need for drugs or surgery
- Stimulating the body's natural healing mechanism, causing natural regrowth of structural tissue
- A low risk of side effects, when performed correctly
- Permanent results when full treatment course is completed

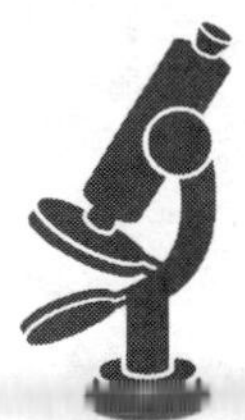

Research into the effectiveness of reconstructive therapy is needed. This type of therapy could provide a revolution in orthopedic medicine by offering regeneration rather than surgery.

The Future of Reconstructive Therapy

Although reconstructive therapy has been used to treat a wide range of musculoskeletal conditions for over forty years, its practice has not become widespread in the United States. In recent years, however, according to Dr. Faber, the number of practitioners has been growing, and currently approximately two hundred physicians practice reconstructive therapy.

"One major reason for the slow growth of reconstructive therapy," Dr. Faber suggests, "may be the fact that the substances used in reconstructive therapy are not patented and therefore would not provide the huge profits that other pharmaceutically-backed drug therapies receive. Reconstructive therapy also requires specialized training, and a serious commitment on the part of the physician to master the procedure."

Reconstructive therapy can play an important role in the medicine of the future. It may well be the first nondrug, nonsurgical approach to result in a much-needed change in medical treatment of long-lasting musculoskeletal problems, currently addressed by orthopedics, neurosurgery, physical medicine, and physical therapy.

"The initial turning point will be the discovery of reconstructive therapy by professional athletes," according to Dr. Faber. "Although reconstructive therapy is well documented in science and through the case histories of thousands of successful patients, the recovery of a single famous athlete by reconstructive therapy is what's needed to bring the therapy into the spotlight it so richly deserves."

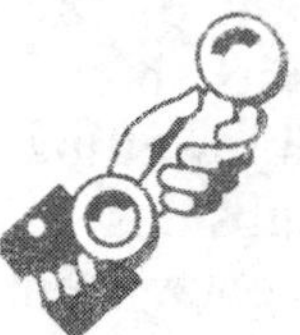

Where to Find Help

When requesting information on reconstructive therapy, refer additionally to sclerotherapy, a term considered synonymous by many associations.

Milwaukee Pain Clinic
6529 West Fond du Lac Avenue
Milwaukee, Wisconsin 53218
(414) 464-7246

Provides reconstructive and other musculoskeletal therapies; training courses in reconstructive therapy available. For additional information send a legal size, self-addressed, stamped envelope.

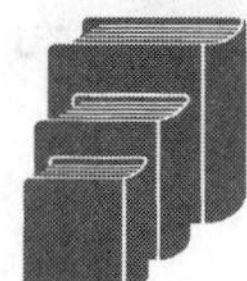

Recommended Reading

Pain, Pain Go Away. Faber, William J., D.O., and Walker, Morten, D.P.M. San Jose, CA: Ishi Press International, 1990.

This book contains information on reconstructive therapy, a physician reference list, symptom lists, and forty-three case histories concerning all areas of the body.

Sound Therapy

Sound and music can have a very powerful effect on one's health. Sound therapy is used in hospitals, schools, corporate offices, and psychological treatment programs as an effective treatment to reduce stress, lower blood pressure, alleviate pain, overcome learning disabilities, improve movement and balance, and promote endurance and strength.

The ability of sound and music to heal has been recognized for thousands of years. The writings of Pythagoras and Plato in ancient Greece, the soothing harp music of young David in the Bible, and the chanted hymns of the Vedas in India, all recognize the healing power of sound. In modern times the therapeutic power of sound was medically noted as early as 1896, when doctors discovered that a young boy's brain, partially exposed due to an accident, responded differently when various types of music were played. Certain music increased cerebral and peripheral circulation, while other music stimulated mental lucidity.[1]

Because the ear is not only the primary organ of hearing, but also has powerful influences on eye movement, the rhythms of the physical body, prebirth brain growth, and general regulation of stress levels in the body, greater emphasis is now placed on the therapeutic union of sound and healing. Recently, much attention has been placed on the negative aspects of sound, either from music played too loudly or from exposure to the hard noise of industrial machinery. "Calling noise a nuisance is like calling smog an inconvenience," states William H. Stewart, former U.S. Surgeon General, who suggests that "noise must be considered a hazard to the health of people everywhere."[2] Accordingly, one study found that more than 60 percent of incoming college freshmen have impaired hearing in high frequency ranges due to prolonged exposure to high auditory levels.[3]

How Sound Therapy Works

Sound therapists recognize that certain sounds can slow the breathing rate and create a feeling of overall well-being; others can slow a racing heart, even soothe a restless baby. Sound can also alter skin temperature,

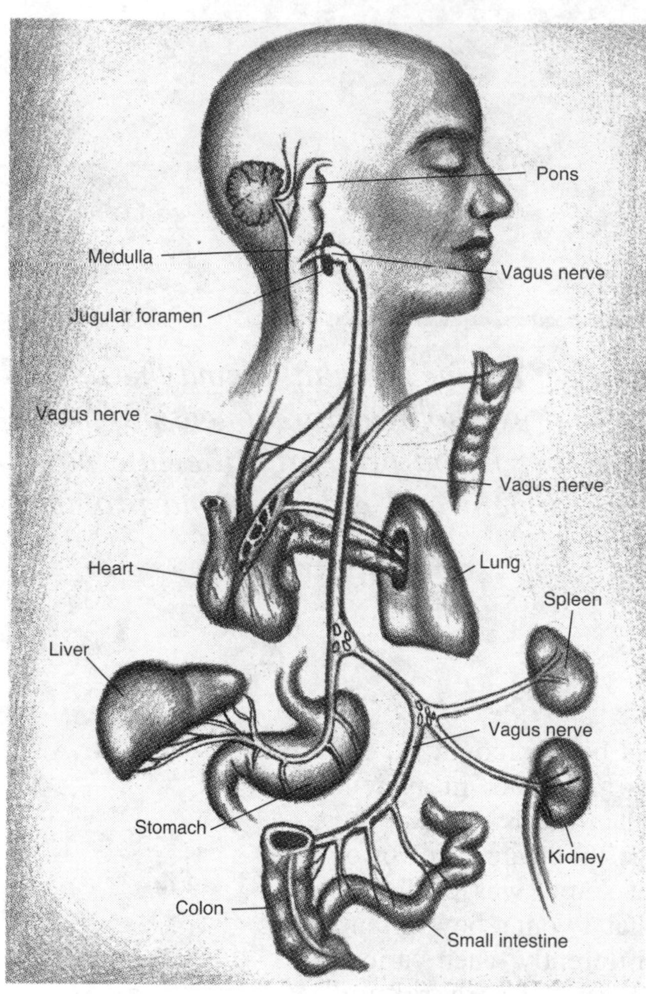

The vagus nerve and its connection to internal organs.

reduce blood pressure and muscle tension, and influence brain wave frequencies. Although some sounds (like ultrasonic waves) are beyond the range of the ear, they can have a profound effect on the human condition.

Defined as "oscillating energy waves within the audible range," sound originates and travels from one source to another as waves, each sound with its own velocity and intensity, and each with its own frequency, pitch, and wavelength. (Music is essentially a pleasurable sequence of sound waves.) The intensity of the vibration, or the loudness of sound, is measured in units called decibels. Although volume is a factor, it is not necessary that one be consciously aware of a sound for it to have an effect because sound creates a response in the entire body, not just the ear.

People respond to sound vibrations in two main ways: via rhythm entrainment and resonance. According to Steven Halpern, Ph.D., of San Anselmo, California, "Rhythm entrainment describes the phenomenon whereby, in the presence of any external rhythmic stimulus, the natural rhythm of the heartbeat will be overridden and caused to pulse in sync with the sound source. This may be the rhythm of drums, or the rhythmic pulse of the music, or it may just be your refrigerator's motor.

"Resonance refers to the physical phenomenon in which different frequencies of sound (different pitches) stimulate the body to vibrate in different areas. Typically, low sound resonates in the lower parts of the body and high sound resonates in the higher parts of the body."

Sound is linked to the physical body by the eighth and tenth cranial nerves. These carry sound impulses through the ear and skull to the brain. Motor and sensory impulses are then sent along the vagus nerve (which helps regulate breathing, speech, and heart rate) to the throat, larynx, heart, and diaphragm. Don G. Campbell, B.M.E.D., Director of the Institute for Music, Health, and Education in Boulder, Colorado, explains, "The vagus nerve and the emotional responses to the limbic system (specific areas of the brain responsible for emotion and motivation) are the link between the ear, the brain, and the autonomic nervous system that may account for the effectiveness of sound therapy in treating physical and emotional disorders."

Various elements of sound influence separate parts of the brain. Rhythm, for example, engages the reptilian or hindbrain (see illustration), while its tempo can alter the sense of time. The human body also has its own rhythmic patterns, and there is growing evidence that the rhythms of the heart, the brain, and other organs enjoy a special synchronicity. Illness can arise when these inner rhythms are disturbed.[4] Tone engages the limbic midbrain (see illustration), which governs emotion. According to Campbell, "The real power of sound is in the way the tonal or harmonic aspects influence our emotions and midbrain functions."

Sound can also be used to help the body regulate its corticosteroid hormone levels, helping to control the severity of spastic muscle tremors, reduce cancer-related pain, and reduce stress in heart patients.[5]

Auditory Integration Training

Alfred A. Tomatis, M.D., who practices in Paris and teaches worldwide, was one of the first to notice a strong interrelationship between hearing, the voice, and psychophysiological development. His early work explored the relationship between sounds in the womb and the development of the brain with regard to memory, language, and learning. Dr. Tomatis discovered a direct connection between hearing impairment and vocal range, and a direct connection between hearing impairment and overall health and well-being.

See Autism, Hearing and Ear Disorders.

In the early 1950s, Dr. Tomatis designed a system that duplicated how a mother's voice sounds to her unborn child. He then played this filtered voice to children with learning disabilities. In one case, a fourteen-year-old autistic boy who had not spoken since age four began to babble like a ten-month-old.

"The human body has its own rhythmic patterns, and there is growing evidence that the rhythms of the heart, brain, and other organs enjoy a special synchronicity. Illness can arise when these inner rhythms are disturbed."

From these experiments, Dr. Tomatis and his colleagues developed the Electronic Ear, a machine that simulates the stages of listening development, used to repattern the hearing range and the attention span.

The Electronic Ear is designed to exercise the muscles of the middle ear and improve the ear's response to all frequency ranges. Special headphones equipped with a bone-conduction transducer (to sense vibrations through the bone) deliver sound to the patient via a sophisticated stereo system linked to tuning and filtering components. As lower frequencies are filtered out, the proper auditory preference is introduced. Dr. Tomatis claims to be able to retrain the ear to stop blocking these frequency ranges of sound. Using the Electronic Ear, sound therapists have been able to teach those with dyslexia, autism, learning dysfunctions, and attention deficit disorders how to focus and listen more effectively. Others have improved their creative skills, musical ability, foreign language learning ability, and organizational ability.

Billie M. Thompson, Ph.D., Director of Sound, Listening and Learning Center in Phoenix, Arizona, used the Electronic Ear as part of her treatment for a hypersensitive six-year-old autisic girl who did not speak and who wore a ski cap twenty-four hours a day to limit outside stimulation. After three days using the device, the girl discarded her cap and went out to a restaurant with her family for the first time. She also went to church and heard an organ without having to leave in pain. Although she still does not speak more than a few words, she is more social now, participating in many of the family's activities, and no longer retreating into the corner in fear of sound anymore.

While the Electronic Ear is currently being used in treatment centers throughout North America, it is only one aspect of the Tomatis method of treatment, according to Dr. Thompson.

"As the ear opens, the individual becomes more receptive and responsive to sound and more motivated to communicate," says Dr. Thompson. "By retraining the ear, people of all ages profoundly improve how they learn and relate to others, as we are creatures of movement, rhythm, and sound. With the ear as a key integrator, organizer, and analyzer of information, sound therapy can profoundly enhance thought and communication skills and can make possible a vastly enhanced level of listening."

"There are sounds that are as good as two cups of coffee."
—Alfred Tomatis, M.D.

According to Dr. Tomatis, longer mental and physical endurance can result from listening to Mozart or Gregorian chants, particularly the recordings from the French Abbey of Solesmes. Using an oscilloscope, he measured the Abbey's dawn and midnight masses for Christmas and the masses for the Epiphany and Easter. He found that the sounds fell within the bandwidth he had already determined was uniquely suited for energizing purposes. "There are sounds that are as good as two cups of coffee," offers Dr. Tomatis. "If I have a long job to do, I always put on Gregorian chanting because it enables me to remain charged without difficulty. I don't put it on loud, but it's always in the background."[6]

Audiotapes based on Dr. Tomatis' work contain enhanced high-frequency sounds that support and enliven the upper register sound of the listener.

Guy Berard, M.D., a French physician, developed a method of retraining, similar to that of Dr. Tomatis, which concentrates on patients who are hypersensitive to high-frequency sounds or who suffer from loss of normal frequency hearing. Often this hypersensitivity can result in behavioral and cognitive problems when certain frequencies are perceived in a distorted manner.

Dr. Berard uses a device called the Ears Education and Retraining System (EERS), which reduces hypersensitivity by optimally allowing all frequencies to be heard with the same comfort and clarity. This device takes music from a sound source (audio tape or compact disc) and filters out the frequencies to which the patient has shown hypersensitivity. The EERS then electronically modulates these frequencies and returns them via headphones to the ears. Dr. Berard has found that after about ten hours of listening to these processed sounds, the listener makes significant progress toward accepting that frequency.

One of Dr. Berard's patients was an eleven-year-old autistic girl who suffered from both a hypo- (low) and hyperacute (high) sense of hearing. Over the course of twenty half-hour sessions using the EERS, Dr. Berard was able to decrease the hyperacute points of the girl's hearing while bringing the deficits up, thus creating a more normal hearing pattern. This also helped correct the girl's dyslexia, attention deficit, and hyperactivity, and today she is a happily married college graduate, working on a University of Oregon research project to help autistic adults.

Toning

For years, the Institute for Music, Health, and Education has researched and trained students to use "toning" (making elongated vowel sounds and allowing them to resonate through the body) as a simple way to release stress, balance the mind/body, improve the ear's ability to listen, and improve the speaking and singing voice.

"Toning is the art of making elongated vowel sounds and sensing where they internally vibrate," says Don Campbell. Toning causes the brain waves to synchronize and balance within three to five minutes, and this greatly influences the sense of physical and emotional well-being.

"Specific areas of the brain are tuned to specific tone frequencies," says Campbell. "The pitch of the vowel sound determines where it will resonate in the brain."

According to Campbell, toning brings more benefit than singing or speaking because singing and speaking "move the vibratory epicenters so quickly there is no time for the body to balance itself with the sound. To sound the voice through toning is to massage ourselves internally. There is no other way to localize oxygenation, energy flow and pulsation noninvasively within such a short period of time."

A voice with good timbre and rich overtones will recharge the individual each time it is used, notes Dr. Tomatis. For example, in the 1970s, when he was asked to investigate why monks in a certain French Benedictine monastery had become depressed, tired, and physically uneasy, Dr. Tomatis learned they had abandoned their former habit of chanting in Latin nine times a day. He recommended they resume their chanting. When they did, their energy increased and their depression and fatigue disappeared.

Therapeutic Uses of Sound Therapy

Today, sound has been incorporated into many different types of therapeutic settings, including hospital surgery, recovery, and birthing wards; the care of patients with Alzheimer's disease, cancer, and AIDS; hospice (for the dying); for birthing; dentistry; and psychotherapy.

In the Hospital

Music in the hospital setting is not a new phenomenon—it is used to reduce pain in surgical, dental, obstetrical, and gynecological procedures. Where music therapy is introduced patients view their hospitalization more positively, report reduced physical discomfort, and experience improvement in mood parameters. Ralph Spintge, M.D., of Germany, Executive Director of the International Society for Music in Medicine, has completed a study of nearly ninety-thousand patients in the peri- and post-operative phases of surgery. Ninety-seven percent of the patients said music during their recovery helped them relax. Other patients found that music enabled them to get by with less anesthesia. Soft, tonal music was found to be especially effective. Patients who listened to slow baroque or classical music a few days before surgery, then had it filtering through the recovery room, found that the music minimized postoperative disorientation.[7]

With Alzheimer's Patients

Music therapy can be particularly healing in Alzheimer's patients. Patients who cannot communicate verbally and are unable to initiate purposeful movement have increased needs for sensory and environmental stimulation that can tap into remote memory. Music and speech patterns (tone and rhythm) are very effective and are utilized not only to provide psychological comfort, but also to enhance communication in an older individual who may be withdrawn, depressed, or institutionalized.

This training to improve communication is proven and recommended.[8] Family members can be trained to improve communication with loved ones using a variety of methods to increase attentiveness, especially for those in the early and midphases of the disease. These include tapping the hand in rhythm with speech, reading poetry to music, and playing music that has language-based phrasing, such as the slow movement of baroque concertos. Music as a time-ordered art form can make music therapy sessions beneficial by helping to reorient patients who become distracted by the symptoms of Alzheimer's. For individuals in the final stages of the disease, music therapy intervention frequently takes a palliative form and can be utilized to provide psychological comfort.

For the Dying

Therese Schroeder-Sheker is an academic musicologist who founded the field of music thanatology. Using voice and harp in a twenty-year clinical practice, she reconstructed the medieval infirmary music once used within monastic medicine to comfort the dying. Her work has been successfully applied in numerous home, hospital, and hospice settings for the treatment of cancer, respiratory illnesses, and AIDS. This "musical-sacramental-midwifery," as Schroeder-Sheker calls it, is being used at St. Patrick Hospital and at the Mountain West Hospice, both in Missoula, Montana, as well as in other programs in the United States and Europe. Other professionals can be of great benefit to the person who is making the transition, as well as to his or her friends and relatives.

For Birthing

"Many parents have discovered the benefits of playing a variety of relaxing music to their babies while still inside the womb," says Dr. Halpern. "But when it comes to actually choosing the soundtrack for the delivery room, the best long-term results, in terms of the health and well-being of the newborn, are coming from births that provide soothing, nurturing soundtracks."

The therapeutic application of music can be beneficial for the expectant mother who may be in a state of confusion during labor. Listening to music during the birth process often enhances feelings of comfort and security, and heightens self-esteem, socialization, and personal control over the situation.[9]

In Dentistry

For more than fifty years, the healing properties of music have been implemented in dentistry and oral surgery. Wallace Gardner, D.M.D., of Boston, Massachusetts, asserts that loud, stimulating music effectively alleviated pain in 65 percent of his patients, and a Boston study found that sound stimulation was the only analgesic agent required in 90 percent of the five thousand dental operations performed.[10] Additional research shows that due to the release of endorphins (the body's own natural pain killers), audio analgesia with dental patients is comparable in effectiveness to morphine.[11]

In Psychotherapy

As early as the 1950s, medical research showed that music can evoke a range of emotions from sadness to joy, and can be used to moderate feelings of anger or depression.[12] When music is enhanced by imagery, one's moods and physical sensations can alter rapidly. Recent experiments by Stanislav Grof, M.D., Jean Houston, Ph.D., and Helen Bonny, Ph.D., all show how music helps to deepen many aspects of the therapeutic process. A combination of music, imagery, and breathing cannot only bring about strong emotional releases, but can tap into realms of the unconsciousness that only the most powerful of drugs have been able to do.

Dr. Bonny, former Director of Music Therapy at the Catholic University of America, in Washington, D.C., had used music to facilitate psychotherapy, but began using music to heal herself when she developed heart disease. From her work, Dr. Bonny developed a technique called Guided Imagery and Music (GIM). "GIM involves listening in a relaxed state to selected music, a programmed tape, or live music in order to elicit mental imagery, symbols, and deep feelings arising from the deeper conscious self," she says. GIM is used in conjunction with psychotherapy for neurotic patients and as a way to lessen pain and anxiety and explore consciousness in mentally healthy people.

Instruments in Sound Therapy

An emerging field in Sound Therapy is the use of devices that utilize specific sound frequencies to achieve therapeutic benefits such as pain reduction or relaxation. Treatments from devices such as cymatic instruments and the Infratonic QGM are currently being used worldwide.

The Infratonic QGM: The Machine That Produces *Qi* Energy

Lu Yan Fang, Ph.D., a senior scientist at the National Electro Acoustics Laboratory in Beijing, China, discovered that *Qigong* masters emitted from their hands high levels of waves called secondary sound. She constructed a machine that simulated this infratonic sound and tested it on over 1,100 hospitalized patients. Numerous therapeutic benefits were noted, including pain reduction, headache relief, increased circulatory functioning, muscular relaxation, alleviation of depression, and increased brain production of alpha waves.[13]

See Energy Medicine, Qigong.

Her instrument, the Infratonic QGM, received awards of recognition from the China Ministry of Health and the National Committee for Traditional Chinese Medicine. In China it is medically recognized as an effective pain management tool. In the United States it is currently pending FDA (Food and Drug Administration) approval for use as a therapeutic massage device.

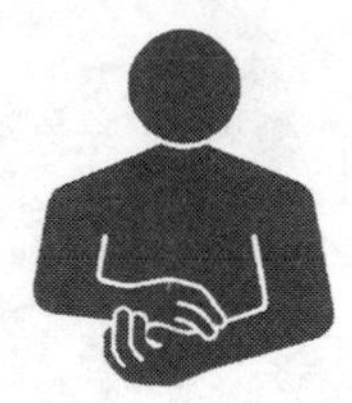

Sound therapy is uniquely suited to self-care. Many new sound devices and tapes can be used at your convenience in the comfort and privacy of your home.

Cymatic Therapy

According to Sir Peter Guy Manners, M.D., D.O., Ph.D., of Worcestershire, England, cymatic therapy, unlike other sound therapies, is not applied through auditory channels, but directly through the skin. Cymatic therapy uses sound waves within the audible range to stimulate natural regulatory and immunological systems, and to produce a near-optimum metabolic state for a particular cell or organ.[14]

"Every object, whether inanimate or alive, possesses a unique electromagnetic field that exhibits antagonistic, complimentary (resonant), or neutral reactions when it interacts with other electromagnetic fields," says Dr. Manners. Resonant equilibrium represents the healthy state (resonance may be defined as the frequency at which an object most naturally vibrates); illnesses is represented by resonant disequilibrium.

Cymatic therapy uses a computerized instrument to establish equilibrium in the body by transmitting resonant frequencies of sound into the body. These signals pass through healthy tissues, but reestablish healthy resonance in unhealthy tissues.

Dr. Manners has researched the signals given out by healthy tissues. By intercepting electrical messages transmitted via the central nervous system to individual cells, this research has allowed the coding of cymatic signals that cells understand. Each tissue has been given an H-factor (harmonic factor) according to the signal emitted. The cymatic instrument adjusts acoustic audible sound frequencies in order to induce beneficial stimulation, activation, and circulation when applied to the body via direct contact with affected areas or by way of acupuncture meridians.

Cymatic therapy does not heal, but simply places the body in a situation so that it can heal itself without pain, surgery, or drugs. According to Dr. Manners, cymatic therapy for humans in the future will likely concentrate on the skin, peripheral nerves, and bone, since these are the areas capable of regeneration. It may also be useful in organ transplantation, balancing the resonance of the transplanted organ with that of the recipient.

Cymatic instruments have been in use worldwide for over twenty-eight years, and have been in use in the United States since the late 1960s. They are used by nurses, chiropractors, osteopaths, and acupuncturists throughout the world. Training is required to become a cymatic practitioner. Cymatic instruments produce no side effects, and the only contraindication for use is for patients with pacemakers.

The Future of Sound Therapy

The emerging field of sound therapy recognizes that through sound, people can help tune themselves to a more fundamentally healthy state of mind, body, and spirit.

Instruments, devices, and systems such as sound tables, auditory floors, brain wave headsets, and numerous audio tapes and compact discs designed to manipulate brainwaves are beginning to appear on the market. "Instruments such as the Electronic Ear," says Dr. Thompson, "have already made great strides in treating patients, such as autistics, whose options were limited with other treatment methods." At the same time, sound therapists who realize that the "listening" components (auditory and psychological) are unique for each individual are beginning to test the use of their voices as instruments for physical adjustments integrated with massage, guided imagery, and physical movement.

Accordingly, many practitioners believe that sound waves will be elemental in the healing process of the future. Sound will not only be used for treatment, but perhaps also for the diagnosis and prescription of certain tones that can bring the patient's health back into balance.

Where to Find Help

For further information on music and sound therapy contact:

The American Association of Music Therapy
P.O. Box 80012
Valley Forge, Pennsylvania 19484
(215) 265-4006

AAMT treats mental illness, including retardation, and provides hospital visits, psychological counseling, music healing, and stress reduction. It also accredits schools, and publishes a newsletter. A nonprofit organization that certifies music therapists, AAMT holds conferences for professional music therapists and the general public. It does not treat medical problems, but does offer referrals to music therapists.

The Chalice of Repose Project
St. Patrick's Hospital
554 West Broadway
Missoula, Montana 59806
(406) 542-0001 Ext. 2810

CORP is a nonprofit, seven-institution medical and educational cooperative that is housed at St. Patrick's Hospital in Missoula, Montana. Offering three degree programs, it is a palliative-medical teaching and clinical organization that conducts research, publishes, holds conferences, certifies music thanatologists, and trains twenty-five resident music thanatology interns each year.

Georgiana Institute
P.O. Box 2607
Westport, Connecticut 06880
(203) 454-1221

Provides education, workshops, consulting, and information on the Berard method.

Guided Imagery and Music
Temple University
Presser Hall 0012-00
Philadelphia, Pennsylvania 19122
(215) 787-8314

This organization teaches the GIM method. Provides a trilevel training program with internship, as well as fifteen programs taught internationally. GIM is also taught in three universities and accredited through the National Association of Music Therapy.

The Institute for Music, Health, and Education
P.O. Box 4179
Boulder, Colorado 80306
(303) 443-8484

The Institute trains students to use "toning" to release stress, balance the mind and body, improve the ear's ability to listen, and improve the speaking and singing voice. Video and audio cassettes are also available and year-long accredited courses are offered by correspondence.

The National Association of Music Therapy
8455 Colesville Road, Suite 930
Silver Springs, Maryland 20910
(301) 589-3300

NAMT is an association for music therapists that provides publicity for music therapy; publishes a journal, books, and videotapes on musical therapy; accredits schools; and sponsors a national annual conference.

Sound, Listening and Learning Center
2701 East Camelback, Suite 205
Phoenix, Arizona 85016
(602) 381-0086

There are over 180 Tomatis Centers in Europe and now over a dozen in North and Central America that provide education, workshops, consulting, therapeutic sessions, and information on the Tomatis method.

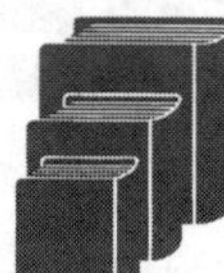

Recommended Reading

About the Tomatis Method. Gilmore, T.; Madaule, P.; and Thompson, B., eds. Toronto: Listening Center Press, 1989.

Presents Alfred Tomatis' research on the ear, brain, and communication. Reveals the role of listening in human communication with specific attention to learning disabilities.

The Conscious Ear. Tomatis, Alfred. Tarrytown, NY: Staton Hill Books, 1991.

An autobiography of Alfred Tomatis, a pioneer in sound therapy, and its effects on learning and behavioral disabilities. He discusses the integration of the whole person and the interdependence on balanced listening. Gives alternatives to medication in the field of learning disabilities.

Mind, Music, and Imagery. Merritt, Stephanie. New York: Plume Press, 1990.

Explores how music can affect human emotions, spirit, and body. Offers a program and forty exercises designed to stimulate creativity, reduce stress, increase memory retention, and promote health.

MusicMedicine. Spintge, Ralph. St. Louis: MMB Music, 1992.

An up-to-date compendium of fine music therapists and researchers. Detailed articles on clinical studies around the world.

Music and Miracles. Campbell, Don. Wheaton, IL: Quest Books, 1992.

Collection of essays from researchers, healers, and musicians about the ability of music to create spiritual, mental, and physical change.

Music: Physician for Times to Come. Campbell, Don. Wheaton, IL: Quest Books, 1991.

A collection of essays by musicians, music therapists, physicians, scientific researchers, and spiritual teachers on the impact of sound vibrations as seen by modern science as well as Eastern, Western, Christian, and esoteric traditions.

The Roar of Silence. Campbell, Don. Wheaton, IL: Quest Books, 1989.
An artistic and scientific look at the healing powers of breath, tone, and music with lessons on using sound as a healing force.

Sound Health. Halpern, Steven. New York: Harper and Row, 1985.
An easy-to-understand book that draws on scientific and medical research, history, art, and psychology to explain the effects of music and sound on body, mind, and spirit.

"No illness which can be treated by diet should be treated by any other means."

—Moses Maimonides (1135-1204)

Traditional Chinese Medicine

Traditional Chinese Medicine is an ancient method of health care that combines the use of medicinal herbs, acupuncture, food therapy, massage, and therapeutic exercise. It has proven effective for many conditions, including chronic degenerative disease, cancer, infectious disease, allergies, childhood ailments, heart disease, and AIDS.

Traditional Chinese Medicine (TCM) has been practiced for over three thousand years and, at present, one-quarter of the world's population makes use of one or more of its therapies. A complete system of medicine, it has been selected by the World Health Organization for worldwide propagation to meet the health care needs of the twenty-first century.[1]

"The philosophy of Traditional Chinese Medicine is more preventive in nature than conventional medicine, and views the practice of waiting to treat a disease until the symptoms are full-blown as being similar to 'digging a well after one has become thirsty."

TCM's approach to health and healing is very different from modern Western medicine. TCM looks for the underlying causes of imbalances and patterns of disharmony in the body, and views each patient as being unique. Western medicine generally provides treatment for a specific illness, whereas Traditional Chinese Medicine addresses how the illness manifests in a particular patient and treats the patient, not just the disease. As Roger Hirsh, O.M.D., L.Ac., Dipl. NCCA, of Santa Monica, California, explains, "The conventional Western physician focuses predominantly on the pathogenic factor (the disease), rather than the response of the patient to the factor."

Fundamentals of Traditional Chinese Medicine

The philosophy of Traditional Chinese Medicine is preventive in nature and views the practice of waiting to treat a disease until the symptoms are full-blown as being similar to "digging a well after one has become thirsty."[2] In line with this, TCM makes a point of educating the patient with regard to lifestyle so that the patient can assist in his or her own therapeutic process. The TCM practitioner educates the patient about diet, exercise, stress management, rest, and relaxation.

As Traditional Chinese Medicine views the human body as a reflection of the natural world—the part containing the whole—the TCM doctor thinks and speaks in analogies with nature. The flows of energy and fluids in the body are spoken of as channels and rivers, seas and reservoirs. A diagnosis might describe the body in terms of the elements—wind, heat, cold, dryness, dampness. Despite this poetic language, TCM is not a folk medicine but a comprehensive professional discipline, based on an alternative, complete system of thought.

The terms *yin* and *yang* are used by the TCM practitioner to describe the various opposing physical conditions of the body. These terms stem from a basic Chinese concept describing the interdependence and relationship of opposites. Much as hot cannot be understood or defined without first having experienced cold, *yin* cannot exist without its opposite *yang*, and *yang* cannot exist without *yin*. Together, the two complementary poles form a whole.

See Acupuncture, Qigong.

Roger Jahnke, O.M.D., of Santa Barbara, California, explains that when applying these concepts to the human body, "*Yin* refers to the tissue of the organ, while *yang* refers to its activity. In *yin* deficiency, the organ does not have enough raw materials to function. In *yang* deficiency, the organ does not react adequately when needed."

These two conditions are forever connected, though, "in a system of interdependence and interrelatedness," adds Maoshing Ni, D.O.M., Ph.D., L.Ac., Vice-President of Yo San University of Traditional Chinese Medicine in Santa Monica, California. For example, says Dr. Ni, a yin deficiency in thyroid hormone levels, the raw material of the thyroid gland, would eventually cause a yang deficiency in the thyroid, as its function becomes impaired by the lack of hormones. Likewise, poor thyroid function, a yang deficiency, would eventually result in a yin deficiency, as the gland's output of hormones decreased.

Traditional Chinese Medicine also introduces a major component of the body, *qi* (also referred to as *chi*), that Western medicine does not even acknowledge. *Qi*, according to Dr. Ni, is difficult to define. "We call it life force, and it is all inclusive of the many types of energy within the body and is essential for life itself," he says. This vital life energy flows through the body following pathways called meridians.

These meridians flow along the surface of the body, and through the internal organs, with each meridian being given the name of the organ through which it flows, such as "liver," or "large intestine." Organs can be accessed for treatment through their specific meridians, and illness can occur when there is a blockage of *qi* in these channels. Therefore it is essential in Traditional Chinese Medicine to keep the *qi* flowing in order to maintain health. The healthy individual has an abundance of *qi* flowing smoothly through the meridians and organs. With this flow, the organs are able to harmoniously support each other's functions.

Five Phase Theory

The interrelationships of the organs to each other is another important concept in Traditional Chinese Medicine. Ten organs are arranged into a system that places each in one of five categories: fire, earth, metal, water, and wood. This system, called the Five Phase Theory, is based on the premise that each organ either nourishes or inhibits the proper functioning of another organ, just as the basic elements also act either adversely or beneficially on each other. "The Chinese have, for thousands of years, watched how things worked around them in order to understand why things happen, why things transform from one thing to another," says Dr. Ni. "They've taken this same conceptual model and applied it to the human body and found it really works well."

For example, as fire melts metal, so does the heart, which is associated with fire, control the lungs, which are associated with metal. Likewise, as metal cuts wood, the lungs control the liver; as wood penetrates the earth, the liver controls the spleen; as the earth dams water, the spleen controls the kidneys; and as water quenches fire, the kidneys control the heart.

The organs are also divided up into two groups of *yin* and *yang* organs. "The heart, spleen, lungs, kidney, and liver belong to the *yin* group, because they are what we call more substantial organs, more

Element	***Yin* Organ**	***Yang* Organ**
Fire	Heart	Small intestine
Earth	Spleen	Stomach
Metal	Lungs	Large intestine
Water	Kidney	Bladder
Wood	Liver	Gallbladder

solid," explains Dr. Ni, "whereas, the *yang* organs are hollow organs like the small intestine, stomach, large intestine, and bladder, where things just pass through. They're more functional—remember, yang is function, action, and yin is more passive, solid, substantial—that's why they're categorized that way."

"In treating a patient, a TCM practitioner first looks for patterns in the details of his or her clinical observations of that patient. This allows the practitioner to discover the disharmony in the system of that individual."

Dr. Ni adds that "there is a synergistic relationship in all the organs," as in all the elements, so the interactions are a little more complex when deciphering disease symptoms. "A patient came to me with stomach ulcers for which the prescribed medication gave some relief, but had a side effect, constipation. He took a laxative to deal with the constipation, but then he developed a cough and chronic bronchitis. The medication prescribed for the bronchitis also had a side effect, a urinary tract infection. He also developed lower back pain. Additional antibiotics for the urinary tract infection then caused liver problems—a congested feeling and pain. Finally he became irritable, emotionally unbalanced, and had difficulty sleeping. This was the point at which he came to me.

"Deficiency in earth (stomach) led to deficiency in both metal organs (large intestine and lungs). As the metal organs weakened, it impacted the water (kidney and bladder), and in turn affected wood (liver) which affected fire (heart)—so that all five organs became involved in the Five Phase Theory sequence. The original problem had been caused by excess stomach cold, due to *qi* deficiency. This had been caused by poor digestion of the raw food diet he had adopted, but the subsequent problems were caused by the medication he had been taking. I took him off the medication and treated him with acupuncture, herbs, and food therapy. After about two and a half months he became healthy."

The Practice of Traditional Chinese Medicine

In treating a patient, a TCM practitioner first looks for patterns in the details of his or her clinical observations of that patient. This allows the practitioner to discover the disharmony in the system of that individual. Familiar with symptoms that are standard to each disease, the doctor also considers what symptoms or behaviors would be especially telling to the individual patient. For example, some people are very active and constantly moving, even red in the face, yet these appearances may not indicate any malady. On the other hand, it is perfectly normal for others to exhibit slowness and inactivity. It is against this individual landscape that the TCM practitioner attempts to correctly assess the pattern of disharmony when an individual becomes ill.

A pattern may be so commonly associated with a certain treatment that the pattern and treatment carry the same name. But often the doctor must develop a strategy by carefully balancing many details. Stomach ulcers, for instance, may originate in very different patterns of disharmony, although the resulting ulcers may appear identical. Because the roots of the disease are diametrically opposed, each type of ulcer may also require a very different type of treatment than the other, and the wrong treatment could make things even worse. "Yet in Western medicine, ulcers are generally treated with whatever anti-ulcer medication there may be, without differentiating," says Dr. Ni. "What Chinese medicine does is it deciphers the response of the patient. How is the patient's body reacting to the illness, to the cause of the illness? It's these patterns that we seek to determine and then treat accordingly." Alternatively, people with different symptoms, but the same pattern of disharmony, can often be treated by the same medicines or therapies.

"The TCM practitioner also looks at the impact of a wide range of personal and environmental factors. Mood influences, activity, sex, food, drugs, weather, and seasons of the year can each affect the healing process."

Methods of Diagnosis

A first-time patient, accustomed to Western medicine, may be surprised that TCM diagnosis does not require procedures such as blood tests, x-rays, endoscopy (the inspection of the inside of a body cavity by an endoscope), or exploratory surgery. Instead, the TCM practitioner performs the four following, noninvasive methods of investigation:

- Inspection of the complexion, general demeanor, body language, and tongue
- Questioning the patient about symptoms, medical history, diet, lifestyle, history of the present complaint, and any previous or concurrent therapies received
- Listening to the tone and strength of the voice
- Smelling any body excretions, the breath, or the body odor
- Palpation (or feeling with the fingers) of the pulse at the radial arteries of both wrists (pulse diagnosis), the abdomen, and the meridians and/or acupuncture points

Through pulse diagnosis, a skilled practitioner can examine the strength or weakness of the *qi* and "blood," which includes lymph and other bodily fluids, and assess how these affect each of the organs, tissues, and layers of the body. The practitioner will also look at the impact of a wide range of personal and environmental factors. Mood influences, activity, sex, food, drugs, weather, and seasons of the year can each affect health and the healing process. "All these factors need to be weighed when making a diagnosis," states Dr. Hirsh, "but the presence of one factor doesn't always warrant a disease outcome."

Similarly, one diagnostic method will not always be able to adequately determine a pattern. The TCM practitioner will use all these various diagnostic tools to cross-check and amplify the other methods until the practitioner is certain that the pattern of disharmony he or she has found is correct.

Dr. Ni explains that what TCM practitioners try to do with all forms of diagnosis is look at illness in the body from the point of view of function. "Too much function or too little function—illness can really be simplified in this way," says Dr. Ni. "Either your body is not having enough of a substance or having too much of it in an illness. Or it's functioning too quickly and too fast, or it's functioning too slowly. If you categorized the body in those simplistic terms, that's what illness is all about. For example, how do you get colds? In Chinese medicine, we recognize that you get colds because your body cannot adjust quickly enough to changes in the environment such as cold weather. This allows the bacteria or virus, whatever it may be, to invade.

"Because of this understanding, TCM treatment, unlike most Western medical practices, will not only treat the inevitable symptoms of the disease, in this case the actual cold, but will also treat the underlying cause, the body's inability to adapt to change quickly enough to resist the invading microbes."

TRADITIONAL CHINESE MEDICINE IN THE TWENTIETH CENTURY

Today, Traditional Chinese Medicine (TCM) is a synthesis of the best of China's scholastic and professional medicine, empirically proven and time-tested folk remedies, and modern technology. Since the early part of the twentieth century, Chinese doctors began to incorporate elements of modern Western medicine, including modern physiology, pharmaceutical medicines, and treatment and modern research protocols. In 1949 a special effort to update TCM began when the post-war communist Chinese government began to revise and unify its standards of practice in an effort to improve public health. National committees of the finest TCM doctors of every medical specialty compared the knowledge gained from their own experience. Seeking new ideas, researchers fanned out into the vast Chinese countryside to interview peasant healers. As a result, many new remedies were added to the repertoire of formally approved TCM treatments.

Treatments in Traditional Chinese Medicine

Historically, a Chinese doctor was known as someone who prescribed herbal medicine, but Traditional Chinese Medicine today incorporates a wide range of methods of treatment, including herbal medicine, acupuncture, dietary therapy, and massage.

Herbal Medicine: Herbs are still a primary part of a TCM treatment. A prescription consists of generous piles of ingredients, distributed in paper packets containing a day or two's dose. The visually intriguing ingredients—perhaps bark, roots, or oyster shell—come from the vegetable, animal, and mineral kingdoms. The formulas may contain from six to nineteen different substances and are assembled with great care. These are prescribed to treat the root of the disease and its manifestation, and the formula must also be balanced within itself.

Although the herbs are taken internally as decoctions (herbs boiled in water), TCM doctors also prescribe pills, powders, syrups, tinctures, inhalants, suppositories, enemas, douches, soaks, plasters, poultices, and salves. Specific foods may also be part of the protocol. "What we do is learn about the healing properties of each food," says Dr. Ni. "For example, ginger. Ginger is warming, and it's pungent. It has a healing property of warming the stomach to dispel cold, arresting diarrhea, and settling the stomach from nausea. When you're armed with knowledge like this, then you can begin to apply a whole system, in a very systematic way, for recommending a particular diet to your patients that would assist in their recovery."

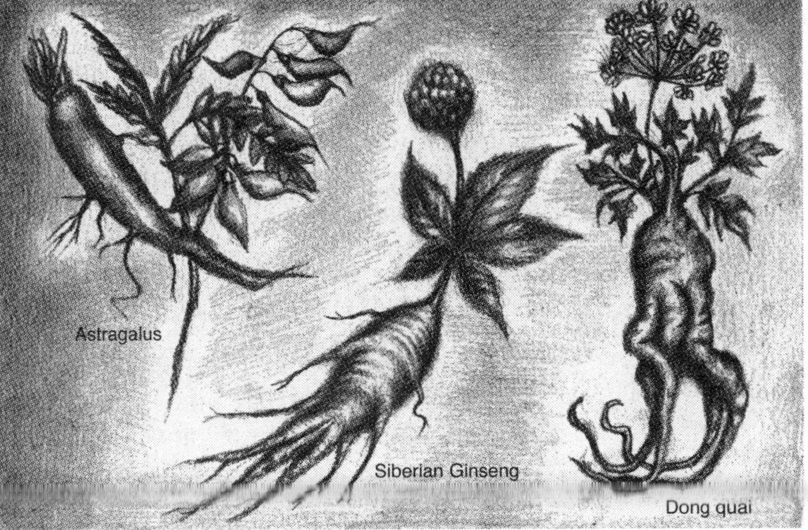

Chinese herbs.

Dr. Ni recalls a patient who came to see him after suffering from three weeks of excruciating hemorrhoid pain that his medical doctor felt could only be relieved through surgery. "He couldn't sit, he couldn't sleep, he couldn't walk, every position hurt him so badly," explains Dr. Ni. "In Chinese medicine, this condition is diagnosed as having spleen *qi* deficiency. In other words, his spleen energy was weak and so the rectum was prolapsing, causing hemorrhoids.

"Realistically, with acupuncture, we have to treat continuously every day or every other day for a week or two, but, he lived far away and couldn't come in. So I said go home and eat four yams a day. Within a week's time—one week—his hemorrhoids completely disappeared, and the pain, of course, went away too.

"When he went back to his doctor, his proctologist, he was told that hemorrhoids don't just go away, as severe as he had them, and that they wouldn't go away from yams. But I know that yams have a healing property for strengthening the spleen *qi* and, therefore, pulling the hemorrhoids back up because that was the cause of his hemorrhoids." Dr. Ni adds, "I wouldn't recommend yams for every hemorrhoid condition, though, because, again, in Chinese medicine, hemorrhoids may have many different causes."

Acupuncture: Acupuncture is also extensively used in Traditional Chinese Medicine. Using the meridian system and its thousands of corresponding surface points, acupuncture uses special needles placed strategically into these "acupoints" to help correct and rebalance the flow of energy within the specific meridian, consequently relieving pain and/or restoring health. Moxibustion is also sometimes used, which is the burning of special "moxa" herbs on or above a specific acupoint.

Massage: Massage and manipulation are also integral parts of the modern practice of TCM, including professional remedial massage therapies such as osteopathic and chiropractic adjustments. "There are many different massages in Chinese medicine," says Dr. Ni. "We have one massage called *Tui Na*, which is a combination of acupressure, massage, and manipulation.

"The purpose of massage is not dissimilar to acupuncture, in that the whole goal is to promote the flow of *qi* and to remove blockages, thereby alleviating any imbalances." Dr. Ni adds that massage is most often used in conjunction with other treatment therapies, such as acupuncture. "They are often used together for musculoskeletal problems such as a sprain."

Qigong and other therapeutic exercises are another aspect of TCM, particularly as a means of stress reduction and preventative therapy. Meditative relaxation, calisthenics, internal energy exercises, and the laying on of hands are all incorporated into the overall Chinese medicine approach, as well as an emphasis on spiritual meditation.

Conditions Treated by Traditional Chinese Medicine

Traditional Chinese Medicine addresses the full range of human illness. While best known for treating chronic illnesses such as asthma, allergies, headaches, high blood pressure, gallbladder disease, lupus, diabetes, and gynecological disorders, TCM also treats acute, infectious illness. Extensive research is continuously being pursued in a wide range of TCM applications and reported on in scores of medical journals published around the world.[3]

Research has also shown that TCM can effectively complement modern Western medicine when the two systems are used in concert for acute, chronic, or life-threatening diseases.[4] In China, a combination of TCM and modern Western medicine has been shown to be more effective for treating liver cancer than Western medicine alone.[5] TCM can also minimize the hazardous side effects of some Western medicines while reinforcing their positive therapeutic effects.

In his practice, Dr. Hirsh sees many patients in conjunction with Western doctors for infertility problems and is able to design acupuncture treatments that complement and support the other medical procedures. He frequently gives acupuncture treatment to women who have just been artificially inseminated, and he works with patients taking Clomid (a fertility drug) to help regulate the woman's fertility cycle. As Dr. Hirsh states, "Traditional Chinese Medicine can increase the success rate of Western medicine, and at the same time slow down the clock on a woman's aging endocrine system."

THE STORY OF MR. HO

Li Shi-zhen, the Chinese doctor revered for reformalizing Traditional Chinese Medicine in the seventeenth century, told the story of Mr. Ho: "Mr. Ho was an old woodcutter, bent over with age. He lived alone in the forest, which was a good thing, because he could hardly cut wood anymore and had to forage for food to supplement his tiny income. One day he came across a large tuber (which looked like a huge potato), scratched it out of the ground, and made a stew of it. This was all he had to eat for several days. But this was very lucky because, to his amazement, he found himself gradually standing up, having more energy and being able to chop more wood. Attributing this to the plant, he consumed it for several months and gained greater energy—so much that he attracted a young woman whom he married and soon they had several children. The tuber he found (Polygonal multiflorum) *was named 'ho-shou wu' in honor of Mr. Ho."*

In Li Shi-zhen's story, the old woodcutter had kidney weakness which gave rise to a weak lower back, poor sexual function, and the symptoms of old age. Ho-shou-wu helps these conditions and it is a major component of 'sho-wu-chih,' a commercially prepared tea that is drunk for health maintenance by millions of Chinese every day.

East Meets West: A Case History

What is known as hypertension in the West is termed liver fire and can be treated by TCM. Dr. Wu, a famous physician in China, was visited by a forty-two-year-old man who had been diagnosed as having hypertension and the early stages of coronary heart disease. He complained of throbbing temples and soreness at the top of his head. An examination identified the following elements: red (not pink) tongue, deep yellow urine, constipation, poor appetite, painful teeth and eyes, insomnia, pain on the right side of the body, and excessive dreaming. His pulse was "wiry and sinking." The man was diagnosed with "constrained liver *qi* accompanied by liver fire ascending to disturb the head."

The treatment called for harmonizing the liver, cooling the liver fire, and transforming mucus. Twelve herbs were given as a tea for three days and another combination for nine additional days. With this treatment, the patient's blood pressure dropped from 180/130 to 130/90, well within normal range, and soon all his symptoms disappeared. A final herbal prescription was then given, which was taken for a longer period of time to ensure that the patient's blood pressure remained normal.

The Future of Traditional Chinese Medicine

According to Dr. Hirsh, "TCM is continually evolving. I believe that diagnostic technology, advanced surgical procedures, electroacupuncture biofeedback testing, and modern homeopathy are aspects of Western tradition that can be integrated with TCM in order to create an 'Integral Chinese Medicine'.

"I see the need for a quantum leap in medical care," Dr. Hirsh adds. "We have a chance with 'Integral Chinese Medicine' to make that leap. Here in America, we have the finest aspects of Western medicine. What we lack is a system of putting this technology together with other diagnostic and treatment techniques, and this is what TCM has to offer. We need to integrate our ability to identify pathogenic [disease-producing] factors with the therapeutic principles that millions of Chinese practitioners have refined after treating billions of patients.

"The real advantage of Integral Chinese Medicine is that you are integrating this great technology with common sense thinking that has allowed the Chinese to evolve an affordable health care system for 1.3 billion people."

Where to Find Help

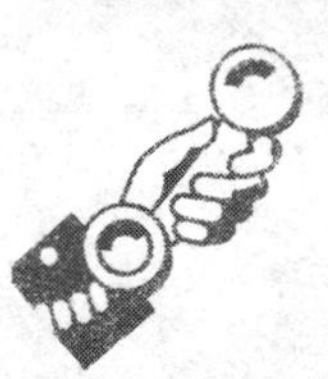

Traditional Chinese Medicine is well suited to anyone looking for safe healing without side effects, answers he or she can understand in everyday human terms, and involvement in and responsibility for his or her own healing. Western patients seeking to avail themselves of the benefits of TCM therapy should contact:

American Association of Acupuncture and Oriental Medicine
4101 Lake Boone Trail, Suite 201
Raleigh, North Carolina 27607
(919) 787-5181

The AAAOM is a national professional trade organization of acupuncturists who meet acceptable standards of competency and can provide you with the names and locations of local members. Referrals by written request only for a five dollar fee.

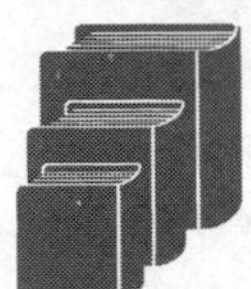

Recommended Reading

Acupuncture Medicine: Its Historical and Clinical Background. Omura, Y. Tokyo: Japan Publications, 1982

In this book, basic concepts of acupuncture points, meridians, and four methods of diagnosis and related topics are explicitly explained. The author provides comments from the viewpoint of Western medicine and sciences.

Between Heaven and Earth: A Guide to Chinese Medicine. Beinfield, H.; and Korngold, E. New York: Ballantine Books, 1991.

Combining Eastern traditions with Western sensibilities, this book addresses three vital areas of Chinese medicine—theory, therapy, and types— to present a comprehensive yet understandable guide to this ancient system.

Chinese Herbal Medicine. Reid, Daniel P. Boston, MA: Shambhala Publications, Inc., 1987.

This large format, highly illustrated book provides the general reader with insight into one of the world's most complex and little-known natural sciences. Describing the art and practice of herbal medicine as applied today, it also highlights the potential to combine modern Western diagnosis and traditional Chinese treatment to form a complete and effective system for both preventative and curative medicine.

***The Essential Book of Traditional Chinese Medicine.* Vols. 1 and 2.** Liu, Y. New York: Columbia University Press, 1988.

The most authoritative works on the subject to be translated into English, these two books represent a unique collaboration between Chinese and American scholars. Volume 1 covers the history, philosophy, and general theory of Traditional Chinese Medicine. Volume 2 addresses the diagnosis, treatment, and prevention of diseases.

Tao of Nutrition. Ni, Maoshing, D.O.M., Ph.D., L.Ac.; and McNease, Cathy. Santa Monica, CA: Seven Star Communications, 1993.

Based on traditional Chinese principles of using food for healing, this book explains the energies and therapeutic properties of foods and details how to create a diet that is most appropriate for health and well-being. Includes sample meal plans, recipes, and dietary recommendations for over forty health conditions.

TAO: *The Subtle Universal Law and the Integral Way of Life.* Ni, Hua-Ching. Santa Monica, CA: Seven Star Communications, 1993.

Provides an introduction to Taoism, the philosophy supporting the concepts of Traditional Chinese Medicine. Also contains much useful information on TCM itself, including techniques for maintaining and enhancing one's health.

The Web That Has No Weaver: Understanding Chinese Medicine. Kaptchuk, Ted. Chicago: Contemporary Books, 1985.

The germinal introduction to Traditional Chinese Medicine for the layperson familiar with Western medicine. It has excellent descriptions of pulse diagnosis, pattern of disharmony, many other concepts, and detailed case histories comparing the TCM view with that of conventional Western medicine.

Zang Fu: The Organ Systems of Traditional Chinese Medicine. Ross, Jeremy. Edinburgh, Scotland: Churchill Livingstone Longman, 1985.

The Zang Fu, the organ systems, are the central core of Traditional Chinese Medicine. This book gives a clear, well organized framework of the theory of Zang Fu, illustrated with many tables, diagrams, and actual case histories, showing how the theoretical principals are applied in clinical practice. It is an essential text for every serious student and practitioner of Traditional Chinese Medicine.

Veterinary Medicine

The principles of alternative medicine are as applicable to animals as they are to human beings. Alternative veterinary medicine is directed toward maintaining natural good health. Animal treatment and healing are achieved using gentle yet effective methods, to treat not only symptoms, but to cure their underlying conditions.

Veterinary medicine has been revolutionized in the past decade. With both domestic and wild animals, veterinarians are now using the same alternative therapy used in humans, such as acupuncture, homeopathy, nutrition, vitamin and mineral supplementation, herbs, electroacupuncture biofeedback testing, and chiropractic, to directly stimulate an animal's immune system, strengthen its vital life force, and alleviate any disequilibrium in the body.

Christopher Day, M.A., Vet.M.B., M.R.C.V.S., Vet.F.F.Hom., who runs an alternative animal clinic in England says, "Medical alternatives such as homeopathy, acupuncture, herbs, aromatherapy, Bach flower remedies, and chiropractic provide a vast therapeutic armory that not only outweighs modern conventional medicine in scope, but also in capability. At our clinic we very rarely need to resort to modern drugs, and then only to provide symptom relief. Alternative medicine provides the key to cure, whereas conventional drugs tend only to suppress."

> *"There is nothing in conventional medicine today that treats chronic degenerative conditions as successfully as holistic therapies."*
>
> —Joanne Stefanatos, D.V.M., President, American Holistic Veterinary Association

According to Joanne Stefanatos, D.V.M., President of the American Holistic Veterinary Medical Association, "There is nothing in conventional medicine today that treats chronic degenerative conditions as successfully as holistic therapies." Dr. Stefanatos has found that holistic veterinary medicine has proven to be the best method of treatment for animal disorders such as feline leukemia; feline peritonitis (inflammation of the membrane lining of the abdominal cavity); radial nerve paralysis (loss of sensation and function in the network of nerves that supply the limbs); distemper; arthritis; cataracts; heart, liver, and kidney disease; chronic skin conditions; hip dysplasia (abnormal development of calcium surrounding the hip); and pesticide, metal, and chemical toxicities.[1]

Other veterinarians, like Richard Pitcairn, D.V.M., Ph.D., of Eugene, Oregon, have found the treatment of chronic disease by allopathic methods to be frustrating and ineffective. "My change to holistic medicine has revitalized my practice," says Dr. Pitcairn. "Success with homeopathy, especially with chronic disease, is very personally rewarding. I have used homeopathy as my primary means of therapy since 1978, emphasizing good nutrition and vitamin and mineral supplements. The reason for my switching to homeopathy is simple: It is much more effective than any other system of medicine I have used before."

The reason for this effectiveness and the consistency of the results can be explained very simply, according to H. C. Gurney, D.V.M., of Conifer, Colorado. "Animals do not have the power to reason whether a treatment is going to work or not, it either will or it won't. A drug placebo [a substance having no pharmacological effect] will not have the same psychological effect on an animal as it might on a human, and, likewise, an animal will not be skeptical of an alternative medical approach, as a person might."

VACCINATING YOUR PET

Although vaccinations are part of a dog or cat's routine health care, pet owners should be aware of the side effects. According to Joanne Stefanatos, D.M.V., of Las Vegas, Nevada, and President of the American Holistic Veterinary Medical Association, the modified live virus used in pet inoculations can cause harmful responses. "Animals can either have an allergic reaction, in which they break out in hives, have diarrhea and/or vomiting, or can develop vaccinosis (a reaction of immune system suppression), which can occur ten days to two weeks after a modified live vaccine is given, causing lethargy." Animals are also sensitive to the formaldehyde and other preservatives in vaccines.

Rabies is the only vaccine required by law for pets in the United States, but vaccinations for contagious illnesses such as parvo, corona, and distemper are also recommended by veterinarians. "I advise pet owners to get these vaccinations for their animals," says Dr. Stefanatos, "but I also suggest using a killed virus (as opposed to a modified live virus), and not giving more than one vaccine in a day." Dr. Stefanatos also supplements vaccines with the homeopathic Thuja *60X injection to prevent reactions.*

An animal's system is so influenced by vaccinations that Dr. Stefanatos recommends using only homeopathic vaccinations for domestic animals over eight years of age, who have been previously vaccinated yearly. "Their systems retain enough of the antibodies to fight against illness for the rest of their lives, even in dogs and cats living to age twenty."

Alternative Veterinary Prevention and Treatments

Alternative veterinarians are making use of the entire range of alternative disciplines available today, with particular emphasis on diet and nutritional concerns, acupuncture, chiropractic, homeopathy, and electroacupuncture biofeedback. Flower remedies (which relieve the emotions) have also proven to be very effective. It is important, though, that a proper diagnosis be made by a practitioner who has experience with these modalities. For example, as cats are particularly sensitive to herbs, felines who are given too strong a dose or the wrong type of herb can be adversely affected.

Diet and Nutrition

Alternative veterinarians agree that diet is the critical cornerstone of a total health care program for any animal or pet. Good nutrition is the key not just in treatment but in the prevention of animal disease.

"Start with diet," urges Dr. Pitcairn. "Is the food fresh and natural or highly processed and of an inferior quality? Will it support health?" Unfortunately pet owners often fail to pay attention to the food they give their pets.

Veterinarians who practice alternative medicine agree that animals should not be fed commercial pet food. "Processed, devitalized food creates disease while energetic, live natural food offers life and good health," says Dr. Stefanatos. Canned pet foods, for example, are often filled with toxic chemicals and additives (often not listed on the can), and may contain potentially harmful by-products. Additives like sodium nitrite, butylated hydroxyanisole (BHA), butylated hydroxytoluene (BHT), lead, artificial flavorings and colors, salt, and sugar should be strictly avoided. Slaughterhouse wastes, known as the four D's—tissues from animals that are dead, dying, disabled, or diseased when they arrive at the slaughterhouse—are a common ingredient to canned pet foods.[2] These wastes can include moldy, rancid, or spoiled processed meats, as well as tissues too severely riddled with cancer to be eaten by people.

"Holistic veterinarians agree that diet is the critical cornerstone of a total health care program for any animal or pet. Good nutrition is the key not just in treatment but in the prevention of animal disease."

Dr. Pitcairn recommends his clients feed their pets fresh, uncooked whole foods like meats, soft vegetables, and fruits along with well-cooked whole grains that can be flavored with broths. Dr. Stefanatos considers the best food for a pet to be natural food, and recommends that clients prepare their pets' diets from scratch.

Raw beef bones are a good choice once a week (no chicken or pork chop bones), but they should be thrown away after four hours to reduce the risk of bacteria. Safflower and olive oils are good, but hydrogenated fats and oils should be avoided. For pets with a sweet tooth, baked yams and dried fruits are canine and feline favorites.

Dr. Stefanatos also recommends that pets be fed twice a day rather than one large meal, as it helps to reduce overeating while promoting digestion. Other tips include:

- Keep food at room temperature.
- Avoid using a microwave to heat food.
- Replace tap water with bottled or filtered, especially with birds.
- Never feed your pet food that has been known to have been irradiated (it not only decreases enzymes and the vitamin/mineral content of the food, but food irradiation has been proven to cause tumors and cancers in laboratory rats and mice).
- Exercise your pet regularly (it's as important as diet), and allow your pet plenty of sunlight.

Wheat, milk, sugar, salt, colorings, flavorings, and preservatives should be avoided, says Dr. Day, and food should be from known organic sources. If an animal is being fed food that is not organic, it is difficult to avoid the risk of antibiotic residues. Also, feeding a single type of food day in and day out is liable to introduce deficiencies and toxicities even if the food is designed to be "complete." The safest way to achieve a balanced diet is to offer plenty of variety.

Food should not be prepared in aluminum pots and plastic feeding bowls should be eliminated. "I once had an epileptic dog I had been unsuccessfully treating for eighteen months," says Dr. Day. "One day its plastic feeding bowl was accidentally broken and replaced with a ceramic one. The fits stopped immediately."

Acupuncture

Founded in the early 1970s to instruct other veterinarians in veterinary acupuncture, the International Veterinary Acupuncture Society has certified over seven hundred veterinarians worldwide to date. Grady Young, D.V.M., of Thomasville, Georgia, a co-founder of IVAS, found that acupuncture did not discriminate between the species. As with human acupuncture, which provides a means of transferring excess energy from certain meridians to other meridians deficient in energy, veterinary acupuncture rebalances the body's total energy system to facilitate healing and health. Veterinarians report that acupuncture has been shown to be effective in treating arthritis, canine hip dysplasia, kidney disorders, metabolic imbalances, allergies, aging disorders, cataracts, and spinal disc problems.

"Veterinarians report that acupuncture has been shown to be effective in treating arthritis, canine hip dysplasia, kidney disorders, metabolic imbalances, allergies, aging disorders, cataracts, and spinal disk problems."

Dr. Gurney states that the majority of the cases he treats with acupuncture fall into various categories of chronic disease. "The real advantage of this procedure is in avoiding the use of drugs, and sometimes surgical techniques, to treat these problems. While these methods may result in short-term gains, it is usually at the expense of long-term quality health."

Dr. Gurney testifies that 85 percent of the animals he treats demonstrate clear improvement after only three acupuncture treatments, but that the most important use of the procedure is for "health maintenance," after the initial crisis is over.

"For example, steroid therapy may well rescue an animal from an acute or life-threatening episode, but the use of steroids to combat long-term chronic illness can also lead to the loss of normal function in the adrenal glands, which regulate many of the body's processes essential for a healthy life."

Dr. Day recounts treating a German shepherd who almost died from steroid therapy. "When it came to me, the dog had already been given massive doses of steroids by a local veterinarian, under university supervision. The dog nearly died. It took us three weeks to revive him properly using homeopathy." A recurrent lameness in its left foreleg, for which the dog had been receiving steroids, was subsequently treated with acupuncture and the dog has been problem-free for over four years now.

See Acupuncture.

In cases such as ligament injuries, skin conditions, vomiting, and diarrhea, veterinary acupuncture can have a truly healing effect. And while veterinary acupuncture cannot cure cancer, John Limehouse, D.V.M., of North Hollywood, California, says he has seen a positive effect on tumors. A young Great Pyrenees was brought in suffering extreme pain from sarcoma of the femur. After four acupuncture treatments, she was walking comfortably and her tumor had shrunk 75 percent. Dr. Limehouse explains that the acupuncture released polypeptides (a union of two or more amino acids) that in turn helped control the inflammation.[3]

Acupuncture can also be a primary modality for the treatment of traumatic injury, according to Dr. Stefanatos. "A two-year-old shepherd-dobie mix fell out of a moving truck, severely bruising his right front leg, resulting in radial nerve paralysis. He hobbled on three legs for several weeks while veterinarians tried steroids, muscle relaxers, and antibiotics to no avail, finally recommending amputation of the leg."

Instead, the dog was brought to Dr. Stefanatos. "After only five acupuncture treatments, the leg was restored to its full, normal use."

Environmental Factors

An alternative veterinarian looks closely at the environment of the owner and his or her pet. Are there problems with the water? Are the water pipes old and rusty? Are there excessive levels of radon or other common environmental hazards? Is the pet chewing on plants that have been sprayed with toxic pesticides?

The major environmental deterrent to an animal's good health is ground level chemicals and toxins. Common yard pesticides are the worst offenders, easily absorbed not only from grasses and soil, but through the skin as well. A good place to begin is to stop using them. According to Dr. Joanne Stefanatos, D.V.M., of Las Vegas, Nevada, the single main cause of the increase in cancer in animals today is from pesticides such as DDT and diazinon. DDT and PCB pesticides are also the main cause of mammary tumors in animals, which is also the main cause of most animal nervous disorders.

Richard Pitcairn, D.V.M., Ph.D., of Eugene, Oregon, states that household wastes and shelf products can pose major problems for pets. Cats and dogs have been known to lick up antifreeze for its sweet taste. Automotive products, poison baits, solvents, cosmetics, disinfectants, medicines, and especially soiled garbage are all a common source of pet poisoning. Also, Dr. Pitcairn cites poisoning from the accumulation of lead and fluoride in water as common and serious matters to a pet's well-being.[4]

Even the water your animals drink can have an adverse effect upon them, says H. C. Gurney, D.V.M., of Conifer, Colorado. He recommends using only purified or distilled water. "Good water can aid our animals, while poor quality water can seriously add to their health problems in terms of adding pollutants or excess chemicals the body is ill-prepared to deal with."

Dr. Gurney continues, "Unless you have gone to the expense of a complete water test, you really don't know for certain what your animal is drinking." Some waters contain nitrate, nitrite, and nitrosamine compounds, which interfere with the proper absorption of vitamin A, which can lead to poor coat quality and breeding problems (small litters, retained placentas, weak puppies, and miscarriages). Other waters have been shown to have a significant concentration of metal isotopes and heavy metal, which can be highly carcinogenic.

Homeopathy

Carvel Tiekert, D.V.M., of Bel Air, Maryland, Executive Director and originator of the American Holistic Veterinary Medical Association, believes that homeopathy has taken on an increasingly important role in alternative veterinary medicine, as it integrates with all other modalities of treatment and allows the animal to heal naturally from the inside out. "At least 75 percent of all animals examined by alternative veterinarians now receive some form of homeopathic treatment," he states.

See Homeopathy.

Dr. Stefanatos has found homeopathy to be a powerful tool in her arsenal of alternative treatments, even in emergency situations. "When I first saw the six-week-old African lioness, Simba Samburu, she appeared to be dying; semi-comatose and convulsing from diazinon pesticide intoxication after ingesting grass that had been sprayed. Homeopathic diazinon 30x saved her life, reviving her just minutes from death. She was blind for three days after the episode, but by the end of the week had made a complete recovery. She is now three years old, beautiful, and very healthy."

Dr. Day presents a stark contrast between the procedures of conventional medicine and those of homeopathy. "An eighteen-month-old West Highland white bitch came in with "dry eye" in one eye. Four months previously, the other eye had been affected, treated conventionally for one month and then been submitted for surgery for a parotid duct transplant. This had relieved the condition but the initial damage to the cornea remained.

"When the second eye became affected it was around Easter, so no surgery time was immediately available. The dog was then brought to me in order to stabilize her condition until the surgery could be scheduled. I started her on a homeopathic injection treatment twice daily plus artificial tears as necessary. It soon became obvious that the artificial tears were needed less and less often until eventually the impending operation was canceled and the artificial tears were stopped altogether. There was no damage to the eye and it is still completely healthy without treatment to date."[5]

Veterinary Energy Medicine

"In the past, medicine has relied on surgery and drugs. The medicine of the future will be energy based," states Dr. Stefanatos. "We are on the verge of a totally new era of understanding of biological processes, medical diagnosis, and a way of therapy based on the electromagnetic environment. Because a change in energy precedes a change in structure, electroacupuncture biofeedback testing can now detect pathological dysfunction in animals before any physical symptoms appear."

Electroacupuncture biofeedback testing is a method of testing based on measurement of the electrical properties of acupuncture points. Using an electroacupuncture biofeedback instrument to detect energy imbalances, veterinarians can then prescribe the proper treatment—be it acupuncture, homeopathy, nutrition, or, as in most cases, a combination thereof. Dr. Stefanatos uses electroacupuncture biofeedback to test healthy animals in order to discover bacteria, viruses, fungi, or pesticides that can be eliminated from their bodies before they become destructive.

See Chiropractic Energy Medicine.

"A champion blood line Akita female brought in for inability to get pregnant was tested by electroacupuncture biofeedback and found to have DDT pesticides and brucella abortus bacteria as her main toxins," says Dr. Stefanatos. "I gave her homeopathic remedies two times daily for one week and then treated her with acupuncture. She became pregnant with her next heat and delivered twelve puppies, all healthy."

"As old as acupuncture and homeopathy are, I believe that bioenergetic medicine is the medicine of the future," agrees Dr. Limehouse. "It will allow us to return to true preventative medicine. We will someday look back on these times and feel like we were in the dark ages of healing."[6]

Chiropractic

Sharon Willoughby, D.V.M., D.C., of Port Byron, Illinois, a veterinarian and a chiropractor, pioneered chiropractic for animals in America. She has treated and adjusted a wide variety of animals ranging from canaries to cats, dogs, cows, horses, and goats. Dr. Willoughby established the American Veterinary Chiropractic Association (AVCA) in 1989 and developed a certification course for veterinarians and chiropractors. So far, the AVCA has certified 150 veterinarians and chiropractors across the country.

Dr. Willoughby works extensively with performance horses in her practice; hunter/jumper, racing, saddlebred, and saddle seat classes, barrel horses, as well as reining and cutting horses. "We run into a lot of gait and performance problems with these animals, such as undiagnosed lameness, gait abnormalities, difficultly moving in a certain direction, a decreased level of flexibility and back pain," says Dr. Willoughby.

"The major environmental deterrent to an animal's good health is ground level chemicals and toxins. Common yard pesticides are the worst offenders, easily absorbed not only from grasses and soil, but through the skin as well."

"With all these horses, the sport requires them to be at the top of their athletic and physical performance ability. Chiropractic can do wonders for these horses both as a preventative to maintain optimal functioning and, when necessary, to treat lameness or other injuries."

Dr. Willoughby also does a considerable amount of work on smaller animals, particularly dogs. "I see a lot of geriatric dogs, that are very stiff, and are having difficulty getting up and down, where their quality of life has decreased considerably. There's a certain amount of acceptance among the public that since they are old, they should be like this.

"With chiropractic we are not restoring them to six months of age but we see these dogs returned to an increased vigor for life. They are happier, they are playing more, they are working with their owners again, they are not sleeping as much, and they are much less stiff than they were."

Dr. Stefanatos has also found chiropractic to work where traditional medical therapy had failed. In a similar case, a Chihuahua was brought in to her for a second opinion with a full set of head and neck x-rays, a complete blood panel, and a CAT scan, because for the last six weeks the dog had had a head tilt and vertigo. A simple chiropractic adjustment during examination corrected the head tilt and restored the head to its proper position.

Another problem addressed by chiropractic is traumatic injury from accidents. Often, according to Dr. Willoughby, the obvious trauma is taken care of, but not the back problems that may continue. "For example, a dog is hit by a car, it gets its laceration sewn up and fracture fixed, but its spine is left unattended. These types of injuries, which can also include whiplash along with general trauma to the spinal column, can be very great. This is another niche that traditional veterinary medicine doesn't address: those residual effects that will undermine the health of the dog or cat or horse hit by a car, for years.

The Future of Alternative Veterinary Medicine

"My goal is to educate the public to start thinking about prevention rather than disease," says Dr. Willoughby. "I don't want to be a disease doctor, I want to be a health doctor."

This, in essence, is the major tenet that separates most alternative physicians, medical and veterinarian alike, from their counterparts in conventional drug-based medicine. With the rising cost of health care for both humans and animals, prevention has become the watchword for the future with the alternative community being seen as a leading advocate and facilitator of this change in health philosophy.

Dr. Stefanatos has seen this evidenced in an ever-increasing public interest in alternative therapies, leading more veterinary schools to incorporate them into their standard curriculums.

"More and more veterinarians are seeking certification in homeopathy, acupuncture, and chiropractic than ever before," adds Dr. Stefanatos, as the benefits of these alternative therapies become widely accepted.

Today, with the emergence of energy medicine, veterinarians have the potential to pinpoint and eliminate disease-producing toxins in the body long before they have an opportunity to become destructive. Many veterinarians, such as Drs. Stefanatos and Limehouse, feel that energy medicine represents the future of holistic medicine and holds the key to true preventative health care for both animals and humans.

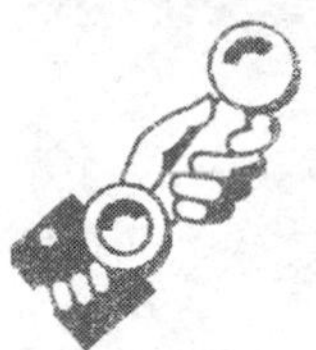

Where to Find Help

To learn more about the use of alternative veterinary medicine, or to locate a veterinarian who employs alternative methods in the treatment of animals, contact:

American Holistic Veterinary Medicine Association
2214 Old Emmorton Road
Bel Air, Maryland 21015
(410) 569-0795
A group of practitioners whose purpose is to function as a forum for the exploration of alternative areas of health care other than acupuncture in veterinary medicine.

American Veterinarian Chiropractic Association
P.O. Box 249
Port Byron, Illinois 61275
(309) 523-3995
Dr. Willoughby is a chiropractor and teaches seminars through AVCA to veterinarians and chiropractors. Also functions as a referral service to the public.

International Veterinary Acupuncture Society
International Journal of Veterinary Acupuncture
2140 Conestoga Road
Chester Springs, Pennsylvania 19425
(215) 827-7245
(215) 827-1366 (Fax)
IVAS offers courses to veterinarians, and provides a list of veterinarians across the country. Proceedings and literature available. A referral service to the public.

Recommended Reading

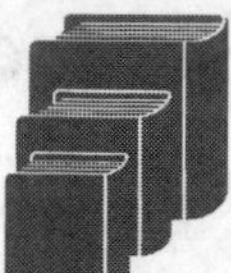

Dr. Pitcairn's Complete Guide to Natural Health for Dogs and Cats. Pitcairn, Richard H., D.V.M., and Pitcairn, Susan Hubble, D.V.M. Emmaus, PA: Rodale Press, 1982.

An excellent book for those who need advice on making a new approach. Diet, exercise, and common pet ailments and their treatments are covered.

Holistic Pet Care Video. Stefanatos, Joanne, D.V.M. Las Vegas, NV: Agape Video Systems, 1325 Vegas Valley Drive, Las Vegas, Nevada 89109, 1991.

A highly informative, two-and-a-half-hour video that covers alternative therapies from acupuncture to vitamin/mineral supplements. Teaches the most common do's and don'ts for animals, and explains how to treat home emergencies.

Keep Your Pet Healthy the Natural Way. Lazarus, Pat. New Canaan, CT: Keats Publishing, 1986.

Written with both the lay person and veterinarian in mind, this book talks extensively about the do's and don'ts of diet. Other chapters deal with arthritis, eye problems, problems with the skin and hair, infectious diseases, heart problems, hypertension, and cancer.

What the Animals Tell Me. Lydecker, Beatrice. New York: Harper & Row, 1989.

Covers pet psychology, emotional problems, the necessity of respect for a pet, and discusses preferred pet products.

Yoga

Yoga is the among the oldest known systems of health practiced in the world today, and research into yoga practices has had a strong impact on the fields of stress reduction, mind/body medicine, and energy medicine. The physical postures, breathing exercises, and meditation practices of yoga have been proven to reduce stress, lower blood pressure, regulate heart rate, and even retard the aging process.

The meaning of the word yoga is "union": the integration of physical, mental, and spiritual energies that enhance health and well-being. First systematically set down in writing by Patanjali in the second century B.C. in the *Yoga Sutras*, yoga teaches a basic principle of mind/body unity: If the mind is chronically restless and agitated, the health of the body will be compromised, and if the body is in poor health, mental strength and clarity will be adversely affected. The practices of yoga can counter these ill effects, restoring mental and physical health.

Many of the original biofeedback studies at the Menninger Foundation in Topeka, Kansas, were conducted on yogis (those adept in the practices of yoga). Their union of mind and body gave them control over functions ranging from thyroid output to heart rate. This first alerted medical doctors and scientists to the link between consciousness and physical functioning. Today, yoga is commonly practiced throughout the world and holds a prominent place in the emerging field of mind/body medicine.

The Eightfold Path of Yoga: A Complete System of Health

Classical yoga is organized into eight "limbs" that provide a complete system of physical, mental, and spiritual health. The eight limbs of yoga are systematically arranged to outline specific lifestyle, hygiene, and detoxification regimens, as well as physical and psychological practices that can lead to a more integrated personal development. Ultimately, yoga helps prepare one for heightened vitality and spiritual awareness.

The first four limbs serve to bring the mind and body into harmony. A strong emphasis is placed upon the necessity of purification and detoxification of the body, and various practices are encouraged to purify the body and the senses, including bowel purification, enemas, nasal cleansing, and cleansing of the eyes. The practices mirror many of the lifestyle changes recommended today by alternative physicians and can be invaluable to maintaining one's quality of health. The first four limbs are comprised of postures and breathing practices. The remaining four limbs deal with stages of meditation.

Yogic Postures (*Asana*)

The most widely known yogic practice is *asana*, often known as Hatha yoga (*asana* means "ease" in Sanskrit). It includes a variety of physical postures and exercises that create immediate changes in the body. There are two main types of *asana* today: meditative and therapeutic.

Meditative *asanas* bring the spine and head into perfect alignment, promoting proper blood flow throughout the body, and bringing the mind into a state of relaxation and stillness that facilitates increased concentration during meditation. At the same time, these *asanas* keep the glands, lungs, and heart properly energized.

Therapeutic *asanas* such as the cobra, locust, spinal twist, and shoulder stand are geared toward improving health and physical well-being, and have been commonly prescribed for patients with back, neck, and joint pain. Originally, therapeutic *asanas* were designed simply to create a condition of ease in the body as a prelude to meditation, and were known as cultural *asanas*, or physical culture asanas. Only within the past fifty to seventy-five years have the postures been applied to specific physical disorders, according to Rudolph Ballentine, M.D., Director of the Center for Holistic Medicine in New York City.

Although yoga postures may involve very little movement, the mind is involved in the performance of every *asana*, to provide discipline, awareness, and a relaxed openness. The discipline and awareness help maintain the posture, and the relaxation and openness help stimulate the circulation of *prana* (life energy), allowing the student to fully experience the power and essence of the posture. According to the *Yoga Sutras*, a properly executed *asana* creates a balance between movement and stillness—exertion and surrender—which is precisely the state of a healthy body. The practitioner learns to regulate autonomic functions like heartbeat and breath, while physical tensions fade into relaxation.

ALTERNATE NOSTRIL BREATHING EXERCISE

Nadi shodhana *(purification of the channels) is a simple* pranayama *exercise that purifies the* nadis *(channels) along which the* prana *flows. It balances the flow of breath in the nostrils and the flow of energy in the* nadis. Nadi shodhana *should be practiced at least twice a day, in the morning and evening.*

Sit upright on a cushion or a firm chair with your head, neck, and body aligned. Breathe in a relaxed fashion from your diaphragm for three complete breaths. Inhalation and exhalation should be of equal length and should be slow, controlled, and free from sounds or jerks. Close your right nostril with the thumb of your right hand and exhale completely through your left nostril. At the end of the exhalation, close your left nostril with your right index finger and inhale through the right nostril.

Repeat this cycle of exhalation with the left nostril and inhalation with the right nostril two more times, always making sure to maintain an equal inhalation and exhalation rate.

At the end of the third inhalation with the right nostril, exhale completely through the same nostril while still keeping the left nostril closed. At the end of the exhalation, close the right nostril and inhale through the left nostril. Repeat the cycle of the exhalation through the right nostril and inhalation through the left nostril two more times. Place the hands on the knees and exhale and inhale through both nostrils evenly for three complete breaths. This completes one cycle of nadi shodhana. *With practice, gradually lengthen the duration of the inhalation and the exhalation.*

Breath Control

Pranayama focuses on regulating the breath (*pranayama* literally means "regulation or control of *prana*, or life force"). Yoga teaches that *prana* circulates throughout in the body in a system of 72,000 subtle nerves or *nadis*. When the flow of *prana* is interrupted through stress, improper diet, or toxins, one's physical, emotional, and mental health are affected. Chronic blockage of the flow of *prana* can eventually lead to illness. *Pranayama* exercises are designed to help remove these blockages and promote a steady and even flow of *prana* throughout the body.

Pranayama is performed in a calm and aware state of mind and can help the practitioner to regulate previously unconscious bodily functions. Studies have demonstrated that the practice of pranayama can aid digestion, cardiac function, and a variety of other physical ailments, and in one study conducted at City Hospital in Nottingham, England, it was found to be particularly effective in reducing the frequency of asthma attacks.[1]

"Studies have demonstrated that the practice of pranayama *can aid digestion, cardiac function, and a variety of other physical ailments, and in one study conducted at City Hospital in Nottingham, England, it was found to be particularly effective in reducing the frequency of asthma attacks."*

The connection of the breath and the mind is a basic principle of yoga. If the mind is calm and focused, the breathing will be steady and rhythmic. If the mind is restless and agitated, the breathing will be restless and agitated. A fundamental instruction in yogic breathing practices is the elimination of any jerkiness in the breathing motion so as to maintain smoothly flowing breath. This will then correlate with subsequent smoothness in the flow of thoughts, making yogic breathing exercises very useful in calming the restlessness of the mind and creating clarity, focus, and heightened energy. Therefore, *pranayama* is often performed as a preparation for meditation.

See Meditation, Mind/Body Medicine.

Meditation

Meditation is a state of focused concentration that may result in a heightened sense of peace and awareness. Meditation is so thoroughly effective in reducing stress and tension that, in 1984, the National Institutes of Health recommended meditation over prescription drugs as the first treatment for mild hypertension.[2] Meditation has also been shown to have a positive effect on immune functions and strengthens the body's defenses against infectious disease.[3] Herbert Benson, M.D., of the Mind-Body Institute at Harvard University, documents how meditation practice can stimulate certain areas of the hypothalamus, affecting breathing rate, oxygen consumption, brain wave rhythm, and blood flow.[4]

"Meditation is so thoroughly effective in reducing stress and tension that, in 1984, the National Institutes of Health recommended meditation over prescription drugs as the first treatment for mild hypertension."

The final stage of yoga is *samadhi*, or spiritual realization, the culmination of a long, disciplined and dedicated practice. In *samadhi*, one is said to enter a fourth state of consciousness, a state of awareness separate from, and beyond, the ordinary states of waking, dream, and sleep.

Conditions Benefited by Yoga

The potential benefits of yoga—health, vitality, and peace of mind—are limited only by one's commitment to its practice. Since the early 1970s, there have been more than a thousand well-designed studies of meditation and yoga, demonstrating their effectiveness in stress and anxiety alleviation, blood pressure and heart rate reduction, improved memory and intelligence, pain alleviation, improved motor skills, relief from addictions, heightened visual and auditory perceptions, and enhanced metabolic and respiratory functions.[5]

Mary Pullig Schatz, M.D., President of the Medical Staff at Centennial Medical Center in Nashville, Tennessee, and author of *Back Care Basics*, reports of a twenty-three year-old diabetic woman who was able to substantially decrease her insulin dependency by a large margin after beginning the practice of yoga. New studies support this anecdotal data,[6] and demonstrate the effectiveness of yoga in the treatment of hypertension, bone marrow depletion, cardiovascular arrhythmia, thyroid disorders, menstrual problems, and other physical ailments.[7]

In several studies, yoga was also shown to significantly reduce both blood pressure and the need for drug therapy in adult patients suffering from hypertension. The patients were also able to maintain these benefits after the cessation of the yoga therapy with only minimal daily relaxation exercises.[8] And in another study dealing solely with the effects of meditation on hypertension, subjects were found to have a reduction in systolic blood pressure after meditative techniques had been taught to them and practiced over a period of twenty weeks. The subjects, though, did not show a reduced need for drug therapy as did those in the yoga study, and when they stopped practicing meditation, their blood pressure returned to its original pretest level.[9]

“Studies have shown that yoga has a beneficial effect on the respiratory system, with results ranging from lowered breathing rates and increased lung capacity to a diminishment of asthma attacks.”

Respiratory functions have been among the most frequently measured variables in scientific evaluations of yoga. Largely because of the emphasis it puts on the breathing system, especially in *pranayama* practices, studies have shown that yoga has a beneficial effect on the respiratory system, with results ranging from lowered breathing rates and increased lung capacity[10] to a diminishment of asthma attacks.[11]

Other studies have suggested that yoga can help reduce serum cholesterol in the blood,[12] and helps fight allergies by increasing levels of histaminase in the blood (an enzyme secreted by the adrenal glands which breaks down histamine, a substance involved in allergic reactions).[13]

An aspect of yoga that distinguishes it from other forms of physical culture (i.e., exercise, sports) is attention to the well-being of the endocrine and nervous systems. These systems are toned and stimulated by Hatha yoga practices in at least two different ways. First, local increases in circulation are brought about in the endocrine glands and nerve plexuses (the network of nerves) through a variety of *asanas*. For example, during *sarvangasana* (shoulder stand), gravitational effects tend to increase circulation in the thyroid gland, and, during *bhujangasana* (cobra position), contraction of the lumbo-sacral musculature increases circulation to the plexus of that region. A second way is during *pranayama*, the manipulation of the breathing system which has a highly beneficial effect on the nervous system.[14]

Another aspect of yoga now being studied is the control of blood flow. In one of the studies at the Menninger Foundation, a yogi exhibited a high degree of control over his blood flow. It has been recently suggested that if blood flow to the tumor region could be restricted, the growth of tumors could be abated.[15]

Children also can benefit from the practice of yoga. A study published in the *Journal of Mental Deficiency Research* reported that when applied to a group of ninety mentally retarded children, yoga helped produce a "highly significant improvement in IQ and social adaptation."[16]

See Ayurvedic Medicine.

Yoga is also an integral part of Ayurvedic medicine. Ayurvedic physicians regularly advise patients in the practice of postures, breathing exercises, and meditation.

In the West, more and more physicians are prescribing Hatha yoga classes, and "yoga therapy" is a growing field in American health care. The therapeutic results of yoga are starting to make converts of the established medical community, with some insurance companies now covering expenses, thus signaling an acceptance of the economic benefits yoga can bring to the health care system as well.

Yoga Therapy

Robin Munro, Ph.D., of Cambridge, England, had a long history of bronchial problems which began with asthma as a child and led to a bronchitis condition as an adult. After a severe bronchial attack at the age of thirty-seven, his condition became chronic and could only be controlled through drugs and repeated courses of antibiotics. The condition became so acute it began to interfere with both his family life and his work.

During the course of exploring alternative therapies for his problem, Dr. Munro met an Indian doctor experienced in yoga therapy. Dr. Munro had already been practicing yoga for over ten years, which, together with deep relaxation, had alleviated his bronchitis, but had not cured it.

The new yogic regime prescribed by the Indian doctor consisted of very simple postures and breathing exercises, together with a short session of vigorous exercise. It was first developed at Kaivalyadhama, near Bombay, India, a yoga institute that has been pioneering scientific research on the therapeutic qualities of yoga for seventy years. During the first few months, acupressure was prescribed to Dr. Munro to overcome acute attacks without medication. After a year the acupressure became unnecessary as well. Three years after beginning his new program, Dr. Munro's chest was virtually normal and has remained so ever since. "I have not taken a single antibiotic since the day I started," attests Dr. Munro. "That's nearly twenty years ago now."

Personally convinced of the effectiveness of yoga therapy, Dr. Munro founded the Yoga Biomedical Trust in 1983. The Trust's first venture was to carry out a survey of people who practiced yoga. High percentages of people with many different ailments said they considered yoga to have helped them. The table below shows the results from the nearly three thousand responses. Subsequent research has begun to substantiate many of these anecdotal findings.

"The Trust has already carried out successful trials on the benefits of yoga for maturity-onset diabetes and rheumatoid arthritis," states Dr. Munro. "And it is currently embarking on a long-term study into the effects of yoga on aging."

According to Dr. Munro's research, yoga is particularly valuable in the prevention and management of stress-related chronic health problems. "Yoga cannot cure every condition," concludes Dr. Munro, "but it can substantially help most of them."

Health Conditions Benefited by Yoga

The 1983-84 Yoga Biomedical Trust survey charted the responses of 3,000 individuals with health ailments who were prescribed yoga as an alternative treatment therapy.

Ailment	Number of Cases Reported	Percent Claiming Benefit
Back Pain	1,142	98
Arthritis or rheumatism	589	90
Anxiety	838	94
Migraine	464	80
Insomnia	542	82
Nerve or muscle disease	112	96
Menstrual problems	317	68
Premenstrual tension	848	77
Menopause disorders	247	83
Hypertension	150	84
Heart disease	50	94
Asthma or bronchitis	226	88
Duodenal ulcers	40	90
Hemorrhoids	391	88
Obesity	240	74
Diabetes	10	80
Cancer	29	90
Tobacco addiction	219	74
Alcoholism	26	100

A Program of Simple Hatha Yoga *Asanas*

While some specific yoga *asanas* can help particular health conditions, the safest and most reliable way to use Hatha yoga therapeutically, says Dr. Ballentine, is to follow a balanced program of postures to achieve an overall normalizing and health-inducing effect. It is best for the beginner to start with a simple program of basic postures. One such beginning yoga program, as suggested by Dr. Ballentine, can be found below and performed in about a half an hour. An initial structured class or instruction is suggested as a foundation for exercises later practiced on one's own.

Corpse (*Shavasana*)

The first posture, called the corpse, is an excellent posture to start a yoga program. The corpse can also be used between postures to help relax and prepare the mind for the next posture in the sequence, and, at the conclusion of the program, to help reduce fatigue.

Lie on your back with your arms spread out about twelve to eighteen inches from your side, palms open and up, and your feet spread about as wide as your shoulders.

Place a folded blanket or towel behind your head and neck. Close your eyes and relax, breathing slowly and deeply, allowing the abdomen to expand with each inhalation and to fall with each exhalation.

Practice this exercise for five to ten minutes.

This exercise has many benefits:

- An excellent relaxation technique that aids circulation and improves the functioning of the nervous system
- Helps relax the skeletal muscles, enabling one to go further into the postures while reducing the likelihood of injuries
- Reduces fatigue

“The safest and most reliable way to use Hatha yoga therapeutically is to follow a balanced program of postures that will have an overall normalizing and health inducing effect.”

—Rudolph Ballentine, M.D.

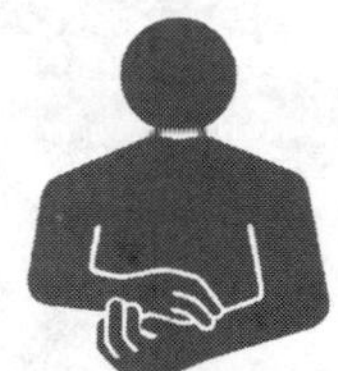

Yoga is ideally suited as an integral part of your personal health maintenance program.

Child's Posture (*Balasana*)

Sit in a kneeling position with the top of your feet on the floor and your buttocks resting on your heels, keeping the head, neck, and trunk straight. Relax the arms and rest the hands on the floor, palms upward and fingers pointing behind you.

Exhaling, slowly bend forward from the hips until the stomach and chest rest on the thighs and the forehead touches the floor in front of the knees. As your body bends forward, slide the hands back into a comfortable position.

In the child's posture the body is completely relaxed and very compact. Do not lift the thighs or buttocks off the legs. Keep the arms close to the body. If you experience discomfort, extend the arms above the head a shoulder's width apart, keeping the arms straight and the palms on the floor.

Do not hold this posture for more than five minutes, as it reduces the circulation in the legs. People with excess weight may find this exercise more comfortable if the knees are spread apart.

Child's posture.

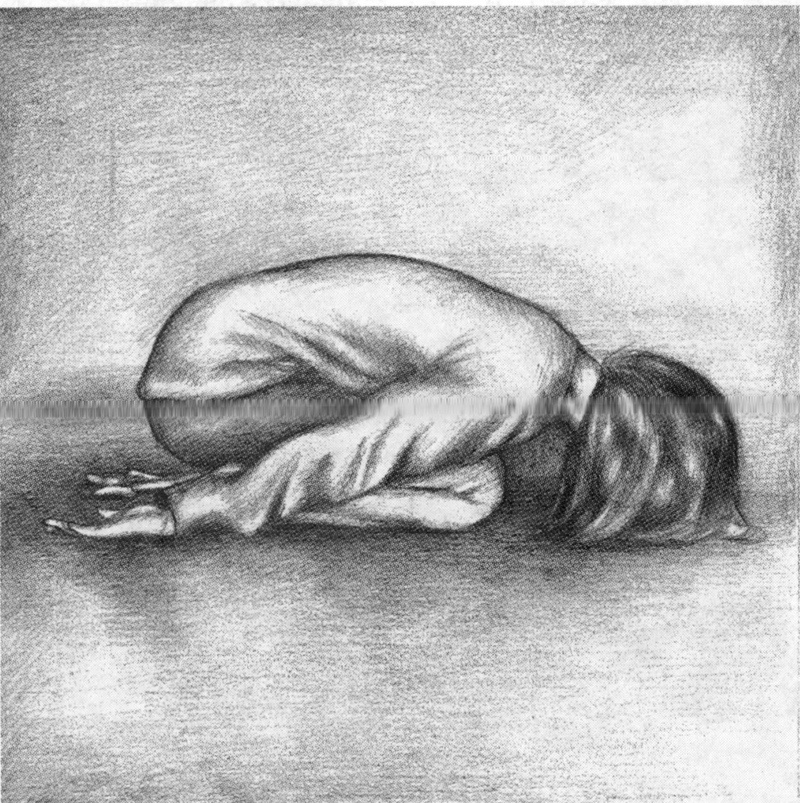

To release the posture, inhale as you slowly lift the head and trunk and return to a kneeling position.

This exercise has many benefits:

- Relaxes the back and promotes healing of back injuries by taking pressure off the intervertebral discs and providing a mild and natural form of traction
- Relieves pain in the lower back that may be caused by other postures. It can be used as a bridge between various asanas if lower back pain persists

Posterior Stretch (Paschimottanasana)

Sit with your head, neck, and trunk straight and your legs together, extended in front of your body. Inhaling, raise your arms overhead, stretch up and expand the chest.

Exhaling, with your back straight and head between the arms, bend forward as far as possible, placing the hands comfortably on the legs. The back of your knees should remain on the floor. Relax, breathe evenly, and hold for five to ten seconds.

To further the stretch: Remain in position, inhale, and stretch forward from the base of the spine to the crown of the head. Exhaling, bring the head further down toward the legs. Relax and breathe evenly.

This exercise has many benefits:

- Stimulates the peristaltic movement (wavelike contractions) of materials through the digestive tract and prevents constipation
- Stimulates the entire abdominal area: kidneys, liver, stomach, spleen, and pancreas
- Relieves indigestion and poor appetite
- May be therapeutic in the treatment of diabetes
- Stretches the hamstring muscles of the thighs and the muscles and ligaments of the back
- Gently massages the intervertebral discs; develops flexibility of the spinal column

Posterior stretch.

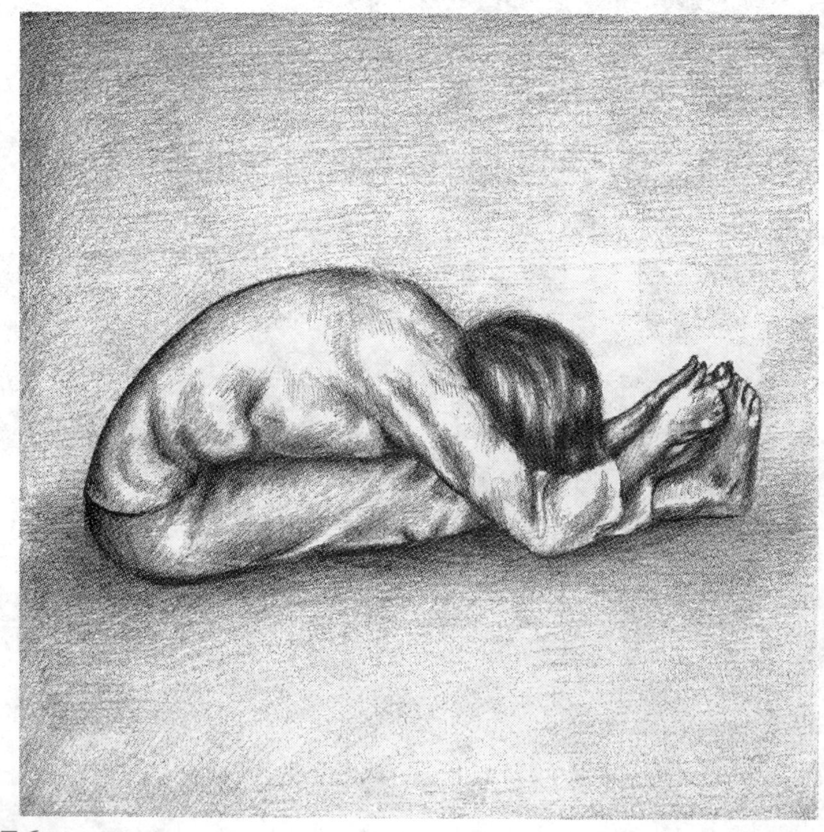

Cobra (*Bhujangasana*)

Lie on your stomach with your forehead resting on the floor, legs and feet together, with your body fully extended and relaxed. Bend the elbows, keeping them close to the body, and place your hands palm down beside the chest, aligning the fingertips with the nipples.

Inhaling, slowly begin to raise

your head, allowing first the nose and then the chin to touch the floor as the head is stretched forward and upward. Without using the strength of the arms or hands, slowly raise the shoulders and chest; look up and bend back as far as possible. Breathe evenly; hold for five seconds.

Exhaling, slowly lower the body until the forehead rests on the floor. Relax.

In this posture the navel remains on the floor. Do not use the arms and hands to push your body off the floor, use the muscles of the back only. Keep the feet and legs together and relaxed.

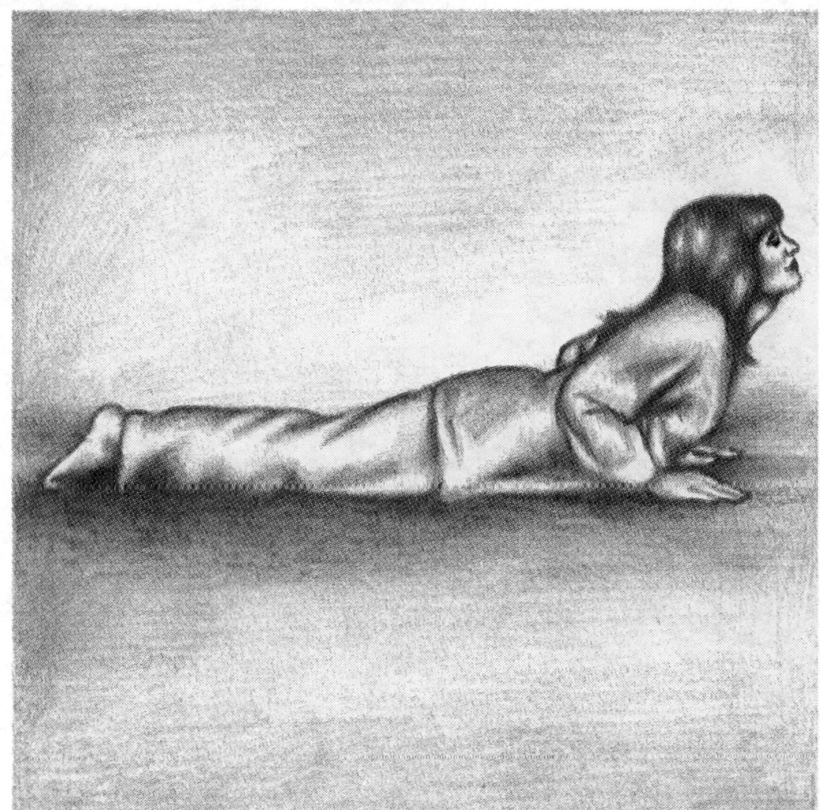

Cobra.

This exercise has many benefits:

- Strengthens the muscles of the shoulders, neck, and back
- Develops flexibility of the cervical vertebrae
- Corrects deviations of the spine
- Improves circulation to the intervertebral discs
- Expands the chest and develops elasticity of the lungs
- May help low back pain, constipation, stomach pains, gas pains, and backaches

Locust (*Shalabhasana*)

Lie on your stomach with your legs together and your arms extended along the sides of your body; place the chin on the floor. Make fists with the hands, placing the thumbs and the forefingers on the floor. Keeping the arms straight, place the fists under the tops of the thighs.

Inhaling, raise both legs as high as possible. Breathe evenly; hold for five seconds.

Exhaling, slowly lower the legs and relax.

This exercise has two primary benefits:

- Strengthens the muscles of the lower back
- Reduces lower back pain tendencies

Half Spinal Twist (*Ardha Matsyendrasana*)

Sit with your head, neck, and torso straight with your legs together, extended in front of your body.

Bend the left leg and place the left foot on the floor at the outside of the right knee. Twist the body toward the left and place the left hand approximately four to six inches behind the left hip, fingers pointing away

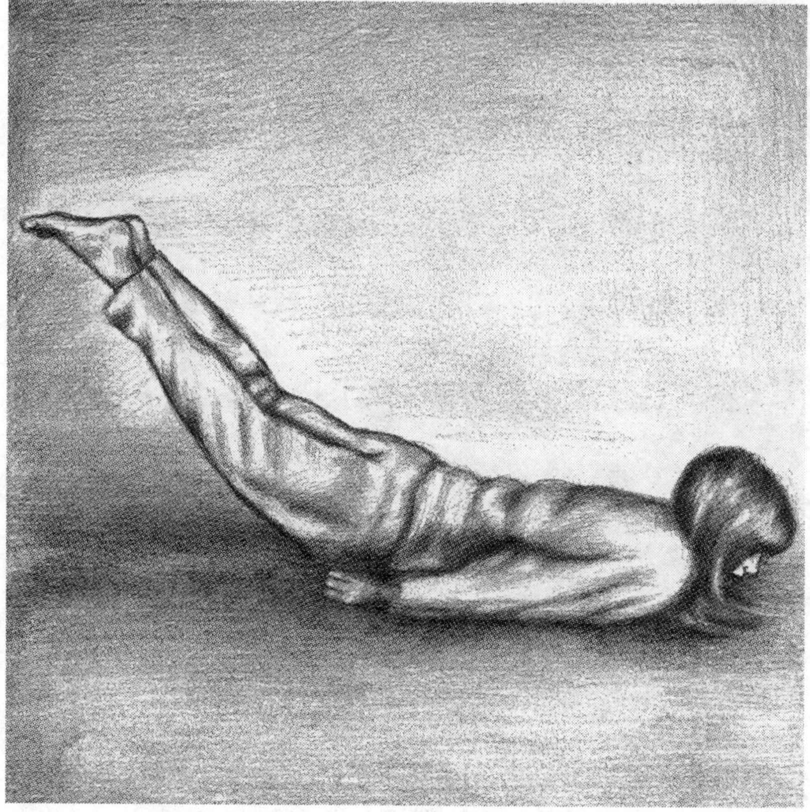

Locust.

Half spinal twist.

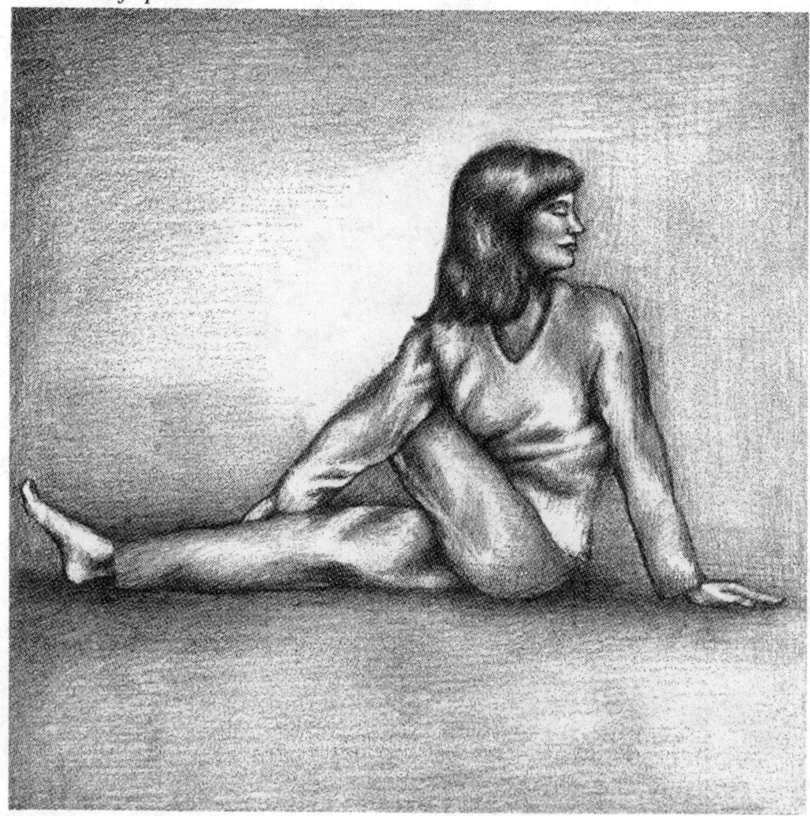

from the body. Bring the right arm over the outside of the left leg and grasp the left foot with the right hand. When bringing your arm over your leg, you may bend slightly forward if necessary; however, do not arch back and then twist your body.

Keeping the back straight, turn to the left, twisting from the lower spine, and look over the left shoulder. Do not use the arms to force your body further into the twist, use them only for balance.

Breathe evenly; hold for five seconds. Repeat on the opposite side.

This exercise has many benefits:

- Provides twist to the spinal column, stretching and lengthening the muscles and ligaments and keeping the spine elastic and healthy
- Alternately compresses each half of the abdominal region, squeezing the internal organs and promoting better circulation through them
- Combats constipation, reduces fat, and improves digestion

Shoulderstand (*Sarvangasana*)

Lie on your back with your legs together, flat on the floor. Bend the elbows and place the hands as close to the shoulders as possible, with fingers pointing toward the small of the back and the elbows firmly on the floor. Raise both legs until they are perpendicular to the floor, lifting the hips toward the ceiling. Press the breastbone against the chin, gently at first and more firmly with experience. Keep the legs straight, relaxed and perpendicular to the floor.

Breathe evenly; hold for twenty to thirty seconds. Slowly increase your capacity until you can hold this posture comfortably for one minute.

This exercise has many benefits:

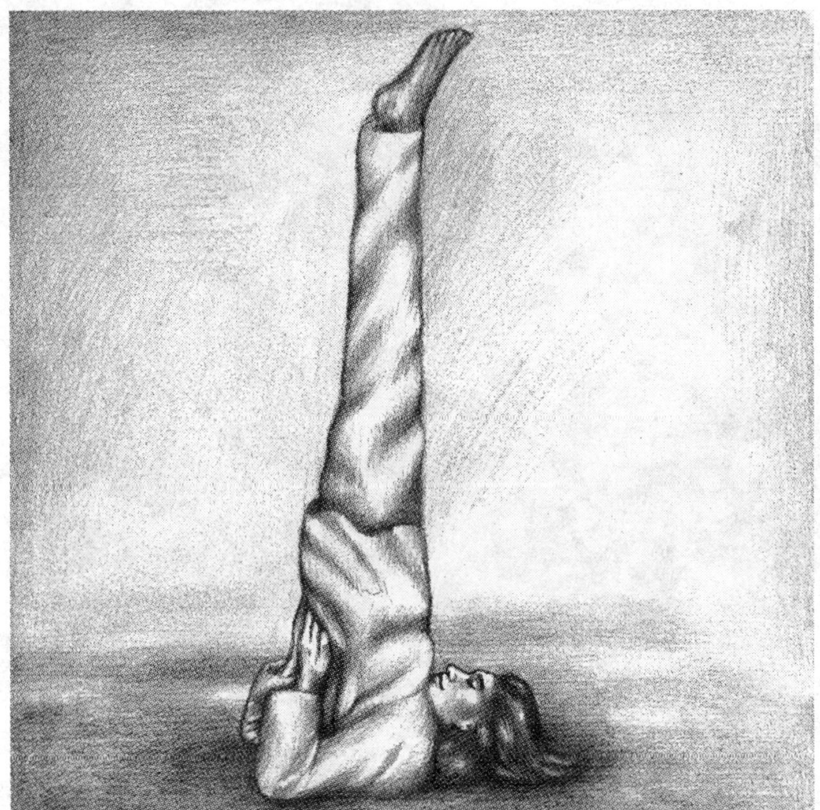

Shoulderstand.

- As implied in the literal translation of sarvangasana, "all member posture" or "entire body posture," this exercise benefits all parts of the body: the shoulders, arms, legs, head, neck, back, and internal organs
- Strengthens arms, chest, and shoulders
- Strengthens the back and abdominal muscles
- Places gentle traction on the cervical vertebrae, keeping this important area healthy and flexible
- Venous drainage of the legs occurs quickly and completely, especially benefiting those persons with varicose veins
- Diaphragmatic breathing is easily observed and learned
- Causes higher blood pressure and simple mechanical pressure in the neck, said to rejuvenate the thyroid and parathyroid glands, making them function optimally
- Reduces the occurrence of acute and chronic throat ailments
- Increases the blood supply to all the important structures of the neck
- Called the "Queen of *asanas*" and considered a panacea for internal organ ailments, especially those associated with old age. Fights indigestion, constipation, degeneration of the endocrine glands, and problems occurring in the liver, the gallbladder, the kidney, the pancreas, the spleen, and the digestive system

Half Fish (*Ardha Matsyasana*)

Sit with your head, neck, and trunk straight, legs together and extended in front of your body. Lean back and place the elbows and forearms on the floor in line with the body and legs. Arch the back, expanding the chest, and stretch the neck backward, placing the crown of the head on the floor. Increase the stretch by further arching your back and pulling your head as far as you can toward the back. Be sure to keep the mouth closed to maintain the stretch in the neck.

Breathe evenly; hold for fifteen to twenty seconds. Gently lower the

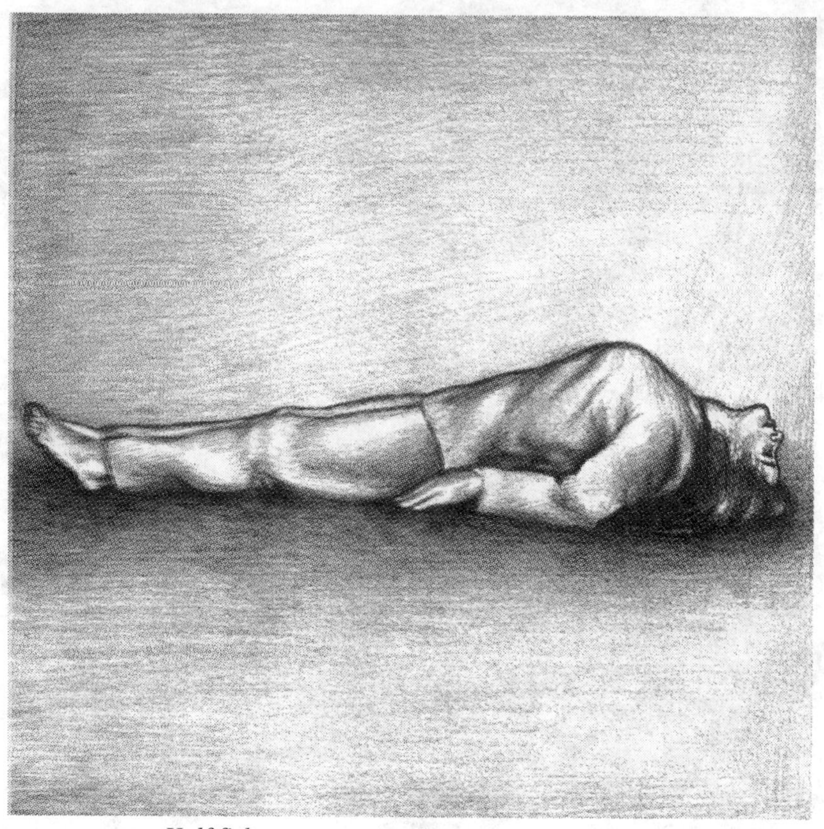

Half fish.

body to a prone position. Relax. Once again, conclude with corpse posture to ensure complete relaxation and prevent fatigue.

This exercise has many benefits:

- Provides a stretch to the cervical vertebrae complementary to that of the shoulder stand. It amplifies the effects of the shoulder stand and eliminates the slight stiffness in the neck and back that results from doing the shoulder stand alone.
- Expands the chest, promoting deep inhalation, giving good ventilation to the top of the lungs and increasing lung capacity

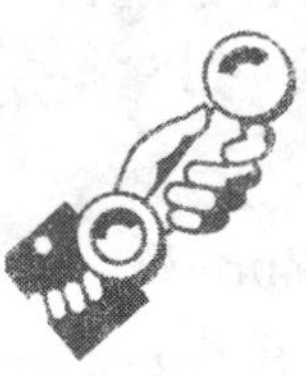

Where to Find Help

There are several forms and schools of yoga available in the West, including: *Ashtanga, Integral, Iyengar, Kriya, Kundalini, Sivananda, Tantra, and Vini*. Each emphasizes a different aspect of the body/mind/spirit relationship.

The telephone book, health food stores, and alternative practitioners are the best sources for referrals. The following organizations may be contacted for further help and assistance.

Himalayan Institute of Yoga, Science, and Philosophy
RRI Box 400
Honesdale, Pennsylvania 18431
(717) 253-5551
(800) 822-4547

The Institute offers classes, a catalogue of more than sixty books, audio cassettes, and videos, and has centers all over the country.

International Association of Yoga Therapists
109 Hillside Avenue
Mill Valley, California 94941
(415) 383-4587

A nonprofit organization emphasizing education and research for yoga and yoga therapy. An international organization with an annual journal, the Journal of the International Association of Yoga Therapists.

Iyengar Yoga
2404 27th Avenue
San Francisco, California 94116
(415) 753-0909

Offers classes, teacher training, a bookstore, a mail order catalog, and referrals.

Samata Yoga and Health Institute
4150 Tivoli Avenue
Los Angeles, California 90066
(310) 306-8845
(310) 306-4632 (Fax)

Samata Yoga and Health Institute specializes in yoga therapy for backs and stress, group classes and teacher training programs. A videotape, Healthy Back, Healthy Mind, *by Larry Payne, Ph.D., is offered through Samata featuring exercises for the lower and upper back .*

Sivananda Yoga
5178 South Lawrence Boulevard
Montreal, Quebec, Canada
H2T 1R8
(514) 279-3545

Has centers worldwide, including in the United States, Canada, Bahamas, India, and Europe. North American centers are in the following cities:

Chicago	*(312) 878-7771*
New York	*(212) 255-4560*
San Francisco	*(415) 681-2731*
Los Angeles	*(310) 478-0202*
Toronto	*(416) 966-9642*

Recommended Reading

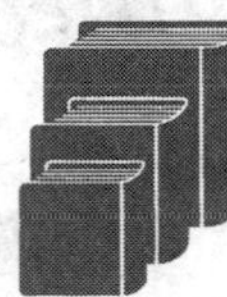

Back Care Basics: A Doctor's Gentle Yoga Program For Back and Neck Pain Relief. Schatz, Mary P., M.D. Berkeley, CA: Rodmell Press, 1992.

Offers a gentle and effective approach to back rehabilitation without drugs or surgery. Uses the therapeutic techniques of Iyengar-style yoga.

The Complete Illustrated Book Of Yoga. Vishnudevananda, Swami. New York: Harmony Books, 1980.

A classic in its field, outlining a complete yoga training program for beginners. Also provides meditative techniques for relaxation and stress release, as well as the philosophy upon which yoga is founded.

Hatha Yoga: Manual I. 2nd Edition. Samskrti and Veda. Honesdale, PA: The Himalayan International Institute, 1985.

An introductory workbook for beginning students in the practice of Hatha yoga. Contains clear-cut explanations of the various postures and breathing exercises, accompanied by easy-to-follow illustrations on the basic principles of Hatha yoga, including stretching, breathing, and relaxation.

Lectures on Yoga. Swami Rama. Honesdale, PA: The Himalayan International Institute: 1979.

The lectures of Swami Rama on a lifelong pursuit of yoga and its far-reaching influences.

***Light on* Pranayama.** Iyengar, B. New York: Crossroad Publishing, 1992.

Techniques of yogic breathing together with a comprehensive background of yoga philosophy.

Light on Yoga. Iyengar, B. New York: Schocken Books, 1987.

Six hundred pictures, detailed descriptive text, and philosophy of yoga practices.

Yoga Journal. 2054 University Avenue, Berkeley, California 94704 (510) 841-9200

A popular magazine found at health food stores and health-oriented bookstores. Also publishes a national directory of six to seven hundred yoga instructors.

"The art of healing comes from nature and not from the physician. Therefore, the physician must start from nature with an open mind."

—Paracelsus

Part Three: Health Conditions

An Important Message

This book is intended as an educational tool to acquaint the reader with alternative methods for the maintenance of good health and the treatment of illness. The publisher hopes the book will enable the reader to improve his or her well-being and to better understand, assess, and choose the appropriate course of treatment for an illness or health condition. Because the methods described in this book are, by definition, **alternative** methods, many of them have not been investigated and/or approved by any government or regulatory agency. National, state, and local laws vary regarding the use and application of many of the treatments that are discussed. Accordingly, this book should not be substituted for the advice and treatment of a physician or other licensed health professional, but rather, should be used in conjunction with professional care. Pregnant women in particular are especially urged to consult with their physician before using any therapy.

Your health is important. Use this book wisely. Discuss the alternative treatment options described herein with your doctor. Ultimately, you, the reader, must take full responsibility for your health and how you use this book. The publisher expressly disclaims responsibility for any adverse effects resulting from your use of the information contained herein.

Addictions

Addictions afflict millions of people in the United States alone. Many alternative physicians believe that conventional methods fail because they do not recognize the genetic and biochemical imbalances that research has shown to be at the heart of addiction. By focusing on readjusting these imbalances through diet and nutritional supplementation, acupuncture, biofeedback, and herbal medicine, alternative physicians are contributing to significant and long-lasting positive change.

Addiction can be defined as any physical or psychological dependence which negatively impacts a person's life. Although a person can be addicted to many forms of behavior such as gambling, over-eating, sex, or reckless behavior, the term "addiction" is most commonly used to refer to dependency on cigarettes, alcohol, and drugs (both legal and illegal). In severe cases, addiction can become so obsessive that it may seem to take on a life of its own, and the individual's true identity can take a second place to the personality of the addiction.

"When someone with addictive behavior is deprived of, or attempts to abandon, his or her addiction, the resulting withdrawal symptoms demand a solution. During withdrawal from the addictive substance, something must be done to keep the painful, sometimes unbearable, symptoms at bay."

According to James Braly, M.D., Medical Director of Immuno Labs, Inc. in Fort Lauderdale, Florida, fundamentally all addictions are biochemically the same. He notes that addictive substances become a "necessary" ingredient of body chemistry, so that withdrawal occurs when the substance is withheld. "Addiction means that the body has made an unhealthy adaptation that must slowly be reversed," Dr. Braly explains. "Until then, nerve impulses are confused and biochemistry scrambled."

When someone with addictive behavior is deprived of, or attempts to abandon, his or her addiction, the resulting withdrawal symptoms demand a solution. During withdrawal from the addictive substance, something must be done to keep the painful, sometimes unbearable, symptoms at bay.

Causes of Addiction

According to Leon Chaitow, N.D., D.O., of London, England, experts are unable to agree on what causes addiction.

Long perceived as a problem of weak willpower, substance abuse is now considered by most researchers in the field to be a "disease," similar in development to diabetes. In other words, according to Dr. Chaitow, a genetic predisposing condition is usually present that is triggered by familial, environmental, societal, and dietary factors. As a result, even when stabilized, an addict must closely monitor the addictive substance throughout his or her lifetime.

Biochemical Imbalances

The body produces its own natural mood enhancers and painkillers, called neurotransmitters, which in healthy individuals work efficiently. Dr. Chaitow cites research into brain function that suggests that the addictive personality may lack these natural stimulants (catecholamines) and relaxants (endorphins) and postulates that the addictive brain may send wrong or garbled messages to the body through malfunctioning neurotransmitters. "Because of this malfunction, addictive personalities may seek alternatives to natural mood enhancers through the artificial stimulus of addictive substances," he says.

Janice Keller Phelps, M.D., author of *The Hidden Addiction and How to Get Free from It*, asserts that addiction stems from individual biochemistry and unique genetic makeup. She believes there is a difference in addictive bodies from birth and that an addictive body may be evident in childhood by the presence of colic, hyperactivity, loss of sleep, irritability, crying, and learning disabilities. Additionally, Dr. Phelps says, "Long before a child can get involved in drugs and alcohol, he's often gotten very addicted to sugar."

Substantiating this line of thought, Dr. Chaitow points to the link between brain chemistry and food addictions. Serotonin (another neurotransmitter) is a calming, analgesic-like substance which is secreted in response to carbohydrate and sugar consumption. "Sugar addiction," she says, "may be a misguided attempt to replenish serotonin in the system." A Massachusetts Institute of Technology study describes groups of people who feel depressed, anxious, and tense—the right conditions for substance abuse—before eating a carbohydrate snack, and who feel peaceful afterward, their bodies sated with calming serotonin.[1]

Kathleen DesMaisons, M.Ed., President of Radiant Recovery in Burlingame, California, believes that many addictive people have an actual biochemical flaw in the way they process sugar and carbohydrates. This flaw in metabolization causes an addict to respond to sugar as if it were alcohol and to white flour products as if they were sugar.

She explains, "Genetically, these people have biochemically sensitive bodies which invite chemical imbalance. Substances like sugar, by creating insulin and rapidly penetrating the cell wall, actually alter the permeability of the cell."

The "normal" person, DesMaisons states, has stronger, more impermeable cells which prevent the rise and fall of blood sugar and the jagged peaks and valleys of violent emotions that plague addictive personalities. "Sugar is like an opiate drug that can make life manageable," DesMaisons says. "The child who used sugar becomes the adolescent who discovers alcohol, which is the perfect drug because, beyond its high sugar content, it has an anesthetic property. The addictive personality moves naturally into other drugs. The whole syndrome is really about pain management."

THE ADDICTION/ALLERGY CONNECTION

James Braly, M.D., Medical Director of Immuno Labs, Inc. in Fort Lauderdale, Florida, believes there is a strong correlation between addiction and allergies. "We become addicted to foods as a way of adapting to allergic reactions to them, and we tend to crave foods we're allergic to because we need them to keep withdrawal symptoms at bay," he explains. When we reach this point and need a particular food in order to feel good, or rather, in order not to feel bad, we are addicted to it. This topsy-turvy phenomenon is called the allergy/addiction syndrome."

Recent research in the field of addiction suggests that excessive craving for any substance indicates an allergic condition in relation to that substance. "According to this theory," says Leon Chaitow, N.D., D.O., of London, England, "by constantly exposing themselves to an addictive substance, addicts prevent themselves from experiencing the more violent displays of allergic symptoms—the substance 'masks' the allergy, in other words."

Furthermore, Dr. Chaitow points out that an addict's withdrawal symptoms are almost identical to the symptoms which occur when an allergic substance is removed from the diet or environment—ranging from tremors to prostration, cramps, vomiting, sweating, and hallucinations. "Any food or drink which is commonly consumed or craved may in fact be an allergic substance for an individual if withdrawal from it makes one feel unwell, or if consumption of it produces euphoria," Dr. Chaitow says. Alcohol is the classic substance fitting this description.[2]

Dr. Chaitow draws another connection between addiction and allergies in alcoholics. He states that the normal population of microorganisms housed in the gut are severely disturbed in alcoholics and may lead to malabsorption of fats, protein, carbohydrates, folic acid, and vitamin B_{12}. This disruption, together with a more permeable or leaky gut, allows foreign and toxic substances to cross the intestinal wall. As a result, allergies may develop and feed alcohol cravings and possible food allergies.[3]

Dr. Braly also points out that many of the foods from which alcohol is made—particularly grains, corn derivatives, sugars, and yeast—are common allergens. He maintains that many alcoholics are also addicted to these foods and thus perpetuate their allergies with excessive drinking.

Following this line of thinking, many researchers believe that addiction may be a way of restoring natural body chemicals through artificial, destructive means. Dr. Chaitow says, "We turn to various substances to enhance or replace the body's diminished capacity to produce the chemicals we crave for energy or relaxation."

Treating Addictions

Over the last decade, substance abuse treatment in the United States has been focused primarily on Twelve-Step support groups and individual "talking" therapies, control by medications such as methadone and antidepressants, expensive month-long hospital stays, and, of course, criminal punishment.

It is still unknown whether these methods, combined or individual, will be successful in the long run. However, a 1980 Rand Corporation study confirmed earlier research which found that the addictive population studied, once sober, or "clean," had less than a 15 to 20 percent rate of continued abstinence.[4] Compared to such low success rates, the following alternative approaches offer great promise.

Diet

Proper diet is essential in treating addictions, according to Kathleen DesMaisons. "My main focus is to reverse symptoms of addiction by changing the clients' neurochemistry and nutrient deficiency through dietary intervention," she says. "This principle is called 'biochemical restoration'. If this is accomplished, then the addictive behavior that has previously been unmanaged can be reversed. Ultimately, the goal is to teach our clients how to recognize and modulate their feelings by paying attention to the foods they eat."

Since DesMaisons finds that most, if not all, addictive people have problems processing sugar and carbohydrates, her approach is to immediately place them on a program of three meals a day, with an emphasis on eating proteins at each meal. "Most people in an addictive state are very protein deficient," she explains. "First of all, normally they haven't been eating regularly, and secondly, they don't have protein when they do eat because their bodies are craving sugar and simple carbohydrates. So by getting them to eat regularly of the protein foods, which are the most complex foods and take the slowest time to break down in the stomach, you start to alter their neurochemistry. They become able to maintain a very stable blood sugar level and a very consistent supply of serotonin and dopamine (another neurotransmitter) to the brain, so that they don't crave the artificial high from alcohol or drugs."

DesMaisons also instructs her clients to keep a food journal of what they eat and how they feel afterward so that they have an actual record of how food affects their moods. "We often have people who have been given antianxiety medication, and no one has bothered to ask them what they eat and drink," says DesMaisons. "They come in not eating regularly while drinking three pots of coffee a day. That is the source of their anxiety symptoms."

DesMaisons suggests meal choices based on the client's lifestyle and ethnic background. Typical choices include fish, poultry, meat, cheese, eggs, tofu, and peanut butter. In addition, complex carbohydrates are permitted, including beans, grains, and vegetables. "We also encourage a little bit of fat, although not from animal products," DesMaisons says, "because healthy fat leads to the body's production of serotonin, creating a sense of well-being and relaxation. Using olive oil, for instance, is one way to achieve this."

Clients who follow this eating plan will normally notice significant changes in how they feel, often within three to four days, according to DesMaisons. "It's simple and sometimes startling," she says. "For example, for a cocaine addict who is feeling suicidal and is trying to get sober, who hasn't eaten in days, sometimes all it takes is a turkey sandwich to stabilize him so he can begin the recovery process."

Once DesMaisons' clients begin to experience a positive change, their caffeine and sugar intake is examined and gradually reduced. DesMaisons also educates them about all of the different sugars that can be found in foods. "Many people are only aware of the overt sugars contained in pies, cakes, cookies, and ice cream," she says. "They have to also be aware of the hidden sugars, particularly the many forms of corn syrup, such as dextrose, multidextrose, sorbitol, and mannitol. I really encourage people to read labels to see what it is they are eating." Because of its high sugar content, fruit is also avoided, particularly grapes, cherries, watermelon, and all fruit juices. Citrus fruits, apples, and strawberries, however, can be permitted due to their lower sugar content. "Interestingly, carrot juice is also avoided," say DesMaisons, "because it's also high in sugar."

One of DesMaisons' clients came to her at age twenty-eight after never being sober for more than a month since she was twelve years old. "She'd been in hospitals repeatedly for attempted suicide and had been drinking since she was nine," DesMaisons says. "One day she got very upset and went out and drank a gallon of Jack Daniels. She had to be hospitalized, but three days later she walked into my office and said, 'All right, whatever you tell me to do, I'll do.'" She was placed on the biochemical food plan and after one month no longer had any cravings for alcohol. After achieving sobriety, she was then able to begin dealing with the emotional issues surrounding her addiction. "Today, she has been sober for four years and her entire life has changed," DesMaisons relates. "She's in a healthy relationship, has been promoted at her job, and is really an example of radiant recovery."

DesMaisons also incorporates acupuncture, counseling, and guided imagery, with a focus on self-awareness and independence. According to her, 75 percent of her clients remain sober two years or more after completing the program.

Nutritional Supplementation

In boosting the body's biochemical defenses against addiction, Dr. Phelps uses nutritional supplements and adrenal supports, such as vitamin C, pantothenic acid (vitamin B_5), and adrenal extracts in her treatment regimen. She also stresses that a patient must remove all addictive substances from the diet, including sugar and caffeine.

Megavitamin therapy is commonly cited as one of the most vital tools for replenishing vitamin deficiency, which, according to Dr. Aesoph, affects more than 50 percent of all alcoholics. She points out that narcotics addicts often suffer from a deficiency of essential minerals, especially magnesium, calcium, and potassium. She explains that since alcohol enhances free radical formation (the molecules held responsible for damaging and possibly aging the body), antioxidants are needed to oppose their effects, such as selenium, zinc, and vitamins C and E. She adds that chromium aids in stabilizing the erratic blood sugar seen in alcoholic hypoglycemia, while choline and folic acid are also commonly cited as important supplements to assist in the body's recovery from addiction.

See Acupuncture, Chiropractic, Mental Health.

Intravenous withdrawal support for severe cases is often used in Dr. Braly's treatment. He states that those with severe withdrawal problems can benefit from three or four consecutive days of intravenous therapy consisting of vitamin C, calcium gluconate, magnesium sulfate, pantothenic acid, and vitamin B_6. "Withdrawal symptoms can often be completely eliminated after one or two days using this approach," Dr. Braly says. Other nutrients that he recommends include evening primrose oil, vitamin B complex, MaxEPA, and glutamine (an amino acid).

Dr. Corazon Ilarina, M.D., of the Bio Medical Health Center in Reno, Nevada, treated a marijuana addict with an intensive program of mineral supplements. By analyzing the patient's hair, Dr. Ilarina determined that the patient was suffering from elevated aluminum, lead, nickel, and beryllium levels. She started the patient on a treatment program that included magnesium, chromium, and manganese supplements, thymus and pancreatic extracts, and high dosages of vitamin C to fight the patient's high toxic levels. After nutritional supplementation, Dr. Ilarina states, "There was a dramatic improvement in lowering the toxicity levels of the patient, and the craving for marijuana and alcohol was alleviated."

Acupuncture and Traditional Chinese Medicine

Michael Smith, M.D., of Lincoln Hospital in New York, has found acupuncture to be the most effective treatment for heroin, cocaine, and crack addictions. Studies have also shown fewer relapses and fewer readmissions to treatment centers for addicts and alcoholics who have had acupuncture therapy.[5] Dr. Chaitow reports that even corporations such as General Motors and Chevron are employing acupuncture to counter-

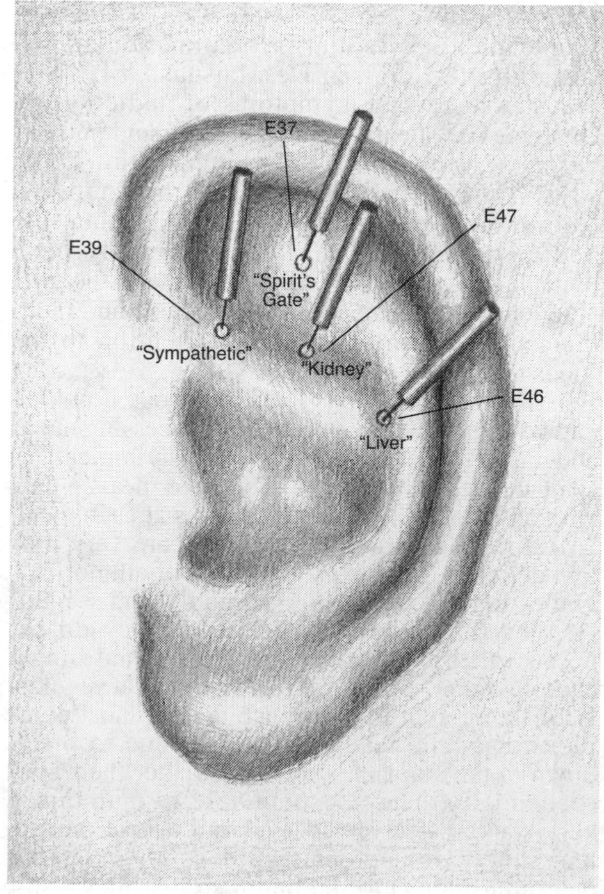

Acupuncture points for addiction.

act cocaine and alcohol abuse, while creating data bases for further research.

According to Pat Culliton, Dipl. Ac. (NCCA), Director of the Acupuncture and Alternative Medicine Program at Hennepin County Medical Center in Minnesota, Oregon law now requires a series of acupuncture treatments before a heroin addict can qualify for a methadone treatment. "The state of Oregon hopes that many people will successfully detoxify with acupuncture and therefore not need to start a methadone maintenance program."

Sir Jay Holder, M.D., D.C., Ph.D., founder and Director of Exodus, an addiction treatment hospital in Miami, Florida, has developed a form of auriculotherapy (ear acupuncture) for addiction treatment. He has used it to successfully treat addictions, as well as obsessive behavior related to work, sex, and gambling. Auriculotherapy, according to Dr. Holder, has over an 80 percent success rate among addicts of nicotine, alcohol, cocaine, heroin, and other drugs.[6]

Dr. Holder explains that each type of addiction correlates to specific ear acupoints. "Every drug has a specific receptor site. We meet the needs of that receptor site by supplying and directing endorphins through acupuncture. This allows the body to turn itself back on again. So, the body is helped through the difficult period of withdrawal, until its natural restorative powers return."

Kathleen DesMaisons also finds acupuncture, particularly auriculotherapy, to be an effective addiction treatment. "Several needles in the ear daily dramatically minimizes detox symptoms," she says. "My clients report a significant decrease in discomfort, heightened relaxation, and a far better ability to maintain their sobriety."

William Michael Cargile, B.S., D.C., F.I.A.C.A., Chairman of Research for the American Academy of Acupuncture and Oriental Medicine, will often use ginger seeds on ear acupoints rather than needles. The serrated seeds, without penetrating the skin, are placed on the ear with medical tape and are distinctly successful in treating cocaine addiction.

Dr. Cargile describes a forty-six-year-old patient who benefited enormously from ginger seed treatment: "She was a mother of eight children by seven different men, and a crack prostitute. We used whole-body acupuncture in twelve treatments and sent her home with ginger seed on the ears, and during the treatment, she had only one relapse. In the last year and a half she's been clean, with consistently clear urine analysis. Today, she holds down two jobs, and has not had a single relapse."

At the Yo San University Clinic in Santa Monica, California, Maoshing Ni, D.O.M., Ph.D, L.Ac., practices Traditional Chinese Medicine, including acupuncture and nutritional guidance. He reports the case of a patient with a twelve-year history of hard drug abuse. He could only walk with difficulty, he suffered from shortness of breath, his balance was off, and he had a multitude of physical maladies.

"The first acupuncture treatments were applied to the patient's ear points, Dr. Ni relates. "This helped him sleep and become calmer. We saw immediate relief, and his drug craving was much diminished. I then started him on a pro-

CHIROPRACTIC AND ADDICTION

Chiropractic is an important adjunct to primary treatments for addiction, according to Sir Jay Holder, M.D., D.C., Ph.D., founder and Director of Exodus, an addiction treatment hospital in Miami, Florida. Dr. Holder, in connection with the University of Miami School of Medicine and the Florida Chiropractic Society, is guiding the first large study of chiropractic adjustment in treating chemical addiction. "The double-blind study has already presented impressive preliminary results with statistics demonstrating a 97 percent retention rate," Dr. Holder says. These figures indicate that an individual receiving chiropractic treatment may be ten times more likely to complete a drug recovery program.

"By removing subluxations that interfere with the normal functioning of the nervous system, a person in a drug treatment center is more likely to complete his or her term of stay because the person now can meet the needs of all the other modalities that are offered as treatment," states Dr. Holder. "We have fewer people with drug detox or withdrawal symptoms. Their physical complaints are almost eliminated and they can now concentrate on why they're in treatment."

Dr. Holder reports that the American College of Addictionology and Compulsive Disorders (ACACD) in Miami has chosen chiropractic as the profession of choice in training for board certification in addictionology. "The ACACD targeted the chiropractic community because chiropractic is a drugless approach," continues Dr. Holder. "People who are chemically dependent must stay away from mood-altering substances their entire lives. And the obvious type of primary care physician who is going to best be able to meet the needs of the recovery community is someone who isn't going to use mood-altering substances."

gram of Chinese herbs to restore the functions of his liver and kidneys since his adrenal glands were depleted. This helped the detoxification and strengthening process. I also put him on a very cleansing, strict high-fiber, low-fat diet. As a result, his mind began to clear, and his appetite returned, and today the patient is recovering well, and has suffered no relapses."

Biofeedback Training and Brain Wave Therapy

Developed by Gene Peniston, Ed.D., A.B.M.P., Chief of Psychology Service at Sam Rayburn Memorial Veterans Center in Bonham, Texas, and Paul J. Kulkosky, Ph.D., Professor of Psychology at the University of Southern Colorado in Pueblo, brain wave therapy is a revolutionary treatment for addiction, using biofeedback and visualization techniques to bring about significant behavioral change by actually altering the addictive personality.

"You're literally changing personal biology, the way someone functions," says Steven Fahrion, Ph.D., of the Menninger Clinic in Topeka, Kansas, where the treatment is also used.

Brain wave therapy involves three separate treatment procedures, says Dale Walters, Ph.D., Director of Education for the Center of Applied Psychophysiology at the Menninger Clinic. "In the first part, alcoholics and addicts learn how to use galvanic skin response biofeedback in association with breathing exercises and relaxation phrases to begin to develop a relaxation response and an orientation to relaxation."

According to Dr. Peniston, this allows a patient's alpha brain waves to rise, while also facilitating the ability to descend into a *theta* state of consciousness (a very deep level of relaxed brain wave activity). This is important, says Dr. Peniston, "because it is only in the *theta* state that long-lasting physiological or mental change can take place."

The next phase of the program is visualization. "This involves the development of alcohol or drug rejection scenarios. Patients visualize themselves standing outside a liquor store or bar, looking in but not going in. They then see themselves walking away and rejecting the purchase of drugs and alcohol.

"Before going on to the brain wave training, it is critical that the person be able to visualize himself in situations where he would ordinarily drink or take drugs, and then see himself turning away from that," says Dr. Fahrion.

Brain wave training is the third part of the treatment and is also the most important. In this phase these new positive images become consolidated and, in effect, stamped on the personality of the patient. Using biofeedback equipment, the patient is further induced into an alpha state and then into a theta state. "Alpha is the bridge to theta," says Dr. Peniston. "It only takes being in the deeper theta state of consciousness about 10 percent of the time during a session for true change to take place. Once a person is in that state, the hippocampus (a ridge along the brain's side cavities) region is activated. This is where all the experiences a person's had in childhood and adulthood, particularly those that were traumatic and anxiety-provoking, are housed. It's during this state that the hypothalamus system (a region of the forebrain that regulates basic body sections) is reprogrammed."

Dr. Fahrion adds, "Because the brain can't discriminate between created visualizations and actual events, it substitutes the image of the person turning away from the addictive substance for the old behavior. So it really changes the way the person thinks about himself."

Dr. Fahrion describes an example of this alteration in self-thought with a patient's account of her visualization. "It's foggy and cold. The air is thick and stuffy, kind of grey. I lean inside my friend's car that smells like cigarette smoke and heavy metal music is playing. They ask me if I want to use. And I say, 'No, I don't want to use.' I turn around and start to walk to school. As I walk, the sun starts to come out, the air is lighter and easier to breathe. Everything begins to clear as I walk away. I'm confident in my decisions, feeling lifted up and good about myself."

See Biofeedback Training, Guided Imagery Hypnotherapy, Neuro-Linguistic Programming.

According to Dr. Peniston, each session lasts about half an hour, with the whole treatment program usually requiring at least thirty sessions, depending on the patient's individual needs and disposition going into therapy. In addition to *alpha-theta* brain wave training, the program also includes instruction in relapse prevention, shame and guilt work, the biology of addiction, spirituality exercises, and self-help groups.

"The thing that's so exciting about this, of course, is the relapse prevention aspect," adds Dr. Fahrion. "Usually there's this revolving door of relapse where a person attends a treatment program and often, before he is even out a week or two, he has relapsed again."

"With our first study we had about an 80 percent success rate," reports Dr. Kulkosky. "With traditional therapy, such as psychotherapy and anticraving medication, after thirteen months there was only a 20 percent success rate, and after five years, it had dropped down to zero.

We're now five or six years past our first study and we're still seeing about a 70 percent success rate."

Part of the reason for the high success rate is that if someone does relapse, the body will immediately reject the alcohol or drug, causing a severe flulike reaction that will usually put the person in bed for several days. "Nobody has an explanation as to why this happens yet," says Dr. Fahrion, "but it's quite consistent all over the country.

"The other thing that happens is the kick, the high from the addictive substance disappears. It just doesn't give the person the boost that it did before, and between these two things, it's not something that she likes to repeat that much."

Using herbs to stop smoking

According to Michael Murray, N.D., of Bastyr College in Seattle, Washington, lobelia is the most notable herb used to combat the effects of nicotine withdrawal. "The active ingredient in lobelia, lobeline, has similar actions to nicotine, but it's gentler, has a longer duration of action, and is a suitable alternative to nicotine chewing gum or the nicotine patch," Dr. Murray says. Lobelia has also been shown to have antidepressant action. "Another herb that's been shown to contain components useful in helping people to quit smoking," adds Dr. Murray, "is Ephedra sinesis *or* ma-huang. *Ephedrine, the active constituent in this herb, decreases the number of cigarettes smoked. Lobelia or lobeline is more effective when it's used with a stimulant. So it's possible that by combining lobelia and ephedra (a stimulant), you'll get better results than if you use either alone."*

Lobelia, however, warns Dr. Murray, is only an interim measure in treating nicotine dependency. Because the patient can become hooked on this herb, it is important to wean the smoker off lobelia over a period of a month. Dr. Murray notes that oat extracts have also induced smokers to decrease the number of cigarettes smoked, even while they claimed to be unaware of the effect.

"It's the most amazing thing to witness," says Dr. Peniston. "You can look at a person that has gone through this, and she looks younger. All the tension has gone out of her face. We've followed the original group for a little better than four years and the change has been phenomenal. Some have gone back to work, some have gone back to college, they've held jobs for the first time, they've had no relapses and no craving or desire for alcohol or drugs. They're just different people."

"What brain wave therapy needs in terms of having a mass impact in the country is a large controlled study. We have a proposal in with the National Institute of Drug Abuse to do a three-year study in which we would treat four hundred addicted individuals. If that grant were to come through I think it would make all the difference," Dr. Fahrion says.

Herbal Medicine

Herbal medicine can play an important role in treating addiction, particularly with regard to the liver, which is one of the body's organs most damaged by substance abuse. As the body's toxins begin to filter out, cleansing and healing the liver is critical. Lauri Aesoph, N.D., of Sioux Falls, South Dakota, recommends treating a faltering liver with milk thistle, which contains some of the most powerful liver protective substances known, and not only protects it from damage, but encourages the growth of new cells.

Since optimal function of eliminative organs, such as the kidneys and liver, is necessary to battle addiction and sustain recovery, blood cleansing herbs are also vital. Dr. Aesoph recommends wild oat extract, burdock root, fumitory, echinacea, and licorice root, which are all useful in this respect.

Like other drugs, the withdrawal symptoms of caffeine, mainly headache, fatigue, and depression, make abstinence difficult. Dr. Aesoph suggests the use of herbs, including feverfew, lime blossom, and chamomile flowers, which can help break the coffee habit.

Oatstraw is one of many herbs useful in addiction treatment, according to Michael Murray, N.D., of Bastyr College in Seattle, Washington. "Oats," he explains, "have long been used in India to treat opium addiction. Evidently, they help rebalance the endorphin levels in the brain."

Siberian ginseng has been shown to normalize the neurotransmitters in the brain. "This demonstrates that it has some sort of balancing effect. I think that would be very important in someone who needs stimulants or some other addictive substance to function," says Dr. Murray.

Dr. Aesoph cites skullcap, valerian, balm, and vervain as natural alternatives to the pharmaceutical sedatives and tranquilizers used to treat anxiety, inside and outside of addiction treatment. "My first choice," says Dr. Murray, "would be using St. John's Wort, due to its antidepressive qualities. Also, it doesn't have strong sedative effects like valerian."

Ayurvedic Medicine

Virender Sodhi, M.D. (Ayurveda), N.D., of Bellevue, Washington, Director of the American School of Ayurvedic Sciences, practices Ayurvedic medicine, which asserts that the three particular human body types all have certain individual weaknesses, which, for different reasons, can lead to addiction. According to Dr. Sodhi, Ayurvedic medicine holds that an individual develops addictive behavior while attempting to cope with fear and anxiety. Each of the three body types, *vata, pitta,* and *kapha*, copes with anxieties differently. Knowing this, the individual can prevent or cope with these inherent tendencies in an orderly and systematic manner. For example, Dr. Sodhi explains that a *pitta* body type (very driven, overachievers) will not be able to tolerate alcohol.

See Ayurveduc Medicine.

Part of the Ayurvedic diagnostic method outlined by Dr. Sodhi is an examination of the pulse, the tongue, and the eyes, which indicates the condition of inner organs and suggests proper herbs and vitamins needed for treatment. *Ghee* is often used in treatment, as are *ashwagandha* and *calamus*.

Dr. Sodhi relates the case history of one female patient addicted for ten years to marijuana. He describes her as "a *kapha* type, slow moving with a tendency to abuse stimulants for energy," who was suffering from depression and disorientation. Her adrenal glands were exhausted. Dr. Sodhi administered gotu kola and put her on a vitamin regime, including B_6, B_{12}, and folic acid injections, as well as amino acids to revive the adrenal glands. Dr. Sodhi states, "Within three months she recovered from the lethargy and depression and soon her glandular functions returned to normal."

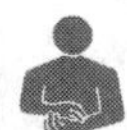
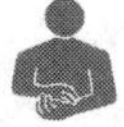

Self-Care

The following therapies can be undertaken at home under appropriate professional supervision:

Alcoholism

Aromatherapy: Fennel rose, juniper, rosemary.

Fasting: Detoxifies the body, but only if not malnourished.

Homeopathy: *Berberis, Nux vomica, Sulphur, Lachesis.*

Hydrotherapy: Steam, sauna, immersion bath, all help rid the body of toxins.

Meditation: Alcoholics who practice Transcendental Meditation show a steady decline in alcohol use as well as a 90 percent sobriety rate after two years.[7]

Smoking

• Biofeedback Training • Fasting • Meditation • Qigong • Yoga

Homeopathy: *Daphne ind., Tabacum.*

Hydrotherapy: One of the following: immersion bath, wet sheet pack, or steam/sauna. Apply one to two times weekly to produce sweating. Also consider enema daily during detox.

Juice Therapy: Two to three week juice fast may be effective for detoxifying the bloodstream from nicotine and to end the craving for cigarettes. Avoid acidifying juices (citrus, tomato).

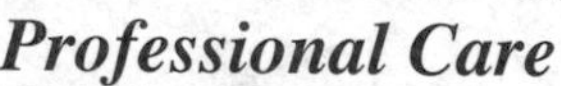

Professional Care

The following therapies should only be provided by a qualified health professional:

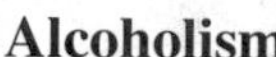

Alcoholism

• Acupuncture • Applied Kinesiology • Biofeedback Training • Chiropractic • Detoxification Therapy • Environmental Medicine • Hydrotherapy • Magnetic Field Therapy • Meditation • Naturopathic Medicine • Orthomolecular Medicine • Osteopathy • Oxygen Therapies

Smoking

• Acupuncture • Detoxification Therapy • Environmental Medicine • Hypnotherapy • Magnetic Field Therapy • Naturopathic Medicine • Neural Therapy

Where to Find Help

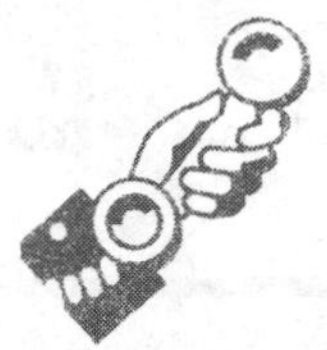

For more information on and referrals for treatment of addictions, contact the following organizations.

American Association of Acupuncture and Oriental Medicine
4101 Lake Boone Trail, Suite 201
Raleigh, North Carolina 27607
(919) 787-5181
The AAAOM is a national professional trade organization of acupuncturists who meet acceptable standards of minimum competency and can provide you with the names and locations of local members.

American Association of Naturopathic Physicians
2366 Eastlake Avenue, Suite 322
Seattle, Washington 98102
(206) 323-7610
Contact them for the location of a licensed naturopathic physician in your area.

American School of Ayurvedic Sciences
10025 NE 4th Street
Bellevue, Washington 98004
(206) 453-8022
This college provides medical training for physicians and health care practitioners, as well as individual courses for lay people. Dr. Virender Sodhi's Ayurvedic, Naturopathic Medical Clinic is also located at this address.

Center for Applied Psychophysiology
Menninger Clinic
P.O. Box 829
Topeka, Kansas 66601-08829
(913) 273-7500 Ext. 5375
One of the pioneering groups in biofeedback. This organization has research, treatment, and workshops in all areas of mind/body medicine, including extensive work with biofeedback and brain wave therapy as a treatment for addicton.

Sitike Counseling Center
1211 Old Mission Road
South San Francisco, California 94080
(415) 589-9305
One of the premier centers for treating addiction through dietary and nutritional intervention using their Biochamical Restoration Program. Also offers acupuncture and counseling, and can provide referrals to similar programs nationwide. Treatment is on an outpatient basis.

Recommended Reading

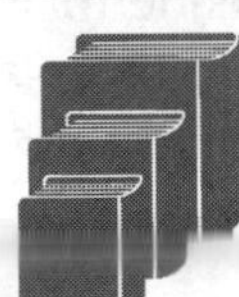

Dr. Braly's Food Allergy and Nutrition Revolution. Braly, James, M.D. New Canaan, CT: Keats Publishing, Inc., 1992.
A comprehensive investigation into food allergies and their link to other illnesses, including addiction. Outlines the factors involved in addiction and how to treat them using diet, nutritional supplements, and exercise.

Encyclopedia of Natural Medicine. Murray, Michael, N.D.; and Pizzorno, Joseph, N.D. Rocklin, CA: Prima Publishing, 1991.
An authoritative guide to naturopathic medicine outlining the basic principles of health and how they can be used to treat over sixty health conditions, including alcoholism. Includes self-help approaches using diet, nutrition, and herbal medicine.

The Hidden Addiction: And How to Get Free. Phelps, Janice, K., M.D., and Nocrse, A. E., M.D.
Two out of five Americans are susceptible to addictions—be it to alcohol, nicotine, sweets, or other drugs—because of their metabolisms. The authors provide a test to discover if you have an addictive personality and offer a detailed treatment program.

AIDS

AIDS, more than any other disease, has been surrounded by stigma and mystery ever since it was recognized over a decade ago. Researchers are still debating its cause, and even whether it is, in fact, a new disease. So far, conventional medicine has offered no answers as to how to treat AIDS. Meanwhile, certain alternative physicians are approaching the disease from a different perspective, and their work is proving that, contrary to popular belief, AIDS is not a death sentence.

A basic premise of alternative medicine is that all diseases, if properly approached and treated in time, are reversible. This includes AIDS (acquired immune deficiency syndrome), as the following stories suggest. A man suffering from AIDS for five years came to Joan Priestley, M.D., of Los Angeles, California. His doctors had told him that his case was terminal and had given him five months to live. He was suffering from severe weight loss and diarrhea and was ravaged by opportunistic infections and Crohn's disease. Today, over one year after beginning agressive treatment with Dr. Priestley, the man, despite a continued low T-cell count, which is considered a marker for AIDS and HIV (human immunodeficiency virus) infection, is symptom free, has regained forty pounds, and lives a productive, engaging life.

“AIDS is defined primarily by what appears to be severe immune deficiency, and is distinguished from virtually every other disease in history by the fact that it has no constant, specific symptoms.”

A patient suffering from night sweats and fever, and diagnosed as HIV positive (HIV is commonly believed to be the cause of AIDS) was weak and faint all of the time as his T-cell count continued dropping. He sought out Robert Cathcart III, M.D., of Los Altos, California, a pioneer in the use of vitamin C therapy as a treatment for illness. Fifteen months after beginning intravenous vitamin C treatments, the patient's T-cell count had risen from under 300 to 600. He felt healthy and for the first time in his life went over a year without having a cold or flu.

In 1984, Jon was diagnosed with Kaposi's sarcoma, a form of skin cancer common to gay men with AIDS. He had also been suffering with hepatitis for a year.. After adopting a protocol of nutritional supplementation, herbs, and diet, under the supervision of Laurence Badgley, M.D., of Foster City, California, his symptoms began to improve. Today, over nine years later, Jon is healthy and working two full-time jobs.

These are just three cases of people with AIDS or HIV who have turned their illness around and are now on the road to health. Other cases will follow as this chapter explains the various methods that are being used outside of the framework of conventional medicine to keep people with AIDS alive. To understand how and why such treatments work, though, it is important to examine what AIDS is and what it is not.

What is AIDS?

AIDS is defined primarily by what appears to be severe immune deficiency, and is distinguished from virtually every other disease in history by the fact that it has no constant, specific symptoms. Once the immune system has begun to malfunction, a broad spectrum of health complications can set in. "AIDS" is an umbrella term for any or all of some twenty-eight previously known diseases and symptoms. When a person has any of these microbial diseases or opportunistic infections, and also tests positive for antibodies to HIV, (thought by most scientists to cause the immune destruction), an AIDS diagnosis is given.

The diseases that mark AIDS differ widely from country to country, and even from risk group to risk group. In the United States and Europe, some of the most common diseases associated with AIDS are Kaposi's sarcoma (a form of cancer), pneumocystis pneumonia, candidiasis, and mycobacterial infections such as tuberculosis, toxoplasmosis (a disease caused by protozoa that damages the central nervous system, eyes, and the body's internal organs), cytomegalovirus, and the herpes virus. Other more general conditions not included in the twenty-eight indicator diseases, but often associated with the disease, include diarrhea, weight loss, night sweats, fevers, rashes, and swollen lymph glands.

"The diseases that mark AIDS differ widely from country to country, and even from risk group to risk group."

THE TROUBLE WITH DEFINING AIDS

By January 1, 1993, extreme alterations were being made to the original definition of AIDS. Previously, in order to be diagnosed as having AIDS, it was necessary to have one or more of twenty-five symptoms listed by the Centers For Disease Control (CDC), as well as being HIV positive. In January, the CDC added three new conditions—cancer of the cervix, bacterial pneumonia, and tuberculosis—which, when found in combination with the HIV virus, would constitute AIDS.

The effect of this decision will be to dramatically and artificially inflate the statistics of people who have AIDS. In the United States alone, the figures will show a rise from 250,000 to 400,000 (from 1982 to date), with a huge increase in the number of women with a sudden AIDS diagnosis. This caused famed British epidemiologist, Dr. Gordon Stewart, to ask the pertinent question: "Will any woman with cervicitis, any man with urethritis, or prostatitis, or genitourinary cancer, or any cancer, or perhaps severe infection, or any other unspecified, wasting, or multiple disease, who happens to be HIV positive, be diagnosed and registered as having AIDS and treated for HIV disease, because those in the business can expand their domain across any diagnostic code and scruple?"[2]

There are some striking differences between the various "risk groups," or groups of people within which AIDS has remained concentrated. Kaposi's sarcoma, for instance, one of the earliest symptoms by which AIDS was diagnosed, is twenty times more common in gay men with AIDS than in all other American AIDS patients.[1]

Tuberculosis, meanwhile, is mainly seen in intravenous drug users. AIDS in Africa, by contrast, lacks the distinction of "risk groups," but is said to be distributed evenly among the population and between the sexes. There, AIDS is defined primarily by diarrhea, wasting, fever, and a persistent cough: symptoms that have all been quite common in Africa for decades and are seen in most tropical diseases.

Because of these and other discrepancies, there is much confusion and dissent about what AIDS really is, and even if it is accurate to classify it as a disease entity. The common factor that all these disconnected symptoms and diseases revolve around is HIV. If HIV antibodies are detected, these diseases converge as AIDS; if not, then they are diagnosed simply for what they are. In other words, any degree of immune suppression, in the presence of HIV, is classified as AIDS. But the same degree of immune suppression, in the absence of HIV, is by definition not AIDS.

This has led to a kind of diagnostic chaos never before seen in medicine. The answer as to who has AIDS and who doesn't may depend on which doctor a person questions. There is also tremendous dispute about whether, in fact, HIV is the cause of AIDS. This question has been argued both in the media, the AIDS community, and in the scientific literature, and still remains unresolved. One camp believes that HIV causes the immune suppression that leads to AIDS, while the other argues that various environmental risk factors such as recreational and pharmaceutical drugs, sexually transmitted diseases, and bacterial infections are the real cause of the immune suppression, and that HIV is just a byproduct of an already suppressed immunity. This also raises questions about how people "get" AIDS. Do they "catch" it or do they "acquire" it over a period of several years? All of these questions need to be resolved before the true nature of the relationship between AIDS and HIV can be fully understood.

"The answer as to who has AIDS and who doesn't may depend on which doctor a person questions. There is also tremendous dispute about whether, in fact, HIV is the cause of AIDS."

The HIV Debate

Most AIDS scientists refer freely to HIV as "the causative agent of AIDS," or the "primary cause of AIDS," but when asked just exactly what body of scientific evidence supports the notion of HIV being the cause of AIDS, they are less certain. Although there is a strong correlation between HIV and AIDS—meaning that most people with AIDS also test positive for HIV—it is not a total correlation, nor is correlation proof of causation.

Though some 60,000 papers have been written on HIV, the evidence that HIV causes AIDS is still tenuous and can best be described as circumstantial; the damage is done, the cells are depleted, and HIV is present at the scene of the crime.[3]

Despite billions of dollars and years of research from around the world, the question remains, how does HIV cause AIDS? Mainstream AIDS opinion asserts that there is no question as to whether HIV causes AIDS—the only question is how—while the dissident view insists that we don't yet know whether HIV causes AIDS.

The HIV/AIDS hypothesis was first announced at a press conference on April 23, 1984. Robert Gallo, M.D., of the National Cancer Institute, stepped up to a podium at the packed press conference in Washington D.C. and announced that the cause of AIDS had been found. It was, he claimed, a new retrovirus (RNA virus with tumor-causing properties), supposedly isolated in his own lab, that he named HTLV-lll (human T-cell lymphotropic virus), and which was later renamed as HIV. At the time of the announcement, this hypothesis was based on nothing more than a strong correlation between AIDS cases and HIV. Most, though not all, of the AIDS patients studied, showed antibodies to HIV. Half of them had detectable live virus. With the help of the world media, Dr. Gallo's hypothesis soon became accepted as fact. The first reports stated that the "probable" cause of AIDS had been found, but very soon the word "probable" was dropped as HIV found its new identity as "the AIDS virus."

"Nobody in their right mind would jump into this thing like they did," says Dr. Kary Mullis, of La Jolla, California, recipient of the 1993 Nobel Prize in Medicine, and inventor of the Polymerase Chain Reaction, that is one of the mainstays of AIDS viral technology. "It had nothing to do with any well considered science. There were some people who had AIDS and some of them had HIV—not even all of them. So they had a correlation. So what?"[4]

In 1987, molecular biologist Peter Duesberg, Ph.D., Professor of Molecular and Cell Biology at the University of California at Berkeley, launched a frontal attack on the HIV-AIDS hypothesis in the journal *Cancer Research*. Dr. Duesberg, a world-renowned scientist and long standing member of the National Academy of Sciences, had helped map the genetic structure of retroviruses, and is known as one of the world's leading experts on retroviruses. After reading every single paper ever written on HIV and AIDS, Dr. Duesberg concluded that the virus was "harmless," pointing out, among other things, that HIV was a latent, inactive virus, which infected very few cells. Dr. Duesberg stated flatly that he "wouldn't mind being injected with it."[5]

Perhaps the most striking point of Dr. Duesberg's critique of the HIV-AIDS hypothesis was that HIV showed very little direct cell killing activity. In fact when he viewed HIV under a microscope, amidst lymphocytes (cells important in the creation of antibodies), it didn't move at

CAN THERE BE AIDS WITHOUT HIV?

Growing numbers of cases of severe immune suppression have been reported that appear to be clinically identical to AIDS, but do not test positive for HIV. Because HIV is not present, these cases are not registered as AIDS. The Centers For Disease Control's rationale for this is simple: AIDS is caused by HIV. Therefore, if HIV is not present, the cases cannot be AIDS.

Although several hundred cases of HIV negative "AIDS" have been documented in the medical literature for years, it was not until the International AIDS Conference in Amsterdam in July of 1992, that the world media reacted with alarm, writing front page stories about the "new disease," and criticizing CDC officials for not taking the "handful" of cases more seriously. A single abstract sparked the uproar, written by an American doctor who reported on six cases of AIDS with no HIV. Upon hearing the doctor's presentation, several more doctors started to volunteer cases of their own that fit the same description.

Seeking to calm the ensuing chaos, the CDC quickly settled on a new name for the "mysterious new disease." It would be called "ICL," which stands for idiopathic CD-4 lymphocytopenia. "Idiopathic" refers to a disease for which the cause is not known. "That's what they should call AIDS," says Harvey Bialy, M.D., scientific editor of the journal BioTechnology, and an outspoken critic of the HIV causation theory of AIDS. "ICL, it's perfect!"[6]

all, and the cells remained perfectly intact. According to Dr. Duesberg, this is to be expected. "Retroviruses are not typically cytocidal, that is, they do not kill cells."[7] The mainstream AIDS community, for its part, contends that direct cell killing is not necessary in order to implicate HIV, believing that the virus kills cells by one of several highly complex indirect mechanisms. One of these is known as *apoptosis*—a mechanism by which HIV is said to program cells to kill themselves in the future. Dr. Duesberg counters that there is no evidence for any of these elaborate mechanisms, and that HIV is far too simple in its genetic structure to be able to perform all these feats. Harvey Bialy, M.D., scientific editor of the journal *BioTechnology*, agrees. "HIV is an ordinary retrovirus," he says. "It only contains a very small piece of genetic information. There's no way it can do all these elaborate things they say it does."[8] Dr. Duesberg further argues that the HIV-AIDS theory fails to fulfill the standard set of rules used to determine whether a particular organism causes a particular disease. These rules, known as "Koch's Postulates," were established by German bacteriologist Robert Koch, who determined the causes of tuberculosis, anthrax, and several other infectious diseases using the following rules:

- The suspected organism has to be present in each and every case of the disease, and in sufficient quantities to cause disease.
- The agent is not found in other diseases.
- After isolation and propagation, the agent can induce the disease when transmitted to another host.

Dr. Duesberg concedes that there are limitations to Koch's Postulates, especially since most pathogens (disease-causing agents) are pathogenic only when the immune system is already below par. However, he argues, HIV has been shown to fail all three postulates, since it has already been established that the virus is not present in every case of AIDS-like disease; because it is found not in one, but in twenty-eight distinct diseases; and because chimpanzees, when inoculated with HIV, have consistently failed to develop AIDS.[9]

There are, at present, 125 to 150 chimpanzees around the world in captivity who have been injected with HIV, some as long ago as ten years. None of the chimps has developed any symptoms of AIDS.[10]

A British study conducted in 1987 also looked at accidental exposure to HIV by medical personnel (scratched with a needle previously used on infected individuals, for example). The study noted, "One surprising and mildly reassuring fact is that when health workers were examined after needlestick wounds only one out of fifteen hundred in the United Kingdom and the United States became infected."[11]

Can A Person Be HIV Positive And Not Get AIDS?

Though many people do become infected with HIV, a great deal of evidence now points to the possibility of a healthy immune system being able to keep the virus in check.[12] Australian researchers have been studying a group of six people who each received contaminated blood products infected by a single common donor. Both the donor and the people infected have now been under scrutiny for up to ten years, and after this length of time both the donor and five of the recipients have remained symptom free, with no decline of CD4 cells (cells involved in immune function and used as a marker for evidence of AIDS) and no sign of the P24 antigen (a specific marker that identifies a cell and causes the production of antibodies to destroy it) in the blood, which is considered a sign of worsening AIDS conditions. One of the six recipients has died of pneumonia (pneumocystis carinii), but she had received massive immunosuppressive treatment for systemic lupus erythematosis (an inflammatory disease causing abnormal growth of blood vessels and connective tissue) and cannot be regarded as a typical individual. In only one of the surviving study group members has it been possible to even isolate HIV. In the others, the researchers were unable to find evidence of the presence of the virus, despite repetitive testing of body fluids.

The researchers have no clear cut answer for their findings, stating, "It is not clear whether the benign course of HIV infection was due to host, viral, or other unknown factors."[13]

Their belief is that this was possibly a less virulent strain of HIV, but credit for the lack of progression to AIDS could just as easily be due to healthier immune systems, with the exception of the immune compromised patient with lupus. Even more significantly, the lack of HIV development could be due to the absence of co-factors.

Co-factors

The AIDS establishment still stands firmly by its conviction that HIV causes AIDS, although they are now finally conceding that HIV alone may not lead to AIDS without the help of one or more co-factors. These can include recreational and pharmaceutical drug use, recurrent infections, chronic use of antibiotics, poor nutrition, and pollution, as well as many psychoneuroimmunological co-factors, such as stress, fear, and despair.

When AIDS was first recognized in 1980-

81, the syndrome was called GRID, for Gay Related Immune Deficiency, since it was initially only found in gay men. The first few hundred cases were seen in male homosexuals who lived in major cities, particularly New York and San Francisco, who had frequently used both recreational and pharmaceutical drugs, and had been exposed to numerous bacterial infections and sexually transmitted diseases. The CDC initially suspected that AIDS was caused by drugs, most specifically amyl nitrates, or "poppers," a drug that was prevalent in gay discos of that era, and which proved to cause Kaposi's sarcoma in rats.

“The AIDS establishment still stands firmly by its conviction that HIV causes AIDS, although they are now finally conceding, that HIV alone may not lead to AIDS without the help of one or more co-factors.”

Other groups, though, soon started showing up as targets for AIDS's host of opportunistic diseases. Hemophiliacs, intravenous drug users, and the third world poor, particularly in Africa, all started coming down with the mysterious disease. As with gay men, all these risk groups shared similar symptoms of immune suppression caused by a number of possible factors, including drug use, frequent exposure to various bacteria and germs (as from a blood transfusion or a dirty needle), unsafe sexual practices, malnutrition, unsanitary eating and living conditions, or a combination of some or all of the above.

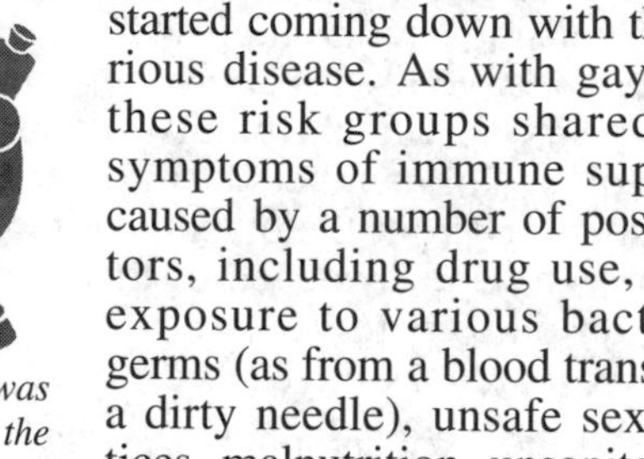
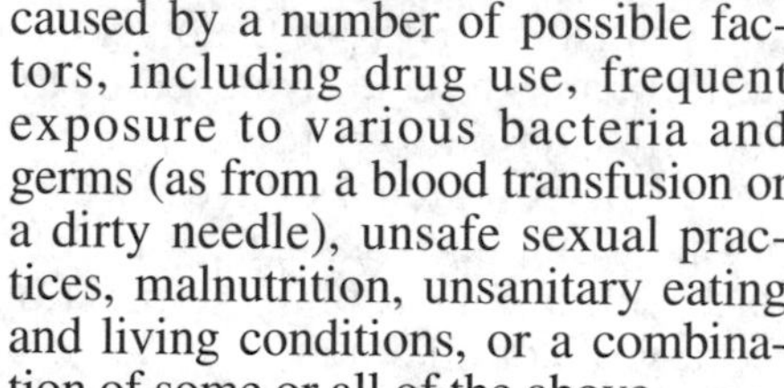

Before HIV was declared to be the single cause of AIDS, many immunosuppressive factors were still being investigated. The government should be urged to renew intensive research into these many potential co-factors.

Before HIV was declared to be the single cause of AIDS, many of these various immunosuppressive factors were still being investigated. In 1984, with the discovery of HIV, these other investigations suddenly stopped. Ten years later, there is a vast amount of research on HIV, and very little on any of the possible co-factors. "We were all forced into a very dogmatic and simplistic view of what caused AIDS," says Michael Lange, M.D., an infectious disease specialist at St. Luke's Roosevelt Hospital in New York City. "Today I think even the greatest proponents of HIV no longer believe that it does all that damage to the immune system by itself. There have to be other factors involved. And because of the HIV hypothesis there's been little or no research done on what those other factors may be."[14]

Immune System Cells and AIDS

AIDS is often accompanied by a steady decline in CD4 immune cells, which in a healthy person should hover between 900 and 1600, but in a person with AIDS can decline to as low as zero. In 1989, a CD4 cell count of less than 500 became the cutoff point after which AZT therapy was advised.

Virtually all AIDS therapies, both mainstream and alternative, have used the CD4 count as a marker for immune suppression. Official doctrine has it that HIV also destroys T4 cells, another critical part of the immune system. T4 cells scout out and identify invading pathogens, and trigger other immune system cells to attack these invaders. With a drastic reduction in T4 cells, the ability to respond against potential disease is reduced. Germs which ordinarily would have no effect on the body become potent enemies.

Another phenomenon in people with AIDS is a curious reversal of the ratio between T4 and T8 cells (another cell type vital for proper immune function). While a healthy person has a high T4 cell count and a low count of T8 cells, a person with AIDS has the opposite ratio. The CDC has now applied for permission to say officially that if the absolute ratio count of T4 to T8 cells in the body falls far below the normal range of 1000 to 200, this, with a positive HIV test, is sufficient for a diagnosis of AIDS.

Alternative physicians, even though they have been successful in reviving overall health in persons with AIDS (PWA's), have struggled with the restoration of full T4 cell counts. It has been observed, however, that high T4 counts do not necessarily correspond with health. Researchers have found people whose T4 counts are almost non-existent (under 10) who show no signs of disease."[15]

“Prior to AIDS, T-cell counts were rarely performed, and scientific understanding of their significance remains unresolved.”

Prior to AIDS, T-cell counts were rarely performed, and scientific understanding of their significance remains unresolved. At the AIDS Conference in Berlin in 1993, researchers stressed that they no longer believed that CD4 counts were a particularly valuable marker for clinical disease progression, because certain drugs had raised CD4s with no improvement in health.

AIDS has thus been simplified by the media, in part, to mean nothing more than a deficiency of these immune system cells. While T-cell loss is certainly one of the markers for AIDS, blood tests of a typical patient reveal a far more complicated picture, a kind of immunological chaos that is commonly referred to as "immune collapse." Some scientists feel it is even more complex than that, that it is a problem of the immune system gone haywire, perhaps even attacking itself in a process known as "autoimmunity." The only thing totally clear at present is that the immune systems of people with AIDS are damaged, and that the most important thing is to explore what treatments may restore the immune system, thereby restoring health.

THE HIV/AIDS TRAP

"I discovered that I was HIV-1 antibody positive in the spring of 1987, while in the process of deciphering what I consider to be non-life threatening but bothersome health problems that I strongly suspected were not AIDS but the result of other stresses on my immune system," says G. Steven Rose. A gay man, Mr. Rose was trying to go through a process of elimination in order to find out exactly what microbial factors and others stressors were causing his recurring bouts of mononucleosis and depression. He found evidence of several microbes, including cytomegalovirus(CMV), Epstein-Barr virus (EBV), and hepatitis B. "Because I tested positive for the HIV antibody, I wound up getting sucked into the AIDS machine. I was put on an AIDS track that seemed to have a mind of its own, winding up in an AZT clinical trial.

"AZT was offered to me as the only hope to deal with HIV infection. I doubted the paradigm from the start, but it took me a while to stand up to it. I finally realized that the AZT was harming me and walked out in disgust. I realized that chasing one killer microbe could not possibly be the way to restore my health, that my health was not as bad as I suspected, and that the only way to heal myself to the degree that I was sick, was to not take toxic drugs. I didn't follow any elaborate alternative methods, relying only on diet, rest, and a simple meditation technique. I simply stopped doing the damage, and gradually, my health returned. Today, as far as I can tell, I'm not dying of AIDS. In fact I've developed a pot belly. I've moved away from the medical model and towards living with myself the way I am and the more I do that, the healthier I become."

AZT[16]

AZT is now the most widely sanctioned medical treatment of AIDS currently in use, although many experts suggest that it is highly toxic and just as likely to kill the user as is AIDS. The reasoning behind its continued use is that AZT is believed to interfere with the process by which HIV-RNA is converted into DNA, thus neutralizing its effectiveness. This does not happen in all the infected cells, though, leaving a reservoir of infection. Also, if HIV is not the major cause of AIDS, this interference might in itself be of limited value, even if all the infected cells were influenced.

While there may be a short term (months rather than years) increase in T-cell numbers, this is usually followed by a rapid decline to a point lower than that before AZT treatment began. Until recently it was believed that there was evidence of a very small increased survival rate in those taking AZT but the results of the recent Concorde study confirmed that the drug neither prolongs life nor staves off symptoms of AIDS in those with HIV but no symptoms.

The supposed benefits of AZT also do not take into account the strong negative trade-offs, in terms of side effects. When viral DNA synthesis is being interrupted by the drugs, it also stops normal healthy T-cells from being able to synthesize DNA. HIV will also rapidly develop a resistance to the drug, mutating into different strains which are not influenced by it.

In addition, most health experts believe that, even when infection is active, at most one T-cell in five hundred is infected with HIV. This means that 499 healthy T-cells are killed by AZT for every one which contains HIV and which is deactivated. Since one of the main medical theories about HIV is that it does its harm through the destruction of T-cells, it becomes clear from the scenario outlined above that AZT is nearly five hundred times more harmful to the immune system's healthy T-cells than is HIV. This theory does not even include the damage done by AZT's admitted toxicity, which suppresses the important tasks of bone marrow, without which immune function collapses, causing anemia, neutropenia (abnormally small number of neutrophils in blood, a white blood cell that protects against infection) and leukopenia (abnormal decrease in white blood corpuscles) in between 20 and 50 percent of people given the drug, with up to half of these requiring transfusions within weeks of commencing its use.

Among other common symptoms resulting from AZT side effects are muscle wasting, extreme nausea, acute hepatitis, headaches, insomnia, dementia seizures, and the appearance of cancerous lymphomas (9 percent of patients).

When comparing AZT treatment studies with the results of the Healing Aids Research Project (HARP) study conducted by Bastyr College in Seattle, Washington which treated HIV-infected patients using alternative therapies such as nutrition, herbs, psychological counseling, and hyperthermia, it was found that, unlike all the published AZT results involving similar patient groups, none of the HARP patients progressed, over a one year period, to AIDS itself, or died,[17] whereas in the AZT studies, the progression rate was between 3 and 7 percent.[18] This points out that alternative methods, which are much cheaper economically, produce at least as good results, over a one year period, as AZT, with no toxicity. A longer HARP study is currently in progress.

Alternative Treatments for AIDS

While the mainstream view of AIDS treatment focuses almost entirely on the elimination of HIV, the alternative view places the emphasis on restoring overall health by first eliminating the co-factors. Prevention of a decline towards AIDS itself, after HIV infection, seems to be dramatically helped by using methods which either retard other infections or which enhance the natural protective, detoxification, and self-healing roles of the body, including the immune system which, together with the other defensive systems, tries to maintain the body's proper balance for health.[19]

Whether the virus can be held in check seems to depend on a number of factors, namely where the individual who is HIV infected is starting from—at what level is immune function, how much previous disease or infection has there been, what other medical problems are there, and how much toxicity is there from drugs, pollution, and other harmful environmental elements. Other important factors include the person's nutritional status, emotional state, and stress coping abilities, as well as "lifestyle" choices, including sexual, that may be helping or harming the defense effort. HIV entering a super-efficient immune system may well be overwhelmed and get nowhere. On the other hand, HIV entering a system already compromised by poor nutrition, other illnesses, and drugs, will find its task that much easier. One only has to look at the previously cited six cases from Australia to see a clear example of this. The immune compromised person succumbed whereas the five with sound immune systems have almost no sign of HIV and no sign at all of ill-health after up to ten years.

There are also many case histories of people who are HIV positive and who have developed advanced signs of AIDS (Kaposi's sarcoma, etc.) and yet who have managed to turn their condition around, regaining relative good health.[20]

Although such stories can be dismissed as "anecdotal," the sheer volume of these anecdotes overwhelms the weight of the dismissive arguments of the skeptics.

Continuing long-term studies at Bastyr College, are also examining the possibility of holding the disease at bay, of keeping people who show early signs of AIDS from degenerating further, and often of turning their condition around so that they become active, productive, and self-sufficient once more.[21]

Some of the alternative methods being used today to improve the health and immune function of individuals with AIDS and HIV-infection include improved nutritional status, detoxification, mind/body medicine, stress reduction therapies, herbal medicine, homeopathy, and ozone and other oxygen-based treatments.

> *"Broad segments of the American population have been proven to be deficient in specific vitamins and minerals, which are critical to immune system function. For example, persons with AIDS are often deficient in folic acid, selenium, zinc, and iron."*
>
> —Lawrence Badgley, M.D.

Diet and Nutrition

"Nutrition is the foundation of natural therapy," Dr. Badgley states. "Broad segments of the American population have been proven to be deficient in specific vitamins and minerals, which are critical to immune system function. For example, persons with AIDS are often deficient in folic acid, selenium, zinc, and iron."

While there is no universal dietary or nutritional prescription for the treatment of AIDS and HIV, since each person has varying needs and histories in terms of diet and nutrition, there are a few general guidelines a person can follow.

- Eat whole foods with as many essential nutrients and as few additives as possible.
- Fresh, organic vegetables, fruits, and proteins (fish and meat) are suggested whenever possible.
- Avoid processed foods.
- Reduce or eliminate refined carbohydrates (sugars, white flour, etc.) and replace with complex carbohydrates (vegetables, whole grains, beans, etc.) rich in nutrients.
- Reduce polyunsaturated and saturated fats and oils.

- Use monounsaturated oils (olive oil) with special emphasis on omega-3 oils (fish and certain plant oils).
- Eat smaller portions, more frequently throughout the day to optimize absorption of nutrients from food.
- Try to keep a balance of food intake which ensures that 65 percent is complex carbohydrates (vegetables, fruits, pulses, and grains), 15 percent protein (fish, yogurt, eggs, and meat), and 20 percent fat.
- Make sure fruits and vegetables are thoroughly clean and free of parasites and bacteria by steaming lightly before eating.
- Eat a wide variety of foods to help avoid becoming sensitized to specific food families through repeated exposure.
- Eliminate chocolate, caffeine, and alcohol.[22]

Because of everybody's biochemical individuality (genetic and environmental differences), each patient will have specific nutrient requirements. A qualified health care professional should always be consulted in order to receive specific, individual guidelines.

Dr. Badgley reports of a patient who has been HIV positive for eight years and was diagnosed with AIDS three years ago, and who claims to have eliminated his symptoms through diet and cleansings. He began a diet of raw organic fruits and vegetables, emphasizing freshness, moderation, and a variety of foods. He also utilizes enemas to rid his system of toxins and to cleanse the colon where the virus is harbored. He avoids foods that are mucous-forming like dairy products, eating only cheeses made from sunflower and pumpkin seeds. The patient reports that his T-cell counts have risen to normal levels and a liver disease with which he had been diagnosed is now also in remission.

Malnutrition is another common problem associated with people who are HIV positive and is almost universal in people with AIDS. This is often due to disruptions in the digestive processes caused by the weakening of the immune system. Raw foods, such as vegetables, can be lightly cooked (steamed, stir-fried, added to soups, stews, etc.) or juiced to better facilitate digestion. Sometimes, though, nutritional supplements taken orally or via injection (intramuscularly or intravenously as appropriate), are the only way to ensure that adequate nutrients get into the body (although with impaired absorption capabilities, the oral route does not always guarantee that what is swallowed arrives where it is needed).

People who are HIV positive and/or who have been diagnosed as having AIDS are most commonly deficient in the following essential nutrients: vitamin B_6,[25] folate,[26] vitamin B_{12},[27] selenium,[28] and zinc.[29] Nutritional supplementation has been shown in clinical studies to offer great benefits to people already seriously ill with AIDS, and it is seen by many as the cornerstone requirement if there is to be recovery. In one six month study, vitamins, minerals, amino acids, and essential fatty acids were all supplemented. Among the observed clinical benefits was a general improvement in well being and a significant decrease in the P24 antigen.[30]

Candidiasis

Candidiasis, or yeast overgrowth in the intestinal tract, is a common feature of anyone who is immune compromised and therefore can be a major problem for people who are HIV positive or have AIDS.

A nutritional strategy that helps discourage yeast overgrowth concentrates on reducing, or cutting out altogether, the intake of simple carbohydrates and sugars, while emphasizing complex carbohydrate intake.[23]

In addition, an anticandidiasis strategy usually employs antifungal foods such as garlic and olive oil, along with the taking of specific substances that kill the yeast, such as caprylic acid (a fatty acid) and aloe vera.

Repopulation of the intestinal tract with friendly bacteria while the yeast is being targeted often involves the use of cultured dairy products such as kefir and live low-fat yogurt, as well as probiotic supplements such as Lactobacillus acidophilus *and bifidobacteria to help colonize the tract with necessary microorganisms.* Lactobacillus bulgaricus, *which is a noncolonizing bacteria, is also sometimes used because of its powerful antifungal and antibiotic potential.*[24]

Along with the above, other nutrients commonly supplemented in HIV positive and AIDS cases are vitamins A (beta-carotene), B-complex, and E. The B vitamins thiamine (B_1), riboflavin (B_2), pantothenic acid (B_5), pyridoxine (B_6), and B_{12} are especially essential for improving a weakened immune system. Vitamin C has also proven to be a powerful antioxidant and inhibitor of viruses and bacteria, as well as having specific and potent immune enhancing effects.[31]

See Candidiasis, Probiotics (in Appendix.)

According to Dr. Cathcart, "Preliminary clinical evidence is that massive doses of ascorbate (a salt of vitamin C) can suppress the symptoms of disease and can markedly reduce the tendency for secondary infections." Working with a group of 102 patients, most of whom were taking vitamin C on their own, Dr. Cathcart reports "considerable improvement" in most of the patients' conditions. Some of the improvements include a reduction of diseased lymph glands and the disappearance of Kaposi's sarcoma lesions.[32]

Supplementation of folic acid, biotin, potassium, magnesium, and manganese is also recommended, as well as amino acids and essential acids, particularly omega-3 and omega-6. A good multivitamin and mineral supplement can take the place of the individual supplements listed above, but the best advice is to always consult with a qualified health practitioner in order to optimize any supplementation regimen.

Always consult with a qualified health practitioner in order to optimize any supplementation regimen.

Dr. Priestley reports good results from placing an HIV positive patient on a regimen of intravenous nutrition with supplements taken three times a week in an IV-nutrient drip. Dr. Priestley also prescribed high doses of oral vitamin C daily and B-complex shots once a week, as well as garlic capsules, Siberian ginseng, beta-carotene, zinc, and aloe vera. The patient also began exercising, meditating, and using acupuncture.

Since beginning treatment, the patient has gained forty pounds and now has much fewer symptoms, despite having a low T-cell count, according to Dr. Priestley, who has continued the patient on a course of nutrients and preventative medicines to guard against infection.

Herbal Medicine

The use of herbal medicines in the treatment of AIDS is widespread today, with additional research ongoing to assess possible further applications and effectiveness. Some of the herbal remedies most often employed include astragalus,[33] carnivora (venus fly trap),[34] echinacea,[35] licorice,[36] and goldenseal.[37] Garlic[38] and isatis root[39] are also commonly used because of their broad antibacterial and antiviral qualities, as is ginseng, for its tonic effects on the thymus gland, in addition to its ability to resist all forms of stress.[40] St. John's Wort (*Hypericum perforatum*) is also used because of its specific retrovirus blocking actions.[41] Chinese bitter melon, monolaurin, and lentinan (extract of *shiitake* mushrooms) have also shown dramatic anti-HIV effects.[42]

See Diet, Herbal Medicine, Nutritional Supplements, Orthomolecular Medicine.

According to Subhuti Dharmananda, Ph.D., Director of the Institute for Traditional Medicine in Portland, Oregon, herbal remedies used in specific combinations can often be much more effective than taking the herbs individually.[43]

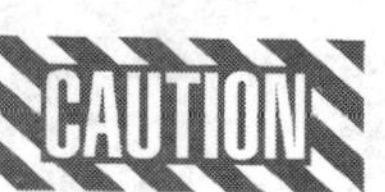

There are many herbal combinations available, but they should only be administered with the advice of a qualified health practitioner, as all herbal compounds and many individual herbs can be toxic if used incorrectly or in excessive amounts.

Dr. Badgley reports that one of his patients, who was diagnosed with Kaposi's sarcoma nine years ago, has had excellent results with a tea brewed from a mixture of the herbs echinacia, red clover tops, chaparral, dandelion, sasparilla, and pau d'arco. The patient reports that the tea, in combination with a whole foods diet and nutritional supplements, stimulates his appetite and helps maintain his strength.

Acupuncture

Acupuncture has been shown to be an effective and vital tool for the treatment of HIV infection and AIDS, particularly when coupled with other alternative therapies such as herbal remedies. Preliminary studies at the Quan Yin Clinic in San Francisco, California have shown acupuncture to increase immune function, white blood cell production, and T-cell production. It also alleviates many of the symptoms related to HIV infection and AIDS. According to a published report, "Many patients report a reduction in fatigue, abnormal sweating, diarrhea, and acute skin reactions after only four to six acupuncture treatments. Many describe an improved sense of well being, some report weight gain, and are able to return to longer hours of work."[44]

William Michael Cargile, B.S., D.C., F.I.A.C.A., Chairman of Research for the American Association of Acupuncture and Oriental Medicine, has worked with AIDS patients for many years, and has been able to increase T-cell counts with acupuncture treatments. "One of these patients had a T-cell count of 30 to 40," he recounts. "We eventually brought it up to 270, and although this is half the level a person is said to need, he's been doing great for the last six months." Dr. Cargile adds that the key to understanding acupuncture's influence on blood values and cell counts lies partly in its ability to minimize stress and strengthen the body's adaptive mechanisms. "I think that if we had more acupuncture and less AZT, we would see a qualitative improvement in these patient's health," he states.

Numerous clinical studies have borne out Dr. Cargile's claims. When two hundred patients in New York with AIDS were treated with acupuncture, it was found to reduce levels of secondary opportunistic infections and to be generally beneficial. Also, at Lincoln Memorial Hospital in New York City, out of twenty-seven people with AIDS who received acupuncture treatments, twenty reported that fatigue was reduced and that night sweats and diarrhea improved after between one and three weeks. Many also gained substantial amounts of weight. Michael Smith, M.D., who oversaw the patients, reports that in some cases T-cell ratios rose dramatically over a two to three month period with acupuncture alone.[45]

> *"I think that if we had more acupuncture and less AZT, we would see a qualitative improvement in these patient's health."*
>
> —William Cargile, B.S., D.C., F.I.A.C.A., Chairman of Research, American Association of Acupuncture and Oriental Medicine

In addition, fifteen patients who attended acupuncture treatments regularly at Somerville Centre near Boston, reported improvement in general symptoms and six reported that acupuncture helped reduce side effects of medical treatment for Kaposi's sarcoma.[46]

Sir Jay Holder, M.D., D.C., Ph.D., founder and Medical Director of the Exodus Treatment Center in Miami, Florida, has also achieved significant results using acupuncture. He describes the case of a man with AIDS, suffering from Kaposi's sarcoma, and given just twenty-two months to live. Within three weeks of treatment with acupuncture and Chinese herbs, his T-cell count returned to normal and his lesions disappeared.

See Acupuncture, Traditional Chinese Medicine.

Most acupuncture treatments for people with HIV or AIDS last approximately forty-five minutes, and are entirely painless, except for a slight pricking sensation when the needles go in. In addition, most acupuncturists today use presterilized, disposable needles to protect both themselves and patients from AIDS, hepatitis, and other infectious diseases.

Bitter Melon

For centuries, in Asian cultures, bitter melon has been used as a treatment for a wide variety of ailments. It is believed that eating bitter melon regularly will clean and purify blood and ward off a variety of infections. Since the early 1980s, bitter melon fruits and seeds have been tested in vitro and in vivo as an effective therapy for cancers, tumors, and HIV.

Stanley Rebultan, a Filipino-American man, who is HIV positive took bitter melon liquid extract for nearly four years as his sole antiviral treatment, and saw his T4 cell count increase by 121 percent (480 to 1060), his T4 to T8 ratio improve by 68 percent (.91 to 1.53), and his CD4 percentage rise by 77 percent (26 percent to 46 percent).

At the Amsterdam International Conference on AIDS in 1992, Quingcai Zhang, a Chinese medical doctor and herbalist presented additional data supporting Rebultan's experience. In Dr. Zhang's study, those who took bitter melon for four months to three years had CD4 counts increase between 33 percent and 285 percent. His findings showed that, in most cases, it normalized T4 to T8 ratios, raised T4 counts over time, and increased energy and a sense of well-being. Dr. Zhang also noted that bitter melon blocked HIV-infected macrophage (immune cells that recognize and ingest foreign antigens), something AZT does not do, as well as infected lymphocytes, such as CD4 cells.[47]

Bitter melon extracts or boiled decoctions can be taken orally or rectally. A rectal retention enema is recommended, though, because the plant is very bitter and unpleasant to drink, and may cause nausea. Using the retention enema method also avoids the breakdown of the bitter melon proteins in the stomach acid, allowing them to instead be absorbed directly into the bloodstream through the colon and large intestines.

While bitter melon has shown remarkable results for those who stick with it, many people quit before the therapy can take effect. Rebultan admits that it took him three months before he felt comfortable with the treatment procedure, but explains, "It's a long-term therapy. You won't gain results overnight. It takes at least six months to see results but if I have to do this my entire life to maintain a normal sense of well-being, then I will. Herbal therapy takes a long time. It's not like the overnight miracles of pill popping that American medicine feels so entitled to."

Hyperthermia

Researchers have proven that HIV is heat sensitive,[48] and will become increasingly inactive as the body temperature is raised progressively above normal (98.6 degrees Fahrenheit) for extended periods of time.[49] Much as a fever is the body's natural defense mechanism against infection and disease, hyperthermia can be used to similar effect by artificially raising the body's temperature above normal. This also stimulates the immune system by increasing the production of antibodies and interferon (a protein substance produced by virus-invaded cells that prevents reproduction of the virus).

Certain forms of hyperthermia can also be employed as part of a self-care regimen. Hot baths are the simplest method of inducing a fever at home, and for viral infections such as HIV, they can be combined with hot drinks and blanket wrapping to stimulate the immune system. After a hot bath, a person can wrap up in dry blankets, with a hot water bottle over the abdomen, in order to perspire heavily for as long as can be tolerated. This may take several hours and should be followed by a cool shower. It is also possible to produce a mild fever with the hot bath by simply wrapping up in the dry blankets after the bath. Again, allow several hours to perspire heavily and follow with a cool shower.

A wet sheet pack may also be used to raise the body temperature. In this case, the patient wraps in a very cold, wet sheet, followed by several blankets. Like the dry pack, it will take several hours to produce a fever, the cold sheet causing reactions in the body that encourage the production of heat. It is often useful to precede this procedure with some kind of heating such as exercise, a hot bath, or a hot shower.

Other more "high tech" methods are also available, such as shortwave or microwave diathermy (the use of high frequency current to generate heat in a part of the body), ultrasound, radiant heating (heat from a light source), and extracorpeal heating (heat administered from a source outside the body), but these are usually administered only in a medical or hospital setting.

At the Natural Health Clinic at Bastyr College, hyperthermia is commonly used in the treatment of HIV infection. Hyperthermia treatment was also included as part of the college's HARP study. Participants were given a series of hyperthermia baths (102 degrees Fahrenheit) for forty minutes. These were administered twice weekly for three weeks at a time, over the course of a year. According to Leanna Standish, Ph.D., N.D., who oversaw the HARP study, when participants in the study were asked what aspect of the treatment had the greatest impact, the overwhelming response was "hyperthermia." There was a reported decrease in night sweats and in the frequency of secondary infections. Also, many of the participants claimed to have a greater sense of well-being after receiving hyperthermia treatments.[50]

See Hydrotherapy, Hyperthermia.

While hyperthermia treatments may not be able to kill every invading virus (with approximately 40 percent HIV inactivation after thirty minutes in a 107.6 degrees Fahrenheit bath), they reduce their number, making it easier for the immune system to handle the remaining viruses. Hyperthermia is also a useful technique for detoxification because it releases toxins stored in fat cells.

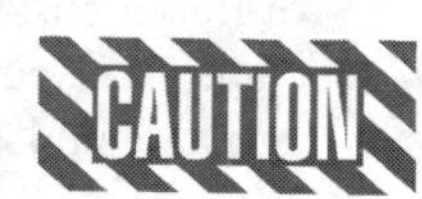

Caution: *Hyperthermia should only be undertaken with proper supervision, because of the possible damage toxins might cause when released, particularly to the kidneys and liver. Certain individuals are also more sensitive to the effects of heat and their conditions should be treated with great care. These include people with anemia, heart disease, diabetes, seizure disorders, and tuberculosis. Overall, however, when used knowledgeably hyperthermia is a safe and effective treatment for HIV infection, with ill effects appearing usually only when body temperature exceeds 106 degrees Fahrenheit.*

Oxygen Therapy

In 1988, Kenneth Wagner, M.D., former head of the Naval Hospital's AIDS unit in Bethesda, Maryland, and Steven Kleinman, M.D., Medical Director of the American Red Cross Blood Services for Los Angeles, along with Michael Carpendale, M.D., of the Veterans Administration Medical Center in San Francisco, California, and Mark Rarick, M.D., an AIDS researcher at the University of Southern California, all came out in support of using oxygen therapy as a primary treatment for AIDS and HIV infection. Their message was direct and simple—oxygen therapy is the safest and most effective method of treating AIDS and its associated infections.[51]

Oxygen therapy uses either ozone or hydrogen peroxide to combat HIV in much the same way as the human immune system uses self-generated oxygen free radicals (a single oxygen atom) to destroy bacterial and viral infections. The extra oxygen atoms in both ozone (O_3) and hydrogen peroxide (H_2O_2) break off and link with the invading molecules, altering their molecular structure, in effect killing the harmful cells and leaving behind only oxygen (O_2) or water (H_2O).

A recent study found that when HIV-infected blood was removed from the body and treated with ozone, the virus was completely deactivated.[52] One current AIDS treatment method mimics this approach, removing blood from the body, infusing it with ozone, and then replacing it. Another approach has been to simply inject a diluted form of ozone into the bloodstream. This treatment can be done daily for several weeks at a time.

French researchers Bertrand Vallancien and Jean-Marie Winkler studied ozone therapy with a group of patients with HIV, herpes, and hepatitis. After nine weeks of transfused ozone, T4 and T8 cells moved toward normal levels in all cases, and the ozone treatments caused no other problems.[53]

Hydrogen peroxide, like ozone, can be administered intravenously, and can also be taken rectally by enema, vaginally, or transcutaneously (absorption by bathing) according to Charles H. Farr, M.D., Ph.D., Medical Director of the International Bio-Oxidative Medicine Association. He advocates the intravenous method of delivery, however. "Some doctors are using combinations of ozone and peroxide and reporting good results as well, because of a synergistic response in the cells," he adds.

See Oxygen Therapy.

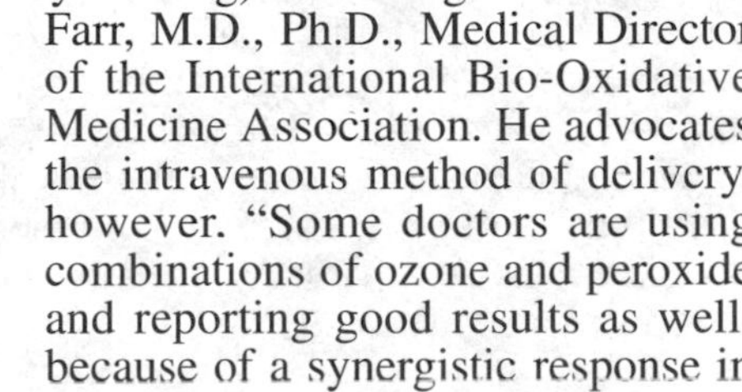

Although hydrogen peroxide can also be taken orally, Dr. Farr, who first characterized the effects of hydrogen peroxide on humans in 1984, recommends against it, because the enzymes of the stomach are unable to process it properly.

While oxygen free radicals are deadly to viruses and bacteria, they can also do damage to healthy tissue if left unchecked. When the body manufactures these oxygen-based defense substances, it follows this immediately by sending protective antioxidant enzymes to quench the process before harm to healthy tissue can take place. Nutritional support is also generally recommended with any oxygen therapy, particularly vitamin C supplementation, which acts as a stabilizing antioxidant agent.

Mind/Body Medicine

There is an absolutely vital relationship between a person's emotional state and their immune system. In cases of AIDS and HIV infection, this relationship has a profound impact on whether the individual maintains or recovers health, or whether he or she slips further down into the disease state.[54]

As with cancer, a tremendous negative mental and emotional burden is initially placed on patients diagnosed HIV positive or with AIDS, because of all the implications which lurk behind these diagnoses. According to Herb Joiner-Bey, N.D., of Bastyr College, without spiritual and mental involvement, people find it difficult to generate the commitment to getting themselves well. This makes the restoration of a positive, realistic outlook that encourages self-reliance, a key ingredient in any alternative approach to HIV infection and AIDS.[55]

Emotions such as guilt, hopelessness, suppressed anger, and fear, which are common among many persons with AIDS, add to the burden of the immune system. Yet, according to Leon Chaitow, N.D., D.O., of London, England, most negative emotions can be resolved with a little effort and attention. "Any stress coping strategy which reduces these negative influences on the nervous system—be this relaxation, meditation, visualization, or some form of psychotherapeutic counseling, treatment, or group work—will help immune function," Dr. Chaitow points out.

Jon Kaiser, M.D., of San Francisco, California, specializes in the practice of alternative therapies and the mind/body connection. Nearly 70 percent of his patients are HIV positive. One of his patients came to him after continually having his anxiety about being diagnosed HIV positive dismissed by his former doctors. In conjunction with a protocol of diet, nutritional supplements, and herbs, Dr. Kaiser addressed the man's stress-related symptoms. As a result, the man regained control over his emotions and his health has improved to the point where he has been asymptomatic for the last four years. Among the points Dr. Kaiser emphasizes to his patients are the following:

- AIDS is not a death sentence.
- Someone who begins a sound, alternative program early on can reasonably consider the possibility of living out a normal life span.
- Maintain a positive attitude.
- Don't panic, or give into the negative programming that the media and the medical establishment promote.
- Follow a balanced, focused treatment program.

Janet Konefal, Ph.D., Associate Professor of Psychiatry at the University of Miami School of Medicine, employs a counseling protocol aimed at "expanding limiting beliefs and altering behaviors among HIV positive individuals." She also places great emphasis on the needs of the therapist in dealing with the distress which permeates AIDS and HIV associated illnesses. Dr.

MASSAGE THERAPY

Massage can have immense benefits for people with AIDS or HIV. The benefits are both physical, such as improved circulation and drainage of blood and lymph, relaxation of muscles, and improved movement for joints; and mental and emotional, including reduced stress and a greater sense of ease and well being.[56]

According to Robert King, L.M.T., past President of the American Massage Therapy Association, massage provides an environment in which emotions relating to issues such as death, dying, and sadness can emerge, as well as acting as a catalyst which reinforces touching and hugging in daily life. Improvement also takes place in relation to self-image and self-esteem after receipt of a caring massage. A person's sense of isolation and loneliness is also broken down.

The resulting stress reduction derived from massage therapy can have a powerful immune enhancing benefit as well. Research at the Miami School of Medicine, Touch Institute, in Miami, Florida, has shown increased natural killer cell activity and other immune system improvements directly related to massage therapy.[57]

Yet, despite the obvious advantages of massage therapy for someone who is HIV positive or has AIDS, it is not always readily available. Due to fear, ignorance, and misinformation about how AIDS is contracted, people with AIDS often suffer from the emotional battering of being social outcasts. The end result is that touch is one of the first things that leave their lives, once they are diagnosed.

Important: People with AIDS who receive massage often have specific requirements. The massage should not be too fast or too deep, to ensure that the adrenal system is not overstimulated, which can challenge the immune system. The person giving the massage should use gentle touch, focusing on relaxation, comfort, and nurturing, rather than on assessing and dealing with postural problems. It is also vital not to release too many toxins into the immune system, and to bear in mind the person's individual symptoms. Massage is always contraindicated for cancer, and those with pulmonary problems (pneumonia) require gentle pats rather than rubs in the affected areas.

It is also important for anyone HIV positive or with AIDS to avail themselves of a licensed massage therapist who has a background in dealing with their condition and emotional state. In many areas free massage is available for anyone HIV positive or with AIDS, with many volunteer organizations offering on site walk-ins.

Konefal's approach is to gradually take the individual—whose negative mental state may carry images of past illness and loss, as well as poor images of future prospects in terms of health, happiness, and survival—toward a position in which positive, hopeful images can start to regularly replace these negative images.

See Bodywork, Guided Imagery, Hypnotherapy, Mind/Body Medicine, Neuro-Linguistic Programming.

In order to achieve this shift, Dr. Konefal employs techniques which incorporate symbolism, imagery, and goal setting in a structured and individualized manner. "The end result is that the patient's dark, morbid, immunosuppressing thoughts give way to light, life-affirming thoughts that foster the will to live, and create an emotionally stronger and far more optimistic individual," she says.

Summary

It is by concentration on the person with AIDS or HIV, rather than on the illness or virus, that many long-term survivors of both conditions have succeeded in maintaining good levels of health. In the long run it is through attention to underlying health through a variety of methods, with a focus on co-factor infections, that both AIDS and HIV may be successfully controlled.

Self-Care Treatment

The following therapies can be undertaken at home under appropriate professional supervision.

- ***Biofeedback Training***
- ***Guided Imagery***
- ***Meditation***

Aromatherapy: tea tree, garlic.

Homeopathy: *Hypericum.*

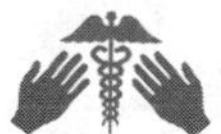

Professional Care

The following therapies should only be provided by a qualified health professional:

• Cell Therapy • Enzyme Therapy • Fasting • Orthomolecular Medicine • Magnetic Field Therapy • Traditional Chinese Medicine

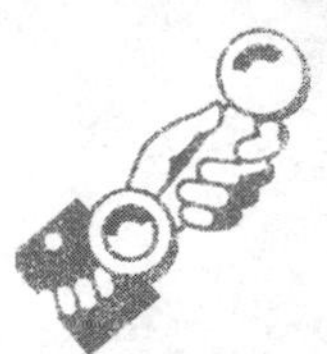

Where to Find Help

For information on, or referrals for, treatment of AIDS contact the following organizations.

AIDS Alternative Health Project.
3223 N. Sheffield Avenue
Chicago, Illinois 60657
(312) 327-6437

An organization staffed by professional volunteers who offer chiropractic, acupuncture, bodywork, nutritional and herbal counseling, and massage therapy to HIV+ individuals. Services are available for a nominal fee, which can be waived for people who are unemployed, or receiving unemployment, social security, or disability benefits.

Cure Now
P.O. Box 29386
Los Angeles, California 90029
(213) 660-7563

Cure Now is a group formed to educate people on positive healing alternatives, and to improve the psychological and spiritual attitudes surrounding AIDS and HIV.

HEAL
16 East 16th Street
New York, New York 10003
(212) 674-HOPE

Offers information to people seeking to strengthen their health and immune systems. Provides information on an alternative approach to health that "precludes toxic, immunosuppressive drugs, but includes physical, emotional, psychological, and spiritual efforts." Also provides referrals to hypnotherapists trained to deal with the fears of an HIV diagnosis.

Immune Development Trust
Gatesden, Cromer Street
King's Cross, London, WC1H 8EA
071-837-2151 (Ph.)/071-837-7742 (Fax)

The Trust accepts without charge anyone who is HIV+, and provides a range of alternative treatments, including acupuncture, herbal medicine, massage therapy, and other types of bodywork.

Quan Yin Healing Arts Center.
1748 Market Street
San Francisco, California 94102
(415) 861-4964

Offers a program for people with AIDS or who are HIV+. Services include acupuncture, herbal medicine, yoga, and massage therapy. Also provides lecture series and discussion groups to provide support and nutritional information. Available on a sliding scale fee basis.

Acupuncture/Traditional Chinese Medicine

American Association of Acupuncture and Oriental Medicine
4101 Lake Boone Trail, Suite 201
Raleigh, North Carolina 27607
(919) 787-5181

The AAAOM is a national professional trade organization of acupuncturists who meet acceptable standards of minimum competency and can provide you with the names and locations of local members. Referrals by written request only. A fee of five dollars is charged.

Herbal

American Association of Naturopathic Physicians
P.O. Box 20386
Seattle, Washington 98102
(206) 323-7610

Provides referrals to a nationwide network of accredited or licensed practitioners. Publishes a quarterly newsletter for both professionals and the general public. Also offers a series of brochures and pamphlets on a variety of subjects.

Hyperthermia

Bastyr University
Natural Health Clinic
1307 North 45th Street, Suite 200
Seattle, Washington 98103
(206) 632-0354

Bastyr University is an accredited educational institution that offers degree programs in the natural health sciences. These include programs in naturopathic medicine; homeopathy; midwifery; acupuncture; nutrition; Chinese herbal medicine; marriage and family counseling; and applied behavioral sciences. Bastyr also offers a limited number of Distance Learning courses in these areas for students unable to attend classes at its Seattle, Washington facility. The physical medicine department of the Natural Health Clinic of Bastyr University uses hyperthermia treatment for detox and in conditions ranging from upper respiratory infection to chronic fatigue syndrome and HIV infection.

National College of Naturopathic Medicine
11231 Southeast Market Street
Portland, Oregon 97216
(503) 255-4860

Offers postgraduate training in naturopathic medicine and support teaching clinics. The teaching clinic uses hyperthermia for a wide variety of conditions.

Massage

American Massage Therapy Association
1130 West North Shore Avenue
Chicago, Illinois 60626-4670
(312) 761-2682

Offers comprehensive information on most areas of massage and bodywork, including an extensive review of scientific research. They also publish the Massage Therapy Journal, *available at many newsstands and health food stores.*

Oxygen Therapy

International Bio-oxidative Medicine Foundation (IBOM)
P.O. Box 13205
Oklahoma City, Oklahoma 73113-1205
(405) 478-IBOM Ext. 4266

The foundation publishes and distributes a newsletter, as well as scientific research data. Supports educational programs that highlight current research and the therapeutic use of oxidative modalities. Encourages basic and clinical research. Membership available.

International Ozone Association
31 Strawberry Hill Avenue
Stamford, Connecticut 06902
(203) 348-3542

A professional scientific organization disseminating information on use and production of ozone through meetings, synopsis, and world congresses. Publisheabooks and journals on ozone.

Medizone International, Inc.
123 East 54th Street
tew York Street
New York NY 10022
212-421-0303

Developers of ozone-based blood purification systems and treatment for diseases caused by lipid enveloped viruses including AIDS, hepatitis B and herpes.

North Carolina Bio-Oxidative Health Center
4505 Fair Meadow Lane,
Suite 111
Raleigh, North Carolina 27607
(800) 473-9812 (U.S. and Canada)
(407) 967-6466 (Outside North America)

Outpatient facility which focuses on metabolic and intestinal detoxification. Comprehensive and synergistic treatment regimens for each patient are developed utilizing therapies such as colon hydrotherapy, intravenous therapies (including ozone), and external ozone hydrotherapy. Supportive elements such as acupuncture and lymphatic massage, as well as techniques to address the psychological/emotional components of health and illness are also part of the program.

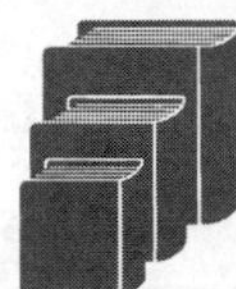

Recommended Reading

AIDS: The HIV Myth. Adams, Jad. New York: St. Martin's Press, 1989.
An exploration of Peter Duesberg's HIV hypothesis that debunks the theory that the virus causes AIDS.

The AIDS War. Lauritson, John. New York: Asklepios, 1993.
Contains the latest information regarding the dangers of using AZT to treat AIDS, as well as information on Peter Duesberg and the censure he received from the conventional medical establishment for his theory that HIV does not cause AIDS. (Available from Asklepios, 26 Saint Marks Place, New York City 10003.)

Healing AIDS Naturally. Badgley, Laurence, M.D. Foster City, CA: Healing Energy Press, 1987.
Outlines Dr. Badgley's protocol for treating AIDS using alternative medicine.

Poison By Prescription: The AZT Story. Lauritson, John. New York: Asklepios, 1990.
An expose of the politics involved in AIDS research and how AZT, a known toxic substance, became the conventional medical establishment's drug of choice for dealing with AIDS and HIV. (Available from Asklepios, 26 Saint Marks Place, New York City 10003.)

Rethinking AIDS. Root-Bernstein, Robert. New York: The Free Press, 1993.
A thorough investigation which indicates that HIV alone does not cause AIDS.

Rethinking AIDS
2040 Polk Street, Suite 321
San Francisco, CA 94109
(415) 775-1984 (FAX)
A monthly newsletter published by the Group for the Scientific Reappraisal of the HIV Hypothesis. (Comprised of over four hundred scientists and physicians worldwide).

Surviving AIDS. Callen, Michael. New York: HarperCollins, 1990.
Outlines the alternative medicine approach to health taken by the author, one of the longest survivors of AIDS.

A World Without AIDS. Chaitow, Leon, D.O., N.D.; and Martin, Simon. London, England: Thorsons Publishing Group, 1988.
A convincing argument that conventional medicine approaches do not "cure" disease, which outlines how AIDS can be treated using methods of naturopathic medicine. Also includes an appendix outlining 21 ways to strengthen the immune system.

Allergies

Allergies are more widespread than most physicians, including allergists, realize, and they can cause far more serious health problems, both physical and mental, than is commonly believed. Allergy sufferers don't need to despair, however. Proper diet and nutrition, combined with other alternative approaches, can relieve and reverse allergies, even after conventional approaches have failed.

An allergy is an adverse immune system reaction to a substance that most people find harmless. Allergies can manifest in a variety of ways. Common examples of an allergic response include headaches, fatigue, sneezing, watery eyes, and stuffy sinuses following exposure to dust, pollens, dust mites, animal dander, chemicals, and a variety of other materials. "The allergic reactions themselves can range from mild to severe depending on the person," explains Richard Wilkinson, M.D., who practices environmental medicine in Yakima, Washington. "Many of the conditions are so common that they are almost considered normal by the people who suffer from them."

Though conventional estimates suggest that 35 million Americans are afflicted with allergies, James Braly, M.D., Medical Director of Immuno Labs in Fort Lauderdale, Florida, places the figure much higher. "Actually the majority of Americans suffer from allergies," he says. "This is particularly true of food allergy, which is, along with undernutrition, the most commonly undiagnosed condition in the United States today."

Types of Allergies

Allergies fall into two categories, those caused by environmental factors, and those caused by food. Either type can result in a wide range of symptoms, and can cause or contribute to asthma, bronchitis, rheumatoid arthritis, diabetes, eczema, migraines and cluster headaches, chronic fatigue syndrome, gastrointestinal disorders, glaucoma, kidney problems, weight gain, seizures, heart palpitations, depression, and even cerebral palsy and multiple sclerosis, among other conditions.

Environmental Allergies

The most common cause of environmental allergies are the pollens of various plants such as trees, weeds, and grass, according to Dr. Wilkinson. House dust, mites, molds, and tobacco smoke are other causes. Less common, but equally serious,

ARE YOUR SYMPTOMS DUE TO ALLERGIES?

The following questionnaire developed by Leon Chaitow, N.D., D.O., of London, England, can help you determine if you suffer from allergies:

- *Do you suffer from unnatural fatigue? 1. Occasionally 2. Regularly (3X a week or more). (Score 1 or 2 depending on your answer.)*
- *Do you at times have weight fluctuations of four or more pounds in a day accompanied by puffiness of the face, ankles, or fingers? (Score 1 if infrequently, 2 if frequent—more than once a month—or severe.)*
- *Do you have hot flashes (apart from menopause) or find yourself sweating for no obvious reason? (Score 1 if infrequently, 2 if several times a week or more.)*
- *Does your heart race or pound strongly for no obvious reason? (Score 1 if infrequently, 2 if several times a week or more.)*
- *Do you have a history of food intolerance causing any symptoms at all? (Score 2 if your answer is yes.)*
- *Do you crave bread, sugary foods, milk, chocolate, coffee, tea? (Score 2 if yes. The maximum score for this is 2.)*
- *Do you suffer from migraine or severe headaches, irritable bowel syndrome, eczema, depression, asthma, or muscle aches? (Score 2 if yes. Maximum score is 2.)*

"The most anyone could score on this test would be 14," Dr. Chaitow explains. "If your score is 5 or higher there is a strong likelihood that allergies are part of your symptom picture."

are products often found in the home. "Cosmetics, perfumes, household cleaning agents, the gas we use for heating and cooking, the fabrics in our clothes, and even the metals used by dentists as fillings can trigger allergy attacks in some people," Dr. Wilkinson says.

Food Allergies

The fact that physical and mental disorders can be caused by allergic reactions to food was first discovered during the 1940s by Theron Randolph, M.D., the founder of environmental medicine. His findings have resulted in a growing number of studies which link food allergies to a wide spectrum of health conditions. Dr. Braly defines food allergies as abnormal or adverse immunological responses to foods that other people eat with impunity. "But food allergies must be distinguished from nonallergic reactions to food, such as enzyme deficiencies or food poisoning," he points out.

Food allergies must also be distinguished from toxic reactions that affect everyone more or less identically, according to Leon Chaitow, N.D., D.O., of London, England, because, while a toxic substance such as cyanide will affect anyone who ingests it, any number of people can eat the same food, and only the persons allergic to it will have a reaction. The foods most commonly found to cause allergies include wheat, corn, milk, and other dairy products, egg whites, tomatoes, soy, shellfish, peanuts, chocolate, as well as food dyes and additives.

What Causes Allergies?

One of the primary causes of allergies is an impaired immune system, which substantially increases the risk of allergic reactions. "This occurs when the immune system becomes stressed due to an overload of toxins," says Charles Gableman, M.D., a practitioner of environmental medicine in Encinitas, California.

Dr. Chaitow, in researching allergies, has found that a number of factors negatively impact the immune system. These include increased toxic burden due to pollution in all its forms; disturbance of infant immune systems through repeated vaccination and immunization; and damage to healthy intestinal flora due to overreliance upon antibiotics and steroids (especially birth control pills).

"The immune system may also be weakened by hereditary problems," states Fuller Royal, M.D., of Las Vegas, Nevada. "Usually this will be reflected in the gastrointestinal tract, so that nutrients are not able to be absorbed and utilized properly. This can then set you up for

Allergies and Childbirth

According to James Braly, M.D., Medical Director of Immuno Labs, Inc., in Fort Lauderdale, Florida, children born of parents who are both prone to allergies have up to a 90 percent chance of developing allergies themselves. "This may occur during pregnancy, particularly with food allergies," Dr. Braly says. "One of the immune mechanisms that mediate allergies, an antibody called IgG, transfers through the placenta from the mother's blood into the fetal blood supply, causing the fetus to passively develop allergies to the same foods that the mother is allergic to."

It has also been shown that babies born of mothers with a personal or family history of Type 1 insulin-dependent diabetes can develop insulin deficiency and Type 1 diabetes within their first six months of life by being bottle fed with cow's milk or breast-fed if their mothers drink cow's milk.[1] "During those first six months the baby's immune system is very immature," Dr. Braly explains, "and very susceptible to lactalbumin, a protein in cow's milk made up of an eighteen amino acid sequence that is identical to the amino acid peptide on the surface of the insulin-producing cells of the baby's pancreas. When the baby is exposed to the cow's milk, his or her immune system will form antibodies against the lactalbumin that will, in turn, attack and destroy the insulin-producing cells of the pancreas. But if the baby is not exposed to cow's milk until after the first six months, this does not occur, due to the maturation of the immune system."

Dr. Braly recommends that women genetically predisposed to diabetes who plan to become pregnant discover what foods they are allergic to before pregnancy and eliminate them from their diet. They should then breast-feed their babies without consuming dairy products for a minimum of six months while still refraining from the foods they are allergic to.

According to Dick Thom, N.D., D.D.S., of Beaverton, Oregon, a mother who smokes during her pregnancy can also increase the likelihood of her baby developing allergies. "The time of year of the birth and weaning are also important factors," Dr. Thom states. "Being born or weaned immediately prior to the peak of pollen season, for instance, can increase the child's risk of becoming allergic to that particular allergen."

ALLERGIES AND CEREBRAL PALSY

People who suffer from cerebral palsy may have sensitivities or allergies to certain foods or elements of their environment that can intensify their symptoms, according to Marshall Mandell, M.D., Medical Director of the New England Foundation for Allergies and Environmental Diseases. "Food can pass through the digestive track into the bloodstream and then to the brain, causing an allergic response that can trigger exaggerated cerebral palsy symptoms," Dr. Mandell explains. He refers to such reactions as "a hay fever of the brain."

In his clinical practice, Dr. Mandell has witnessed intermittent and unpredictable flare-ups of cerebral palsy occurring in patients, due to allergies aggravating what he calls the patients "biological weak spots," or areas of the body that may have healed to a degree but are still highly sensitive to outside irritations.

Two patients Dr. Mandell treated illustrate his findings. The first involved a woman with cerebral palsy who experienced sudden exaggerated symptoms of her condition for no discernible reason, under circumstances that normally did not cause her problems. Dr. Mandell conducted a series of tests on her and discovered that she was allergic to tomatoes. Upon being questioned, the woman admitted that prior to each of her attacks she had included tomatoes with her meals. Once she eliminated tomatoes from her diet, her flare-ups stopped, as well.

The second patient was an eleven-year-old boy from Canada, whose doctors advised be institutionalized due to his extreme spasticity. "When the boy's mother brought him to see me, his condition was so aggravated that his muscles were in a continuous state of spasm," Dr. Mandell says. "I tested the boy and determined that food allergies were responsible. Once his diet was adjusted so that the offending foods were no longer included, the boy's condition dramatically improved, to the point where his mother describes him as being a totally different person."

These are but two examples of numerous cerebral palsy patients Dr. Mandell has treated whose conditions were found to be aggravated by food or other allergies, and which improved once their exposure to the offending allergens was eliminated. His findings suggest a need for further research into the role allergy might play in contributing to cerebral palsy.

food allergies." Dr. Royal also agrees that antibiotics can cause allergic reactions and feels that in many cases their use is unnecessary. "Antibiotics further add to the confusion the immune system is facing," he says, "until the immune system is no longer able to tell friend from foe. When that happens, it starts reacting to all sorts of things which are not foes, that then become treated as allergens. This lead to fatigue and allows viruses, bacteria, and so forth to come in and play havoc."

Other causes of food allergies include nutritional deficiencies, a repetitive and monotonous diet, chemicals in the food chain due to pesticides and preservatives, and chronic intestinal yeast overgrowth (candidiasis), according to allergy specialist John Mansfield, M.D., of England.[2]

"A repetitive diet can contribute greatly to the development of allergies," says Marshall Mandell, M.D., Medical Director of the New England Foundation for Allergies and Environmental Diseases. Dr. Randolph has found that diets of allergy patients normally consist of thirty foods or less, which they eat repeatedly. "These thirty foods then become the basis for the most common food intolerances," says Dr. Mandell. "If someone eats bread every day, for instance, he could easily develop a wheat allergy due to the immune system's continuous exposure to it."

"Leaky gut syndrome", or excessive permeability in the digestive tract, is another major factor that can lead to allergies, according to Dr. Braly. "In these cases," he explains, "the immune system reacts to the particles of partially digested foodstuffs (macromolecules) that leak into the bloodstream through the gut as if they were foreign material." Among the causes of leaky gut syndrome, Dr. Braly cites poor digestion, alcohol consumption, the use of nonsteroidal anti-inflammatory drugs (NSAIDS), viral and bacterial infections, parasitical infestation, vitamin, mineral, amino acid and/or essential fatty acid deficiencies, excessive stress, antibiotics, premature birth, candidiasis, and radiation. "These are all factors that one should consider and bring under control as part of an overall approach for treating allergies," he advises.

Allergies and Addiction

As early as the 1940s, practitioners of environmental medicine, led by Dr. Randolph, found that people with food allergies are often addicted to the very foods they are allergic to. According to Dr. Randolph, an allergic reaction to food can last for up to three or more days, making the addiction to the food difficult to discover. This is because the symptoms that a person normally experiences when undergoing withdrawal from an addictive substance can actually improve or be suppressed if the person eats more of the food he or she is addicted to.

"The relationship between food allergy and food addiction is both extremely close and subtle," Dr. Wilkinson explains. "If people are allergic to coffee, for instance, they won't usually break into a rash or start sneezing when they drink it. Instead, symptoms such as a headache might occur hours after the coffee is consumed, or they might later experience severe exhaustion if they refrain from having another cup. But most people will tend to drink coffee regularly and thus get relief from their symptoms without realizing that it is the coffee that is causing them."

See Addictions.

The suppression of symptoms caused by addictive/allergenic foods when they are eaten has been termed "masking" by Dr. Randolph, as the foods will mask, or camouflage, the actual allergic symptoms.

"The likelihood of having an allergic reaction to any given food is directly proportional to how often a person eats it," says Dr. Gableman. "This is not true in all cases, but as a rule the foods that we eat the most as a culture tend to be the ones we are most allergic to."

A FOOD ALLERGY TIMETABLE

Michael Lesser, M.D., of Berkeley, California, has created a timetable based on patient case histories which can be used to determine the foods or liquids you may be allergic to.[3] When experiencing the symptoms below, notice if they began within the given time frame. If so, they may be due to food allergies.

Symptom	Time after food was eaten
Indigestion or heartburn	30 minutes
Headache	Within 1 hour
Asthma, runny nose	Within 1 hour
Stomach bloat/diarrhea	3 to 4 hours
Rashes or hives	6 to 12 hours
Weight gain by fluid retention	12 to 15 hours
Fits, convulsions, mental disturbance	12 to 24 hours
Mouth ulcers, joint/muscle pain, backache	48 to 96 hours

Treatment of Allergies

"In order for true healing of allergies to occur, it is necessary to address their cause rather than just treat the outward manifestations or symptoms," says Dr. Wilkinson. "This involves identifying the substances a person is allergic to and eliminating them from the diet and environment. At the same time, the body needs to be purged of toxins and the immune system needs to be stimulated. Since no two people are exactly alike, therapeutic approaches will vary, and usually a combination of therapies is the best course of action."

Among the therapies which have proven most effective in treating allergies are diet and nutrition, herbal medicine, acupuncture, Ayurvedic medicine, and homeopathy.

Diet and Nutrition

"Proper diet is the foundation from which to deal with allergies of all types," says Dick Thom, N.D., D.D.S., of Beaverton, Oregon. "If the body is continually being stressed by the foods that are meant to nourish it, there will be less reserves left over for the immune system to deal with other 'foreign' substances." One way to ensure that the body is receiving a greater supply of nutrients from food, while at the same time minimizing the risk of exposure to allergenic foods, is to increase the variety of foods eaten and rotate them so that they aren't eaten too frequently. This is known as a "rotation diet."

According to Dr. Braly, a rotation diet is one of the simplest and most effective measures anyone can take to both prevent and deal with the problems of food allergies. "Normally I would rotate the foods every four days," he advises. "This means that you are not eating any one food more often than every four days. You might be able to have the same food more than once in a day, but then you wouldn't have it again until four days later. Some people may need to go longer than that, but usually four days is pretty close to ideal."

Dr. Braly also suggests adopting a lifestyle that includes a wide variety of nonallergenic fresh fruits and vegetables, seeds and nuts, and low-fat, nondairy animal protein in your diet. "Grains are important too," he says, "although due to my experience I make it a general policy to avoid the gluten grains such as wheat, rye, barley, white rice, and oats, which many people are not able to tolerate, either. I would stick to grains like brown rice, millet, amaranth, and corn, as examples."

TESTING FOR ALLERGIES

Currently, a variety of tests are available for identifying allergies. Regardless of which method is used, Richard Wilkinson, M.D., Director of Yakima Allergy Clinic in Yamika, Washington, points out that it is always necessary to demonstrate a cause and effect relationship between the suspected allergen and the outbreak of symptoms if the test is to be effective.

Skin testing: *"Skin testing is one of the most consistent methods of testing people for pollen, mold, dust, chemical, and other environmental allergies," Dr. Wilkinson says. He especially recommends Serial Endpoint Titration or SET testing, which enables a physician to quantitatively evaluate how a person reacts to allergens in the environment. "Based on the testing result, allergy shots or drops can then be formulated that will usually bring on noticeable improvement for the patient within a few weeks." SET testing is also a more accurate method of evaluation than the commonly used scratch test, in which the outer layer of skin is pierced and minute amounts of the suspected allergens are placed within the surface break, where antibodies can react to them. "It's not unusual for patients to take shots based on scratch testing for a year or more before any benefit is derived," Dr. Wilkinson says.*

The IgG ELISA and FICA test: *According to James Braly, M.D., Medical Director of Immuno Labs, Inc., in Fort Lauderdale, Florida, testing for food allergies can be far more difficult than determining environmental reactions, because most food allergies are dealt with in the body by IgG antibodies, while most allergy tests only measure the presence of IgE antibodies. The IgG ELISA and FICA (Food Immune Complex Assay) test, a recent breakthrough in the field of food allergy testing, offers new hope for food allergy sufferers, however.*

"We know that one of the fundamental causes behind food allergies is the penetration of undigested or partially digested food from the digestive tract into the bloodstream," Dr. Braly explains. "With the FICA and IgG ELISA test, we can measure the actual presence of specific foods and their specific IgG antibodies in the blood to precisely determine which foods a person is allergic to."

The IgG ELISA and FICA test is also convenient, automated, and currently the only commercially available test of its kind for delayed food allergies. It involves taking a blood sample that is then tested for the presence of IgG antibodies against over one hundred foods. The results are computer analyzed to determine which foods the patient is allergic to. The test can be done through the mail, as long as samples reach testing labs within seventy-two hours after the blood is drawn.

Electroacupuncture biofeedback: *This form of testing is widely used in Europe to screen for both food and environmental allergies, and to determine what remedy to use to properly neutralize the allergic reaction. "A small current of electricity is introduced at specific acupuncture points on the patient," explains Fuller Royal, M.D., of Las Vegas, Nevada. "Various allergens are then introduced into the circuitry, enabling the physician to determine any change in the way the patient reacts to the current."*

According to Dr. Royal, a healthy reading would be fifty on a scale of zero to one hundred. "Allergens cause the reading to be far above fifty," he says. "As they are found, various treatment doses are also added into the circuit. The correct treatment will cause the reading to climb down to a reading of fifty." Dr. Royal states that using electroacupuncture biofeedback allows him to accurately test for a full spectrum of allergens, and that the entire battery of tests can be done in an hour.

Ray C. Wunderlich, Jr., M.D., of St. Petersburg, Florida, had a patient whose history illustrates the importance of a proper diet in relation to allergies. She was a twenty-nine-year-old mother of a young child, who came to Dr. Wunderlich complaining of chronic exhaustion. She was also suffering from chronic sinus congestion and taking allergy shots for mold, pollen, and dust.

The woman's sinus congestion had developed one year after her child was born and worsened once she began taking the allergy shots. "Lab tests revealed that she had extensive nutrient deficiencies combined with food allergies to many of the foods she ate frequently," Dr. Wunderlich recounts. He discontinued her allergy shots and placed her on a diet that avoided all of the foods she was allergic to while still meeting her need for proteins, fats, and complex carbohydrates. Nutritional supplementation was also undertaken. "She responded promptly to that treatment regimen," says Dr. Wunderlich, "and experienced a marked increase in energy. And her sinus congestion, which she thought was caused by mold, dust, and pollen, but was actually due to the foods she had been eating, cleared up as well."

According to Dr. Braly, if digestive disorders are compounding the allergies, which is usually the case, they will also need to be corrected before any significant improvement can occur. "I find that many people with such complaints suffer from deficiencies in vitamin A, certain B vitamins, zinc, magnesium, and/or essential oils," Dr. Braly says. "Some people, especially as they get older or if their allergies are severe, also require digestive assistance in the form of pancreatic enzymes and/or hydrochloric acid, so supplementing each meal with them can be helpful as well."

Both zinc and vitamin A play an important role in the production of secretory IgA, a gastrointestinal antibody secreted from the salivary glands in the mouth and from cells that line the digestive tract. "The IgA antibody latches on to what is perceived in the body as allergens or potential allergens in the foods that we eat," Dr. Braly explains. "It [IgA] results in a protective coat of mucous being formed around these allergens and prevents them from being absorbed into the bloodstream. If you're zinc and vitamin A deficient, you produce less secretory IgA, and therefore your susceptibility to food allergies increases. Zinc also plays a role in the production of the body's hydrochloric acid (HCI), which the body needs as well for proper digestion to occur."

Another group of nutrients that Dr. Braly employs to treat allergies is vitamin P or certain bioflavonoids. "Certain bioflavonoids are some of the most effective antiallergy nutrients that I've come across," he says. "Many of my patients who are allergy prone, both to their diet and their environment, over a period of time stop having allergic reactions once these bioflavonoids start taking effect. Quercetin, my favorite bioflavonoid, taken orally along with bromelain, vitamin C, and glutamine, has produced wonderful results."

Finally, vitamin C in high doses can have a dramatic effect in improving allergy symptoms, particularly hay fever and asthma, due to its ability to counteract the inflammation responses that are part of such conditions. "Vitamin C is one of nature's miracles," Dr. Mandell says. Robert Cathcart, M.D., who pioneered the technique of taking vitamin C to bowel tolerance, also recommends its use for allergies. His own seasonal symptoms of hay fever were blocked upon taking sixteen grams of vitamin C orally during a twenty-four-hour period, following exposure to pollen. In cases of more severe exposure, he advises that the dose of vitamin C be increased as well. Dr. Cathcart bases his recommendations on clinical experience with over one thousand patients with allergies, the vast majority of whom gained significant relief from this approach.[5]

THE HUNTER-GATHERER DIET

Research by Boyd Eaton, M.D., and Melvin Konner, Ph.D., has clearly established the fact that our Stone Age ancestors ate large amounts of animal protein and even larger quantities of fruits and plants, with very few milk products or cereal grains in their diet.[4] Leon Chaitow, N.D., D.O., of London, England, speculates that the change away from this diet over the centuries may have a lot to do with the upsurge in allergies worldwide. "We humans became agricultural beings only around ten thousand years ago," he says. "In terms of our evolution, that is a very fleeting moment in time. It's quite likely that our change in feeding patterns has occurred much faster than our adaptation mechanisms have been able to handle."

Lending weight to this theory is the fact that it is precisely those foods which our Stone Age predecessors didn't eat—cereal grains and dairy products—that most frequently provoke allergic reactions. "This has led to what is called the primary allergy approach, first developed in Sweden by Ursulla Jonsson," Dr. Chaitow reports. The approach, which is now being used to treat allergies throughout Europe, adopts a "no cereals, no dairy products" diet as a first step in treating all allergies, whether caused by food or the environment. "The results are impressive," Dr. Chaitow says. "In the majority of cases, most allergy problems vanish after a few weeks of eating this way. And in many cases, a gradual reintroduction of the offending foods is possible on a rotating diet basis, once the person has become desensitized."

Herbal Medicine

There are a variety of herbs that offer relief from allergies, according to Dr. Thom. Among those he employs are anticatarrhals, such as goldenseal, red sage, and goldenrod, to help eliminate mucous; and astringents such as yarrow and myrrh to help contract inflamed tissues and reduce secretions and discharges.

To strengthen immune response, Paul Yanick, Jr., Ph.D., of Neversink, New York, recommends echinacea, astragalus root, golden seal root, and *Pfaffia paniculata* (suma or Brazilian ginseng), a Brazilian herb which numerous studies prove is effective and safe for treating weakened immune systems.[6]

One of Dr. Braly's favorite herbs is cayenne pepper. "I love it," he says, "and I love its active

ALLERGIES AND PROBIOTICS

Due to environmental toxins, the prevalence of pesticides and preservatives in foods, and the overreliance on antibiotics and other drugs, the normal bowel flora of the digestive tract can be damaged. "When this occurs," says Leon Chaitow, N.D., D.O., of London, England, "it sets the stage for colonization of opportunistic parasites and yeast overgrowth, or candidiasis. The boundary between the intestinal tract and the rest of the body is also broken, which allows for many allergenic substances to enter into the bloodstream. This, in turn, triggers an allergic reaction by the immune system."

*Imbalances of intestinal flora are common among allergy sufferers. To normalize this situation, Dr. Chaitow stresses the need to restore bowel flora balance with a daily program of probiotics, or the use of friendly bacteria that inhabit the intestines under healthy conditions. "*Lactobacillus acidophilus, Lactobacillus bulgaricus *and the bifidobacteria are the key players in this process," Dr. Chaitow says. "But care must be taken to select the proper strains," he cautions. "To be effective, probiotic supplements should be freeze-dried, contain only the declared and desirable strains of the species, and have concentrations of the friendly bacteria of about 1 billion parts per gram. They should also be kept refrigerated."*

ingredient, capsaicin, which is a strong 'dual' anti-inflammatory agent. This makes cayenne a particularly effective remedy for treating allergies, especially as it is also very inexpensive and readily available." Dr. Braly has reversed allergies, including asthma, simply by instructing his patients to sprinkle liberal amounts of cayenne pepper on their meals. "In some instances, I've been able to reverse the condition overnight," Dr. Braly says.

See Candidiasis, Parasitic Infections, Probiotics (in Appendix).

One such case involved a man who had suffered from nightly asthma attacks which were often so bad that his coughs and wheezing would force him to sit up in bed, making sleep extremely difficult. Dr. Braly suggested that the man use cayenne with his food for a few days and then report back to him. "Four days later, he told me that after the first day of sprinkling the cayenne on his food he was symptom free for the first time in thirteen years," Dr. Braly reports.

Using herbs to treat allergies involves an individual approach, however, according to Dr. Thom. "No one herb will work for all allergy sufferers," he says. "Patients whose conditions are severe would do best to consult with a trained herbalist or naturopath."

Acupuncture

Allergies are considered a symptom of immune dysfunction in acupuncture theory, according to William Michael Cargile, B.S., D.C., F.I.A.C.A., Chairman of Research for The American Association of Acupuncture and Oriental Medicine. "In treating allergies, it's vital that we restore the immune system on a systemic level," he says. "Acupuncture is ideally suited to accomplish this."

Dr. Cargile treats environmental and food allergies with equal success. One of his patients was a fifty-one-year-old man who came to him with a severe milk allergy. "He had reached a point where he would have immediate diarrhea and other gastrointestinal complaints whenever he had milk, and it had endoscopically been verified that he had a stomach ulcer as result," Dr. Cargile relates.

After only two acupuncture treatments given to enhance his immune function, the man was again endoscopically diagnosed and it was found that his ulcer had disappeared. Moreover,

Acupressure point for allergy relief.

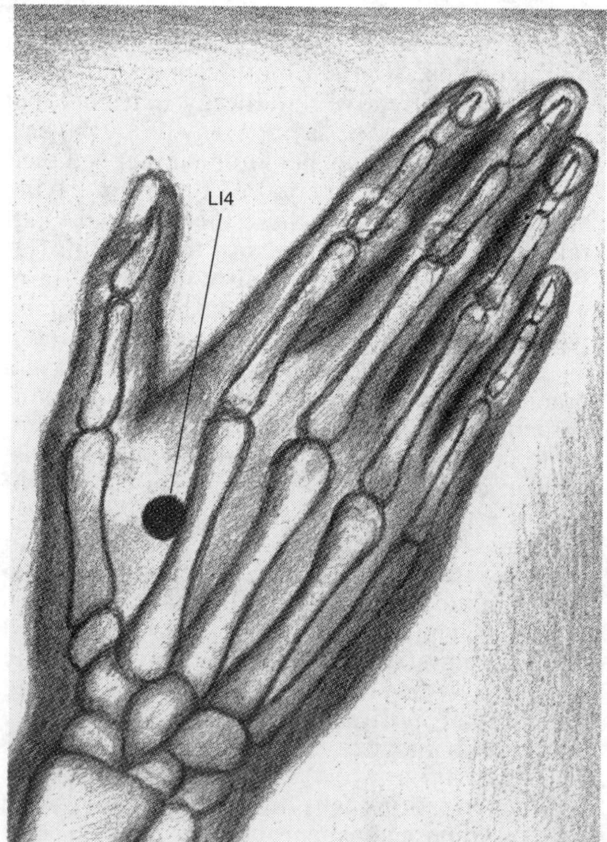

he gained immediate relief from his allergies, despite making no change to his diet. "In fact," says Dr. Cargile, "his diet got worse because he began drinking milk again. Instead of experiencing a recurrence of symptoms, he is now able to drink milk without a problem."

Another of Dr. Cargile's patients was a six-year-old boy who had had extensive allergy tests which showed him to be allergic to nearly fifty substances, both in his environment and in his food. "A year before I saw him," says Dr. Cargile, "he had fallen from a swing and hit his neck on an oak root. Because he didn't break any bones, his doctor sent him home and said that he was okay. In reality, though, he had incurred whiplash, and it was soon after this that his allergies began."

Dr. Cargile employed chiropractic to treat the boy's whiplash, which had impaired his digestive abilities due to subluxations along the boy's spine. This was followed by a course of acupuncture to restimulate the boy's digestive and immune systems. The child had suffered from migraines almost daily, and also had chronic sinusitis due to his condition. After his first treatment, his headaches ceased, and by the third treatment he was free of sinusitis and other allergic symptoms. "I now see him three or four times a year on a maintenance basis, but otherwise he's fine and now able to eat freely and not have any reaction to his environment," Dr. Cargile says.

USING ACUPRESSURE TO RELIEVE AN ALLERGY—A SELF-HELP APPROACH

Michael Reed Gach, Ph.D., Director of the Acupressure Institute in Berkely, California, has found that allergic reactions can often be relieved through the use of acupressure, the use of fingertips in place of needles to stimulate acupoints. Dr. Gach explains, "As soon as you begin experiencing an allergic reaction, apply pressure on the point in the center of the webbing of your hand, between your thumb and index finger. (See point LI4 on illustration opposite.) Gradually apply firm pressure onto the point, angling the pressure toward the bone that connects with the index finger," Dr. Gach instructs. He recommends keeping a constant pressure for at least two minutes while taking slow, deep breaths. Then repeat the process to the same point on your other hand. "This point works like an antihistamine," Dr. Gach further explains. "I have found that this simple technique can often arrest an allergy attack very quickly, making it a very useful self-help remedy that anyone can use."

Ayurvedic Medicine

In Ayurvedic medicine, allergies are viewed as a result of impaired digestion. "This is known as an *ama* condition," explains Virender Sodhi, M.D. (Ayurveda), N.D., in Bellevue, Washington. "In other words, the person with allergies is having trouble digesting his proteins, carbohydrates, or fats, and this leads to a breakdown in the system that eventually creates the allergy."

From the Ayurvedic perspective, Dr. Sodhi points out that the digestive system has a link to all allergies, not just those caused by food. "Proper digestion aids the body to clear out toxins," he says. "When digestion becomes impaired, a greater threshold of toxins have to be dealt with and eventually the body becomes overwhelmed. This is what leads to the allergies. So, in Ayurvedic medicine we always start with the digestive system in order to treat allergies."

Dr. Sodhi advises patients with allergies to adopt a rotation diet, while taking steps to enhance their production of secretory IgA, an immune antibody common to the mucus membranes of the gastrointestinal tract. "There are many good herbs to stimulate the IgA," he says. Among the herbs he uses are ginger, garlic, onion, cayenne pepper, black pepper, and long pepper. Dr. Sodhi suggests that people with allergies take the herbs one-half hour before their meals. "This will help produce more IgA and stimulate the digestion," he says.

Another herb that Dr. Sodhi recommends is *triphala*, which can be taken daily both as a treatment and as a preventative approach to allergies. "I use *triphala* a lot," he says, "because it is very effective in both aiding the digestion and helping to eliminate toxins from the body. It's also good for killing off bugs in the intestinal tract." He recommends that *triphala* be taken three times a day in tablet form, either before or after each meal.

See Acupuncture, Ayurvedic Medicine, Homeopathy.

To further aid the body's journey back to health, Dr. Sodhi will also often place his patients on a *pancha karma* program of cleansing and detoxification. This consists of full body massages of herbs and oils, followed by an herbal steam sauna. "The massage allows the herbs and oils to penetrate through the skin, where they bond with the toxins and then draw them out through the pores. The sauna completes the process, as the toxins continue to circulate and be eliminated as the person perspires."

A number of massage treatments are usually called for, then the person is often placed on a program of fasting, using fruit and vegetable juices, and sometimes herbal teas. The duration of the fast varies according to the severity of the case, but usually runs from two days to a week. Herbal laxatives are given in addition, to further clean out the small intestine, spleen, and liver, followed by colonics or enemas to treat the large intestine. Dr. Sodhi has found the *pancha karma* program to be most effective for dealing with allergies, but warns that it should only be undertaken under the guidance of a trained Ayurvedic physician.

One of Dr. Sodhi's patients illustrates how effective the program can be. When she first came to him, she had to wear a respiratory mask, due to the severity of her allergies. "She had to be very careful about her environment and the air that she breathed, or she would have an attack," Dr. Sodhi says.

Before coming to Dr. Sodhi, the woman had tried conventional medical approaches without success and her condition was continuing to worsen. Dr. Sodhi placed her on the *pancha karma* program for a period of three months, during which time she was carefully monitored and tested. At the end of this time, the woman was able to once again breathe freely and her energy was much improved. "If she encounters a very strong chemical, she may still use her respirator mask," Dr. Sodhi says, "but under normal conditions she can function fully now and it's been over a year since I treated her."

Homeopathy

Homeopathy has widespread applications for the treatment of allergies, because in many situations minute, diluted doses of the very substance a person is allergic to can be prepared as homeopathic solutions that trigger the body's natural ability to heal itself. "For instance," says Dr. Royal, "if someone has a problem with ragweed pollen, a diluted solution of it, given sublingually or by injection, will often neutralize the person's reaction to it." Dr. Chaitow confirms this, citing the fact that in Europe during hay fever season, hay fever sufferers have been shown to reduce or prevent their reactions by beginning a course of homeopathic pollen supplements a few months before the pollen count rises.

Homeopathic remedies are best prescribed by a competent homeopath. Self-diagnosis is discouraged due to the variety of factors that must be considered before the appropriate treatment is selected.

Homeopathic remedies are best prescribed by a competent homeopath. Self-diagnosis is discouraged due to the variety of factors that must be considered before the appropriate treatment is selected. "You have to take an overview of the entire patient and can't afford to overlook anything," Dr. Royal says. He regularly screens his allergy patients for dietary and environmental factors that may be causing their condition, including testing for hydrocarbons, formaldehyde, mold spores, house dust, pollens, monosodium glutamate, and artificial food dyes. From this, he is able to prescribe the most appropriate choice of remedy, and reports a high degree of success using this protocol.

Self-Care

The following therapies can be undertaken at home under the guidance of a physician:

• Fasting • Guided Imagery

Aromatherapy: To calm stress and soothe allergic reactions: lavender, melissa, and chamomile.

Juice Therapy: • Carrot, beet, and cucumber juice • Carrot and celery

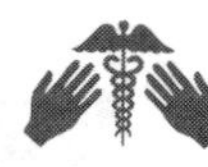

Professional Care

The following therapies should only be provided by a qualified health professional:

• Acupuncture • Applied Kinesiology • Cell Therapy • Chelation Therapy • Environmental Medicine • Hypnotherapy • Neuro-Linguistic Programming • Orthomolecular Medicine • Osteopathy

Biological Dentistry: Hal A. Huggins, D.D.S., reports the improvement or disappearance of food allergies after removing toxic dental amalgams. He believes that food allergies can be caused by the absorption of mercury by food as it is ingested.

Bodywork: Reflexology, *shiatsu*.

Craniosacral Therapy: Nasal allergies.

Magnetic Field Therapy: Exposure to negative magnetic field helps to neutralize the acidity of the blood associated with allergies and make it more alkaline.

Oxygen Therapy: Hydrogen peroxide therapy.

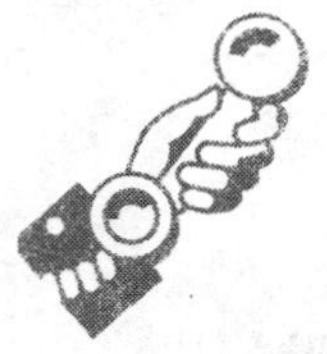

Where to Find Help

For more information on, and referrals for, treatment of allergies, contact the following organizations.

American Academy of Environmental Medicine
P.O. Box 16106
Denver, Colorado 80216
(303) 622-9755
The academy offers extensive training for physicians interested in learning more about environmental medicine.

American Association of Acupuncture and Oriental Medicine
4101 Lake Boone Trail, Suite 201
Raleigh, North Carolina 27607
(919) 787-5181
The AAAOM is a national professional trade organization of acupuncturists who meet acceptable standards of competency and can provide you with the names and locations of local members. Referrals by written request only.

American Association of Naturopathic Physicians
2366 Eastlake Avenue, Suite 322
Seattle, Washington 98102
(206) 323-7610
Contact them for the location of a licensed naturopathic physician in your area.

American School of Ayurvedic Sciences
10025 NE 4th Street
Bellevue, Washington 98004
(206) 453-8022
This college provides medical training for physicians and health care practitioners, as well as individual courses for lay people. Dr. Virender Sodhi's Ayurvedic, Naturopathic Medical Clinic is also located at this address.

Immuno Labs, Inc.
1620 West Oakland Park Boulevard
Suite 300
Fort Lauderdale, Florida 33311
(800) 231-9197
Specialized allergy and immunology testing for physicians around the world. Provides referrals worldwide to physicians who do allergy testing.

International Foundation for Homeopathy
2366 Eastlake Avenue East
Suite 301
Seattle, Washington 98102
(206) 324-8230
Provides educational courses for both homeopathic professionals and the general public. Offers referrals to homeopathic health professionals.

National Center for Homeopathy
1500 Massachusetts Avenue NW, Suite 42
Washington, D.C. 20005
(703) 548-7790
Provides a referral list of health professionals who practice homeopathy as well as information on homeopathy. Gives courses for lay people and professionals and organizes study groups around the country.

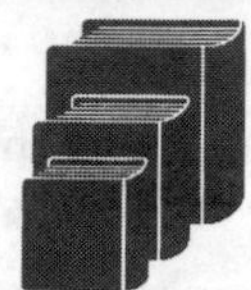

Recommended Reading

An Alternative Approach to Allergies. Randolph, Theron, M.D.; and Moss, Ralph, Ph.D. New York: Harper Perennial, 1990.
A comprehensive guide to staying well and allergy-free in a polluted world by a pioneer in the field of environmental medicine.

Brain Allergies: The Psychonutrient Connection. Philpott, William H., M.D.; and Kalita, Dwight, Ph.D. New Canaan, CT: Keats Publishing, Inc. 1980.
A comprehensive look at the role nutrition and orthomolecular medicine can play in treating brain allergies, including a self-help protocol and a special appendix for physicians.

Dr. Braly's Food Allergy and Nutrition Revolution. Braly, James, M.D. New Canaan, CT: Keats Publishing, Inc., 1992.
A valuable self-help approach for recovering from food allergies. Includes the latest research on the subject, testing methods, and a detailed treatment method based upon diet and nutrition. Also includes treatment protocols for some forty illnesses linked to food allergies, and provides a recipe section and meal plan for restoring health.

No More Allergies. Null, Gary, Ph.D. New York: Villard Books, 1992.
A detailed investigation into the causes of allergies related both to food and the environment, as well as their link to other illnesses, such as asthma, arthritis, chronic fatigue syndrome, and diabetes. Also outlines testing methods, treatments, and a diet plan to restore immune function.

"A dedicated physician can only be sure about the healing properties of a medicine when it is made as pure and perfect as possible."

—Samuel Hahnemann (1755-1843)
Founder of Homeopathy

Alzheimer's Disease and Senile Dementia

A devastating illness with no known single cause or cure, Alzheimer's disease is said to afflict 4 million American adults.[1] However, some estimates suggest that up to 40 percent of these patients are misdiagnosed and actually have other forms of senile dementia. Many alternative physicians report success in treating those with Alzheimer's-like dementia by addressing the various causes and symptoms underlying the condition.

Alzheimer's disease is a progressive, degenerative disease that attacks the brain, resulting in impaired memory, decreased intellectual and emotional functioning, and ultimately complete physical breakdown. It was first identified in 1907 by German physician Alois Alzheimer who, during postmortem examinations, discovered abnormal formations of plaque on nerve endings and tangles of nerve fibers in the brain tissue of individuals who had exhibited symptoms of senile dementia. This plaque was found primarily in the hippocampus, the part of the brain related to memory and intellectual function.

> *"The best estimates are that 40 percent of the people diagnosed with Alzheimer's do not, in fact, have Alzheimer's."*
> —Abram Hoffer, M.D.

Alzheimer's disease is the most common form of senile dementia, afflicting approximately 10 percent of those over the age of sixty-five and almost 50 percent of those over the age of eighty-five.[2] Symptoms vary, from depression, fatigue, and occasional forgetfulness to disorientation and aggressive or paranoid behavior. This range of symptoms, coupled with the fact that a definite diagnosis can be obtained only in postmortem examination, causes frequent misdiagnosis.

According to Abram Hoffer, M.D., a pioneer of orthomolecular and nutritional medicine, "There are really a number of factors in senile dementia. The best estimates are that 40 percent of the people diagnosed with Alzheimer's do not, in fact, have Alzheimer's. It has come to the point that anyone over the age of sixty-five with the slightest memory loss is in danger of being labeled with Alzheimer's. Therefore, we should not let the title deter us from developing a treatment approach."

> *"The automatic diagnosis of Alzheimer's can be a real danger. Any type of toxic reaction, even alcoholism, can produce symptoms of dementia."*
> —Abram Hoffer, M.D.

Causes of Alzheimer's Disease and Other Forms of Senile Dementia

Currently, the medical establishment spends millions of dollars each year attempting to isolate a single cause of Alzheimer's. Because other forms of senile dementia sometimes mimic the symptoms of Alzheimer's, Dr. Hoffer and other alternative physicians stress the importance of eliminating other possible causes of dementia before arriving at an Alzheimer's diagnosis. "The automatic diagnosis of Alzheimer's can be a real danger," says Dr. Hoffer. "Any type of toxic reaction, even alcoholism, can produce symptoms of dementia."

Joseph Pizzorno, N.D., President of Bastyr College in Seattle, Washington, explains that two treatable conditions capable of causing senile dementia are often confused with Alzheimer's—pernicious anemia (a severe form of blood disease marked by a progressive decrease in red blood cells, muscular weakness, and gastrointestinal and neural disturbances) and cerebral vascular insufficiency (a lack of blood supply to the brain due to constricted arteries). Among the possible causes of senile dementia that can appear as Alzheimer's are multiple strokes, Parkinson's disease (a disease where the cells that normally produce the neurotransmitter dopamine die off, resulting in a loss of muscle control), Huntington chorea (a hereditary disease of the central nervous system, characterized by progressive dementia and rapid, jerky motions), thyroid disorders, brain tumors, and head injuries. Other causes of senile dementia include drug reactions, environmental toxins, nutritional deficiencies, allergies, candidiasis, depression, alcoholism, and infections such as meningitis, syphilis, and AIDS.

Alzheimer's research is beginning to uncover multiple factors that may contribute to the disease. This indicates that the search for a single cause may be unfounded. Possible contributing factors include genetic tendencies, as well as environmental influences and nutritional deficiencies.

Genetic Tendencies

Researchers have discovered a link between genetic predisposition and Alzheimer's disease. In many families, people in succeeding generations develop Alzheimer's. A specific connection has also been uncovered between Alzheimer's and Down syndrome (a variety of mental retardation). Individuals suffering from Down syndrome often exhibit Alzheimer's-like memory problems or dementia in their thirties and forties. Postmortem examinations of the brains of older Down patients have revealed many of the characteristic abnormalities of Alzheimer's, such as nerve plaques and nerve fiber tangles in the brain.[3]

See Biological Dentistry.

Environmental Influences

Gary Oberg, M.D, past President of the American Academy of Environmental Medicine, treats patients suffering from environmental illness. "Toxins such as chemicals in food and tap water, carbon monoxide, diesel fumes, solvents, aerosol sprays, and industrial chemicals can cause symptoms of brain dysfunction which may lead to an inaccurate diagnosis of Alzheimer's or senile dementia," says Dr. Oberg.

Studies have shown that a susceptibility to toxins such as aluminum and mercury are linked to the onset of Alzheimer's and senile dementia.

Aluminum: Research indicates that, because of the high levels of aluminum found in the brain cells of Alzheimer's victims, this metal may be a causal factor in the development of the disease.[4] While the source of aluminum toxicity in the body has not yet been proven, aluminum can enter the body through inhalation (by factory workers in certain industries) and by oral ingestion. It has been suggested that aluminum ions may leach into the body from aluminum cooking utensils, cans, and foil, as well as underarm deodorants, antacid pills, and other common products, many of which contain traces of aluminum.[5]

"Toxins such as chemicals in food and tap water, carbon monoxide, diesel fumes, solvents, aerosol sprays, and industrial chemicals can cause symptoms of brain dysfunction which may lead to an inaccurate diagnosis of Alzheimer's or senile dementia."
—Gary Oberg, M.D.

Mercury: A study involving postmortem examination of brain tissue from Alzheimer's victims has also indicated the presence of high levels of mercury.[6] Another study makes a clear connection between the presence of mercury in brain tissue and the presence of "silver" amalgam dental fillings, which contain approximately 50 percent mercury as well as silver, tin, copper, and zinc.[7]

"In a recent test of seven thousand patients, we found 90.3 percent to be sensitive to mercury," says Hal A. Huggins, D.D.S., of Colorado Springs, Colorado. "What this means is, that while different people will react in different ways to mercury, in 90.3 percent of the people with amalgam fillings, the mercury will significantly suppress the immune system."

Reactions to high levels of mercury in the body can range from nervousness and depression to suicidal tendencies and severe neurological diseases such as multiple sclerosis, Lou Gehrig's disease (a syndrome marked by muscular weakness and atrophy due to degeneration of motor neurons of the spinal cord, medulla, and cortex), and Alzheimer's. "How you are going to react depends on your genetics," says Dr. Huggins. "A person with very strong stock will last a very long time before his immune system breaks down. But susceptibility also depends on lifestyle and exposure to other stressors such as poor nutrition and environmental factors."

According to Dr. Huggins, metal fillings also create low levels of constant electrical activity that is conducted directly to the brain, creating aberrant behavior. While the electrical mechanism created by a combination of metals in the mouth does not itself directly suppress the immune system, Dr. Huggins cautions that it does enable metals to come out of the fillings faster, to be absorbed through the cheeks and tongue into the blood supply.

Nutritional Deficiencies

Reduced levels of certain vitamins, minerals, and amino acids have been tentatively linked with Alzheimer's,[8] including folic acid, niacin (vitamin B_3), thiamine (vitamin B_1), vitamin B6, vitamin B_{12}, vitamin C, vitamin D, vitamin E, magnesium, selenium, zinc, and tryptophan.

DRUGS ASSOCIATED WITH A HIGHER INCIDENCE OF MENTAL CONFUSION

According to the Physicians Desk Reference *the following drugs are associated with side effects of mental confusion.[11] (Statistics refer to the percentage of individuals affected.)*

- *Anestacon Solution (Among most common)*
- *Atrofen Tablets (1-11%)*
- *Clozaril Tablets (3%)*
- *Desyrel and Desyrel Dividose (4.9-5.7%)*
- *Dilantin Infatabs, Kapseals, Parenteral (Among most common)*
- *Dilantin-30 Pediatric/Dilantin-125 Suspension, Dilantin with Phenobarbital Kapseals (Among most common)*
- *Duragesic Transdermal System (10% or more)*
- *Eldepryl Tablets (3 of 49 patients)*
- *Foscavir Injection (More than 5%)*
- *Hylorel Tablets (14.8%)*
- *IFEX (Among most common)*
- *Intron A (Up to 12%)*
- *Lioresal Tablets (1-11%)*
- *Marplan Tablets (Among most frequent)*
- *Nipent for Injection (3-10%)*
- *Permax Tablets (11.1%)*
- *Roferon-A Injection (8%)*
- *Sinemet CR Tablets (3.7%)*
- *Stadol Injectable, NS Nasal Spray (3-9%)*
- *Tonocard Tablets (2.1-11.2%)*
- *Wellbutrin Tablets (8.4%)*
- *Xanax Tablets (9.9-10.4%)*
- *Xylocaine Injections, with Epinephrine Injections (Among most common)*

Treating Alzheimer's Disease and Senile Dementia

According to Dr. Hoffer, "When a doctor is examining a person who is experiencing symptoms of dementia, the first thing he needs to do is to make an accurate diagnosis and determine what is behind the symptoms. He should not automatically assume it is Alzheimer's. This should be followed by a survey of all the possible underlying factors. If you are unable to find an explanation, then you can finally assess with greater probability that it is Alzheimer's."

Alternative treatments focus on nutritional supplementation, herbal medicine, detoxification (including mercury dental amalgams and aluminum), as well as treating food allergies and candida overgrowth.

Nutritional Supplements

Nutritional supplementation is one effective approach in treating Alzheimer's. Studies in Japan have shown that daily supplements of coenzyme Q10, vitamin B_6, and iron returned some Alzheimer's-diagnosed patients to "normal" mental capacity.[9] In another study, Alzheimer's patients who took a daily regimen of evening primrose oil, zinc, and selenium showed significant improvements in alertness, mood, and mental ability.[10]

Dr. Hoffer employs a nutritional approach to senile dementia, noting that while the majority of Alzheimer's patients he has treated over the past thirty years have not responded to vitamin therapy, he has observed remarkable improvement in patients with cardiovascular problems who exhibit Alzheimer's-like symptoms. "I find that if an elderly patient is losing memory or ability to concentrate due to some cardiovascular problems, nutritional supplementation can be very helpful. If they have had a stroke, you can't ever bring them completely back to normal, but vitamins can play an important role in restoring some function."

Dr. Hoffer combines niacin, which improves circulation and lowers cholesterol levels, with large doses of vitamins C and E. He also recommends folic acid, noting that 40 percent of all senile patients are deficient in this B vitamin. Recently, Dr. Hoffer has begun to use a comprehensive vitamin approach with low daily doses of aspirin, and reports an initial positive response with a few Alzheimer's patients. "In small doses, aspirin is really quite safe, and it may help to prevent the platelets from sticking to each other and improves circulation to the brain," he says.

Sandra Denton, M.D., Director of Alaska Alternative Medicine in Anchorage, also uses a program of nutritional supplements to build the immune systems of Alzheimer's patients and those with senile dementia. Her program is based on individual need and normally includes vitamins C, E, and B_{12}, as well as the herb *Ginkgo biloba* to increase circulation in the brain. Dr. Denton notes that many chronic health conditions improve once the gastrointestinal tract regains its functional integrity. She also stresses the importance of maintaining healthy function of the gastrointestinal tract in order to ensure proper vitamin and mineral absorption.

Herbal Medicine

Ginkgo biloba has been shown to improve circulation and increase mental capacity in several clinical trials. In particular, the herb has been effective for treating problems associated with cerebral circulation, neurotransmission (the energetic impulse of nerve cells), neuron membrane lesions caused by oxygenated free radicals (highly reactive destructive molecules), and neuronal metabolism (all physical and chemical changes taking place in a nerve cell) threatened by lack of oxygen.[12]

David L. Hoffmann, B.Sc., M.N.I.M.H., of Sebastapol, California, past President of the American Herbalist Guild, reports success with the use of *Ginkgo biloba* with Alzheimer's patients and those with senile dementia. "The herb is quite safe, even in doses many times higher than those usually recommended, and clinically it seems to be effective for patients with vascular disorders for all types of dementia; and, because of its beneficial effects on mood, for patients suffering from cognitive disorders secondary to depression because of its beneficial effects on mood. For people who are just beginning to experience deterioration in cognitive function, ginkgo might enable them to maintain a normal life."

Environmental Medicine

In addition to taking a comprehensive history, Dr. Oberg screens all his patients for dietary and environmental sensitivities capable of producing symptoms. Food sensitivities are determined by using an elimination diet. According to Dr. Oberg, if symptoms disappear when a particular food is avoided and then reappear when it is reintroduced into the diet, the person is sensitive to that food and should avoid it. Dr. Oberg notes that when toxic substances are removed from the diet, symptoms will often disappear.

To diagnose environmental sensitivity, he uses a technique called maximum tolerated intradermal dose testing to determine how much of a particular substance is toxic to the patient. The patient can then be desensitized to the substance by being injected with the largest dose of that substance which does not produce a response (such as a skin wheal).

According to William G. Crook, M.D., of Jackson, Tennessee, a pioneer in the field of environmental medicine, overgrowth of the yeast *Candida albicans* in the gastrointestinal tract can contribute to food allergies and poor absorption of nutrients, and may be related to a number of health and behavioral problems, including depression, hyperactivity, irritability, and "brain fog." Says Dr. Crook, "One of the most common complaints I receive comes from women in their thirties who feel like they're getting Alzheimer's because they can't remember things. I often find these symptoms are related to a candida overgrowth in the intestines. Although I don't know the exact mechanism—whether the candida produces toxins which interfere with brain function, contributes to food allergies, or a combination of things—treatment for candida and a change in diet generally help."[13]

Dr. Crook's treatment for patients with candida-related health problems, including Alzheimer's and cerebral dysfunction symptoms, is relatively simple. After performing a thorough physical examination and taking their age into consideration, he puts patients on an elimination diet. Patients whose histories include antibiotic drugs, a high-sugar diet, or birth control pills are treated for candida or yeast overgrowth in the intestines. After the candida is under control, Dr. Crook recommends following a sugar-free diet, including acidophilus (as a supplement, or as found in some yogurts) to restore intestinal flora.

See Candidiasis, Environmental Medicine.

Chelation Therapy

Garry F. Gordon, M.D., co-founder of the American College of Advancement in Medicine, reports that chelation therapy can benefit memory in patients with Alzheimer's-like dementia by improving blood flow to the brain. Chelation therapy uses chelating agents (such as EDTA—ethylenediaminetetraacetic acid) administered intravenously to restore proper cir-culation by removing the calcium content of plaque from arterial walls. Dr. Gordon cites numerous studies showing an increase in cerebrovascular circulation using EDTA chelation therapy.[14] Chelation therapy may also be beneficial to patients with senile dementia by removing aluminum, mercury, and other heavy metals from the body.

Charles Farr, M.D., Ph.D., co-founder of the American Board of Chelation Therapy, success-

> *"Chelation therapy can benefit memory in patients with Alzheimer's-like dementia by improving blood flow to the brain."*
> —Garry F. Gordon, M.D.

fully uses chelation therapy in cases of senile dementia that are due to either atherosclerosis (hardening of the arteries) of the cerebral arteries or toxins in the body. "When a patient comes in and is not functioning well, having trouble concentrating and remembering things, we have no immediate way of measuring whether it is a circulatory problem, toxicity, or an Alzheimer's-like situation."

In cases of senile dementia, Dr. Farr recommends ten to fifteen chelation treatments, alternating with intravenous hydrogen peroxide, in order to more quickly stimulate the circulatory system. If the patient has atherosclerosis, or is suffering from environmental toxins, a turnaround by ten to fifteen treatments is expected. If not, Dr. Farr assumes it is Alzheimer's.

Dr. Farr recounts the case of his mother, a nurse, who was in a progressively deteriorating situation when in her early sixties. She had reached a point where she could not work, had lost her memory, and was not aware of what was going on around her. Still, she was not interested in receiving chelation therapy. When she got to the point where she could no longer function, and did not even know where she was, her family physically carried her into the clinic and started chelation treatments. Within four months her symptoms completely disappeared. Dr. Farr says she was able to go back to work for another fifteen years, remaining lucid until she died at the age of eighty-eight.

See Chelation Therapy, Oxygen Therapies.

Biological Dentistry

At the Huggins Diagnostic Center in Colorado Springs, Colorado, Dr. Huggins uses a multidisciplinary approach to treat patients with Alzheimer's and senile dementia. He combines the removal of amalgam fillings with numerous other therapies, including dietary supplements and nutritional counseling, acupressure, massage, movement therapy, and psychological support. "What we do is balance chemistry," Dr. Huggins explains. "Our goal is to increase the total efficiency of the chemistry of the body, and to accomplish that, we bring more oxygen into the diseased areas, enabling the body to do the healing."

Removing amalgam fillings is the first step. This process is supported by IV (intravenous) drips of vitamin C and other solutions to protect the immune system from stress. Silver fillings are replaced with fillings made of materials that have been tested for biocompatibility.

After the fillings are removed, detoxification is performed to remove residues of mercury and other poisons from the body. According to Dr. Denton, an expert in the field of chelation therapy who served for two years as Medical Director of the Huggins Diagnostic Center, "There are several agents, including EDTA, which have the ability to bind tightly to other substances and carry them out of the body. Vitamin C, to some extent, can also take heavy metals out of the body."

Mercury poisoning is recognized as a serious risk to the body, but Dr. Huggins stresses that "removing the fillings is only 5 to 10 percent of the solution. The rest of the picture is extremely complex, but can lead to remarkable recovery. Once you get started, however, the one thing that will destroy your recovery is improper nutrition. Eating just one food to which an individual is allergic can significantly interfere with recovery."

The Huggins Diagnostic Center says it has been able to achieve success with 85 percent of its patients, and in some cases has brought about rapid improvement in people suffering from Alzheimer's and senile dementia. One of Dr. Huggins's patients, a woman who had been diagnosed with advanced Alzheimer's disease, hadn't spoken for fourteen years. "She just sat and glared angrily and looked as if she was ready to beat somebody up," says Dr. Huggins. "We started taking fillings out of her mouth, and on the twelfth day of our fourteen-day program, she started to mumble something. Her husband said, 'What did you say?' and she snapped at him, 'Nothing!' The patient continued to improve, and recently her husband even called to jokingly request one or two fillings be put back in because she was talking so much."

See Biological Dentistry.

Dr. Huggins cautions, however, that improvement in Alzheimer's patients is usually slower. "Hers is an unusual case," he notes. "Most of the time you do not see much progress until perhaps at the end of a month or two; at that point the patient can tie his or her shoes, and perhaps a year or two later is out driving a car. That's slow improvement, but it's pretty good when compared to how far he or she could be going in the other direction."

Traditional Chinese Medicine

While Alzheimer's disease and senile dementia are chronic illnesses that appear to have become widespread only in the last couple of decades, healing therapies that are thousands of years old have demonstrated some success in treating the disease. Maoshing Ni, D.O.M., Ph.D., L.Ac., Vice-President of Yo San University of Traditional Chinese Medicine in Santa Monica, California, has been treating patients with Alzheimer's and senile dementia for the past six years. He comments, "When we can catch Alzheimer's disease in the first six months to a year, when the symptoms are relatively mild, we seem to be able to stem the progression of the illness. When it's more progressed—when a person cannot walk well without help, speech is slurring, and memory is going—then degeneration is at a point where we may be able to improve symptoms to a certain degree, but recovery is disappointing."

To halt the advance of the disease in the early stages, Dr. Ni employs a combination of acupuncture with Chinese herbs, nutrition, and an exercise program, the latter of which is critical. "In China, we use a form of therapeutic exercise called *qigong* [pronounced chee-kung] that is unique. It is a simple-to-do deep-breathing exercise that aids in healing by improving cardiovascular delivery and oxygenating the body." Because it also combines concentration and visualization, Dr. Ni points out *qigong* exercises the brain and balances the body in various ways.

A seventy-two-year-old man who had been diagnosed with Alzheimer's came to see Dr. Ni. He was weak, with slurred speech, and would occasionally blank out from time to time, making it difficult for him to remember where he was and why he was there. Over the course of two weeks, Dr. Ni performed four treatments of "scalp acupuncture" to stimulate the energy channels (meridians) in the scalp. Once the needles were placed, Dr. Ni had the man exercise lightly for twenty minutes. This included moving his limbs, walking, stomping his feet, and singing. By the fourth treatment the patient had regained clarity of speech and claimed to feel better than he had in over a year. Dr. Ni explains that scalp acupuncture can actually clear pathways through the plaque that has accumulated in the brain, and therefore alleviate many of the senility problems

CASE STUDY: TOM WARREN

While physicians throughout the country describe successes with various patients afflicted with this "incurable" disease, perhaps the most vivid success story is that of Tom Warren who wrote a book about his recovery from an Alzheimer's-diagnosed illness.

Tom was diagnosed with Alzheimer's in June 1983, after undergoing a CAT (computer-assisted tomograph) scan. "Several doctors read my x-rays, but the diagnosis was always the same," he recounts. "I was fifty, and I had been experiencing symptoms such as memory loss and fatigue for five years. I was so exhausted; there were times when I had to crawl up the stairs. My head ached. My handwriting deteriorated. Conversation became difficult. Some days all I could do was sit and look at my shoes."

Tom began reading everything he could find that might provide a clue to the cause, and a cure. "Sometimes I couldn't remember something I'd read thirty seconds earlier," he says, "but I would somehow know it was important and would mark the passage."[16] When his wife, a pharmacist, came home, she would help interpret his notes and assist Tom with implementing some of the things he discovered.

In his search for a cure, Tom read more than fifty books and sought out a number of medical specialists. Finally a pattern emerged, and he determined that Alzheimer's and other chronic diseases may be caused by toxic metals and chemicals in the patient's immediate environment. He began a program that included the removal of all amalgam fillings, full testing for food allergies, and a switch to an organic, whole foods diet. Additionally, Tom followed a nutritional supplementation program, including niacin (vitamin B_3), a regular exercise regime, and a complete avoidance of household chemical pollutants. On April 4, 1987, a new CAT scan indicated the disease process had reversed. "Once more I could appreciate sunsets, remember names, drive a car, converse with friends, think, and plan. More importantly, however, I returned to work after an absence of eleven years."

Says Tom, "In one way or another everything I read and learned pointed to: one, remove poison from the body; two, learn how to live in your environment; three, balance body chemistry; four, avoid junk food as if it were poison; five, exercise, and in time the body will heal itself."

Over the years, Tom Warren has received thousands of telephone calls from people who have read his book and followed its advice to have amalgam fillings removed, follow a program of nutritional supplementation, and adhere to an organic, whole-foods diet. He notes that those who continued to have problems refused to or were unable to remove gas heating and cooking from their homes, and stresses that an Alzheimer's-diagnosed patient cannot live in a chemically contaminated environment. "Getting well again is up to you," says Tom.[16]

associated with Alzheimer's. Other treatments included the herbs ginseng, *dong quai*, and *ho-shou-wu* to enhance vitality and mobility.

Some practical hints believed to reduce susceptibility to Alzheimer's and senile dementia include: Stop smoking (smokers have four times the risk of developing Alzheimer's); avoid products with aluminum, make every effort to purify living environment of toxins, and avoid foods containing preservatives and artificial colors.

Ayurvedic Medicine

Virender Sodhi, M.D. (Ayurveda), N.D., Director of the American School of Ayurvedic Sciences in Bellevue, Washington, says he has also had some success applying Ayurvedic practices to patients with Alzheimer's disease and senile dementia. "I had an elderly eighty-four-year-old patient, a woman who was brought in by her daughter," says Dr. Sodhi. "She was generally confused, and every time you tried to talk with her, she would only talk about her legs. She had a son and a daughter, and, as it often happens, they began fighting over who would control the money and who would write the checks. Six months after beginning treatment their mother began to get better and one day she said, 'Now stop fighting. I can live by myself.' She began making her own decisions about what she would eat, what she would do. It was a great improvement."

Dr. Sodhi combines Ayurvedic therapies with basic homeopathic medicine to help alleviate Alzheimer's symptoms. Using a metabolic-type analysis, he prescribes a regimen of dietary and herbal remedies, and also recommends a cleansing program, noting estimates that as many as 80 percent of Alzheimer's patients suffer from environmental toxicity. As part of the program, liver herbs are used to cleanse the liver, along with a compound called Livit 2. Dr. Sodhi also uses *triphala*, a combination of three herbs, and gotu kola, which he says is very good for increasing brain cell function. For circulation, he prescribes the herbs *Ginkgo biloba* or macunabrure. Dr. Sodhi also gives supplements of thiamine (vitamin B_1) and niacin (vitamin B_3), though he cautions that patients with liver damage must be careful not to overload the liver with niacin.

See Acupuncture, Ayurvedic Medicine, Qigong, Traditional Chinese Medicine.

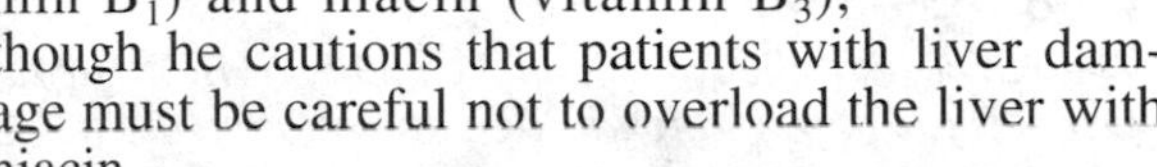

Treatment varies depending on each patient's blood chemistry and individual needs. "My main criterion, however, is to work out digestion and elimination—because if you don't have good digestion and elimination, it doesn't matter what you put into your body, it all goes down the drain," says Dr. Sodhi.

Self-Care

The following therapies can be undertaken at home under appropriate professional guidance:

Hydrotherapy: Constitutional hydrotherapy may be applied two to five times weekly.

Professional Care

The following therapies can be provided by a qualified health professional:

• ***Cell Therapy*** • ***Naturopathic Medicine***

Detoxification Therapy: Depending on the condition of the person.

Oxygen Therapy: Hydrogen peroxide therapy (IV).

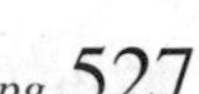

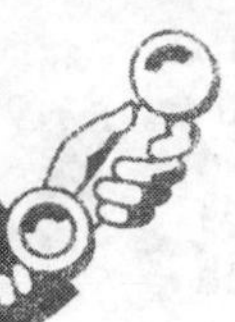

Where to Find Help

For more information on, or referrals for, treatment of Alzheimer's disease, contact the following:

American Academy of Biological Dentistry
P.O. Box 856
Carmel Valley, California 93924
(408) 659-5385

The purpose of the American Academy of Biological Dentistry is to promote biological dental medicine, which uses nontoxic diagnostic and therapeutic approaches in the field of clinical dentistry. They publish a quarterly journal, Focus, *and hold regular seminars on biological diagnosis and therapy.*

American Academy of Environmental Medicine
P.O. Box 16106
Denver, Colorado 80216
(303) 622-9755

The academy offers extensive training for physicians interested in learning more about environmental medicine. For information on physicians practicing environmental medicine send a self-addressed, stamped envelope stating your request.

American Association of Acupuncture and Oriental Medicine
4101 Lake Boone Trail, Suite 201
Raleigh, North Carolina 27607
(919) 787-5181

The AAAOM is a national professional trade organization of acupuncturists who meet acceptable standards of competency and can provide the names and locations of local members. Referrals by written request only.

American Association of Naturopathic Physicians
2366 Eastlake Avenue, Suite 322
Seattle, Washington 98102
(206) 323-7610

Provides a directory of naturopathic physicians and offers referrals to a nationwide network of accredited or licensed practitioners. Publishes a quarterly newsletter for both professionals and the general public. Also offers a series of brochures and pamphlets on a variety of subjects.

American College of Advancement in Medicine
P.O. Box 3427
Laguna Hills, California 92654
(714) 583-7666

This pioneer organization seeks to establish certification and standards of practice for chelation therapy, providing training and education and sponsoring semi-annual conferences for physicians and scientists. ACAM provides referrals and informational material, including a directory listing of all physicians worldwide who have been trained in preventative medicine as well as in the ACAM protocol for chelation therapy. The directory is updated monthly. The organization also provides a copy of the ACAM protocol for chelation to the public.

American Holistic Medical Association
4101 Lake Boone Trail, Suite 201
Raleigh, North Carolina 27607
(919) 787-5181

A professional organization for holistic practitioners, the AHMA offers information and services for its members and lobbies for holistic issues. It also provides referrals for the public. Requests must be in writing.

American School of Ayurvedic Sciences
10025 NE 4th Street
Bellevue, Washington 98004
(206) 453-8022

This college provides medical training for physicians and health care practitioners, as well as individual courses for lay people. Dr. Virender Sodhi's Ayurvedic, Naturopathic Medical Clinic is also located at this address.

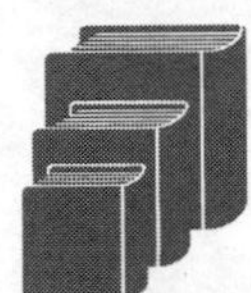

Recommended Reading

An Alternative Approach to Allergies. Randolph, Theron G., M.D.; and Moss, Ralph W., Ph.D. New York: Bantam Books, 1990.
This is an excellent overview, co-authored by the man generally regarded as the father of environmental medicine.

Beating Alzheimer's. Warren, Tom . Garden City Park, NY: Avery Publishing Group Inc., 1991.
The author's account of his experience with, and recovery from, Alzheimer's. Warren investigates the diagnosis and treatment of food allergies, toxic amalgam "silver" dental fillings, and mineral and vitamin deficiencies. Includes documented research that explains why Warren's treatment worked and why it may work for others.

Brain Allergies: The Psychonutrient Connection. Philpott, William, H., M.D; and Kalita, Dwight K., Ph.D. New Canaan, CT: Keats Publishing, 1980.
Has excellent material on allergies and the benefits of "supernutrition."

Detecting Your Hidden Allergies. Crook, William, G., M.D. Jackson, TN: Professional Books; Future Health, 1988.
Gives specific instructions on how to use an elimination diet to determine food allergies.

It's All in Your Head. Huggins, Hal A., D.D.S.; and Huggins, Sharon A. Tacoma, WA: Life Sciences Press, 1989.
Dr. Huggins' critique of the use of mercury, a toxic element and environmental hazard, in dentistry. For those suffering mercury poisoning, the book examines a number of conventional and alternative treatments.

The Yeast Connection. Crook, William, G., M.D. Jackson, TN: Professional Books, 1986.
One of the first and best books giving practical advice regarding what has come to be known as the candida or yeast problem.

"A wise man ought to realize that health is his most valuable possession."

—Hippocrates

Arthritis

Millions of people suffer from some form of arthritis. Because arthritis is commonly believed to be incurable, the standard medical response has been simply to prescribe medication to reduce the symptoms. Substantial evidence, however, now shows that the pain and disability caused by arthritis can be alleviated, and even prevented, through diet, nutritional supplementation, stress reduction, and other alternative therapies.

Arthritis is an inflammation of the joints, surrounding tendons, ligaments, and cartilage. Among the oldest known afflictions of human beings, it can affect virtually every part of the body: from the feet, to the knees, back, shoulders, and fingers. According to the National Institutes of Health (NIH), arthritis effects range from slight pain, stiffness and swelling of the joints, to crippling and disability. Arthritis affects people of all ages. The NIH reports that about 15 percent of the population today is afflicted with arthritis or a related disorder, and that two hundred thousand children in the United States have some form of the disease.[1]

Types of Arthritis

There are a variety of arthritic conditions, with the three most common forms of the disease being osteoarthritis, rheumatoid arthritis, and gout.

Osteoarthritis

Osteoarthritis is a degenerative disease of the large weight-bearing joints, often associated with old age, in which small bony growths, calcium spurs, and occasional soft cysts appear on bones and in the joints. As the disease progresses, the joint cartilage deteriorates, finally interfering with movement. The National Institute of Arthritis and Musculoskeletal and Skin Diseases reports that about one-third of adults in the United States have x-ray evidence of osteoarthritis in the hand, foot, knee, or hip, and by age sixty-five as much as 75 percent of the population has x-ray evidence of the disease in at least one of these sites.[2]

See Chronic Pain.

The symptoms of osteoarthritis include: mild early-morning stiffness, stiffness following periods of rest, pain that worsens on joint use, loss of joint function, local tenderness, soft tissue swelling, creaking and cracking of joints on movement, bony swelling, and restricted mobility.

Rheumatoid Arthritis

Rheumatoid arthritis, while less common than osteoarthritis, is a serious and very painful joint disease, often resulting in crippling disabilities for young and old alike. It incapacitates the synovial tissue, which is the membrane that lines joints and secretes the lubricant which normally allows bones to move painlessly against other bones. With this condition, joints—most commonly the small joints of the hand—become tender, swollen, even deformed. Night sweats, depression, and lethargy are among the other symptoms. Over time, the condition can also spread to other parts of the body.

“ The National Institute of Arthritis and Musculoskeletal and Skin Diseases reports that about one-third of adults in the United States have x-ray evidence of osteoarthritis in the hand, foot, knee, or hip, and by age sixty-five as much as 75 percent of the population has x-ray evidence of the disease in at least one of these sites. ”

Rheumatoid arthritis affects about 2.1 million people in the United States —most often women.[3] The condition usually starts between the ages of twenty and fifty, although it can begin at any age. Symptoms of rheumatoid arthritis include: fatigue, low grade fever, weakness, joint stiffness, and vague joint pain. These symptoms can lead to the appearance of painful, swollen joints within several weeks.[4]

Gout

Gout is a type of arthritis caused by a buildup in the body of uric acid, which is found in meats and other foods and also produced by the body. When this production is out of balance or there is inadequate elimination of uric acid, gout occurs.[5]

When the level of uric acid rises to unhealthy levels in the body, it crystallizes in the joint cartilage and synovial tissue and fluid, causing sharp, needle-like pain in the joints, as well as fever, chills, and loss of mobility.[6] Some of the health problems caused by gout include constipation, indigestion, headaches, depression, eczema, and hives, and those who suffer gout also run a much higher risk of heart and kidney problems.

In 50 percent of gout cases, the first attack is characterized by intense pain in the first joint of the big toe. If the attack progresses, fever and chills will appear. Initial gout attacks usually strike at night and are preceded by a specific event such as excessive alcohol ingestion, trauma, certain drugs, or surgery. Subsequent attacks are common, with most patients experiencing another attack within one year. However, nearly 7 percent of gout sufferers never have a second attack. The condition affects approximately three out of every thousand adults and is primarily a disease of adult men, 95 percent of gout sufferers being males over the age of thirty.[7]

Causes ofArthritis

Arthritis is caused by a variety of factors, including joint instability, age-related changes, altered biochemistry, hormonal factors, and genetic predisposition. Yet other environmental and psychological factors have also been found to bring on the condition.

"Five to ten years ago, it would have been heresy to state that allergens could induce arthritis, and that, by the elimination of those allergens, the arthritis would go into remission," says James Braly, M.D., Medical Director of Immuno Labs, Inc., of Fort Lauderdale, Florida. "Now it's accepted among most rheumatologists and allergists that some people do have allergy-induced arthritis."

Stress can disrupt the body's hormonal balance as well. When stress interferes with the production of progesterone and thyroid hormone, menopausal difficulties increase. This accounts for the fact that a great many women develop osteoarthritis at this time. Raymond Peat, Ph.D., of Eugene, Oregon, also points out that stress-induced cortisone deficiency can be a factor in some forms of arthritis.[8] When stress occurs, body systems release adrenalin and cortisone, a process that weakens the immune system. In this way, bacteria and other detrimental organisms such as *Candida albicans* spread throughout the body.[9]

Causes of Osteoarthritis

Osteoarthritis is considered by many to be a natural result of the aging process. To a large degree this is true, with nearly everyone over the age of sixty showing some signs of the disease.[10] Dr. Braly cites age, excess weight, general wear and tear, and a lifetime of inadequate diet and exercise as the chief causes of osteoarthritis. Other research has found additional causes to be skeletal defects, genetic factors, and hormonal deficiencies—as evidenced by the many women who suffer osteoarthritis after menopause.[11] Yet many people with osteoarthritis never suffer from the aches, pain, and stiffness associated with the disease.[12] Even for sufferers, there is much that can be done to restore arthritis-stricken bodies to functional health, when the underlying, systemic causes of the disease are identified and addressed.[13]

"Five to ten years ago, it would have been heresy to state that allergens could induce arthritis, and that, by the elimination of those allergens, the arthritis would go into remission. Now it's accepted among most rheumatologists and allergists that some people do have allergy-induced arthritis."

—James Braly, M.D.

Causes of Rheumatoid Arthritis

Rheumatoid arthritis, on the other hand, is classified as an autoimmune disease in which the body attacks its own tissue. "A primary cause of most rheumatoid arthritis appears to be delayed food allergy and the often related problem of abnormal permeability of the intestinal wall," says Dr. Braly.

According to Dr. Braly, this abnormal permeability allows incompletely digested food particles to pass through the walls of the digestive tract and into the bloodstream, where, if not cleared, they are eventually deposited in tissue. There they can cause an inflammatory reaction, and, because the body is allergic to the deposited food particles, an autoimmune disturbance in which the body's own immune system begins to attack the tissue around the joints.

Other causes of rheumatoid arthritis include genetic susceptibility, lifestyle factors, nutritional factors, food allergies, and microorganisms. There may also be an association between rheumatoid arthritis and abnormal bowel function.[14]

Causes of Gout

The underlying cause of gout is unknown, yet research has found that it can basically be attributed to metabolic or renal problems. Increased production of uric acid may be the result of enzyme defects, metabolic defects, chronic anemia, kidney disease, or other complex conditions.[15]

> *"The traditional conception of gout as an 'affluent' condition, has some basis in reality since meats, particularly organ meats, increase production of uric acid, while alcohol inhibits uric acid secretion by the kidneys."*

While "high living" may not be the primary cause of gout as it is currently understood, proper diet, nutrition, and metabolic balance all play crucial roles in the prevention and treatment of this disease today. In fact, the traditional conception of gout as an "affluent" condition, has some basis in reality since meats, particularly organ meats, increase production of uric acid, while alcohol inhibits uric acid secretion by the kidneys.[16]

Treatment and Prevention of Arthritis

The primary keys for treating and preventing arthritis are proper diet and nutrition, detoxification, and stress reduction. Special care should also be taken to avoid substances that might cause allergic reactions in the body, and, when needed, hormonal supplementation and replacement is essential.[17] Pain management and correction of skeletal/postural problems can also be addressed through a variety of other modalities, including herbal medicine, environmental medicine, bodywork, chiropractic, acupuncture, and Ayurvedic medicine.

Diet and Nutrition

For decades, medical researchers, including those with the Arthritis Foundation itself, refused to acknowledge that diet, nutrition, and food allergies could play a role in immune function and arthritis. Today, however, proper diet and nutrition are believed to be key elements in the prevention of all types of disease, including arthritis. An important first step in treating arthritis lies in

DRUGS ASSOCIATED WITH A HIGHER INCIDENCE OF ARTHRITIS

According to the Physicians Desk Reference *the following drugs are associated with side effects of arthritis. (Statistics refer to the percentage of individuals affected.)*[22]

TheraCys BCG Live (Intravesical) (1.0-7.1%)
Tonocard Tablets (4.7%)
Videx Tablets, Powder for Oral Solution, & Pediatric Powder for Oral Solution (1-11%)
Wellbutrin Tablets (3.1%)

achieving normal body weight, as excess weight puts increased stress on weight-bearing joints affected with arthritis.[18] A diet rich in fresh vegetables, fruits, nuts, and whole grains is recommended for maximum nutritional benefit. Cold water fish and other sources of essential fatty acids are also valuable for the prevention of arthritis, because of the anti-inflammatory characteristics of such foods.[19] Michael Murray, N.D., of Seattle, Washington, suggests particularly the consumption of cold water fish such as mackerel, herring, sardines, and salmon, which are believed to significantly reduce inflammatory/allergic response. Studies have also shown that arthritis patients showed major clinical improvement when supplementing their diets with cod liver oil, which also may reduce the inflammatory process.[20]

See Detoxification Therapy.

According to Dr. Braly, fatty meats, eggs, margarine, shortening, and dairy products should be dramatically cut down or eliminated from the diet. He also advises the same for caffeine, alcohol, tobacco, and sugars. Patients should also be tested for food allergies.

Robert Bingham, M.D., Medical Director at the Desert Arthritis and Medical Clinic in Desert Hot Springs, California, reports that approximately one-third of those who suffer from rheumatoid arthritis are sensitive to solanines, or nightshade plants, which include potatoes, peppers, eggplant, tomatoes, and tobacco. These should be eliminated from the diet.[21] Furthermore, Dr. Murray reports that some patients with rheumatoid arthritis have benefited from fasting, although he stresses that this should be done only under direct medical supervision.

WATER, NOT MEDICATION, TO RELIEVE ARTHRITIC PAIN

"The most important life-giving substance in the body, and the one that the body desperately depends on, is water," says Fereydoon Batmanghelidj, M.D., of Falls Church, Virginia author of Your Body's Many Cries for Water. *Yet the body has no water storage system to draw on in times of need, according to Dr. Batmanghelidj, who points out that the parts of the body that suffer most from a shortage of water in the body are those without direct vascular circulation, especially the joint cartilages in fingers, knees, and the vertebrae.*

Chronic pains of the body are often indicators of chronic dehydration, adds Dr. Batmanghelidj. "When any of your joints begin to signal aching pains that come and go, the first thought that should occur to you is, 'my body is severely short of water.'" Often, though, when the signs of water deficiency in joint cartilages are not recognized for what they indicate, painkillers are prescribed, frequently resulting in a dependence on addictive medication, and possible permanent damage to cartilage separation of the joint bones.

"Rheumatoid joint pain is a direct signal of local water deficiency," explains Dr. Batmanghelidj. "If water intake is consciously and regularly adjusted to the needs of that particular body, in most cases, these pains will gradually disappear. Local swelling of joint surfaces will possibly disappear too. What is more important, the joint structure will begin to repair itself."

Nutritional Supplements

Many researchers believe a proper balance of vitamins and minerals is essential in the treatment of arthritis. Linus Pauling, Ph.D., of the Linus Pauling Institute for Science and Medicine, in Palo Alto, California,[23] and Robert Cathcart, III, M.D., of Los Altos, California,[24] both recommend large quantities of vitamin C. Vitamins A, B_1, B_6, E, and niacinamide (a form of vitamin B_3 which helps improve joint flexibility) have also proven effective in treating and preventing arthritis.[25]

Other dietary supplements which have anti-inflammatory and antioxidant effects[26] important for arthritis prevention and treatment include boron,[27] zinc, copper, selenium, manganese, pantothenic acid, methionine, superoxide dismustase,[28] proteolytic enzymes (enzymes that catalyze oxidative reactions), flavonoids, L-phenylalanine, tryptophan, and sulfur (cysteine). Bee pollen, royal jelly (another bee product rich in pantothenic acid), and evening primrose oil are also beneficial in alleviating arthritis symptoms, especially among rheumatoid arthritics. All these supplements, though, should be taken only under proper medical supervision.

Julian Whitaker, M.D., of Newport Beach, California, notes that glucosamine sulfate supplementation can be especially effective in helping reverse arthritis. According to Dr. Whitaker, glucosamine plays an integral part in stimulating the production of connective tissue and new cartilage growth essential to the repair of arthritis damage.

Calcium and magnesium are also vital nutrients in the fight against arthritis. Calcium is essential for bone, joint, muscle, and ligament health, while magnesium is necessary for calcium's proper incorporation into bone, by preventing a buildup of calcium in the soft tissues and joints. Most people, though, consume too much calcium and not enough magnesium. High protein diets, which are normal for many Americans, contain a lot of phosphorus, which binds up magnesium and makes it unavailable for the body's use.

See Fasting.

The Rheumatoid Disease Foundation suggests the use of boron to treat osteoarthritis, rheumatoid arthritis, and osteoporosis. Boron apparently plays a role in the retention of calcium and also positively stimulates hormonal factors for both men and women, contributing to healthy bones. The parathyroid gland contains more boron than any other tissue. Boron enhances parahormone activity and the parathyroid gland is the primary organ controlling mineralization of bones.

Dietary treatment for gout sufferers is intended to maintain the production of uric acid at normal levels. Gout patients should eliminate alcohol intake, which both increases uric acid production and reduces uric acid excretion in the kidneys. Reports indicate that elimination of alcohol is all that is needed to reduce uric acid levels and prevent gout in many individuals.[29]

Gout sufferers should also maintain a low-purine diet, which completely omits organ meats, meats, shellfish, yeast (brewer's and baker's), herring, sardines, mackerel, and anchovies. Foods with moderate levels of protein, including dried legumes, spinach, asparagus, fish, poultry, and mushrooms, should also be curtailed. To control uric acid levels, refined carbohydrates and saturated fats should be kept to a minimum. Dr Murray advises weight reduction in obese individuals, using a high-fiber, low-fat diet. Liberal fluid intake should also be maintained, which keeps urine diluted and promotes the excretion of uric acid.

For gout patients, Dr. Murray recommends the following nutritional supplements: 1.8 grams a day of eicosapentaenoic acid (EPA), 400 to 800 IUs a day of vitamin E, 10 to 40 milligrams a day of folic acid (under a doctor's supervision), and quercetin (with bromelain), 125 to 250 milligrams three times a day between meals.[30]

Herbal Medicine

According to David Hoffmann, B.Sc., M.N.I.M.H., of Sebastopol, California, past President of the American Herbalist Guild, many anti-inflammatory and alternative herbs help in alleviating the symptoms of arthritis. Of the many possible combinations this is a safe mixture that can be taken over a long period of time: combine the tinctures of meadowsweet, willow bark, black cohosh, prickly ash, celery seed, and nettle in equal parts and take one teaspoonful of this mixture three times a day. In cases of rheumatoid arthritis add wild yam and valerian to the mixture and take one teaspoonful of this mixture three times a day.

According to Dr. Murray, yucca and devil's claw may possess positive anti-inflammatory and analgesic effects for arthritic patients. In clinical trials on gout patients, devil's claw was found to relieve joint pain, as well as reduce serum cholesterol and uric acid levels. For gout sufferers, Dr. Murray recommends a dosage of devil's claw of 1 to 2 grams three times a day of dried powdered root; 4 to 5 milliliters three times a day of tincture (1:5); or 400 milligrams three times a day of dry solid extract (3:1).

See Herbal Medicine.

Other recommended herbs include licorice and alfalfa.[31] Feverfew has also been found to be effective in inhibiting the synthesis of pro-inflammatory compounds and decreasing the body's inflammatory response. Other herbal remedies that have proven effective for rheumatoid arthritis include tumeric, ginger, skullcap, bupleurum, and ginseng.[32]

Dr. Murray recommends that arthritis and gout sufferers consume half a pound of fresh or

THE ARTHRITIS VACCINE

According to Robert Bingham, M.D., Medical Director at the Desert Arthritis and Medical Clinic in Desert Hot Springs, California, the use of the yucca plant as a vaccine has proven highly successful as a nonspecific immune stimulator which reduces infection and inflammation.

Yucca extract is made from an extract of the yucca plant found in the Southwestern deserts and in Mexico. Its main therapeutic agent is a high concentration of the steroid saponin, which improves circulation in the intestinal tract, while reducing any abnormal fat content in the blood. One of the main benefits of this "natural medicine" is that it has no harmful side effects, unlike most of the pharmacological medicines prescribed for arthritis.[33]

Standard dosage is two tablets taken three times a day with meals, according to Dr. Bingham. Results are usually felt within three weeks, with the maximum effect being felt after four months. The yucca extract is safe enough to take for longer periods of time to prevent any recurrence of symptoms and can be purchased today without a prescription.[34]

Dr. Bingham's clinic has conducted several successful clinical studies of yucca extract and its approval as an herbal food supplement by the Food and Drug Administration (FDA). Today, it is already being used by close to three thousand physicians across the United States, and thousands of patients worldwide. It is available in Japan, Korea, England, Germany and, to some extent, Canada.

SEA CUCUMBER

According to studies cited by Morton Walker, D.P.M., marine organisms known as sea cucumbers emit defensive toxins which have been found useful in the alleviation of some human diseases, dysfunctions, and disorders. Taken orally, sea cucumber toxins have been found to be a definite anti-inflammatory agent for the symptomatic relief of rheumatoid arthritis, osteoarthritis, tendinitis, sports injuries, and associated conditions.

According to Dr. Walker, clinical experience indicates that in homeopathic dilutions, sea cucumber toxins are about twenty-five times more effective than aspirin in reducing inflammation and have a greater lasting effect. An August 1992 study conducted by the University of Queensland found that sea cucumber was not only anti-inflammatory but also antiarthritic, attacking the disease process itself rather than the symptoms.

Sea cucumber has been approved by Australia's Department of Health as an effective arthritis treatment. In addition, Mitchell Kurk, M.D., D.O., O.D., Medical Director of the Biomedical Revitalization Center of Lawrence, New York, has found that the conditions of approximately 70 percent of his arthritic patients have improved with use of sea cucumber.[35]

canned cherries per day. Cherries, hawthorn berries, blueberries, and other dark red-blue berries are rich sources of compounds that have been found to favorably affect collagen metabolism and prevent and reduce inflammation of joints.[36]

Environmental Medicine

"Allergic and allergy-like sensitivities are very important factors in a large percentage of arthritis cases," states Marshall Mandell, M.D., Medical Director of the New England Foundation for Allergic and Environmental Diseases. "Allergies may or may not cause arthritis, but they definitely play a major role in a majority of cases because they often aggravate and perpetuate the condition. When the substances to which the arthritic patients are sensitive are eliminated, avoided, or contacted less frequently, the arthritis is relieved or eliminated."

The link between arthritis and allergic reactions to different environmental chemicals and foods was first pointed out by Theron G. Randolph, M.D., of Batavia, Illinois, the founder of environmental medicine. Dr. Randolph tested over one thousand arthritis patients with commonly eaten foods and chemical substances ranging from natural gas, auto exhaust, paints, perfume, and hair spray to insecticides, tobacco, and smoke to find out which of these substances caused their symptoms.[37] The connection between arthritis and allergies was found to be quite significant.

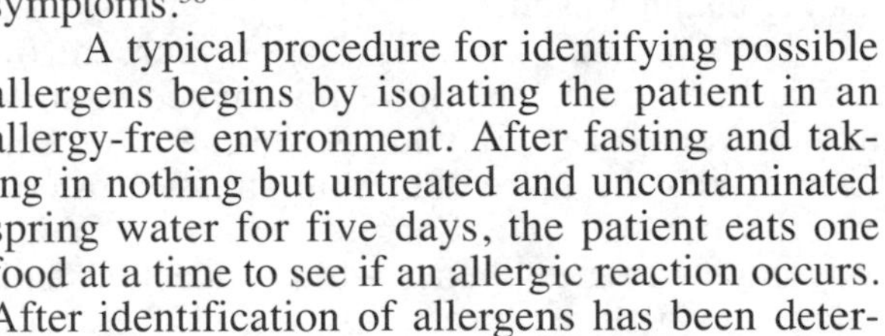

See Bodywork, Environmental Medicine.

In his own tests of over six thousand patients, Dr. Mandell found foods, chemicals, grasses, pollen, molds, and other airborne substances caused allergic reactions in the joints of nearly 85 percent of the arthritics he tested. Numerous other studies have shown various foods and food additives, as well as foreign invaders like protozoa, bacteria, yeast, and fungus, can also trigger or aggravate arthritic symptoms.[38]

A typical procedure for identifying possible allergens begins by isolating the patient in an allergy-free environment. After fasting and taking in nothing but untreated and uncontaminated spring water for five days, the patient eats one food at a time to see if an allergic reaction occurs. After identification of allergens has been determined, the patient returns to normal life, with the knowledge of which foods and elements to avoid altogether or to take or use very sparingly.[39]

Bodywork

Osteoarthritis is directly related to skeletal and postural difficulties. Tendons and ligaments can be torn or stretched as a result of injury, exercise, or aging. The fascial tissues (thin sheets of connective tissue which hold muscles, joints, and organs together) tend to thicken and rigidify from overuse. When the body tries to compensate, bony spurs may appear in joints, and on bones.

Bodywork can alter postural difficulties. Restoration of proper, natural posture through deep massage and movement reeducation can

BATTLING ARTHRITIS PAIN WITH SHARK CARTILAGE

I. William Lane, Ph. D., an independent consultant specializing in marine resources, reports that shark cartilage in capsule form is now being used successfully to combat the pain of arthritis. Shark cartilage contains large amounts of mucopolysaccharides (carbohydrates that form chemical bonds with water) which stimulate the immune system. This reduces the pain and inflammation of arthritis. Since cartilage is living tissue, oral dosages are believed to actually help repair damaged human cartilage, according to Dr. Lane.[40]

Additional research shows the angiogenesis-inhibiting properties of shark cartilage work synergistically with the mucopolysaccharides to stop new blood vessel invasion of cartilage. This eliminates degradation of functioning cartilage. Clinical trials and practical application have shown that shark cartilage orally administered before meals is effective in reducing the pain score for many arthritic patients. Eighty percent of osteoarthritis patients at Comprehensive Medical Clinic in Southern California responded well. The percentage of response for rheumatoid arthritis patients studied in other research was 50 to 60 percent.[41]

Patients completing the various studies showed a decrease in pain by 5 to 6 points on a scale of 10, with 10 being unbearable pain. Some, who had suffered pain performing physical activities before using shark cartilage, no longer experienced such pain after just three weeks of treatment.[42]

Arthritic patients should not expect instant results from taking cartilage extracts, however. Since human cartilage does not have a blood supply, it is difficult to get new building materials into the joint areas. Also, during the healing process, joints continue to be subjected to activity and stress-bearing. Therefore, the benefits of cartilage supplementation tend to be gradual.[43]

enable arthritic sufferers to free themselves from the pain and limitations of the disease.

Rolfing, for example, has been found to help many arthritis sufferers. The procedure was originally devised by Dr. Ida Rolf, a biochemist who used her technique to rid herself of arthritis. She realized conditions causing arthritic disturbance could be changed by stretching fascial tissues. Such a procedure repositions the body in balanced alignment with gravity. "Many diagnoses of 'arthritis' reflect nothing more serious than a shortened or displaced muscle or ligament resulting from a recent or not-so-recent traumatic episode," said Dr. Rolf.[44]

Chiropractic

Chiropractic is an increasingly popular, drug-free treatment for arthritis which has proven highly effective for many who suffer from the disease. Certain cases of arthritis, particularly of osteoarthritis, are false diagnoses with the symptoms actually caused by misalignment, or 'subluxation' of vertebrae and joints. When this is the case, chiropractic adjustments can restore a full range of movement and free the body from pain.

According to William Michael Cargile, B.S., D.C., F.I.A.C.A., Chairman of Research of the American Association of Acupuncture, osteoarthritic patients can often be treated successfully with a combination of chiropractic and acupuncture. With osteoarthritic cases, he has generally found abnormalities in the bladder meridian region of the spine, along with abnormalities in the bladder channel itself.

Dr. Cargile estimates that 95 percent of osteoarthritic cases also have misaligned or subluxated vertebrae. "If your vertebrae is out of position and there are abnormal stresses, osteoarthritis occurs," Dr. Cargile explains. "Your body begins to grow bones—little stalactites and stalagmites between levels, fusing itself." He recommends regular preventative chiropractic treatment to keep these stresses on bones from occurring.

Acupuncture

According to Dr. Cargile, rheumatoid arthritis is a result of an immuno-chemical problem which prohibits white blood cells from being able to recognize the joint surface as part of itself. "Acupuncture reduces the aggressiveness of the body against its own tissue and enhances its recognition of the joint surface," he says.

Dr. Cargile uses acupuncture as a whole-body system, utilizing an individual, case-by-case approach to stimulate the immune system. "We are not just affecting arthritis in the hands, we are actually affecting the spleen because of its role in the lymphatic system, and its production of white blood cells," he explains.

Dr. Cargile cites the use of acupuncture on a fifty-six-year-old woman with a twenty-year-old case of medically diagnosed rheumatoid arthritis. She had become almost totally bedridden and was being treated with methotrexate, a toxic drug used in chemotherapy for cancer. The combination of her condition and the drug's extreme toxicity had her near death, but her fear of needles had kept her away from acupuncture. When she finally agreed to try it, she was delighted to discover she felt no pain from the needles.

See Acupuncture, Ayurvedic Medicine, Chiropractic.

Treatments took place three times a week initially, then two times a week after the second month, and finally, once a week after the third month. She improved dramatically, with a marked decrease in inflammation, and a much improved range of motion. Her pain decreased as well as all the associated symptomatic conditions of her arthritis. The patient, formerly a very successful Realtor, was able to go back to work. Today, she is again productive with her own business.

Dr. Cargile has also found much success using a combination of acupuncture with chiropractic for the treatment of arthritis, particularly in cases of osteoarthritis.

ARTHRITIS AND DENTAL AMALGAMS

Hal Huggins, D.D.S., of Colorado Springs, Colorado, a leading authority on biological dentistry, has found arthritic symptoms are often associated with mercury dental amalgams. He notes that once the amalgams are removed, the symptoms usually disappear.

Dr. Huggins recalls treating a patient, a professional pianist, with arthritis in her hands so pronounced she could no longer perform. She had also suffered from other medical problems for years, including tachycardia, candidiasis, stuttering, and mononucleosis. Dr. Huggins found she had two mercury fillings and a bridge with a metal base. Both the bridge and mercury amalgams were removed. The patient quickly regained her former energy, and the swelling and pain in her fingers subsided. She was able to play the piano in concert again within two months.

Ayurvedic Medicine

According to Virender Sodhi, M.D. (Ayurveda), N.D., Director of the American School of Ayurvedic Sciences, of Bellevue, Washington, Ayurvedic medicine attributes arthritis to problems in the digestion of carbohydrates, proteins, and fats which create production of intermediate molecules called *ama* and a condition called "leaky gut syndrome." This digestive disorder triggers immune and allergic responses and results in the inflammation of the body's joints. Dr. Sodhi describes osteoarthritis as a "complete metabolic dehydration with no fluid left in the joints."

Ayurvedic medicine treats the digestive problems by working with diet and nutrition. Dr. Sodhi recommends that arthritic patients avoid foods that can cause indigestion, like broccoli, cauliflower, and lettuce. He advises patients to take herbs which enhance digestion, such as ginger, cayenne, black pepper, long pepper, and tumeric. Patients are further advised to avoid proteins, especially from animal sources such as beef, chicken, shellfish, and pork (fish protein is acceptable), and to avoid alcohol, coffee, and tea. One liquid he recommends for arthritic patients is pineapple juice with a pinch of tumeric which helps the body combat "leaky gut syndrome."

Dr. Sodhi also tests his arthritic patients for food allergies and for bacterial parasites that can cause joint inflammation. Other Ayurvedic herbs are recommended to promote digestion and the immune system. In particular, *triphala* helps cleanse the intestine and aids in the proper digestion of food. To increase joint mobility and protect joints from further damage, he recommends flaxseed, fish oils, and *boswellia.* Oil massages are very beneficial, using sesame or even olive oil. For swollen joints, massaging with castor oil helps pull toxins out of the system.

Breathing exercises to relieve the stiffness of the joints and to increase oxygenation are also important according to Dr. Sodhi. He prescribes a regimen of breathing patterns, flexes of the hands, feet and elbow, and *pranayama* yoga positions for arthritic patients. After exercising, he recommends a soak in hot water enhanced with baking soda or salt, ginger, peppermint, and eucalyptus. He states that Ayurvedic treatment for many patients can turn their condition around in three to four months.

One of Dr. Sodhi's patients was a twenty-eight-year-old man diagnosed with rheumatoid arthritis who had been taking conventionally prescribed cortisones with little success. Dr. Sodhi changed his diet, eliminating milk, meat, wheat, and all nitrates (a salt of nitric acid found in hot dogs and other cured meats). The patient was also put on a program of Ayurvedic herbs which reduced inflammation, cleansed the liver, and supported the adrenal glands. Additionally, he began a regimen of breathing exercises to coordinate his biological clock and trigger the nighttime secretions of growth hormones. The patient was slowly weaned off his medication and became pain free.

Another sixty-year-old female with severe osteoarthritis in her hands and shoulders was taking anti-inflammatory drugs with little effect. Dr. Sodhi placed her on a therapeutic diet and prescribed Ayurvedic herbal medicines and massages. Within six months, the patient's flexibility so improved that she could fully rotate her arms and shoulders and was able to begin walking two miles a day.

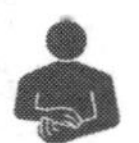

Self-Care

The following therapies can be undertaken at home under appropriate professional supervision:

Osteoarthritis

• Flower Remedies • Guided Imagery • Yoga

Aromatherapy: • Dissolve camphor, mint in rubbing alcohol or sesame oil and apply externally. • Lemon, marjoram

Juice Therapy: • Celery juice during acute inflammatory stage • Carrot, celery, and cabbage juice • Carrot, beet, and cucumber

Rheumatoid Arthritis

• Guided Imagery • Yoga

Aromatherapy: Detoxify with cypress, fennel, and lemon. Massage affected joints with rosemary, benzoin, chamomile, camphor, juniper, lavender.

Hydrotherapy: Constitutional hydrotherapy: apply two to five times weekly. Or heating compress: apply once daily to affected areas.

Leon Chaitow, N.D., D.O., of London, England, reports that the neutral bath [patient immersed in water (35 degrees centigrade) for two hours] has been effective in reducing the swelling of joints in rheumatoid patients.

Juice Therapy: • Carrot, celery, and cabbage juice. Add a little parsley. • Potato juice • Cherry juice • Take juice of half a lemon before every meal and before going to bed. • Carrot, beet, and cucumber • During acute stage, one pint to one quart celery juice daily • Radish, garlic • No tomato.

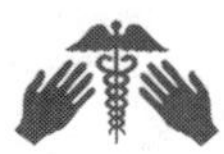

Professional Care

The following therapies should only be provided by a qualified health professional:

Osteoarthritis

• Acupressure • Applied Kinesiology • Cell

Therapy* • *Chelation Therapy* • *Craniosacral Therapy* • *Enzyme Therapy* • *Light Therapy* • *Orthomolecular Medicine* • *Osteopathy* • *Reconstructive Therapy* • *Reflexology

Bodywork: • Rolfing • *Shiatsu*

Rheumatoid Arthritis

• Applied Kinesiology • Chelation Therapy • Enzyme Therapy • Magnetic Field Therapy • Naturopathic Medicine • Orthomolecular Medicine • Osteopathy • Oxygen Therapies • Sound Therapy

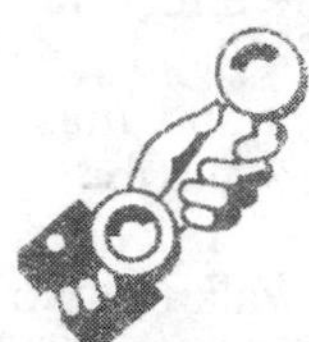

Where to Find Help

For more information on, and referrals for, treatment of arthritis, contact the following organizations.

American Association of Acupuncture and Oriental Medicine
4101 Lake Boone Trail, Suite 201
Raleigh, North Carolina 27607
(919) 787-5181

The AAAOM is a national professional trade organization of acupuncturists who meet acceptable standards of competency and can provide you with the names and locations of local members. Referrals by written request only.

American Association of Naturopathic Physicians
2366 Eastlake Avenue, Suite 322
Seattle, Washington 98102
(206) 323-7610

Contact them for the location of a licensed naturopathic physician in your area.

American Chiropractic Association
1701 Clarendon Boulevard
Arlington, Virginia 22209
(703) 276-8800

A major source for information on chiropractic. Monthly publication and newsletter. Provides referrals on request.

American School of Ayurvedic Sciences
10025 NE 4th Street
Bellevue, Washington 98004
(206) 453-8022

This college provides medical training for physicians and health care practitioners, as well as individual courses for lay people. Dr. Virender Sodhi's Ayurvedic, Naturopathic Medical Clinic is also located at this address.

Immuno Labs, Inc.
1620 West Oakland Park Boulevard
Suite 300
Fort Lauderdale, Florida 33311
(800) 231-9197

Specialized allergy and immunology testing for physicians around the world. Provides referrals worldwide to physicians who do allergy testing.

International Chiropractors Association
1110 North Glebe Road
Suite 1000
Arlington, Virginia 22201
(703) 528-5000

The original chiropractic association founded by B. J. Palmer, the son of the founder of chiropractic, Daniel David Palmer. Programs and services to meet the needs of chiropractors, patients, students, and the public. Concerned with legislation, health care policy, public relations, continuing education, skills development, publications, and interprofessional relations.

The Rheumatoid Disease Foundation
5106 Old Harding Road
Franklin, Tennessee 37064

They have a listing of more than two hundred physicians who use one or more of the various recommendations for osteoarthritis, rheumatoid disease, and gout. They are nonprofit, charitable, tax-exempt, so send a contribution to help defray the cost of services requested.

World Chiropractic Alliance
2950 N. Dobson Road, Suite 1
Chandler, Arizona 85224
(800) 347-1011

An international association of chiropractors with the purpose of promoting and advancing the profession. Offers guidance and assistance to professionals. Emphasis on vertebral subluxation correction. Provides public education and information. Publishes two newspapers for professionals and provides referrals for chiropractors nationwide.

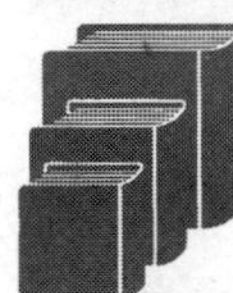

Recommended Reading

Arthritis: The Allergy Connection. Mansfield, John, M.D. Wellingborough, England: Thorsons Publishers Ltd., 1990.
Outlines the factors which contribute to arthritis, including food and environmental allergies, and candidiasis.

The Arthritis Helpbook. Lorrig, Kale; and Fries, James. Reading, MA: Addison-Wesley Publishing Co., 1990.
A self-care program for coping with arthritis that includes diet, nutrition, exercise, and mind/body techniques such as guided imagery and meditation.

Arthritis Relief At Your Fingertips. Gach, Michael Reed, Ph.D. New York: Warner Books, 1989.
A self-help guide for relieving arthritis pain through exercise and acupressure massage by a leader in the field.

Taking Care of Arthritis. Kantrowicz, Fred, M.D. New York: Harper Perennial, 1991.
A comprehensive overview of the types of arthritis, the factors which cause them, and the best methods of treatment.

How to Deal with Back Pain and Rheumatoid Joint Pain. Batmanghelidj, Fereydoon, M.D. Global Health Solutions, 1991.
These pains as two of the newly exposed thirst signals of the body are explained in this book. The physiology of pain production and its direct relationship to chronic regional dehydration of some joint spaces is explained: Special movements that would create vacuum in the disc spaces and draw water and the displaced discs into the vertebral joints are demonstrated.

Your Body's Many Cries for Water. Batmanghelidj, Fereydoon, M.D. Falls Church, VA: Global Health Solutions, Inc., 1992.
A fascinating discussion about the importance of water in the body, and how simply increasing the amount of water consumed per day can significantly improve arthritic and other pain conditions. (Available from Global Health Solutions, Inc., P.O. Box 3189, Falls Church, Virginia 22043.)

"Medicine is a collection of uncertain prescriptions, the results of which taken collectively, are more fatal than useful to mankind. Water, air and cleanliness are the chief articles in my pharmacopeia."

—Napoleon Bonaparte

Autism

Autism is a severe, lifelong behavioral disorder with no known single cause or cure. Alternative treatment programs, including diet, nutritional supplementation, and auditory training, have been helpful in allowing some autistic individuals to participate in society with some degree of success.

Autism is a mysterious illness which has long baffled the medical community. A permanent condition that usually begins shortly after birth, and always before age two and a half, autism occurs in approximately five out of every ten thousand children, and is characterized by withdrawal and an inability to communicate in a normal manner. Autistic individuals often form strong attachments to a particular object rather than to people, display compulsive behavior such as rocking or arm flapping, and avoid eye contact. While some autistic individuals are mute, others exhibit a bizarre, ritualistic speech pattern. They are often institutionalized, particularly if the individual is subject to violent or self-destructive episodes. However, despite severely limited learning capacity, some autistic children show extraordinary talent in a specific area such as music or mathematics.

Causes of Autism

According to Bernard Rimland, Ph.D., Director of the Autism Research Institute in San Diego, California, "Autism is not a disease with a specific cause, but rather a syndrome with a combination of abnormal behavioral characteristics. Although a genetic basis for many cases of autism has long been suspected, only recently have researchers been able to tie specific genes to autism."

Metabolic disorders have been found in some cases of autism. And defects in the breakdown of peptides (simple proteins such as insulin, endorphins, and other neurotransmitters) during the digestive process, as indicated by an increased level of urinary peptides, have been found in autistic children.[1]

Other possible causes of autism include:

- **Fetal alcohol syndrome:** In a Canadian study, one in fifty-four children with fetal alcohol syndrome (birth defect, characterized by deficiencies in growth and mental deficiencies) also had autism.[2]
- **Brain stem defects:** Studies have linked brain stem defects (significantly decreased brain stem size) to autism.[3]
- **Lead poisoning:** Elevated blood levels of lead have been found in some autistic children.[4]
- **A defect in the myelination process (insulation of nerve fibers):** This may account not only for autistic symptoms, but also for the frequent development of epilepsy in older autistic children.[5]
- **Unusual blood flow patterns in the brains of adults with infantile autism:** Total brain blood flow has been found to be significantly decreased in autistic children.[6]
- **Viral infections:** Rubella (German measles) or cytomegalovirus (related to the herpes virus) during the mother's pregnancy, and severe infections during infancy, may be associated with the onset of autism.[7]
- **Food allergies:** Reports suggest that sensitivities to certain foods, especially wheat, sugar, and cow's milk, may contribute to behavioral symptoms.[8] Because many autistics have food allergies, these allergens need to be identified and eliminated from the diet.[9] Most traditionally trained allergists are not aware that allergies can affect the brain, so a specialist in environmental medicine should be sought.
- **Infant vaccinations:** Harris L. Coulter, Ph.D., of Washington, D.C., a medical historian, believes that autism and many other brain disorders are caused by infant vaccinations, particularly with the pertussis (whooping cough) vaccine.[10] Incidences of autism rose in the 1950s, which coincides with the time vaccinations became popular in the United States, according to Dr. Coulter.

- **Yeast infections caused by antibiotic treatment for repeated ear infections:** Many children develop autism following antibiotic treatment for repeated ear infections, according to William Crook, M.D., of Jackson, Tennessee.[11] Dr. Crook believes that chronic use of antibiotics destroys the normal bacteria living in the intestinal tract, leading to overgrowth of the yeast *Candida albicans* as well as to "leaky gut syndrome," in which undigested food particles get into the circulation, sparking off autoimmune reactions and food allergies, all of which are common in autistics.
- **Parasites, yeast infections, and a deficiency of digestive enzymes:** Constantine A. Kotsanis, M.D., of Grapevine, Texas, believes that autism has a multifactorial cause and that parasites, yeast infections, food allergies (yellow, red, and green food dyes), and a deficiency of digestive enzymes all may play a role.

Treating Autism

The conventional methods of treating autism consist of drugs and behavior modification. While behavioral approaches incorporating a firmly structured, purposeful educational program have proven to be highly beneficial in many cases, alternative physicians claim increasing success using a combination of other therapies. These include nutritional supplementation, the elimination of food allergies, auditory integration training, and craniosacral therapy.

Nutritional Supplements

High-dosage (megavitamin) nutritional supplementation is playing an increasingly important role in the treatment of autism. Dr. Rimland states that, "Researchers both in the United States and abroad have demonstrated very clearly that 30 to 60 percent of autistic children and adults show significant behavioral and other benefits from the administration of large amounts of vitamin B_6 and magnesium."

Magnesium is employed because the body cannot effectively use vitamin B_6 without adequate magnesium. According to Dr. Rimland, some studies show not only behavioral improvement, but normalization of brain waves and of metabolism. He adds that this approach is far safer, more rational, and more helpful than the use of any drug. A magnesium deficiency has also been shown to cause hearing hypersensitivity and hyperirritability, both associated with autism.[12] Dr. Rimland also recommends the supplementation of zinc, as well as the other B vitamins in his program.

Vitamin C has also been shown to significantly reduce autistic behavior such as rocking, spinning, and hand flapping, according to a recent study.[13] Dimethylglycine (DMG), a nontoxic chemical found in minute amounts in foods, has also proved helpful in treating autism, according to Dr. Rimland. Many parents have reported that within days of starting DMG, their autistic child's behavior improved noticeably, and better eye contact was observed, as well as an improvement in the child's speech, adds Dr. Rimland.

Diet

Diet is an important factor in treating autism. Dr. Kotsanis recommends that autistic individuals eat a diet of whole, unprocessed, alkalinizing foods such as vegetables, since many autistic's blood is overly acidic. "Canned, packaged, and frozen foods contain preservatives and other food additives which can have adverse effects on autistics," he adds. "Dairy products should be avoided because of their mucous-producing properties, as should processed sugar, due to the chemicals used in refining. Foods with yellow, red, and green dyes should be completely eliminated from the diet as well as aspartame (an artificial sweetener found in Equal® or NutraSweet®) because at high heat aspartame can potentially break down into formaldehyde."

> *"Researchers both in the United States and abroad have demonstrated very clearly that 30 to 60 percent of autistic children and adults show significant behavioral and other benefits from the administration of large amounts of vitamin B_6 and magnesium."*
>
> —Bernard Rimland, Ph.D.

Another dietary factor to consider when treating autism has to do with the peptides contained in cow's milk and gluten-derived products. According to a recent study, when milk and gluten-derived peptides were removed from the diet, language, social interactions, and behavior all improved.[14] In this particular study, fifteen autistic children and adults, aged six to twenty-two, were treated by restricting or eliminating cow's milk and gluten-derived products from their diets. According to the study, "These patients were socially isolated, were resistant to learning, showed peculiar attachment to certain objects, showed fear of unusual items and situations, and demonstrated both repetitive motor behavior and severe problems with emotional expression. Language problems and disturbed attention were also common."

Urine analysis samples showed that patients had increased levels of cow's milk and gluten-derived peptides. Depending on the specific pattern of peptides in the urine, three types of diets were prescribed to reduce overall peptide levels. Some patients received a gluten-free and milk-reduced diet, others received a milk-free and/or gluten-reduced diet, and a third group received a milk- and gluten-free diet.

See Allergies.

Milk reduction was achieved by eliminating milk and cheese, and gluten reduction was achieved by giving only gluten-free bread and cakes. After one year, all the study subjects had changed in the direction of the normal spectrum; they were less psychotic, more communicative, and showed less bizarre behavior. Other statistically significant changes included improved attention and social integration, improved motor ability and skills, and a decrease in irrational emotional outbursts. Especially noteworthy was the decrease in resistance to learning demonstrated by all cases.

Dr. Crook says he has noticeably improved the behavior of autistic children by using an elimination diet. Any food normally consumed more than once a week is removed from their diets. As symptoms improve, each food is added back to the diet one at a time. One of Dr. Crook's patients became more alert, less hyperactive, and more sociable after wheat, sugar, corn, and eggs were removed from his diet.[15]

William Philpott, M.D., and Dwight Kalita, Ph.D., report of an autistic patient who exhibited agitation, aggressiveness, and hyperactivity after eating corn. This same patient became extremely agitated when given either raisins, honey, or bananas. In addition to food allergies, this patient exhibited heavy metal toxicity (cadmium) and several nutritional deficiencies. Fasting and the elimination of the above foods helped him become more calm, alert, and self-confident, and to speak with less effort.[16]

Autism and Auditory Integration Training

"Many autistic individuals are highly sensitive, and can hear far beyond the normal human range," according to Dr. Kotsanis. "To an autistic individual, rain sounds like rocks falling on a roof.

"This hypersensitivity can result in a number of problems, including blocking out other sounds, fear of noises and people, and an inability to concentrate."

Auditory training has been reported to bring about a wide range of improvements in speech and behavior in many autistic individuals. The technique is based on the work of two French doctors, Alfred Tomatis, M.D., and Guy Berard, E.N.T. Both the Tomatis and Berard methods provide stimulation to the listener.

Berard training involves listening to ten hours of music (in twenty half-hour sessions) played through Berard's electronic modulating device, known as the Ears Education & Retraining System (EERS). An audiogram is first performed to detect frequencies to which the patient is hypersensitive so that they may be screened out of the music. Then the EERS is used to take music from a sound source, filter out specific frequencies found to cause the individual discomfort, modulate the sound electronically in an unpredictable manner, and finally send the sounds back to the ears through headphones to exercise the entire hearing apparatus.

> *"Many autistics have highly sensitive hearing and can hear far beyond the normal human range. To an autistic individual, rain sounds like rocks falling on a roof. This hypersensitivity can result in a number of problems, including blocking out other sounds, fear of noises and people, and an inability to concentrate."*
>
> —Constantine A. Kotsanis, M.D.

See Diet, Nutritional Supplements, Orthomolecular Medicine.

The Berard method asserts that behavioral and cognitive problems may arise when people perceive sounds in an unequal manner. Certain frequencies, in other words, may be better comprehended than others, leading to some sounds becoming distorted to the listener, who then may have comprehension and behavior difficulties. Berard claims that his approach can reduce distorted hearing and hypersensitivity to specific frequencies and that, ideally, all frequencies can be perceived equally well.

Favorable results from the Berard method are often achieved within a matter of days. One extremely hyperactive nine-year-old boy overturned furniture and switched equipment on and off on his initial visit to Dr. Kotsanis' office.

After two months of auditory training, the patient sat quietly in the reception area reading while waiting for the doctor. Dr. Kotsanis considers auditory integration training to be the most important factor in his treatment for autistic individuals.

The Tomatis method establishes a connection between listening, language, and learning. According to Billie Thompson, Ph.D., Director of the Sound, Listening and Learning Center in Phoenix, Arizona, the Tomatis method focuses on listening, which involves more than just hearing. Following a listening test, a program to improve auditory processing, audio-vocal control, and desire to communicate is developed. Auditory hypersensitivity is lessened, attention is increased, and the nervous system becomes more balanced notes Dr. Thompson.

> *"Auditory training gives autistic children the desire to communicate. It allows them to hear sounds in a different way and can profoundly affect the way they learn and relate to others."*
>
> —Billie Thompson, Ph.D.

The Tomatis method program often, though not always, uses the filtered sounds of the mother's voice as the child would have heard it in utero. This is done in order to reintroduce the rhythm and intonation of language and the curiosity and desire to tune in. Both bone and air conduction are stimulated, and Tomatis' own device, the patented Electronic Ear, is used to control filtering, balance, timing, and emphasis of different frequencies. Mozart, Gregorian chants, and children's nursery and folk songs are used in different stages of the program. Dr. Thompson notes that research done by Dr. Tomatis shows that high frequency sounds, achieved through filtering, provide a great deal of cortical stimulation which helps children and adults access this energy for improved thinking and processing.

Dr. Tomatis tells about a fourteen-year-old autistic boy, who had not spoken since age four, who began to babble like a ten-month-old on hearing the sound of his mother's filtered voice. Dr. Thompson describes a hypersensitive six-year-old autistic girl who did not speak and who wore a ski cap twenty-four hours a day to limit outside stimulation. "After three days she discarded the cap, went out to a restaurant with her family for the first time, and went to a church and heard an organ without leaving in pain. Though she still does not speak more than a few words, she is more social, does more activities with the family, and does not go to the corner in fear of sound."

Says Dr. Thompson, "To begin the Tomatis method is given for two hours a day for fifteen days. It then continues for at least two additional eight-day intensives. Auditory training gives autistic children the desire to communicate. It allows them to hear sounds in a different way and can profoundly affect the way they learn and relate to others. Our goal is to help the person learn to listen, when possible, to speak, and to have more awareness and self-control."

Craniosacral Therapy

Craniosacral therapy manipulates the bones of the skull and the underlying membranes to alleviate pressure and restrictions. The Upledger Institute in Palm Beach Gardens, Florida, uses craniosacral therapy to help treat autism. John Upledger, D.O., Medical Director of the Upledger Institute, reports that over one hundred autistic children have been treated at the Institute. In these children, he found a pattern of cranial restrictions in autistic individuals consistent with developmental distortions of the brain, spinal cord, and the bones of the skull. Manipulation seeks to improve the range of motion in the craniosacral system (brain, spinal cord, surrounding membranes, as well as the bones of the skull and spine) in people with autism, and produces improvements in behavior.

See Craniosacral Therapy.

"As corrections are made, self-abusive behavior such as head banging abates entirely or reduces in severity," says Dr. Upledger. He believes that the effectiveness of the craniosacral treatments may be due to alleviating long-standing internal head pain.[17] According to Bill Stager, D.O., of the Upledger Institute, "The light touch, hands-on therapy reduces antisocial and self-destructive behavior. It takes two to three treatments for the patient to get familiar with the therapist and begin to respond. After that, progress is quite rapid." Substantial changes are seen within ten to twenty sessions, given weekly. A concentrated, two-week program, with sessions eight hours a day for five days, is also available for out-of-town patients. Therapy must be continued over the years to maintain the benefits.

Leon Chaitow, N.D., D.O., of London, England, also reports that a combination of cranial osteopathy (a form of craniosacral therapy) and nutritional treatment offers an effective therapy for autistic children.

A Multifactorial Approach to Treatment

Dr. Kotsanis has developed a multifactorial approach to treating autism. Although this treatment method has been in use for only a short time, he reports that it has shown dramatic results. Because he has found parasites and yeast infections to be prevalent in autistic individuals, Dr. Kotsanis begins by prescribing a bowel cleansing program. This consists of Chinese herbs, biocidin (an antifungal agent made of various herbs), citrus extract, oil of oregano, nystatin, and nyzoral (antifungal medications). Many autistics are also deficient in digestive enzymes, adds Dr. Kotsanis, and thus must supplement these at every meal. Furthermore, most of these children have "leaky gut syndrome," where there is permeability in the intestinal cell wall allowing undigested food particles into the bloodstream. To correct this he uses butyric acid (a fatty acid derived from butter), L-glutamine (an amino acid), and beta-carotene. He also believes it is necessary to replenish the normal flora of the digestive system. For this Dr. Kotsanis recommends acidophilus, aloe vera extract, and garlic extract. Vitamins A, B, C, and E, along with calcium, magnesium, zinc, and selenium are also important elements in his treatment protocol, as well as essential fatty acids and antioxidants.

See Energy Medicine, Light Therapy, Sound Therapy.

Another key element in Dr. Kotsanis' program lies in addressing inhalant, food, and chemical allergies and sensitivities. In this phase, offending foods and chemicals are eliminated, and the patient is placed on allergy injections for pollen, mold, and animal dander allergies, if these are present. In addition, the patient's surroundings are made as free from irritants (e.g., feather pillows, harsh laundry detergents, cigarette smoke, pesticides, etc.) as is possible. And it is recommended that the patient eat whole, unprocessed, organic foods, and drink purified water.

Next, Dr. Kotsanis utilizes auditory integration therapy twice a day for ten days and, if necessary, repeats it after six months. He considers this the most important aspect of the treatment program. At the present time, he is investigating the effect of combining sound and color therapy with voice vibration therapy for the treatment of autism.

Dr. Kotsanis also notes that strong psychological support and involvement by the family of the autistic is important for the treatment to be most effective. Although he prefers to treat children of young age, his program is applicable to all age groups.

Dr. Kotsanis has treated thirty-six autistic children with this multifaceted approach and reports a high degree of success. Thirty of the thirty-six, or 83 percent, had an increase in language and speech. Additionally, thirteen of fourteen who were sound sensitive had a decrease or complete elimination of sound sensitivities. One nonverbal eleven-year-old was so sensitive to light and sound prior to treatment that he spent all day hiding in a closet. After ten days in Dr. Kotsanis' program, he began to speak, and within two to three months, he was playing and engaging in social interactions in a normal manner. According to Dr. Kotsanis, some common remarks made by parents and friends concerning the children treated were that they were calmer, more attentive, exhibited better overall behavior, were more affectionate, and showed a better retention of information and memory.

Dr. Kotsanis stresses that while auditory integration therapy is an extremely important part of the treatment plan, every element mentioned contributes to a positive outcome. He feels that this multidisciplinary approach yields a more optimal result than any single discipline can offer alone.

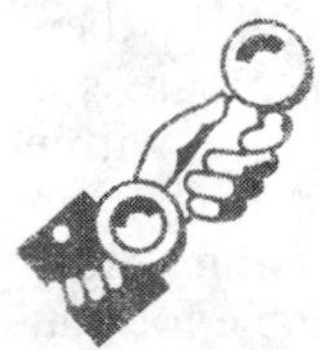

Where to Find Help

For additional information on, and referrals for, autism treatment, contact the following organizations:

Autism Research Institute
4182 Adams Avenue
San Diego, California 92116
(619) 281-7165
(619) 563-6840 (Fax)

The Autism Research Institute conducts research on the causes, diagnosis, and treatment of autism and publishes a quarterly newsletter that reviews worldwide research. Literature on causes and treatment available. Refers patients and families to health care professionals and clinics offering alternative treatment for autism and other childhood behavior disorders. Maintains a list of auditory training practitioners. Provides information on the B_6 megavitamin approach, as well as on DMG at no cost. (The Autism Research Center provides information only: it is not a clinic or treatment center.)

Autism Services Center
Prichard Building
605 9th Street
P.O. Box 507
Huntington, West Virginia 25710-0507
(304) 525-8014
(304) 525-8026 (Fax)

The Autism Services Center assists families of autistic children and acts as an advocate with technical assistance in designing appropriate therapy. Publishes a six page quarterly newsletter with news of the center's treatment facilities and stories of autistics who have benefitted from different therapies.

Autism Society of America
8601 Georgia Avenue, Suite 503
Silver Springs, Maryland 20910
(301) 565-0433
(301) 565-0834 (Fax)

The society has 160 chapters throughout the United States and will provide answers to questions on autism. Annual membership includes a quarterly newsletter with supportive information and research news. Makes available a wide range of books on dealing with autism.

The Georgiana Organization, Inc.
P.O. Box 2607
Westport, Connecticut 06880
(203) 454-1221

The Georgiana Organization provides education, workshops, consulting, and information on the Berard method.

Sound, Listening and Learning Center
2701 E. Camelback, Suite 205
Phoenix, Arizona 85016
(602) 381-0086

The Sound, Listening and Learning Center provides education, workshops, consulting, therapeutic sessions, and information on the Tomatis method.

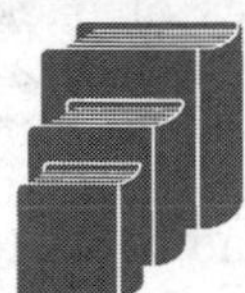

Recommended Reading

Autistic Adults at Bittersweet Farms. Giddan, Norman S., Ph.D.; and Giddan, Jane J., M.A. Binghamton, NY: The Haworth Press, 1991.
A detailed view of Bittersweet Farms, an eighty-acre residential program for autistic adults and adolescents in northwest Ohio. The Bittersweet program is based upon the premise that autistic adults need special care and training throughout their lives, which can be satisfying and productive.

Brain Allergies: The Psychonutrient Connection. Philpott, William H., M.D.; Kalliat, Dwight, Ph.D. New Canaan, CT: Keats, 1980.
An exploration of the ecological influences and organic causes of illness, as well as the benefits of supernutrition.

Children with Autism: A Parent's Guide. Powers, Michael D. Psy.D., ed. Rockville, MD: Woodbine House, 1989.
A complete introduction to autism which will ease the family's concerns while showing how to cope with the child's disorder.

Nobody Nowhere. Williams, Donna. New York: New York Times Books, Random House, 1992.
The autobiography of a partially-recovered autistic.

Nutritional Influences on Mental Illness. Werbach, Melvyn, M.D. Encino, CA: Third Line Press, 1991.
A comprehensive, professional guide to the current medical research on nutrition and mental illness.

The Ultimate Stranger: The Autistic Child. Delacato, Carl H., Ed.D. Novato, CA: Arena Press, 1984.
Offering convincing evidence that autism is a neurological rather than psychological disorder, Dr. Delacato suggests that the condition is a consequence of the malfunction of one or more of the five senses and describes a treatment plan.

Vaccination Social Violence and Criminality—The Medical Assault on the American Brain. Coulter, Harris L. Berkeley, CA: North Atlantic Books, 1990.
The author argues that vaccination has produced a generation of neurologic defectives and changed the tone and atmosphere of modern society.

Back Pain

Back pain is the leading cause of disability for people under the age of forty-five, with 80 percent of all Americans suffering from back pain at some point in their lives. Most people, though, are completely unaware of all the things they habitually do that contribute to this problem. Alternative medicine offers a number of systems for healing aching backs, and a variety of approaches designed to prevent future problems and pain.

Back pain can be divided into two basic categories, acute and chronic. Acute pain comes on quickly, either immediately or over a period of several hours. It is often the result of a sudden motion or injury that may come from something as simple as lifting up a heavy object, or from an accident or fall. On the other hand, chronic back pain comes on slowly and remains for a very long time, sometimes lasting for months or even years. It may come and go, but it is never far from one's mind, preventing one from enjoying the things one wants to do.

While acute and chronic back pain can manifest in different ways, oftentimes they are interrelated, with the acute problem leading to a chronic one, or, just as commonly, with a chronic condition, which can be hidden for long periods of time, setting off the acute symptoms. "What often happens," says Doug Lewis, N.D., Chairperson of the Physical Medicine Department of Bastyr College in Seattle, Washington, "is a person may have leaned over and picked up a box, or been vacuuming, twisting back and forth, something like that, and that's the event that sets it off. What set it up to begin with, though, was some sort of postural dysfunction that already existed and actually created a weak spot in the spine."

All too often, according to Dr. Lewis, the pain is treated without regard for the underlying cause. "The site of the pain is rarely the site of the dysfunction," he adds. "You may make the pain subside, but you're not correcting the dysfunction that caused the pain in the first place. If you leave the pain alone and treat the cause, then you have the pain as a monitor for whether or not your therapy is working."

Causes of Back Pain

In order to understand the causes of back pain, says Mary Pullig Schatz, M.D., Medical Staff President at Centennial Medical Center in Nashville, Tennessee, it is also important to understand the anatomy of the spine and its relationship to the rest of the body. "The spine affects and is affected by every movement your body makes," she explains. "The way you stand, the way you sit, the way you move, the way you pick up and carry objects—all these things have the potential to help or hurt your back."[1]

These are some of the physical factors that can be caused, or contributed to, by poor posture and movement, all of which can affect the proper functioning of the spinal column, inevitably leading to back pain, according to Dr. Schatz.

- Foot, knee, and leg alignment
- Muscle strength in legs, buttocks, back, and abdominal wall
- Abdominal protrusion such as from a beer belly or pregnancy
- Hip flexibility
- The position of the pelvis, especially if it is tilted forward, back, or to either side
- The position of the neck in relation to the shoulders
- Shoulder carriage and the mobility of the arms at the shoulder joints
- The shape and flexibility of the lumbar (lower back), thoracic (upper back), and cervical (neck) spinal curves[2]

"One of the most common postural problems leading to back pain," says Dr. Lewis "is a twist in the pelvis due to a leg-length discrepancy. This can be anatomical, where the legs actually are different lengths, or it can be functional, in which case the legs are at different lengths because the pelvis is twisted. This can produce a lateral, or side to side, curvature of the spine, or scoliosis, when it becomes pronounced enough.

"Anyone who has broken a leg automatically must assume there is a leg-length difference," adds Dr. Lewis. "Also, quite frequently, any injury to a leg during childhood or puberty, before the growth plates have fused, can cause a leg-length discrepancy because it doesn't allow normal growth of the leg."

Leg, buttocks, back, and abdominal muscles, when they become too contracted or too tight on one side or the other, can also produce similar pelvis twists and leg-length discrepancies, according to Dr. Lewis, as well as other postural deviations and spinal misalignments that can lead to extreme pain and physical impairment.

Eugene Kozhevnikov, M.D., O.M.D., of St. Petersburg, Russia, notes that back pain can also be caused by muscle problems which keep the vertebrae in misaligned positions. He claims that if muscles in acute cases are not relaxed, the back problems become chronic. Back pain can also be caused by stress, both mental and physical, because during stressful situations, the muscles tense and can exaggerate postural strains or musculoskeletal misalignments.

Organic problems can also lead to back pain symptoms. "For example," says Maoshing Ni, D.O.M., Ph.D, L.Ac., Vice-President of Yo San University in Santa Monica, California, "gallstones, kidney stones, infections, uterine fibroid tumors, and ovarian cysts can all result in severe back pain because the nerves that go to these organs come from the spine."

Dr. Lewis recounts a patient he had who came to him with lower back pain. "I treated her for the seeming indications of her pain, and she'd go away and feel great for two or three days, and then, by the following week she'd be back in, with exactly the same complaint, exactly the same intensity," says Dr. Lewis. "We did this several times, with the same result, until finally I said to her, 'I think you should see a gynecologist.'

"She went in and had an exam, discovered a grapefruit-sized cyst on her right ovary, which was removed, and immediately all of her back pain went away.

"The reverse situation can also occur" Dr. Lewis notes. "If there's a chronic dysfunction in the musculoskeletal part of the system, that can negatively influence what happens with the organs. Quite often when I have patients with severe or even mild dysmenorrhea (pain associated with menstruation), I will treat the lower back and that will relieve the dysmenorrhea."

Dr. Lewis has also found a lot of back pain in smokers, which he believes is related to the destruction of vitamin C in the body as a result of smoking.

Because there are so many different factors that contribute to back pain, it is not only important to identify what the problem is, but how the problem arose. This will allow the healing practitioner to apply the most appropriate form of treatment for a person's ailing back.

Treating Back Pain

"When you're dealing with back pain, the type of therapy someone gets often depends on the type of doctor he or she goes to see," says David Bresler, Ph.D., L.Ac., Director of Program Development at the Los Angeles Healing Arts Center and former Director of the UCLA Pain Center. "When you see an orthopedist, you'll get physical therapy and cortisone, maybe even surgery. If you see a physiatrist, you'll get exercises and maybe some physical therapy. If you see a chiropractor, you'll get adjusted, and if you see an acupuncturist, you'll get needled. It's a rather arbitrary way to determine what's best for a patient." Dr. Bresler tailors his approach to the specific needs of each patient, and if it seems appropriate, he will refer the person to someone else.

Today, people with back pain can choose from any number of alternative approaches, including all the various physical manipulation techniques and movement awareness therapies, mind/body medicine, energy medicine, acupuncture, and naturopathy. Each of these modalities has been proven effective in some cases, but not in all. Ideally, an alternative practitioner will help the patient explore all the treatment possibilities available and encourage him or her to take an active role in the treatment process.

Prevention: The Most Effective Solution for Back Pain

Because most cases of back pain are muscular in origin, the pain usually occurs as a result of the way a person uses, or misuses, his or her body. Faulty habits in the ways a person sits, stands, and walks strains the back, pushing and pulling the spine out of alignment and causing weakness, spasms, and sprains in tendons, ligaments, and muscles. The end result is pain, which can be felt either in the back or referred through the nervous system to other parts of the body.

Most back pain can be avoided by taking the simple preventative step of staying in good physical condition. Research has shown that exercise can also be of benefit in the treatment of low back pain and injury. Of particular value are exercise programs that maintain and enhance proper function of the lower back and spine.

These include aerobic exercises, stretches, and strengthening exercises such as sit-ups. These both help to stabilize the pelvis and progressively increase the free range of movement of the back.[3]

Proper movement is another key to a strong and healthy back. Often, for example, when walking, one inadvertently overtightens the muscles in the arms, legs, neck, and back with every step taken. This excess strain can eventually lead to chronic pain and illness—both physical and psychological—and can only be corrected when the patient learns how to use his or her body more efficiently, and to maintain new habits and postures through an ongoing process of exercise and self-awareness.[4]

Physical Manipulation Techniques

Physical manipulation techniques aim to move the various parts of the body—muscles, connective tissues, and vertebrae—into proper functional alignment, and can often correct serious problems relating to stress and physical pain.

Dr. Lewis uses a physical manipulation technique known as neuromuscular releasing. "This is a soft-tissue manipulation for releasing tissue texture alterations such as knots, edema (excess of fluid in body tissues), fibrosis (abnormal formation of fibrous tissue), and scarring from various muscle tissue and from the layers between muscles.

"Oftentimes people think of this as simply massage, but it is a much more specific technique than massage," says Dr. Lewis. It involves using thumb pressure on the tissues to sweep through them in order to break up and release any tissue texture alterations which may be inhibiting muscle movement and contributing to back pain problems.

STRETCHING FOR RELIEF OF BACK PAIN

"Without a doubt, stretching is far more important for the relief of back pain than strengthening exercises," says Doug Lewis, N.D., Chairperson of the Physical Medicine Department of Bastyr College in Seattle, Washington. "We really focus too much on strengthening muscles and I think it's a mistake. It's a mistake at least until we've done a good job of stretching them."

The key for Dr. Lewis is to find what muscles or muscle groups are asymmetrically tight or imbalanced, causing postural problems and strain leading to back pain. One of the most common muscles associated with this kind of back pain problem is the rectus femoris, which is the muscle that runs from above the hip down through the kneecap and into the front of the tibia (the inner, longer bone of the leg between the knee and ankle). "If the muscles in both legs are tight, it can produce an anterior pelvic tilt, where the whole pelvis leans forward. This oftentimes creates a lordosis in the back, which is an excess amount of lumbar curve, commonly referred to as sway back," says Dr. Lewis.

In order to stretch these muscles out to correct the problem, Dr. Lewis instructs patients to stand and put the knee of the leg they want to stretch on the seat of a chair, while holding the back of the chair with the opposite hand for balance. "The idea is to pull the heel of the leg you want to stretch to the buttocks, and push forward with the pubic bone," he says. "This will push the pelvis backward, and you'll feel the stretch all the way from the knee, up the leg, to the front of the thigh."

The Pelvic Rock is another easy stretch to help with low back pain, according to Dr. Lewis, and can be done sitting in a chair. "Simply sit up straight, back against the chair back so that you have the normal low back curve. Then just allow your pelvis to roll back as if you were going to slouch into the chair. Hold that for a few seconds and then come back up into the straight position with the normal lumbar curve."

Dr. Lewis also advocates the "Cat-Cow" yoga position, "where you're on your hands and knees, and you alternately drop your back into a sway back position, and then arch it like a cat.

"There is one other stretch that is frequently quite useful, especially when there is extreme acute back pain, where the person can't move much, as well as for people who are stiff in the morning and have trouble getting out of bed. While lying flat on the back, perhaps with a pillow under the knees so as not to put too much of a strain on the lower back, alternately push one foot out and then the other. You don't actually have to be pushing against anything, rather, as you're pushing out with your heel, it's as if you're trying to make your leg longer. What you're doing actually is rocking the pelvis back and forth instead of from front to back as in the Pelvic Rock.

"As you do each stretch, hold the stretch, don't bounce. Hold it for five to ten seconds, then release and relax for five to ten, then go back into the stretch and hold it for five to ten seconds. Another essential factor to remember is that any muscle you are going to stretch must absolutely be relaxed. I can't emphasize this enough. It must be relaxed in order for it to stretch at all."

"Following that, it is essential to relax and stretch these muscles back out again because it is generally my opinion that most dysfunction comes from excessive muscle tension, rather than weak muscles." Dr. Lewis illustrates this by explaining that muscles always work in pairs. "When a muscle contracts, the antagonist to that muscle will be held in relaxation. For example, in order to lift something with your forearm, the biceps muscle will contract while the triceps on the opposite side of the arm must relax, otherwise we would simply tighten up and not be able to move at all.

"In cases of low back pain, though, one of the most common things is to have a person do sit-ups to strengthen the abdominal muscles. Yet, quite often the abdominal muscles are not weak, but are being held in relaxation because the muscles in the back are in spasm. So if you can get these muscles in the back to relax, they'll stop inhibiting the tone of the abdominal muscles."

Other forms of physical manipulation techniques that are used for the treatment of back pain include chiropractic, osteopathy, bodywork, and yoga.

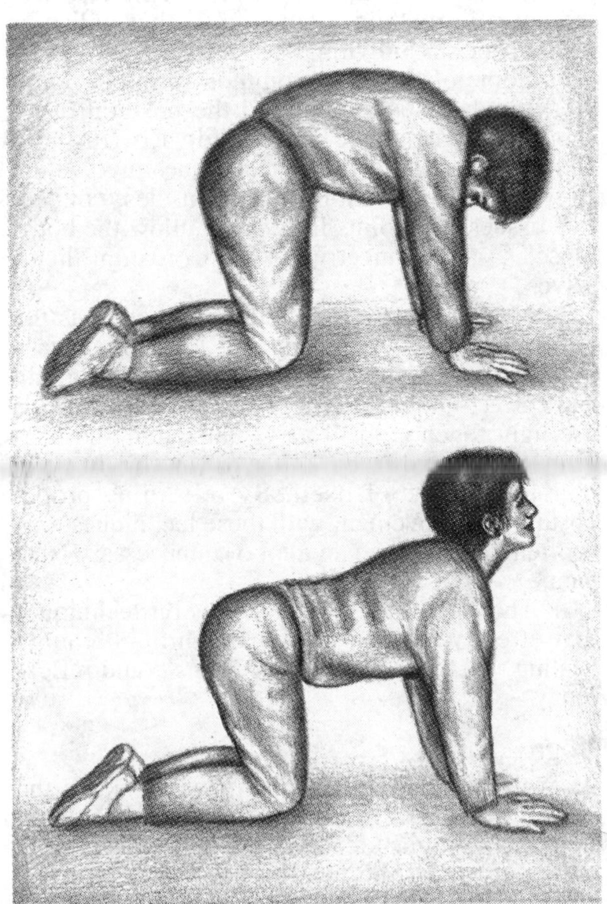

Cat-Cow position.

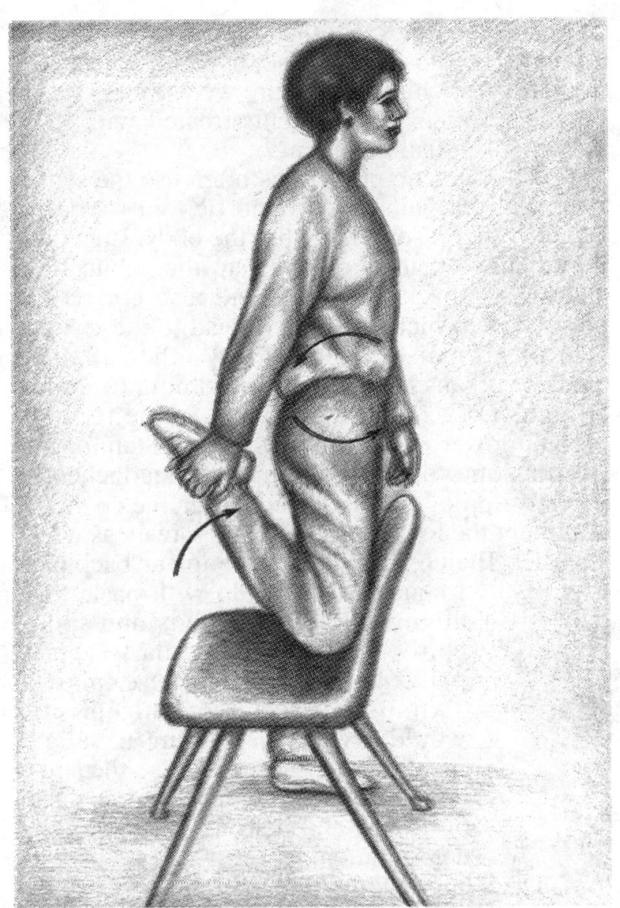

Exercise to stretch the rectus femoris muscle.

Chiropractic: Chiropractors specialize in the manipulation of joints and the vertebrae in the back and neck. Chiropractic theory holds that back pain is often due to subluxations, which are misalignments of the vertebrae. A misaligned vertebra can press on a nerve and produce pain not only in the back but in areas fed by the nerve. Thus, this "referred" pain can be felt in other parts of the body, like the arm or the leg, or can even affect the functioning of organs throughout the body.

Chiropractic treatment has been found to be more beneficial to patients with persistent back and neck complaints than other forms of manipulation.[5] Other research in Great Britain found chiropractic to provide "worthwhile, long-term benefits" for patients with low back pain in comparison to hospital outpatient management. This study also found chiropractic benefits to persist for a three-year period, indicating long-term benefits.[6] For patients with uncomplicated, acute low back pain, chiropractic has also been found to be effective.[7] Finally, a cost comparison study of back-related injuries showed the number of work days lost for patients treated with chiropractic to be nearly ten times less than that of patients treated under medical care. Also, average compensation costs for chiropractic care were $68.38, compared to $668.39 for patients treated with standard, nonsurgical treatment.[8]

Chiropractic physicians often use the symptoms of back pain as a diagnostic tool for determining other disorders within the body. Likewise, they believe that by clearing up the subluxation causing the back pain, they will also correct the nerve flow, which will in turn lead to the restoration of normal function of any other affected areas or organs of the body. According to Robert Blaich, D.C., of Los Angeles, patients with chronic lower back pain who undergo chiropractic for some other problem like headaches or digestive problems often find that in the course of treatment the lower back pain goes away as well.

Dr. Blaich states that since lower back pain frequently has to do with basic misalignments of the pelvis and spine, chiropractic is a particularly appropriate treatment. As he explains, "Almost all forms of chiropractic would involve correcting misalignments which in turn reduce the stress on joints, help to reduce wear and tear on joints, and help to minimize joint deterioration."

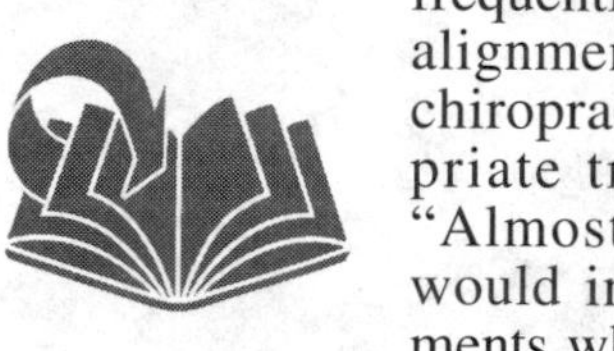

See Bodywork, Chiropractic, Osteopathy.

Dr. Blaich states that chronic lower back pain usually stems from a preexisting weakness. At a minimum, he advises chiropractic treatment every three to six months, although many people benefit from more frequent visits to maintain proper alignment and safeguard against injury to disks. The frequency of visits depends on a myriad of predisposing factors, including the condition of one's body and lifestyle. As Dr. Blaich puts it, "When you own a car, you wouldn't go two hundred thousand miles without getting your tires aligned. And if your tires were wearing out prematurely you would replace the shock absorbers. With alignment, your tires will wear better. That is very similar to what we do in chiropractic as preventive maintenance for the back."

Osteopathy: By being able to combine methods from both traditional and alternative medicine, the osteopath is in a unique position to help in the treatment of ailing backs. There are also a wide range of different osteopathic manipulative approaches which can be applied as treatment for back pain, notes Leon Chaitow, N.D., D.O., of London, England. This allows patients the opportunity to choose between several different options in order to find the one most appropriate for their specific needs.

Osteopathic techniques can be used for both chronic and acute back pain, as well as for either joint or soft-tissue problems. The methodology ranges from gentle joint mobilization to specific thrust methods similar to those used in chiropractic. The difference between osteopathic and chiropractic methods, however, lies in variations in basic concepts as well as in the forms of manipulation most commonly used.

While some osteopaths may manipulate the spine and other joints of the body to relieve back pain and restore alignments, they are also licensed to give injections in order to relieve painful inflammation in the joints. Additionally, they may apply electrical stimulation and various forms of mechanical therapy in order to trigger muscle relaxation, including gentle "muscle energy" techniques, and functional and positional release techniques, all unique to osteopathic medicine.

Bodywork: Bodywork includes all the various forms of massage, deep tissue, and movement awareness therapies that can be applied to the treatment of back pain. Once again, because there is such a wide choice of techniques available to choose from, the patient is able to select the specific method, or methods, that will best meet his or her individual needs.

Some of the more common forms of bodywork used for back pain and the postural problems that can cause it, include Rolfing and Hellerwork. Both of these techniques involve the strenuous manipulation of the muscles, connective tissues, and joints in order to allow the body, muscles, and connective tissue to realign themselves.

Movement awareness therapies such as the Feldenkrais Method™ and the Alexander technique have also proved effective for realigning and correcting the body's posture. These methods use light touch as well as visualization and suggestion in order to reprogram the body's ingrained image of itself. By relearning proper posture and movement with these techniques, one is often able to alleviate a lot of unnecessary back pain.

There are many other hands-on techniques that effectively treat back pain through energy healing, such as acupressure, *shiatsu,* and reflexology.

Yoga

As well as being an excellent way to keep the body limber and in shape, the yoga breathing exercises and postures also have the potential to reduce much of the tension and stress that can contribute to back pain. A primary focus of yoga

SELF-AWARENESS, SELF-HELP

The following exercise is a variation on a typical Feldenkrais exercise that can greatly benefit an aching back.

Lie on your back and take a few deep breaths. Notice how your spine is resting on the carpet. Do all the vertebrae touch, or are there spaces between your back and the floor? Does one side of your back touch the floor differently than the other? Does one side feel heavier than the other?

Bend both legs, putting your feet flat on the carpet. Gently drop your knees to one side, noticing how far down they seem to go. Bring them back to center and drop them once again to the same side, noticing any differences. Repeat this twenty-five times and then rest, stretching your legs back out. How does your back now touch the floor? Does your breathing seem any different than before?

Bend your legs again and drop them to the other side, noticing how far they seem to go. How does this side compare to the other? Bring your legs back to center and rest. Now imagine doing this movement in the most relaxed and fluent manner. Do this in your mind ten times, and then actually bend your knees to that side. Is the movement easier and fuller than before? Do this movement another twenty times, paying attention to how it makes your head move. When your legs drop, does your chin move toward or away from your chest? How does this movement affect your breathing?

Now stretch your legs back out and rest, noticing how your back now touches the ground. What differences do you notice in your breathing, neck, and head? Stand up, and walk around slowly, noticing how your body moves and feels.

Many people will notice surprising differences in their movement and posture. Indeed, some people find that their backs now lie completely flat on the ground for the first time in their lives, and those with chronic pain may find the problem completely alleviated from this simple five-minute exercise.

is therapeutic relaxation through gentle exercise and meditation. Yoga teachers believe that by focusing the mind inward, one is able to profoundly relax and revitalize the body and achieve a greater sense of harmony and well-being.

"When your attention is directed inward, your body receives messages that you are safe and secure and that it is appropriate to relax," explains Dr. Schatz. "So muscles relax, blood pressure drops, nerves are calmed, anxiety is decreased, immunity is heightened, and healing is enhanced."[9] All of these things can greatly improve one's ability to deal with both the symptoms and causes of back pain. Likewise, a regular yoga regimen can help to prevent back pain in the first place.

Mind/Body Medicine

According to Dr. Bresler, the connection between mind and body is well established in the rapidly developing field of psychoneuroimmunology—the study of the interaction between emotions, the nervous system, and the immune system. In applying this perspective to healing, Dr. Bresler uses a combination of guided imagery, relaxation, and biofeedback. In the case of treating back pain, his patients are encouraged to form an image about what's going on in their backs. "They give the pain a voice," says Bresler, "asking it, 'What do you want? Why are you here? What do you have to offer?' The pain may indeed have something to offer, like not going to work, or not having to make love to one's spouse. When we get an answer, we ask it if there's a way the patient can get what he or she needs without having a painful back." In this way, "we honor the body's inner wisdom and intelligence.

See Mind/Body Medicine, Yoga.

"Another technique that integrates the body and mind is biofeedback, which teaches how to consciously control heartbeat, respiration, muscle tension, and brain waves. By using this awareness, it is possible to learn how to consciously relax those muscles that are causing one to experience pain."

Melvyn Werbach, M.D., Director of the Biofeedback Medical Clinic in Tazana, California, tells of a mother of two infants who was suffering from chronic back pain. "She had had two failed spinal fusions, and lifting two babies put her in agony. We used Biofeedback-Assisted Relaxation Training (BART), and it was very successful, far more so than the surgery. Most of the pain disappeared and the rest she was able to control. Several years later, her back pain was still under control.

BART also seems to affect the immune system and other functions, adds Dr. Werbach, and it can also lower the perception of pain. Biofeedback can also affect secondary muscle spasms, and thereby reduce muscle tension which is often the primary cause of pain.

Energy Medicine

Energy medicine techniques such as ultrasound have also been used to treat back pain.

"Ultrasound helps to break up local edema as well as local fibrosis where there's been inflammation," states Dr. Lewis. "Also, if there's been an injury and there's been some kind of scarring between the muscle layers, the ultrasound can break that up to a certain extent. It will also warm the tissues, which helps to relax the muscles. It can also reduce the nerve conduction velocities, which means that the rate at which a pain impulse is conducted along a nerve pathway to the brain is slowed down, causing a pain-relieving effect."

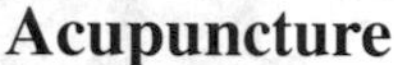

See Acupuncture, Energy Medicine, Naturopathic Medicine.

Energy devices such as the TENS unit (Transcutaneous Electrical Nerve Stimulator) are also used for the relief of back pain. The TENS, which can be used at home, works by simply applying an electrical current to the affected nerves in the area of the back pain, causing conduction to be blocked and pain to be relieved. TENS units and other similar energy devices are also believed to stimulate the production of endorphins, the body's own natural painkillers.

Acupuncture

"Many studies have shown the effectiveness of acupuncture for treating back pain," states Dr. Bresler. "At UCLA, we researched the different styles of acupuncture, comparing Korean, Vietnamese, Japanese, Chinese, and American acupuncturists, and found them equally effective." Dr. Ni, adds that Traditional Chinese Medicine recognizes that psychophysiological problems can also trigger back pain, and that "acupuncture works to release the stress that has been internalized into the body."

Back pain that is the result of nerve-pinching conditions like arthritis and osteoporosis can also be treated through acupuncture, which helps to restore the flow of blood and energy that is needed to bring essential healing nutrients such as calcium, to the injured back. "Acupuncture can also relax muscle spasms or strengthen weak back muscles," states Dr. Ni.

For back pain, Dr. Kozhevnikov uses acupuncture both to relax muscles and to release muscle contractions caused by related damaged organs. Dr. Kozhevnikov claims that 90 percent of herniated disk cases could and should be treated with this program first rather than undergoing surgery. His treatment also involves electroacupuncture, physical manipulation, and various energy medicine devices.

Naturopathic Medicine

Naturopathic physicians are especially well-equipped to treat back pain because they are able to provide nutritional support for strengthening and repairing the tissues, herbal and homeopathic remedies, and hydrotherapy for relieving inflammation, as well as soft tissue and joint manipulation for correcting postural dysfunctions.

The use of nutritional supplements can be very helpful for the treatment and prevention of back pain, according to Dr. Lewis. "Vitamin C and bioflavonoids are extremely important for strengthening the connective tissues, especially in smokers who have depleted their vitamin C resources." He recommends taking two to three thousand milligrams of each daily, spread out through the day.

"Calcium-magnesium supplements should also be taken for muscle relaxation, particularly in instances where there's muscle spasm and twitching," adds Dr. Lewis. He recommends five hundred milligrams of a calcium-magnesium supplement daily, preferably in a citrate form, "because it allows for much better absorption."

Dr. Lewis also counsels his patients on a variety of home therapies for relieving back pain, including slant boards, inversion boots for hanging upside down, and back swings. "All these devices apply some sort of traction to the tissues in the back," adds Dr. Lewis, "and that can be very helpful."

Another important tool are shoe lifts for correcting any anatomical leg-length problems. "I tend to be very aggressive about using shoe lifts, especially if the patient is young," says Dr.

ICE: AN IMMEDIATE HOME REMEDY

For years, the standard prescription for any pain was aspirin, a heating pad, and plenty of rest. Although these may have offered minor relief, today, most doctors and health practitioners recommend a far more effective home remedy.

"Ice is probably the most effective method for treating back pain, particularly acute cases," says David Bresler, Ph.D., L.Ac., Director of Program Development at the Los Angeles Healing Arts Center and former Director of the Pain Clinic at the UCLA Medical Center. This is especially true when there is swelling, heat, or redness surrounding the painful area. Ice allows the blood to reabsorb the fluids and chemicals that surround the injured area, and is particularly effective during the first few days of treatment.

A standard treatment for back pain is to apply ice for ten minutes, heat for five minutes, then reapply ice, heat, and ice once more for the same amount of time. This can be repeated as often as needed throughout the day. However, if the swelling and pain continues, consult a doctor immediately.

Lewis, "and I rarely find that they produce any negative response for the patient. They may be sore as their body adapts to the change, but in almost all cases I find it very, very positive." Orthotics, which help to correct flat-footedness plus other inversions and eversions of the foot, are also helpful for back pain, as they correct and balance the foot which is the foundation of all good posture, according to Dr. Lewis.

Self-Care

The following therapies can be undertaken at home under the guidance of a physician:
• Fasting • Guided Imagery • Qigong • Yoga

Acupressure: To relieve back pain briskly rub the backs of your hands over B23 and B47 (for an illustration of these point numbers please see the acupressure chart on pages 874-875) in your lower back for one minute. If your back pain is up higher or in deeper, lie down on two tennis balls that are one inch apart wrapped in a towel or sock. Place the balls underneath the tightest parts of your back muscles as you breathe deeply for one minute. Then roll on to another area that is tight or painful and continue to breathe deeply for another minute. Next, put the balls aside and firmly bring your knees into your chest several times with your head on the ground. Immediately afterward, cover yourself on your back with your legs bent, feet flat on the floor and deeply relax with your eyes closed for ten minutes. Repeat this two or three times daily to prevent and relieve back pain.

Aromatherapy: • For muscular fatigue: lavender, marjoram, rosemary, clary sage. • For acute pain: black pepper or ginger, birch.

Ayurveda: *Kaishore guggulu* 200 mg., generally taken twice a day after lunch and dinner with warm water. *Dashamoola basti*: one pint *dashamoola* tea with one-half cup sesame oil three times a week and massage locally with *mahanarayan* oil.

Herbs: The cause of the pain must be identified before appropriate herbs can be prescribed. For example, if related to physical strain or rheumatic problems drink an infusion of meadowsweet three times a day and rub the area with lobelia and cramp bark (see Muscle Cramps). If associated with menstruation, combine equal parts of skullcap and cramp bark tinctures, taking one teaspoonful as needed.

Homeopathy: *Arsen alb., Arnica, Actea rac., Rhus tox., Calc fluor., Natrum mur., Ruta grav.* Consult a physician if pain persists.

***Hydrotherapy*:** Contrast application: apply daily to affected area. Lower back: hot moist compresses (with water and hot apple cider vinegar) to lower back. Follow with alternating hot and cold percussion shower on painful area.

Lifestyle: In dealing with back pain it is important to improve posture and to learn proper body use. Regular exercise can dramatically decrease back discomfort.

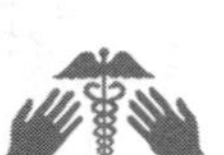

Professional Care

The following therapies should only be provided by a qualified health professional:
• Applied Kinesiology • Colon Therapy • Craniosacral Therapy • Environmental Medicine • Hypnotherapy • Neural Therapy • Reconstructive Therapy

Bodywork: Acupressure, massage, Reflexology, Trager.

Cell Therapy: For spinal disorders.

Detoxification Therapy: Detoxification is indicated. Back pain is often associated with congestive organs, stress, and referred pain.

Oxygen Therapy: If caused by injury, hyperbaric oxygen therapy may be helpful.

Traditional Chinese Medicine: Cupping is an ancient Chinese therapy which helps to regulate the flow of energy and blood. Suction is created over the painful area on the body by introducing fire in to a cup and placing the cup on the desired point. The amount of suction can be regulated according to the treatment and the age of the patient.

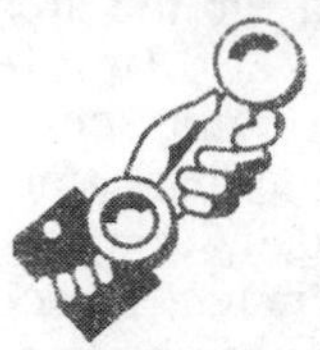

Where to Find Help

For more information on, or referrals for, treatment of back pain, contact the following organizations:

Acupuncture

American Association of Acupuncture and Oriental Medicine
4101 Lake Boone Trail, Suite 201
Raleigh, North Carolina 27607
(919) 787-5181

The AAAOM is a national professional trade organization of acupuncturists who meet acceptable standards of competency and can provide you with the names and locations of local members.

Biofeedback

Association for Applied Psychophysiology and Biofeedback
10200 West 44th Avenue
Suite 304
Wheat Ridge, Colorado 80033
(303) 422-8436

Provides names and phone numbers of chapters in your state. (Formerly Biofeedback Society of America.)

Bodywork

North American Society of Teachers of the Alexander Technique
P.O. Box 3992
Champagne, Illinois 61826-3992
(217) 359-3529

For information, referrals, and training.

Feldenkrais Guild
P.O. Box 489
Albany, Oregon 97321
(503) 926-0981

For information, practitioner directory, training, and certification.

The Rolf Institute
P.O. Box 1868
Boulder, Colorado 80306
(303) 449-5903

For information, practitioner directory, training, and certification.

Chiropractic

American Chiropractic Association
1701 Clarendon Boulevard
Arlington, Virginia 22209
(703) 276-8800

A major source for chiropractic information. Monthly publication and newsletter. Clinical councils with specialization in sports injuries and physical fitness, mental health, neurology, diagnosis and internal disorders, nutrition, orthopedics, physiological therapeutics, diagnostic imaging, and occupational health.

International Chiropractors Association
1110 North Glebe Road
Suite 1000
Arlington, Virginia 22201
(703) 528-5000

The original chiropractic association founded by B. J. Palmer, the son of the founder of chiropractic, Daniel David Palmer. Programs and services to meet the needs of chiropractors, patients, students, and the public. Concerned with legislation, health care policy, public relations, continuing education, skills development, publications, and interprofessional relations.

World Chiropractic Alliance
2950 N. Dobson Road, Suite 1
Chandler, Arizona 85224
(800) 347-1011

An international association of chiropractors with the purpose of promoting and advancing the profession. Offers guidance and assistance to professionals. Emphasis on vertebral subluxation correction. Provides public education and information. Publishes two newspapers for professionals and provides referrals for chiropractors nationwide.

Naturopathic Medicine

American Association of Naturopathic Physicians
2366 Eastlake Avenue, Suite 322
Seattle, Washington 98102
(206) 323-7610

Provides referrals to a nationwide network of accredited or licensed practitioners.

Osteopathy

American Academy of Osteopathy
3500 DePauw Boulevard
Suite 1080
Indianapolis, Indiana 46268
(317) 879-1881
(317) 879-0563 (Fax)

The American Academy of Osteopathy (a practice affiliate of the American Osteopathic Association) represents D.O.'s who provide skilled osteopathic manipulative treatments as part of their practices.

Yoga

International Association of Yoga Therapists
109 Hillside Avenue
Mill Valley, California 94941
(415) 383-4587

A nonprofit organization emphasizing education and research for yoga and yoga therapy. An international organization with an annual journal, the Journal of the International Association of Yoga Therapists.

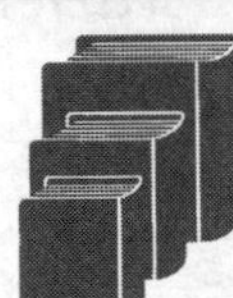

Recommended Reading

The Alexander Technique. Barlow, Wilfred. New York: Alfred A. Knopf, 1973.

The founder of the Alexander Institute shows how to reduce mental stress and muscular tension by becoming more aware of balance, posture, and movement in everyday activities.

Awareness through Movement. Feldenkrais, Moshe. New York: Harper and Row, 1977.

This is a genuine self-help guide to improved posture, flexibility, breathing, health, and functioning through twelve easy-to-follow Awareness through Movement lessons.

Back Care Basics: A Doctor's Gentle Yoga Program for Back and Neck Pain Relief. Schatz, Mary Pullig, M.D. Berkeley, CA: Rodmell Press, 1992.

Offers a gentle and effective approach to back rehabilitation without drugs or surgery. Uses the therapeutic techniques of Iyengar style yoga.

Free Yourself from Pain. Bresler, David E. Topanga, CA: The Bresler Center, 1992.

This self-help book for managing chronic pain and depression includes several chapters illustrating the use of guided imagery for pain control. (Available from The Bresler Center, 115 South Topanga Canyon Boulevard, Suite 158, Topanga, California 90290. (310) 455-3634.)

Pain Erasure. Prudden, Bonnie. New York: M. Evans and Co., 1980.

This book explains Bonnie Prudden's method for pain relief using myotherapy. Her method has been hailed by doctors and patients.

Rolfing: The Integration of Human Structures. Rolf, Ida. New York: Harper and Row, 1977.

The mother of Rolfing explains, "Once free of the muscular rigidity imposed by past experience, the body structure can be put back into natural alignment with the forces of gravity, a process necessary for physical well-being."

Mind Over Back Pain. Sarno, John, M.D. New York: Berkeley Books, 1986.

An exploration of the role mind/body medicine can play in alleviating back pain caused by excess mental stress and tension.

Life Without Pain. Linchitz, Richard, M.D. Reading, MA: Addison-Wesley Publishing Co., 1987.

A self-help approach for eliminating chronic pain, including back pain, using diet, nutrition, exercise, and mind/body techniques.

Cancer

Despite over twenty years of research, with billions of dollars spent each year, the conventional medical establishment's "war on cancer" has been a dismal failure. Today, we are no closer to understanding the underlying causes for the rapid rise of cancer rates or to finding safe and effective treatments. Most people continue to equate cancer with death, or, at the very least, an excruciating journey back to health filled with physical debilitation and pain. However, a variety of alternative therapies exist which have proven safer, gentler, and more effective at reversing, and preventing cancer, than standard conventional techniques.

Cancer is a disease in which healthy cells stop functioning and maturing properly. As the normal cycle of cell creation and death is interrupted, these newly "mutated" cancer cells begin multiplying uncontrollably, no longer operating as an integrated and harmonious part of the body. They also become parasitic, and can develop their own network of blood vessels to siphon nourishment away from the body's blood supply. This process, if unchecked, will eventually lead to the formation of a cancerous tumor. As the abnormal cells circulate within the bloodstream, the cancer can also spread to other parts of the body. This can cause the formation of more tumors and further sap the body's energy supply, weakening and eventually poisoning the patient with toxic byproducts.

Cancer is almost always fatal if left untreated. This year alone, it will claim the lives of more than half a million Americans, with over one million additional new cases being reported, and one out of every three persons developing cancer within their lifetime.[1] The figures are no less frightening for the rest of the world, as cancer rates continue to climb steadily, particularly among the industrialized nations.[2]

With cancer claiming so many lives each year, the search for a cure has become a global industry. Yet, as enticing as the idea of a "magic bullet" for cancer may seem, because of the multiple factors related to the disease, conventional medicine may never be able to offer the same sort of protection against cancer that it has been able to offer, for example, against polio and tetanus. Still, there is hope, with much of it coming today from the field of alternative medicine.

This chapter will examine the most promising alternative treatments for the prevention and treatment of cancer. Because of the stranglehold that conventional medicine has had over the cancer debate, many of these therapies have been suppressed, despite their proven effectiveness. This chapter will also highlight stories of actual cancer survivors—men and women who have beaten the odds and returned to health using a variety of alternative medical methods.

Types and Causes of Cancer

Every cell in the body has the ability to turn cancerous, and many do so on a daily basis. Normally, the immune system is able to protect the body by destroying these cells or reprogramming them back to normal functioning. If the body's defense systems have been damaged, however, this process cannot happen, allowing the cancer to establish itself.[3] If the cancer cells do not spread beyond the tissue or organ where they originated, the cancer is considered to be localized. If the cancer spreads to other parts of the body, it is then said to have metastasized.

"Every cell in the body has the ability to turn cancerous, and many do so on a daily basis."

While there are more than one hundred different types of cancer, affecting virtually every part of the body, cancer is usually broken down into five basic categories: carcinomas, sarcomas, myelomas, lymphomas, and leukemias.

- **Carcinomas**, the most common cancers, are tumors which originate in tissues which cover a surface, or line internal organs. Lung, breast, prostate, skin, and intestinal cancers are all carcinomas.
- **Sarcomas** originate in connective tissues and muscles, attacking bones, muscles, cartilage, or the lymph system. They are the most rare malignant tumors, and also the most deadly.
- **Myelomas** are also rare tumors, and they start in the plasma cells which are found in the bone marrow.
- **Lymphomas** are cancers of the lymph system, a series of glands which act as a filter for the body's impurities. Lymph glands, or nodes, are found in the neck, the groin, the armpits, and the spleen. Hodgkin's disease and non-Hodgkin's lymphomas are the two most prevalent types of lymphoma in the United States. Burkitt's lymphoma, while rare in the United States, is another form of the disease that is common in Central Africa.
- **Leukemias** are cancers which originate in the tissues of the bone marrow, spleen, and the lymph nodes. Leukemias are not solid tumors, and exhibit an overproduction of white blood cells.

Each of these types of cancers can be caused by a variety of factors, ranging from air pollution and tobacco smoke, to environmental radiation and industrial chemicals such as asbestos, benzene, and vinyl chloride, to naturally occurring substances such as aflatoxins (toxins produced by fungus commonly found in peanuts, corn, milk, and other foods), as well as the body's own production of oxygen free radicals.

Though the causes of cancer are still being debated, science is much closer today to understanding the fundamental factors involved in the process. For some time it has been clear that tumors arise as a result of a series of changes or rearrangements of information coded in the DNA within sin-

CANCER INCIDENTS AND DEATH PER YEAR IN MEN AND WOMEN

According to the American Cancer Society, the incidence of cancer among men and women in the U.S. by site is as follows:[4]

Men		Women	
Prostate	165,000	Breast	182,000
Lung	100,000	Colon and rectum	75,000
Colon and rectum	77,000	Lung	70,000
Bladder	39,000	Uterus	44,500
Lymphoma	28,500	Lymphoma	22,400
Oral	20,300	Ovary	22,000
Melanoma of the skin	17,000	Melanoma of the skin	15,000
Kidney	16,800	Pancreas	14,200
Leukemia	16,700	Bladder	13,300
Stomach	14,800	Leukemia	12,600
Pancreas	13,500	Kidney	10,400
Larynx	10,000	Oral	9,500

The American Cancer Society also lists the following cancer deaths by site and sex.

Men		Women	
Lung	93,000	Lung	56,000
Prostate	35,000	Breast	46,000
Colon and rectum	28,800	Colon and rectum	28,200
Pancreas	12,000	Ovary	13,300
Lymphoma	11,500	Pancreas	13,000
Leukemia	10,100	Lymphoma	10,500
Stomach	8,200	Uterus	10,100
Esophagus	7,600	Leukemia	8,500
Liver	6,800	Liver	5,800
Brain	6,600	Brain	5,500
Kidney	6,500	Stomach	5,400
Bladder	6,500	Multiple myeloma	4,600

gle cells.[5] Scientists also believe that cancers are generated in two steps, initiation and promotion.

Factors which start the initiation process are called initiators, or triggers. They interact directly with the cellular DNA to start the cell damage process. Initiators can take the form of carcinogens (cancer-causing substances), such as tobacco smoke, environmental pollution, pesticides, heavy metals, and industrial chemicals; as well as specific viruses; radiation; oxygen free radicals; and hormones, particularly estrogens.[6]

Initiation of a cancer cell can occur in various ways. For example, low-fiber diets may prolong the residence time of body wastes in the gut, leading to greater exposure of the intestinal lining to cancer-causing agents. A breakdown of metabolic function can also lead to initiation when enzymes, which normally deactivate cancer-causing substances, start to function improperly. This causes them to activate the carcinogens instead, allowing the enzymes to react directly with cellular DNA.[7] In other cases, cellular reproduction may be so accelerated that cells reproduce too quickly, leaving little or no time for repair. This allows defects in the DNA to become imbedded into the genetic materials passed from one cell to the next as a permanent mutation. DNA repair may also be interrupted by initiators. For example, toxic metals such as lead, mercury, and cadmium can prevent DNA from being repaired.[8]

“After the initiation of the cancer process, the disease will often lie undetected for many years.”

After the initiation of the cancer process, the disease will often lie undetected for many years, according to the American Institute for Cancer Research.[9] Factors which promote the disease process during this latent period are called promoters. While promoters do not directly interact with the cellular DNA, they can further the cellular damage, allowing cancer cells to continue spreading abnormally. Promoters may also hamper the removal of initiated cells, by damaging the body's defense systems, particularly the immune system. Lastly, promoters can alter certain tissues of the body in order to make them more favorable for tumor growth. This is usually accomplished by enhancing the conditions for establishing the blood supply necessary for nourishing the tumor cells.

The following are among the most common factors associated with the initiation and promotion of cancer:

Diet and Nutritional Factors

These are considered the primary agents for initiation and promotion of cancer today. According to the National Academy of Sciences, 60 percent of all cancers in women and 40 percent of all cancers in men may be due to dietary and nutritional factors.[10] Likewise, diet and nutrition are also the principle preventative measures against cancer, and the ones over which people have the most control.

“According to the National Academy of Sciences, 60 percent of all cancers in women and 40 percent of all cancers in men may be due to dietary and nutritional factors.”

Fat intake is one of the key risk factors linked to cancer, especially animal fat, which has been consistently implicated with higher cancer rates.[11] The cancers most closely associated with high fat intake include breast, colon, rectum, uterus, prostate, and kidney.[12] Partially hydrogenated oils, which are commonly found in processed foods, are also considered to be a major contributor to the carcinogenic effect of fats.[13] It is interesting to note that in breast cancer studies conducted on laboratory mice, tumor growth was enhanced by a high-fat diet only after a chemical carcinogen was introduced.[14] This suggests that fat is not an initiator, but a promoter, of cancer and that it acts as a repository for carcinogenic toxins.

“Many cancer-causing pesticides and industrial chemicals found in the environment and in our foods tend to accumulate in fatty tissues, whether in fish, cattle, fowl, or people,” states Samuel Epstein, M.D., Professor of Occupational and Environmental Medicine at the University of Illinois School of Public Health. “Although these chemicals for the most part have been banned or strictly regulated, they are very durable and remain in the environment for a long time. Crops grown in soil contaminated with these chemicals will pass on their residue to the animals that are fed them, where they will accumulate in the fatty tissue. If persons choose foods with the highest

“Many cancer-causing pesticides and industrial chemicals found in the environment and in our foods tend to accumulate in fatty tissues, whether in fish, cattle, fowl, or people.”
—Samuel Epstein, M.D.

concentrations of these chemicals, then they, too, will build up higher and higher concentrations of the same chemicals in their own fatty tissue." This process is known as bioaccumulation, and, according to Dr. Epstein, these fat-soluble carcinogens are found in highest concentrations in the body's fattiest tissues, such as the brain, sexual organs, and breasts.

The high intake of animal protein has also been associated with an increased risk of breast, colon, pancreatic, kidney, prostate, and endometrial cancer, although such risks are usually closely linked to fat content, since many sources of protein are also high in fat.[15] Sugar is also believed to have a direct effect on cancer growth, as well as acting to nullify the positive effects of protective foods such as fiber.[16] In addition, it can significantly add to the risk of breast cancer, says veteran cancer researcher, Wayne Martin, of Fairhope, Alabama. "When someone eats sugar, the body produces insulin, and insulin can cause breast cancer just as estrogen does," he explains.

Iron is another possible risk factor for cancer, according to Martin. "Much of the cancer in our population today is caused by doctors. At their insistence we have iron added to our bread, rice, and pasta," says Martin, citing a recent study by the National Cancer Institute which found that men with lower iron stores suffered less cancer.[17]

Smoked, pickled, and salt-cured foods contain several known carcinogenic substances, including nitrosamines and polycyclic aromatic hydrocarbons, which have been linked to cancer of the stomach and esophagus. Additionally, potentially cancer-causing substances are also produced when meat, chicken, or fish are fried, broiled, or barbecued for a long time at high temperatures.[18]

Caffeine, which is found in coffee, tea, colas, and chocolate, is thought to be a factor for cancer of the lower urinary tract, including the bladder. Studies have found the rates for these cancers to be significantly higher in people who drink more than three cups of coffee a day.[19] Caffeine is also known to damage cellular DNA and to impair its normal repair, thereby adding to the potential risk for cancer.[20] Several studies also associate the intake of alcohol, including beer, with increased cancer risk.[21]

Food additives are another potentially cancer-causing hazard. Among the most common are saccharin and cyclamates, both used as artificial sweeteners and linked to greater incidences of bladder cancer; butylated hydroxytoluene, used as a preservative and linked to liver cancer; and tannic acid, found in wines and fruits and linked to liver cancer. Aflatoxins, which are found in milk, cereals, peanuts, and corn, have also been linked to liver, stomach, and kidney cancer.[22]

Smoking and Tobacco Use

It is estimated that 350,000 deaths occur each year in the United States as a result of tobacco use. One third of these deaths occur from smoking-related lung cancer alone, making it the single major cause of cancer death, accounting for 30 percent of all deaths. (Diet accounts for a higher percentage, but is not considered a singular cause.) While cigarette smoking may be the principal culprit, other forms of tobacco use, such as cigar and pipe smoking, and smokeless tobacco, are also factors. And, in addition to lung cancer, smoking has been linked to cancers of the head and neck, mouth, throat, vocal cords, bladder, kidney, stomach, cervix, and pancreas, as well as some leukemia. Additionally, smokeless tobacco has been linked to cancers of the lip and tongue.[23]

See Detoxification Therapy, Diet.

Secondary smoke, or passive smoke, is also a dangerous carcinogen, according to a recent United States Environmental Protection Agency (EPA) report, which listed it in the same category as benzene, radon, and asbestos. It causes 20 percent of all lung cancers in the United States not attributed directly to smoking, accounting for about three thousand lung cancer deaths each year among non-smokers. This risk is doubled for non-smoking spouses of smokers.[24]

According to John A. Sherman, N.D., of Portland, Oregon, cigarettes contain over four thousand known toxic poisons. Tar, which is formed when organic compounds are burned, is the leading cancer-causing chemical found in tobacco smoke. Carbon monoxide is also released during smoking, reducing the amount of oxygen to organs like the brain, lungs, and heart.

Nicotine, an alkaloid found in tobacco, is highly addictive, and is extremely poisonous if ingested directly. While only a small amount of nicotine is absorbed during smoking, this can still cause an adrenaline release, greatly increasing heart rate and blood pressure. Nicotine also acts as a promoter, making it easier for cancers of all kinds to spread throughout the body.[25]

See Respiratory Conditions.

In addition, a direct link has been found between lung cancer and flue-dried tobacco, especially that to which sugar has been added, while no significant correlation between traditional sugar-free, air-dried tobacco and cancer has been established. Studies show that England

THE "PILL" AND CANCER

According to a recent study, women who have taken oral contraceptives for more than four years are almost twice as likely to get breast cancer at age fifty as non-users. This study is consistent with three other studies, all linking birth control pills with a greater risk for breast cancer. The risk continues to increase as the length of use goes up, climbing to 80 percent for women using the pill for over four years.[26]

and Wales, which have the highest male lung cancer rate in the world, also have the highest sugar content in cigarettes, about 17 percent. France, where tobacco is air-dried and contains only 2 percent sugar, has one-third less lung cancer. The United States, where sugar in tobacco averages 10 percent, has about half the male lung cancer death rate as in Great Britain.[27]

Environmental Toxicity

"Environmental toxicity is one of the most important areas of cancer causation and cancer prevention and it is yet to receive adequate recognition from the cancer research establishment," Dr. Epstein notes. "Neither the National Cancer Institute or the American Cancer Society have ever given scientific testimony before Congress or any regulatory agency on the importance of avoiding exposure to toxic chemicals." This, despite significant evidence that environmental carcinogens in the home and the workplace are one of the primary causes of cancer.

"We have more than enough scientific information on the relationship between environmental and occupational toxins and increasing cancer rates," Dr. Epstein adds. "The problems are economic and political. Industry, with its powerful lobby, has moved heaven and earth to prevent increased emphasis on the phase out of toxic and carcinogenic chemicals in air, water, food, and the workplace."

> *"Environmental toxicity is one of the most important areas of cancer causation and cancer prevention and it is yet to receive adequate recognition from the cancer research establishment."*
> —Samuel Epstein, M.D.

For example, while researchers have continued to promote the link between fat intake and cancer, especially breast cancer, they have steadfastly chosen to ignore the fact that adipose (fatty) tissue is the chief repository for chemical toxins, such as pesticides, absorbed by the body. "In all the studies on fat consumption funded by the NCI, none have even bothered to consider this issue," Dr. Epstein notes, "even though, as far back as 1968, independent researchers had already found evidence of a link between elevated pesticide concentrations in adipose tissues and cases of carcinoma."

Additionally, in 1976, a research team at the Department of Occupational Health at Hebrew University-Hadassah Medical School in Jerusalem completed a study of women with breast cancer that compared cancerous breast tissue with healthy breast tissue from the same woman. What the study found was significant in that the concentration of toxic chemicals, including pesticides such as DDT, and industrial chemicals such as PCB's, was "much increased in the malignant tissue when compared to the normal breast and adjacent adipose tissue."[28]

In 1978, following public outcry and threatened legal actions, Israel banned many of the chemicals cited in the 1976 study, resulting in a significant decrease in the level of toxic chemicals found in breast milk. Over the next decade the rate of breast cancer mortality also declined sharply, with a more than 30 percent drop in deaths among Israeli women under forty-four years old, and a drop of 8 percent overall. This, in spite of the fact that every other known risk factor for breast cancer, such as alcohol consumption, fat intake, lack of fruits and vegetables in the diet, and the age women gave birth for the first time, increased dramatically. The only answer researchers could come up with to account for this stunning drop in cancer rate, was the greatly reduced level of environmental toxicity. During this same period, the rate of breast cancer deaths worldwide rose by an overall rate of 4 percent.[29]

> *"As far back as 1968, independent researchers had already found evidence of a link between elevated pesticide concentrations in adipose (fatty) tissues and cases of carcinoma."*

Subsequently, independent researchers in the United States, supported with a grant from the U.S. National Institute of Environmental Health Sciences, conducted a similar study. Their findings verified that high concentrations of PCB's and other common toxins found in drinking water and household products exist in the breasts of women with cancer. But these same chemical concentrations were not found in the breasts of women with only fibroid cysts or benign tumors.

One of the main problems with environmental toxicity is that the chemicals associated with cancer can be found almost anywhere, including in our air, our water, our workplaces, and our homes. Even chemicals such as DDT, which have been banned from use for years, still show up in the environment today. These chemicals are very durable and do not break down easily. Their residues can stay in the soil or water for years, to be passed on indefinitely through the food chain as they go from soil or water to plant to animal to human consumption.

The use of home and garden pesticides is another major source of toxicity and has been linked to a variety of cancers, including childhood leukemia and brain cancer. In a recent study, indoor pesticide use was found to result in a risk factor four times higher than normal for childhood leukemia. This risk became seven times higher for the children of parents who used garden pesticides, and continued to climb in both cases, as the frequency of pesticide use went up.[30]

“One of the main problems with environmental toxicity is that the chemicals associated with cancer can be found almost anywhere, including in our air, our water, our workplaces, and our homes.”

Childhood brain cancer has been directly associated with the use of chemical pesticides, such as diazinon and carbaryl, in the garden or orchard, as well as with various herbicides used to control weeds. Pesticides used to control pests in the home have also been implicated in this disease, including those found in no-pest strips, termite pesticides, home pesticide bombs, and flea collars for pets.[31]

No-pest strips may seem innocuous, but they emit continuous vapors of DDVP (the active ingredient used in most strips), a highly carcinogenic chemical associated with an increased risk for all types of cancer in children and adults alike, according to the EPA. People who use these strips as directed and are exposed to them over a lifetime have a greatly increased chance of getting cancer. This can be as high as one in one hundred, which is ten thousand times the risk that the EPA considers to be of significant concern. The EPA also estimates that members of a household using the pest strips face a cancer risk ten times greater than even pest control workers who apply DDVP thousands of times a year without wearing protective clothing.[32]

The cancer danger of the use of some pesticides extends to pets who come into close contact with contaminated soils, lawns, and plants. Flea collars with DDVP put pets at a similarly increased cancer risk.[33]

Also, in our industrial age of plastics, chemicals, and metals manufacturing, it is common to find a higher incidence rate of cancer in any group of workers which are overly exposed to any of these carcinogens. Arsenic and vinyl chloride have been found to cause liver and lung cancers in smelting, tanning, and plastic workers. Asbestos has been linked to lung cancer in miners, glass and pottery workers, and iron workers. Painters and dye workers have been found to have a higher incidence of bone marrow cancers and leukemia because of their exposure to benzene. It is estimated that 10 percent of all cancers are attributable to job-related exposure to carcinogens.[34]

INDUSTRIAL TOXICOLOGY

Industrial toxicology is an emerging technology which enables people to quantify the level of dangerous toxic chemicals absorbed into their bloodstream and bodily tissues via exposure at the workplace. One of the leading scientists in this field is Hildegarde L. A. Sacarello, Ph.D., founder and past President of the International Academy of Toxicological Risk Assessment.

Dr. Sacarello monitors the level of various contaminants in the workplace by obtaining tissue samples from workers and comparing the levels found to the recommended maximum safety levels. (She is also able, in the case of male workers, to determine levels of toxins by analyzing semen.) Her expertise in this area enables her to determine the risk which a particular worker faces of developing environmentally induced illness, including cancer, and to advise that person accordingly. In some cases the employee is advised to totally avoid any further exposure.

For example, a seventy-five-year-old man was diagnosed with prostate cancer. Dr. Sacarello analyzed specimens of the cancerous tissues. These tissues showed abnormally high levels of a variety of carcinogenic chemicals, including arsenic, chlordane, and DDT, causing toxic overload and liver dysfunction in the patient. After three months of a detoxifying herbal and vitamin therapy, the patient's tumor shrunk by about a third.

Industrial toxicology offers the chance for workers to limit damaging exposure in the workplace, as well as a way for them to determine what factors may affect their health in the future.

Indoor pollution, found in offices and homes, can also contain contaminants which lead to cancer. Some examples include formaldehyde fumes from pressed wood furniture and cabinets; fumes and vapors produced by cleaning products, air fresheners, paints, hobby supplies (glues, varnishes, etc.), and improperly vented gas stoves and dryers; lead and other chemicals found in drinking water; office or home air systems which fill the air with bacteria, mildew, and viruses; and radon gas infiltration. The EPA estimates that indoor radon pollution may cause as many as ten thousand cancers a year in the United States.[35]

The established link between cancer and toxins in the home, workplace, and environment indicates the need for further research concerning the threat these toxins pose to overall health. To support the use of goverment funds for research in this field, write your elected represenive.

The disinfection of drinking water with chlorine, which is standard practice throughout the United States, has also added to the toxic level of carcinogens Americans are exposed to on a daily basis. While the EPA tries to downplay the cancer risk from chlorinating drinking water by asserting that the known risk of water-borne disease in humans, if water is not disinfected, is much greater than the theoretical risk of developing cancer, a recent study conducted jointly by the Medical College of Wisconsin and Harvard University, has found a very definite link between chlorine and cancer. The study found that the consumption of chlorinated drinking water accounts for 15 percent of all rectal cancers and 9 percent of all bladder cancers in the United States, or an additional 6,500 cases of rectal cancer and 4,200 cases of bladder cancer each year. Additionally, people drinking chlorinated water over long periods of time have a 38 percent increase in the chance of contracting rectal cancer and a 21 percent increase in the risk of contracting bladder cancer.[36]

See Biological Dentistry, Energy Medicine.

Fluoride is another chemical which is routinely added to the water system today, even though it was first linked to cancer back in 1975. A comparison of ten large U.S. cities that fluoridated their water with ten cities that did not found an increase of approximately 10 percent in cancer deaths in the cities with fluoride in their water. As a result of this study, tests were ordered by Congress which confirmed that fluoride added to water causes cancer in laboratory animals,[37] but the government has yet to change its policy on fluoridation.

Environmental Radiation

According to a 1991 EPA study, there is growing evidence of a link between heavy electrical currents and cancer.[38] Studies in recent years have suggested a higher incidence of leukemia and brain tumors among people exposed to electrical fields on the job.[39] A 1987 study found that children living near electric power lines faced five times the risk of all forms of cancer compared to children who did not.[40] Even more disturbing, is the fact that ordinary household appliances generate larger overall electromagnetic fields (EMFs) than power lines, even the 500 kilovolt long distance power transmission lines. Although the appliance EMFs drop off after roughly sixteen feet, many people stand or sit closer than five meters to their appliances.[41]

In addition, there is concern about people who live or work near nuclear power plants. In

DENTAL FACTORS AND THEIR LINK TO CANCER

Alternative health practitioners knowledgeable in energy medicine and biological dentistry have noted for some time a link between dental problems and degenerative illness. When a tooth is infected or otherwise affected, it can block the energy flow along one or more of the body's acupuncture meridians, causing the deterioration of a corresponding organ or tissue, which may in time lead to cancer.

These blockages can also be caused by the use of dental amalgam material, namely the silver fillings most people have in their mouth. "These so-called silver fillings actually contain 50 percent mercury and only 25 percent silver," says Joyal Taylor, D.D.S., of Rancho Santa Fe, California, President of the Environmental Dental Association. This makes such fillings especially harmful, since mercury is a noted carcinogen, as well as having the ability to impair immune function and create blockages.

Practitioners in the field of energy medicine have been able to use this relationship between certain teeth and various organs and tissues of the body in order to diagnose cancer in its earliest stages. Also, by removing or correcting the dental problems which may have helped lead to the cancer formation in the first place, they are able to aid in the treatment of the disease as well. In addition, dentists in the field of biological dentistry advocate the proper removal and replacement of all toxic amalgams as a preventative measure, regardless of the patient's current health.

the United Kingdom, a higher rate of leukemia was been reported in children living near nuclear facilities.[42] Another study of over eight thousand men working at the Oak Ridge National Laboratory in Tennessee, who were exposed daily to EMFs, found that they had a much higher risk of cancer, particularly leukemia.[43] Radiologists have also historically had higher incidences of cancer, as have other workers exposed to low-dose radiation.[44]

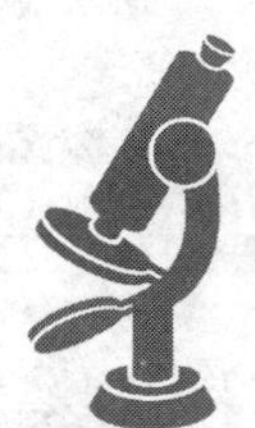

The results of studies that explore the immediate cancer risk associated with environmental radiation indicate the need for further research into this area.

Solar radiation, or sunlight, particularly ultraviolet-B radiation (UV-B), is another common carcinogen, accounting for over 400,000 skin cancers a year. Fortunately, most of these are curable, with only a small percentage developing into truly dangerous melanomas.[45]

Oxygen Free Radicals

Toxic pollution, tobacco smoke, nuclear and ultraviolet radiation, exercise, and many other seemingly disparate substances and activities can all generate damaging oxygen free radicals, which are unstable molecules that circulate within the body. Free radicals are dangerous because they are extremely potent biochemically and have a tendency to attack and destroy the fragile membranes which surround cells, making the body more vulnerable to various cancer initiators and promoters. In addition, the oxygen free radicals themselves may interact with cellular DNA causing mutations which can lead to cancer formation.[46]

Geopathic Stress

"While it is well known that the earth has a magnetic field, it is much less well known that there is a vertical field going from the ground up to the sky," says Anthony Scott-Morley, M.D. (Hon.), Ph.D, of the Institute of Bioenergetic Medicine in Dorset, England. "It has been assumed that the vertical field holds the same intensity throughout fairly large areas," continues Dr. Scott-Morley. "Actual readings with the magnetometer, however, indicate wide variability in field strength within short distances. It is thought that this variability constitutes geopathic stress, in which the body is unable to adapt to the large changes in field strength within short distances (there can be 40,000-70,000 nanotesla in just six inches), leading to a disruption of homeostasis [the body's normal function of regulating health]." In sensitive individuals geopathic stress can disrupt the body's ability to maintain homeostasis, according to Dr. Scott-Morley. "Ionizing radiation from the earth is another form of geopathic stress," Dr. Scott-Morley adds. "This can be given off by certain types of rock structures such as granite."

In 1971, the theory of geopathic stress was supported by investigations of such disturbed geological areas which showed the presence of gamma rays, soil radiations which are hazardous to a person's health. The investigations also showed that subterranean water flows, especially water flows that crossed, produced measurable increases in magnetic anomalies, in electrical conductivity of the soil and air, in acoustics, in field strength of UHF waves, and in the intensity of infrared radiation.[47]

While these geopathic stress sites can be very small, "perhaps no more than ten inches by ten inches," according to Dr. Scott-Morley, medical researchers in the United States and Europe, have linked them to the development of many serious illnesses, including cancer and birth defects. One large scale study published by the United States Department of Health, Education, and Welfare in 1979, reported that geopathic stress may be a factor in between 40 and 50 percent of all human cancers, accounting for between 60 and 90 percent of all cancers attributed to environmental radiation.[48]

Geopathic stress in home and work environments is a key factor in the onset of disease, as well as in the failure of some patients to respond to treatment. Yet, because geopathic stress zones can be so small, merely relocating a bed or a desk can have dramatic results, according to Dr. Scott-Morley.

To locate geopathic zones, the services of a "dowser" can be employed. A dowser uses a forked stick as a measuring instrument to search out these areas in the home or office which are being affected by geopathic stress. Referrals to dowsers can generally be found by contacting well drillers, who often make use of their services to locate underground waterbeds.

In addition to these rudimentary "divining rods," measuring instruments have been developed in Germany (such as the Geomagnetometer) which record the existence of geopathic stress. This will remove the element of human error associated with a measurement being taken by the person doing the dowsing.

Oxygen Deficiency

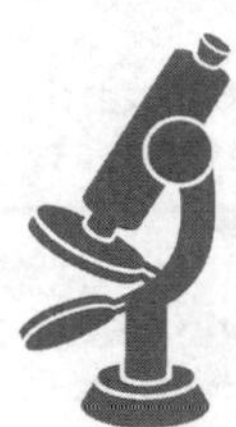

The goverment should examine the wealth of existing studies on oxygen therapy as a treatment for cancer. If approved by the FDA, oxygen therapy could save thousands of lives annually.

One of the most well known theories of cancer causation was originally put forth by two-time Nobel laureate, Dr. Otto Warburg of Germany, a biochemist who won his first Nobel Prize in 1931 for his discovery that oxygen deficiency and cell fermentation are part of the cancer process. "From the standpoint of the physics and chemistry of life, the difference between normal and cancer cells is so great that one can scarcely picture a greater difference," Dr. Warburg wrote almost half a century ago. "Oxygen gas, the donor of energy in plants and animals is dethroned in the cancer cells and replaced by an energy yielding reaction of the lowest living forms, namely, a fermentation of glucose."[49]

According to Dr. Warburg's theory, when cells are deprived of oxygen, they can become "primitive" and enter into glucose reactions, deriving energy, not from oxygen, as normal plant and animal cells do, but rather from the fermentation of sugar. This primitive survival mode is thought to be the way that organisms existed first on earth, before they began using oxygen. It is also a much more inefficient method, as the rapid reproduction of the cancer cells uses up large amounts of glucose, breaking it down into lactic acid, a waste product which puts a severe drain on the body. This also causes an imbalance in the body's acid/base ratio, or pH level. As the acidity of the body rises, it becomes even more difficult for the cells to respire (use oxygen) normally. Medical studies have shown that cancerous tumors contain as much as ten times more lactic acid than healthy human tissues.[50]

See Oxygen Therapy, Stress.

One possible reason for the dramatic increase in cancer rates over the past several hundred years, according to Dr. Warburg's theory, may be the dwindling oxygen supply brought about by rampant deforestation, exploding population, and the burning of fossil fuels. By contrast, according to this same oxygen deficiency theory, cancer cells cannot exist in an oxygen-rich environment. Therefore, if sufficient oxygen is provided, the frenzied glucose fermentation stops and normal aerobic, or oxygen, respiration returns.

Stress and Related Psychological Factors

Even as far back as the second century A.D., the Greek physician Galen noted that melancholic women were more likely to develop cancer. Today, the effects of emotions and stress are increasingly being examined for their link to the development of cancer.

According to Leon Chaitow, N.D., D.O., of London, England, when psychological and emotional changes occur in a person, stress is often produced, resulting in increased adrenaline levels, hormonal changes, and decreased immune function. "Usually, the body can adapt itself, continuing to function during this temporary condition before returning to normal," Dr. Chaitow

THE TYPE C PERSONALITY

The term "Type C personality" is used in much the same way to describe people at risk for cancer, as the term "Type A personality" is used for people at risk for heart disease. While there is no clear consensus on what exactly makes up a Type C personality, or even if such a thing exists, researchers have found a significant amount of anecdotal and suggestive evidence to support certain psychological features that can greatly increase a person's risk for cancer.

The main psychological aspect associated with cancer is loss, either loss of a loved one, or loss of hope. Many cancer patients feel a profound sense of hopelessness and despair, particularly about the meaning of their own existence. Often this feeling has been present as far back as the patient can remember.

The other psychological aspect commonly associated with a cancer personality is the suppression, or repression, of emotions, especially anger. This is seen in people who deny their own needs by holding in their emotions from an early age.

These two characteristics often combine into a third feature of the Type C personality, that of loneliness. This loneliness is usually characterized at an early age by a lack of closeness to one or both parents that later carries on into adulthood as a lack of closeness with friends or a fulfilling relationship.

Most people experience one or all of these traits at some various times in their lives. This is normal, if it does not become a chronic condition. The people who are most at risk from these psychological factors are those who began showing these signs at an early age, then carried them into adulthood. Researchers have found that these psychological patterns, along with stress, can greatly add to a person's cancer risk.[56]

says. "But when the stress is too severe, or if it becomes chronic, chemical changes begin to occur in the body, creating an environment which may increase the risk of serious disease, including cancer." Additionally, the increased adrenal levels, hormone imbalance, and loss of immune function, are all factors in cancer formation.

Over the last seventy-five years, numerous studies have linked stress, and its related psychological components, to a person's susceptibility to cancer.[51] Several recent studies have also linked stressful changes in a child's life, including personal injury or the loss of health of another family member, with the onset of cancer.[52] Other studies found adults who had recently lost a loved one, or were widowed, divorced, or separated, to have the highest cancer rates.[53]

In addition, a basic inability to cope with stress was found to account for a significant rise in cancer incidences.[54] How people dealt with illness, especially cancer, has also been shown to have a dramatic impact on disease recovery.[55]

Genetics

The basic mechanisms that account for the development of cancer reside in the cellular genetic material, primarily the DNA, according to cancer researcher David A. Steenblock, D.O., of Lake Forest, California. "This genetic material can either be inherently programmed to be vulnerable to the onset of cancer due to the passage of faulty genes from one generation to the next (such as in some instances of breast, colon, and lung cancer), or, as is usually the case, the healthy DNA is altered by an initiator—usually a carcinogenic toxin," Dr. Steenblock explains.

See AIDS.

These altered genetic materials are now referred to as "cancer genes," or *oncogenes*, which can turn on a cell's proliferative capacity if a cancer promotor comes into contact with it. "In other cases these changes to the genetic structure will simply result in faulty metabolism leading to gradual energy loss, triggering the cell to divide in an attempt to repair itself," Dr. Steenblock says. "Unfortunately, the divided cells, or 'daughter cells,' inherit the same, or worse, genes. Because of this, the metabolism remains poor, resulting in another round of cell division, and another round of faulty daughter cells."

Viruses

Originally, when cancer genes were discovered in viruses, it was believed that viruses were a major cause of cancer. Subsequently, however, oncogenes have been found in human and animal cells, making it apparent that the viruses were merely integrating the damaged genes into their own cellular material, and were not actually transmitting the gene to their host.

Despite this fact, there are still several viruses which have been linked directly to cancer. These include the hepatitis B virus, which is linked to primary liver cancer; Epstein-Barr virus, which is linked to Burkitt's lymphoma, nasopharyngeal cancer (cancer of the nose and pharynx), and Hodgkin's disease; herpes simplex 2, which is linked to cervical cancer; papilloma viruses (viruses associated with genital warts), which are linked to cervical, vaginal/vulva, and penile cancer; HTLV (human T-cell lymphotropic virus, a retrovirus in the same family as HIV), which is linked to various leukemias and lymphomas; CMV (cytomegalovirus), which is linked to Kaposi's sarcoma (a cancer of the skin); and HIV, which is linked to AIDS and Kaposi's sarcoma. While none of these are known to be transmitted through casual contact, several, including HIV, are sexually and/or blood transmittable.[57]

> *"By going to a physician who subscribes to the pleomorphic theory, and who uses the kind of microscopy that enables the observation of the pleomorphic forms, one can be diagnosed with a disease such as cancer up to eighteen months before it would be diagnosed by even the most sensitive of conventional methods."*

Pleomorphism

Although roundly criticized and dismissed by mainstream practitioners, one of the most fascinating lines of cancer research, largely suppressed and unknown in the United States, is the pleomorphic theory of cancer. This theory, which states that microrganisms can change and take on multiple forms during a single life cycle, actually dates back more than a century to French scientist Antoine Bechamp, a rival of Louis Pasteur. A doctor, chemist, and professor at the University of Toulouse, Bechamp discovered tiny molecular granules called microzymas, or "small ferments," which could change size and shape and become disease causing bacteria. Pasteur refuted this discovery, claiming that all disease was caused by external, preexisting, never-changing microbes that invaded the body.

With the advent of sophisticated, high-tech microscopic equipment, however, scientists were able to get a better view of the microorganisms in the body. German scientist Robert Koch, a Nobel Prize laureate for his discovery of the tuberculin bacillus bacterium, made note of the pleomorphic nature of the typhoid bacillus bacterium. In California in the 1930s, researcher Royal Rife used a light microscope with thirty thousand magnification to show the presence of pleomorphic organisms in human cancer specimens. And in the late 1940s, Virginia Livingston, M.D., of Newark, New Jersey, isolated what she claimed to be the cancer-causing microbe, having found this microbe present in all cases of cancer.[58]

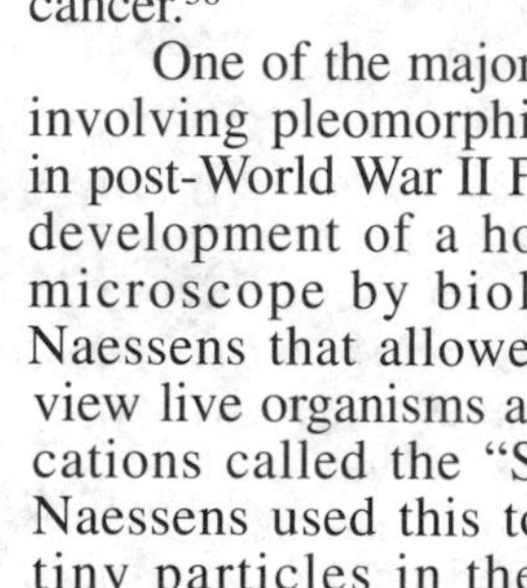

The results of studies that explore pleomorphisms and its role in the process of cancer and other illnesses indicate the need for further research into this area. To support the use of goverment funds for research in this field, write your elected representive.

One of the major breakthroughs involving pleomorphic theory came in post-World War II France, with the development of a homebuilt optic microscope by biologist Gaston Naessens that allowed scientists to view live organisms at high magnifications called the "Somatoscope." Naessens used this tool to uncover tiny particles in the blood never before seen, although earlier researchers had surmised their existence. Naessens named these particles *somatids*, meaning "tiny bodies." "I have since become convinced that the somatid is the smallest unit of life, the precursor to DNA, capable of transforming energy into matter," Naessens says.

Naessens' research revealed that these somatids normally went through a three stage micro-cycle: somatic, spore, double spore. But when the human immune system became stressed or damaged by pollution, sickness, emotional distress, or other causes, the somatids evolve through a macro-cycle of thirteen additional forms. These various forms have been associated with diseases like cancer, multiple sclerosis, lupus, AIDS, and other disorders.

German zoologist and bacteriologist, Guenther Enderlein, discovered similar microorganisms to Naessens' somatids. He named them *protits*, and found that these tiny, protein-based microorganisms flourished in the blood cells, plasma body fluids, and tissues, living in harmony with the body in a symbiotic or mutually beneficial relationship. But when there was any severe change or deterioration in the body's internal environment, these protits, like Naessen's somatids, would pass through several different stages of cyclic development, advancing from harmless agents to disease-producing bacteria or fungi.[59]

Dr. Enderlein believed that a diet rich in animal fats and proteins could trigger these normally harmless microbes to change into the higher, toxic forms that cause diseases ranging from cancer and leukemia to AIDS. According to his research, radiation and other carcinogenic influences could also initiate this change.[60]

It is important to note that many mainstream microbiologists and cancer specialists adamantly deny the pleomorphic theory of cancer. They assert that such somatid and protit forms are mere laboratory anomalies, and that, even if they do exist, they play no role in cancer. Still, other researchers, who also work in the mainstream of conventional medicine, believe that there is something to the pleomorphic theory. Raymond Keith Brown, M.D., a physician and former fellow at the Sloan-Kettering Institute for Cancer Research in New York City, asserts, "Pleomorphic organisms are demonstrable as the silent stage of a gamut of infections, and they've been found in not only cancer patients, but those individuals afflicted with arthritis, multiple sclerosis, and other diseases."[61]

"Prevention is the most important, and most reliable, cancer-fighting tool that exists today, and there is much that an individual can do to prevent cancer."

Pleomorphic microorganisms do not cause disease, however. "They are simply witnesses to a weakening of the natural defenses of the body, and sign posts that can be used for early diagnosis of disease," Naessens says. By going to a physician who subscribes to the pleomorphic theory, and who uses the kind of microscopy that enables the observation of the pleomorphic forms, a person can be diagnosed with a disease such as cancer up to eighteen months before it would be diagnosed by even the most sensitive of conventional methods. This kind of early warning can give the patient the greatest chance for recovery and survival.

Prevention

Prevention is the most important, and most reliable, cancer-fighting tool that exists today, and there is much that an individual can do to prevent cancer. It is especially vital for a person to maintain a strong and healthy immune system. This can be accomplished in a number of ways, including through a diet that ensures the optimal intake of immuno-enhancing nutrients while decreasing the intake of immunosuppressing foods. Living a life free from continual emotional or mental distress is also important, as well as avoiding carcinogenic toxins in the home and in the environment.

Diet and Nutrition

With up to 60 percent of all cancers being related to dietary factors,[62] diet and nutrition are perhaps the most important aspects of any cancer prevention regimen. This is evidenced by the fact that in 1988, the U.S. Surgeon General called for the reduction of dietary fat as a top priority for the prevention of chronic diseases, including cancer.[63]

A diet which consists largely of organically grown fresh fruits, vegetables, and whole grains, with little or no fat or meat (particularly grilled, charred, smoked, or cured meats[64]), is highly recommended, especially for women who wish to decrease their risk of breast cancer.[65] The National Cancer Institute recommends that Americans reduce their fat intake to no more than 30 percent of total calories, while increasing their consumption of fresh fruits and vegetables.[66]

Additionally, it is essential to avoid highly processed foods, as they can contain partially hydrogenated fats,[67] as well as chemical additives that are potentially carcinogenic.[68] Cutting down on sugar,[69] caffeine,[70] and alcohol[71] is also highly recommended.

Eating organically grown foods is extremely important, as recent studies have shown that organic foods are not only far more free from carcinogenic pesticide contaminants than conventionally grown foods, they are also richer in the essential nutrients and trace elements necessary for cancer prevention, including beta-carotene, vitamin E, and selenium.[72] In a recent five-year study of nearly thirty thousand rural Chinese, researchers from the National Cancer Institute found that daily doses of these three nutrients reduced cancer deaths by 13 percent.[73]

The following is a list of these and other important cancer-fighting nutrients and elements, along with their sources:

Beta-carotene: The precursor of vitamin A, beta-carotene is found in carrots, sweet potatoes, spinach, and most leafy green vegetables. Another recent study found that a diet high in carotenes, especially beta-carotene, was protective against all cancers.[74] Beta-carotene is particularly important for women as a deterrent to cervical cancer.[75]

Beta-carotene has also been shown to protect the lungs against both tobacco smoke and smog, inhibiting lung cancer.[76] In addition, another study found that ex-smokers who daily ate green and yellow vegetables high in beta-carotene also decreased their risk of stomach cancer as well as lung cancer.[77]

Vitamin B_6: Found in bananas, leafy green vegetables, carrots, apples, organ meats, and sweet potatoes, vitamin B_6 is essential for maintaining optimal immune function, and helps maintain healthy mucous membranes which line the respiratory tract, providing a natural barrier to pollution and infection. It is also a valuable protection against cervical cancer.[78]

Vitamin C: Found in citrus fruits, cantaloupe, broccoli, green peppers, and many other fruits and vegetables, vitamin C is integrally involved in the maintenance of a healthy immune system, as well as protecting against a variety of cancers.[79]

Vitamin E: Found in dark green vegetables, eggs, wheat germ, liver, unrefined vegetable oils, and some herbs, vitamin E is a powerful antioxidant that can directly reduce the damage done by ozone and other substances found in smog. It can also help protect against bowel cancer.[80]

Selenium: An essential trace mineral found in fruits and vegetables, selenium helps the body produce glutathione, an enzyme essential for detoxification. Low dietary levels of selenium have been correlated with higher cancer incidence, therefore supplementation of this nutrient acts as a deterrent against cancer in general.[81]

Additional nutrients which have been shown to be protective against cancer, or whose deficiency can increase cancer risk, include:

Folic Acid: Protects against cervical cancer,[82] and necessary for proper synthesis of RNA and DNA. Found in beets, cabbage, dark green leafy vegetables, eggs, dairy products, citrus fruits, and most fish.

See Nutritional Supplements, Orthomolecular Medicine.

Calcium: Protects against colon cancer,[83] and vital for proper bone and tooth formation, blood clotting, and cellular metabolism. Found in dark green vegetables, most nuts and seeds, milk products, sardines, and salmon.

Iodine: Protects against breast cancer,[84] and needed for proper energy metabolism and the growth and repair of all tissues. Available in seafood and sea vegetables such as kelp, dulse, and iodized salt.

Magnesium: Protects against cancer in general,[85] and necessary to maintain the pH balance of blood and tissue, as well as the synthesis of RNA and DNA. Found in most nuts, fish, green vegetables, whole grains, and brown rice.

Zinc: Protects against prostate cancer,[86] and necessary for the formation of RNA and DNA, as well as healthy immune function. Contained in whole grains, most seafoods, sunflower seeds, soybeans, and onions.

Garlic: Protects against cancer in general.[87]

Omega-3 Fatty Acids: May inhibit cancers, especially breast cancer,[88] and essential for the proper functioning of all tissue and every cell in the body. Contained in fish such as salmon, mackerel, sardines, haddock, and cod; evening primrose oil; and flaxseed and linseed oils.

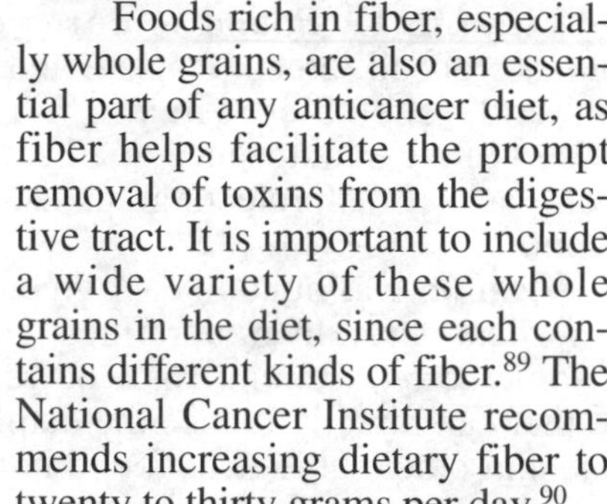

Our power as consumers can have a direct effect on industry and manufacturing. A grassroots boycott of products known to contain carcinogens can hasten their elimination from the marketplace.

Foods rich in fiber, especially whole grains, are also an essential part of any anticancer diet, as fiber helps facilitate the prompt removal of toxins from the digestive tract. It is important to include a wide variety of these whole grains in the diet, since each contains different kinds of fiber.[89] The National Cancer Institute recommends increasing dietary fiber to twenty to thirty grams per day.[90]

It is also important to drink only pure, filtered water, in order to avoid any carcinogenic toxins, such as chlorine and lead, which might be lurking in public water systems. Likewise, well water, unless it has been adequately tested, is not to be trusted. Pesticides from farms, as well as industrial runoff, can leach through the soil into underground wells.

Avoid Toxins in the Home

It is extremely important to be wary of the carcinogenic chemicals and contaminants found in everyday consumer items, including household products, cosmetics, foods, and beverages. Such common items as furniture polishes, car interior cleaners, and even common cleansers contain carcinogens ranging from formaldehyde to crystalline silica. While none of these products alone may present a critical carcinogenic exposure, when many little exposures are added together, they become cumulative, stressing the body's immune system and damaging cells until eventually, over time, cancer sets in.[91]

In addition, at present, many chemicals used in cosmetics, pesticides, and other products do not require full safety testing before they are allowed to be marketed and used by millions of consumers. Therefore, it is important to gain as much information as possible about the products to which a person's family will be exposed. For example, among the two leading brands of kitchen cleansers, Ajax contains high amounts of crystalline silica while its competitor, Comet, does not.[92]

"This sort of conscientious buying will enable people to vote with their dollars for an environmental clean-up of all carcinogenic substances used in manufacturing and industry, including those found in pesticides," Dr. Epstein states.

Dr. Epstein also recommends boycotting all consumer products containing carcinogens. "There are a number of substitutes available," he explains. "For example, a combination of plain water mixed with distilled white vinegar and a small amount of baking soda, borax, and lemon juice can clean the home and bathroom as effectively as many higher-priced cleaners."

Informed consumerism such as this can also bring pressure to bear on the government to require that all products and chemicals be proven safe before they are allowed to be sold to an unsuspecting public.

Reduce Exposure to Electromagnetic Fields (EMFs)

The United States Congress' Office of Technology Assessment recommends a policy of prudent avoidance of EMFs. Prudent avoidance means measuring electromagnetic fields and acting to reduce all other exposure. To measure electromagnetic radiation in the home or office, one should use a Gauss Meter, a device which measures the amount of gauss, or magnetic flux density, occurring in the home or workspace. It is easy to use and shows which places are safe from chronic exposure and which places are not. In addition, before buying or moving into a new house, apartment, or office, always test for high electromagnetic field levels. Also avoid living or working in areas with close proximity to power lines and generating stations. Computer shields should always be used as well.

Stress Reduction

In line with the growing body of research regarding stress and its link to serious illnesses, many physicians believe that treating an individual's mental and emotional states is as important as treating any cancerous tumors which may be a result of such conditions. Lifestyle change is another factor that needs to be looked at closely, including examining a person's job, major relationships, living situation, and sexual habits.

"There is overwhelming evidence that people who have few social contacts are more likely to get sick and less likely to recover from an illness," says Erik Peper, Ph.D., Associate Director of the Institute of Holistic Healing Studies at San Francisco State University. One long-term study found that people with the lowest amount of social ties were two to three times more likely to die of all causes than those with the most social connectedness.[93]

This can be especially true in instances of cancer diagnoses. David Spiegel, M.D., a psychiatrist at Stanford University, demonstrated that women with breast cancer who participated in a weekly support group lived twice as long as those who did not.[94]

The letting out of emotions linked to a person's condition, especially for cancer patients, can be very therapeutic. Several studies have shown a clear connection between people who expressed high levels of anger toward their disease and increased survival lengths.[95]

Early Detection

Early detection is imperative for the most effective treatment of cancer. By learning about their body and recognizing the telltale signs of cancer, a person can do a great deal to ensure that cancer is detected at an early stage.

"Early detection is imperative for the most effective treatment of cancer. By learning about our bodies and recognizing the telltale signs of cancer, we can do a great deal to ensure that cancer is detected at an early stage."

According to Dr. Epstein, there are seven symptoms which should be noted by every health-conscious individual:

A Change in Bowel or Bladder Habits: Continuing urinary difficulties, constipation, diarrhea, gas pains, rectal bleeding, or blood in the stool, should not be ignored and should be a warning to seek professional help.

Chronic Indigestion or a Difficulty in Swallowing: Difficulties in swallowing, continued indigestion, nausea, heartburn, bloating, and loss of appetite may all be symptoms of colon cancer or cancer of the esophagus.

Unusual Bleeding or Discharge: The early stages of uterine cancer and later stages of cervical cancer exhibit signs of unusual bleeding or discharge. Prompt attention to these symptoms will afford the patient a better chance of catching cancer at its most treatable stage. In the case of cervical cancer, Pap tests can detect problems before the later stages of bleeding.

Thickening of or Lumps in the Breast or Testicles: Self-examination of the breast and testicles offers women and men the best protection against breast and testicular cancer. A lump or thickening in the breast, or noticeable change in the testicles, are early warning signs and should not be ignored.

Nagging Cough or Voice Hoarseness: Coughs which become chronic, especially for smokers, should be checked. If there is a cancer in the air passages into the lungs, they may be partially obstructed or irritated. Coughing may be a sign of this obstruction or irritation.

Changes in Warts or Moles: Changes in warts or moles, or sores which do not heal, may be indicative of melanoma. Skin cancers may appear as dry, scaly patches, as pimples which never go away, or as inflamed or ulcerated areas. Warts or moles which grow or bleed should be checked, as should sores in the mouth which persist.

Sore Throat Which Does Not Heal: Persistent hoarseness, a persistent lump in the throat, soreness in the neck, or difficulties in swallowing are signals that your body may be harboring a cancer. Cancer of the larynx exhibits these symptoms, yet is treatable when caught early.

There are also many different methods for early detection. These include:

Prostate Specific Antigen (PSA): The PSA is used for early detection of prostate cancer. Many physicians, both mainstream and alternative, recommend that the PSA be used annually. However, they also warn of lab variability. They also caution physicians not to overreact, noting that many men with prostate cancer do not necessarily die of it.

Electroacupuncture Biofeedback: The prospect of detecting life-threatening diseases such as cancer at the earliest stage has led some alternative medical practitioners to investigate energy medicine, based on the belief that an individual's energy field alters with the onset of disease. This changing energy field can be diagnosed using electroacupuncture biofeedback devices, leading to early detection.

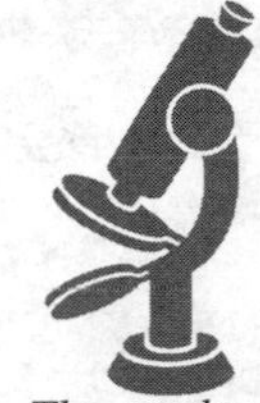

The results of studies that explore the effectiveness of electroaccupuncture biofeedback and other energy-based devices as tools for early screening for cancer indicate the need for further research in the area. If approved by the FDA these devices could save the lives of thousands annually.

Electroacupuncture biofeedback instruments were first used in Europe in the early 1970s, and have been used in the United States since the 1980s. As controversial as they are, their use is becoming increasingly widespread as physicians seek better ways to screen for a wide variety of illnesses that can be used along with traditional methods.

Alternative Treatments for Cancer

It is important that the cancer patient initially consider the value of both conventional and alternative treatments before making a decision about which approach to health to follow. Conventional cancer physicians view cancer as a tumor which, if not caught quickly enough, will spread its poison throughout the body and eventually cause death.

MAMMOGRAPHY: BENEFITS AND RISKS

While the use of mammography is commonly recommended to detect breast cancer, it is important that its drawbacks be noted, as well. First, x-rays can cause cancer. There is clear evidence that the breast, particularly in premenopausal women, is highly sensitive to radiation, with estimates of increased risk of up to one percent for every RAD (radiation absorbed dose) unit of x-ray exposure. "Even for low dosage exposure of two RADs or less, this exposure can add up quickly for women having annual mammographies," notes Samuel Epstein, M.D., Professor of Occupational and Environmental Medicine at the University of Illinois School of Public Health. "More recent concern comes from evidence that one percent of women, or over one million women in the United States alone, carry a gene that increases their breast cancer risk from radiation fourfold."

Secondly, mammography provides false tumor reports between 5 and 15 percent of the time.[96] False positive results cause women to be re-exposed to additional X rays and create an environment of further stress, even possibly leading to unneeded surgery.

"Furthermore." says Dr. Epstein, "while there is a general consensus that mammography improves early cancer detection and survival in post-menopausal women, no such benefit is demonstrable for younger women." Still, the American Cancer Society recommends annual or biannual mammography for all women ages forty to fifty-five.

In addition, mammography may also fail to detect advanced tumors measuring less than two centimeters in diameter. Yet a tumor can be felt manually when it reaches about one centimeter (approximately one half inch) in diameter, and with training in self-examination, women can detect even smaller tumors.[97] In view of this, women should take self examination all the more seriously.

Many experts believe that early detection through manual examination provides the best all-around results, as well. "It is certainly the safest, least expensive, and least invasive preventive action available to women," Dr. Epstein points out. "It also enables women to become familiar with their breast tissue, natural lumps and all, and to report early on any noticeable changes."

For the time being, mammography's place in breast cancer detection is secure. But it is a passing technology, which will soon be replaced by safer testing methods. Two such methods already available include transillumination with infrared light scanning, and the Antimalignane Antibody in Serum (AMAS) test. Transillumination is based on the concept that light will shine through most breast tissue but will be blocked by lumps. Its advantage is that it does not use radiation. The AMAS test measures serum levels of AMA, an antibody found to be elevated in most patients in the early stages of active nonterminal malignancies.[98]

At present, the three major treatments employed by conventional physicians to treat cancer are chemotherapy, radiation, and surgery. Each of these treatments is highly invasive and can pose severe side effects, and each may actually shorten the cancer patient's life, rather than saving it. For example, the chemicals used in chemotherapy are themselves toxic and carcinogenic, and may destroy the body's immune system, which is why some patients die of chemotherapeutic drugs before they actually succumb to cancer. Alan Levin, M.D., of the University of California Medical School, points out, for instance, that women with breast cancer are likely to die faster with chemotherapy than without it.[99] And John Cairns, M.D. of the Harvard University School of Public Health notes that of the approximately half a million people who die each year of cancer, only about 2 to 3 percent of them actually gain any benefit from chemotherapy.[100]

Surgery to remove cancerous tumors grew out of the premise, since discarded, that localized tumors were isolated manifestations of the disease and that removal of the diseased body part, if caught in time, would prevent the cancer from spreading. Surgery removes as much of the cancer as possible (very often leaving dangerous cancer cells behind), but does not correct the underlying cause of the cancer. Consequently, the tumor often re-occurs. Physicians now know, as well, that a cancer may already have spread to distant parts of the body long before it becomes detected elsewhere as a lump. This has been borne out by studies which show that mastectomy (the removal of breast tissue, underlying muscle, and all lymph modes in the armpit) presents no advantage, in terms of survival, over a lumpectomy and radiation.[101]

Radiation also poses inherent health haz ards. Patients who receive radiation often experience painful sores of the mouth, throat, genitals, and other parts of the body, as well as the onset of ulcers, diarrhea, gastrointestinal disorders, reproductive problems, and birth defects. Ironically, they can also develop further cancer, because patients who undergo radiation therapy face a significantly increased risk of leukemia.[102]

Conventional medicine rarely treats cancer as a systemic illness. Alternative medicine, by contrast, regards cancer as the manifestation of an unhealthy body whose defenses are so imbalanced that they can no longer destroy cells that turn cancerous, as would normally occur in a state of health. Its essential premise is that healthy bodies do not develop cancer, and that cancer is a reflection of the body as a whole, rather than a localized disease in one particular part of the body. Therefore, alternative therapies seek to strengthen the immune system of the cancer patient, and generally shun the use of highly toxic modalities, such as radiation and chemotherapy. Instead, they prefer to heal the entire body, and employ a multifaceted, nontoxic approach to doing so, incorporating treatments which rely on biopharmaceutical, immune enhancement, metabolic, nutritional, and herbal, nontoxic methods.

“The essential premise of alternative medicine is that healthy bodies do not develop cancer, and that cancer is a reflection of the body as a whole, rather than a localized disease in one particular part of the body.”

Because cancer is a disease with multiple causes, it is important to realize that the best chance of treating it lies in an approach which addresses all of the factors involved. The therapies which follow are among the ones which offer the most promise as cancer treatments. Bear in mind that some of them may work well for certain types of cancers and not for others. Still, they all merit attention.

Caution: *The information presented in this chapter is not to be used in any manner in the non-professional treatment of cancer, nor should people with cancer attempt to undertake any of these methods without medical supervision. The material which follows is meant solely as a first step in the education process concerning cancer and the factors involved in its treatment.*

Biopharmaceutical Therapies

Biopharmaceutical therapies include antineoplaston therapy, the work of Gaston Naessens, the use of hydrazine sulfate, shark cartilage, vitamin C therapy, and laetrile. Each of these therapies has been developed by highly credentialed physicians and medical researchers. What they have in common is the use of nontoxic, naturally-derived compounds that rebalance the body's biochemical functioning. Yet, each therapy has been condemned by the orthodox medical establishment.

Antineoplaston Therapy

General Background: Stanislaw Burzynski, M.D., Ph.D., based in Houston, Texas, is a graduate of the Lublin Medical Academy in Poland, where he graduated first in his class in 1967. A year later, at the age of twenty-five, he earned a Ph.D. in biochemistry. Dr. Burzynski's treatment is based on the theory that the body has a parallel biochemical defense system independent of the immune system. Dr. Burzynski, who is credited with discovering this system, refers to it as the Biochemical Defense System (BDS). “The mechanism of defense in this system is completely different than in the immune system,” Dr. Burzynski explains. “It is a reprogramming of defective cells. It's no longer killing of the cells, but changing the program inside the defective cell, which means that the cell will begin to function normally. In the case of cancer, for instance, if all of the cancer cells will be reprogrammed and function normally, then, ultimately, we won't have cancer anymore.”[103]

Dr. Burzynski has found that the BDS consists of short-chain amino acids, known as polypeptides, that are able to inhibit cancer cell growth. He has named these polypeptides *antineoplastons* (meaning anti-new growth).

According to Dr. Burzynski, cancer is largely a disease caused by a malfunction in information processing. “The cell develops according to the program for cellular differentiation,” he notes. “Millions of cells are differentiated in the human body every day, bringing up the possibility of errors in the program for differentiation. Taking under consideration such large numbers of cells undergoing differentiation, it is more than likely that a significant number of these cells will develop toward neoplasia [tumor growth].”[104] Antineoplastons, he claims, are able to reprogram cancer cells to restore this process to normal. They interact with the DNA of the cells, actually becoming part of the DNA and taking the place of carcinogens which would otherwise occupy the same spots on the DNA strand. As this

INTEGRATING TREATMENT METHODS

Perhaps the best illustration of what needs to be done when a person is diagnosed with cancer comes from the experience of Neal Dublinsky. In November 1987, Neal, then twenty-four-years-old and recently embarked upon a career as a corporate attorney in Los Angeles, was diagnosed with the most advanced stage of non-Hodgkin's lymphoma Stage IV. The bulky tumor had spread to his entire abdomen and there was fluid build-up in his lungs. "I was shocked when I got the diagnosis, and was in extreme physical pain," Neal recalls. "My doctor told me that I had to undergo chemotherapy if I wanted to live. I didn't know better, so I did it."

Neal received chemotherapy for four months. The treatments reduced the tumor but the reduction was short-lived. They also caused traumatizing side effects, including total hair loss, a feeling of being poisoned, and high level gastrointestinal distress. "During this time, I was taking an aggresive combination of six different drugs, and every three weeks I received more chemotherapy," Neal says. "Afterwards, I was completely incapacitated, and each time I returned for another treatment, it got worse."

After the fourth month, Neal underwent radiation therapy for three more weeks. "The radiation only took a minute," Neal notes. "But within an hour I would be violently ill and retching from my core, and I could no longer eat solid foods. After the daily radiation treatments ended, Neal then underwent a bone marrow transplant using his own bone marrow.

"That was the worst time of my life," Neal continues, "but once it was over, it looked like I would be all right." Only four months later, though, a new tumor emerged in his pelvic area that was beginning to compress his right kidney. At this point, all Neal's doctors could offer him was the prospect of another series of even harsher chemotherapy to buy him a little more time, but with no hope of a cure.

Neal had lost faith in what conventional medicine could do for him by this point. "The physician who performed my bone marrow transplant knew everything about transplants, but almost nothing about other treatment options," he says. "It was that way with each of my doctors. Even though they meant well and were experts in their fields, none of them were able to put it all together and see the big picture."

Instead of giving up, Neal contacted alternative cancer associations, including the International Association of Cancer Victors and the Cancer Control Society. He also bought books and read voraciously, educating himself about every alternative therapy he could find. In addition, he phoned over twenty cancer survivors to learn about their experiences with the therapies he was discovering.

Neal was particularly intrigued by the antineoplaston therapy developed by conventionally-trained physician Stanislaw Burzynski, M.D., Ph.D., of Houston, Texas. "I spoke with ten of Dr. Burzynski's former patients," he relates. "They had all responded well to his therapy and had suffered from similar kinds of cancer as my own. They spoke of Dr. Burzynski in glowing terms and encouraged me to see him. I decided to follow their advice, but ultimately my decision to go was a leap of faith, because my doctors' attitudes about alternative therapies was dismissive. I figured if I was going to die, I was going to die fighting."

In December, 1988, Neal began treatment. The first thing he noticed was that it was not painful. Dr. Burzynski put him on an IV drip of antineoplastons that ran ten hours a day. For ten months, Neal remained on the drip as an outpatient. "Within weeks of beginning the treatment, my biochemical profile improved," he reports. His liver and kidney function progressed, and he started to feel better. His tumor was gradually regressing, showing slow and steady improvement.

After the ten months, Neal received four injections of antineoplastons a day, together with oral capsules. Six months later, he achieved complete remission. He stayed with the treatment for another eighteen months, taking the capsules for maintenance, then he was taken off the medicine altogether. During this time he also adopted a dairyless, vegetarian diet, augmented with nutritional and herbal supplements. He underwent a series of localized hyperthermia treatments and colonic irrigations, as well, and had his mercury amalgam fillings removed from his mouth. "I began to incorporate elements of many health programs, because I wanted to survive," he says.

He has. Today Neal continues on in good health. When asked about his experience with conventional medicine, he becomes angry. "I feel I was ripped off," he says. "I should have been told about antineoplastons in the first place. The chemotherapy may have temporarily shrunk my tumor, but it did not resolve my underlying problem. It was only after I met Dr. Burzynski that I started to make progress. I'm eternally grateful to him, because as far as I'm concerned, he saved my life."

Neal's suggestion to others diagnosed with cancer is simple. "Learn about all the alternative therapies," he says. "You should know more than you will ever use. Read, explore, and research everything, keeping an open mind. Visit the clinics. Consult with the doctors. Interview patients, especially those whose histories, type of cancer, stage, and background are most like your own, because different therapies have better track records for different types of cancer. Most importantly, don't become passive. Your treatment is a choice. Don't let others make it for you. Take charge and face it head on."

occurs, the antineoplastons redirect the DNA back into normal reproduction.

The body of the cancer patient has only about two or three percent of the amount of antineoplastons of the body of a healthy person. Because of this, the BDS becomes deficient against the chemical and physical carcinogens, viruses, and other cancer-causing agents, leading to the development and continued growth of cancer.[105]

Antineoplastons can be extracted from blood serum and urine, and manufactured synthetically. Approximately 95 percent of Dr. Burzynski's patients receive synthetic antineoplatons. Over 2,000 patients have been treated at the Burzynski Research Institute (BRI), most of them diagnosed with advanced or terminal cancer. The majority of them have benefited from antineoplaston therapy, experiencing complete or partial remission, or stabilization of their conditions. In addition, few side effects have been noted. The range of cancers which Dr. Burzynski has treated include lymphoma, breast cancer, leukemia, bone cancer, prostate cancer, lung cancer, colon cancer, and cancer of the bladder.[106]

"In the case of cancer, if all of the cancer cells will be reprogrammed and function normally, then, ultimately, we won't have cancer anymore."
—Stanislaw Burzynski, M.D., Ph.D.

Despite these well-documented successes, including a 1977 study which found that 86 percent of advanced cancer patients given antineoplastons improved,[107] and the nontoxic nature of anti-neoplaston therapy, the American Cancer Society placed Dr. Burzynski's work on its Unproven Methods list in 1983. In Europe, Japan, and other areas of the world, however, Dr. Burzynski's work is heralded as an important breakthrough in cancer treatment. In addition, he regularly is invited to share his research on cancer treatments at symposiums worldwide, including most recently at the July, 1993, 18th International Congress of Chemotherapy in Stockholm, Sweden. There, along with fellow M.D.'s and Ph.D.'s from the United States, Brazil, The Netherlands, Poland, and Japan, he presented the latest results in cancer treatment based on his work.[108]

Phase II clinical trials investigating different forms of antineoplaston treatment, such as capsules or injections, in groups of 15 to 35 patients diagnosed with a specific type of cancer, such as breast or prostate, were conducted from 1988 through 1990. The first trial was with patients with *astrocytoma*, a highly malignant form of brain tumor. Most of these patients' tumors had progressed to Stage IV before the trials began. Previously, these patients had undergone surgery, radiation therapy, and/or chemotherapy, yet their tumors were still growing. Each night, for six weeks, they received seven hours of intravenous drip. The majority of the patients were treated on an outpatient basis, and most of them improved rapidly, to the point where, after six weeks, some of the adults were able to resume working part-time, and the children were going back to school. According to Dr. Burzynski, 80 percent of the patients experienced "objective response", meaning complete or partial remission, or stabilization of their tumors.[109]

In October, 1991, the National Cancer Institute (NCI) sent investigators to conduct an on-site investigation at Dr. Burzynski's Institute. Based on their findings, the NCI issued an official statement approving Dr. Burzynski's documentation of seven out of eight patients who recovered from advanced, inoperable brain tumors.[110] Thereafter, the NCI issued its approval for Dr. Burzynski to undertake four phase II outside clinical trials involving various forms of brain tumors. In 1989, the FDA had previously allowed Dr. Burzynski to clinically test antineoplastons in breast cancer patients.

Antineoplastons may be especially effective in cases where cancer is diagnosed quite early, and in the prevention of cancer, according to Dr. Burzynski. Patients generally are treated on an outpatient basis. The treatment of benign tumors, such as fibrocystic breast disease, benign brain tumors, and genital warts, is also possible with antineoplastons . In such cases, Dr. Burzynski points out that the antineoplastons can be taken orally.[111] Antineoplaston therapy can be used with conventional modes of therapy, as well, including chemotherapy or immunotherapy. The advantage is that the destructive effects of chemotherapy are minimized because only lower doseages are necessary, and because the antineoplastons stimulate bone marrow function.[112]

Case History: In 1989, one of Dr. Burzynski's patients, a ten year old boy, was diagnosed with *glioblastoma*, the most highly advanced brain tumor. He underwent radiation therapy that proved largely ineffective and in fact damaged the viability of his growth-related pituitary gland. His mental function was also diminished by the therapy, according to his mother. Despite harsh criticims from his physicians, the boy began antineoplaston treatments with Dr. Burzynski in the spring of 1990. Within one month, the tumor mass began to break down. By November 1990, he was in complete remission, and he remains cancer free.[113] A July, 1993 segment of CBS's "Street Stories" on Dr. Burzynski showed the boy visibly healthy and playing basketball with his friends.

714X

General Background: Developed by biologist Gaston Naessens, the 714X treatment consists of three consecutive series of twenty-one days of injections of nitrogen-rich camphor and organic salts directly into the lymphatic system. Jacinte Levesque, O.M.D., of Montreal, Quebec, Canada, and a close associate of Naessens, and owner of a holistic health care clinic, notes that this therapy was developed when Naessens observed that cancer cells required and used up a lot of nitrogen, often stealing it from healthy cells. "In order to do this, cancer cells excrete a poisionous compound called the 'co-cancerogenic K factor,'" Levesque says, "which paralyzes the immune system, allowing the cancer cells to draw the needed nitrogen from the healthy cells.

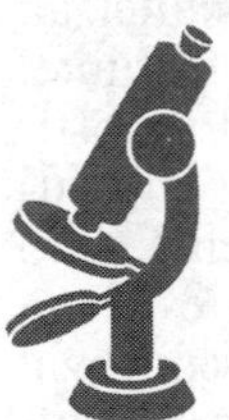

The results of studies that explore the benefits of antineoplaston therapy and 714X indicate the need for further research into their effectiveness as treatments for cancer. To support government funds being used for this purpose, write your elected representatives.

"When the 714X is introduced into the system, it acts as an attractor for the cancer cells, because of the high level of nitrogen in the camphor. Now, because the cancer cells are getting their nitrogen from the camphor molecules, they no longer have to excrete the K co-factor to immobilize the healthy cells' defensive systems.

"It's like a distraction, because the 714X doesn't kill the cancer cells, but rather attracts them and feeds them in order to liberate the immune system," Levesque adds. "So while the 714X is engaging the cancer cells, the immune system starts to pick up, and is able to do its job once again since it isn't paralyzed by the co-factor anymore."

Another major benefit of the treatment, notes Levesque, is its additional effect on the lymph system. "The first thing that the 714X actually does, because of the action of the organic salts when it is injected into the lymphatic system, is to liquify the lymph, allowing toxins to be flushed out," she says. "This is important because one of the consequences of cancer, due to the fact that cancer cells put out so many toxins, is that the lymph system becomes clogged up. This also helps the immune system because one of its main jobs is to take toxins out of the body so it can function properly."

According to Naessen's protocol, the 714X preparation is injected into the lymphatic nodes of the groin, with injections given once a day for periods of twenty-one consecutive days followed by a break of two days, to allow the patient to rest while the natural defenses of the body are restored. People with advanced cases of cancer, though, can receive a more intense and prolonged therapy, since 714X has no harmful side effects.

"714X can be used as an adjunct to other treatments as well," adds Levesque, "but patients receiving it should not take vitamin E or vitamin B_{12} at the same time." Harvey Bigelson, M.D., of Scottsdale, Arizona, treats cancer with a combination of 714X and other alternative therapies, and reports that he is achieving between 60 and 80 percent effectiveness.

In May 1989, Naessens was put through a criminal trial by the Quebec Medical Corporation of Physicians, who charged him with practicing dangerous and illegal therapies, fraud, and criminal negligence. He was acquitted. Today his formula is still available in Canada, as well as in Mexico, and Western Europe.

Case History: A forty-year old woman diagnosed with breast cancer was strongly advised by her doctor to have a mastectomy. She refused, and instead took three consecutive twenty-one day series of 714X injections. "Since then I have had a tremendous feeling of well-being, even a renewed 'lust for life,'" the woman states. "And when, at my own initiative, I went back to the clinic where I was first diagnosed, for tests, I was told that I had no trace of cancer left in my body."[114]

Former U.S. Congressman Berkley Bedell, of Iowa, who spoke on this subject before the U.S. Senate subcommittee special hearing on alternative medicine, attributes his recovery from prostate cancer to his treatments with 714X as well.[115]

Hydrazine Sulfate

General Background: Often, cancer patients die not from the disease itself but from a process called *cachexia*, a condition in which the body becomes malnourished and the patient simply wastes away. In 1968, Dr. Joseph Gold, Director of the Syracuse Cancer Research Institute in Syracuse, New York, discovered that the chemical hydrazine sulfate could reverse cachexia, providing the body with extra strength to fight the disease.

Although not touted as a "cure," hydrazine sulfate has been documented to shrink tumors and even cause them to completely disappear. It also seems to work at every stage of disease, particularly for cancers of the rectum, colon, ovaries, prostate, thyroid, breast, and lung, as well as for Hodgkin's disease, melanoma, and lymphoma.

Weight gain, as well as the disappearance of tumors and symptoms, are some of the benefits of hydrazine sulfate therapy.

At the Petrov Research Institute of Oncology in Leningrad, scientists followed the progress of 740 terminal cancer patients over a fifteen year period, all of them suffering from a broad range of tumors. No matter what form of cancer had triggered the condition, nearly 50 percent saw an improvement in their cachexia, with 14 percent seeing pronounced benefits. In addition, 10 percent had their tumors regress and all saw a stabilization of the disease process.[116] Rowan Chlebowski, M.D., Ph.D., replicated these results in a double-blind, placebo-controlled study of terminally-ill lung cancer patients suffering from cachexia at the Harbor-UCLA Medical Center.[117]

While hydrazine sulfate can be toxic, the form used in cancer treatment differs from industrial grade versions in that it has been highly purified. Side effects are limited to occasional nausea, dizziness, itching, drowsiness and euphoria. Although there have been occasional reports of patients experiencing numbness in their extremities, these conditions have been alleviated through the use of vitamin B_6.

Shark Cartilage

General background: One of the reasons tumors grow is because they develop their own blood supply. Most tissues and organs also do this in a process known as *angiogenesis*. Cartilage though, a tough, elastic, connective tissue, found in most animals, including sharks and humans, does not develop a blood supply, because it contains an "anti-angiogenic" substance which stops the blood supply from developing, according to I. William Lane, Ph.D., of New Jersey, one of the leading proponents of shark cartilage therapy.[118]

The basis for shark cartilage therapy is that if the blood supply to tumors can be interrupted, they will stop growing and eventually die. Research has demonstrated that cartilage's anti-angiogenic properties can do just this.[119] Robert Langer, Ph.D., of the Massachusetts Institute of Technology, has further demonstrated that shark cartilage contains one thousand times more of the angiogenesis inhibitor than any other type of cartilage.[120]

Testing with shark cartilage has been successful on animals and most recently on terminally ill cancer patients. The first human study was conducted in conjunction with Dr. Ernesto Contreras Jr. of the Hospital Ernesto Contreras in Tijuana, Mexico. The patients chosen suffered from a variety of cancers, including cervical, colon, and breast, and all had a life expectancy of only three to six months. Shark cartilage—the sole form of cancer treatment—was administered via retention enema, and after the first month, seven out of eight of the patients experienced tumor reductions ranging from 30 to 100 percent. In all cases symptomatic improvements were noted as well, including pain control, weight gain, improved energy, and attitude.[121]

Another clinical study using shark cartilage was done with nineteen terminal cancer patients in Cuba, with the cooperation of Dr. Lane. After sixteen weeks of treatment there were no toxic side effects, and in every case, the tumors stopped growing, with many shrinking from between 15 percent and 58 percent. These patients were all terminal with wide metastasis to other parts of the body, and had received prior treatments that had all failed.[122]

Dr. Lane has also been working with Renato Martinez, M.D., and naturopathic consultant Dante Ruccio, N.D., both from Bloomfield, New Jersey, in a study involving ninety-four advanced or terminal cancer patients. According to Dr. Ruccio, twelve are reported in complete remission and all but two are still under shark cartilage treatment and receiving positive benefit.[123]

Since March, 1993, NCI-trained oncologist and immunologist Charles B. Simone, M.D., of Laurenceville, New Jersey, has been monitoring patients with advanced cancers who are using shark cartilage as food supplement. Of the twenty patients he monitored over the initial eight weeks, he reported the complete elimination of tumors in four patients and a reduction in three others.[124]

Case History: Dr. Ruccio recalls that the first cancer remission he observed as a result of shark cartilage therapy was in a "distinguished looking elderly minister" suffering from prostate cancer which had spread into his bones. A prestigious New York cancer center had given the minister only three to six months to live. Over a period of time on shark cartilage, the minister's specific antigen blood marker, PSA, which had originally indicated the cancer activity in his prostate, dropped by about 98 percent from its previous level of 2100, to a count of 5 or 6, indicating almost no cancer activity. The shark cartilage also returned the minister's outward appearance to its normal, healthy, pink glow, and he no longer had to urinate using a catheter.[125]

Laetrile

General Background: Known technically as *amygdalin*, or vitamin B_{17}, Laetrile was first synthesized in 1924.[126] Much of the experimental work on Laetrile has been conducted by Harold

W. Manner, Ph.D., Chairman of the Biology Department at Loyola University, Chicago, whose work is considered to be among the first unbiased studies of the overall value of Laetrile. He reported that Laetrile is virtually nontoxic and that, when used along with vitamin A and certain enzymes, it stimulates the production of antibodies against spontaneous breast tumors in mice. There was complete regression in 76 percent of the mice treated which had mammary carcinomas.[127]

Vitamin C therapy can be an important part of a health maintenance program and can reduce long-term health costs.

The best results using Laetrile are usually obtained when it used in conjunction with proteolytic enzymes, diet, vitamin A and other vitamins and minerals.[128]

Laetrile is a good example of a therapy which is sometimes effective and sometimes not. Between 1975 and 1977, fourteen patients were interviewed in an informal study, as to the benefits derived from Laetrile. Of the twelve responding to the study, three were cured, two were materially helped using Laetrile in conjunction with chemotherapy and/or surgery, and seven died from two to seventeen months after treatment.[129]

Case History: No physician has had more clinical experience with Laetrile than Ernesto Contreras, Sr., M.D., of the Contreras Hospital in Tijuana, Mexico. Dr. Contreras has used Laetrile clinically for more than thirty years on thousands of mostly terminally diagnosed patients with impressive results.

"The best results using Laetrile are usually obtained when it used in conjunction with proteolytic enzymes, diet, vitamin A and other vitamins and minerals."

Many of Dr. Contreras' cases have been reviewed by Alex Duarte, O.D., Ph.D., of Grass Valley, California, a Fellow of the International Academy of Medical Preventics. According to Dr. Duarte, one of Dr. Contreras' patients was a man suffering from severe colon cancer. Using Laetrile alone, Dr. Contreras was able to arrest the cancer, and the man has since been in remission for over fifteen years.

Immune Enhancement Therapies

Immune enhancement therapies are frequently used by alternative physicians to treat cancer. A strong immune system is one of the keys to the delay and prevention of cancer, but the combination of poor nutrition and exposure to pollutants and natural toxins can cripple immune function, as can the aging of the thymus gland.

Immune enhancement therapies seek to restore the immune system to optimum function so that the body can then subdue the cancer. In alternative medicine, this is accomplished without the side effects associated with conventional therapies.

VITAMIN C THERAPY

Cancer tissue liberates an enzyme called hyaluronidase, which dissolves hyalouronic acid (a protective agent of the connective tissue) and allows for the spread of tumors.[130] This observation led two time Nobel laureate Linus Pauling, Ph.D., of Palo Alto, California, to conclude that vitamin C would be of value in curing cancer based on the premise that more collagen fibrils (small, insoluble protein fibers that are often components of a cell) would be formed, providing a more effective wall against the spread of the tumor.[131] A controlled study provided startling evidence that megadoses of vitamin C increased survival time in cancer patients. Patients treated with vitamin C lived an average of 300 days longer than patients who were not given supplemental amounts of vitamin.[132] Perhaps the greatest evidence of the value of large doses of vitamin C in fighting cancer comes from the combined work of Abram Hoffer, M.D., Ph.D., of Victoria, British Columbia, and Dr. Pauling. In a recent study, forty patients with cancer of the breast, ovary, uterus, or cervix continuously received large daily doses of ascorbic acid and other vitamins. Another sixty-one patients with other kinds of cancer followed the same regimen, while thirty-one patients received no vitamin supplements and served as the control group. The control group lived an average of 5.7 months. Of the others, 80 percent of the patients with cancer of the breast, ovary, cervix, or uterus, had a mean survival time of 122 months; while forty-seven patients with the other kinds of cancer lived for an average of seventy-two months. This study shows that the length of life for those using vitamin C was thirteen to twenty-one times longer, than those who did not receive it..[133]

Immuno-Augmentative Therapy (IAT)

General Background: During the 1960s, the late Lawrence Burton, Ph.D, a former senior oncologist at St. Vincent's Hospital in New York City, isolated the four blood protein components used in the immuno-augmentative therapy (IAT), which he developed. Dr. Burton demonstrated that an imbalance in these four blood protein components would lead to the development of cancer. He labeled the four protein components the *tumor antibody*, which destroys cancer cells; the *tumor complement*, which activates the tumor antibody; the *blocking protein*, which inhibits the tumor antibody; and the *deblocking protein*, which neutralizes the blocking protein.

When these four components are balanced, the body is able to subdue cancer cells as part of its normal activity. But if any of the components are out of balance, the body cannot adequately defend itself. For example, if there is too much of the blocking protein, the tumor antibody will be inhibited and unable to vanquish cancer cells. "All cells, when they die, release a blocking protein," Dr. Burton explained. "This prevents further activation of the antibody by its complement, which, in the case of cancer, would be the tumor cell."[134]

The proportions of the four components used in IAT are determined by daily blood analyses. Dr. Burton discovered that by injecting certain amounts of the components into his patients, he could bring about remissions in many forms of cancer, including in patients who were classified as terminally ill. He was quick to point out, however, that his treatment was not a cure for cancer. "It is just like using insulin for diabetes," he said. "It controls the cancer and the patient can live a normal lifespan."[135]

Despite Dr. Burton's low-key approach, by his own admission IAT has achieved tumor reduction, and even complete remission, in 40 to 60 percent of patients. Particularly impressive are the recoveries of patients with advanced colon cancer and *mesothelial* cancer (cancer of the abdomen). According to the NCI, there is a virtual zero five-year survival rate for both of these diseases, with patients with mesothelial cancer normally not surviving longer than four to seven. "We are the court of last resort," Dr. Burton once joked, noting that the patients who came to him had tried everything else first, with their conditions only becoming worse. "Yet, on an overall basis, we are still sending four to six out every ten people home improved." One of his patients who suffered from mesothelial cancer, for example, received IAT treatments for four years. Three years after he finished his treatments, his cancer remained in complete remission.[136]

IAT has also shown good results as a treatment for cancers of the bladder, prostate, and pancreas, as well as for lymphomas. Furthermore, since the IAT process builds on the body's own natural anti-cancer immune function, it is virtually nontoxic. Dr. Burton did admit, however, that IAT was normally unsuccessful in treating bone cancer.

Although Dr. Burton passed away in 1993, IAT is still offered today at the clinic he founded in Freeport on Grand Bahama Island. Gustavo Andrade, M.D., of Tijuana, Mexico, is another physician who has had extensive clinical experience using the IAT method.

Case History: One of Dr. Burton's patients is a seventy-eight-year-old woman, who credits her long-term survival to IAT. In 1968, the woman was diagnosed with endometrial (concerning the mucous membrane that lines the inner surface of the uterus) and uterine cancer. Her physician recommended a hysterectomy (removal of the uterus), which she underwent. She also received radiation therapy. In 1979, she was diagnosed with infiltrating ductal carcinoma of the breast, which had spread to her lymph nodes. Although the breast tumor was very large, she refused to undergo a masectomy. She received further radiation therapy, with only partial results. In 1981, she began IAT treatments with Dr. Burton, and achieved complete remission of her condition. Twelve years later, she remains cancer free, and each year has an annual checkup at the clinic Dr. Burton founded in Freeport.

"Dr. Burton discovered that by injecting certain amounts of the components he discovered into his patients, he could bring about remissions in many forms of cancer, including in patients who were classified as terminally ill."

Livingston Therapy

General Background: In the 1940s, the late Virginia Livingston, M.D., discovered a bacterium which she called *Progenitor cryptocides*. According to Dr. Livingston, this bacterium exists in all of us from the moment of conception until the moment of death, and she claimed that it is responsible for cancer. Like other pleomorphic microorganisms, *Progenitor cryptocides* can change size and shape, becoming as small as a virus and as large as a bacterial microbe. It can be viewed in all of its forms under a darkfield microscope. Dr. Livingston discovered that the bacterium caused cancer in experimental animal studies, and she found it in virtually all human and animal cancers.

Foods can also be contaminated with Progenitor cryptocides, including beef, chicken, eggs, and milk, according to Dr. Livingston. This means that eating such foods can provide a basis for the infectious transmission of cancer. Because of this, the Livingston diet emphasizes fresh, raw or lightly cooked plant foods.

The basis of Livingston therapy is restoration of the immune system using a diet of vegetarian raw foods, vaccines, and nutritional supplements. The vaccines are derived from a culture of the patient's own bacteria "It comes from the patient's own tissues, either from the tumor, the urine, the blood or the pleura [lung fluid], and it's specific for each person" Dr. Livingston explained.[137] The Bacillus Calmette-Guerin (BCG) vaccine is also used, which is a mild tuberculin vaccine that stimulates the immune system. According to Dr. Livingston, BCG helps stimulate white blood cells to kill cancer cells. It's important to be certain that the patient has enough white blood cells to receive the vaccine, she noted, otherwise a waiting period is necessary for the white blood cell count to rise.

Dr. Livingston also discovered that pleomorphic microbes secrete a hormone that is remarkably similar to *human chorionic gonadotropin* (HCG). During pregnancy, HCG coats the placenta, safeguarding the fetus from being destroyed by the mother's immune system. Dr. Livingston theorized that when a cancer cell forms, stimulated by Progenitor cryptocides, it is protected by a similar hormone. Her research, though initially ridiculed, was proven accurate through the work of researchers at Rockefeller University, Princeton Laboratories, and Allegheny General Hospital who found that all cancer cells do indeed contain HCG.[138]

Another key to Dr. Livingston's program was her discovery that naturally occurring *retinoid abscisic acid* (a plant hormone and derivative of vitamin A) neutralizes HCG production. According to Dr. Livingston, abscisic acid is a plant growth regulator which "causes seedlings to go to sleep in the Fall."[139] Similarly, Dr. Livingston found, abscisic acid may cause cancer microbes to go to sleep. Her research has shown that cancer patients tend to have low levels of this naturally occurring anti-cancer chemical. Foods rich in abscisic acid include carrots, green leafy vegetables, nuts, seeds, and cereals. Unfortunately, the liver must be functioning optimally in order to convert vitamin A to abscisic acid, and the acid can be destroyed by cooking. However, the liver function of cancer patients is often subpar. To help counteract this condition, Dr. Livingston recommended drinking carrot juice with liver powder, noting that the enzymes present in the liver powder break down the vitamin A into abscisic acid. She also advocated eating a near raw foods diet as a method of preserving their abscisic acid content. No sugar or refined flours, or high-sodium foods are allowed, and few, if any, animal foods, because of their high likelihood of being contaminated.[140]

Dr. Livingston reported success with advanced breast cancer patients, as well as individuals with cancer of the esophagus (which had spread to the liver), colon cancer, Hodgkin's disease, and melanoma. Many of these cancers had spread to other portions of the body, and the patients were considered terminal. Although she passed away in 1990, Dr. Livingston's work is being carried on by other physicians. Using the Livingston vaccine, they have noted shrinkage or disappearance of tumors, as well as complete remissions in patients with lymphocytic leukemia and malignant lymphoma.[141]

According to Neil Nathan, M.D., who carries on Dr. Livingston's work at the Livingston Foundation in San Diego, California, the success of the Livingston therapy depends on whether or not the cancer has metastasized. "When we work with people whose tumors are localized, such as in the prostate or the breast, and who haven't received chemotherapy or radiation, the remission rate ranges from 70 to 95 percent," he says. "If the cancers have moved into the bone, local lymph nodes or other areas that we consider signs of metastasis, then the remission rate drops down to 40 to 50 percent. And in cases that are considered terminal, meaning the cancer has spread to the major organs, and the patient has maybe three months to live according to conventional standards, we have about a 20 percent rate of remission. But even that rate is still better than what conventional medicine offers."

Case History: One of Dr. Livingston's patients was a woman diagnosed with an inoperable inflammatory carcinoma of the breast, which is usually rapidly fatal. Two days after beginning Dr. Livingston's treatment, the woman's breast returned to its normal pink color. She returned home, and her doctors could not understand how the tumor had become operable. Knowing that here cancer was an extremely vicious type of cancer, the woman chose to have a mastectomy as a safeguard. But when her doctors did the pathology report, the tumor that had been diagnosed in the previous biopsy was found to be completely gone, and her lymph nodes were clear. Today, the woman reports that she feels better than she has in years, due to following the Livingston program.

Metabolic Therapies

The practitioners of metabolic therapies feel that, because many factors are involved in the onset of cancer, no one therapy will be enough to treat it. Metabolic treatments include an eclectic mix of diet and nutritional supplementation, herbal medicine, detoxification, immune stimulation, and enzyme therapy. The therapeutic goal of such therapies is to rebuild and revitalize all of the body's life-sustaining functions, thereby eliminating all traces of disease.

Issels' Whole Body Therapy

General Background: Josef Issels, M.D., of Germany, came to the conclusion that the only way to attack cancer was not to attack the local manifestation—the tumor—as most conventional therapies do, but rather to strengthen the entire body. "Dr. Issels believes that chronic and especially malignant diseases can only develop if the metabolism and the natural resistance of an organism is negatively changed by various so-called 'causal factors,'" says Wolfgang Woppel, M.D., of Germany, an associate of Dr. Issels. "These include genetic traits, microbes, dental amalgams and infections, abnormal intestinal flora, faulty diet, neural interferences, chemical toxins, and radiation."

From this realization Dr. Issels developed his *"ganzheitstherapie,"* or whole body therapy, combining many different modalities in a single protocol to improve the body's natural defense systems. One of the first things his program recommends is the removal of infected teeth and dental amalgams (mercury amalgams), because these are a tremendous source of toxic stress on the body.

A patient's diet is also closely addressed, particularly the removal of tobacco, coffee, tea, and other harmful substances from the diet. Organic whole foods are stressed, along with proper digestive support, in the form of acidophilus. Dr. Issels therapy also addresses the patients' emotional state, by having patients unload toxic emotions like stress and anger. This is accomplished through a form of informal psychotherapy.

On top of this framework, Issels' program employs oxygen therapies such as the haemotogenic oxidation therapy. In this therapy, blood is drawn from the patient and oxygen is bubbled through it. Ultraviolet rays are then applied and the blood is left to settle for up to an hour, then returned to the patient by intravenous drip. This procedure sterilizes and reactivates the blood causing an aggressive immune response to be unleashed on the cancer.

Dr. Issels whole body therapy also uses various hyperthermia techniques to reenergize the immune system. By provoking a fever in the body, Dr. Issels found that he could increase the number of disease-destroying leukocytes (white corpuscles) in the bloodstream. His program also employs vaccines for specific types of cancer, using ultrafiltrates of cancer tissues in much the same way as modern vaccines use infectious agents to stimulate antibody production.

In one long-term study, Dr. Issels' treatment protocol was applied to 252 terminal patients who had previously undergone conventional surgery and radiation therapy. After five years, 16.6 percent were still alive and functioning. After fifteen years on the program, though, over 92 percent of the original survivors were still alive and showed no signs of cancer.[142]

In another study, 370 cancer patients, with various types and in various stages of the disease, followed Dr. Issels' program. After five years, 87 percent were still alive and showing no signs of the cancer recurring. Further research showed the relapse rate to be only 13 percent with Dr. Issels' whole body therapy.[143]

Since Dr. Issels has retired, there are two doctors keeping his work going, Dr. Woppel and Ahmed Elkadi, M.D., of Panama City, Florida. Dr. Elkadi employs Dr. Issels' program with his own refinements, such as the use of the herbal compound *Nigella sativa*, or black seed spice. With this herb Dr. Elkadi has observed a 55 percent enhancement of the helper T-cells and the suppressor T-cells, and a 30 percent enhancement of natural killer cells activity.

Case History: A patient with cancer of the lymph glands, and multiple sclerosis had tried many remedies. None of them worked until he met Dr. Issels, who examined his mouth and teeth. Dr. Issels told the man there were two things wrong; he had too many fillings in his mouth, and his tonsils needed to be removed. As soon as the fillings and tonsils were removed, the toxins in the man's body began to drain again, and his lymph nodes, which were the size of Easter eggs, began to shrink. Today, the patient is much improved and continues to work in the publishing industry.

Revici Therapy

General Background: One of the underlying principles of Revici therapy is that the health of the body depends on a state of balance between the building processes (anabolic), such as cell growth, and the breakdown processes (catabolic), such as digestion. Developed by Emanuel Revici, M.D., of New York City, this therapy employs the use of selenium, as well as other elements such as calcium, copper, and oxygen, to re-balance the body's chemistry. These elements are administered intravenously in a lipid (fat) form. This also allows for greater penetration of membranes, more efficient transportation in the circulatory system, greater concentration in the tumor, and a slow, but persistent reaction. This also allows for megadoses of these compounds to be taken without causing any toxicity, and serves as a tumor targeting and antiviral agent as well.

At the 1981 ACS Science Writers Forum, it was reported that "the results of recent experiments demonstrate that selenium supplementation to the diet of mice significantly inhibits both viral and chemical carcinogen-induced tumor formation in the mammary gland." Other experiments also found selenium to inhibit "tumors in the skin, liver, and colon." In addition, a clinical trial of Dr. Revici's methods was conducted in Belgium by Professor Joseph Maisin, Director of the Cancer Institute of the University of Louvain, and President of the International Union against Cancer, on twelve advanced cancer patients. Professor Maisin reported dramatic improvements in nine of the twelve patients (75 percent), including the regression of tumors and metastases.[144]

In spite of these studies, Dr. Revici nearly had his medical license revoked by the state of New York in the 1980s. However, intensive lobbying in the state capitol led to a 1988 hearing held by Congressman Guy Molinari to address the issue of alternative cancer therapies, particularly the work of Dr. Revici. Among those testifying was Seymour Brenner, M.D., a radiation oncologist who practices in New York State. Dr. Brenner wrote to Congressman Molinari, detailing some ten patients' histories of successful treatment with Revici therapy.[145] As a result, Dr. Revici was able to retain his medical license.

Case History: A thirty-four-year-old man who had undergone above-the-knee amputation of his left leg because of bone cancer, subsequently had the cancer spread to both sides of his lung, as well as to both of his kidneys. In October, 1980, the patient began Dr. Revici's program, and immediately gained back twenty pounds in weight. A chest x-ray in 1981 showed stabilization of the tumors in his lungs, while other tests showed that the tumor in his right kidney had almost completely disappeared and that the tumor in his left kidney had also decreased in size. As of 1988, the patient was reported to be "currently well, with no progressive disease," according to Dr. Brenner.[146]

Gerson Therapy

General Background: The Gerson therapy was developed by Max Gerson, M.D., a German doctor who emigrated to the United States in the 1930s. Shortly after graduating from medical school, Dr. Gerson began to experience severe migraine headaches. He reasoned that he could alleviate his problem by reworking his diet. After succeeding in doing so, he found that he able to successfully treat tuberculosis patients with diet alone as well. He then took the next leap, which was to treat cancer patients with his diet. He also treated both Dr. Albert Schweitzer and his wife for various health problems, including diabetes. A grateful Dr. Schweitzer said of Dr. Gerson, "I see in him one of the most eminent geniuses in medical history."

Dr. Gerson believed that cancer would not occur in bodies with properly balanced and functioning livers, pancreases, thyroid, and immune systems. He found that he could reverse the majority of cancer in patients that came to him with his dietary regime, which consisted of a low-salt vegan diet, supplemented ten times a day with freshly crushed fruit (primarily apple) and vegetable (primarily carrot) juices, taken at hourly intervals. This acts to innundate the body with the nutrients from nearly twenty pounds of fresh, organic foods. In addition, patients take three or four coffee enemas a day for detoxification and pain relief. There is also supplementation with various substances such as pepsin, potassium, lugol's solution (a source of supplementary iodine), niacin, pancreatin (a digestive enzyme culled from bovine pancreas), and thyroid extracts, which are taken to stimulate various organ functions, especially the liver and thyroid.

What Dr. Gerson discovered was that cancer patients had an excess of sodium, far outweighing the potassium in their bodies. The sodium acts as a poison in the body, because it is an enzyme inhibitor, whereas potassium is an enzyme activator. The fruits and vegetables in the diet are used to correct this sodium and potassium imbalance. This in turn helps revitalize the liver so it can begin to rid the body of malignant cells again. The coffee enemas then aid in the elimination of these dead cancer cells.

> *"I see in [Max Gerson] one of the most eminent geniuses in medical history."*
>
> —Albert Schweitzer

Many of Dr. Gerson's cancer patients, whom he treated in the 1940s and 1950s, are documented to have lived on in good health for many decades after their treatment period.[147] Although Dr. Gerson passed away in 1959, his work is being carried on by his daughter, Charlotte, and her staff at the Gerson Institute in Tijuana, Mexico.

Case History: A woman in her early forties was diagnosed with advanced melanoma and cervical cancer. Six months after beginning the Gerson therapy, a second biopsy revealed that her cervical cancer had completely disappeared. Similarly, her melanoma vanished. That was over twelve years ago, and she has been free of cancer since.

Kelley's Nutritional-Metabolic Therapy

General Background: Individual nutrition, detoxification, and supplemental pancreatic enzymes make up the therapy that was advanced by William Donald Kelly, D.D.S., now retired to Washington State. A dentist by training, Dr. Kelley developed his protocol in response to his own pancreatic cancer, which he faced in the late 1960s.

One of the main points of Dr. Kelley's therapy is that cancer is often caused by the body's inability to effectively metabolize protein. This inability can be linked to improper amounts of proteolytic enzymes, according to Dr. Kelley, who asserts that these protein-digesting pancreatic enzymes are the body's first defense against tumors, rather than the immune system. Dr. Kelley's theory is supported by research which has shown that not only does the pancreas secrete digestive enzymes into the small intestine, it also secretes them into the bloodstream where they can reach all cells in the body, including cancer cells which they digest and subdue.[148]

Dr. Kelley's metabolic detoxification therapy calls for the restriction of protein intake, while emphasizing a diet of whole grains, fruits, and vegetables. This is additionally supplemented with proteolytic enzymes as well as raw juices. Each person, though, has different nutritional needs and different capacities for the absorption of food and therefore needs to be dealt with on an individual basis, according to Dr. Kelley's theory, which divides patients into ten different metabolic types, with slow-oxidizing vegetarians at one end and fast-oxidizing carnivores at the other. Thus, for each patient, a different version of Dr. Kelley's program may be indicated. Dr. Kelley also recommends coffee enemas as a detoxifying agent.

Nicholas Gonzalez, M.D., of New York City, a classically trained immunologist, currently employs a cancer treatment which to a large extent is based on Kelley's therapy. Dr. Gonzalez' protocol includes six basic concepts first put forward by Dr. Kelley—an appropriate diet for each individual, intensive nutritional support, photomorphogen (raw beef organs and glands) support, digestive aids such as hydrochloric acid, proteolytic enzyme supplementation, and detoxification.[149]

Dr. Gonzalez did not just blindly adopt Dr. Kelley's work though. Rather, his belief that some of Kelley's protocols were valid came as a result of a five hundred-page, five-year study of Dr. Kelley's cancer patients. The study was conducted under the auspices of Robert Good, M.D., Ph.D., former President of Memorial Sloan-Kettering Cancer Center.

Dr. Gonzalez originally tracked fifty of Dr. Kelley's patients, ages ranging from twenty-one to seventy-one, all of whom were diagnosed as terminal or with extremely poor prognosis, encompassing twenty-five different types of cancer. The results were astonishing as Dr. Gonzalez discovered the average survival time for the group was ten years and climbing.

"The ultimate goal for all of us is to try and get trials so we can get our therapies tested. Then if it really does work, the world will have the documented facts to confirm it."
—Nicholas Gonzalez, M.D.

To further test Dr. Kelley's results, Dr. Gonzalez decided to track twenty-two of his patients who had been diagnosed with pancreatic cancer, since this form of cancer had a five-year survival rate with conventional medical therapies of nearly zero percent, as well as a life expectancy of only two to three months. Ten of the patients who only consulted with Dr. Kelley once and then did not follow his treatment program survived only an average of sixty-seven days, or just over three months. Seven who followed his program only partially survived an average of 233 days, or nearly eight months. The five patients who followed his program closely though, had a median survival rate of nine years as of 1987; four of the five were still alive and one had died of Alzheimer's disease.[150]

Dr. Gonzalez, in his own practice today, has found that about 80 percent of his patients do well on his application of Dr. Kelley's therapy. "It is essential, though, that each patient comply 100 percent with their individual program in order for them to survive," says Dr. Gonzalez, adding that most of his patients "usually have already received radiation and chemotherapy, and may have been told they have only a few months to live by their previous physicians."

While Dr. Gonzalez' 80 percent success may be accurate and encouraging, it still needs to be verified through controlled trials. According to Dr. Gonzalez the NCI is currently reviewing his patient record in view of just such a trial. "The ultimate goal for all of us is to try and get trials so we can get our therapies tested," says Dr. Gonzalez. "Then if it really does work, the world will have the documented facts to confirm it."

Case History: A twenty-eight year old lawyer suffering from leukemia was brought to Dr. Gonzalez. Her leukemia was in its most advanced stage referred to as "blast crisis," and she had been told by her previous doctors that she had only a few days to live. Dr. Gonzalez kept her alive, and after three months on his protocol, she became noticeably better. A year later, she was in complete remission and resumed her career.

American Biologics

General Background: One of the largest metabolic treatment center is the American Biologics Hospital in Tijuana, Mexico, which is headed by Robert Bradford, D.Sc. The Medical Director is Rodrigo Rodriguez, M.D. and the Information Officer is Michael Culbert, D.Sc. American Biologics (AB) offers a multifactorial array of cancer therapies. According to Dr. Culbert, AB treats the human not the tumor. One of the primary modalities used is Laetrile, since AB is one of the pioneering institutes in Laetrile use. Dr. Culbert points out that various indigenous populations have been cancer free because the natural components of their diet contain significant Laetrile content.

Diet is another factor addressed by AB, including the elimination of sugar, excess animal protein, refined carbohydrates, and stimulants such as caffeine. "We also incorporate those foods that are rich in Laetrile, such as apricot kernals, cherry stones, and bitter almonds," says Dr. Culbert. "Nutritional supplementation is given ,as well, in the form of vitamin C and other antioxidants to scavenge free radicals."

In addition, AB uses embryonic live cell therapy to bolster the patient's endocrine system. Cerebral and adrenal tissue are used, among many things, to replenish DHEA, a hormone necessary for the proper function of the immune system. Finally, detoxification therapy is used through enemas and colonic irrigation.

In 1987, AB presented to the Office of Technology Assesment, an arm of the United States Congress, an overview of their first 5000 cancer cases. More than 90 percent of these cases were supposedly terminal. Of these cases, AB achieved a five year survival rate with few or no symptoms of about 20 percent.

Case History: A male patient at American Biologics had a very serious tumor. "He was an engineer with *rhabdomyosarcoma* (a type of bone cancer) of the thigh the size of a bowling bowl," Dr. Culbert relates. "His doctors told him that he would have to have his leg and part of his groin removed, and have to undergo radiation. We placed him was on a total metabolic program, and ozone gas was also infused directly into the tumor on intermittent days with herbal poultices also applied. Over a couple of months, the tumor became soft. Then it popped open and oozed out. At last report, ten years later, the patient was still doing well."

Evers Therapy

General Background: The International Medical Center (IMC) in El Paso, Texas and Juarez, Mexico, is another major metabolic treatment center. This clinic was the brainchild of H. Ray Evers, M.D., a pioneering alternative physician who spent most of his practice in Alabama. therapy. Dr. Evers passed away in 1990 at the age of seventy-seven. Treatment at IMC incorporates various alternative medicine protocols which Dr. Evers developed for various conditions, including cancer. His hand picked successor is Francisco R. Soto, MD.

According to Dr. Soto, patients at IMC receive a thorough physical examination, biochemical profile, bioelectrical profile, complete blood count (CBC), CAT and MRI scans, and ultrasound. When appropriate, a biopsy is done to determine the stage of the disease. "Treatments rest on a foundation of nutrition, oxidative therapy (hyperbaric oxygen, ozone, and Koch vaccination), and antioxidant Eversol chelation therapy," Dr. Soto says. "In addition, cell therapy is administered, in the form of frozen live cell, thymus, and whole cell injections, as well as magnetic field therapy, Laetrile, shark cartilage, and a detoxification program."

Case History: In August 1987, William Carson, a retired commercial banker was diagnosed with a Stage IV bladder cancer. A biopsy showed that the tumor was growing directly on the lining of his bladder and there was strong indication that it had invaded the muscle wall of the bladder. His urologist advised him to have his bladder removed within the next two weeks. Instead, Carson went to Dr. Evers. He received chelation therapy, along with megadoses of vitamin C. In addition, he was placed in a hyperbaric oxygen chamber to increase the oxygen content of his blood and to enhance the effectiveness of the chelation therapy. His bladder cancer went into a complete remission within 20 days. Nearly six years later, Carson remains cancer free and is now the U.S. Director of IMC.

Herbal Therapy

For the greater part of human history, nature has provided medical professionals with their pharmaceutical agents. And nature's pharmacy continues to play an integral role in the healing profession. Taxol, a promising new chemotherapy agent, is derived from the Pacific yew tree. Penicillin is derived from a mold. Aspirin, although now made synthetically, was first derived from the bark of the willowgreen tree. Digitalis comes from foxglove. Some 3,000 or more plant species have been used in the healing of cancer. In fact, the anticancer drugs *vincristine sulfate* and *vinblastine sulfate* were discovered by looking at the healing plants of native healers of Madagascar who used the herb periwinkle.

In China, *Fu Zheng* therapy relies upon ginseng and astragalus, among other herbs. The Journal of the American Medical Association, reported that life expectancy doubled for patients with rapidly advancing cancers when Chinese herbs were added to their treatment plan. JAMA noted that in general, "Patients who received Fu Zheng therapy survived longer and tolerated their treatment better than those patients who were treated by Western medicine alone. In addition, the five year survival rate was twice as high among patients with nasopharyngeal [nasal passage and pharynx] cancer (53 percent versus 24 percent)."[151]

Hoxsey Therapy

General Background: Perhaps no therapy has had as colorful a history as that of the late Harry Hoxsey. An herbal folk healer with a fanatical following, Hoxsey's herbal therapies date to the 1840s and his great-grandfather who bred horses in Illinois. One of his horses had cancer on its leg and was put to pasture to die. Instead, the horse began grazing on certain plants in the pasture, and was cured. Hoxsey's great-grandfather later mixed the plants into a salve and used it to treat horses. Hoxsey's father, who was a veterinarian, also used the salve. Harry Hoxsey, who assisted his father, also learned how to make the salve.[152]

The Hoxsey therapy is a mix of internal and external herbal preparations, including an emphasis on diet, vitamin and mineral supplements, as well as personal counseling. Although vigorously attacked by the ACS, Hoxsey herbal remedies were also used by Native Americans to treat cancer and the formula contain herbs with established anticancer properties.[153]

Among the herbs used in the Hoxsey external formula is *Sanguinaria canadensis,* also known as bloodroot, which has been used by Lake Superior Native Americans to treat cancer. Doctors using bloodroot paste in the 1960s healed cancers of the nose, external ear, and other organs.[154] The major component of the internal tonic is potassium iodide. The herbs include red clover, buckthorn bark, burdock root (which has known antimutagenic properties[155]), *stillingia root*, berberis root, poke berries and root, licorice root, *Cascara amarga*, and prickly ash bark. Actual proportions and methods of extraction have been kept secret.[156] Patients taking the tonics are cautioned to avoid tomatos, alcohol, processed flour, and vinegar, because of their ability to negate the tonic's effect. Cancers which have responded most favorably to the Hoxsey tonics include lymphoma, melanoma, and skin cancer. The Hoxsey method was placed on the ACS Unproven Methods List in 1968. The Hoxsey Clinic, located in Tijuana, Mexico, estimates that 80 percent of the patients who use the Hoxsey formula benefit substantially.

Case History: In 1979, a fifty-six-year-old woman was sent home to die after her surgeons found a tumor the size of a ping pong ball in her right ovary. Exploratory surgery had shattered the tumor into several pieces, causing it to spread throughout her body. Her colon and liver were particularly affected.

The woman visited the Hoxsey Clinic to begin treatment. Taking the tonic daily, she began to feel better within a few weeks. She continued the treatment for six years, at which point she was able to discontinue taking the treatments, due to full restoration of her health. Today, fourteen years after receiving a death sentence from her doctor, she remains vigorously healthy.

Self-Care

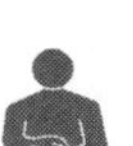

• Biofeedback Training • Guided Imagery • Light Therapy • Meditation

Hydrotherapy: Hyperthermia: apply one to two times weekly. Constitutional hydrotherapy: apply two to five times weekly.

***Juice Therapy*:** • Carrot, beet (roots and tops) • Fresh raw cabbage and carrot juice. • Grape, black cherry, black currant • Wheatgrass juice • Asparagus juice • Fresh apple juice • Carrot, celery • Carrot, spinach • Carrot, cabbage

Professional Care

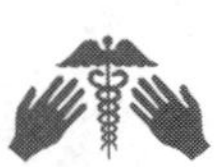

• Cell Therapy • Chelation Therapy • Enzyme Therapy • Fasting • Magnetic Field Therapy • Traditional Chinese Medicine

Oxygen Therapy: Hydrogen Peroxide Therapy, Ozone Therapy

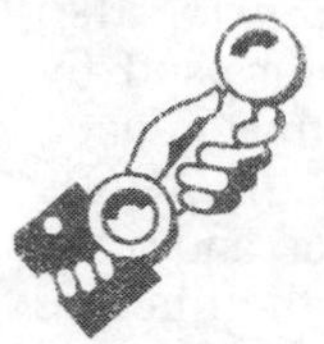

Where to Find Help

The following organizations provide information about the alternative therapies discussed in this chapter. They can also provide referrals to patients.

The Alliance for Alternative Medicine
P.O. Box 59
Liberty Lake, WA 99019
(509) 255-9246
A political action group for freedom of choice in medicine. Also provides information about alternative treatment centers and support groups.

Arlin J. Brown Information Center
P.O. Box 251
Fort Belvoir, VA 22060
(703) 752-9511
A clearinghouse for information regarding alternative cancer therapies. Information available upon request.

Cancer Control Society
2043 North Berendo Street
Los Angeles CA 90027
(213) 663-7801
Provides listings and information on alternative cancer treatment centers and patients who have recovered from various cancers using alternative therapies. Particular emphasis on metabolic therapies. Also sponsors an annual convention showcasing 40-50 alternative practitioners who treat cancer.

Foundation for Advancement in Cancer Therapy
P.O. Box 1242
Old Chelsea Station
New York, NY 10113
(212) 741-2790
A clearinghouse for information regarding alternative cancer therapies, emphasising nutritional and metabolic approaches.

International Association for Cancer Victors and Friends
7740 West Manchester Avenue
Suite 110
Playa del Rey, CA 90293
(310) 822-5032
Provides information and listings on alternative cancer treatment centers and patients who have recovered from cancer using alternative methods. Focus is on cancer treatments and scientific research conducted around the world.

People Against Cancer
P.O. Box 10
Otho, Iowa 50569
(515) 972-4444
A nonprofit, grassroots membership organization dedicated to cancer prevention and medical freedom of choice. Provides counseling and information on alternative cancer treatments.

World Research Foundation
15300 Ventura Boulevard
Suite 405
Sherman Oaks, CA 91403
(818) 907-5483
Large research library of alternative medicine. Library is open to the public. Provides a computer search and printout of specific health issues for a nominal fee.

Resources for Specific Therapies

714X

C.O.S.E., Inc.
5270 Fontaine
Rock Forest, Quebec, Canada J1N3B6
(819) 564-7883

Antineoplaston Therapy

Burzynski Clinic
6221 Corporate Drive
Houston TX 77036
(713) 777-8233

Chelation Therapy

American College of Advancement of Medicine
23121 Verdugo Drive
Suite 204
Laguna Hills, CA 92653
(714) 583-7666
(800) 532-3688

Gerson Therapy

Gerson Institute
P.O. Box 430
Bonita, CA 91908
(619) 472-7450

Centro Hospitalario Internationale del Pacifico, S.A.
Playa, Tijuana, Mexico

Hoxsey Therapy

Bio-Medical Center
P.O. Box 727
615 General Ferreira
Colonia Juarez
Tijuana, Mexico 22000
011 52 66-84-9011
011 52 66-84-9081
011 52 66-84-9082
011 52 66-84-9376

Hydrazine Sulfate

Syracuse Cancer Research Institute
Presidential Plaza
600 East Genesee Street
Syracuse, NY 13202
(315): 472-6616

Immuno-Augmentative Therapy (IAT)

Immuno-Augmentative Therapy Center
P.O. Box F-2689
Freeport, Grand Bahama
(809) 352-7455

IAT Patients Support Group
Mr. Frank Wiewel
P.O. Box 10
Otho, IA 50569-0010
(515) 972-4444

Issel's Whole Body Therapy

Akbar Clinic
4000 East 3rd Street
Panama City, FL 32404
(904) 763-7689

Kelley's Nutritional-Metabolic Therapy

Nicholas Gonzales, M.D.
737 Park Avenue
New York, NY 10021
(212) 535-3993

Laetrile and Shark Cartilage

Hospital Ernesto Contreras
Paseo Playas de Tijuana, No. 19
Tijuana, B.C., Mexico
011 52-66-80-1850
(800) 262-0212 (California)
(800) 523-8795 (Rest of U.S.A.)

Livingston Therapy

Livingston Foundation Medical Center
3232 Duke Street
San Diego, CA 92110
(619) 224-3515

Revici Therapy

Emanuel Revici, M.D.
26 East 36th Street
New York, NY 10016
(212) 685-0111

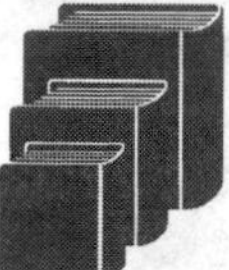

Recommended Reading

Beating the Odds. Marchetti, Albert, M.D. Chicago, IL: Contemporary Books, 1988.
An overview of alternative cancer treatments that have proven successful in treating cancer.

Cancer and Nutrition. Simone, Charles B., M.D. Garden City Park, New Jersey: Avery Publishing Group, 1992.
An authoritative overview outlining a ten point plan for the prevention and treatment of cancer using nutrition. Includes a discussion of the various risk factors which contribute to cancer and how to minimize them.

The Cancer Industry. Moss, Ralph, Ph.D. New York: Paragon House, 1989.
A thorough exploration of the political and economical forces behind the suppression of alternative treatments for cancer.

Cancer Therapy. Moss, Ralph, Ph.D. New York: Equinox Press, 1992.
An in-depth review of alternative medicine therapies used to treat cancer, including contact addresses and phone numbers.

The Complete Guide To Cancer Prevention. Dreher, Henry. New York: Harper and Row, 1988.
A comprehensive guide to preventing cancer using nutrition in combination with preventative environmental and psychological measures.

The Conquest of Cancer. Livingston-Wheeler, Virginia., M.D. New York: Franklin Watts, 1984.
An outline of Livingston Therapy as it applies to treating cancer. Includes the role of diet and the use of the Livingston vaccine.

Options: The Alternative Cancer Therapy Book. Walters, Richard. Garden City Park, New Jersey: Avery Publishing Group, 1993.
A complete and up-to-date overview of all available alternative cancer therapies, including an explanation of how they work and quidelines for selecting an appropriate treatment. Also includes a comprehensive resource guide.

The Persecution and Trial of Gaston Naessens. Bird, Christopher. Tiburon, CA: H. J. Kramer, 1991.
Highlights the work of Gaston Naessens in the field of cancer and other illnesses, including 714X, and the trial he faced because of his discoveries.

Sharks Don't Get Cancer. Lane, I. William, Ph.D., and Comac, Linda, Garden City Park, NY: Avery Publishing Group Inc., 1992.
This book describes new evidence concerning the cancer preventative properties of cartilage. Shark cartilage appears to slow the growth of blood vessels which are essential for the rapid growth demonstrated in most malignant tumors.

Third Opinion. Fink, John M. Garden City Park, New Jersey: Avery Publishing Group, 1988.
An international directory of alternative therapy centers for the treatment and prevention of cancer.

Candidiasis

Although widespread, candidiasis, or yeast overgrowth, is generally overlooked by the medical establishment because its symptoms so closely mimic those of other conditions. Alternative physicians, however, recognize the seriousness of candidiasis, and where conventional medicine has often been ineffective in treating candidiasis, various alternative methods offer much hope for success.

Everyone has candida, a form of yeast (*Candida albicans*) normally confined to the lower bowels, the vagina, and the skin. In healthy individuals with strong, functioning immune systems, it is harmless and kept in check by "good" bacteria, called bifidobacteria and acidophilus. But if the balance of the intestinal environment is altered by a compromised immune system or other factors, then opportunistic candida proliferates, infecting other body tissues. The candida becomes pathogenic, transforming from a simple yeast into an aggressive (mycelial) fungus that can severely compromise one's health. This condition is known as candidiasis.

According to James Braly, M.D., Medical Director of Immuno Labs, Inc., in Fort Lauderdale, Florida, the fungal form of candida appears to permeate the gastrointestinal mucosal lining and break down barriers to the bloodstream. "When the fungal form of candida occurs in the body, allergic substances can penetrate into the blood more easily, where they form immense complexes, and perhaps even promote food allergy reactions," Dr. Braly says. Since their symptoms are often interrelated, he emphasizes that candidiasis should usually be treated together with food allergies.

See AIDS, Allergies, Chronic Fatigue Syndrome, Constipation, Female Health, Gastrointestinal Disorders, Male Health, Mental Health, Respiratory Disorders.

Candidiasis can affect areas of the body far removed from candida colonizations in the gastrointestinal tract and vagina. Its symptoms cover a broad spectrum and the condition can cause a number of diseases ranging from allergies, vaginitis, and thrush (a whitish fungus in the mouth or vagina), to an invasion of the genital-urinary tract, eyes, liver, heart, or central nervous system. At its most destructive, candidiasis is involved in autoimmune diseases such as Addison's disease and AIDS. Other symptoms of candidiasis, according to Dr. Braly, include digestive problems such as bloating, cramping, gas and diarrhea, respiratory problems, coughing, wheezing, earaches, central nervous system imbalances, generalized fatigue, and loss of libido.

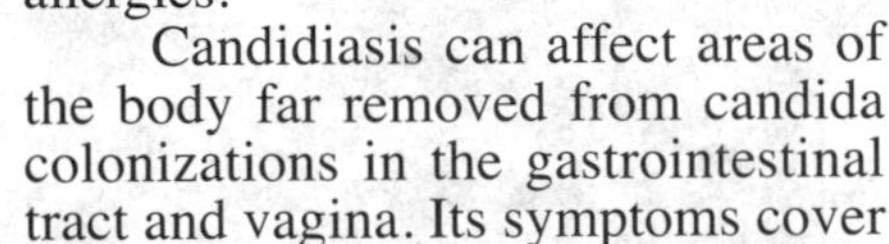

Symptoms of Candidiasis

There is a wide array of candidiasis symptoms depending on individual age, sex, environmental exposures, and immune systems. These include (but are not limited to):[1]

- *Chronic fatigue, especially after eating*
- *Depression*
- *Gastrointestinal problems such as: bloating, gas, intestinal cramps, chronic diarrhea, constipation, or heartburn*
- *Rectal itching*
- *Allergies (including both food and airborne)*
- *Severe premenstrual syndrome*
- *Impotence*
- *Memory loss, severe mood swings, and feeling mentally "disturbed"*
- *Recurrent fungal infections such as "jock itch," athlete's foot, or ringworm*
- *Extreme sensitivity to chemicals, perfumes, smoke, or other odors*
- *Recurrent vaginal or urinary infections*
- *Prostatitis*
- *A feeling of being lightheaded or drunk after minimal wine, beer, or certain foods*

These symptoms worsen in moldy places (such as basements) or in damp climates, and after eating or drinking yeast or foods containing sugar.

Causes of Candidiasis

Since many of its symptoms are shared with other conditions, candidiasis must be diagnosed by examining predisposing factors in a thorough personal medical history. Leon Chaitow, N.D., D.O., of London, England, describes the likely candidate for candida overgrowth as someone whose medical history includes: steroid hormone medication (such as cortisone or corticosteroids), often prescribed for skin conditions such as rashes, eczema, or psoriasis; prolonged or repeated use of antibiotics which are frequently given for urinary and ear infections, sinusitis, bronchitis, and other infections; ulcer medications (such as Tagamet and Zantac); or oral contraceptives. Certain illnesses such as diabetes, cancer, and AIDS can also increase susceptibility to candida overgrowth.

“Since yeast infections enter the body easily through the vagina, and yeast festers in estrogen, women of child-bearing age are more vulnerable to candidiasis.”
—Murray Susser, M.D.

As Leyardia Black, N.D., of Lopez Island, Washington, points out, “Candidiasis is basically a twentieth century disease, a disease resulting from medical developments like antibiotics, birth control pills, and estrogen replacement therapy. And it can be triggered at a very young age, when children are first being treated with antibiotics.”

Dr. Chaitow agrees. “Fully 35 percent of women using birth control pills have associated cases of acute vaginal candidiasis,” he says, “and there are undoubtedly many others who have less pronounced evidence of yeast overgrowth as immune competence is gradually compromised by the hormonal onslaught.”

Murray Susser, M.D., of Santa Monica, California, points out that since yeast infections enter the body easily through the vagina, and yeast festers in estrogen, women of child-bearing age are more vulnerable to candidiasis. Also, women who have been pregnant are susceptible, since hormonal changes encourage candida overgrowth. When men develop candidiasis, antibiotics, high sugar intake, or immune suppression (from illness, toxins, and stress) are usually the root cause.

Frequently, candidiasis is caused by a combination of factors. As Dr. Chaitow explains, “All too often more than one influence is operating. Over a few years, a patient may have had several series of antibiotics for a variety of conditions, while using steroids as well, perhaps in the form of the contraceptive pill. If the patient—most commonly a young woman—also happens to be living on a diet which is rich in sugars, then the candida is very likely to have spread beyond its usual borders into new territory.”

As Dr. Chaitow points out, when the immune system is completely suppressed (as in AIDS), yeast proliferates freely and colonizes the body and bloodstream, leading to septicemia (blood poisoning). In less drastic but more prevalent cases, the immune system is temporarily suppressed and T-helper cells (lymphocytes which pass into the bloodstream to help fight infection) are destroyed. Such immune suppression can be due to any number of factors, such as poor diet (including ingestion of pesticides and preservatives), alcohol use, chemotherapy, radiation, exposure to environmental toxins, antibiotics which

See Antibiotics (in Appendix), Parasitic Infections.

Candidiasis and Parasites

Leon Chaitow, N.D., D.O., of London, England, reports that the presence of parasites in many patients can make candidiasis very difficult to treat, and that parasite infestation encourages yeast overgrowth. When treatment results for candidiasis are poor, Dr. Chaitow recommends testing for coincidental parasitic infection. Before treatment for candidiasis, all parasitic infections must first be successfully treated. Researchers believe that candidiasis can become resistant to treatment because of parasites such as Giardia lamblia, amoebas, nematodes, and cestodes.[2]

Parasites can be identified by means of blood, urine, and fecal testing as well as electroacupuncture biofeedback. According to Dr. Chaitow, this method is also useful for revealing how well the body will tolerate any medications which may be prescribed.

To get rid of identified parasites, Dr. Chaitow advises pursuing a comprehensive herbal medicine approach rather than medication. “In many cases, antiparasitic prescriptive drugs have not proved to be lastingly effective,” he points out. “They may diminish symptoms for one or two months, but the symptoms later return with full force.” Parasites can be fought with high dosage probiotic substances such as Lactobacillus acidophilus, *bifidobacteria, and* Lactobacillus bulgaricus. *Treatment may last from eight to twelve weeks. Dr. Chaitow reports an 80 percent success rate in cases of seriously ill people afflicted with parasites and yeast overgrowth using this method.*

injure or destroy the T-cells, and stress. Consequently, conditions are created for opportunistic infections—and yeast—to grow.

Antibiotics

According to Dr. Susser, antibiotics, life-saving cures for so many diseases, may be the single greatest cause of candidiasis, because antibiotic treatment for infections is nondiscriminatory, killing the "good" intestinal chemistry-balancing bacteria, as well as the "bad" infection-causing bacteria.

Both acidophilus and bifidobacteria produce natural antifungal substances (as well as antibacterial materials) as part of their control mechanism over yeast.[3] One of the activities of "good" bacteria is the manufacture of a B vitamin, biotin, which exerts control over yeast. When biotin is lacking, as a result of damage by antibiotics to acidophilus, bifidobacteria, and the microflora ecology, yeast has a chance to change from its simple yeast form into a different organism, an encroaching mycelial (vegetative) fungus.[4]

> *"Antibiotics, life-saving cures for so many diseases, may be the single greatest cause of candidiasis."*
> —Murray Susser, M.D..

Antibiotics can cause the altered imbalanced intestinal environment that candida requires to change into its mycelial form. Dr. Chaitow explains, "Candida puts down minute rootlets which penetrate the tissues on which the yeast is growing. When this happens to be the inner wall of the intestines, it breaks down the barrier which exists between the closed world of the bowel and the body. Toxic debris, yeast waste products, and partially digested proteins are allowed into the bloodstream, resulting in allergic and toxic reactions."

Healthy bifidobacteria and acidophilus intestinal colonies can usually withstand one or two short episodes of antibiotics without serious harm. If, however, use of antibiotics is frequent or prolonged (as with a course for acne treatment or an infection), then the spread of candida becomes inevitable.

"A vicious cycle may develop as a result," Dr. Chaitow says. "Antibiotics alter the balance of intestinal flora and suppress the immune system. An individual with suppressed immune function is much more susceptible, not only to candidiasis but to bacterial infections, which are then treated with antibiotics, which, in turn, increase the growth of candida, and so on."

Diet

According to Dr. Susser, sugar in the diet can greatly contribute to candida overgrowth. When sugar is eaten, intestinal fermentation creates a toxin called acetaldehyde which affects all of the body's physiological functions, including digestion and hormonal processes. Yeast thrives on sugar in order to grow, therefore, a high-sugar diet is one of the predisposing factors for candidiasis.

Alcohol

Candidiasis patients should also stay away from all alcohol since it is composed of fermented and refined sugar. It is also more toxic than sugar and feeds yeast. According to Dr. Susser, alcohol suppresses the immune system, disturbs the whole adrenal axis, and "you can say empirically that it makes anyone with candida worse."

Some candidiasis sufferers will feel, and appear to be, intoxicated. An unusual symptom of certain people with severe candidiasis is the presence of alcohol in the bloodstream even when none has been consumed.[5] First discovered in Japan, and called "drunk disease," this condition creates strains of *Candida albicans* which turn acetaldehyde (the chemical created by sugar and yeast fermentation) into ethanol. This is a process well understood by distillers of homemade brew. These candidiasis patients whose yeast turns sugar into alcohol are chronically drunk.[6] They have developed what is only half-jokingly called "auto-brewery syndrome."

A medical test has been developed in which, after an overnight fast, the individual is given one hundred grams of pure sugar. Blood samples taken both before the sugar loading, and an hour after, are measured for alcohol. An increase of alcohol indicates yeast "auto-brewery" intoxication.[7]

Another connection between alcohol and candidiasis has been found in a study of 213 alcoholics at a recovery center in Minneapolis. Test and questionnaire results indicated that candidiasis is a common complication of alcoholism due to the combination of high sugar content in alcohol and the inability of alcoholics to assimilate nutrients. Additionally, female alcoholics with candidiasis were significantly sicker than nonalcoholic women with candidiasis.[8]

Many of the symptoms exhibited in alcoholism such as insomnia, depression, loss of libido, headaches, sinusitis/postnasal drip, digestion, and intestinal complaints, overlap with those in candida overgrowth. Obviously, drinking alcohol increases levels of sugar in the system. But other habits of alcoholics are also at fault. Many alcoholics tend to be smokers, for instance, and so are at risk for respiratory infections which are treated with antibiotics.

Treating Candidiasis

Successful treatment of candidiasis first requires the reduction of factors which predispose a patient to candida overgrowth. Secondly, the patient's immune function must be strengthened. Diet, nutritional supplements, herbal medicine, Ayurvedic medicine, and acupuncture are some of the choices alternative physicians use to accomplish these ends.

Diet

In order to overcome candidiasis, sugar must be avoided in all its various forms. These include: sucrose, dextrose, fructose, fruit juices, honey, maple syrup, molasses, milk products (which contain lactose), most fruit (except berries), and potatoes (whose starch converts into sugar). Dr. Black says, "In treating candida, my basic dietary taboos are sweets, alcohol, and refined carbohydrates."

See Ayurvedic Medicine, Herbal Medicine, Nutritional Supplements.

Many candidiasis sufferers also have allergies and sensitivity to various foods. Although *Candida albicans* yeast is not synonymous to yeast in foods, such as bread, a cross-reaction between food yeast and candida frequently occurs. As a result, foods containing or promoting yeast, such as baked goods, alcohol, and vinegar, should be avoided until possible sensitivities are clearly diagnosed.

Dr. Black states that some of her patients are very sensitive to yeast and do better staying away from yeast-containing foods. To test for such sensitivity, she takes patients off all yeast-containing foods for a week. Then she adds such foods back in the diet, one at a time. If the symptoms reappear, then clearly yeast-containing foods should be avoided.

Similarly, Dr. Braly employs a "rotation" diet when he suspects food allergies. On this regimen, patients avoid certain suspected allergic foods and rotate nonallergic food every four or more days. They are then later reintroduced to the suspected foods after three to six months to see if symptoms are provoked. Other foods which may have an allergic potential are also rotated, that is, eaten only every four days, in order to avoid further allergic developments. As a result, a greater variety of food is eaten and more nutrients absorbed, while possible allergic reactions are avoided.

Molds are another aspect of candida sensitivity, according to Dr. Susser. These include food molds (found in cheeses, grapes, mushrooms, and fermented foods), and environmental molds (found in wet climates, in damp basements, in plants, and outdoors). Mold and yeast can also exchange forms. Therefore, the ingestible molds of cheeses and fermented foods should be avoided. Avoiding food yeast and mold does not attack the candida yeast itself, but is an attempt to ease stress on the immune system caused by substances which can trigger allergies.[10]

Even so, food yeast and mold avoidance should be considered case by case for each individual as, in some cases, it may not be necessary. As Dr. Susser says, "My personal opinion is that most anticandida diets are too strict. It is unnecessary to take candida patients off of vinegar and mushrooms unless they are allergic to these things."

Dr. Susser also advises patients to avoid yogurt because of its high sugar content, despite its high concentration of lactobacilli, which suppress "bad" bacteria and keep other organisms under control. He finds that freeze-dried acidophilus supplements in capsule form are more effective in combating bacteria than even unsweetened raw yogurt.

Candida growth can also be fostered in the diet through consumption of meat, dairy, and poultry products due to the heavy use of antibiotics. Traces of antibiotics given to dairy cows can later show up in milk. Meat eaters should make sure that meat is free of antibiotic contamination. Organic (hormone and antibiotic-free) meat and poultry should be consumed whenever possible. For candidiasis patients, seafood (free of mercury toxins) and vegetable protein are preferable, since they are not only antibiotic-free, but lower in fat.

According to Dr. Chaitow, both bifidobacteria and acidophilus should be supplemented dur-

Diagnosing Candidiasis

When symptoms are chronic rather than acute or sudden, Leon Chaitow, N.D., D.O., of London, England, has found that a yeast infection is often to blame. Additionally, if specific symptoms have been treated with little or no success, the diagnosis usually suggests candida. Many physicians have pointed to blood tests showing elevated candida antibodies. However, since most people have candida organisms in their systems, tests will usually show an antibody presence even if the patient is not suffering from candidiasis.[9] Stool specimens and physical examinations are clearly in order, but since there is no single diagnostic test, the individual's complete medical history and response to treatment is the key to proper diagnosis.

ing candidiasis treatment to help repopulate the bowel, and for antifungal activity. This "good" bacteria supplementation is called probiotics. Dr. Chaitow also recommends that other probiotic products, such as *Lactobacillus bulgaricus*, be used to assist the colonizing activities of bifidobacteria and acidophilus.

Nutritional Supplements

According to Dr. Chaitow, a general nutritional support program is frequently needed to help build up immune function and digestive efficiency, which may have become severely depleted or compromised after months or years of chronic candidiasis.

Specific nutritional supplementation can be helpful in rebuilding weakened immune function. Recommended supplements include individual B vitamins (which increase antibody response and are used in nearly every body activity), vitamin C (which stimulates adrenaline and is essential to immune processes), vitamin E (the lack of which depresses immune response), vitamin A (which builds resistance to infection and increases immune response), and beta-carotene (a vitamin A precursor which increases T-cells). Antioxidant immune-boosters, such as selenium, calcium, and zinc, are also very useful in combating candidiasis. Other adrenal stimulants are chromium, magnesium, and glandular adrenal (an extract). Essential fatty acids (such as evening primrose oil) may be considered as well.[11]

> *"In order to overcome candidiasis, sugar must be avoided in all its various forms."*

As routine supplementation, Dr. Braly offers the following regimen: vitamin C (8 to 10 grams daily), vitamin E (one 400 IU capsule daily), evening primrose oil (six to eight capsules daily), max EPA (six capsules daily), pantothenic acid (250 milligrams daily), taurine (500 to 1,000 milligrams daily), zinc chelate (25 to 50 milligrams daily), goldenseal root extract with no less than 5 percent hydrastine (250 milligrams twice a day), *Lactobacillus acidophilus* (one dry teaspoon three times daily; if allergic to milk, use nonlactose acidophilus).

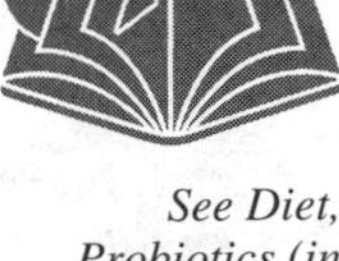

See Diet, Probiotics (in Appendix).

Dr. Braly also recommends supplementation of hydrochloric acid (HCl). He notes that aging, alcohol abuse, food allergies, and nutrient deficiencies create a lack of HCl in the stomach which prevents food from digesting and permits candida overgrowth. Such supplementation, he says, helps restore the proper balance of intestinal flora. Dr. Braly recommends one capsule of HCl and pepsin at the start of meals, increasing cautiously to two to four capsules with each meal if needed.

> **DRUGS AND CANDIDIASIS**
>
> *The use of drugs to treat candidiasis is the accepted practice in the medical community. These drugs can be exorbitantly expensive (as high as fifteen dollars a pill) and toxic, with dangerous side effects.*
>
> *Virender Sodhi, M.D. (Ayurveda), N.D., of Bellevue, Washington, points out that the most popular of these drugs, Nystatin, cannot rid the body of candida because of candida's ability to mutate when under attack into different, eluding strains. Dr. Sodhi formerly used Nystatin with patients but found that even after a year of using it, he was not getting results. According to Dr. Sodhi, Nystatin does not effectively get rid of harmful candida; it only causes* Candida albicans *to mutate into another species of yeast. Therefore, Nystatin treatment can continue for long periods and still have little effect. Meanwhile, Dr. Sodhi claims, Nystatin lingers in the intestine and kills other potentially helpful organisms.*

Herbal Medicine

Herbs are often used to kill harmful yeasts and shore up immune function. They are used in teas, dried in capsules or tablets, or taken in suppository form. Herbs which contain berberine (an alkaloid found in the berbercia family) have proven particularly useful anticandida agents. These include goldenseal, Oregon grape, and barberry.

Berberine fights candida overgrowth, normalizes intestinal flora, helps digestive problems, has antidiarrheal properties, and stimulates the immune system by increasing blood supply to the spleen. Soothing to inflamed mucous membranes, it can be taken as a tea, or in other fluid and dry forms.[12] Other antifungal and antibacterial herbs include German chamomile, aloe vera, ginger, cinnamon, rosemary, licorice, and tea tree oil.[13] Fennel, anise, ginseng, alfalfa, and red clover are also effective.

Dr. Braly's first line of attack on candidiasis is caprylic acid, only after which, if there is no improvement, will he use drugs. Since caprylic acid is readily absorbed into the system, it should be taken in enteric or sustained release forms. Dr. Braly also likes goldenseal root extract, standardized to 5 percent or more of its active ingredient, hydrastine, 250 milligrams twice daily. In a recent study goldenseal seemed to work better in killing off candida than other common anticandida therapies, adds Dr. Braly. Other fatty acids derived from olives (oleic acid) and castor beans have also been found to be useful.

Dr. Susser points out, however, that caprylic acid is far from a panacea. "It's most useful," Dr. Susser says, "when you combine it with a good diet, allergy care, the right nutrients, acidophilus, and other treatments."

Garlic, a well-known folk remedy, is a particularly effective antifungal agent. It has been shown to be effective against some antibiotic resistant organisms and can be taken in capsule and deodorized form. In cases of vaginal candidiasis, it can used as a suppository or douche.

Pau d'arco bark, obtained from a tropical tree native to Brazil, has long been used to treat infections, intestinal complaints, and genital ailments (cystitis, prostatitis). It is reported to be an analgesic, an antiviral, a diuretic, and a fungicide. However, many products claiming to contain pau d'arco have only trace amounts, or even none, of the herb. These products also may use a part of the tree other than the bark, or may have been damaged in production and shipping.[14] When purchasing products with pau d'arco, be sure that they contain lapachol, an organic compound known for its antibiotic action.

Plant Enzymes

The use of plant enzymes should be considered, especially in the early stages of recovery, to help reduce sensitivity reactions, according to Lita Lee, Ph.D, of Eugene, Oregon, who uses plant enzymes with great success. Many of her candidiasis patients come to her after unsuccessfully trying Nystatin, probiotics (the use of friendly bacteria to restore gastrointestinal health), herbs, homeopathics, and fatty acids of many kinds. According to Dr. Lee, "Certain cellulose enzymes will digest the common kinds of yeast, whereas other yeasts sometimes yield to amylase enzymes. I use a very potent probiotic that contains acidophilus, bifidus, and certain cellulose enzymes, which digests yeast and reestablishes 'friendly' bowel bacteria."

Along with this formula, Dr. Lee uses another one containing protease, calcium, and magnesium to cleanse the blood of toxic debris. Dr. Lee states, "This is the best and fastest working treatment for candidiasis I have tried. It also works very well in combination with homeopathics and herbals, and I do not hesitate to add those to the enzyme protocol when needed."

Ayurvedic Medicine

According to Virender Sodhi, M.D. (Ayurveda), N.D., Director of the American School of Ayurvedic Sciences, in Bellevue, Washington, Ayurvedic medicine considers candidiasis to be a condition caused by *ama*, the improper digestion of foods. Dr. Sodhi attributes candidiasis to the widespread use of antibiotics, birth control pills, and hormones and to environmental stresses, as well as to society's addiction to sugar in the diet.

"Ayurvedic medicine believes that these stresses on the system cause carbohydrates to be digested improperly," he says. "Furthermore, the immune system in the gut becomes worn down."

See Acupuncture, Ayurvedic Medicine, Enzyme Therapy.

From an Ayurvedic perspective, Dr. Sodhi believes that successful treatment of candidiasis depends on strengthening the immune system and improving digestion through stimulation of the secretory IgA. This can be accomplished through a combination of treatments. Grapefruit seed oil and tannic acid are useful in treating candida overgrowth, since, according to Dr. Sodhi, they act as antifungals and antibiotics. He uses, additionally, long pepper, *trikatu*, ginger, cayenne, and *neem* before meals to increase immunoglobulin and digestive functions. "These herbs increase the mucous by stimulation of the globular cells in the stomach," Dr. Sodhi says.

Dr. Sodhi begins dosage with a quarter teaspoon of herbs, about thirty minutes before each meal, with dosage increasing gradually to eight to ten teaspoons of herbs a day.

Dr. Sodhi also uses acidophilus, and recommends that his patients cleanse toxins from their systems using the *pancha karma* program, which involves dietary modification and the use of herbs. Results from Dr. Sodhi's approach usually occur within four to six months.

Acupuncture

William Michael Cargile, B.S., D.C., F.I.A.C.A., Chairman of Research for The American Association of Acupuncture and Oriental Medicine, has successfully used acupuncture on patients with candidiasis. He advises, "I would start by using meridians which influence genital function, spleen, and stomach. These are *yin* meridians and they correspond to areas of immune system enhancement. You want to normalize the metabolism of the cells in that part of the body." But Dr. Cargile adds that treatment is "a waste of time" if the patient doesn't also pay attention to nutrition, which he calls "a significant solution."

Dr. Cargile cites a forty-one-year-old female patient who suffered from severe candidiasis. She was a single mother of three children, who had chronic low-grade sore throats and was taking five antibiotic prescriptions. "This had been going on at least three years," Dr. Cargile says. "She was constantly bloated, had colonic distension, and had oral thrush so bad it looked like cotton sticking down her throat. She had clearly destroyed the balance of her intestinal flora."

Dr. Cargile gave her a gargle solution of tea tree oil which reduced the pathogens. He had her change her diet and douche with liquid acidophilus, and gave her acupuncture treatments through meridians which reached the larynx and throat. "After three treatments over a period of three weeks, she was 90 percent better," he states. "She had no oral candida like before, and was well on the road to recovery."

Recovery

Although self-help is therapeutic for candidiasis, a health regimen should be undertaken with the guidance of a practitioner who understands the condition and is willing to try a variety of treatment options.

Recovery from chronic candidiasis seldom takes less than three months and is usually well advanced by six months, but it can take longer to recover completely. Medical studies show that until bowel candida is under control, local manifestations will continue to appear (such as vaginal thrush). Local treatment alone (for thrush, or other symptoms) is not enough.

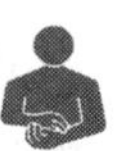

Self-Care

The following therapies can be undertaken at home under appropriate professional supervision:

Aromatherapy: Tea tree oil.

Hydrotherapy: Constitutional hydrotherapy: apply two to five times weekly.

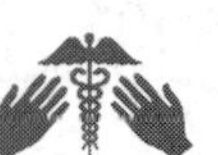

Professional Care

The following therapies should only be provided by a qualified health professional:

• Colon Therapy • Fasting • Magnetic Field Therapy • Orthomolecular Medicine • Traditional Chinese Medicine

Oxygen Therapy: Hydrogen peroxide therapy (IV).

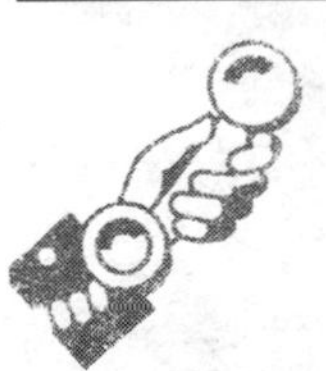

Where to Find Help

For more information on, or referrals for, treatment of candidiasis, contact the following organizations.

American Association of Acupuncture and Oriental Medicine
4101 Lake Boone Trail, Suite 201
Raleigh, North Carolina 27607
(919) 787-5181

The AAAOM is a national professional trade organization of acupuncturists who meet acceptable standards of competency and can provide you with the names and locations of local members.

American Association of Naturopathic Physicians
2366 Eastlake Avenue, Suite 322
Seattle, Washington 98102
(206) 323-7610

Contact them for the location of a licensed naturopathic physician in your area.

American School of Ayurvedic Sciences
10025 NE 4th Street
Bellevue, Washington 98004
(206) 453-8022

This college provides medical training for physicians and health care practitioners, as well as individual courses for lay people. Dr. Virender Sodhi's Ayurvedic, Naturopathic Medical Clinic is also located at this address.

The College of Maharishi Ayur-Veda Medical Center
P.O. Box 282
Fairfield, Iowa 52556
(515) 472-5866

The center provides referrals to health centers, which offer methods of prevention and treatment of a broad range of illnesses. They also train practitioners and provide information to the lay public.

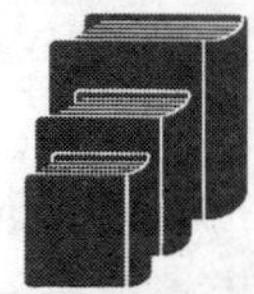

Recommended Reading

Dr. Braly's Food Allergy and Nutrition Revolution. Braly, James, M.D. New Canaan, CT: Keats Publishing, Inc., 1992.
A valuable self-help approach for recovering from food allergies. Includes the latest research on the subject, testing methods, and a detailed treatment method based upon diet and nutrition. Also includes treatment protocols for some forty illnesses linked to food allergies, including candidiasis, and provides a recipe section and meal plan for restoring health.

***Encyclopedia of Natural Medicine*.** Murray, Michael, N.D.; and Pizzorno, Joseph, N.D. Rocklin, CA: Prima Publishing, 1991.
An authoritative guide to naturopathic medicine outlining the basic principles of health and how they can be used to treat over sixty health conditions, including candidiasis. Includes self-help approaches using diet, nutrition, and herbal medicine.

The Missing Diagnosis. Truss, C. Orian, M.D. Birmingham, AL: Missing Diagnosis, Inc., 1985.
A comprehensive overview of candidiasis and how to treat it by a pioneer in the field. (Available from Missing Diagnosis, Inc., P.O. Box 26508, Birmingham, Alabama 35226.)

Solving the Puzzle of Chronic Fatigue Syndrome. Rosenbaum, Michael, M.D.; and Susser, Murray, M.D. Tacoma, WA: Life Sciences Press, 1992.
Although primarily a book about CFS, this comprehensive study also provides a detailed overview of candidiasis, including its causes and best approaches for treatment.

***The Yeast Connection*.** Crook, William, M.D. New York: Vintage Books, 1986.
A landmark book in the field of candidiasis. Provides general information as to the causes of the disorder and outlines an effective treatment plan for dealing with it.

"The significant problems we have cannot be solved at the same level of thinking we were at when we created them."

—Albert Einstein

Children's Health

Natural and alternative approaches can be very effective in maintaining a child's health, as well as treating common childhood illnesses with fewer harmful side effects than conventional medicine. Certain standard medical treatments such as the extensive use of antibiotics and immunizations are being challenged by researchers, physicians, and government officials with regard to their safety and overall effectiveness.

Caring for children is a demanding and sometimes difficult task for parents. When sickness arises, parents may feel frustrated by not being able to identify what is wrong with the child, as well as in not being able to determine the severity of the condition. When dealing with a childhood illness, parents need to evaluate the condition of the child and decide what steps to take. Today, physicians and parents have many options in caring for children, especially in the area of alternative medical care.

Attention to diet as well as nutritional supplementation, and the appropriate use of herbs can have a very beneficial effect on a child's health. In addition, homeopathy, Traditional Chinese Medicine, naturopathic medicine, and Ayurvedic medicine all offer comprehensive approaches to children's health. Though no single approach is meant to replace the advice and supervision of a qualified health care practitioner, safe alternatives to conventional medical care allow parents to make informed decisions about the types of treatment their children should receive.

Raising a Healthy Child

All parents want their children to be healthy and vibrant. Caring for a child is an all-consuming job for parents, one that practitioners of alternative medicine understand as having several important components. These include a stable and loving environment, a comprehensive understanding of what constitutes proper diet and nutrition, and a thorough knowledge of parental health rights, particularly when choosing a health care professional, obtaining and retaining medical records, and deciding whether or not to immunize a child.

Providing a Loving Environment

According to Lendon Smith, M.D., a pediatrician in Portland, Oregon, and author of numerous books on children's health, the physical, mental, and emotional well-being of a child is dependent upon the child's sense of security and self-esteem as provided by the parents. As a result, says Dr. Smith, "The foundation for a child's health may well begin with the parents' relationship, even before conception. Following that, the most important thing for the child, is to be held, massaged, loved, smiled at, and essentially told that he or she is accepted and worthwhile."

Dr. Smith explains that spending time with a child, especially listening to him or her, is vital. Parents would do well to avoid using too many "commands and questions" in speaking to their children. Dr. Smith points out that, "If children only hear commands and questions that act as challenges to a child's behavior, such as, 'What are you doing in there?' or 'Don't get yourself dirty,' they tend to develop a low self-image."

Virender Sodhi, M.D. (Ayurveda), N.D., Director of the American School of Ayurvedic Sciences in Bellevue, Washington, agrees. "A child's sense of security is very fragile. When parents fight, a child's whole world seems threatened. This creates great stress for the child and the result can be a breakdown in the immune system, followed by recurring illnesses." Dr. Sodhi maintains that "growing children should be given a lot of physical affection and verbal encouragement and validation. "This does not spoil the child," he says, "rather, it helps him or her build good self-esteem."

> *"Growing children should be given a lot of physical affection and verbal encouragement and validation. This does not spoil the child, rather, it helps him or her build good self-esteem."*
> —Virender Sodhi, M.D. (Ayurveda), N.D.

Diet and Nutrition

Proper nutrition not only helps to create a strong defense against illness, it is crucial to a child's well-being. For instance, Dr. Smith notes that a majority of early childhood illnesses and infections are due to food allergies, especially the early introduction of cow's milk and/or other allergy-producing food products into a child's diet.

Breast-feeding: Breast-feeding decreases the likelihood of the development of allergic sensitivities to certain foods later in life, according to both Dr. Smith and Dr. Sodhi, who explains that, "Children who are breastfed not only take in vital nutrients from the mother's milk, but they also receive the antibodies necessary to protect them against childhood illnesses such as ear infections and certain types of measles."

Dr. Smith emphasizes that nursing for at least eight to ten months contributes to the child having fewer allergies, better jaw formation, good teeth, and a good dental arch. He mentions that, "If babies are given anything other than breast milk in the first few months of life, food sensitivities may develop. Their intestines are not meant to digest anything other than breast milk. The immature cells lining the intestines will allow foreign food particles to pass through undigested. These bits are antigenic (material that causes immune reactions) and may set up an allergenic or antibody response that the child will never outgrow."

See Allergies, Pregnancy and Childbirth.

Both Drs. Sodhi and Smith recommend that a child be breastfed until he or she no longer wants to nurse, which may take place anywhere from six months to two years of age, or later.

Solid Foods: Dr. Smith notes that when a child is ready to eat solid foods, usually sometime between four and six months, parents can introduce fresh fruits and vegetables, grains and legumes, and low-fat proteins like chicken and fish. Organically grown products are the best choice as they contain fewer environmental toxins, and it is a good idea to avoid foods that are high in processed sugars, fats, or other additives, such as many baby foods, most breakfast cereals, candy, soda, and "fast food." However, as children reach

Check with your pediatrician to determine the proper order of introducing solid foods into your baby's diet.

ALTERNATIVES TO BREAST-FEEDING

If a mother is unable to breast-feed, for whatever reason, Lendon Smith, M.D., a pediatrician from Portland, Oregon, recommends seeing a lactation consultant. He also suggests that the mother try to breast-feed again after one month, as women sometimes find they are able to breast-feed successfully at that time. Dr. Smith has found that goat's milk is a good alternative to breast-feeding for the first ten to twelve months. He suggests diluting the goat's milk with pure water (three parts goat's milk to one part water). Dr. Smith recommends that parents be sure to use goat's milk that is supplemented with folic acid, as goat's milk has been associated with a type of anemia related to low folic acid content in the milk. The label on the carton will reveal if the milk contains folate.

Maoshing Ni, D.O.M., Ph.D., L.Ac., Vice-President of Yo San University of Traditional Chinese Medicine, in Santa Monica, California, also recommends goat's milk as an alternative to breast-feeding. If the child develops colic from goat's milk, Dr. Ni suggests boiling it with ginger root and citrus peel to make it more digestible.

Soybean milk is another popular alternative to cow's milk when breast-feeding is not possible. But because soybeans have found their way into the American diet, soy has become a common food allergen. Other options are amino acid milk, almond milk, and rice milk. However, Eric Jones, N.D., a naturopathic pediatrician in Seattle, Washington, points out that these milks by themselves do not provide full nutrition to infants. Dr. Smith has seen babies who have developed eczema from cow's milk, asthma from soy milk, diarrhea from almond milk, and irritability from goat's milk. He suggests rotating these milks to prevent babies from reacting to any particular one of them.

school age, it may be more difficult to control their diet, so Dr. Smith recommends keeping the diet at home as healthy and "junk free" as possible in order to offset habits picked up from schoolmates or in other homes. Usually the example of healthy eating set by the parents will win out in the long term, says Dr. Smith.

Maoshing Ni, D.O.M., Ph.D., L.Ac., Vice-president of Yo San University of Traditional Chinese Medicine in Santa Monica, California, says that the biggest problem today with the eating habits of children is their large intake of sugar. In his practice, he suggests that parents take their children off sugar completely. Dr. Ni recommends that a child's diet include a good proportion of beans and legumes, which contain calcium, minerals, and protein. He also recommends soy milk and soy products and discourages using dairy products.

"Today the biggest problem with the eating habits of children is their large intake of sugar."
—Maoshing Ni, D.O.M., Ph.D., L.Ac.

Dr. Ni notes that, according to Traditional Chinese Medicine, the kidney system is the most important system in the developmental stages of the child. For this reason, Chinese doctors use herbs such as lycium berries, as well as massage techniques to tone and fortify the kidneys and liver.

See Diet, Environmental Medicine.

In Traditional Chinese Medicine, bone marrow soup is believed to promote the development of a child's brain and increase the child's intellect. Dr. Ni suggests a soup made with sheep bones, including the marrow, or chicken soup with herbs, for the strengthening qualities they provide to a child. Lycium berries may also be added to this soup to help strengthen a child's mental acuity. *Ginkgo biloba* is another herb that is often given to children, and it is used with alpinia seed (ginger lily). Any and all of these herbs can be added to a fortifying soup.

David L. Hoffmann, B.Sc., M.N.I.M.H., of Sebastopol, California, past President of the

PARENTAL HEALTH RIGHTS

Lauri M. Aesoph, N.D., a natural health writer and educator from Sioux Falls, South Dakota, believes that parents, as health care consumers, have certain rights when seeking medical treatment for themselves and their children. Here are her suggestions:

Ask questions of your doctor: *Ask the physician what he or she finds during an examination and exactly what it means. Ask why lab tests are ordered and what the results indicate. If you're uncomfortable about the choice of treatment, press for an explanation. If you've read about an alternative therapy you'd like to try, share that information with your doctor. Anytime you feel your doctor has missed something or hasn't asked pertinent questions, say so. Remember, you know your child better than anyone—including your doctor.*

Feel free to change doctors: *It is a good idea to interview several physicians before choosing the one whom you feel can provide your child with the best possible care. Ideally, parents should join the physician in becoming active members of the health care team. It is also important to remember that your doctor provides your family with a service, and both you and your child should be comfortable with him or her. If your child is uneasy with your choice of physician, consider looking for another, as it is difficult for a doctor to examine or diagnose an anxious child. Your child should trust your health care provider, not dread a trip to the doctor's office.*

Obtain copies of medical records and laboratory reports: *Ask for copies of your child's medical notes, as well as x-rays, blood tests, and other procedures, and maintain an accurate file on the health of your child for future reference. You can save valuable time by collecting medical records, and you will be more knowledgeable about your child's medical history.*

Learn about your child's condition: *Take time to read about your child's current or past illnesses. Educating yourself on the symptoms, as well as the conventional and alternative treatments available, provides you with the tools to ask your doctor relevant questions. This will also place you in a better position to decide if you need to seek a second opinion.*

Consider an alternative treatment or practitioner: *There is more than one way to view and treat an illness. Even clinicians who practice similar types of medicine may disagree about the appropriate treatment for a particular disease. Your health care professional need not necessarily be an M.D.; naturopathic physicians, osteopathic doctors, homeopaths, chiropractors, acupuncturists, and other practitioners of alternative medicine use methods that may be effective in treating your child's disorders. More and more medical doctors are now also seeking training in various alternative modalities such as Ayurvedic medicine, Traditional Chinese Medicine, herbal medicine, and homeopathy.*

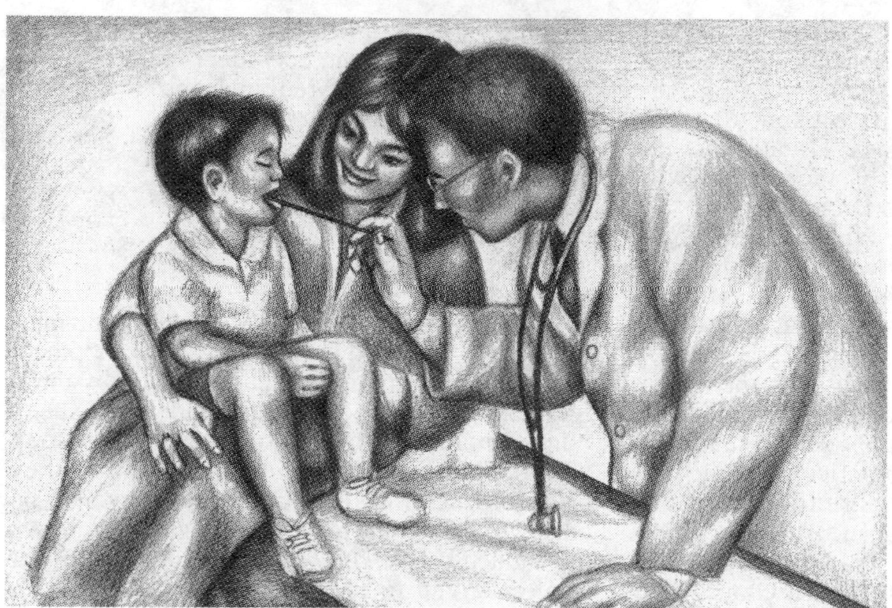

American Herbalist Guild, believes that children can greatly benefit from herbs in their diet. Nettle, like spinach, is an excellent fortifier for children. He suggests that parents be creative with salad greens, substituting them for lettuce, which he says contains virtually no nutrients. Though Hoffmann understands that it is sometimes difficult to get children to eat raw vegetables, herbs can be incorporated into a child's diet in other ways. Instead of letting children eat jellies and jams that contain large amounts of sugar, Hoffmann recommends that parents experiment with other fruits and herbal berries. Bilberries can be made into a syrup or jam and are used to treat children with eyesight problems. Likewise, hawthorn berries are recommended by herbalists to treat children with congenital heart problems or whose family has a history of cardiovascular disease.

Factors Influencing Children's Health

Parents concerned about maintaining the health of their children can take measures toward preventing diseases by making sound medical choices. "Conventional medical practices, such as the blanket use of immunizations and antibiotics, have been proven to adversely affect the immune systems of both children and adults," says Dr. Smith. "Allergies to foods and medications have also been shown to impact a child's ability to fight diseases." Alternative treatments, because they work by strengthening the immune system rather than attacking a virus or removing a symptom, may provide better long-term health with fewer potentially dangerous side effects.

Allergies

Researchers and physicians have drawn a link between repeated ear infections and allergic conditions such as hay fever, asthma, eczema, and hives.[1] Allergies to particular foods such as dairy and wheat may also encourage ear infections in some children, according to both Drs. Smith and Sodhi. In such cases, young patients can often be successfully treated by the elimination of the offending foods from their diet.[2] When treating an allergic person, the doctor's goal should be to remove as much of the allergenic load (substances the child is allergic to) as possible. In this way, the child's immune system, weakened from fighting the allergens, can recuperate and fend off illnesses more effectively.

Antibiotics

The conventional treatment for an ear infection is a course of antibiotics, which begins to relieve the pain in eight to ten hours. Antibiotics are usually prescribed for ten days and, once started, the course must be completed, as the bacterial infection can recur and is more difficult to treat the second time around.

However, recent pediatric literature is full of studies indicating the disappointing results for antibiotic treatment of ear infections.[3]

Drs. Marcus and Bertil Diamant from the University of Copenhagen in Denmark, have written that "eighty-eight percent of patients never need antibiotics, and that the frequency of recurrence of otitis media [ear infections] in the untreated group is low compared with those treated with antibiotics." They conclude that if children are

"Alternative treatments, because they work by strengthening the immune system rather than attacking a virus or removing a symptom, may provide better long-term health with fewer potentially dangerous side effects."

treated for an ear infection with an antibiotic within the first day or two of the onset of symptoms, they are much more likely to get another ear infection within a month. These researchers also discovered that, out of the 10,500 patients they treated over a fourteen-year period, only fifteen required surgical implantation of ear tubes to alleviate congestion.[4] According to Dr. Smith, antibiotics upset the natural balance between the healthy bacteria in the intestines, and chronic antibiotic use can lead to yeast infections.

See Antibiotics, Probiotics (in Appendix).

Immunizations

Vaccinations are developed to guard children and adults against potentially lethal and previously prevalent childhood diseases such as diphtheria, pertussis (whooping cough), tetanus (lock jaw), polio, measles, mumps, rubella, and Hemophilus influenza type B. The United States government and most conventional physicians pressure parents to start childhood vaccinations as early as two months. Proponents say that vaccines are the safest and most effective protection against serious childhood illness for both individuals and the community at large. The possible side effects of immunization, including rashes, fever, diarrhea, sore arms, and even death have been considered to be minimal when compared to the benefits. Supporters maintain that, because parents cannot control their child's activities all the time, immunization is needed to protect the child during exposure to contagious bacteria and viruses.

"The potentially devastating side effects associated with immunizations, combined with the fact that there are too many unanswered questions regarding their safety and effectiveness, are causing many health care experts to now object to blanket immunization."

However, the potentially devastating side effects associated with immunizations, combined with the fact that there are too many unanswered questions regarding their safety and effectiveness, are causing many health care experts to now object to blanket immunization. Today, many parents and physicians are choosing not to automatically pursue a series of immunizations for their children. At the same time, many doctors are advising against certain vaccinations they consider unnecessary and, in some cases, potentially dangerous to children.

Dr. Smith followed the standard pediatric rules for immunization from 1950 to 1975. "During that period I insisted that the children who were brought to me received the required immunizations. We [the medical profession] were the experts in preventive care; we knew what we were doing. We were behind the pressure on the legislators to pass a law: 'No shots, no school'. That was medical bigotry at its arrogant best."

Harris Coulter, Ph.D., a medical historian and author of two books on vaccinations, notes that immunization began as an experiment.[5] "Doctors didn't really know what they were doing. It was a tremendous propaganda campaign by the medical profession." Dr. Coulter does not feel all vaccines are necessary and points out that it is important to distinguish between individual vaccines rather than opting for blanket immunization. Of particular concern to many physicians are the Diphtheria-Pertussis-Tetanus (DPT), Measles-Mumps-Rubella (MMR), and polio vaccines.

Diphtheria-Pertussis-Tetanus (DPT): According to Dr. Smith, as a result of the undesirable side effects caused by administering the shot to some infants, DPT has received the most adverse publicity.

Most pediatricians see six to eight cases of pertussis (whooping cough) a year. Yet, Dr. Smith points out that some children who have had the complete series of DPT shots and even a booster at eighteen months still contract whooping cough. "I began to have mixed feelings about the efficacy of the DPT vaccine," he says, "especially when so many parents reported related fevers and irritability for a day or so after the shots." He suggests that a child be immunized against diphtheria and tetanus, but that parents forego the pertussis vaccine, as it is not as efficient as it should be and is potentially dangerous to the health of the child.

Dr. Coulter agrees. "Tetanus and diphtheria shots are not as dangerous as pertussis," he says. "However, I don't think the diphtheria shot is really needed because we have but two or three cases of diphtheria in the United States every year. And if we stopped vaccinating children it wouldn't make any difference because diphtheria comes from contaminated drinking water. Because our drinking water is not contaminated we're not going to get diphtheria." He feels that vaccination against tetanus is a valuable asset, but he recommends that the shot be delayed until the child is walking. He points out that tetanus is caused by improperly cleansed wounds, and that it is unnecessary to immunize a two-month-old baby, who is unlikely to suffer from a penetrating wound.

Caution: *If an unimmunized child catches diphtheria, an antitoxin to the disease must be given the first three days, or death is likely, particularly in very young children. If therapy is not instituted immediately, the incidence of nerve damage is very high. Tetanus can cause severe brain damage and can also be lethal in young children.*

Measles-Mumps-Rubella (MMR): For parents who choose to vaccinate their children against measles and German measles, Dr. Smith recommends that they follow the protocol to counteract side effects outlined under the heading, Taking Precautions During Immunizations. However, he feels it is better to contract these diseases naturally and be protected by the nutritional protocol he outlines in the treatment section for measles in this chapter.

Caution: *Encephalitis (inflammation of the brain) occurs once in one thousand to two thousand cases,[6] and is a serious side effect of measles. One child in eight who gets encephalitis will die, and half will have central nervous system damage. Bronchopneumonia, otitis media, mastoiditis, brain abscesses, and even meningitis are not rare. Death is also a possibility, though rare. Measles can be a serious disease in adults who have not been vaccinated against it as a child. Parents may want to take this into consideration when deciding whether or not to vaccinate their children against measles. Measles can also lead to severe hearing loss in children.*

If a mother plans on having another child, she should be vaccinated before she gets pregnant. This way, if her first child catches rubella, her unborn child will not be affected.

Polio: Dr. Coulter feels that it is important to vaccinate children against polio. "I had polio myself as a child, a serious case," says Coulter, whose right leg remains slightly paralyzed. "Polio is a dangerous disease. I have no objections to oral polio vaccinations, although there can be associated side effects."

Methods of Immunization: The immune system mounts differing defenses to different diseases, depending on the mode of infection. Dr. Smith explains: "Because the polio virus enters the system through the alimentary canal, it makes sense to give oral polio drops to the child to create an immunity that is as naturally obtained as possible." Dr. Coulter agrees, adding that he believes the oral polio vaccination is also safer than the injectable one.

In the cases of measles, mumps, and rubella, the viruses are airborne and enter the body through the nose and throat passages. After being processed through the tonsils, adenoids, and the lining cells of the lungs, they move throughout the body to the blood, the lymph tissue, the spleen, and liver. Because the vaccine for these viruses is shot into the muscle, it induces antibody production but not cellular immunity, and this may mean that the vaccination is less effective overall.

Taking Precautions During Immunizations: In his book *Every Second Child*, Archie Kalokerinos, M.D., outlines his experiences with a vaccine program designed by the Australian government to improve the health of the native Aborigine people. Following the implementation of this program, one in two children immunized with DPT died within a few days of the shots. Dr. Kalokerinos became convinced that the sudden deaths were related to the DPT shots. Concerned about the seriousness of the situation, he gave every child vitamin C supplements of one hundred milligrams per day, and consequently no children on his vitamin regimen died after being immunized.[7]

"I think immunization should be voluntary. Compelling parents to have their children vaccinated will not be tolerated too much longer in American society."
—Harris Coulter, Ph.D.

Dr. Coulter claims that a mild case of encephalitis may occur after a DPT shot, followed in some instances by residual damage. "In my opinion, this damage can include epilepsy and seizure disorders, hyperactivity, dyslexia, attention deficit disorder, sudden infant death syndrome, anorexia, and many of the conduct disorders, such as violent behavior."

Preparation of the immune system prior to immunizations is important in helping the body counteract the side effects of the vaccines. Dr. Smith injects his young patients with a mixture of B complex/vitamin C. "Recently," he says, "I have administered the following orally: one thousand milligrams of vitamin C, five hundred milligrams of calcium, and fifty milligrams of vitamin B_6 to the child the day before, the day of, and the day after DPT. This mixture needs to be stored up temporarily in the immune system, prior to the inoculation, to the point where the body can process the vaccination in an efficient and safe way. Children following this regimen seem to have no trouble with the shot."

"Homeopathic remedies may also help reduce the side effects of vaccinations," says Jacqueline Wilson, M.D., D.Ht., of Escondido, California, past President of the American

Institute of Homeopathy. "The remedies are prescribed according to the individual and are specific for the side effects exhibited, such as rash, fever, or diarrhea."

The Future of Immunization: The United States government has finally begun to recognize that vaccinations are not completely safe. In 1986, Congress adopted the National Vaccination Compensation Act. The purpose of this program, monitored by the Food and Drug Administration and the Centers for Disease Control, is to gather information from physicians regarding adverse reactions to vaccinations. Although only 10 percent of doctors responded during the first twenty-month collection period, as of September 1992, 17,221 negative reactions to vaccinations were reported. These numbers included 2,525 serious cases and 360 deaths. Compensation is provided for families with well-founded complaints.[8]

"I think immunization should be voluntary," says Dr. Coulter. "Compelling parents to have their children vaccinated will not be tolerated too much longer in American society."

Common Childhood Ailments and Their Treatments

In using alternative therapies for children, caution should be exercised when dispensing any substance, natural or otherwise. Eric Jones, N.D., the Dean of Academic Affairs at Bastyr College in Seattle, Washington, and a naturopathic pediatrician, believes that herbs should never be given to a child except under the guidance of a trained health care practitioner. Likewise, any natural therapy such as Ayurvedic medicine, Traditional Chinese Medicine, or homeopathy, should be undertaken only under the supervision of a licensed expert in that field. Lastly, when using vitamins, minerals, or other natural substances, ask a health care professional what dosage is appropriate for the child in question.

"Herbs should never be given to a child except under the guidance of a trained health care practitioner. Likewise, any natural therapy should be undertaken only under the supervision of a licensed expert in that field."

—Eric Jones, N.D.

Colic

Colic refers to spasmodic pains in the abdomen seen in young infants or children, and is accompanied by irritability or crying. Colic also refers to conditions of gas or other digestive irritability in infants up to three months old. According to Dr. Smith, colic is often due to an alkaline, high-sodium internal condition, but it can also be caused by overfeeding, swallowing air, or emotional upset. Though breast milk is recommended for a baby, colicky, breastfed babies may have cramps because of a sensitivity or an allergy to some food the mother is eating. A sensitizing food will create a red ring of inflammation on the skin at the anal opening of the baby. The most common offending foods are milk, soy, corn, wheat, and eggs. Garlic, onions, cabbage, and beans are common gas-makers for both mother and baby. All these foods should be avoided by nursing mothers, according to Dr. Smith.

"Up to 50 percent of infants are sensitive to cow's milk which can precipitate not only colic, but diarrhea, rashes, ear infections, asthma, and other conditions."

—Lendon Smith, M.D.

For babies who are not breastfed, prepared formula may contribute to colic. Cow's milk, found in formulas such as SMA, Similac, and Enfamil, is often the culprit. According to Dr. Smith, up to 50 percent of infants are sensitive to cow's milk, which can precipitate not only colic, but diarrhea, rashes, ear infections, asthma, and other conditions. Prepared cow's milk formulas may also include many additives such as high fructose corn syrup, which can cause problems for infants, says Dr. Jones.

To treat colic, Dr. Smith recommends giving the baby between one tablespoon and one ounce of a mixture of apple cider and water (one teaspoon of apple cider per eight ounces of water). Dr. Smith has found this remedy to be safe and effective.

Ayurvedic Medicine: An Ayurvedic approach, according to Dr. Sodhi, would be to give the child a tea made of fennel or anise seeds (one teaspoon of the herb to one cup of water). One-half teaspoon of this infusion taken every hour will relieve the colic. A paste made of *asafetida* (one-eighth of a teaspoon of the herb to one teaspoon of water) rubbed on the child's abdomen is used as a treatment.

Traditional Chinese Medicine: Dr. Ni stresses that in Traditional Chinese Medicine, the treatment for colic may vary depending on whether the problem arises from a cold, the flu, indigestion, or an allergy. Once the source has been established and treatment begins, there are many things a parent can do at home. Dr. Ni recommends applying acupressure to the webbed area between the child's thumb and index finger, and massaging that area. Another effective acupressure point is the spot located a distance the width of four of the child's fingers above the navel. A gentle massaging of that area, and the corresponding area along the child's spine, may bring the child relief. Also, a tea (made of ginger, fennel, a little bit of citrus peel, and some scallions) boiled, cooled, and fed to the child, should help to settle the colic, says Dr. Ni.

Homeopathy: Richard Moskowitz, M.D., a homeopathic physician in Watertown, Massachusetts, suggests that mothers who are breast-feeding stop eating dairy products until the child has outgrown the colic, which usually happens at about three months of age. If the colic persists, he recommends the child be given homeopathic remedies such as *Chamomilla*, *Colocynthis*, *Nux vomica* and *Magnesium phosphorica*.

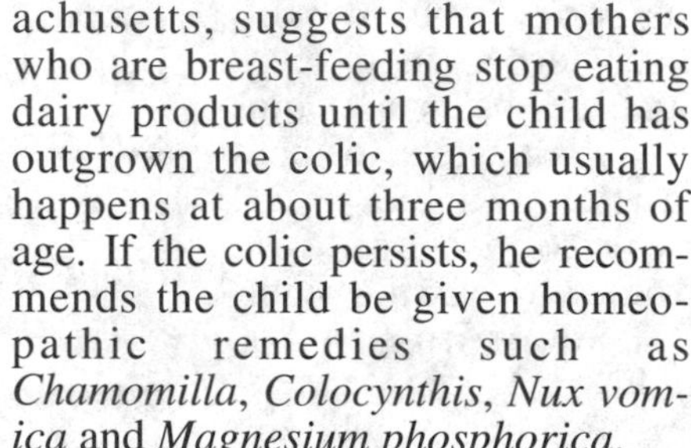

See Ayurvedic Medicine, Herbal Medicine, Traditional Chinese Medicine.

Herbal Medicine: In Europe, according to David Hoffmann, parents use a treatment for colic called grippe water which is simply water that has been infused with dill seed. It is also sold in drugstores in Canada. Though this remedy exists in the *United States Pharmacopeia*, it is rarely used in the United States. Other herbs believed to help alleviate colic are fennel seed and chamomile. All these herbs contain oils known as carminatives, which reduce inflammation in the bowels and can lessen the production of gas. They are also mildly antimicrobial (destroying or preventing the growth of microorganisms), and antispasmodic (relaxing muscle spasms). These remedies may be effective for older children and even adults with stomach ailments, though they are most effective in younger children.

Stomachaches

Even as children grow, stomachaches continue to be a common complaint. Stomach pains stem most commonly from emotional and food-related causes. "For older children," says Dr. Jones, "one of the first things to look at is their emotional state." He estimates that abdominal pains in 80 to 90 percent of children are due to functional causes (related to the functioning of the organ, and not actual damage) rather than any physical disease process. Occasionally, says Dr. Jones, when a child has an upper respiratory infection, he or she may develop a stomachache from swallowing mucous and phlegm.

Eating habits, including how a child eats, may contribute to stomachaches. As with adults, when a child eats too fast and on the run, indigestion may result. Consuming foods containing excessive amounts of additives, sugar, salt, and fats can disrupt digestion. Food allergies or intolerances should also be considered.

If the stomach pain is accompanied by other symptoms, such as vomiting, diarrhea, loss of appetite, a change in weight, fever, bloody stools, or pain during urination, a visit to the doctor is warranted. It is also important for a parent to remember that a stomachache does not necessarily mean that the problem lies in the stomach; abdominal pain may indicate illness elsewhere.

Ayurvedic Medicine: According to Dr. Sodhi, the Ayurvedic remedies that work for colic in babies can be offered to older children in larger doses. Fennel and anise teas can be drunk in the amount of one tablespoon every hour. The herb *asafetida*, used topically for infants, can be taken orally by children suffering from stomachaches. An Ayurvedic doctor should be consulted for a prescription.

Traditional Chinese Medicine: A physician practicing Traditional Chinese Medicine will determine if stomach pain is caused by a specific illness, such as a common cold or flu, and then prescribe herbs to treat that specific illness with the appropriate herbs. According to Dr. Ni, the same remedy used for colic can be applied for any general stomach upset in an older child.

Homeopathy: The homeopathic remedies Dr. Moskowitz uses for colic can also benefit older children suffering from stomach pain. These homeopathics are standard remedies and are adjusted depending on the circumstances of the child's illness, such as whether the symptoms come on at a certain time of the day or whether they are associated with a certain emotional problem.

CAUTION

If the stomach pain is accompanied by other symptoms, such as vomiting, diarrhea, loss of appetite, a change in weight, fever, bloody stools, or pain during urination, a visit to a physician is warranted.

Herbal Medicine: David Hoffmann states that the older the child is, the less responsive he or she may be to certain herbal remedies. He suggests that parents try the remedies he has outlined for colic, but if children over the age of five experiencing stomachaches do not respond to those remedies, he recommends using herbs such as chamomile, peppermint, lemon bar, and anise. If these treatments don't work, it may be that the stomachache is due to an infection or diarrhea. Infections should be treated individually. If diarrhea is associated with the stomachache, Hoffmann recommends the herb meadowsweet.

Ear Infections (Otitis Media)

The eustachian tube, a structure that allows for the equalization of the air pressure between the middle ear and the back of the throat, provides a pathway through which bacteria can enter the ear. Ear infections usually occur following a cold, when the eustachian tube becomes blocked and infected. The pus buildup formed by the bacterial infection causes extreme pain which can be accompanied by a high fever. Dysfunctional eustachian tubes may also contribute to the problem.[9]

Eighty percent of children have at least one ear infection during their first five years. A child suspected of having an ear infection should be examined by a physician. Although antibiotics are usually prescribed for ear infections by conventional doctors, there are many strategies for parents who are interested in a more natural approach to treating infections.

CAUTION

Any problems that persist or worsen should be referred to a physician or licensed health professional.

Breast-feeding has proven to protect against ear infections. Recent studies show that the longer a baby is nursed, the less likely he or she will be to contract otitis media and other infections.[10] Possible reasons for this are that mother's milk contains antibodies that protect against disease, and that nursing precludes the use of cow's milk, an irritant to the eustachian tubes and a common allergen.[11]

"Breast-feeding has proven to protect against ear infections. Recent studies show that the longer a baby is nursed, the less likely he or she will be to contract otitis media and other infections."

Treatments geared toward boosting the immune system can help children prone to ear infections. According to Dr. Smith, "We now know that if a patient is allowed to mobilize his own immune system with an approach such as a cold socks treatment, mullein flower oil ear drops, one thousand milligrams of vitamin C every hour or two, along with the herbal remedy echinacea as well as an appropriate homeopathic remedy, he may not get sick for another year. These treatment modalities often work faster than the antibiotics and are very safe. Once the immune system has been primed and the body learns how to fight off these ear infections without antibiotics, repeated infections are rare." Dr. Smith maintains that antibiotics should only be used if the ear infection moves to the mastoid bone, found behind the ear, or the meninges (three membranes covering the brain and spinal cord).

Ayurvedic Medicine: Dr. Sodhi suggests an Ayurvedic technique of lymphatic drainage massage for ear infections. He teaches the parents how to massage the child's lymphatics (a system of vessels and nodes throughout the body which carry the lymph fluid and help to remove toxins from the body—see page 162 for diagram of the lymphatic system), which will help to drain the inner ear tubes into the mouth. This is a technique that he performs in his office and that can easily be done at home. Massaging the child's lymph nodes daily may help keep the infections from recurring. Dr. Sodhi also recommends vitamin C and garlic; the latter is best given to children in the form of garlic oil capsules.

Traditional Chinese Medicine: Dr. Ni says that in the case of a chronic ear infection, usually seen in children who have been given large doses of antibiotics, one must treat the infection itself while addressing the problem of an immune system weakened by the repeated use of antibiotics. He prescribes herbs that are powdered and then administered to the child in juice or applesauce. Gentian root, honeysuckle flower, and forsythia are examples of herbs that would be combined together under one prescription, as most Chinese remedies tend to be.

"Eighty percent of children have at least one ear infection during their first five years."

Homeopathy: According to Dr. Moskowitz, a critical factor in the long-term treatment of otitis media is the effect of vaccinations on the immune system. He strongly advises parents against vaccinating their children until they are completely over the cycle of ear infections. Many parents don't realize what an added stress a series of vaccinations, such as the DPT booster, poses to the child's weakened immune system, he says. Dr. Moskowitz has seen many children who are nearly cured of a chronic ear infection have the cycle return following a routine immunization.

See Homeopathy.

When treating a child homeopathically for an ear infection, one must consider the child's "constitutional structure," the personality traits of the child. These may include a child's tendency to have certain types of symptoms, such as a tendency to become hot or cold, to perspire in a certain way or area, or to sleep in a certain way. In keeping this basic constitutional profile in mind, it is usually possible to both find a remedy that will help the long-term development of the child and to break the cycle of infection. On top of the homeopathic remedies, Dr. Moskowitz recommends putting four or five drops of hot vegetable, sesame, or mullein flower oil, in the child's ear and keeping it in with a cotton ball, which greatly relieves the pain of the earache.

See Hydrotherapy.

Herbal Medicine: Herbal remedies for ear infections include the internal use of echinacea, as well as garlic oil capsules, says David Hoffmann. He also recommends drops of mullein flower oil in the ear, as long as there is no perforation of the ear drum.

Hoffmann tells of a six-year-old boy who was diagnosed as having neurological deafness (damage to the auditory nerve in both ears) by the Children's Hospital in West Wales, Great Britain. Though the child was not in any pain, he had not been hearing well in class. He came to Hoffmann with his family, all of whom suffered from severe sinus problems. The herbs prescribed to the family members—goldenrod, echinacea, and raw garlic—helped reduce excessive secretion of mucous. Since there are no herbs that can cure neurological deafness, Hoffmann did not expect the child's hearing loss to improve. However, in treating the whole family for sinus blockage, with a low-mucous diet and the prescribed herbs, the boy's sinus problem cleared up and his hearing did improve. Hoffmann concluded that the child had been misdiagnosed and that 50 percent of his hearing problem had been due to mucous buildup resulting from a prolonged infection in the middle ear and was not related to nerve damage.

Strep Throat

Often when a child complains of a sore throat, parents worry that it may be strep throat (an infection due to streptococcal bacteria). While this is not true in all cases, there is some reason for concern. Most cases of strep throat are short-lived. However, a very small number may, if untreated, progress to rheumatic fever and/or cause heart, kidney, brain, skin, or joint problems. If the infection is not fully cleared, it may return again and again, therefore thorough treatment of strep throat is necessary.

Most sore throats are caused by viruses that begin slowly over two or three days. Other factors can be environmental, such as a dry atmosphere, cigarette smoking, pollution, or even yelling. Strep throat, on the other hand, comes on

Cold Socks Treatment

Randall Bradley, N.D., a naturopath from Omaha, Nebraska, frequently uses the cold socks treatment, a long-standing naturopathic therapy for stimulating the immune system.[12]

Dr. Bradley finds this treatment to be effective in relieving the symptoms of many upper respiratory conditions such as head and chest colds, earaches, the flu, sore throats, and even allergies. With this procedure, he says, relief is often seen within thirty minutes. If it is not, one can repeat the treatment while the patient remains covered and in bed. After four hours or usually by morning, the wet socks should be totally dry, the feet warm, and the symptoms gone or much improved. Dr. Bradley says it is effective with both children and adults.

Step 1: *Soak the foot part of a pair of 100 percent-cotton socks in very cold water and wring them out thoroughly.*

Step 2: *Put the child's feet into a basin or bathtub of hot water, as hot as is tolerable without burning. Have the bath deep enough to cover the ankles, have the child sit on a chair or the edge of the bathtub, and keep the rest of the body warm. Soak the feet for about five to eight minutes until they are hot and pink.*

Step 3: *Remove the feet from the hot water and pat them dry with a towel.*

Step 4: *Immediately put on the cold wet cotton socks, and then a pair of dry wool socks over those. At this point the patient should be covered and kept warm.*

Step 5: *Have the child go directly to bed, keeping the feet covered throughout the night. According to Dr. Bradley, this therapy will fail if the feet are uncovered, or if the patient walks around or sits in a chair uncovered.*

Dr. Bradley believes that this home remedy works hemodynamically (by moving the blood to a specific area of the body—in this case the feet). He suggests that when the blood is drawn away from the head to warm the feet, pressure in the head is relieved. As a result, the symptoms of the illness may disappear, and children usually fall asleep immediately. People who try this remedy will not only feel better the next day, but the treatment may actually boost their immune system, moving them through the illness faster, says Dr. Bradley.

suddenly along with a fever, headache, nausea, and general ill feeling. Strep throat is not usually accompanied by cold symptoms, such as a cough and runny nose. Naturopathic physicians are well trained in the diagnosis and treatment of this condition. Some choose to use naturopathic therapies first and monitor the patient's progress. If these treatments are not effective, then the patient may be referred for antibiotics.

CAUTION

Most cases of strep throat are short lived. However, a very small number may, if untreated, progress to rheumatic fever and/or cause heart, kidney, brain, skin, or joint problems.

Dr. Jones says, "I tend to take a conservative approach on strep because of the potential consequences, particularly in the high-risk group between ages five and thirteen." After discovering the typical signs and symptoms of strep, he performs a rapid strep test (a recently developed screening test for strep throat) on his young patients, a procedure which he says is between 85 and 90 percent accurate, and a complete blood count. If strep throat is confirmed, Dr. Jones recommends antibiotics. However, he also treats his strep throat patients with a tincture containing goldenseal, calendula, echinacea, a small amount of oil of bitter orange, and, if the glands are affected, *Galium aparine* (cleavers), along with other immune system-enhancing remedies. Depending on the child's age, the patient is asked to gargle and then swallow the mixture. Acidophilus is also prescribed to offset the effects of the antibiotics on the intestinal tract. Dr. Jones stresses that it is important to determine whether the illness began because of contact with a carrier, or if it is a chronic problem with other underlying causes. The key is early diagnosis and proper treatment.

Traditional Chinese Medicine: For infections of the throat such as strep, Dr. Ni prescribes a combination of honeysuckle flower and forsythia. Isatis roots and leaves can be very effective as well, he says. He also recommends eating large amounts of watermelon and drinking watermelon juice to cool the "hot" condition associated with strep throat. In his experience, Dr. Ni has been able to treat strep throat without resorting to the use of antibiotics. He stresses, though, that when beginning treatment with a doctor practicing Traditional Chinese Medicine, one should stay with that doctor through the entire treatment procedure as these natural remedies may be slower in producing results. He has seen parents become impatient with the healing process and hurry to get antibiotics for their children, not realizing that TCM heals by working from the underlying cause out toward the symptoms. This means that symptoms may linger for a short time after the patient has otherwise recovered from the illness.

Homeopathy: When treating bacterial infections, it is important to realize that a whole new generation of bacteria can evolve in about six hours, genetically selected for those organisms that are resistant to the antibiotic. Like other bacterial organisms, the streptococcus organism is one that people have been taught to be afraid of unnecessarily, according to Dr. Moskowitz. In fact, like all bacteria, it exists throughout the human body and in the environment and may be one of the normal inhabitants of a healthy throat. For this reason, Dr. Moskowitz feels it does not make sense to wage war against the bacteria using heavy doses of antibiotics, as this will also kill the natural flora in the child, lessening resistance to fungus, yeast, candida, and other chronic illnesses. A better solution is to fight the invading organism by strengthening the child's own immune system and by helping the child tolerate the symptoms by providing homeopathic remedies particular to the condition.

Herbal Medicine: One herbal treatment for strep throat that David Hoffmann says works extremely well is osha root (*Ligustieum porteri*). He says that holding this root in the mouth and chewing on it can be very beneficial for infections in the throat, and can be used for adults as well. The problem is in getting children to use it, as the taste of the osha root is quite horrible, according to Hoffmann. "Unfortunately, all the things that work well for strep throat taste pretty rotten," he says. He also recommends that children gargle or slowly sip a tea made of sage. Other internal herbal medications might include echinacea and cleavers, which can be made into a tea or a tincture. Teas can be sweetened with honey and tinctures can be added to juice.

Fever

Conventional doctors have been taught to treat every symptom that comes to their attention. For instance, medication is often prescribed to reduce childhood fever. Yet fever is the body's mechanism for destroying viruses and bacteria. "If we do no more than take the edge off the fever to make the child comfortable," says Dr. Smith, "we may be prolonging the illness."

Alternative therapies take a different approach. Their goal is to bolster and support the child's immune system so that it can learn to recognize and respond quickly to any invading organisms. In fact, according to Dr. Moskowitz, certain childhood infections may be valuable in challenging the child's immune system and consequently strengthening it. He believes it is important for the child to contract certain diseases for this very reason.

During his thirty years of practice, Dr. Smith has found that if parents are able to lower fever temporarily with fever-reducing medicines such as Children's Tylenol and a comfortable hot bath (96 degrees Fahrenheit), then the underlying illness was most likely an innocuous virus. However, if such remedies are unable to control the fever and the child's distress, parents believe that they need to take their children to be examined by a family physician or pediatrician.

As an alternative to aspirin or Tylenol, homeopathic remedies for fever and sickness are useful, safe, inexpensive, and have no side effects, says Dr. Smith. In addition, he adds, many herbal preparations, such as echinacea, not only enhance the immune system but act as antimicrobials, killing both bacteria and viruses. In most cases, he feels that antibiotics are not required. Besides, antibiotics fight only bacteria, not viruses. When antibiotics are used during a viral infection, the prescribing doctor may be trying to avert a secondary bacterial infection. Consult a physician regarding the instances in which an antibiotic may be indicated.

A high fever can cause severe brain damage. Check with your doctor before deciding how best to respond to a fever.

Homeopathy: Dr. Moskowitz sees fever as one of the basic acute responses of a child to any kind of outside influence that might make him or her sick. According to Dr. Moskowitz, producing a fever is one of the signs of a healthy child. As children's immune systems develop, they are able to respond acutely and vigorously to infections, which, according to Dr. Moskowitz, is the best way to deal with the situation. If parents are worried as to whether or not a fever or infection should be treated by a doctor, Dr. Moskowitz believes that the best thing to do is for them to ask themselves: How sick is the child? What is the child doing during this fever? Is the child vomiting, howling in pain, not eating or not responding at all? Or is the child playing video games or making mischief with a sibling? Dr. Moskowitz answers that if the child seems to be coping, the parents may feel confident that the child's immune system will be able to handle the illness with the help of homeopathic remedies.

> *"Many herbal preparations, such as echinacea, not only enhance the immune system but act as antimicrobials, killing both bacteria and viruses."*
>
> —Lendon Smith, M.D.

The remedies Dr. Moskowitz recommends do not take away fever, but rather help the immune system to finish its job of healing. These remedies might include *Aconite*, *Belladonna*, *Ferrum phos*., *Gelsemium*, *Pulsatilla*, and *Bryonia*.

Ayurvedic Medicine: Dr. Sodhi also considers a fever below 102 Fahrenheit degrees to be beneficial in a child, and he does not like to give children medication such as aspirin or Tylenol for it. He does recommend a light, nutritious diet, and cold sponging or homeopathic remedies such as *Belladona*, *Aconite*, and *Sulfur*. He points out that sometimes a fever can be a reaction of fear or anger on the part of the child, and in these cases, it is helpful for the parent to spend time talking or playing quietly with the child.

Traditional Chinese Medicine: According to Dr. Ni, Traditional Chinese Medicine treats a fever by inducing sweating and treating the accompanying infection. A hot bath can be used to induce a fever.

Herbal Medicine: David Hoffmann believes that a fever may be beneficial in a young child, and that a low-grade fever does not need to be reduced. The child should be given a lot of support and comfort along with plenty of fluids. Herbal teas such as peppermint, elder flower, and even yarrow will help the body cope with the fever, but will not suppress it the way aspirin does. If one wants to bring the fever down, he offers meadowsweet, but he suggests that the parents seek advice from a skilled practitioner.

Viral and Bacterial Infections: Most viral infections manifest themselves as fever for seventy-two hours. When the fever dissipates, a watery nose, a strange, croupy cough, or diarrhea appears as the body tries to eliminate the dead virus. The whole disease process lasts about seven to ten days. "If a child gets worse after the first three days, or the problem lasts longer than seven to ten days, specific attention and treatment are necessary," says Dr. Smith. If a fever returns and/or if previously clear mucous changes to a thick, pus-like green or yellow color, a secondary bacterial infection is likely. If the mucous remains clear and watery, but the symptoms continue, an allergy is usually the cause."

> *"Vitamin C is a very effective immune booster and probably the safest first line of defense for infection."*
>
> —Lendon Smith, M.D.

During viral or bacterial infections the immune system needs support. Immune system-supporting therapies such as homeopathic and herbal remedies, including echinacea and goldenseal, may be used. Vitamin C is a very effective immune system booster and probably the safest first line of defense. One thousand milligrams every hour or two over a period of twenty-four hours should produce a favorable result, according to Dr. Smith. Most therapists push the amounts until the patient has an occurrence of loose stools during a bowel movement. This is called "treating to bowel tolerance."

Vitamin A and zinc also feed the immune system. Rest and allowing the child to participate in enjoyable, quiet activities can also speed healing. Dr. Smith recommends limiting sugar consumption, including fruit juices, as well as encouraging the drinking of fluids such as diluted vegetable juices and soups. If fruit juice must be given to the child, says Dr. Smith, dilute it with water.

Traditional Chinese Medicine: In the case of a viral or bacterial infection, before prescribing herbs, Dr. Ni will identify the infection as either a cold type (*yin*) or a hot type (*yang*). For a *yin* type of infection, he will prescribe herbs like cinnamon and ginger, spicier types of herbs that will warm a cool condition. In the case of a *yang* type of illness, which needs to be cooled, herbs like chrysanthemum flowers and peppermint are very effective, Dr. Ni says. To bring down a fever naturally, Dr. Ni recommends a tea made of boiled gypsum.

Homeopathy: Dr. Moskowitz reiterates that, in homeopathy, it doesn't matter whether the organism is viral or bacterial. What matters is the way in which the infected individual responds to it, and the pattern of that response. A homeopath will analyze the symptoms, asking questions like: Is there a discharge? What does it look like? What does it smell like? Is there an accompanying emotional reaction? Sensitivity to the child on the part of the doctor and the parents goes a long way toward narrowing down the appropriate treatments.

Measles

There are two distinct strains in the measles family: rubella and rubeola. They are viruses and need not cause serious illness if the child's immune system is strong. They can be treated like any other viral infection.

Rubeola: Rubeola, or hard measles, is still around despite the shots to protect children against it. It is severe in those with a debilitated immune system, but extra vitamin C can limit it to a minor irritation, says Dr. Smith. The disease begins with a slight fever and dry cough that accelerates over five days, a rash breaking out at the height of the cough and fever along with red rims around the eyes. The rash begins at the head and reaches the feet within twenty-four hours. When the fever falls, the rash fades. Ear infections, bronchitis, and bleeding in the skin are possible complications. "Large doses of vitamin A for a short period of time can be protective," says Dr. Smith, "but one must be careful to avoid vitamin A toxicity. Be sure to consult a health care provider for the correct dosage."

Rubella: Also called German or three-day measles, rubella is a mild viral infection. It is of serious consequence only to unborn babies whose mothers contract the disease in the first trimester of pregnancy, before all the organs are formed, causing birth defects. Rubella is characterized by a low-grade fever, red cheeks, and a fine rash all over the body. The lymph glands located behind the ears will usually be swollen.

Ayurvedic Medicine: Like other viral infections, the body's response to measles is to get rid of the virus by running a high fever and producing the rashes. Dr. Sodhi recommends that the best thing for parents to do is to ride out the cycle of the virus while making the child as comfortable as possible. To this end, Dr. Sodhi suggests that his young patients drink a lot of ginger or clove tea to hasten the progress of the disease.

Traditional Chinese Medicine: Dr. Ni's approach is similar. He maintains that inducing the eruptions of the skin will quicken the resolution of the disease. To do this he prescribes herbs like bupleurum *(chai hu)* and peppermint. He also uses a remedy called cicada, which is the ground-up empty shell shed every seven years by the insect of the same name. Dr. Ni says this is a very effective Traditional Chinese Medicine prescription.

Homeopathy: Dr. Moskowitz is opposed to measles vaccinations for children. In fact, he feels that the best way to handle illnesses such as the measles is to expose children to them when they are about five or six years old. At this age, children will come down with the illness and their immune system will be strengthened at an age where the potential side effects are relatively minor. Measles becomes more dangerous in adolescents and young adults, and poses the most serious threat to women of childbearing age. If measles are contracted in the first few months of a mother's pregnancy, there is a possible risk of deafness to the baby. Vaccinations given to young children have a ten-year life span and so may not protect children when they reach the age of greatest risk. He feels measles is an example of a disease that helps to build a child's immune system for later life. The ability of the body to mount and recover from an illness such as the measles is the prime way the immune system matures in a healthy child, according to Dr. Moskowitz. He feels a disservice is done to the child by not allowing that natural process to happen.

In treating children with a disease like the measles, Dr. Moskowitz will take notes on the "totality" of the symptoms and the way in which the individual responds. This response will dictate the homeopathic remedy appropriate for that child. However, a common homeopathic remedy for the measles is *Pulsatilla*.

Herbal Medicine: David Hoffmann says that there are no herbs that specifically fight the measles, though there are many herbs that will control or alleviate the symptoms. One herbal preparation he recommends to help the itching is distilled witch hazel. To ease the discomfort in the eyes he recommends an eyewash made from a thoroughly filtered infusion of eyebright.

Ayurvedic Medicine: Dr. Sodhi recalls treating a fourteen-month-old child who was suffering from an full-blown case of the measles and had a temperature of 105 to 106 degrees Fahrenheit. His parents had taken him to a doctor who had prescribed antihistamines and antibiotics, but the child was so sick that he could not swallow this medication and would vomit whenever it was administered. In desperation, they called Dr. Sodhi. Upon examining the child, Dr. Sodhi recommended a concoction containing the herb *khubkalan* (one teaspoon to every two cups of water) combined with raisins, to be boiled and taken every hour. He also told the parents to soak the child in a bath of lukewarm water to which one-half cup of baking soda had been added, to reduce the itching. Following this regimen immediately produced marked results. Within one day, the child's rash had begun to improve, his fever was down, and he was sleeping properly. In addition, the child never developed a secondary infection, which is very common with a disease like measles.

Chickenpox

Chickenpox, also called varicella after the varicella-zoster virus, is highly contagious. It is usually a mild illness with a low-grade fever and a blistery rash. Chickenpox is most infectious the day before the rash breaks out. Following that, blisters appear continually for about five days, and consequently, there will be blisters in different stages of development across the entire body: some just starting; some with heads; some turning milky; and those that are fading and crusty. These blisters are incredibly itchy. The older the child, the worse the illness. Adults can develop shingles from the same virus if exposed to a child with chickenpox, says Dr. Jones.

Ayurvedic Medicine: During a case of the chickenpox, it is important to watch for a fever over 102 degrees Fahrenheit, which can be kept down with a cool sponge bath, says Dr. Sodhi. Soaking in an alkaline bath containing baking soda will help relieve itching, as will aloe vera applied to the rash.

Herbal Medicine: David Hoffmann says swabbing the blisters with witch hazel works best in the case of chickenpox. One can also combine equal parts of dried rosemary leaves and calendula flowers and infuse (boil in water) this mixture. Once the infusion is cooled, it can be applied with a wet cloth by gently dabbing the child's skin where needed.

Traditional Chinese Medicine: Dr. Ni will treat a case of the chickenpox with the same treatment he uses for the measles. A seven-year-old boy was brought to Dr. Ni in the early stages of chickenpox by his mother. The child's own pediatrician had told the mother to simply "wait it out," but when the child ran a high fever, suffered from loss of appetite, and experienced severe itching, she wanted to relieve the child's suffering. Dr. Ni's approach was to use herbs to induce the eruptions, which has the effect of speeding the process of the disease and promoting healing. He recommended that the child be given peppermint and bupleurium as well as a prescription of twelve herbs, some to reduce swelling, others to relieve itching, including an herbal cream. The next day the mother, very concerned, called Dr. Ni to report that the child had broken out in spots everywhere. Dr. Ni assured her that this was exactly the pattern he had expected and noted that the child's fever was down. TCM works by forcing the toxins out of the system, he told her. The mother and child followed through with Dr. Ni's recommendations and in two to three days the worst was over. In less than a week, the disease had passed and the child returned to school.

“During a case of the chickenpox, it is important to watch for a fever over 102 degrees Fahrenheit, which can be kept down with a cool sponge bath.”

—Virender Sodhi, M.D. (Ayurveda), N.D.

Homeopathy: Dr. Moskowitz feels that often chickenpox need not be treated at all, but notes that common homeopathic treatments to relieve the symptoms and discomfort of chickenpox include *Antimonium tart.*, *Pulsatilla*, *Sulphur*, and *Rhus tox*.

Mumps

Mumps is characterized by fever and very swollen salivary glands. The glands around the earlobe are those most often affected; however, the sublingual glands found under the tongue may also swell. David Hoffmann feels that the mumps need medical attention as they may become serious. Internally, he recommends the herb cleavers.

Ayurvedic Medicine: Dr. Sodhi explains that with an illness like mumps, it is important that the symptoms not be suppressed but be fully expressed so the disease can "get out" of the body. Swelling is therefore desirable and can be encouraged by drinking "raisin water" made by boiling twenty to thirty raisins in one to two cups of water. According to Dr. Sodhi, taking several cups of this mixture a day helps express the mumps, keeps the virus under control, and aids in nutrition, as many children with this illness find eating difficult. Mustard packs on the glands may be helpful if the disease is not fully expressed. Likewise, a sandalwood pack may reduce swelling if the symptoms are acute and need to be controlled.

Traditional Chinese Medicine: Besides letting a case of the mumps run its course, Dr. Ni prescribes herbs like dandelion, used internally as a tea or externally ground into a powder and made into a poultice with some aloe and applied to the lumps. This will help reduce the swelling.

Homeopathy: Homeopathic remedies for mumps symptoms are *Apis mel.*, *Belladonna*, *Bryonia*, and *Pulsatilla*, according to Dr. Moskowitz.

Childhood Parasites

The problem of parasites in children can provoke fear and embarrassment in parents, but neither response is necessary according to Dr. Smith. He refers to parasites as a children's social disease, as children only acquire them through their interaction with other children.

Pinworms: Dr. Smith notes that 80 percent of children between two and ten years of age at some time contract a case of pinworms. Common symptoms include irritability, night wakefulness, teeth grinding, an itchy anal area, and stomachaches. The eggs are carried by children to everything they touch, including the mouth. Eggs are then swallowed and hatch in the lower colon where the worms mate. The pregnant female crawls out at night and lays thousands of eggs around the rim of the anus and the cycle is repeated. The parasites are transmitted from one child to another in social settings.

Dr. Smith recommends that a parent inspect the child's rectal area at night when the child is sleeping for evidence of the parasite. One way to diagnose this problem is to perform a scotch tape test. To do this, pat the sticky side of the scotch tape against the area around the child's anal opening first thing in the morning. Fold the tape together with the smooth side out, and send or bring the tape to your physician to be tested.

To treat childhood parasites, Dr. Smith recommends a garlic enema. Place two cloves of garlic in a quart of water. Boil the water for a few minutes, cool the liquid and place the fluid in an enema bag. Bring a chair to the edge of the bathtub and have the child lie face down on the chair, with his or her legs hanging into the tub. Lubricate the anal opening, slide the enema tube in for just an inch or so. Let the fluid run in and then out into the tub.

Herbal Medicine: David Hoffmann suggests peeling a clove of garlic, pricking it with pins so that the oils will leak out, and inserting the clove in the anus of the infected child. This remedy may also work for adults, but can be irritating for children, and they may not be able to tolerate it.

Traditional Chinese Medicine: Dr. Ni approaches parasites by trying to find out why they are present in the first place. If the immune system is weak, he will work on strengthening it. He sometimes uses pumpkin and watermelon seeds ground into a powder and taken with aloe juice on an empty stomach every morning.

Homeopathy: In treating pinworms, Dr. Moskowitz prescribes the pharmaceutical drug Vermox. He explains that natural remedies for treating pinworms can take a long time to be effective and the process can be very trying for both parent and child. "Vermox is one of my few prescriptions. It's the kind of drug I really like. One dose of it, and the pinworms are gone for good."

Ayurvedic Medicine: Bitter melon, eaten as a vegetable, is very effective in killing parasites naturally, says Dr. Sodhi. Berberine taken orally also helps, according to Dr. Sodhi, as will tomatoes, eaten with ground black pepper.

Head Lice: Lice are another common infestation among young children, particularly those of school age, and are usually caused by the child's contact with other children. The most noticeable symptom is a persistent scratching of the scalp. Upon close inspection, parents may find tiny, grey-colored insects crawling among the hairs. These are the adults. The lice eggs (nits) are white in color and adhere to the hair shafts about one-quarter of an inch from the scalp. The nits have a seven- to fourteen-day incubation period, so patience and strict adherence to recommended treatment are key.

If the child attends school or day-care, a set of treatment guidelines will be required to eliminate all lice and eggs from the child before he or she can return to school. This usually involves washing the child's head with special head lice shampoo (either over-the-counter formula or prescription) and combing out all the nits with a fine-toothed comb. In addition, all clothing, towels, and bed linens used by the infected child must be washed in hot (160 degrees Fahrenheit) water. Nonwashable items, such as pillows, may be dry cleaned, set aside in a plastic bag for five to seven days, or placed in a freezer for two to three days. All carpets, upholstery (including car upholstery), and mattresses must be vacuumed, and the vacuum bag discarded outside. Any hair care items or accessories, such as combs, brushes, or barrettes, need to be washed and soaked in medicated shampoo or very hot water. As the condition is extremely contagious, all other members of the household must be examined daily, along with the infected person, for at least two weeks. Pets do not need to be treated.

Lice shampoos such as Kwell, which is recommended by Dr. Moskowitz and David Hoffmann are usually effective instantaneously, since they are essentially insecticides. However, it is recommended that they not be used more than once every seven days. Some parents choose to use natural remedies first. One remedy suggested by Dr. Jones is to use one part essential oil of lavender mixed with three parts olive oil. After scrubbing the child's scalp with the mixture of oils, a vinegar rinse helps to loosen the nits from the hair shaft. Dr. Jones stresses that this must be followed by a thorough combing and removal of the eggs, as well as the usual cleaning procedures.

Hyperactivity

Hyperactivity is a complicated and often misunderstood condition. It has been categorized with conditions such as hyperkinetic syndrome, minimal brain dysfunction, and attention deficit disorder (ADD). A child who is inattentive, overly talkative, impulsive, excessively irritable, and is hyperactive for his or her age is labeled as ADD. Natural health practitioners recommend several alternative treatments for this complicated condition.

"The first thing I look at," says Dr. Jones, "is if the child has actually been diagnosed as having attention deficit disorder." According to Jones, at least 50 percent of ADD children have been misdiagnosed. In his practice, he estimates this number to be between 80 and 85 percent. "It is essential to have an accurate diagnosis made through cognitive function testing and other developmental testing. Ask a physician where to have this done."

Hyperactivity may be caused by a learning disability, an unstable home life, food allergies, food additives, excessive sugar ingestion, heavy metal toxicity, or even the need for glasses. Dr. Jones remarks that at least half of his ADD patients improved when taken off sweeteners such as sugar and corn syrup. A recent study performed at Yale University School of Medicine provided a possible reason as to why sugar induces hyperactive reactions in some children. The investigation revealed that, when ingested by children, sugar releases twice the amount of the stimulant hormone adrenalin into the bloodstream as it does in adults.[14]

> *"'The first thing I look at,' says Dr. Jones, 'is if the child has actually been diagnosed as having attention deficit disorder.' According to Jones, at least 50 percent of ADD children have been misdiagnosed."*

Eliminating sugar from the diet does not by itself usually solve the problem. Often, environmental factors can exaggerate a condition such as hyperactivity. Dr. Moskowitz saw a young girl, termed a hyperactive child, who was so sensitive to fragrances that if she smelled a bottle of perfume in the store she would be, in his words, "bouncing off the walls for the rest of the day." Through Dr. Moskowitz's long-term treatment, which included trying various homeopathic remedies, the child's condition improved greatly and she was able to better tolerate these kinds of aggravating stimulants.

Caffeine is found in several brands of soda pop. In a survey involving eight hundred school children, those consuming sodas containing caffeine were more likely to be labeled as hyperactive by their teachers than those who drank caffeine-free soda.[15]

Approximately five thousand food additives are used in food products in the United States.[16] Benjamin Feingold, M.D., conducted extensive research on the possible link between attention deficit disorder, food additives, and naturally occurring salicylates and phenolic compounds. Studies have both supported[17] and dismissed[18] this theory. However, the National Institutes of Health Consensus Development Conference on Defined Diets and Childhood Hyperactivity had decided that further investigation into the role food additives may play in ADD is warranted.[19] Most recently, a joint project between German and British researchers has suggested that food intolerance or allergies may contribute to hyperactivity.[20]

See Diet.

Ayurvedic Medicine: Dr. Sodhi recommends that all children, especially those with hyperactive tendencies, be taken off sugar. He feels that a nurturing, positive environment in which they get a lot of attention and very little criticism can positively affect very active, nervous children. Dr. Sodhi feels that the relationship between the parents can greatly affect the child's behavior. A calming herb like *Macuna prurens* works very well with hyperactive children, notes Dr. Sodhi, who has seen three children who, with the help of this herb, were able to stop taking the prescription drug Ritalin. Another herb he recommends is *ashwagandha*. An Ayurvedic expert should be consulted before using any of these remedies.

Traditional Chinese Medicine: Dr. Ni treats individual cases of hyperactivity according to their manifestations. In Traditional Chinese Medicine, the heart and the liver are the two systems which are addressed in cases of hyperactivity. Herbs such as schisandra berries, biota seed, and zizyphus seed are used to calm the spirit. He also points to a poor diet as a probable cause of hyperactivity and suggests that a nourishing diet be implemented. Dr. Ni recommends parents reduce or eliminate a child's intake of simple sugar, and instead provide a diet high in complex carbohydrates, especially beans.

Homeopathy: Dr. Moskowitz also links conditions of hyperactivity with diet, as well as with other chemical stimuli in the environment such as perfumes, heavy metal pollutants, and cigarette smoke. He attributes these ailments to a chronic depression of the immune system, sometimes as a result of vaccinations, congenital problems that originate in early pregnancy, or a birth injury. In other cases it may be caused by an illness such as meningitis. He stresses that a condition such as hyperactivity tends to be a very complicated mixture of things, and is one that requires a dedicated relationship with the child on the part of the professional.

Herbal Medicine: David Hoffmann feels that the diagnosis of "hyperactivity" itself is problematic. "I think our culture, especially teachers and harassed parents, have found a new label in hyperactivity to try and control very active, very creative, very alive children," he says. For the child experiencing hyperactivity, there are herbs that may be helpful, provided that psychological factors are being addressed and that dietary irritants are avoided. Those herbs include linden flower (especially effective when used in a bath before bed to relax the child) and chamomile for the nervous system, and red clover and milk thistle for the liver and detoxification. He also recommends that the parents of such children find a way to alleviate their own stress and exhaustion.

Self-Care

The following therapies can be undertaken at home under appropriate professional supervision:

Chickenpox

Aromatherapy: Tea tree, bergamot, eucalyptus, chamomile.

Hydrotherapy: Constitutional hydrotherapy: apply two to five times weekly. Heating compress wet sock treatment: several times daily for head or chest congestion, replace socks when dry.

Juice Therapy: • Orange, lemon juice
• Carrot and watercress juice during acute stage.

Colic

Aromatherapy: Peppermint, chamomile, fennel.

Practical Hints: Burping the baby, and keeping the abdomen warm by application of a warm water bottle will often bring relief.

Fever

Aromatherapy: To cool the system: peppermint, bergamot, eucalyptus. To induce sweating: basil, tea tree, lavender, rosemary, cypress, chamomile, peppermint.

Hydrotherapy: To augment a fever that is low. Hyperthermia: apply once to encourage the fever. To lower a fever that is too high: wet sheet pack or immersion bath. A neutral application to reduce fever to a manageable level.

Juice Therapy: • Lemon, grapefruit juice
• Citrus, apple, pineapple, grape, carrot, celery; in combination or alone.

Topical Treatment: To lower fever: poultice of echinacea root • Cold compress to forehead and cold pack to trunk • Rub body with apple cider vinegar.

Measles

Aromatherapy: Spray or vaporize the room: eucalyptus, tea tree, chamomile, lavender.

Hydrotherapy: Constitutional hydrotherapy: apply two to five times weekly. Heating compress wet sock treatment: several times daily for head or chest congestion, replace socks when dry.

Juice Therapy: • Pineapple, pear juice
• Acute stage: orange, lemon, carrot and watercress • Burdock, garlic, celery.

Mumps

Aromatherapy: Lemon, tea tree, lavender.

Hydrotherapy: Constitutional hydrotherapy: apply two to five times weekly. Heating compress wet sock treatment: several times daily for head or chest congestion, replace socks when dry.

Juice Therapy: • Orange, lemon juice • Carrot and watercress

Hyperactivity

Hydrotherapy: Immersion bath or wet sheet pack: neutral application as needed for sedation.

Viral Infections

Hydrotherapy: Constitutional hydrotherapy: apply two to five times weekly. Hyperthermia: apply one to two times weekly.

Juice Therapy: Carrot, celery, beet, garlic.

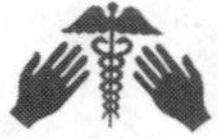

Professional Care

The following therapies can only be provided by a qualified health professional:

Colic

• Applied Kinesiology • Cell Therapy • Chiropractic • Colon Therapy • Fasting • Environmental Medicine • Magnetic Field Therapy • Naturopathic Medicine • Neural Therapy • Osteopathy • Traditional Chinese Medicine

Orthomolecular Medicine: Injection of potassium. As little as a gram of potassium activates the intestinal walls, enhancing digestive abilities.

Fever

• Craniosacral Therapy • Environmental Medicine • Fasting • Traditional Chinese Medicine

Measles

• Fasting • Magnetic Field Therapy • Naturopathic Medicine • Traditional Chinese Medicine

Oxygen Therapy: Hydrogen peroxide therapy (IV).

Chickenpox

• Craniosacral Therapy • Magnetic Field Therapy • Naturopathic Medicine • Traditional Chinese Medicine

Environmental Medicine: According to Marshall Mandell, M.D., chickenpox is a virus infection in which a small number of cases have been considerably relieved by the use of neutralizing doses of influenza vaccine. It has been reported to relieve itching and shorten the course of the illness.

Osteopathy: According to Leon Chaitow, N.D., D.O., osteopathic attention to the child includes gentle "spleen pump" techniques which increase immune activity through enhanced release of white blood cells into the bloodstream, speeding up resolution of the infection.

Oxygen Therapy: Hydrogen peroxide therapy (IV).

Mumps

• Magnetic Field Therapy • Naturopathic Medicine • Traditional Chinese Medicine

Osteopathy: Treatment of mumps may be helped by osteopathic attention to the child which includes gentle spleen pump techniques in an effort to increase immune activity through enhanced release of white blood cells into the bloodstream, speeding up resolution of the infection.

Oxygen Therapy: Hydrogen peroxide therapy (IV).

Hyperactivity

• Applied Kinesiology • Light Therapy • Traditional Chinese Medicine

Behavioral Optometry: Hyperactivity often is tied to sensory dysfunction leading to short attention and loss of context. Behavioral optometry seeks to calm hyperactivity by integrating perception and sensory/motor timing. This results in sustained focus and emotional stability.

Orthomolecular Medicine: The common nutrients which are helpful are niacinamide or niacin, using dosages from 1.5-3 grams per day, the same quantity of vitamin C, and particular attention to pyridoxine which may be used in dosages of 100-250 mg. per day. Zinc may also be required as well, using a zinc citrate, if available, at 15 mg. per day.

Viral Infections

• Cell Therapy • Detoxification Therapy • Environmental Medicine • Enzyme Therapy • Fasting • Guided Imagery • Magnetic Field Therapy • Naturopathic Medicine

Oxygen Therapy: • Hydrogen peroxide therapy (IV) • Hyperbaric oxygen therapy • Ozone inactivates lipid enveloped viruses (Herpes, mumps, measles, retroviruses—HIV, hepatitis, polio, echo virus, coxsackievirus).

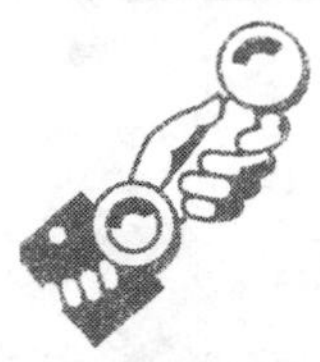

Where to Find Help

For more information on children's health, or to find a qualified practitioner in your area, contact the following organizations.

American Association of Acupuncture and Oriental Medicine
4101 Lake Boone Trail, Suite 201
Raleigh, North Carolina 27607
(919) 787-5181

The AAAOM is a national professional trade organization of acupuncturists who meet acceptable standards of competency and can provide you with the names and locations of local members. Referrals by written request only.

American Association of Naturopathic Physicians
2366 Eastlake Avenue, Suite 322
Seattle, Washington 98102
(206) 323-7610

Provides a directory of naturopathic physicians and offers referrals to a nationwide network of accredited or licensed practitioners. Publishes a quarterly newsletter for both professionals and the general public. Also offers a series of brochures and pamphlets on a variety of subjects.

American School of Ayurvedic Sciences
10025 NE 4th Street
Bellevue, Washington 98004
(206) 453-8022

This college provides medical training for physicians and health care practitioners, as well as individual courses for lay people. Dr. Virender Sodhi's Ayurvedic, Naturopathic Medical Clinic is also located at this address.

International Foundation for Homeopathy
2366 Eastlake Avenue East, Suite 301
Seattle, Washington 98102
(206) 324-8230

Provides educational courses for professionals and the general public. Offers referrals to homeopathic health professionals.

International Health Foundation, Inc.
P.O. Box 3404
Jackson, Tennessee 38303
(901) 427-8100

Originally established by William G. Crook, M.D., to respond to the overwhelming need of information about candida-related disorders, IHF is now also focusing on hyperactivity and learning problems in children and the possible link of chronic ear infections and the repeated use of antibiotics. This foundation collects and disseminates information about these health problems in children and is working to encourage further research on the subject.

Maharishi Ayur-Veda Medical Center
P.O. Box 282
Fairfield, Iowa 52556
(515) 472-5866

The center provides referrals to health centers, which offer methods of prevention and treatment for a broad range of illnesses. They also train practitioners and provide information to the lay public.

National Center for Homeopathy
801 North Fairfax, Suite 306
Alexandria, Virginia 22314
(703) 548-7790

Provides a referral list of practicing homeopaths and information. Gives courses for lay people and professionals, and organizes study groups around the country.

National Vaccine Information Center
512 W. Maple Avenue, Suite 206
Vienna, Virginia 22180
(703) 938-0342
(703) 938-5768 (Fax)

The National Vaccine Information Center (NVIC), operated by Dissatisfied Parents Together (DPT), is a national, nonprofit, educational organization dedicated to preventing vaccine injuries and deaths through public education. NVIC/DPT represents vaccine consumers and health care providers, including parents whose children suffered illness or died following vaccination. NVIC/DPT supports the right of vaccine consumers to have access to the safest and most effective vaccines as well as the right to make informed, independent vaccination decisions.

Recommended Reading

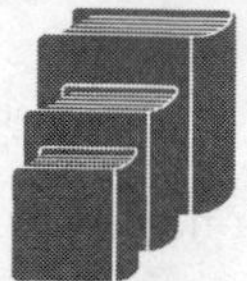

Beyond Antibiotics: Healthier Options for Families. Schmidt, Michael, D.C. Berkeley, CA: North Atlantic Books, 1992.

An overview of ways to boost immunity and avoid antibiotics. Provides a range of alternative health measures, including vitamins, herbal medicines, and "50 ways to boost immunity and avoid antibiotics."

Childhood Ear Infections: What Every Parent Should Know. Schmidt, Michael, D.C. Berkeley, CA: North Atlantic Books, 1992.

A guide to helping control and eliminate ear infections in children. Other topics include the use of antibiotics, the unnecessary removal of adenoids, and the implantation of tubes into ear drums.

The Dao of Nutrition. Ni, Maoshing D.O.M., Ph.D., Santa Monica, CA: SevenStar Communication, 1993.

This book defines Chinese nutrition as "the science that deals with the healing properties of foods to correct disharmonies within the body." Here Dr. Ni breaks down various foods by their healing nature, includes preparation methods and lists remedies for common health conditions.

Divided Legacy: A History of the Schism in Medical Thought, Volume Four: The Bacteriological Era 1870-1990. Coulter, Harris. Berkeley, CA: North Atlantic Press, 1993.

Concluding volume of Coulter's history of medical philosophy, from ancient times to today. Covers the origins of bacteriology and immunology in world medicine, from the founders through the history of twentieth century medicine. Describes the clash between orthodox and alternative medicine, especially in immunology and therapeutics, and investigates the concept of "scientific" medicine.

Every Second Child. Kalokerinos, Dr. Archie. Keats Publishing Co., New Cannan, CT., 1981.

A thorough investigation of the crucial role of nutrition in preventing infant crib death.

Feed Your Kids Right. Smith, Lendon H., M.D. New York: McGraw-Hill, 1978.

This book covers most of the health problems associated with childhood and the more natural methods of treating them.

Help for the Hyperactive Child: A Good Sense Guide for Parents. Crook, William G., M.D. Jackson, TN: Professional Books, 1991.

A large-print, easy-to-read book for parents and children that simply describes options and approaches to dealing with what have come to be known as hyperactivity, attention deficit disorder, and other behavior and learning problems.

How to Raise a Healthy Child . . . In Spite of Your Doctor. Mendelsohn, Robert S., M.D. New York: Ballantine Books, 1987.

A practical and informative guide that demystifies medical treatments for children. This book helps parents to determine what ailments require an office visit and which can be dealt with at home. In the book, Robert Mendohlson, M.D., dissects this problem and calms parents' fears with sound advice on childhood illnesses.

Natural Child Care: A Complete Guide to Safe and Effective Remedies and Holistic Health Strategies for Infants and Children. Riggs, Maribeth. NY: Crown Publishing Group, 1988.

A book devoted to raising children by natural, drug-free methods, this comprehensive, easy-to-use guide includes charts showing the uses of sixty readily available medicinal herbs.

The New Holistic Herbal. Hoffmann, David. Shaftesbury, England: Aliment Books, 1990.

This is a comprehensive, introductory guide to the use of herbal medicine. It covers health and wellness as well as treatments for a range of different conditions and recipes for the preparation of herbal medicines.

A Shot in the Dark. Coulter, Harris, Ph.D.; and Fisher, Barbara. Garden City, NY: Avery Publishing Group, 1991.

A comprehensive, well-referenced discussion of vaccinations, including an examination of the sometimes lethal effects of the pertussis (whooping cough) component of the DPT vaccine, a vaccine required by law for all children. The book is meant to be a guide for concerned parents.

Solve Your Child's Sleep Problems. Ferber, Richard, M.D. New York: Simon & Schuster Inc., 1985.

An invaluable book on the common sleep problems of children, from babies to teens, that offers clear explanations and common sense solutions.

Solving the Puzzle of the Hyperactive Child. Crook, William G. M.D., Professional Books: Jackson, TN, 1987.

An excellent book which summarizes the many things that can make children hard to raise and provides workable solutions.

Vaccination and Immunization: Dangers, Delusions, and Alternatives. Chaitow, Leon. UK: Saffron Walden, 1987.

Discusses the short- and long-term dangers of vaccination and the possible alternatives.

Vaccinations: Mothering Special Edition. *Mothering Magazine*, Santa Fe, NM: 1989.

Articles and commentary on the pros and cons of vaccinations.

Vaccines: Are They Really Safe and Effective. Miller, Neil Z. Santa Fe, NM: New Atlantean Press, 1992.

Evaluates "mandated" and many newer vaccines to determine their safety and both short- and long-term effects.

Vegetarian Baby. Yntema, Sharon K. Ithaca, NY: McBooks Press, 1984.

This book gives information on the basics of a healthy diet, how to prepare vegetarian foods, and when to introduce different types of foods; includes recipes.

Chronic Fatigue Syndrome

Dismissed for many years as an imaginary ailment, chronic fatigue syndrome (CFS) has only recently been accepted as a medical condition. While conventional medicine has acknowledged only limited results in treating CFS, alternative physicians are proving that the illness can be successfully treated by taking a multidisciplined approach specific to the needs of each individual patient.

Chronic fatigue syndrome (CFS) is a mysterious infectious illness which, according to Murray R. Susser, M.D., of Santa Monica, California, afflicts an estimated 3 million Americans and 90 million people worldwide. The National Institutes of Health estimates that most CFS sufferers are middle-class and white and at least two-thirds are women.[1]

While not defined by the Centers for Disease Control in Atlanta, Georgia, until 1988, CFS has probably been around for centuries, although known under different names. Its symptoms resemble those of "the vapors," common in the eighteenth century; and "soldier's heart," suffered by World War I veterans.[2] Medical researchers have sought in vain to find a single cause for CFS, at times attempting to link it to Epstein-Barr virus, candidiasis, and herpes viruses. Alternative practitioners such as Dr. Susser, on the other hand, believe CFS is caused by multiple simultaneous infections which must be treated individually, while building up overall immune defenses.

According to Leon Chaitow, N.D., D.O., of London, England, CFS consists of extreme fatigue accompanied by a cluster of symptoms, which seem to develop together fairly suddenly, often following an infection. No standard medical tests exist to detect CFS today. "A careful medical history, a physical examination, and laboratory tests can pinpoint specific infections, and perhaps the surest way to detect the disease's existence is to inventory the pattern of symptoms," Dr. Chaitow says.

These symptoms, according to Dr. Susser, can include deep fatigue unrelieved by sleep; muscle and joint pain or weakness; headache; memory loss; mental confusion and poor concentration; digestive problems; recurring infections; low grade fever (often in the afternoon); swollen lymph glands; food and environmental allergies/sensitivities; severe exhaustion from minor activity; and depression. Other possible symptoms include allergies, autoimmune reactions, dizziness, anxiety attacks, night sweats, rashes, breathing irregularities, hypersensitivity to heat and cold and to light and sound, and irregular heartbeat. The Centers for Disease Control stipulates that a continuance of a number of the above afflictions for six months is a strong indication that CFS is present.[3]

> *"A careful medical history, a physical examination, and laboratory tests can pinpoint specific infections, and perhaps the surest way to detect the disease's existence is to inventory the pattern of symptoms."*
>
> —Leon Chaitow, N.D., D.O.

Dr. Susser firmly believes that CFS results from combined infectious conditions. He points out that the principle of the syndrome is that patients suffer from several ongoing, simultaneous infections which weaken the immune system. He explains, "The medical establishment talks as if there's only one infection at a time in a person, but there is lots of evidence that more than one can happen. In CFS, we often get hidden, concomitant parasite, yeast, and viral infections which are results of a weakened immune system. One infection puts demand on the immune system which can't kick it, and another infection may join in, leading from one to another in a domino effect."

OTHER TYPES OF FATIGUE

According to Leon Chaitow N.D., D.O., of London, England, fatigue can result from a variety of conditions other than chronic fatigue syndrome. These include:

- *Adrenal insufficiency caused by the overuse of stimulants (tea, coffee, chocolate, cola, alcohol, tobacco, drugs) and/or excessive stress.*
- *Allergies.*
- *Anemia (low levels of iron or vitamin B_{12} in the blood result in anemia, and a blood test can verify this diagnosis).*
- *Candidiasis, which is often misdiagnosed as CFS in women.*
- *Cardiovascular causes (if breathlessness and or chest pain on exertion accompanies fatigue, the heart may be involved).*
- *Chronic ill-health (many chronic diseases have fatigue as a symptom).*
- *Depression.*
- *Diabetes.*
- *Headaches.*
- *Hypoglycemia (low blood sugar).*
- *Infections (if fatigue is accompanied by elevated temperature, then an infection is likely to be the cause).*
- *Nutritional deficiency.*
- *Obesity.*
- *Premenstrual syndrome (the connection will be obvious if it occurs at the same time of the monthly cycle).*
- *Sleep disturbance or inadequate sleep.*
- *Stress.*
- *Thyroid problems (over- or underactive thyroid activity can lead to fatigue).*
- *Toxicity (increasing amounts of environmentally acquired toxins such as lead, aluminum, and mercury can lead to chronic states of fatigue).*

According to Dr. Susser, the degree and severity of symptoms often fluctuate, not only over a period of weeks or months, but even from day to day, and a cyclical pattern of illness and reasonable health can emerge. Frequently, after a severe bout of CFS, a patient resumes normal activity and exercise, only to relapse into extreme fatigue after a period of time.

Dr. Susser reports new developments which have made CFS easier to diagnose. For instance, after exercise, brain circulation in CFS patients gets worse, unlike what happens with healthy persons. Therefore, he tests patients after exercise for decreased brain circulation. In addition, he tests the cortisone levels in the blood, which decrease in CFS patients after exercise. Low levels of this hormone (which is vital in dealing with stress) can indicate the likelihood of CFS.[4]

See Allergies, Candidiasis, Diabetes, Female Health, Headaches, Sleep Disorders, Stress.

Causes of Chronic Fatigue Syndrome

According to Dr. Susser, CFS develops as a combined result of nutritional deficiency; acquired toxicity (from environment, food, and drugs); poor stress-coping abilities; acquired systemic infections (often as a result of excessive use of antibiotics causing candidiasis, and parasite overgrowth); and a vicious cycle of lowered immune function, allergy, more infection, and further depleted energy reserves. Individuals with CFS are continually dragged down in a spiral of decreasingly lower levels of energy.

Other factors that can contribute to CFS, according to Dr. Chaitow, include recurrent viral and bacterial infections (such as acne, sinusitis, cystitis); the reaction of immune system to vaccination and immunization; bowel toxemia and infestation of fungi, protozoa, and parasites; lifestyle factors (inadequate exercise, sleep, and relaxation); hormonal imbalances (particularly in the thyroid); increased muscle tensions and breathing pattern changes (hyperventilation); genetic factors; alcohol, drug, and tobacco abuse; and mercury toxicity from dental amalgams. Many experts in the field also believe that a depressed level of immune function lies at the heart of the problem—though whether as cause or result remains a major area of debate.[5]

According to Dr. Chaitow, the conventional medical establishment's search for a single cause of CFS is misguided. He explains, "There has been a search for bacterial, viral, or fungal activity, and in fact, since many of these are commonly found to be present (active or dormant) in people with CFS (ranging from Epstein-Barr virus to herpes simplex and candidiasis), whatever was found was considered to be 'the cause' of the entire syndrome." Dr. Chaitow believes that CFS is a multisymptomatic condition which he describes as being "similar to an onion in which each peeled layer reveals another layer, or another symptomatic factor."

> *"Chronic fatigue syndrome is a multisymptomatic condition 'similar to an onion in which each peeled layer reveals another layer, or another symptomatic factor.'"*
> —Leon Chaitow, N.D., D.O.

Dr Susser agrees. "I think that the cause of chronic fatigue is infections, similar to the cause of colds and flu syndromes," he says. "And CFS can start with ordinary viral infections like those that cause respiratory infections like the common cold and flus. There are 2,300 viruses which can cause a cold or flu and if one of those hits you and your body isn't able to get rid of it, then you have a chronic infection. That's really what chronic fatigue behaves like, the flu that never got better. I sometimes call it, 'the flu that became always.'"

Chronic Fatigue Syndrome and Biological Dentistry

According to Bill Wesson, D.D.S., of Aspen, Colorado, chronic fatigue syndrome (CFS) can be due, at least in part, to amalgam fillings in the teeth, which contain over 50 percent mercury, a highly toxic substance. He cites the case of a female patient who suffered from CFS for nearly two decades. After undergoing a variety of treatments which all proved useless, she agreed to undergo electrogalvanizing. Dr. Wesson removed silver amalgam fillings in fourteen of her teeth, replacing them with gold and a synthetic substance called gutta percha. Afterwards, the patient reported great overall improvement, with her depression, stomach problems, and fatigue particularly alleviated. "Before I removed her fillings," says Dr. Wesson, "she could hardly walk around the block. Now she's riding her bike, hiking in the mountains, and cross-country skiing, and her fatigue is completely gone."

Dr. Wesson chooses replacement material for fillings according to strength of a patient's immune system. He tests the compatibility of various elements with the patient's blood serum to determine the best material to use for each patient, and he states that new composite plastic resins are the best options for most patients.

Crimson Crescents

One of the primary setbacks to treating chronic fatigue syndrome (CFS) has been the lack of a specific medical "marker" that would indicate a clinical way to diagnose the syndrome. Burke A. Cunha, M.D., Chief of the Infectious Disease Division of Winthrop-University Hospital in Mineola, New York, has discovered arch-shaped, bright red, membrane tissue in the back of CFS patients' mouths. Located on both inner sides of the mouth next to the back molars, these "crimson crescents," as Dr. Cunha calls them, intensify in color as the patient's condition worsens, and fade as the patient improves.

Dr. Cunha states that the crescents appear in 80 percent of CFS patients but show up in less than 5 percent of non-CFS patients with sore throats, and not at all in patients with mononucleosis or strep throat. He states, "If your patient has crimson crescents, you now can say his condition is probably chronic fatigue syndrome."[6] Although Dr. Cunha's findings are recent and have not been confirmed by other health practitioners, the existence of such a marker for CFS bears further investigation.

Viruses

A number of viruses have been implicated in CFS. The herpes family of viruses (which includes the Epstein-Barr virus and oral and genital herpes viruses) has been a primary focus of interest for the medical profession. The Epstein-Barr virus (EBV), the cause of infectious mononucleosis, has received the most attention since its symptoms are duplicated in CFS sufferers, who also have very high EBV antibody levels. Yet even the National Institutes of Health (NIH) reports that there is no clear-cut evidence that the Epstein-Barr virus, or any other virus, is the primary cause of CFS. NIH also reports that recent studies found that a drug called acyclovir, which blocks multiplication of the Epstein-Barr virus, is not effective on CFS patients.[7]

According to Dr. Susser, CFS has a pattern of illness that includes more than EBV alone. While he concedes that EBV may indeed be a major factor in CFS cases, he rejects it as being the sole cause. He also points out the possibility that EBV might be reactivated due to other weaknesses in immune function.[8] Dr. Susser also reports that recent research has also linked CFS to retroviruses, a group which includes the leukemia and AIDS viruses.[9]

"If different virus activity is found in different research efforts, this may mean that it is not the particular virus which matters, but that many different viruses seem capable of continued activity if immune function cannot control them," comments Dr. Chaitow. "Therefore, focus on immune function would be more beneficial than focus on the virus, which is simply taking advantage of the situation."

Psychological Factors

Some in the traditional medical establishment argue that CFS is a psychogenic, or at least, psychosomatic ailment. Dr. Chaitow acknowledges, "In some instances mental-emotional factors might lie behind the condition, since there is ample evidence showing that negative emotions and depression lower immune function."

There is no doubt that a positive or negative attitude greatly affects physical health. Nonetheless, the Centers for Disease Control states, "Many say depression and anxiety developed after the onset of CFS and are secondary reactions to CFS."[10] And Dr. Susser points out that most patients with CFS lead well-adjusted and very active lives prior to the disorder. Furthermore, he reports that many conditions, including heart attacks and cancer, result in depression.

"A reactive depression to the extreme fatigue of CFS should not be surprising," says Dr. Chaitow. "Those with CFS have often been suffering debilitating symptoms for a number of years, barely acknowledged by the medical establishment, and have been offered little appropriate treatment other than a 'chin up' attitude and handfuls of antidepressants."

Treating Chronic Fatigue Syndrome

According to Dr. Susser, CFS is a mixed infection syndrome which will best benefit from a sustained and multipronged approach to healing. Although traditional medical practice has had some success using pharmaceutical drugs to treat CFS, they are prohibitively expensive, and can have severe side effects and unknown toxic effects on the body.

In treating CFS, Dr. Susser looks for infections that are the result of toxicity and nutritional deficiency. Dr. Susser explains, "The most common infections we find are yeast and parasites. We also find hidden bacterial infections such as lyme disease and abscesses in the teeth and sometimes chronic prostatitis, chronic sinusitis, and chronic gastritis." By treating these infections and boosting the patient's nutritional intake with good diet and proper supplementation, Dr. Susser reduces the burden on the immune system.

Diet and Nutrition

Diet is crucial to building the immune system and conquering CFS. According to Michael Murray, N.D., of Seattle, Washington, a healthy diet avoids "empty" foods low in nutrients and high in sugar and fat. Instead, it concentrates on high-nutrient, high-protein, complex carbohydrate foods—vegetables, grains, beans, fish, and poultry (care should be taken to avoid mercury toxins in fish, and antibiotics in poultry). Dr. Murray points out the importance of eliminating all allergic foods and, if one is highly allergic, the rotating of nonallergenic foods. He also advises drinking eight to ten glasses of pure water daily.

> *"Chronic fatigue syndrome is a mixed infection syndrome which will best benefit from a sustained and multipronged approach to healing."*
> —Murray Susser, M.D.

For chronic fatigue syndrome patients suffering from candidiasis, all forms of sugar, including milk products (lactose) and fruit, should be avoided. Caffeine, alcohol, and refined carbohydrates (white flour, white rice) should be completely avoided.

Dr. Murray also advises CFS patients to take a good basic multivitamin/mineral supplement in the most bioavailable and easily absorbable form with adequate amounts of trace minerals. He particularly recommends the following nutritional supplements for CFS patients: beta-carotene, 100,000 IUs a day; vitamin C, 3,000 milligrams a day; pantothenic acid, 150 milligrams a day (not at bedtime); zinc, 15 milligrams a day (picolinate form); multiple vitamin and mineral supplement; adrenal extract, one to two tablets three times a day; thymus gland extract, one to two tablets three times a day.

See Candidiasis.

Magnesium deficiency may also be a problem for CFS patients. According to a recent study, when twenty people with CFS were compared with twenty healthy volunteers, the CFS patients' magnesium content of the blood was shown to be lower. In another study, thirty-two patients with CFS were given intramuscular injections of magnesium. Eighty percent of those receiving the mag-

Drugs Associated with a Higher Incidence of Chronic Fatigue Syndrome

According to the Physicians Desk Reference *the following drugs are associated with side effects of chronic fatigue syndrome. (Statistics refer to the percentage of individuals affected.)*[11]

Accutane Capsules (Approximately 1 in 20)
Actimmune (14%)
Alferon N Injection (6-14%)
Anafranil Capsules (35-39%)
Aredia for Injection (Up to 12%)
Atrofen Tablets (2-4%)
Blocadren Tablets (3.4-5%)
BuSpar (4%)
Cardura Tablets (12%)
Cartrol Tablets (7.1%)
Catapres-TTS (4-6%)
Centrax Capsules (11.6%)
CHEMET (succimer) Capsules (5.2-15.7%)
Combipres Tablets (About 4%)
Cordarone Tablets (4-9%)
Dantrium Capsules (Among most frequent)
Depo-Provera Contraceptive Injection (More than 5%)
Desyrel and Desyrel Dividose (5.7-11.3%)
DynaCirc Capsules (0.4-3.9%)
Engerix-B Unit-Dose Vials (14%)
Epogen for Injection (9.0-25%)
Ergamisol Tablets (6%)
Ethmozine Tablets (3.1-5.9%)
Fludara for Injection (10-38%)
Foscavir Injection (More than 5%)
Hismanal Tablets (4.2%)
Hivid Tablets (Less than 1-34%)
Hylorel Tablets (25.7-63.6%)
Hytrin Tablets (11.3%)
Intron A (18-84%)
Kerlone Tablets (2.9-9.7%)
Lariam Tablets (Among most frequent)
Leucovorin Calcium for Injection (2-13%)
Levatol (4.4%)
Lopid Tablets (3.8%)
Lopressor Ampuls, Tablets (10%), HCT Tablets (10 in 100 patients)
Lozol Tablets (Greater than or equal to 5%)
Ludiomil Tablets (4%)
Marplan Tablets (Among most frequent)
Mesnex Injection (33%)
Mexitil Capsules (1.9-3.8%)
Mykrox Tablets (4.4%)
NebuPent for Inhalation Solution (53 to 72%)
Neupogen for Injection (11%)
Nipent for Injection (29%)
Nolvadex Tablets (3.8%)
Normodyne Injection, Tablets (2-10%)
Norpace Capsules, CR Capsules (3-9%)
Norvasc Tablets (4.5%)
Parlodel Capsules, SnapTabs (1-7%)
Polygam, Immune Globulin Intravenous (Human) (3-6%)
Prinivil Tablets (3.3%)
Prinzide Tablets (3.7%)
Procardia XL Extended Release Tablets (5.9%)
Procrit for Injection (9-13%)
Proleukin for Injection (53%)
Prozac Pulvules & Liquid, Oral Solution (4.2%)
Reglan Injectable, Syrup, Tablets (10%)
Roferon-A Injection (89-95%)
Rowasa Rectal Suppositories, Rectal Suspension Enema (3.44%)
Rythmol Tablets (1.8-6.0%)
Sectral Capsules (11%)
Seldane Tablets (2.9-4.5%)
Supprelin Injection (1-10%)
Tambocor Tablets (7.7%)
Tegison Capsules (50-75%)
Tenex Tablets (3-12%)
Tenoretic Tablets (0.6-26%)
Tenormin Tablets and I.V. Injection (0.6-26%)
Toprol XL Tablets (About 10 of 100 patients)
Trandate Injection (1-10%), Tablets (2-11%)
Valrelease Capsules (Among most common)
Vaseretic Tablets (3.9%)
Visken Tablets (8%)
Wellbutrin Tablets (5.0%)
Xanax Tablets (48.6%)
Zebeta Tablets (6.6-8.2%)
Zestoretic (3.7%)
Zestril Tablets (3.3%)
Zoloft Tablets (10.6%)

nesium had reduced symptoms and improved energy while less than 20 percent of those on placebo injections reported improvement.[12]

Additionally, a New Zealand study found that injection of vitamin B_{12} in CFS patients helped normalize imbalances in their red blood cells.[13]

Supplemental Infusions and Injections

In treating CFS, Dr. Susser also uses infusions of intravenous minerals and vitamins, especially vitamin C, as well as antibiotics, antifungals, antiparasitics, and sometimes even antivirals (which he states are not generally effective). He states that injections of gamma globulin, the fraction of the blood containing antibodies, and of

Kutapressin, an extract of liver which is an effective immune system booster, are becoming standard treatment for CFS.

Dr. Susser says, "Using gamma globulin and Kutapressin together has marked benefit in CFS patients." Given intravenously, gamma globulin is very expensive ($500-$1,000 a shot, of which several are needed over a period of months) and inaccessible to most people, Dr. Susser notes, but given intramuscularly, its cost is moderate. According to Dr. Susser, in most cases treatment should be weekly for several months.

Herbal Treatment

Matt Van Benschoten, O.M.D., M.A., C.A., of Reseda, California, uses herbal medicine to treat the viral infections and immune suppression found in CFS patients. To diagnose CFS, he uses Omura's test (Omura's bi-digital O-ring test), a test of grip strength between the middle finger and thumb on the patient's right hand. Different acupuncture points are stimulated to determine which are the weakest areas in the system (usually the lymph nodes, liver, and brain). Omura's test can also be used to verify the appropriate herbs to clear the virus, says Dr. Van Benschoten. Prescriptions are individualized for each patient.

Dr. Van Benschoten primarily uses antiviral herbs, combined with herbs which stimulate the immune system. "The initial therapy has to be focused on antiviral measures. Once that's accomplished and the virus is fairly well eliminated, you can begin to address some of the secondary factors that cause the weakness in the immune system, such as stress-induced weakness, problems in the intestinal tract, heavy metal poisoning (such as dental mercury), and low-level pesticide poisoning," he says.

Using herbal medicines as the primary therapeutic modality, Dr. Van Benschoten sees a response in 85 to 90 percent of his patients. "The time necessary to completely resolve the situation can vary from as short as four to six weeks to as long as twelve to eighteen months," says Dr. Van Benschoten, "depending upon the duration of the illness and other accompanying health problems."

Dr. Murray recommends herbal regimens for both the acute infectious phase of CFS and the convalescent phase of the syndrome. During the acute phase, he advises using echinacea, goldenseal, and licorice in the following dosages, taken three times a day: as dried root (or tea), 1-2 grams; as freeze-dried root, 500-1,000 milligrams; as tincture (1:5), 4-6 milliliters (one to one and a half teaspoons); as fluid extract (1:10), 0.5-2.0 milliliters (one-quarter to one-half teaspoon); as powdered solid extract (4:1), 250-500 milligrams. Dr. Murray warns that if licorice is to be used for a long time, it is necessary to increase the intake of potassium rich foods. During the acute phase of CFS, he also recommends *Phytolacca de candra/Phytolacca de Americana* (dried root), 100-400 milligrams three times daily; and *Baptisia tinctoria* (dried root), 0.5-1.0 grams three times a day.

For the convalescent or chronic phase of CFS, Joseph Pizzorno, N.D., President of Bastyr College in Seattle, Washington, recommends: goldenseal (in dosages as above); astragalus (dried root), 5-15 grams, three times daily; licorice (in dosages as above); and Siberian ginseng, as dried root or as tea, 2-4 grams three times daily; as fluid extract (1:1), 2-4 milliliters (one-half to one teaspoon) three times daily; as solid extract (20:1), 100-200 milligrams three times daily.

In the recovery phase of CFS, Dr. Pizzorno recommends: *Panax ginseng*, as dried root, 1.5-2.0 grams three times daily; as extracts, equivalent to 25-50 milligrams ginsenosides daily; and Siberian ginseng (dried root), in dosages as above.

Acupuncture/Traditional Chinese Medicine

William Michael Cargile B.S., D.C., F.I.A.C.A., Chairman of Research for the American Academy of Acupuncture and Oriental Medicine, has treated CFS patients using acupuncture alone, concentrating specifically on building the immune system. He says, "If you have an energy depression, it has to do with the immune system, because the immune system is fighting a disease."

Dr. Cargile notes that the immune system uses 60 percent of the body's energy storage compound called ATP (adenosine triphosphate), which manufactures proteins to make immune antibodies. As he explains, "You don't have enough energy because your immune system is using all the ATP and it has shifted the use of ATP to the immune system for the production of antibodies, so there is none left, and that is why you feel so bad."

See Acupuncture, Herbal Medicine, Traditional Chinese Medicine.

Dr. Cargile treats CFS using the acupuncture points which relate to autoimmunity and all the meridians (energy channels) in the body. He also strongly advises patients to undergo allergy testing before acupuncture treatment so they can rid their diets of allergens which are harmful to treatment.

One of Dr. Cargile's patients, a fifty-four-year-old woman with chronic fatigue, was diagnosed with idiopathic chronic fatigue, meaning her condition did not have a known cause such as cancer, thyroid, or endocrine abnormalities. Dr. Cargile states, "She had a thirteen-year history, with no relief, and a continuous worsening of the condition. She literally did not have the motivation to walk to the kitchen more than once a day." Dr. Cargile used acupuncture to stimulate both the woman's immune system and the production of ATP in her body. Within five treatments, the woman, who previously had spent up to twenty hours a day in bed, was walking three miles a day, with her energy level restored.

Maoshing Ni, D.O.M., Ph.D., L.Ac., Vice-President of the Yo San University in Santa Monica, California, also reports successful treatment of CFS He says, "The people who come to see me have been bounced from one internist to another. They've been through the mill, rejected by the Western medical establishment." The key to CFS, says Dr. Ni, is in improving autoimmunity. "People with CFS have a compromised immune system which is weak and at the same time hyperactive. My objective is to strengthen and simultaneously desensitize, normalize, and regulate the immune system."

Over a three-month period, Dr. Ni uses a combination of acupuncture, Chinese herbs, and lifestyle changes, including diet, exercise, rest, and meditation. He explains, "Herbs are used to support immune functions. They are easily assimilated and adapted by the body. And I implement a low-stress diet. Up to 30 to 40 percent of the body's energy goes to digestion. So we want to conserve it." Patients reportedly experience a 65 to 80 percent relief of symptoms after the treatment period and are able to return to a normal life. After a three-month follow-up treatment, Dr. Ni reports that 90 to 95 percent of his patients have recovered from CFS. According to Dr. Ni, "Acupuncture reprograms the body and the herbs support that reprogramming."

One of Dr. Ni's patients, a singer, was so exhausted that she would sleep all day, get up to sing for three hours at night, and then go back to bed. He claims that after three months of treatment she felt substantially stronger. Furthermore, after the three-month follow-up treatment, she entered acupuncture school, eventually taking on full-time work in addition to her class work and singing. "I reminded her that this high-stress pattern was what got her into trouble in the first place, so she readjusted her schedule to work part-time, and committed herself to becoming an acupuncturist," Dr. Ni says "I describe my patients as people who, before treatment, were gulping coffee. After treatment, they learn how to sip tea."

Ayurvedic Medicine

Using the principles of Ayurvedic medicine, Virender Sodhi, M.D. (Ayurveda), N.D., Director of the American School of Ayurvedic Sciences, in Bellevue, Washington, treats CFS by improving digestion and eliminating toxins and allergies. Dr. Sodhi puts patients on diet modification and cleansing programs to get rid of toxins and also works on psychosomatic elements to improve sleep patterns. Dr. Sodhi states, "If patients don't sleep well, growth hormones don't get triggered and the body cannot be repaired." Some of the herbs used in Dr. Sodhi's treatment include *ashwaganda*, *amla*, *bala*, *triphala*, and *lomatium* which are combined according to each patient's particular needs. Acidophilus is also part of the program. According to Dr. Sodhi, *vata* body types are more susceptible to CFS.

See Ayurvedic Medicine, Hyperthermia.

A forty-five-year-old female patient of Dr. Sodhi had been progressively experiencing fatigue for five years, to the point where she could not work at all. After being tested by hospitals and doctors, she was told nothing could be done for her and she was put on antidepressants. The patient refused the medication and came to Dr. Sodhi.

Dr. Sodhi placed the patient on a diet especially prepared for her specific medical history and body type. The diet consisted of vegetables, fruits, and fish with no meat or dairy products. Dr. Sodhi explains, "Within three months of treatment, we were able to bring her test results down to normal. Now, she is working and functioning normally."

Hyperthermia

Bruce Milliman, N.D., of Seattle, Washington, reports success using artificial hyperthermia as the central element in a treatment program for CFS. Dr. Milliman's treatment involves artificially inducing fever in order to augment the body's ability to fight viral infections. Patients must commit to a three-week course of treatment during which they stay home, get total bed rest, and undergo the fever treatment three times daily. To induce hyperthermia, the patient soaks in a bath (as hot as is tolerable) for a full five minutes, while drinking a twelve-ounce glass of tepid water mixed with two thousand milligrams of vitamin C.

Emerging from the bath, the patient quickly dries off and gets into a bed prepared with flannel sheets and wool blankets, placing a hot water bottle under the breast (women) or over the liver (men), and remaining under the blankets for twenty minutes. This procedure stimulates a natural fever response and the body will sweat profusely in its attempt to return to normal body temperature.

According to Dr. Milliman, fever is one of the immune system's natural adaptive mechanisms, and "turning up the thermostat" enhances immune response. He reports a 70 to 75 percent success rate with his patients who follow this protocol for the full three weeks. Dr. Milliman reports that most failures in fever therapy occur in individuals unwilling or unable to address simultaneous disorders such as yeast infections, dental amalgam reaction (to mercury), and hypothyroidism.

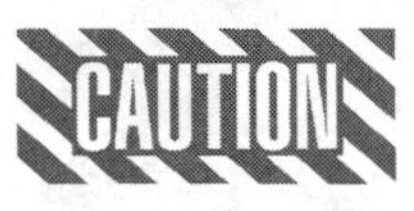

Caution: *This treatment is intended for extreme cases of CFS in which the patient is virtually incapacitated. This protocol may also be contraindicated for certain conditions, such as high blood pressure, diabetes, or endocrinological problems. The program must be carried out under the guidance of a qualified physician.*

Self-Care

The following therapies can be undertaken at home under appropriate professional supervision.

• ***Fasting*** • ***Flower Essences***

Hydrotherapy: Cold friction rub: apply two to seven times weekly •Alternating hot and cold applications.

Juice Therapy: Wheatgrass juice.

Professional Care

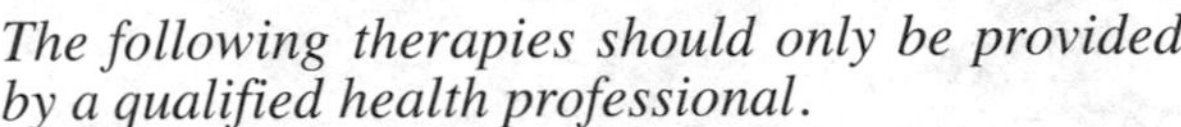

The following therapies should only be provided by a qualified health professional.

• ***Applied Kinesiology*** • ***Chelation Therapy*** • ***Chiropractic*** • ***Colon Therapy*** • ***Environmental Medicine*** • ***Magnetic Field Therapy***

Oxygen Therapy: • Hydrogen peroxide therapy • If the chronic fatigue syndrome is based on Epstein-Barr infection, ozone is reputed to be helpful, applied in autohemotherapy.

Bodywork: Lymphatic massage, Feldenkrais

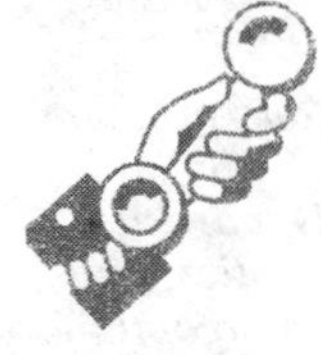

Where to Find Help

The following organizations are good resources for obtaining further information on chronic fatigue syndrome.

American Association of Acupuncture and Oriental Medicine
4101 Lake Boone Trail, Suite 201
Raleigh, North Carolina 27607
(919) 787-5181
The AAAOM is a national professional trade organization of acupuncturists who meet acceptable standards of competency and can provide you with the names and locations of local members.

American Association of Naturopathic Physicians
2366 Eastlake Avenue, Suite 322
Seattle, Washington 98102
(206) 323-7610
Contact them for the location of a licensed naturopathic physician in your area.

American School of Ayurvedic Sciences
10025 NE 4th Street
Bellevue, Washington 98004
(206) 453-8022
This college provides medical training for physicians and health care practitioners, as well as individual courses for lay people. Dr. Virender Sodhi's Ayurvedic, Naturopathic Medical Clinic is also located at this address.

CFIDS Association, Inc.
P.O. Box 220398
Charlotte, North Carolina 28222-0398
(800) 442-3437
(900) 988-2343 (Information line)
(704) 365-9755 (Fax)
The largest nonprofit organization dedicated to funding research and disseminating information on chronic fatigue and immune dysfunction syndrome. Publishes a journal, CFIDS Chronicle, *provides a nationwide referral list of physicians and CFIDS associations, and maintains a computer bulletin board with daily updates on CFIDS research.*

CFIDS Buyer's Club
1187 Coast Village Road, #1-280
Santa Barbara, California 93108
(800) 366-6056
Publishes a quarterly newsletter and offers nutritional supplements at substantial discounts. Call for a catalog listing of all products and prices.

The College of Maharishi Ayur-Veda Medical Center
P.O. Box 282
Fairfield, Iowa 52556
(515) 472-5866

The center provides referrals to health centers, which offer methods of prevention and treatment of a broad range of illnesses. They also train practitioners and provide information to the lay public.

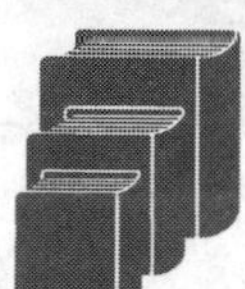

Recommended Reading

Chronic Fatigue Syndrome and the Yeast Connection. Crook, William, M.D. Jackson, TN: Professional Books, 1992.
An overview of CFS, its causes, and how to treat the illness using diet and nutrition.

Dr. Braly's Food Allergy and Nutrition Revolution. Braly, James, M.D. New Canaan, CT: Keats Publishing, Inc., 1992.
A valuable self-help approach to recovering from food allergies. Includes the latest research on the subject, testing methods, and a detailed treatment method based upon diet and nutrition. Also includes treatment protocols for some forty illnesses, including chronic fatigue linked to food allergies, and provides a recipe section and meal plan for restoring health.

Hope and Help for Chronic Fatigue Syndrome. Feide, Karyn. New York: Fireside Books, 1990.
The official book of the CFS Network. A practical approach to overcoming CFS that outlines the disease's symptoms, history, and self-help remedies including nutrition, homeopathy, biofeedback, guided imagery, reflexology, and mind/body medicine. Also provides a listing of organizations nationwide who specialize in providing information on and/or treatment for CFS.

Recovering from Chronic Fatigue Syndrome. Collinge, William, M.P.H., Ph.D. New York: The Body Press/Perigree Books, 1993.
A very comprehensive self-help guide for dealing with CFS, including diet, nutrition, mind/body medicine, and qigong.

Solving the Puzzle of Chronic Fatigue Syndrome. Rosenbaum, Michael, M.D.; and Susser, Murray, M.D. Tacoma, WA: Life Sciences Press, 1992.
A thorough investigation of the causes and problems of CFS, exploring the various co-factors which play a role in the illness, including candidiasis, parasites, viruses and retroviruses, bacteria, antibiotics, and chemical and environmental pollution. Also outlines a comprehensive treatment protocol that combines the best of both alternative and conventional medicine.

Chronic Pain

Chronic pain has become the United States' most common health disorder, affecting nearly one out of three Americans, and costing nearly $40 billion a year in medical bills and lost wages.[1] Today, many alternative therapies are available which have proven effective at both reducing chronic pain symptoms and alleviating their causes. Numerous self-help methods can also be utilized, thus reducing the cost of treating chronic pain as well.

Everyone has experienced pain at some point in his or her life. A person stubs a toe and feels pain, a person is injured in an accident and feels pain. Yet, for some types of pain, there seems to be no underlying reason. It is just there, every day, interfering with one's daily pursuits and the enjoyment of life. This type of pain is categorized as chronic pain.

According to David Bresler, Ph.D, L.Ac., former Director of the Pain Control Unit at the UCLA School of Medicine, pain is generally broken up into chronic and acute pain. "Acute pain refers to any pain from an immediate trauma or condition, and usually acts as a warning system for the body to tell a person something is wrong and needs attention," Dr. Bresler explains.

"Chronic pain, on the other hand, refers to any continual pain problem that has lasted longer than six months. While acute pain is mostly useful, even vital, in a protective way, chronic pain does not seem to offer any clear purpose. It is very often and in most senses of the word, useless, having long since served its purpose as a warning," continues Dr. Bresler. "Pain which lingers long after an injured area has healed is a common example of chronic pain, as well as recurring migraines and headaches, arthritis, recurring back pain, and other neurological disorders. This type of useless, chronic pain constitutes a major part of the pain problem today, involving enormous costs in terms of medication and therapy, as well as causing a vast degree of misery and disability."

> *"While acute pain is mostly useful, even vital, in a protective way, chronic pain does not seem to offer any clear purpose. It is very often and in most senses of the word, useless."*
> —David Bresler, Ph.D, L.Ac.

The Pain Experience

Pain is caused by the stimulation of special sensory nerve endings that respond to bodily irritation, pressure, heat, cold, injury, stress, and disease. However, each person perceives pain differently, and that perception can be influenced by any number of factors including emotional and mental attitudes, previous experiences, and other health conditions. Social, cultural, and ethnic differences also can affect how one perceives and reacts to pain, as well as early learning and developmental predispositions.[2]

"What we think about pain, how afraid or anxious we are about it, what we believe it represents in health terms, all influence how much pain we report," says Leon Chaitow, N.D., D.O., of London, England. "Aches and pains following exercise can usually be laughed off because we know that they will vanish in a day or so, while the same discomfort caused by a wasting disease or an arthritic condition might be complained of as unbearable."

See Arthritis, Back Pain, Headaches, Stress.

Dr. Bresler emphasizes this fact, stating that there is not necessarily a direct relationship between the actual sensation of pain and the way people perceive it.[3] "It is important to recognize the complex subjective experience of pain, which involves physical, perceptual, cognitive, emotional, and spiritual factors," says Dr. Bresler. "Pain is an intensely personal experience, and even if no physical explanation for it can be found, all pain is real."

Many people who suffer from chronic pain also feel helpless concerning their condition, an attitude that is very often reinforced by medical doctors who say, "You'll just have to learn to live with it; nothing more can be done." Unfortunately, the ensuing feelings of depression and hopelessness tend to heighten the experience of pain by causing increased heart rate, blood pressure, respiration, sweating, and muscle tension.[4] This can have an ever-increasing spiral effect on people suffering from musculoskeletal pain, as the increased muscle tension augments the sensation of pain, which further increases the anxiety, which in turn, produces even greater tension and pain.

“Pain is an intensely personal experience, and even if no physical explanation for it can be found, all pain is real.”
—David Bresler, Ph.D, L.Ac.

Coping with Chronic Pain

According to Dr. Chaitow, experts have traditionally been divided on the best approach to understanding and treating chronic pain. Some feel it is best dealt with at the physical, nervous system level, while others tend to emphasize the importance of its emotional and psychological characteristics. "The truth is that both physical and psychological elements are usually intimately combined in most cases of chronic pain, and both require attention when dealing with long-term pain," says Dr. Chaitow.

“Central to whatever is done to and for a person in pain is the need for that person to start to take some degree of control of the situation, to feel empowered to influence the processes at work and to not feel him- or herself to be a mere object, simply the helpless recipient of other people's efforts.”
—Leon Chaitow, N.D., D.O.

"Central to whatever is done to and for a person in pain is the need for that person to start to take some degree of control of the situation, to feel empowered to influence the processes at work and to not feel him- or herself to be a mere object, simply the helpless recipient of other people's efforts. When a person suffering pain understands the causes, nature, mechanisms, and role of that pain, a vital step has been taken in the successful handling of the problem."

Self-help methods therefore become very important in this process, although they cannot simply be picked at random. They need to be a part of a total therapeutic approach, decided upon mutually by patient and doctor, and designed to meet the needs of the individual and his or her specific problem. Dr. Bresler adds that one of the most important aspects in evaluating a subjective experience such as chronic pain is the personal rapport established between patient and doctor.

Change can also be fundamental in the treatment of chronic pain. Often a review of the patient's lifestyle will show certain patterns that contribute to the experience of pain. Sometimes a person can even perpetuate his or her own pain in order to receive certain benefits associated with it. For example, a person in pain often attracts positive, caring attention from others that was missing in his or her life before. Or, in the case of Workmen's Compensation benefits, the sufferer may receive financial rewards, and if the person does not particularly care for the type of work he or she had been doing, the continuation of pain can keep that person out of an unpleasant work situation. The only way to alleviate these type of chronic pain conditions is to reduce the needs that the pain seems to be able to fill. This kind of change can often only be accomplished through some form of professional counseling.

Any time pharmacological remedies are used to treat chronic pain, which is the standard tactic of conventional medicine, there is a risk of developing a dependency. This, in and of itself, can perpetuate the pain symptoms in order to facilitate and rationalize one's now-addictive need for the pain-suppressing drugs.

In addition, any time pharmacological remedies are used to treat chronic pain, which is the standard tactic of conventional medicine, there is a risk of developing a dependency. This, in and of itself, can perpetuate the pain symptoms in order to facilitate and rationalize one's now-addictive need for the pain-suppressing drugs. Fortunately, nondrug methods of pain relief are available.

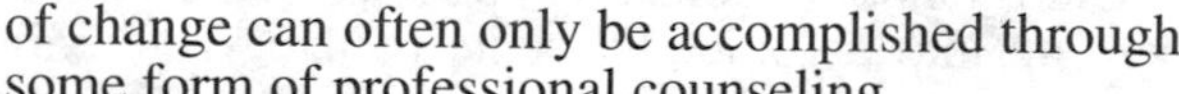

Alternative Treatments for Chronic Pain

Much as a cut heals and a broken bone mends without any external help, the body has made a provision for pain to be eased by natural means, such as the production of endorphins which can produce euphoric and painkilling effects when released. Rather than just suppressing the symptoms of pain, as drug therapy does, doctors and pain therapists using alternative modalities try to utilize and activate these natural healing properties of the body.

Also, recognizing the complexities of chronic pain, with its physical and psychological components, alternative health practitioners employ a wide variety of treatment methods tailored specifically to the individual. These can include diet and nutrition, hypnotherapy, guided imagery, biofeedback, acupuncture, energy medicine, magnetic field therapy, and hydrotherapy. This multidisciplinary approach also includes educating patients about the nature of pain and showing them that they can control their pain.

Diet and Nutrition

According to James Braly, M.D., Medical Director of Immuno Labs, Inc. in Fort Lauderdale, Florida, diet and nutrition can both play important roles in the treatment of chronic pain. "I have seen patients who have tried just about everything to relieve their pain, only to finally find relief when they made changes in their diet and added supplements with proven pain-relieving properties," he says.

Dr. Braly points out that inflammation, one of the principle mechanisms related to chronic pain, is often caused by an allergic reaction. "Often the reactions are due to food allergies," Dr. Braly notes. "If chronic pain symptoms seem to have no other discernible cause, testing for food allergies is advisable."

Once the allergic foods have been determined, Dr. Braly recommends that they be completely eliminated from the diet for a minimum of three months. After that, they can be reintroduced as part of a rotation diet, with no one food being eaten more than once in any four-day period. Dr. Braly also recommends limiting foods high in saturated fats, including red meats, dairy products, warm-water shellfish, partially hydrogenated oils, as well as avoiding alcohol and severely limiting caffeine. He suggests a diet high in fiber and nonallergenic complex carbohydrates. "Organic, free-range poultry, cold sea-water fish, and sources of vegetable protein are also good," he says, "while margarine, shortenings, and other sources of partially hydrogenated oils should be omitted. Simple or refined sugars, including fruit juices, sodas, and pastries, are also culprits."

Along with diet, Dr. Braly suggests the following nutritional supplements be taken daily when in pain: vitamin C to 90 percent of bowel tolerance; evening primrose oil and MaxEPA, both of which supply essential fatty acids which reduce inflammation and decrease pain; vitamin E; magnesium glycinate; and the amino acid, DL-phenylalanine. "DL-phenylalanine is one of the more exciting and important nutritional supplements I have found for relieving pain," Dr. Braly says, noting that it has proven effective in increasing blood levels of endorphins and reducing inflammation in about 80 percent of his patients suffering from chronic pain. "The most exciting new supplement in the treatment of chronic pain of arthritis is glucosamine sulfate, which actually relieves pain by healing and/or regenerating new connective tissues that have been weakened or destroyed with inflammation."

One of Dr. Braly's patients suffered from painful back spasms for years without being able to gain relief. He tested positive for food allergies. The allergic foods were eliminated, along with alcohol, and he began to follow a rotation diet. "After starting the program, he became pain free for the first time in years," Dr. Braly relates. "He couldn't believe that such dramatic relief could occur without drugs or surgery. But after about eighteen months, he strayed from our protocol. Soon thereafter, his back spasms returned. We retested him for allergies, got him back on track, and his pain once more disappeared."

Hypnotherapy

Hypnotherapy has been approved by the American Medical Association as a clinical adjunct in the management of chronic pain, and is currently taught in several medical schools. Although there are numerous ways to induce a hypnotic state, according to Gerald Sunnen, M.D., Associate Clinical Professor of Psychiatry at the New York University Bellevue Medical Center, they all begin by encouraging the patient to enter a deep state of relaxation. The patient may then be given simple suggestions to experience the sensation of pain in a different way, perhaps as a warm or tingly feeling. "This technique is known as symptom substitution, and is used to show the patient that it is possible to control the pain," Dr. Sunnen explains. "This can result in a more positive, hopeful attitude toward one's condition."

See Allergies, Diet, Hypnotherapy, Nutritional Supplements.

When chronic pain is the result of an earlier accident or trauma, the hypnotherapist may also use regression to help the patient remember the incident. By reexperiencing the pain and suffering of the past event, the patient can confront and reevaluate the experience. This helps to alleviate anxiety and fear and will often significantly reduce the present experience of pain.

Hypnosis has been used to help alleviate back pain, abdominal pain, joint pain, burn pain, and headache and migraine pain.[5] However, Dr. Sunnen notes that hypnosis should always be conducted by a trained hypnotherapist in order to avoid any potential retraumatization or the triggering of a psychotic reaction.

Guided Imagery

The imagination can be a powerful tool for overcoming pain, and in the past ten years numerous techniques have been devised to harness this power. These techniques, know as guided imagery, encourage more active participation of the patient, which can help the patient feel more in control of his or her problem. Guided imagery can be particularly effective when other pain management approaches have failed.

One common exercise used by Dr. Bresler involves visualizing the pain in physical terms, such as a burning fire or a terrible monster gnawing on one's bones. "By mentally extinguishing the flames, or taming the monster, the patient will usually experience an immediate reduction in pain," Dr. Bresler says.

"Another very powerful exercise involves the use of an imaginary inner doctor or advisor. First, the patient is taught how to deeply relax, and then asked to imagine being in some beautiful, restful location. Then the patient is invited to visualize an advisor, who may appear in any form imaginable. It could be an animal, or a religious figure, or an old woman in a cave. Then, through dialogue with this inner advisor, important information about the pain can emerge, and creative solutions to its elimination explored."

See Biofeedback Training, Guided Imagery.

Jon Kabat-Zinn, Ph.D., Director of the Stress Reduction Clinic at the University of Massachusetts Medical Center, tells his patients to focus on their pain when it comes up, and to meditate upon the sensations. "By watching the sensations come and go, very often you will find that they change, and that the pain itself has a life of its own," he says. "When you learn how to work with the pain, to listen to it, and to honor it, you discover that it's possible to experience your pain differently. And sometimes, this can result in the sensations actually going away."

Biofeedback Training

Biofeedback training is a technique that uses electronic devices to help a patient learn to regulate various physiological functions such as body temperature, muscle tension, and pulse rate. Through trial and error, the patient learns how to use his or her mind to relax and alter these various bodily functions which can greatly affect chronic pain symptoms. With proper training, many types of pain can be controlled.

George von Hilsheimer, Ph.D., of Maitland, Florida, Diplomate of the American Academy of Pain Management, regularly employs biofeedback when dealing with patients with chronic pain. One of his patients was a forty-two-year-old woman who came to him suffering panic attacks, headaches, and pain in her arm and chest due to an automobile accident she had been involved in three years earlier. "The panic attacks began six weeks after her accident," Dr. von Hilsheimer recounts, "after she was already enduring severe headaches all along the left side of her head and the top of her head. And this was accompanied by pain down her left arm and hand and behind her left breast."

By the time the woman came to him, she was in such a state of panic that she was barely able to leave her home, and had to be driven to his office by her mother. Prior to her visit, the woman had seen an orthopedic surgeon and a chiropractor, both of whom had been unable to help her. Using biofeedback equipment, Dr. von Hilsheimer was able to determine that the nerves and muscles of the woman's left side were overactive, while being underactive on her right. "Her accident had violently rotated her to the right as her car careened left," explains Dr. von Hilsheimer. "As a consequence, her left side muscles had been stretched and activated, and her right side muscles had been compressed and turned off."

Dr. von Hilsheimer had the woman mentally relive her accident and write about it and discuss

THE PLACEBO EFFECT

A placebo is defined as a substance that normally has no physiological effect upon the body, but when given to a patient under the pretext of treatment promotes a healing effect upon the body. This phenomena adds evidence to the notion that a person's beliefs can strongly influence the healing processes of the body.

Numerous studies have indicated that placebos provide relief for a variety of pain related disorders including arthritis, angina, digestive tract pain, and other chronic pain problems.[6] In fact, placebos can be nearly as effective as prescriptive medication. In one study, 82 to 87 percent of chronic headache sufferers responded to analgesic drugs, whereas 60 percent responded to a placebo.[7] In another study, 72 percent of patients suffering from postoperative pain responded to morphine, while 40 percent responded equally as well to placebo injections.[8] Chronic back pain and cancer pain have responded to placebos as well as, if not better than, conventional pain medications.

One explanation for this phenomenon is that the administration of a placebo produces a reduction of chronic anxiety, which helps to decrease the perception of pain.[9] Placebos can play an important part in the medical intervention of pain, and may even help to wean drug-dependent patients from their pain medications.

her feelings regarding the trauma it had caused her. "She repeated this process until the emotional sting of the accident was relieved," Dr. von Hilsheimer says. "At that point her panic attacks ended."

Dr. von Hilsheimer then employed biofeedback training to address the woman's pain. "I had her view a screen which vividly portrayed images of her brain wave activity and she quickly learned how she could speed up the waves," he says. "Then I had her watch the electrical signals from her muscles on a television monitor. These signals showed her how her posture and defensive movements worsened the imbalance between her muscles to cause pain." Dr. von Hilsheimer then taught her exercises and stretches to relieve the pain, and learned to enhance her performance of them by again watching the monitor. Soon she was able to consciously make her muscles produce more or less electricity, to the point where, after three sessions, she could change the signal simply by deciding to. "As a result," Dr. von Hilsheimer says, "without the use of any invasive procedures or medicines, the woman now enjoys a complete restoration of easy movement and freedom from fear and pain, which she maintains by following a home program of exercise, stretching, and biofeedback."

Acupuncture

Acupuncture has been found to be highly effective in the treatment of chronic pain. "Although the mechanism by which it works is not yet fully understood it is known that it can have two separate pain-relieving functions," Dr. Bresler says. Acupuncture stimulates the release of endorphins and enkephalins (the body's own natural painkillers). At the same time, it can block pain messages from getting through to the brain. The acupuncture needles (or acupressure) trigger nerve reactions which travel along thicker and faster nerve channels than the pain sensations do, effectively "shutting the gate" to the brain before the pain messages can even get there.

To date, hundreds of studies worldwide have substantiated acupuncture's effectiveness in treating and managing chronic pain. According to Dr. Bresler, acupuncture was found to be of tremendous benefit, particularly in the treatment of musculoskeletal pain and spasm, arthritis, bursitis, and other similar conditions.

Acupuncture is also helpful in relieving anxiety and depression associated with chronic pain, as well as in helping people reduce their dependence on narcotics and other addictive drugs.

Energy Medicine

One of the most commonly used energy medicine devices for chronic pain is the TENS (Transcutaneous Electrical Nerve Stimulator), a small battery-operated device that produces various frequencies and voltages of mild electrical stimulation. By applying the electrodes to the affected parts of the body, the TENS electrical current acts upon the nerves, causing conduction to be blocked and pain to be relieved. TENS units are also believed to stimulate the production of endorphins. Patients are often taught how to self-administer this treatment. TENS has been used in the management of postsurgical pain, sports injuries, and other neuromuscular pain disorders.

The Electro-Acuscope™ is another energy device used to reduce pain. It uses a lower electrical current than the TENS unit, and works by stimulating tissue repair instead of the nerves. The current is continuously adjusted to match the resistance given off by the damaged tissue in order to facilitate healing. The Electro-Acuscope, because of its prolonged effects on tissue repair, can be applied to a wide range of painful conditions, including arthritis, bursitis, sprains and strains, neuralgia, and bruises. It is also effective in treating acute and chronic pain caused by musculoskeletal disorder, including automobile accidents, lower back sprains, and sports injuries.[10]

See Acupuncture, Energy Medicine, Magnetic Field Therapy.

Magnetic Field Therapy

According to biomagnetic researcher William H. Philpott, M.D., of Choctaw, Oklahoma, magnetic field therapy has many applications for the relief of pain. "The negative magnetic field (traditional south seeking pole) provided by magnetic therapy is ideal for relieving pain symptoms due to its ability to quickly normalize the metabolic functions that create the conditions in the first place," Dr. Philpott says. He points out that the negative magnetic field does not act as a painkiller, or analgesic. Instead, it is a "normalizer of disordered metabolic functions."

One of Dr. Philpott's patients was a woman in her seventies who came to him suffering from a fibrous clot in her left groin that made climbing stairs painful due to the way it impinged on the blood flow of her left leg. Dr. Philpott had her sleep on a negative field magnetic pad with magnets also placed at the crown of her head. After one year of treatment, the woman was climbing stairs freely without pain and it was discovered upon further examination that the clot, which had been present for over thirty years, was healed despite the fact that it had never been treated directly.

Dean Bonlie, D.D.S., of Calgary, Alberta, Canada, a colleague of Dr. Philpott, also employs magnetic field therapy to treat a variety of chronic pain conditions. One of his patients was a retired member of the Canadian Armed Forces who had been released from service on medical grounds for being 48 percent disabled due to three injuries to his lower back. His condition was so severe that he had been operated on and received a spinal fusion. He had also tried medication, heat treatments, chiropractic and physiotherapy, all without long-term results.

Dr. Bonlie applied a four by six inch negative North Pole magnet directly on the injured section of the man's back for twenty-five minutes and the man experienced substantial pain reduction. Moreover, upon standing up, for the first time in years, he did not experience the flash of burning pain down his upper right leg that had previously been one of his symptoms. Dr. Bonlie suggested he begin sleeping on a magnetic sleep pad and the man soon confirmed that, after twenty-five years, he was finally free of his pain.

Hydrotherapy

According to Doug Lewis, N.D., Chairperson of the Physical Medicine Department of Bastyr College in Seattle, Washington, hydrotherapy, including compresses and various contrast (hot and cold) techniques, offers a simple and efficient way of treating a variety of factors which contribute to chronic pain. Hydrotherapy can also be used at home.

"Cold applications are helpful in reducing the sensitivity of the nerve endings which signal pain sensations," Dr. Lewis explains. "Pain generated by inflammation can be eased by use of ice, or alternating hot and cold applications. General anxiety which increases the perception of pain can also be helped enormously by use of a neutral bath or wet sheet pack."

Blockages in circulation, which can result from inactivity or increased muscle tension and lead to poor oxygenation of tissues and pain, can be assisted by techniques such as contrast bathing, cold douches, and hot and cold applications, Dr. Lewis notes.

"Heating compresses that go on cold and are then warmed up are also effective. The congestion and swelling caused by a buildup of fluids, as well as muscle stiffness, can be eased as well, with heating compresses, and a variety of alternating hot and cold applications or immersions," Dr. Lewis says. "Generally, though, cold is more helpful than hot for injuries and inflamed areas, and any hot hydrotherapy methods should almost always end with a short cold application."

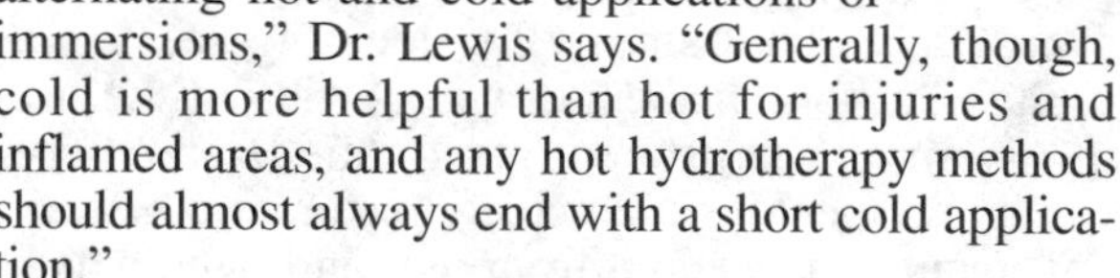

See Aromatherapy, Hydrotherapy.

Using different substances in water can assist in pain relief, too, including Epsom salts and a wide range of essential oils. Steam can also be used to reduce the pain of chest and sinus congestion, with or without suitable additions of aromatic herbs and/or oils.

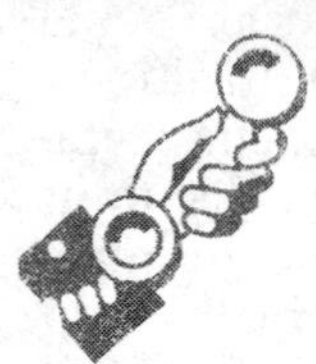

Where to Find Help

For additional information on chronic pain and referrals for treatment, contact the following organizations.

The Academy for Guided Imagery
P.O. Box 2070
Mill Valley, California 94942
(800) 726-2070

The academy trains health professionals to use Interactive Guided Imagery[SM], offering a 150-hour certification program. They publish a directory of imagery practitioners. They also carry books and tapes for professionals and lay people, specifically relating to imagery in medicine and healing. Send for free catalog.

American Association of Acupuncture and Oriental Medicine
4101 Lake Boone Trail, Suite 201
Raleigh, North Carolina 27607
(919) 787-5181

The AAAOM is a national professional trade organization of acupuncturists who meet acceptable standards of minimum competency and can provide the names and locations of local members.

American Association of Naturopathic Physicians
2366 Eastlake Avenue, Suite 322
Seattle, Washington 98112
(206) 323-7610

Provides referrals to a nationwide network of accredited or licensed naturopathic physicians for health professionals and the general public; supported by members and corporate sponsors. It hosts an annual convention, and works to move legislature and licensure in various states.

The American Society of Clinical Hypnosis
2200 East Devon Avenue, Suite 291
Des Plaines, Illinois 60018
(708) 297-3317
Membership is comprised of M.D.'s and dentists trained in the use of hypnosis for treating health conditions. Send a stamped, self-addressed envelope for referrals to practitioners in your area.

Association for Applied Psychophysiology and Biofeedback
10200 West 44th Avenue, Suite 304
Wheat Ridge, Colorado 80033
(303) 422-8436
Provides names and phone numbers of chapters in your state. (Formerly Biofeedback Society of America.)

Center for Applied Psychophysiology
Menninger Clinic
P.O. Box 829
Topeka, Kansas 66601-08829
(913) 273-7500 Ext. 5375
One of the pioneering groups in biofeedback, this organization has research, treatment, and workshops in all areas of mind/body medicine, including extensive work with biofeedback, which includes the Biofeedback and Psychophysiology Clinic.

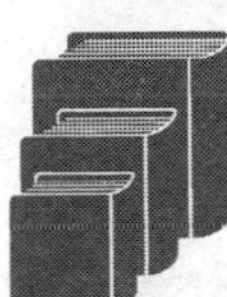

Recommended Reading

Dr. Braly's Food Allergy and Nutrition Revolution. Braly, James, M.D. New Canaan, CT: Keats Publishing, Inc., 1992.
An authoritative book about the role food allergies can play in a variety of illnesses, including chronic pain. Includes testing methods, treatments, and an extensive selection of recipes useful in creating a diet of optimum health.

Free Yourself from Pain. Bresler, David E. Topanga, CA: The Bresler Center, 1992.
This self-help book for managing chronic pain and depression includes several chapters illustrating the use of imagery for pain control. (Available from The Bresler Center, 115 South Topanga Canyon Boulevard, Suite 158, Topanga, California 90290. (310) 455-3634.)

Killing Pain Without Prescription. Gelb, Harold, D.M.D. New York: Harper Perennial, 1982.
An outline of treatments to deal with chronic pain, including diet, nutrition, applied kinesiology, osteopathy, and bodywork. Also includes a resource guide of organizations offering help nationwide.

Life Without Pain. Linchitz, Richard, M.D. Reading, MA: Addison-Wesley, 1987.
A self-help approach for eliminating pain through the use of diet, nutrition, mind/body medicine, and exercise.

Pain Erasure. Prudden, Bonnie. New York: M. Evans and Co., 1980.
This book explains Bonnie Prudden's method for pain relief using myotherapy. Her method has been hailed by doctors and patients.

Colds and Flu

The common cold and the flu are believed by most physicians to be caused by exposure and susceptibility to a variety of common viruses. Yet not everyone "catches" a cold or flu when he or she is exposed to such viruses. For this reason, alternative physicians emphasize treating and preventing the common cold and the flu by strengthening a person's immune system, thereby safeguarding it from susceptibility.

All of us have experienced the sore throat, runny nose, aching, and general sense of misery that announce the onset of the common cold. Other familiar signals include a cough, headache, and dry, sore, or sensitive breathing passages. In a given year, nearly half of the United States population will "catch" a cold and 40 percent will develop influenza, or the flu.[1] The symptoms of both the common cold and the flu are often used somewhat interchangeably because both are caused by the same family of respiratory viruses. According to John Hibbs, N.D., of Seattle, Washington, the distinction between the two depends on how severe the infection is and the range of symptoms. The flu, however, is usually more severe, develops quickly, and involves more of the body than a cold. A cold also occurs at any time of year while the flu, by contrast, usually develops in epidemics, normally in late fall and winter.

"Beyond respiratory inflammation," says Dr. Hibbs, "the flu produces a moderate to high fever, aching muscles, and acute fatigue. Vomiting and diarrhea may also develop and, in extreme cases, the flu may lead to pneumonia in particularly susceptible individuals. Other complications of the flu, although rare, include inflammation of the brain (encephalitis) or heart (myocarditis), Reye's syndrome (a syndrome primarily affecting children, involving abnormal brain and liver function), and croup."

Causes of Colds and Flu

Viruses are commonly thought to be the cause of the cold and flu. However, William Michael Cargile, B.S., D.C., F.I.A.C.A., Chairman of Research for the American Academy of Acupuncture and Oriental Medicine, counters this belief. "When everyone in the workplace and at home seems to have a cold or the flu, why do some of my patients not get it?" he asks. "I treat people with the flu all day. Why don't I get it?"

Dr. Cargile believes some patients can resist viral attacks, while the immune systems in others are weakened and run down to such a degree that they become susceptible to a viral assault. He says, "It comes down to available energy. The chemicals in the body which regulate stress are deficient and as a result the ability to adapt to stress is diminished. These are the kinds of people who are much more susceptible to getting the flu every year."

If any complications or severe worsening of either a cold or the flu develop, particularly when the person is in the vulnerable group described, a physician should be contacted immediately.

Emmanuel Cheraskin, M.D., D.M.D, of Birmingham, Alabama, agrees. "Three healthy people can breathe the same germs at the same moment," he notes. "One may develop pneumonia, another sniffle his way through a cold, and the third goes unscathed. After all, in the case of most epidemics, those people who succumb represent only a fraction of the number of people exposed."[2] This suggests an ebb and flow in immune levels in each individual, dependant on stress, diet, rest, and other factors.

"It's time to lay to rest the notion that germs jump into people and cause diseases," Dr. Cheraskin continues. "The evidence is adequate that microbes challenge the internal milieu. The end result depends upon the organism's ability to resist by means of its army of defense systems."[3]

Some physicians go a step further, stating that a cold or flu can actually be one of the ways the body detoxifies itself. "Seen from this viewpoint," says Dr. Hibbs, "you can say that the virus causing the cold or flu is an accessory to a natural process." He notes that both the common cold and the flu are primarily caused by improper diet and toxicity, and represent the body's attempt to rid itself of toxins through fever, coughing, and the discharge of mucous. "Nature is very homeostatic," he says. "When we run our immune systems down, a cold or flu can arise to detoxify ourselves and bring us back into balance."

Diet

Paying attention to the foods a person eats can help him or her avoid creating the imbalances and toxicity in the body that lead to illness of all sorts, including the common cold and flu, according to Dr. Hibbs. He recommends avoiding all foods that decrease immune function, especially simple sugars, which have been shown to reduce the function of white blood cells.[4] "These are principally the refined sweeteners, cane sugar, corn syrup, and beet sugar," he explains. "But also included are the more 'natural' sources of sugar such as honey and concentrated fruit sugar found in dried fruit and fruit juice, as well as the sugars in alcohol."

> *"It's time to lay to rest the notion that germs jump into people and cause diseases. The evidence is adequate that microbes challenge the internal milieu. The end result depends upon the organism's ability to resist by means of its army of defense systems."*
>
> —Emmanuel Cheraskin, M.D., D.M.D.

Foods that cause difficulties in digestion or that contain high amounts of toxins, and all junk foods, should also be eliminated. "Meats and animal products in general are notoriously difficult to digest, and contain toxins such as bacteria, hormones, pesticides, and antibiotics," Dr. Hibbs points out. "If you do eat meat, make sure your digestion is strong and buy organic, free-range meat products."

Nonfood additives such as synthetic colors, synthetic sweeteners, and synthetic flavorings, preservatives, and synthetic oils found in margarine can also toxify the body and stress mucous membranes and the immune system, Dr. Hibbs notes.

Finally, overeating and improper food combinations can also lead to an accumulation of toxins in the body. "The most common and damaging food combining error people make is consuming foods high in protein, such as meats, milk, eggs, and nuts, with fruit, sugars, and other sweet foods," Dr. Hibbs says.

Allergies

Cow's milk, wheat, and all their derivative foods are often described as "mucous producing." "Whether this mucous production is caused by the alleged high mucous content of food or by an irritation or allergy response that the body has to it is debatable," Dr. Hibbs says. "But the increased congestion of the mucous membranes that these foods can cause correlates with more frequent respiratory infections. Most people who avoid dairy products while recovering from the cold or flu generally have less nasal congestion and throat phlegm. And any food or nonfood (such as monosodium glutamate) to which one is sensitive can cause congestion and susceptibility."

See Allergies, Stress.

Airborne allergies may also play a role in the cold and flu by decreasing resistance and permitting viral infections in the respiratory tract. Dust, pollen, molds, and pet hair all aggravate susceptibility to the cold and flu, just as food allergies can. Inflamed, congested membranes in the nose, sinuses, and throat are more vulnerable to viral attack. Although allergies often share the same symptoms as colds, allergies usually have a seasonal history, and are not accompanied by fever or infection as are the cold and flu.

DRUGS ASSOCIATED WITH A HIGHER INCIDENCE OF THE COMMON COLD AND THE FLU

According to the Physicians Desk Reference *the following drugs are associated with side effects of the cold and flu. (Statistics refer to the percentage of individuals affected.)*[5]

Actimmune (Most common)
AeroBid Inhaler System (10%)
Aerobid-M Inhaler System (10%)
Alferon N Injection (30%)
Asacol Delayed-Release Tablets (3%)
CHEMET (succimer) Capsules (5.2-15.7%)
Intron A (37-79%)
Lopressor HCT Tablets (10 in 100 patients)
Nipent for Injection (3-10%)
Permax Tablets (3.2%)
ProSom Tablets (3%)
Rowasa Rectal Suppositories, Rectal Suspension Enema (5.28%)
Videx Tablets, Powder for Oral Solution, and Pediatric Powder for Oral Solution (Less than 1-7%)

Stress

Stress is another factor that can increase susceptibility to the common cold and flu. During times of stress, hormones are released in the body that cause the thymus gland to shrink, reducing immune activity.[6] The more stress one is under, the greater the chance of viral infection.

This effect was demonstrated in a study that evaluated 420 people for occurrences of stress during the previous year. Job loss, divorce, death, and relocation were among the events included, and fear, sadness, anger, and nervousness were among the emotions monitored. The group was then exposed to one of five cold viruses and tested for antibodies one month later. Of those under the greatest amount of stress, 90 percent became infected, as compared to 74 percent of those under the least stress.[7] Another study of 100 people showed that those who experienced particularly high degrees of anger and tension were four times more likely to develop a cold or bacterial infection than were those who did not experience such emotions.[8]

Treating the Common Cold and the Flu

Maintaining a healthy immune system is generally considered to be the key to avoiding the cold and flu. Proper diet, along with nutritional supplements, and the avoidance of alcohol and tobacco, contribute to enhanced immune functions.

The cold and flu are always best treated at the onset. Caught early, many of the remedies described below can stop the cold or the flu in its tracks.

Diet

"We have between four and five thousand microbes of bacteria, viruses, and fungi, living in and on every pore and hole in our bodies," says Dr. Cargile. "The real key to health lies in limiting their populations through dietary control and eating the right foods."

In addition, Dr. Hibbs notes that getting extra sleep, cutting simple sugar intake, and drinking large amounts of herb tea, water, vegetable juices, and broths for a dehydrated respiratory tract, will strengthen immune function and enhance detoxification.

"Water," says Dr. Hibbs, "flushes the system of toxins." He recommends drinking several glasses of pure water a day all year round and eating generously of fruits and vegetables. "Green and orange vegetables are high in beta-carotene," he says. "Vegetables highest in beta-carotene are leafy greens, carrots, and orange-

NATURAL ANTIBIOTICS

According to Garry F. Gordon, M.D., of Tempe, Arizona, an effective treatment at the first sign of cold or flu symptoms is to take high doses of vitamin A, vitamin C, and garlic.

"The effective dose of vitamin C for a 150-pound adult is normally between 10,000 to 20,000 milligrams divided three to six times during a twenty-four-hour period," Dr. Gordon says. "In some cases, though, the dose can go as high as 50,000 to 100,000 milligrams, depending on the severity of the conditions. This dose is continued until any signs of infection have subsided, usually for a minimum of two to five days." Dr. Gordon recommends using a powdered mineral ascorbate form of vitamin C to minimize excess gas or bowel cramping.

Dr. Gordon stresses the importance of taking high doses of vitamin A at the same time as the vitamin C, usually for a period of not less than three and not more than five days. "High doses," he explains, "means that as long as a person's weight is over 120 pounds and there is no serious liver condition, you may safely use four 25,000 unit capsules three or four times a day, for a total of 300,000 to 400,000 units." Dr. Gordon states that no documented evidence exists of serious toxicity due to high doses of vitamin A as long as it is used only for a short period of time. "It's only when these high doses are used for several weeks or months that signs of toxicity develop," he says. "Even then, all reported side effects are completely reversible once supplementation of the vitamin A is discontinued. And certainly vitamin A in high doses is safer than taking larger doses of aspirins or antibiotics, both of which have many possible side effects."

Dr. Gordon emphasizes the importance of taking vitamin A directly rather than supplementing with beta-carotene, which is synthesized in the liver to form vitamin A. Attempting to synthesize an adequate amount of vitmain A from beta-carotene would overtax the liver, adds Dr. Gordon.

Garlic in high doses, also taken at the same time as the vitamins, is the third part of Dr. Gordon's protocol. "It's the allicin content in garlic that's important," Dr. Gordon says. For this reason, he recommends using garlic capsules or liquid garlic extract, both of which provide higher, more concentrated doses of allicin than does eating garlic cloves. Also, these forms eliminate the odor problem common to many garlic eaters. If taking garlic capsules, he recommends taking ten in the first six hours.

colored squash. During cold and flu seasons, have at least one of each every day."

Garlic (*Allium sativum*), historically a folk remedy, is a strong antimicrobial and antiviral plant. Fresh and powdered garlic have been found to have efficient antibiotic effects, even controlling bacteria which are resistant to commonly used antibiotics. In other medical studies, garlic has been shown to protect against flu viruses and enhance antibody production.[9]

The essential enzyme in garlic which gives it its pungent odor, allicin, is rendered inactive by heat. Cooked garlic is not only less odorous, but it has also lost much of its medicinal properties. To receive garlic's optimum health benefits, it should be taken raw.[10] Deodorized, capsule forms are also available at health food outlets.

Nutritional Supplements

Many nutritional supplements can be valuable aids in dealing with the cold and flu, due to their ability to stimulate immune functions and protect the body from the effects of stress.

The most well-know nutrient for combatting colds and flu is vitamin C. Numerous studies have shown that people taking megadoses of vitamin C (amounts far larger than the U.S. RDA standards) report reductions in "the incidence, severity, and duration of colds.[11]" After several double-blind trial studies, researchers found "that vitamin C supplementation may be useful for lessening the severity of disease as well as reducing transmission of viruses."[12]

> *"We have between four and five thousand microbes of bacteria, viruses and fungi, living in and on every pore and hole in our bodies. The real key to health lies in limiting their populations through dietary control and eating the right foods."*
> —William Michael Cargile, B.S. D.C., F.I.A.C.A.

Beyond its antiviral and antibacterial properties, vitamin C acts as an immunostimulant. It enhances white blood cell production, increases interferon (a group of proteins released by white blood cells that combat a virus) levels and antibody responses, promotes secretion of thymic hormones, and improves connective tissue.[13]

Garry F.. Gordon, M.D., of Tempe, Arizona, also recommends zinc throat lozenges, another important nutrient for maintaining the immune system, and thymus extract, which enhances the protective effect of the thymus gland.

Herbal Medicine

Herbs have a long history of use as a treatment for the cold and flu, due to their ability to stimulate immune functions, as well as their antiviral, anti-inflammatory, and anticatarrhal properties. Herbs which bolster the immune system include echinacea, goldenseal, licorice, elder, St. John's Wort, and astragalus.[14]

"Lomatium deserves special mention as a flu remedy," says Dr. Hibbs. "It's an antiviral and it stimulates the immune system. I find it to be the most effective flu remedy in the herbal pharmacy." In patients taking the herb for full-blown flu symptoms, he has observed full recovery on numerous occasions within twenty-four to forty-eight hours. Although relatively unknown, lomatium is available in some health food stores and herbal outlets.

One of Dr. Hibbs' patients came to him with the flu. "He had nausea but no vomiting, and a 102 degrees Fahrenheit fever for two or three days. He felt very achy and tired with moderate coughing and sneezing, and minimal congestion, but it was obviously the flu and not a cold. I simply put him on a lomatium tincture mixed with the herbs ligustium and echinacea. He took it three or four times a day and was told to drink lots of fluids, get plenty of rest, avoid alcohol and sugar. Within less than forty-eight hours, he was 90 percent better." Dr. Hibbs cautions, however, that lomatium can cause an itchy measles-like rash on the skin of sensitive patients or those who take too large a dose.

See Herbal Medicine.

Mary Bove, N.D., Chair of Botanical Medicine at Bastyr College, in Seattle, Washington, recommends the following herbs for general use in the treatment of colds and flu:

- **Yarrow**, calming to an upset digestive tract, is also an anti-inflammatory and diaphoretic. These qualities make yarrow particularly useful in influenza and respiratory infections associated with fever, malaise, and decreased appetite.
- **Eyebright**, an anticatarrhal and anti-inflammatory, is useful in respiratory conditions, specifically the nasal pharynx and the sinuses.
- **Elecampagne** is a soothing, relaxing, yet stimulating expectorant for irritating coughs and bronchial irritations.
- **Elderflower**, immune-stimulating, anti-inflammatory, anticatarrhal, and diaphoretic, it is a good all-purpose herb for the flu and common cold.

Dr. Bove notes that these herbs can be easily combined or used singly as teas or tinctures.

Homeopathy

Doctors are using both traditional and modern methods in homeopathic treatments for the cold and flu. Contemporary methods include injection of homeopathic remedies intramuscularly or intravenously. This approach is employed by Leonard Haimes, M.D., of Boca Raton, Florida, who injects his patients with a homeopathic preparation containing *Viscum album*, a plant that is known for its antiviral and antitumor properties. Along with the preparation, Dr. Haimes gives other herbs, homeopathic formulas, and large doses of vitamin C.

Dr. Hibbs prescribes the following additional homeopathic remedies:

- ***Aconitum napellus*** for sudden cold or flu symptoms which begin after exposure to cold, and in which the patient is chilled, but feels better in the open air and worse after midnight. These types of symptoms may include anxiety and extreme thirst.
- ***Natrum muriaticum*** for the patient with a profuse, thin, watery, nasal discharge. Symptoms include thirst, sneezing, and loss of taste and sense of smell.
- ***Allium cepa*** for patients whose eyes and nose stream with watery, burning discharge and who sneeze frequently.
- ***Nux vomica*** for patients who have nasal congestion, especially at night. During the day, the nose can be quite runny and burning, and the person may be impatient and irritable.
- ***Eupatorium perfoliatum*** for patients who have deep bone ache, are thirsty, cough with chest soreness, and feel worse in cold air.

Other homeopathic treatments Dr. Hibbs prescribes include *Belladonna*, *Baptisia*, and *Bryonia*.

Acupuncture/Traditional Chinese Medicine

Dr. Cargile believes that weakened immune systems in people with a cold or flu are a result of depletion of energy, ATP (adenosine triphosphate— the energy product of cellular respiration), and p-cortisol (a stress adaptation hormone from the adrenal cortex) levels. To rechannel energy levels in treatment of his patients, Dr. Cargile uses acupuncture meridians related to endocrine functions, digestion, lungs, and other organs. "With these meridian points used in conjunction with each other, we have been able to significantly affect the body's immune system and redirect energy action in the direction needed," he says.

Dr. Cargile says that after treating several patients with acupuncture as a preventative, "people who have had longstanding chronic flu symptoms have not had them now for two years."

See Acupuncture, Homeopathy, Traditional Chinese Medicine.

Traditional Chinese Medicine offers another approach to understanding and treating the cold and flu. According to Marian Small, N.D., L.Ac., of Seattle, Washington, the common cold can be caused by six different environmental factors: wind, heat, cold, dampness, dryness, and summer heat. "When these factors are strong enough or when a person is in a susceptible state, then there is an invasion and illness occurs," notes Dr. Small. "Wind usually affects the throat, lungs, and head. Cold weather can create white or clear discharge of body secretions. Heat can manifest as fevers, thirst, dry stools, rashes, and secretions that are yellow and sticky."

Some Traditional Chinese Medicine formulas recommended by Dr. Small to combat the common cold and flu are:

- ***Yinqiao***, good in the first stage of a cold or flu, it expels wind and heat from the exterior layers of the body. Symptoms can include sore throat, fever with chills, body aches, or headache. It can also be used in certain rashes.
- **Natural herb loquat syrup,** as an expectorant for coughs with phlegm and sinus congestion.
- ***Bo ying powder***, for infants and children with a wide range of childhood diseases, including: fever, headache, cough, upset stomach, diarrhea, or vomiting. It can be mixed with food.
- ***Bi yan pian***, useful for sneezing, sinus congestion, itchy eyes, facial congestion, or hay fever.

Since ephedra increases blood pressure and heart rate, it should be avoided by those with cardiac conditions, high blood pressure, and women who are pregnant.[15]

Another herb, Chinese ephedra (*ma-huang*), has been used in China for thousands of years to treat colds, asthma, bronchitis, fever, and other ailments. Ephedra contains ephedrine which, synthesized, is extensively used in Western medicine both in over-the-counter and prescription remedies for conditions such as hay fever and rhinitis. Ephedra roots and branches, taken in a tea, can be very effective in the treatment of cold and flu symptoms.

> ### Hydrotherapy
> *Outbreaks of the common cold and flu often coincide with dramatic changes of temperature, humidity, and season. Hydrotherapy is another method of strengthening and detoxifying the body and immune system. When done on a regular basis, contrast hydrotherapy, which consists of exposing the body to sudden shifts of hot and cold water temperature, will keep the body and immune system acclimatized. It can be as simple as running the last thirty to sixty seconds of a morning shower at a colder temperature.*

Ayurvedic Medicine

Virender Sodhi, M.D. (Ayurveda), N.D., Director of the American School of Ayurvedic Sciences in Bellevue, Washington, employs a number of Ayurvedic approaches to treat patients with the cold and flu. The objective of Ayurvedic medicine, according to Dr. Sodhi, is to rid the body of indigestible toxins which attract viruses and compromise the autoimmune process. To increase digestion, he uses herbs such as ginger, cayenne pepper, black pepper, long pepper, and holy basil. "I have my patients drink lots of warm water and ginger tea throughout the day, and prescribe breathing exercises which help them to expectorate mucous," he says. "When people know they have an allergy or the flu, they usually use antihistamines which dry up the mucous. So you are stuck with a problem. The body wants to expel the mucous, but the use of antihistamines prevent that from happening."

Dr. Sodhi believes it is important to expectorate during a cold or flu in order to clean out nasal passages. He uses an exercise called the nasal douche for this purpose. "To perform this is very easy," Dr. Sodhi says. "Take a teapot and fill it with sea salt and warm water. Let the water flow from the spout through one nostril and into the other. You should feel the nasal passages clearing within a brief time."

Hyperthermia

Hyperthermia can be used to stimulate immune response and detoxification through sweating. "The enhancement of the body's natural tendency to fever during a cold or flu has beneficial effects," says Dr. Hibbs, "including a dramatic stimulation of detoxification through the skin." Though uncomfortable, fever produces a natural antibiotic effect within the body, and additionally appears to shorten the duration of infection.[16] Dr. Hibbs recommends that fever treatments be coupled with a very clean, simplified diet featuring large amounts of water, steamed vegetables, vegetable juice, or broth.

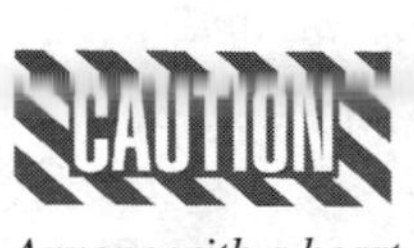

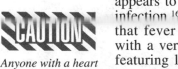

Anyone with a heart condition should consult his or her physician before undertaking this preventive technique.

Dr. Hibbs describes the treatment on a five-year-old patient. "She had come down with flu symptoms a few hours earlier, including lethargy and fatigue, a fever of 101.5 degrees Fahrenheit, a headache, and a sore throat. She was not hungry and was just encouraged to drink liquids. I gave her a single ninety-drop dose of a 50:50 mixture of tinctures of echinacea and lomatium, and she was then given a fever treatment at home. The home treatment consisted of placing her in a hot bath in a very warm bathroom. In the bath, she drank a cup of hot yarrow tea.

"She was attended constantly by an adult and her temperature was taken every two to three minutes orally. When her temperature reached 103 degrees Fahrenheit, which took ten to fifteen minutes, she was quickly toweled dry and clothed in heavy cotton pajamas. She went immediately to bed, fell into a deep sleep, and woke the next morning feeling completely well and was able to attend school as usual without relapse."

Dr. Hibbs notes, however, that hyperthermia should be used with caution in a patient who already has a fever. "The body temperature should never be permitted to rise above 104 degrees Fahrenheit," he says. "If it does, cool water sponging or medication can be used to reduce it. Medications may also be needed to control fever, particularly in small children. But it should be kept in mind that these drugs interrupt the normal immune response and, while reducing the symptoms, may lengthen infections."

Self-Care

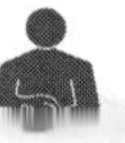

The following therapies can be undertaken at home under appropriate professional supervision:

• Biofeedback Training • Fasting • Guided Imagery • Yoga

Aromatherapy: Inhalations and baths with camphor, eucalyptus, lavender, lemon, peppermint, pine, rosemary, tea tree.

Flower Remedies: For emotional states as appropriate.

Juice Therapy: • Lemon, orange, pineapple, black currant, elderberry juice • Carrot, beet, tomato, green pepper, and watercress. Add small doses of onion or garlic juice to vegetable juices. • Carrot, celery • Carrot, spinach • Carrot, beet, cucumber

Topical Treatment: For head cold: spray throat and nasal passages with witch hazel.

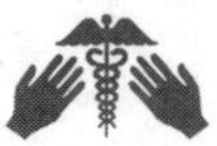

Professional Care

The following therapies should only be provided by a qualified health professional:

• Applied Kinesiology • Chiropractic • Colon Therapy • Environmental Medicine • Magnetic Field Therapy • Orthomolecular Medicine • Osteopathy

Bodywork: • Acupressure • Reflexology • *Shiatsu* • Percussion massage to break up cold

***Oxygen Therapy*:** Hydrogen peroxide

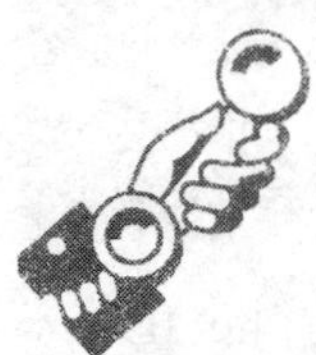

Where to Find Help

For additional information on colds and the flu, contact:

American Association of Acupuncture and Oriental Medicine
4101 Lake Boone Trail, Suite 201
Raleigh, North Carolina 27607
(919) 787-5181

The AAAOM is a national professional trade organization of acupuncturists who meet acceptable standards of competency and can provide you with the names and locations of local members.

American Association of Naturopathic Physicians
2366 Eastlake Avenue, Suite 322
Seattle, Washington 98102
(206) 323-7610

Contact them for the location of a licensed naturopathic physician in your area.

American Holistic Medical Association
4101 Lake Boone Trail, Suite 201
Raleigh North Carolina 27607
(919) 787-5181

Provides referrals, for a fee. Publishes a bimonthly magazine, several publications, and guidelines for nutrition and fitness. Sponsors conferences on holistic medicine for the holistic professional.

American School of Ayurvedic Sciences
10025 NE 4th Street
Bellevue, Washington 98004
(206) 453-8022

This college provides medical training for physicians and health care practitioners, as well as individual courses for lay people. Dr. Virender Sodhi's Ayurvedic, Naturopathic Medical Clinic is also located at this address.

The College of Maharishi Ayur-Veda Medical Center
P.O. Box 282
Fairfield, Iowa 52556
(515) 472-5866

The center provides referrals to health centers, which offer treatment or prevention for a broad range of illnesses. They also train practitioners and provide information to the lay public.

International Foundation for Homeopathy
2366 Eastlake Avenue, East, Suite 301
Seattle, Washington 98102
(206) 324-8230

Provides educational courses for professionals and the general public. Offers referrals to homeopathic health professionals.

National Center for Homeopathy
801 North Fairfax, Suite 306
Alexandria, Virginia 22314
(703) 548-7790

Provides a referral list of practicing homeopaths and information. Gives courses for lay people and professionals, and organizes study groups around the country.

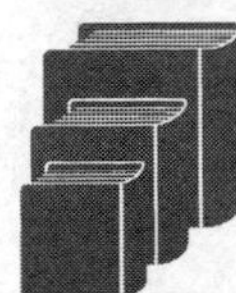

Recommended Reading

Breathe Free. Gagnon, Daniel; and Morningstart, Amadea. Wilimot, WI: Lotus Press, 1990.
A nutritional and herbal medicine self-help guide to treating a full range of respiratory conditions, including colds and flu.

The Common Cold and Common Sense. Alexander, Dale. New York: Fireside Books, 1981.
A practical approach to treating colds and flu based on diet and nutrition.

Encyclopedia of Natural Medicine. Murray, Michael, N.D.; and Pizzorno, Joseph, N.D. Rocklin, CA: Prima Publishing, 1991.
An authoritative guide to naturopathic medicine outlining the basic principles of health and how they can be used to treat over sixty health conditions, including colds. Includes self-help approaches using diet, nutrition, and herbal medicine.

***Vitamin C: Who Needs It*.** Cheraskin, Emmanuel, M.D. Birmingham, AL: Arlington Press, 1993.
An informational book on the nutritional benefits of vitamin C.

"Oh, the powers of nature! She knows what we need, and the doctors know nothing."

—Benvenuto Cellini

Constipation

Each year Americans spend billions of dollars on laxatives to deal with some form of constipation. Despite this fact, conventional medicine gives little attention to this growing national problem, preferring to prescribe medicine that treats symptoms rather than the root causes of the condition. Alternative medicine takes a different view, and offers a variety of approaches to help cleanse the colon and return it to a natural state of health.

Constipation refers to a difficulty or infrequency in the passage of stools due to sluggish action of the bowels. This can be a serious condition that can result in headaches, fatigue, depression, pain, and other digestive problems. According to James Braly, M.D., Medical Director of Immuno Labs, Inc., in Fort Lauderdale, Florida, constipation can undermine the whole body system, affecting digestion, the clearing of toxins from the system, energy level, and the absorption of nutrients.

There is a wide discrepancy between conventional and alternative health communities concerning what constitutes regular bowel movements. According to the *Physician's Manual for Patients*, "Daily bowel movements are not essential to health."[1] This view represents the conventional medical outlook. However, alternative practitioners strongly disagree with this idea, feeling that two or three bowel movements a day are ideal for health maintenance.

"Constipation can undermine the whole body system, affecting digestion, the clearing of toxins from the system, energy level, and the absorption of nutrients."
—James Braly, M.D.

Still, Leon Chaitow, N.D., D.O., of London, England, points out that different physical body types have very different tendencies which require different considerations. For example, he has found that stocky individuals very often have superb bowel function and a rapid transit time. In contrast, Dr. Chaitow has found that lean individuals, whose diets are more vegetarian, often have a sluggish and slow bowel pattern. He notes that people are different biochemically and emotionally and must be treated on an individual basis.

Regardless of such individual differences, however, it is now known that irregular bowel movements are directly related to serious health conditions. In 1981, a study published in *The Lancet* reported that women who have less than three bowel movements per week have four times the risk of breast disease than those who have one or more bowel movements per day.[2] Furthermore, colon cancer accounts for over 56,000 deaths each year.[3]

Causes of Constipation

According to Patrick Donovan, N.D., of Seattle, Washington, constipation can be caused by a number of different factors and conditions, including poor diet and nutrition, food allergies, lack of exercise, poor posture, emotional upsets and anxiety, imbalances of estrogen and progesterone, imbalances in the autonomic nervous system, a variety of drugs and medications, and the misuse of laxatives and enemas. Constipation for many patients can also alternate with diarrhea and abdominal cramps in a common condition known as irritable bowel syndrome.

Dr. Donovan notes that many older patients' dependence on laxatives and enemas leads to relaxed gut muscles which make elimination more difficult. He stresses that proper elimination is necessary to avoid a buildup of toxins in the body, a condition that can lead to chronic inflammatory/autoimmune diseases such as rheumatoid arthritis, lupus, ankylosing spondylitis, Crohn's disease, and ulcerative colitis. Improper elimination may even cause a state of toxemia in which toxins are leached back into the bloodstream. This is called "autointoxication," which in turn brings about a great variety of symptoms and ailments.

Diet

Dr. Braly points to poor diet as the most significant cause of constipation. Highly processed foods, fast foods, fatty foods, sugars, and salt all contribute to a variety of digestive problems, he notes.

See Allergies, Diet, Female Health, Male Health.

Perhaps the single most important cause of constipation is a lack of fiber in a person's diet. The *British Medical Journal* recently summarized studies on this fact and stated that "fiber increases stool bulk, holds water, and acts as a substrate [catalyst] for colonic microflora," all of which "decreases transit time, reduces intracolonic pressure, and produces a softer stool."[4]

The dietary ideal is a proper balance of proteins, carbohydrates, vitamins, mineral salts, roughage, and fluids. Dr. Chaitow recommends a "60/40" diet, where 60 percent of the total food consumption is fruits and vegetables and the remaining 40 percent is made up from carbohydrates (20 percent derived from bread, cereals, and grains), proteins (15 percent), and fats (5 percent). The relative acidity or alkalinity of food is also important to diet and health. Foods that are too acidic—such as meats, dairy, and sugar—can interfere with the functioning of the colon, while alkaline foods (like vegetables and fruits) have a natural laxative effect upon the digestive tract, according to Dr. Chaitow.

"Perhaps the single most important cause of constipation is a lack of fiber in a person's diet."

Additionally, Dr. Chaitow points to the possibility that food sensitivities and allergies can cause constipation, with dairy products being a common offender.

Misuse of Laxatives

The use of some form of over-the-counter laxative is widespread in the United States. Yet, according to Dr. Braly, laxatives are only effective as a treatment for occasional constipation. He has found that when laxative use by patients becomes chronic, the laxatives only aggravate the condition. Most drugstore laxatives contain ingredients that provide abnormal stimulation of the intestines and slowly paralyze them by damaging intestinal nerves.

Stress

According to Dr. Braly, anxiety, fear, worry, grief, and frustration have all been known to affect the digestive tract, causing ulcers, diarrhea, or constipation. In some serious cases, peristalsis (the wavelike contractions and dilations of the colon muscles that expel waste matter) becomes extremely weak and the colon becomes severely dysfunctional. When stressed, the nervous system becomes enzyme deficient, saliva flow decreases, and lactic acid accumulates, causing stomach pain and indigestion.

See Environmental Medicine, Stress

Drugs, Chemicals, and Environmental Toxins

Constipation may also result as a side effect from the use of literally hundreds of common medications, including some antibiotics and anti-inflammatories, muscle relaxants, opiates, analgesics, antacids, anticonvulsants, antidepressants, antipsychotics, antihypertensives, diuretics, and anaesthetics.[5] In addition, the intake of bismuth and iron salts, and exposure to toxic metals (arsenic, lead, mercury) found in the earth's air and water are contributing factors to constipation.[6]

Treatment of Constipation

In treating constipation, Dr. Donovan's aim is to normalize bowel movements, which he believes is absolutely necessary for good health. "The first three things I think of in treating constipation are fluid, fiber, and exercise," he says. "When someone is constipated, it is usually due to an insufficiency of these three things."

Diet and Nutrition

Since poor diet is a major cause of constipation, a healthy diet is a key to elimination. The general recommendation is to change to a high-fiber diet rich in carbohydrates, vegetables, and fruits. Dr. Donovan emphasizes that increasing dietary fiber increases the frequency and quantity of bowel movements.

Major sources of fiber include wheat bran, whole grain products, and beans. The addition of as little as twenty grams (0.7 ounces) of bran each day can increase fecal weight by 127 percent and decrease transit time by 40 percent,[8] two factors that are essential in alleviating constipation and keeping the colon healthy. A 1978 *The Lancet* study showed that an equal quantity of cabbage, carrots, or apples would produce a similar but smaller effect.[9]

Sometimes people avoid increasing fiber because they find it less palatable than the highly refined diet they have grown used to. Others object to the increase in flatulence and bloating that resulted from taking in too much bran too fast. According to Dr. Donovan, this problem can be easily corrected by increasing fiber intake gradually or using more mucilaginous (thick, sticky) forms of bran such as psyllium seeds or linseed (flax).

The amount of fluids people drink is another important consideration in the treatment of constipation. Dr. Braly recommends a minimum of six to eight glasses of pure water per day. In order to promote proper digestion, however, high liquid intake should occur away from mealtimes, because consuming excessive liquids with food reduces digestive functions.

According to Steven Bailey, N.D., of Portland, Oregon, raw juice therapy can be helpful for constipation. One approach involves drinking sixteen ounces of one of the following juice combinations throughout the day. Choose from any of the following formulas:

• Eight ounces of carrot combined with eight ounces of apple

DRUGS ASSOCIATED WITH A HIGHER INCIDENCE OF CONSTIPATION

According to the Physicians Desk Reference *the following drugs are associated with side effects of constipation. (Statistics refer to the percentage of individuals affected.)*[7]

Anafranil Capsules (22-47%)
Anaprox and Anaprox DS Tablets (3-9%)
Aredia for Injection (Up to 15%)
Asacol Delayed-Release Tablets (5%)
Asendin Tablets (12%)
Atrofen Tablets (2-6%)
Calan SR Caplets, Tablets (7.3%)
Clinoril Tablets (3-9%)
Clozaril Tablets (More than 5-14%)
Colestid Granules (1 in 10)
Combipres Tablets (About 10%)
Cordarone Tablets (4-9%)
DHC Plus Capsules (Among most frequent)
Daypro Caplets (3-9%)
Desyrel and Desyrel Dividose (7.0-7.6%)
Dilacor XR Extended-Release Capsules (3.6%)
Duragesic Transdermal System (10% or more)
Empirin with Codeine Tablets (Among most frequent)
Habitrol Nicotine Transdermal System (3-9% of patients)
Hivid Tablets (Less than 1-6.4%)
Hylorel Tablets (21.0%)
Intron A (Up to 10%)
Isoptin Oral Tablets, SR Sustained Release Tablets (7.3%)
Limbitrol DS Tablets, Tablets (Among most frequent)
Lioresal Tablets (2-6%)
Ludiomil Tablets (6%)
Lupron Injection (5% or more)
MS Contin Tablets (Among most frequent)
MSIR Oral Solution, Oral Solution Concentrate, Tablets (Among most frequent)
Marplan Tablets (Among most frequent)
Mepron Tablets (3%)
Mevacor Tablets (2.0-4.9%)
Mexitil Capsules (4%)
Nalfon 200 Pulvules & Nalfon Tablets (7%)
Naprosyn Suspension, Tablets (3-9%)
Neupogen for Injection (5%)
Nicoderm Nicotine Transdermal System (3-9%)
Nipent for Injection (3-10%)
Norpace Capsules, CR Capsules (11%)
Oramorph SR (Morphine Sulfate Sustained Release Tablets) (Among most frequent)
Orudis Capsules (Greater than 3%)
Paraplatin for Injection (6%)
Parlodel Capsules, SnapTabs (3-14%)
Paxil Tablets (13.8%)
Permax Tablets (10.6%)
Procardia XL Extended Release Tablets (3.3%)
Proleukin for Injection (5%)
Prozac Pulvules & Liquid, Oral Solution (4.5%)
Questran Light, Powder (Most common)
Relafen Tablets (3-9%)
Retrovir Capsules, Syrup (6.4%)
Rythmol Tablets (2.0-7.2%)
Sanorex Tablets (Among most common)
Sectral Capsules (4%)
Stadol Injectable, NS Nasal Spray (3-9%)
Tambocor Tablets (4.4%)
Tenex Tablets (1-16%)
Triaminic Expectorant DH (Among most frequent)
Trilisate Liquid, Tablets (Less than 20%)
Velban Vials (Among most common)
Verelan Capsules (7.3%)
Videx Tablets, Powder for Oral Solution, & Pediatric Powder for Oral Solution (Less than 1-16%)
Voltaren Tablets (3-9%)
Wellbutrin Tablets (26.0%)
Xanax Tablets (10.4-26.2%)
Zofran Injection (11%), Tablets (5-7%)
Zoloft Tablets (8.4%)

• Eight ounces of carrot, four ounces of celery, and four ounces of apple

• Twelve ounces of carrot combined with four ounces of spinach

Dr. Donovan recommends combining the intake of fiber and fluids through fruit smoothies. He advises patients to blend a mix of high pectin fruits like apples, peaches, pears, and berries, with a quarter cup of oat bran and a quarter cup of flaxseed powder or flaxseed meal. If there are no dairy allergies, a few tablespoons of yogurt may be added as well.

Donald Brown, N.D., of Bastyr Naturopathic College in Seattle, Washington, states that for treating constipation one of the most important nutrients is magnesium, which is naturally found in vegetables and fruits.

Although there are a number of effective bulking agents that one can find in health food stores that help with constipation, Dr. Brown has noted that many people who use them become bloated and still remain constipated. "With these individuals, I usually prescribe a therapeutic dose of magnesium—eight hundred milligrams daily for adults—and this is often enough to get the plumbing going again. Once this has happened, we can begin work on diet and other bowel conditions," he says.

Dr. Brown also emphasizes the importance of fluid intake and the use of folic acid, particularly with women. Treatment includes a complete medical history which may show that the problem relates to the use of various drugs and antibiotics. He recommends a stool analysis to check for yeast overgrowth, and pays close attention to the function of the liver which, he notes, is critical to normal bowel function. Following Dr. Brown's treatment, a patient is able to establish healthy, regular bowel movements in three to four weeks, which can then be maintained through improved diet and regular exercise.

Dr. Braly recommends routine nutritional supplementation for constipated patients. Additionally he advises using vitamin C to 90 percent bowel tolerance, taking six to eight capsules daily of evening primrose oil, and increasing dosages of MaxEPA (a form of essential fatty acids) to three to six capsules daily.

Herbal Medicine

As alternatives to possibly harmful conventional laxatives, a number of natural laxatives are available. Dr. Braly advises every day adding one or two teaspoons of psyllium or ground flaxseed to breakfast cereal or mixed into a beverage. He warns, however, it is possible for some patients to develop severe allergic reactions to psyllium, in which case it should be avoided.

For constipation, Dr. Brown regularly recommends the use of herbs such as aloe, *Cascara*

The Mayr Cure for Constipation

As an alternative to high liquid intake, Leon Chaitow, N.D., D.O., of London, England, cites a naturopathic cure for digestive problems which involves "reeducating" the digestive system. This diet cure promotes the maximal amount of chewing of food; it involves eating dry bread rolls, each morning and before each meal, in order to stimulate salivary flow.

During the cure, each mouthful of food is chewed ideally fifty times, until food becomes a paste. This is intended to stimulate the "satiety" center in the brain and also for marked enzyme mixing with the food, according to Dr. Chaitow.

The breakfast meal consists of a stale (three-day-old or dry toasted) roll. Small bites of the dry food should be eaten, with no fluids consumed at all. When the bite of roll has become a paste in the mouth, place one teaspoonful of live yogurt into the mouth. Chew this mixture a few more times (making it a total of fifty chews), and then swallow. Continue following the mouthful of bread paste with teaspoons of yogurt until the roll is consumed. Dr. Chaitow recommends having nothing else for breakfast but points out that patients will not feel hungry.

Thirty minutes after breakfast, Dr. Chaitow advises drinking herbal tea, either pau d'arco, lemon verbena, linden blossom, fennel, or sage.

Lunch consists of another dry roll, consumed as above, then follows with lightly cooked vegetables accompanying either a vegetarian, fish, or lean meat dish. Again, no liquid is consumed with the meal, but herbal tea should follow thirty minutes later.

The evening meal consists of another dry roll, followed with live yogurt, herbal tea, and cooked vegetables.

During the Mayr cure, Dr. Chaitow advises having no fruit, raw vegetables, fatty foods, alcohol, coffee, or sugar. According to Dr. Chaitow, the key to success in this program is the length of time spent chewing food, which is encouraged by the dry roll.

If the bowels aren't moving after starting the diet, Dr. Chaitow recommends taking a level teaspoon of Epsom salts in a cup of hot water a half hour before breakfast. After three to five days, he predicts that the bowels should start to function efficiently.

Acidophilus and Constipation

Natural supplements are also used to help facilitate the rebuilding of flora and the growth of "friendly bacteria" in the colon. Leon Chaitow, N.D., D.O., of London, England, recommends daily supplementation of a half teaspoon of Lactobacillus acidophilus *in high potency (over 1 billion microorganisms per gram) accompanied by one-eighth teaspoon of* Bifidobacteria bifidum *taken in a four to one ratio, twenty minutes before meals. He also recommends one-half teaspoon daily of* Lactobacillus bulgaricus *taken with meals to enhance the resident friendly bacteria.*

A female patient of John Hibbs, N.D., of Seattle, Washington, came to him wanting relief from lifelong constipation. She was motivated, and agreed to lifestyle changes including diet, exercise, and increased fluid intake, but none of these helped the constipation. Tests for parasites, yeast overgrowth, and digestive problems were negative. As a general measure, Dr. Hibbs prescribed Lactobacillus acidophilus, *one-eighth teaspoon twice daily. After taking the supplement for four months, the patient's bowel movements became quite regular.*

sagrada, senna, and rhubarb. He also advises using dandelion root and silymarin, which help stimulate normal liver functioning and alleviate constipation.

Dr. Donovan also uses the medicinal herb blackthorn, which has long been used as for its laxative properties. According to him, it acts in the large intestine to increase peristalsis.

Stress Reduction

Proper exercise and relaxation also play a role in reducing and eliminating constipation, a fact that is recognized by both conventional and alternative physicians alike. Exercise tones the abdominal muscles, stimulates the peristaltic action of the colon, decreases emotional stress, and increases breathing and oxygenation of the body, all essential steps in rejuvenating the body and achieving exceptional health. The best exercise, according to Dr. Braly, is a brisk daily walk of at least thirty minutes after a meal, combined with aerobic exercises four to five times weekly.

Eating foods slowly, moderately, and in a relaxing environment can also reduce susceptibility to constipation. According to Dr. Hibbs, when a person eats in a relaxed state, a signal is sent from the parasympathetic nervous system to the bowel to empty out any stool, hence the rationale for a bowel movement after each meal.

Dr. Hibbs describes a male patient suffering from many effects of stress, including fatigue and constipation. The patient relied heavily on coffee to keep him going physically and had developed chronic adrenal fatigue. Dr. Hibbs took him off caffeine and sugar, which are both stimulants and were taxing his system. Appropriate exercise and dietary changes were made and he was put on adrenal supportive supplements containing glandular tissue, herbs, and nutrients twice a day. His bowel habits normalized quickly and remained that way when he stopped the adrenal supplement several months later.

See Bodywork, Chiropractic, Herbal Medicine, Osteopathy.

Another type of stress, the misalignment of the spine, can also contribute to constipation. Lumbar spinal adjustments by a chiropractor may be helpful, as well as other forms of bodywork. Dr. Chaitow recommends treatments such as osteopathic manipulation and *shiatsu* massage to improve spinal mechanics.

Ayurvedic Medicine

To treat constipation Ayurvedic medicine recommends colon detoxification, according to Vasant Lad, M.A.Sc., Director of the Ayurvedic Institute in Albuquerque, New Mexico. "One method is to use a medicated enema made up of a concoction of *dashamoola*, a traditional combination of ten herbs," Dr. Lad explains. He recommends boiling one tablespoon of dashamoola powder in one pint of water for ten minutes,

Constipation and Allergies

According to James Braly, M.D., Medical Director of Immuno Labs, Inc., in Fort Lauderdale, Florida, food allergies can often be a factor in constipation. He cites the case of one of his patients, a banker in his mid-forties, who complained of fatigue, lower back pain, dizziness, nausea, weight gain, high blood pressure, headaches, and severe constipation. The patient was dependent on laxatives and also taking two prescription medicines and six to eight aspirins daily. Dr. Braly changed the patient's diet, eliminating key allergic foods, and within ten days his chronic constipation disappeared, along with all the other conditions except lower back pain. The patient was able to give up all his medications and had lost eight pounds. Dr. Braly states, "No amount of bran or other fiber would have done the trick alone. The elimination of allergies was the crucial factor."

strain, cool, and add one half cup of warm sesame oil. Use this mixture for basti, during the vata time of day, (in the early morning six to seven o'clock and six to seven o'clock in the evening until bowel function is improved.

Triphala can also be used according to Dr. Lad using one half to one teaspoon of its powdered form in a warm glass of water before bedtime. "Some people may experience a diuretic effect from triphala," Dr. Lad says. "In these cases, they can steep the mixture overnight, and strain and drink it in the morning. Senna leaves are also used in Ayurvedic tradition to treat constipation, taking one half teaspoon or less with ginger tea. During pregnancy, however, triphal and senna should not be used. Instead, one may take one cup of hot milk with a teaspoon of *ghee* (clarified butter) before bedtime. This usually acts as a mild laxative during pregnancy. It is also important that there should be some amount of roughage in the diet on a regular basis, such as wheat or oat bran, notes Dr. Lad.

For children with constipation, Virender Sodhi, M.D. (Ayurveda), N.D., Director of the American School of Ayurvedic Sciences in Bellevue, Washington, recommends drinking almond oil with a dash of sugar added to increase peristalsis. *Acacia fistula*, a sweet fruit high in vitamin C and fiber which can also be used, mixed with sugar, honey, and rose petals.

The diet of one patient suffering from constipation was found by Dr. Sodhi to be deficient in fruits and vegetables. Dr. Sodhi changed the patient's diet and had him drink eight glasses of water daily. He was also given *triphala*. Soon the patient's constipation was relieved and his digestive function returned to normal.

See Acupuncture Ayurvedic Medicine, Traditional Chinese Medicine.

Acupuncture/Traditional Chinese Medicine

Maoshing Ni, D.O.M., Ph.D., L.Ac., Vice-President of Yo San University in Santa Monica, California, recommends a combination of herbs, and exercise in addition to dietary changes when treating constipation. "Acupuncture," he states, "can restore the natural peristaltic action of the colon, as can exercise, deep breathing, and massage." Rhubarb root, aloe vera, and senna leaf are often given as a tea by Dr. Ni to alleviate constipation and to help rehydrate the intestines.

"But the use of herbs is more complex," Dr. Ni says, "and must be matched to the conditions and constitution of the individual. An elderly or frail person would be given a different herbal compound than someone else, perhaps a mixture of seed lubricants like sesame, apricot kernel, and peach kernel."

In Traditional Chinese Medicine, diet is also a highly individualized matter. Dr. Ni generally recommends a high-fiber diet. "Beets and cabbage have done wonders," he adds, "particularly for people who may find that bran is too harsh."

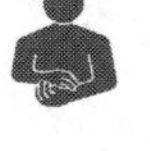

Self-Care

The following therapies can be undertaken at home under appropriate professional supervision:

• Fasting • Qigong • Yoga

Acupressure: To relieve constipation, firmly press CV6 (for an illustration of this point number please see the acupressure chart on page 874) by placing all of your fingertips three finger widths below the belly button between your naval and pubic bone. Gradually press in one inch deep or until you can lightly touch something firm. Maintain this firm pressure for three minutes while you breath deeply and keep your eyes closed.

Aromatherapy: Massage clockwise around abdomen with rose, marjoram, camphor, fennel, black pepper, rosemary.

Homeopathy: *Alumina, Bryonia, Graphites, Natrum mur., Nux vomica, Silicea.*

Hydrotherapy: Constitutional hydrotherapy: apply two to five times weekly. Enema/colon irrigation: apply daily as needed.

Take a cool sitz bath for five minutes. Spastic constipation: take a hot sitz bath for more than ten minutes. Keep cold compress on forehead and drink water. Hot and cold shower: alternate long hot streams and short cold streams on abdomen. Chronic constipation: cold compress on abdomen covered with large dry towel.

Juice Therapy: • Carrot, beet, or celery juice with one teaspoon of garlic or yellow onion juice • Chronic constipation: add garlic, yellow onion, black radish, spinach, watercress, or dandelion to carrot, beet, celery, cabbage, cucumber, tomato • Lemon juice • Apple juice • Carrot, apple • Carrot, celery, apple • Carrot, spinach

Lifestyle: Take a brisk walk early in the morning.

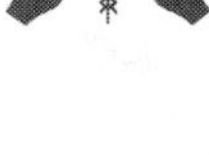

Professional Care

The following therapies should only be provided by a qualified health professional:

• Biofeedback Training • Chiropractic • Colon Therapy • Craniosacral Therapy • Environmental Medicine • Hypnotherapy • Magnetic Field Therapy • Orthomolecular Medicine • Osteopathy

Bodywork: Reflexology, *shiatsu*, Trager.

Where to Find Help

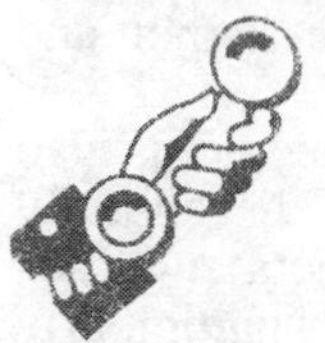

For more information on, or referrals for, treatment of constipation, contact the following organizations.

American Association of Acupuncture and Oriental Medicine
4101 Lake Boone Trail, Suite 201
Raleigh, North Carolina 27607
(919) 787-5181

The AAAOM is a national professional trade organization of acupuncturists who meet acceptable standards of minimum competency and can provide you with the names and locations of local members.

American Association of Naturopathic Physicians
2366 Eastlake Avenue, Suite 322
Seattle, Washington 98102
(206) 323-7610

Contact them for the location of a licensed naturopathic physician in your area.

American School of Ayurvedic Sciences
10025 NE 4th Street
Bellevue, Washington 98004
(206) 453-8022

This college provides medical training for physicians and health care practitioners, as well as individual courses for lay people. Dr. Virender Sodhi's Ayurvedic, Naturopathic Medical Clinic is also located at this address.

Ayurvedic Institute
11311 Menaul NE, Suite A
Albuquerque, New Mexico 87112
(505) 291-9698

The Institute, directed by Dr. Vasant Lad, trains people from all walks of life in most of the aspects of Ayurveda.

Recommended Reading

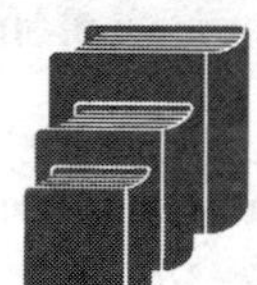

Dr. Braly's Food Allergy and Nutrition Revolution. Braly, James, M.D. New Canaan, CT: Keats Publishing, Inc., 1992.

A comprehensive investigation into food allergies and their link to other illnesses, including constipation. Outlines the factors involved in constipation and how to treat them using diet, nutritional supplements, and exercise.

Encyclopedia of Natural Medicine. Murray, Michael, N.D.; and Pizzorno, Joseph, N.D. Rocklin, CA: Prima Publishing, 1991.

An authoritative guide to naturopathic medicine outlining the basic principles of health and how they can be used to treat over sixty health conditions, including constipation. Includes self-help approaches using diet, nutrition, and herbal medicine.

What Your Doctor Won't Tell You. Heimlich, Jane. New York: Harper Perennial, 1990.

This compelling look at the world of alternative medicine includes a comprehensive chapter on constipation, including the illnesses it can contribute to. Also provides a treatment program based diet, nutritional supplements, herbal medicine, and colonic irrigation.

Diabetes

According to the U.S. Department of Health and Human Services, nearly 6 million people in the United States suffer from diabetes, which is now the seventh leading cause of death among Americans. Practitioners of alternative medicine combine diet, exercise, and weight loss to help control diabetes and prevent or delay the onset of serious complications.

Diabetes mellitus, more commonly referred to simply as diabetes, is a chronic degenerative disease caused by a lack of, or resistance to, the hormone insulin, which is essential for the proper metabolism of blood sugar (glucose). Normally blood sugar rises after a meal as glucose is absorbed into the bloodstream, causing the pancreas to produce enough insulin to return the blood sugar level to its normal range. Diabetic individuals are either unable to produce insulin, or their cells have become resistant to insulin and they are unable to move glucose from the bloodstream to the cells, and thus cannot maintain a normal blood glucose level.

Excess glucose in the bloodstream is toxic, according to Peter H. Forsham, M.D., of Evergreen Hospital, in Kirkland, Washington, noting that excess glucose in diabetics can diminish the biological effectiveness of various proteins in the body. For example, when glucose binds to hemoglobin (the iron-containing pigment of the red blood cells), the oxygen-carrying capacity of hemoglobin is reduced.[1]

Types of Diabetes

There are two major forms of diabetes mellitus: insulin-dependent juvenile diabetes (Type I); and non-insulin-dependent adult-onset diabetes (Type II).

In Type I diabetes, the body is unable to produce insulin. As a result, glucose builds up in the bloodstream and spills over into the urine, while the body literally "starves" to death because the cells cannot get the nourishment, which is provided by glucose, to produce energy to carry out their normal functions. Symptoms of Type I diabetes include excessive thirst, hunger, urination, and dehydration, often accompanied by weight loss. Insulin injections are currently the only known method to control Type I diabetes but are not considered a cure. Injections must be taken daily (sometimes several times a day, usually before meals), and must be timed so that the peak action of the insulin will occur when the sugar from the meal elevates the blood glucose to its highest level. Type I diabetes usually begins in childhood, but it may occur later in life if the pancreas is damaged due to injury or disease. Five to 10 percent of those diagnosed with diabetes are Type I diabetics.[2]

Most diabetics, however, have Type II diabetes, which usually occurs in middle age. Symptoms are the same as for Type I, with the exception of weight loss. In Type II diabetes, the pancreas still produces insulin, but the cells are resistant to its action and therefore cannot absorb the glucose produced by food intake. The cells of the body may also be unable to properly utilize insulin in the absorption of glucose from the bloodstream. Often Type II diabetes can be remedied by dietary management, exercise, and weight control. Oral medications prescribed to stimulate the body to produce more insulin can also be used until blood sugar levels are brought to normal and stabilized. When the insulin levels in a Type II diabetic are out of control as a result of dietary abuse and lack of exercise, however, insulin injections may be temporarily required to restore balance. Once diet and weight are under control, the insulin shots are usually no longer needed.

"Diabetes can lead to heart and kidney disease, atherosclerosis, hypertension, strokes, cataracts, retinal hemorrhages, neuropathy, gangrenous infections of cuts or sores, loss of hearing, blindness, and even death."

Gestational Diabetes

A third type of diabetes, gestational diabetes, is found in pregnant women and is a temporary condition. Characterized by excessive hunger, thirst, and the need to urinate, it is a mild condition and often goes unnoticed, but it is an important condition to treat because elevated blood sugar levels can damage the fetus. Gestational diabetes can usually be controlled with diet but may require insulin. It has been found to respond well, and even to resolve, with a combination of diet and exercise.[3] Jonathan Wright, M.D., Director of the Tahoma Clinic in Kent, Washington, says he has had success treating, and even curing, gestational diabetes with diet and nutritional supplements, particularly vitamin B_6.

Either type of diabetes, when poorly controlled, can lead to heart and kidney disease, atherosclerosis, hypertension, strokes, cataracts, retinal hemorrhages, neuropathy (nerve damage), gastroparesis (loss of peristaltic action in the gastrointestinal tract), gangrenous infections of cuts or sores (with possible amputation of the feet or legs), loss of hearing, blindness, and even death. These complications are easier to avoid in both types of diabetics if blood sugar levels are kept as close to the normal range as possible.

Causes of Diabetes

Although a genetic predisposition appears to govern susceptibility to both types of diabetes, a number of other factors can also be involved. Diet and obesity are key elements in the cause of Type II diabetes. Autoimmune processes, in which antibodies created to fight allergies or viral infections, react against the body itself, may also play a role in causing both types of diabetes.

Type I Diabetes

In Type I diabetes the insulin-producing cells of the pancreas have been destroyed and are unable to produce any more insulin. Seventy-five percent of Type I diabetics have antibodies to their own pancreatic cells, as opposed to 0.5 to 2.0 percent of individuals without diabetes, supporting the theory of an autoimmune cause of the disease.[4]

Viral infections may also be responsible for initiating an autoimmune disease process in Type I diabetes. Viruses that may induce an autoimmune reaction include the pertussis (whooping cough) virus, hepatitis virus, rubella virus, coxsackievirus, Epstein-Barr virus, cytomegalovirus, and herpes virus 6.[5] Also, some patients with Type I diabetes have been shown to have antibodies to the albumin (a simple protein) in cow's milk which are capable of reacting with the insulin-producing cells in the pancreas.[6]

Susceptibility to Type I diabetes may also be genetically predetermined. Every individual has a specific "tissue type"—similar to a blood type—which is inherited from the person's parents. Ongoing immunology research shows that many diseases, including Type I diabetes, seem to occur predominantly among persons with specific tissue types.[7]

Type II Diabetes

Diet, obesity, allergies to certain foods, viral infections, and stress are all factors that can contribute to the onset of or aggravate Type II diabetes.

An estimated 85 percent of all Type II diabetics are overweight when diagnosed.[8] After completion of a worldwide study sponsored by the United Nations, Australian scientist Kelly West, M.D., Ph.D., concluded, "The cause of Type II diabetes is usually obesity; the preventative, and often the cure, is leanness."[9]

Dr. Ernest Pfeiffer, Professor of Medicine at Ulm University in Germany, concurs. "It's almost a law that any person 30 percent overweight for thirty years will become a [Type II] diabetic."[10]

The main cause of obesity is a poor diet, and the key factor is not *how much* but *what* is consumed. Largely at fault are processed, concentrated foods which are high in calories and stripped of valuable fiber and essential nutrients, according to Jonathan Wright, M.D., Director of the Tahoma Clinic in Kent, Washington.

A poor diet, in and of itself, is also a major contributing factor for Type II diabetes, as exemplified by what has happened over the years on the Pacific island of Nauru. Until recently, Type II diabetes was unknown in Nauru, where the islanders ate a simple diet consisting mainly of bananas and yams. When phosphates were discovered and mined on the island, the inhabitants attained wealth and settled into a life of leisure, which included adopting a Western diet high in sugar, fat, and carbohydrates. With this change in lifestyle, many began to develop Type II diabetes. Now, according to a study by the World Health Organization (WHO), up to one-half of the urbanized Nauru population in the age range thirty to sixty-four years old has diabetes, illustrating that adult-onset diabetes may be triggered by poor diet rather than genetic makeup. The WHO concludes that an apparent epidemic of diabetes

Complications of Diabetes

Complications with Type I and Type II diabetes can occur when blood sugar levels are not properly controlled. These include ketoacidosis and hyperosmolar nonketogenic coma. When blood sugar levels are not controlled over long periods of time, circulatory problems can occur causing damage to the small capillaries which supply the small nerves, resulting in retinopathy (damage to the retina), neuropathy (nerve damage), nephropathy (kidney disease), and foot ulcers.

Ketoacidosis: *When insulin-dependent (Type I) diabetics do not take sufficient insulin, glucose builds up in the bloodstream. The body must then break down fats for energy, but this process produces ketones, which are toxic to the body and can induce a state of acidosis (excessive acidity in the body). Large doses of insulin are needed to overcome the insulin resistance in this state and hospitalization is often necessary.*

Hyperosmolar nonketogenic coma: *When severe dehydration occurs (from deficient fluid intake, high blood sugar levels, or physical stress such as infection or surgery), it may result in a condition known as hyperosmolar nonketogenic coma (coma from dehydration). This is a medical emergency requiring hospitalization, as it is fatal in 50 percent of cases.*

Diabetic retinopathy: *Damage to the retina of the eye in diabetics is one of the leading causes of blindness in the United States.*[15] *In poorly controlled diabetes, fragile new blood vessels are formed in the retina in an attempt to bring more oxygen to the eye. However, these vessels often break, hemorrhaging into the eye. Laser treatments help to stop the bleeding, but in doing so destroy much of the retina, which is essential for sight.*

Diabetic neuropathy: *Damage to the peripheral nervous system is characterized by pain and numbness, most frequently occurring in the feet and legs. It is usually due to severe damage to the capillaries supplying the peripheral nervous system.*

Diabetic nephropathy: *Damage to the kidneys is a leading cause of death in diabetics. It is primarily due to damage to the capillaries supplying the kidneys.*

Diabetic foot ulcers: *A lack of oxygen supply and peripheral nerve damage due to destruction of capillaries are the main causes of foot ulcers in diabetics. Without proper treatment, gangrene can form, necessitating amputation. To prevent this, the feet should be kept clean, dry, and warm. Diabetics should never go barefoot, as injuries such as cuts and bruises may not be noticed because of numbness from nerve damage, and ulcers may also occur.*

has occurred—or is occurring—in adult people throughout the world, a trend which appears to be strongly related to lifestyle and socioeconomic change, and the fact that populations in developed communities in the industrialized countries, now face the greatest risk.[11]

Another telling example of the role of diet in diabetes occurred in England during World War II. When food shortages and rationing removed white flour, sugar, excessive meat protein, and fats from the typical English diet, the death rate from diabetes fell 50 percent.[12]

See Obesity and Weight Management.

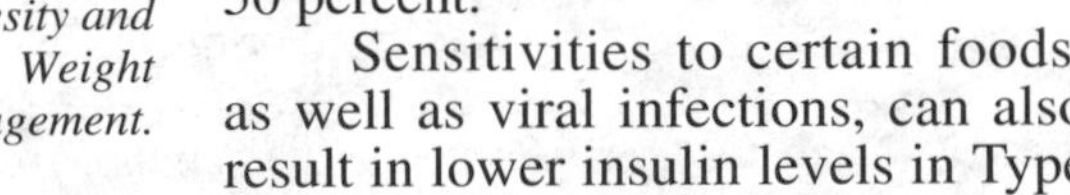

Sensitivities to certain foods, as well as viral infections, can also result in lower insulin levels in Type II diabetics, causing inflammation and ensuing autoimmune damage to the insulin-producing cells of the pancreas.[13] Stress and an individual's ability to manage stress are also important factors affecting the course of diabetes and insulin requirements.[14] Stress can result in the production of adrenalin, which increases blood sugar and thus interferes with diabetic control.

Treating Diabetes

The goal for any doctor or patient in treating diabetes is to bring high blood sugar under control and, as much as possible, to stabilize it at a normal level. This can best be achieved by a treatment approach that encourages diabetics to become actively responsible for their own health.

According to Dr. Wright, for Type I diabetics, who are usually permanently insulin-dependent, a proper diet and a moderate amount of regular exercise are essential for lowering the overall blood sugar level, which reduces the amount of injected insulin required. Type II diabetics can adequately control their blood sugar levels by experimenting with various foods, frequency and size of meals, and other aspects of their lifestyle such as exercise and stress reduction.[16] They may even be able to forego insulin or oral medicine entirely when blood sugar levels are stabilized by weight reduction, exercise, and a sensible food plan. In either case, lowered insulin intake means the likelihood of fewer complications from the disease.[17]

Diet

According to Dr. Wright, a diet emphasizing foods high in complex carbohydrates and fiber, such as whole grains, legumes, and vegetables, reduces the need for insulin by controlling the release of glucose into the bloodstream. The fiber in plant foods can also be beneficial for diabetics by absorbing water in the body, and forming a natural "sponge" in which food particles are suspended. Dr. Wright suggests that diabetics avoid simple carbohydrates (such as fruit juices), and foods containing refined sugar (such as processed foods, cookies, and pastries) because these raise the blood sugar rapidly, thereby requiring a sudden rise in insulin levels which places stress on the pancreas.

James Anderson, M.D., of the Department of Veterans Affairs, at the University of Kentucky in Lexington, has found that eating a high-fiber, high-complex carbohydrate diet helps control Type II diabetes and allows the patient to reduce insulin requirements.[18] Dr. Anderson says that patients on oral hypoglycemics (compounds that cause a decrease in blood sugar) and those taking less than forty units of insulin respond particularly well, as do those who are overweight.

His nutrition plan calls for 55 to 60 percent of the daily calorie intake to be derived from carbohydrates (two-thirds of these from complex carbohydrates), 14 to 20 percent from protein (minimum forty-five grams daily), and 20 to 25 percent or less from fat (10 percent or less from saturated fat), with only two hundred milligrams or less of cholesterol daily, plus forty to fifty grams total dietary fiber daily (ten to fifteen grams of this as soluble fiber). According to Dr. Anderson, this plan lowers fats in the bloodstream and thus reduces the risk of cardiovascular disease in diabetics.

Dr. Anderson points out that since the average American diet contains between eleven and twenty-three grams of fiber daily, some diabetics would need to double or triple their fiber intake. He suggests doing this slowly by adding one high-fiber food per week, particularly whole grains and beans, and increasing fluid intake to help the body adjust to the increased gas production, a common side effect of added fiber.[19]

Dr. Wright has found that eating beans for breakfast keeps the blood sugar under control for the first half of the day, and believes two servings of beans a day have a considerable effect in controlling blood sugar all day. He suggests that sensitive individuals soak the beans overnight in water containing six drops of iodine to help reduce the gas they cause.

A vegetarian diet of whole grains, whole fruits, and vegetables (rather than juices, which are rapidly absorbed) can be helpful for many diabetics. The American Dietetic Association has published research showing that a vegetarian lifestyle reduces the incidence of diabetes and heart disease.[20]

With Type II diabetics, however, Dr. Wright feels that it is necessary to restrict total carbohydrate intake. He recommends moderate amounts of fish and lean meats as sources of protein, along with unsaturated fats and supplementation with vitamins C and E, B-complex vitamins, magnesium, chromium, and zinc. He also suggests small, frequent meals. A daily diet of three small meals, plus mid-morning, mid-afternoon, and bedtime snacks, is the ideal, according to Dr. Wright.

He cites the case of a forty-seven-year-old man who had recently been diagnosed with a mild case of diabetes. An extensive family history of diabetes included his father, whose condition had led to two cataract surgeries, and two uncles who had suffered heart attacks as a result of diabetes. His previous doctor had suggested that he cut down on sugar and salt and get more exercise, but said there was little more he could do.

Dr. Wright's first recommendation was a change in eating habits, and he used as a model the so-called "caveman diet"—complex carbohydrate intake combined with moderate amounts of protein and little or no processed foods. To deal specifically with the patient's concern about cataracts, Dr. Wright advised him to use bioflavonoid supplements to inhibit the enzyme aldose reductase, which has been implicated in

Dietary Guidelines for Diabetics

Jonathan Wright, M.D., Director of the Tahoma Clinic in Kent, Washington, recommends the following dietary control measures for all diabetics:

- *Totally eliminate refined sugar and sugar products.*
- *Avoid "junk" foods.*
- *Eat snacks of protein between meals.*
- *Eat carbohydrates such as whole grains, fresh fruits, and vegetables, which release their natural sugars more slowly and evenly into the bloodstream.*
- *Reduce or eliminate the intake of alcohol, tobacco, and caffeine.*
- *Take off excess weight through exercise and calorie reduction.*

the formation of cataracts. In addition, Dr. Wright suggested nutritional supplementation, specifically vitamins C, E, and B_6, as well as cod liver oil, to slow the process of blood platelet clumping, which is associated with various diabetic complications. This, combined with the rest of Dr. Wright's regimen, normalized his platelet aggregation (blood clotting) time, and eventually all symptoms of diabetes were alleviated.

Food Intolerances: Dr. Wright recommends that diabetics should be thoroughly tested for food intolerances which may be contributing to their disease by causing inflammation and autoimmune destruction of the insulin-producing cells of the pancreas. Foods that often are associated with diabetes-related problems include corn, wheat, chocolate, and dairy-related products.

William H. Philpott, M.D., of Choctaw, Oklahoma, has observed the cause of insulin resistance in Type II diabetes to be edema (swelling) of body cells mostly due to reactions to foods, and to a lesser extent, to chemicals and inhalants.[21] This evidence was achieved by examining blood sugar before and after test meals of single foods. When the offending foods were removed, the diabetic reaction vanished. This reversal of the diabetic reaction occurred immediately upon withdrawal of the offending foods, before any weight reduction or nutritional supplementation. Reactions to foods, chemicals, and inhalants as the cause of insulin resistance in Type II diabetes was confirmed by several statistical research studies.[22] These reactions include immunologic allergic reactions, nonimmunologic allergic-like maladaptive reactions, and addictive reactions.

“A diet emphasizing foods high in complex carbohydrates and fiber, such as whole grains, legumes, and vegetables, reduces the need for insulin by controlling the release of glucose into the bloodstream.”
—Jonathan Wright, M.D.

Dr. Philpott's system of examination for diabetes Type II includes an initial five days of eating foods seldom consumed by the subject, followed by four weeks of test meals of single foods, including monitoring for symptoms and for blood sugar before and after the test meal. Treatment consists of a four-day diversified rotation diet which leaves out the offending food for three months. This is followed by the gradual addition of these foods back into the rotation diet.

Due to the danger of medical complications, food testing cannot be carried out with Type I diabetics, so their food sensitivities need to be determined by skin testing or antibody testing. Dr. Philpott finds that most diabetics he has treated, both Type I and Type II, cannot tolerate cow's milk. In Type I, this intolerance initiates an autoimmune reaction which destroys the insulin-producing cells of the pancreas.

Nutritional Supplements

Dr. Philpott prescribes nutritional supplements based on a patient's laboratory tests. He notes that while every patient has different needs, the most common deficiencies are vitamin B_6, folic acid, riboflavin (vitamin B_2), magnesium, calcium, zinc, manganese, and the amino acids cystine, taurine, and arginine. Dr. Philpott also gives his patients supplements of cod liver oil and either Evening Primrose oil or safflower oil.

Abram Ber, M.D., of Phoenix, Arizona, treats diabetics with nutrition and nutritional supplementation, and feels this is an essential part of diabetic therapy. He uses supplements of vitamin B_6 and biotin, chromium, magnesium, vanadium, essential fatty acids, and flaxseed oil. He also recommends Jerusalem artichokes as part of the diet and uses a mixture of Chinese herbs for his patients. According to Dr. Ber, this treatment can prevent and even reverse the complications of diabetes (such as neuropathy, retinopathy, and nephropathy). He cites the case of a Type I diabetic who had lost most of his eyesight due to diabetic retinopathy and was unable to drive. Over a period of approximately six months on Dr. Ber's supplement program, he regained his vision, and is now able to drive and continues to do well.

See Allergies, Diet, Nutritional Supplements.

There are many nutrients that have proven valuable in treating diabetes.

B Vitamins: Levels of vitamin B_6 in the body drop sharply after the age of fifty, when Type II diabetes is most likely to occur.[23] Vitamin B_6 taken daily can reduce insulin needs and improve basic health.[24] Type II diabetics regained normal blood sugar levels with doses of one hundred milligrams daily of vitamin B_6 in tests by John Ellis, M.D., who recommends fifty milligrams daily for maintenance.[25] Symptoms of diabetic neuropathy were reduced or totally eliminated by vitamin B_6 supplements in studies at the Thordek Medical Center in Chicago.[26]

Biotin, a component of the vitamin B complex, works synergistically with insulin and helps in glucose utilization.[27] Research has shown that biotin is also beneficial for preventing and managing peripheral neuropathy in diabetics.[28]

According to Dr. Wright, diabetic neuropathy also responds well to vitamin B_{12} when it is used in conjunction with topical application of capsicum, a cayenne pepper extract which relieves the pain of neuropathy. Capsicum works by removing substance "P," a pain mediator, from the skin. Dr. Wright also finds that niacinamide (vitamin B_3) can be very beneficial in the early stages of Type I diabetes.

Vitamin C: A high intake of vitamin C has been found to reduce insulin needs, maintain eye health, and help prevent cataracts.[29] It is also important in helping to fight infections, to which diabetics are particularly prone. Megadoses of vitamin C have also been shown to prevent or delay the vascular complications of diabetes by promoting the production of collagen, which strengthens the blood vessels. However, renal (kidney) function should be tested first because megadoses of vitamin C can be toxic in a diabetic with renal insufficiency. A deficiency of vitamin C has been shown to cause degeneration of the insulin-producing cells of the pancreas.[30]

Vitamin E: According to Evan Shute, M.D., co-founder of Canada's Shute Foundation for Medical Research, vitamin E is essential for the treatment of diabetes.[31] Vitamin E is a powerful antioxidant, and has a significant anticlotting effect which may be a factor in preventing premature atherosclerosis and the development of vascular complications such as damage to the eyes and kidneys seen frequently in diabetes.[32] Supplementation of vitamin E has freed some Type II diabetics from taking insulin, and has also been shown to reduce the rate of blood clotting in Type II diabetes.[33]

Chromium: The body's chromium stores are mobilized immediately when either glucose or insulin enters the bloodstream. According to Dr. Philpott, even the slightest deficiency of chromium upsets the body's tolerance to glucose. The lack of chromium in the modern American diet is acute[34] and is aggravated by consumption of refined sugar, which robs the body of stored chromium.[35]

Chromium supplements are effective in treating hypoglycemia (low blood sugar) and act as a "normalizer" of glucose for insulin-dependent diabetics.[36] Exercise appears to increase the levels of chromium in the tissues and increases the number of insulin receptors on cells in Type I diabetics.[37]

Chromium has been shown to restore normal insulin function in Type II diabetics.[38] In a group of Type II diabetics, normal glucose tolerance was restored by 50 percent with daily doses of 150 micrograms of trivalent chromium (the only type of chromium believed to be biologically active in the human body).[39]

Magnesium and Potassium: Deficiencies of magnesium and potassium create a greater glucose intolerance and contribute to damage to organs and the nerves that supply them due to disturbed cell function.[40] Magnesium is essential for the maintenance of a healthy cardiovascular system as well.[41] It reduces plasma lipids (fats in the bloodstream) and serum cholesterol (cholesterol circulating in the blood), is an effective vasodilator (used to widen blood vessels), and helps prevent retinopathy and atherosclerosis. Diabetics who have experienced ketoacidosis are particularly likely to be magnesium deficient. Insulin administration also induces hypokalemia (low blood potassium levels), while potassium supplementation helps improve insulin sensitivity, responsiveness, and secretion.[42]

For older diabetics and diabetics who have problems with absorption of nutrients due to damage to the digestive system, it may be necessary to take minerals and trace elements, such as those listed in the section, "Digestive Enzymes", by intravenous infusion, or transdermally, using dimethylsulfoxide (DMSO), a solvent that facilitates the absorption of medicines through the skin.[48] These methods can be very effective for lowering blood sugar levels, insulin requirements, and high blood pressure, but should not be done without first consulting one's regular physician.

Zinc: Zinc is essential for the normal production of insulin and the digestion of proteins,[43] and has antiviral effects. To confirm a need, ask a doctor for a white blood cell or saliva test, as serum zinc level tests are unreliable, according to Dr. Wright.

Coenzyme Q10: Coenzyme Q10 stimulates production of insulin.[44] Andrew Weil, M.D., suggests taking eighty milligrams a day for at least three months to stabilize blood sugar levels.[45]

Amino Acids: These assure the body's supply of raw materials for manufacture of insulin, which is composed of fifty-one amino acids.[46]

Digestive Enzymes: The use of pepsin and the digestive enzymes protease, amylase, and lipase is sometimes recommended to aid in the digestion and absorption of nutrients, especially in cases of diabetes where the pancreas is not functioning optimally.[47] Dr. Wright reports often finding undigested fat and vegetable material in the feces of Type I diabetics, indicating a need for pancreatic enzyme supplementation.

Exercise and Stress Reduction

Stress leads to the production of adrenalin, which raises the blood sugar level. Relaxation and stress reduction techniques such as yoga, meditation, guided imagery, and massage are therefore recommended for diabetics.

Regular exercise should also be a priority in any diabetic's lifestyle, as it lowers blood sugar, helps control weight, oxygenates tissues, and stimulates metabolic functions. Aerobic exercises are preferred to weight lifting, and walking is ideal. If foot problems exist, a road or stationary bicycle can be a viable alternative.

Diabetics on insulin should monitor their blood sugar level before exercising and plan on having a snack to prevent hypoglycemia when the exercise lowers the blood sugar level. This is necessary because, once an insulin injection is given, there is no way to neutralize the insulin, and it will continue to act to lower the blood sugar level even if the level has naturally dropped below normal as a result of the exercise. Also, before beginning any strenuous exercise program, always consult a doctor for a thorough cardiovascular examination.

Herbal Medicine

According to David L. Hoffman, B.Sc., M.N.I.M.H., past President of the American Herbalist Guild, there are many plants with proven hypoglycemic properties that have much to contribute to a comprehensive management program of non-insulin-dependant diabetes. However, herbs will not replace insulin therapy where it is necessary. Some of the herbs traditionally used in the treatment of diabetes include bilberry, goat's rue, fenugreek, bitter melon, garlic, mulberry leaves, olive leaves, and ginseng.[49]

The appropriate application of hypoglycemic herbs is very important as they can sometimes have a rapid impact on blood sugar levels, and the effect can vary from patient to patient. Their safe use can only occur when utilized as part of a comprehensive diabetes management program that is specifically suited for each individual. It is essential that very close observation be kept on urine and blood signs. This necessitates skilled practitioners training the patient. Preventive work to avoid the long-term complications may be undertaken quite safely, even if no attempt is made to deal with insulin levels. Heart and vascular tonics are appropriate for long-term use, especially hawthorn berry and ginkgo.

"Regular exercise should be a priority in any diabetic's lifestyle, as it lowers blood sugar, helps control weight, oxygenates tissues, and stimulates metabolic functions."

Chelation Therapy

According to Garry F. Gordon, M.D.(H.), of Tempe, Arizona, co-founder of the American College of Advancement in Medicine, chelation therapy is effective in preventing complications of diabetes. Chelation therapy uses chelating agents such as EDTA (ethylenediaminetetraacetic acid), administered intravenously to restore proper circulation by removing the plaque from arterial walls. "Over twenty years of clinical experience has shown me that people with diabetes who receive intravenous EDTA chelation therapy have less amputations, less blindness, less renal dialysis, and other complications of diabetes, than those on conventional treatments," reports Dr. Gordon. He also advocates lifelong use of oral chelators such as garlic, vitamin C, zinc, and certain amino acids like cysteine and methionine, to protect the cardiovascular system.

"Over twenty years of clinical experience has shown me that people with diabetes who receive intravenous EDTA chelation therapy have less amputations, less blindness, less renal dialysis, and other complications of diabetes than those on conventional treatments."
—Garry F. Gordon, M.D.

Additionally, in a Canadian study involving diabetic patients with unusually high levels of iron, Dr. Paul Cutler chelated thirty-two patients with deferoxamine (a chelating agent used to remove iron), resulting in twenty-four patients being totally free of medication in eight to thirteen weeks. Dr. Cutler believes that chelating with deferoxamine could cure one-third of adult cases of diabetes.[50]

Traditional Chinese Medicine (TCM)

Maoshing Ni, D.O.M., Ph.D., L.Ac., Vice-President of Yo San University of Traditional Chinese Medicine in Santa Monica, California, treats Type I and Type II diabetics with acupuncture and a combination of herbs including astragalus, wild yam, and rehmannia. With Type I diabetes, treatment must begin in the early stages of the disease for Traditional Chinese Medicine to be of any help, but it is quite effective, he says, especially at the beginning and intermediate stages of Type II.

See Chelation Therapy, Herbal Medicine, Traditional Chinese Medicine.

According to Dr. Ni, Traditional Chinese Medicine can improve circulatory problems and slow down the process of neuropathy. Dr. Ni reports the case of a patient with Type II diabetes who came to his office with painful, swollen legs resulting from neuropathy. After a few treatments, the inflammation, pain, and swelling were reduced and no further symptoms of neuropathy were evident. TCM may also help to stabilize blood sugar levels in Type II diabetics by restoring balance to the endocrine system.

William Cargile, D.C., L.Ac., F.I.A.C.A., Chairman of Research, American Association of Acupuncture and Oriental Medicine, says he has been very successful in his treatment of diabetes with acupuncture. He has found that treatment of the spleen/pancreas point has effects which reduce the autoimmune component of diabetes. He also notes that acupuncture is helpful in reversing the neuropathy commonly found in long-term diabetics. In one case, he used acupuncture to treat a ninety-year-old patient who had been bedridden for years and had no feeling in his feet. After the third session, the patient was able to walk again, and eventually increased his exercise regimen to three miles a day. His insulin requirements were also lowered by 90 percent and he regained feeling in his feet.

Dr. Cargile also uses laser acupuncture to treat diabetes, and, for Type II diabetics, he uses ear acupuncture to stimulate the sympathetic and autonomic nervous systems. Dr. Cargile stresses that acupuncture alone is not sufficient treatment for diabetes, and always insists his patients have concurrent nutritional and conventional medical care.

Ayurvedic Medicine

Virender Sodhi, M.D., (Ayurveda), N.D., Director of the American School of Ayurvedic Sciences, in Bellevue, Washington, does not differentiate in his treatment of Type I and Type II diabetes. The first thing he addresses is diet modification, eliminating sugar and simple carbohydrates, and emphasizing complex carbohydrates. Protein is limited, since excessive intake can damage the kidneys. Fat is also limited because there is often a deficiency of pancreatic enzymes, making fat digestion difficult. Since many diabetics have autoantibodies (antibodies which are antagonistic to their own bodies), a cleansing program is instituted. Dr. Sodhi uses an Ayurvedic method called *pancha karma*, which begins with herbal massages and an herbal steam sauna, followed by fasting to cleanse the body. This is followed by an herbal purge for the liver, pancreas, and spleen. Colon therapy is next, first to cleanse the digestive tract and then to reconstitute the system.

See Ayurvedic Medicine.

Dr. Sodhi also recommends several herbal preparations for diabetics. "The Indian herb *Gymnema sylvester* stimulates the pancreas to produce more insulin and also blocks sugar absorption from the gut. Bitter melon and *neem*, both lower thc blood sugar, stimulate the pancreas, and also act as liver tonics. A liver tonic is needed, because, if the liver is not cleansed, diabetics tend to form gallstones," he says.

Exercise is another key factor, notes Dr. Sodhi, especially for Type II diabetics. He adds that chromium and nutritional supplements are also necessary, as in other forms of diabetic treatment. Dr. Sodhi's program is not a cure for diabetes, though, and the treatment must be continued long-term for the diabetic to remain healthy.

Self-Care

The following therapies can be undertaken at home under appropriate professional supervision:

• Massage • Reflexology • Qigong • Yoga

Aromatherapy: Rub essence of juniper and olive oil over spleen area.

Hydrotherapy: Constitutional hydrotherapy: applied two to five times weekly.

Juice Therapy: Under doctor's supervision: • String beans, parsley, cucumber, celery, watercress • Carrot, celery, parsley, spinach • Lettuce, spinach, carrot (add a clove of raw garlic) • Sip one glass three times daily.

Topical Treatment: Dry brush massage twice daily to improve circulation.

Professional Care

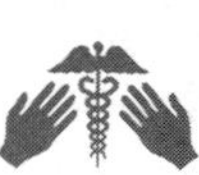

The following therapies can only be provided by a qualified health professional:

• Biofeedback Training • Cell Therapy • Guided Imagery • Magnetic Field Therapy • Osteopathy • Ozone Therapy • Stress Reduction

Hydrogen Peroxide Therapy: Charles Farr, M.D., President of the International Bio-Oxidative Medicine Foundation, reports great success in treating Type II diabetes using intravenous hydrogen peroxide therapy. He says he gets best results with patients on whom he makes the primary diagnosis—and who have never been treated with insulin or any other type of diabetic drug—often being able to reverse their condition and return them to normal.

Where to Find Help

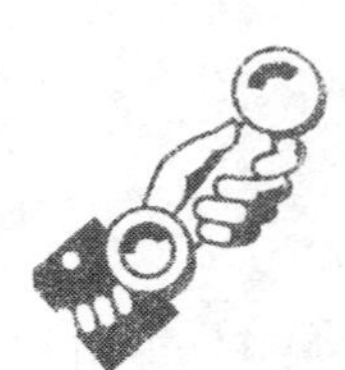

For more information on, or referrals for, the treatment of diabetes, contact the following organizations.

American Academy of Environmental Medicine
P.O. Box 16106
Denver, Colorado 80216
(303) 622-9755
The academy offers extensive training for physicians interested in learning more about environmental medicine.

American Academy of Orthomolecular Medicine
The Huxley Institute for Biosocial Research
900 North Federal Highway
Boca Raton, Florida 33432
(800) 847-3802
This resource serves as a clearinghouse for information and as a referral service for physicians practicing orthomolecular medicine.

American Association of Acupuncture and Oriental Medicine
4101 Lake Boone Trail, Suite 201
Raleigh, North Carolina 27607
(919) 787-5181
The AAAOM is a national professional trade organization of acupuncturists who meet acceptable standards of competency and can provide you with the names and locations of local members. Referrals by written request only.

American Association of Naturopathic Physicians
2366 Eastlake Avenue, Suite 322
Seattle, Washington 98102
(206) 323-7610
Provides a directory of naturopathic physicians and offers referrals to a nationwide network of accredited or licensed practitioners. Publishes a quarterly newsletter for both professionals and the general public. Also offers a series of brochures and pamphlets on a variety of subjects.

American College of Advancement in Medicine
P.O. Box 3427
Laguna Hills, California 92654
(714) 583-7666
This pioneer organization seeks to establish certification and standards of practice for chelation therapy, providing training and education, sponsoring semiannual conferences for physicians and scientists. ACAM provides referrals and informational material, including a directory listing of all physicians worldwide who have been trained in preventative medicine as well as in the ACAM protocol for chelation therapy. The directory is updated monthly. The organization also provides a copy of the ACAM protocol for chelation to the public.

American Holistic Medical Association
4101 Lake Boone Trail, Suite 201
Raleigh, North Carolina 27607
(919) 787-5181
A professional organization for holistic practitioners, the AHMA offers information and services for its members and lobbies for holistic issues. It also provides referrals for the public.

American School of Ayurvedic Sciences
10025 NE 4th Street
Bellevue, Washington 98004
(206) 453-8022
This college provides medical training for physicians and health care practitioners, as well as individual courses for lay people. Dr. Virender Sodhi's Ayurvedic, Naturopathic Medical Clinic is also located at this address.

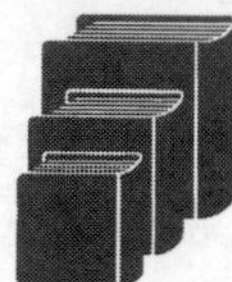

Recommended Reading

Encyclopedia of Natural Medicine. Murray, Michael, N.D.; and Pizzorno, Joseph, N.D. Rocklin, CA: Prima Publishing, 1991.

A definitive guide for the layperson on naturopathic medicine. Includes a chapter on diabetes.

Psyching Out Diabetes: A Positive Approach to Your Negative Emotions. Rubin, Richard, et al. Los Angeles: Lowell House, 1992.

Offers realistic strategies for dealing with the emotional issues associated with diabetes. Diabetics can learn to integrate diabetes into their lives rather than segregating it.

Reversing Diabetes. Whitaker, Julian M., New York: Warner Books, 1987.

Dr. Whitaker argues that conventional treatments are unnecessary, or even dangerous, and shows how diabetics can naturally control their condition through diet and exercise.

Victory Over Diabetes. Philpott, W.H., M.D.; and Kalita, D.K., Ph.D. New Canaan, CT: Keats Publishing Inc., 1992.

In this thorough and well-researched book, Dr. Philpott provides a guide for lifestyle and nutritional changes with the potential of healing diabetics' disordered metabolism. It outlines a nutritional protocol designed to allow patients to reduce insulin dependence.

Female Health

Female health care focuses on helping a woman maintain optimal health as her reproductive system develops and matures. Alternative medicine helps to educate women in a variety of preventative steps to maintain overall health, as well as providing natural treatments for symptoms and diseases related to hormonal and physiological imbalances.

Conventional approaches to women's health have often used invasive medical procedures to deal with common physiological functions, such as the hormonal imbalances experienced during menopause. Alternative medicine offers a variety of therapeutic approaches such as diet, nutritional supplementation, herbal medicine, homeopathy, naturopathic medicine, Traditional Chinese Medicine and Ayurvedic medicine, which can be safely used to address the diverse symptoms of premenstrual syndrome and menopause, as well as diseases of the uterus, vagina, bladder, and breasts.

In turn, women need to make informed choices about diet, exercise, and stress management when taking care of their bodies, says Susan M. Lark, M.D., of Los Altos, California. "These changes alone can produce great results. I've been very impressed in my own practice by how much women can really modify their health problems, just by modifying their lifestyle."

Life Cycles

Throughout her life, a woman's reproductive system follows rhythmic patterns of change, monthly cycles, and the completion of those cycles with menopause. By becoming acquainted with the needs, characteristics, and problems of each phase, a woman can make informed choices about lifestyle and health care.

Menstruation

The reproductive organs mature during puberty, the stage during which a girl becomes a woman and menstruation begins. A woman menstruates an average of five hundred times during her life. Yet there are many misconceptions about menstruation, and some have been repeated so often that they are considered fact. Most notable is the assumption that the average menstrual cycle is twenty-eight days, neatly paralleling the cycles of the moon. While women's bodies do have an observable rhythm, the menstrual cycle actually has a wide range of lengths that can be considered normal. Says Toni Weschler, M.P.H., of Seattle, Washington, "The twenty-eight-day cycle is a complete myth. Cycles vary anywhere from about twenty-four to thirty-seven days. If a woman uses the twenty-eight-day cycle as a point of reference and her cycle is different," Weschler notes, "she may think there's something wrong with her."

While two or three generations ago women began to menstruate at around fifteen or sixteen years of age, today puberty begins at age twelve or thirteen. Menstruation begins when body estrogen reaches a certain level, and Christiane Northrup, M.D., of Yarmouth, Maine, past President of the American Holistic Medical Association and Director of Women to Women, cites several factors that may prematurely increase the body's supply. "High-fat diets help the body produce more estrogen," she says. "Then there are the hormones in beef and chicken [that are] used to speed up their growth process and which we eventually consume. Antibiotics in meat (50 percent of the antibiotics in this country are fed to livestock) can change intestinal flora and slow proper elimination. Some estrogen, instead of being excreted, simply recycles."

The monthly menstrual cycle results from coordinated hormonal interplay among the hypothalamus, the pituitary gland, and the ovaries. Each month, at the start of the cycle, estrogen is secreted by the ten to twenty eggs growing in the ovaries. The estrogen triggers the thickening of the lining of the uterus (the endometrium) with blood vessels, glands, and cells in anticipation of new life, and causes a fertile cervical fluid to be produced. This opens up the cervical opening to

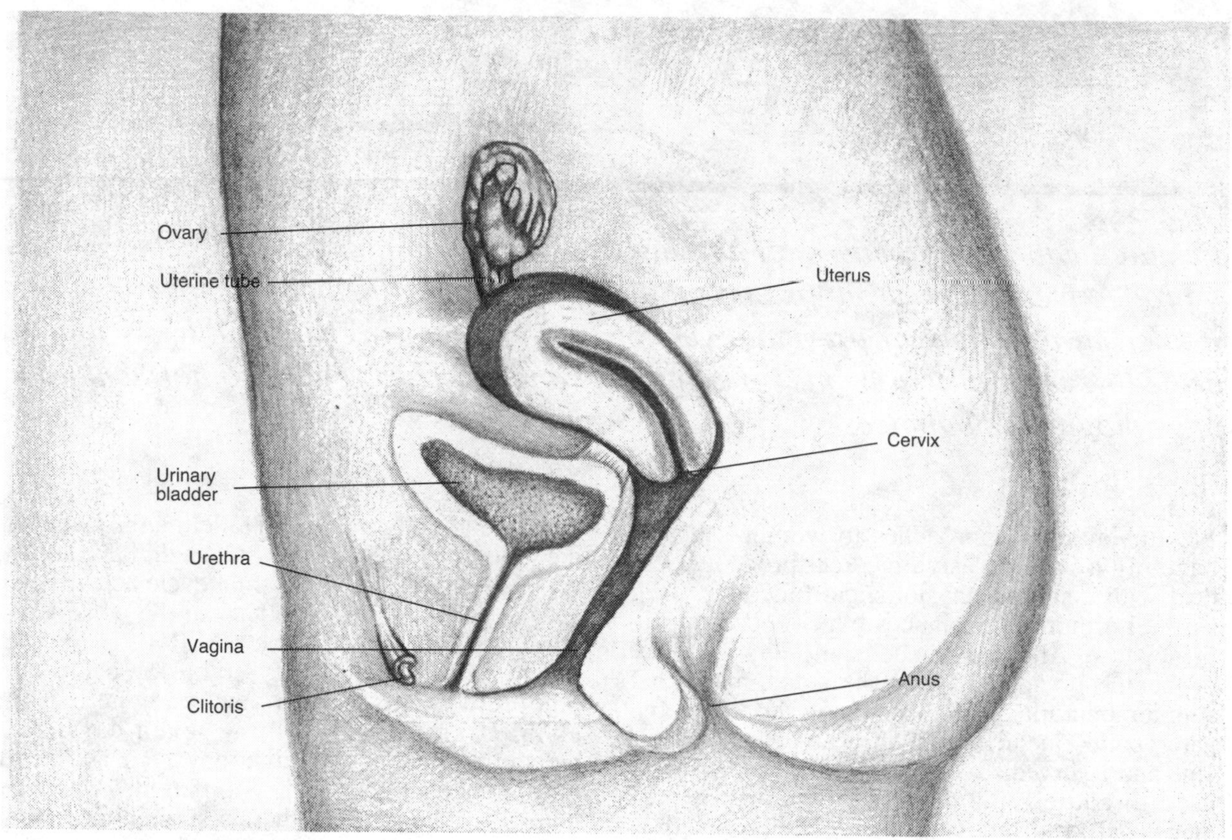

Female reproductive system.

sperm and enhances the sperms' survival. Once the mature egg has left the ovaries, it can be fertilized in the fallopian tubes.

Next, estrogen production subsides and progesterone production increases. This second hormone forms a thick cervical mucous plug in the cervix to prevent sperm or bacteria from entering, and maintains the endometrium in a nutritious, blood-rich stage in anticipation of the egg's fertilization by the sperm, i.e., conception. If conception does not occur, all hormone levels drop, some of the endometrial layer is released, or "shed," and this is called menstruation. The cycle then starts over.

> *"While women's bodies do have an observable rhythm, the menstrual cycle actually has a wide range of lengths that can be considered normal."*

If fertilization does occur, progesterone secretion continues to increase, maintaining the uterine lining and pregnancy until the placenta takes over secreting progesterone and other hormones at about three months' gestation.

Getting to Know Your Cycle: It is important for each woman to become familiar with the patterns of her monthly cycle. Dr. Northrup advises that, premenstrually, "a woman needs to take a little retreat time, moving slower and even resting her mind." When a woman is aware of her cycle, she might be able to plan her days accordingly.

The monthly cycle can also be used as a guide in maintaining general health, because, as research is now suggesting, a woman's immune system peaks before ovulation and decreases afterward.[1] One piece of evidence is the higher incidence of vaginal yeast and chlamydial infections just before menstrual periods.[2] There is a reason for this oscillation in immunity: The dip at this time is necessary so that the foreign sperm and the fertilized egg will be accepted by the woman's body, and an immune boost prior to ovulation cleanses the body of germs before possible pregnancy.[3]

See Pregnancy and Childbirth.

Suzannah Doyle, a certified fertility educator from Corvallis, Oregon, says research now shows that vaccinations, surgery, and prescription drugs have fewer harmful effects when used on a woman before ovulation. Women are even more easily affected by alcohol consumed premenstrually versus during the fertile time. Doyle adds, "In the future, a woman's own observed fertility

Natural birth control

Understanding a womans' menstrual cycle is instrumental in using natural birth control effectively. Contrary to popular belief, several methods of natural contraception are useful and safe, although some purported forms are unreliable, such as douching and withdrawal. The most notorious of these is the rhythm method, which involves predicting when the fertile phase "should" occur and abstaining from intercourse during this time. But, as Toni Weschler, M.P.H., of Seattle, Washington, states, "The rhythm method is based on women having regular cycles, which is why it does not work. The only way to determine when a woman is fertile and when she is not is to identify her fertility signs on a daily basis: basal body temperature (BBT), cervical fluid, and cervical position."

There are two natural birth control methods that employ observation of one's fertility signs: Natural family planning (NFP), says Weschler, "assumes a couple is abstinent [from sexual intercourse] during the woman's fertile time," and barrier methods are not used; fertility awareness method (FAM), gives a couple the option of using barrier methods during fertile periods. "The difference between NFP and FAM is philosophical," notes Weschler.

Fertility observation is used in the ovulation or Billings method, which relies specifically on checking cervical mucous rather than the cervix itself, and in the symptothermal method, which employs all three available fertility signals. Both of these methods must be carefully learned in order to be effective; however, when used scrupulously, the failure rates can be as low as 2 to 3 percent.[4]

Breast-feeding, which may suppress ovulation, has received mixed reports on its effectiveness as a contraceptive. Its reliability depends on how often a baby nurses and whether it is supplemented with other liquids or foods.[5] If a woman wants to use lactation to control fertility, NFP or FAM can be used as a backup method.

Natural barrier methods include the diaphragm, the male condom, the female condom, and the cervical cap—a small latex dome placed over the cervix. (Some may not consider diaphragms natural because of the spermicide jelly or cream that should be used with them.) Like the diaphragm, the cervical cap must be professionally fitted. Advantages of the cap include no spermicide use and the ability to leave it in the vagina longer than the diaphragm.

Another option in birth control is the female condom, which lines the vagina, protecting against transfer of virus and bacteria as well as sperm. This barrier device consists of a soft, thin, polyurethane sheath with two flexible rings. One ring lies inside the closed upper end of the sheath and holds the condom in place after insertion, while the other, on the opposite, open end, remains outside the vagina. This outer portion covers the labia and the base of the penis during intercourse. Among the objections to the female condom is the aesthetic issue of having part of the condom hanging outside the vagina during intercourse, but the advantages of the condom may override this objection. For one thing, the protection provided by the female condom places a woman in greater control of her own sexual health.

Although the female condom has been approved by the Food and Drug Administration, clinical trials have not demonstrated a high efficacy rate, especially in comparison to male condoms. In the United States, 12.2 percent of the participating women became pregnant.[6] While the condom is already being sold in the United Kingdom, Switzerland, and Austria, the Unites States market awaits further testing.

Male condoms can be used alone, or with any of these female barriers to increase contraceptive success. When condoms are used properly, their effectiveness increases dramatically. Other advantages of barrier methods in general is that they protect against sexually transmitted diseases and somewhat against AIDS. Latex condoms should be used rather than lambskin, which permit a high percentage of virus leakage because the material is so porous[7]; however, there is also some risk with latex condoms.[8]

signs will enable doctors to actually adjust drug dosages for their patients. Fertility signs are already being used by some health care providers to increase the effectiveness and accuracy of surgeries, drug therapies, and procedures such as PAP smears and diaphragm fittings."

Menopause

Strictly defined, menopause is the end of all menstrual bleeding. Generally, women experience menopause between age forty-eight to fifty-two, but some women cease menstruating as early as their late thirties and early forties while others stop in their mid-fifties. According to the 1991 U.S. Census Bureau, the number of menopausal women, age forty-five to fifty-four, numbered 13 million and is expected to grow by 73 percent between 1990 and 2010. The aging baby boom population means that thirty-five hundred American women enter the "menopausal years" every day. Yet, because women are healthier now, menopause no longer indicates the onset of old age, and women can expect to live one-third of their adult lives after menopause.[9]

Menopause is caused by the ovaries no longer producing estrogen. Perimenopause is the period before menopause, which occurs approximately between the ages of thirty-five to fifty, but is more commonly thought of as the five to ten years before menopause. It is characterized by several years of irregular cycles with no ovulation since the ovaries are at the end of their egg supply. Without an egg's presence, progesterone is no longer produced and therefore perimenopause is frequently characterized by estrogen dominance, with side effects ranging from water retention, weight gain, and mood swings, to fibrocystic breasts, breast cancer, fibroids, or endometrial cancer.

With the onset of menopause, however, estrogen levels do not drop to zero. Some estrogen is still produced in fat cells, the supporting tissue around the ovaries, and in the intestinal tract using precursors (a substance from which another substance is formed) produced by the adrenals. Weight gain after menopause can be the body's attempt to take advantage of this. Estrogen is also made through other chemical pathways in the body.[11] It is this reserve of estrogen that many natural therapies draw on for their effectiveness.

WOMEN AND MEDICAL RESEARCH

Currently, women's health care amounts to two-thirds of the United States' annual medical bill; however, the bulk of medical research has been done on male subjects. Many studies on the benefits of aspirin in preventing heart attacks, for example, have involved thousands of men and not one woman.[10]

According to Katherine A. O'Hanlan, M.D., Assistant Professor and Associate Director, Gynecologic Cancer Service, Stanford University Medical Center, California, "Older women are dying at much higher rates of heart disease than men, and yet, until about five years ago, the research had only been done on men."

In 1993, the Women's Health Initiative, under the auspices of the National Institutes of Health and the Clinton Administration, began a number of studies on cardiovascular disease, cancer, and osteoporosis in postmenopausal women. Between 150,000 and 160,000 women will be studied through forty-five clinical centers to assess the effectiveness of dietary, behavioral, and drug interventions in the prevention and treatment of these conditions.

Although these changes are encouraging for women, the results of studies begun now will not be available for at least another five to ten years. In the meantime, doctors are often making important diagnostic decisions based on materials that are not completely accurate.

While the bigger issues need to be resolved, each woman should take control of her own health and can start by choosing physicians who provide her with the proper respect and care. According to Dr. O'Hanlan, "A woman needs to pick a doctor that listens to her. Do not hire somebody who doesn't respect you, and this respect needs to be palpable." This alternative approach to female health challenges women to be well informed, to ask questions, and to form good partnerships with health care professionals while exploring a variety of therapeutic approaches.

Potential Health Problems and Treatments

In the early years following puberty, it is common for menstrual periods to be irregular due to hormonal imbalances. Irregular bleeding, spotting, bleeding too much, clots, or a total absence of blood are all signs that a woman's reproductive system needs attention. Women may also experience symptoms such as cramping, headaches, and mood changes. Changes in diet and lifestyle, as well as professional treatment, can significantly relieve these conditions, and a variety of alternative therapies have long traditions of treating the range of female health problems, both chronic and acute. Conditions addressed include those related to the menstrual cycle and menopause, as well as diseases of the uterus, vagina, bladder, and breasts.

Menstrual Cramps (Dysmenorrhea)

As many as 30 to 50 percent of all women suffer from pain during their menstrual period,[12] though until recently the medical community has considered this a "minor" complaint, with the implication that it was "all in a woman's head." New thinking takes menstrual cramps seriously, and, in terms of hormones, proposes that primary dysmenorrhea is caused by excess production of prostaglandins (hormone-like fatty acids) by the endometrium following a decline in progesterone levels.[13]

At least 10 percent of younger women have symptoms so severe that they cannot participate in their normal activities.[14] Besides lower abdominal pain, cramp sufferers may also experience backache, pinching, and pain sensations in the inner thighs, as well as many of the symptoms of premenstrual syndrome. According to Dr. Lark, primary spasmodic dysmenorrhea is the type most commonly found in women in their early teens to late twenties. As she explains, "This is characterized by sharp, viselike pains that are caused by a constriction and tightening of the uterine muscle. Blood circulation and oxygenation of uterine muscle and blood vessels is diminished and waste products of metabolism, such as carbon dioxide and lactic acid, build up and the pain and discomfort are intensified."

In contrast, primary congestive dysmenorrhea produces a dull aching in the low back and pelvic regions, often accompanied by bloating, weight gain, breast tenderness, headaches, and irritability. Says Dr. Lark, "Unlike spasmodic cramping, these symptoms don't improve with age. Some of the worst symptoms are seen in women in their thirties and forties. Excessive amounts of estrogen can worsen these symptoms, since estrogen increases fluid and salt retention in the body."[15]

Diet: Dr. Lark recommends eating whole grains, legumes, fruits and vegetables, and seeds and nuts such as ground, raw flaxseed and pumpkin seed, while avoiding dairy products, saturated fats, salt, alcohol, sugar, and caffeine. For spasmodic symptoms specifically: Choose fish such as trout, mackerel, and salmon; avoid meat, poultry, dairy products, and eggs. For congestive symptoms: Avoid sugar, alcohol, salt, dairy foods, and wheat.

Nutritional Supplements: Dr. Lark recommends vitamin B_3, vitamin B_6, vitamin C, calcium, magnesium, potassium, zinc, and essential fatty acids.

Herbal Medicine: According to David L. Hoffmann, B.Sc., M.N.I.M.H., past President of the American Herbalist Guild, painful cramps associated with menstruation or ovulation can be eased by combining the tinctures of skullcap, black haw, and black cohosh in equal parts and taking one to two teaspoons of this mixture as needed. For water retention, Hoffmann recommends dandelion leaf. "This is a rich source of potassium and, though this herb promotes excretion of urine, which also causes potassium loss, this herb simultaneously replaces the mineral. Take one teaspoonful of the tincture three times a day, or an infusion of the fresh leaves three to five times a day." Dr. Lark also recommends ginger, *Ginkgo biloba*, white willow bark, red raspberry leaf, cramp bark, chamomile, hops, and chaste tree berry.

Homeopathy: According to Lauri Aesoph, N.D., natural health writer and educator from Sioux Falls, South Dakota, *Sepia* and *Lachesis* are common treatments for cramps, and, she notes, "the cramps that are relieved by a hot water bottle or heating pad can also be helped by *Chamomilla*."

Traditional Chinese Medicine: According to Honora Lee Wolfe, Dipl. Ac., of Boulder, Colorado, "Menstrual cramps are due usually to either *qi* stagnation (when the vital energy is unable to move freely through the body) in the lower abdomen, or blood stasis, or a combination of both." Treatment can involve the use of both acupuncture and herbs according to the individual patient's needs.

Craniosacral Therapy: According to Joyce Frye, D.O., F.A.C.O.G., of Philadelphia, Pennsylvania, craniosacral therapy is very effective at controlling and eliminating pain associated with cramping. Explaining the treatment, Dr. Frye states, "There is a primary cranial rhythm which has its own rate and is separate from the pulmonary respiratory rate and cardiac rate, which involves the pumping of the cerebrospinal fluid throughout the areas surrounding the brain and spinal cord, bathing it and having a nutritional and metabolic effect. Craniosacral therapy removes some of the restrictions to that flow, allowing normalization of nerve function."

See Craniosacral Therapy.

Absence of Menstruation (Amenorrhea)

There are many types of amenorrhea, but one in particular, which is experienced by some young athletes, is often misunderstood, according to Dr. Northrup. "It is a common assumption that regular strenuous exercise can cause a young woman to miss her period. In fact, these women are also restricting caloric intake and they are, in fact, anorexic just like every other woman who is addicted to a cultural ideal that is impossible for 90 percent of women to achieve. The nutritional needs for supporting the metabolic demands of the exercise are simply not being met. In my practice, I have found that, if women eat at least five hundred calories more per day than they have been, their periods become reestablished."

Herbal Medicine: According to David Hoffmann, herbs for amenorrhea include chasteberry, false unicorn root, blue cohosh, rue, pennyroyal, and tansy.

Excessive Menstruation (Menorrhagia)

Abnormally profuse menstrual flow is called menorrhagia. In this condition, a woman may lose up to 92 percent of her total menses in the first three days, giving her the impression that she is losing more blood than she actually has. Abnormalities of the endometrium, iron and vitamin A deficiencies, hypothyroidism, and intrauterine devices are all considered possible causes.[16]

Nutritional Supplements: Iron, vitamin C with flavonoids, and vitamin A may be beneficial. For bleeding between periods mixed bioflavonoids may be helpful.[17]

Herbal Medicine: To treat excessive bleeding, Silena Heron, R.N., N.D., of Sedona, Arizona, uses astringent herbs such as partridge berry (squaw vine), yarrow, and lady's mantle.

Premenstrual Syndrome

One of the most common hormone-related conditions of otherwise healthy women is premenstrual syndrome (PMS). For ten to fourteen days before menses, women may experience a wide variety of symptoms, some of which include mood swings, headaches, abdominal bloating, depression, sugar craving, cramps, irritability, and weight gain. These will last through two to three days of menstruation, sometimes longer. According to Dr. Northrup, "Sixty percent of women have enough symptoms due to PMS to suffer. This is far too many women to be suffering from a normal physiological function."

"A good diet for PMS includes fresh fruits, vegetables, whole grains, legumes, nuts, seeds, and fish."
—Tori Hudson, N.D.

Theories on the causes of PMS vary, but hormonal, nutritional, and psychological factors are all possibilities,[18] as are the stresses of Western culture.[19]

Dr. Northrup contends that the underlying cause of PMS is that "we have all been socialized into thinking that menstruation is one of the most awful things we women have to put up with. Given the unity of the mind/body, if you have been brought up to believe this, it doesn't take a scholar to figure out why so many women suffer from a normal body function."

In her *PMS Self-Help Book: A Woman's Guide*,[20] Dr. Lark outlines the four basic types of PMS defined by expert Dr. Guy Abraham, former Clinical Professor of Obstetrics and Gynecology at the University of California at Los Angeles. Type A is characterized by anxiety, irritability, and mood swings; Type C by sugar cravings, fatigue, and headaches; Type H by bloating, weight gain, and breast tenderness; and Type D by depression, confusion, and memory loss. She defines two other common subgroups: Acne, characterized by pimples and oily skin and hair; and Dysmenorrhea, with cramps, low back pain, and nausea. (She notes that many doctors do not consider dysmenorrhea part of PMS.)

There are many ways a woman can help reverse her symptoms of premenstrual syndrome, and formal treatment procedures can also be useful.

Diet: According to Tori Hudson, N.D., Academic Dean at National College of Naturopathic Medicine, in Portland, Oregon, a good diet for PMS includes fresh fruits, vegetables, whole grains, legumes, nuts, seeds, and fish, while foods to be avoided include refined sugars, high amounts of protein, dairy products, fats, salt, caffeine, and tobacco.

Nutritional Supplements: Vitamin A has diuretic and anti-estrogen properties. Vitamin B complex and B_6 are helpful in combating depression and acting as a diuretic. Increasing calcium and magnesium intake to five hundred milligrams two to three times a day alleviates spasmodic and congestive discomfort.[21] Vitamin E and zinc have been shown to be effective in alleviating the symptoms of PMS.[22] In one study, evening primrose oil was shown to decrease irritability, swelling, breast tenderness, and tiredness.[23]

See Homeopathy.

Herbal Medicine: David Hoffmann recommends chasteberry for general, long-term treatment of PMS. For specific short-term complaints he also suggests skullcap for irritability/anxiety symptoms, dandelion for water retention, and cramp bark for cramping.

Homeopathy: "Since the causes of women's health problems are often multisystemic, homeopathy is particularly suitable as a treatment because it addresses the physical, mental, and emotional origins of disease," say Jennifer Jacobs, M.D., M.P.H., Director of the Evergreen Center for Homeopathic Medicine, and a member of the NIH Panel on Alternative Medicine. "We treat a range of these deep constitutional imbalances and give less attention to the ways these manifest in body or mind."

Traditional Chinese Medicine: In Chinese medicine, PMS is considered a blood stagnation problem. Nailini Chilkov, Lic.Ac., O.M.D., of Santa Monica, California, explains how Chinese medicine views irregular periods. "If you are less than twenty-one days, that is because you have too much heat in your system, you are bleeding too much. If your periods are very stretched out, thirty-three to thirty-five days, then we say your system is too cold." Acupuncture and herbs are given to correct these conditions.

Ayurvedic Medicine: Ayurveda's approach to treating PMS relies on basic principles that, once understood, can also shed light on other female health disorders. Nancy Lonsdorf, M.D.,

Medical Director of the Maharishi Ayurveda Medical Association of Washington, D.C., a practitioner of Ayurvedic medicine, explains, "All female disorders are caused by imbalances that fall into three categories of diagnosis: the balance of the *doshas* (or bodily humors)—*vata* (responsible for movement), *pitta* (for metabolism), and *kapha* (for structure); biological rhythm; and purification. All treatments address these three areas of body health." In Ayurveda, the individual can do much for herself through dietary and lifestyle changes. In turn, the practitioner provides the diagnosis and sets the direction of self-care, and can provide herbs to balance the interaction of the *doshas*.

See Ayurvedic Medicine.

Dr. Lonsdorf provides the following guidelines for Ayurvedic self-care based on predominant symptoms:

- **Balance of the doshas:** *Vata energy* is responsible in menstruation for the flow of blood and the endometrial lining. An imbalance manifests as mood swings, a tendency to cry, insomnia, anxiety, and constipation. To correct an imbalance, establish regular daily routines, reduce workload, increase rest and sleep, meditate, and add to the diet a little more oil, sweet-tasting foods (but not refined sugars), salt, and cooked warm foods such as cereal and stews.

  Pitta energy is responsible in menstruation for hormonal changes. An imbalance manifests as anger, irritability, skin rashes, and diarrhea. To correct an imbalance, reduce "Type A" behavior or overactivity and overperformance, establish regular daily routines, meditate, and avoid spicy foods, greasy foods, artificial ingredients, chocolate, caffeine, and alcohol.

  Kapha energy is responsible in menstruation for the contents of the menstrual flow. An imbalance manifests as fluid retention, swollen breasts, weight gain, and lethargy. To correct an imbalance, increase exercise, avoid sour and sweet foods, and increase spicy foods and legumes.
- **Biological rhythm:** Dr. Lonsdorf recommends as a general good habit going to bed at 10:00 P.M. and rising at 6:00 A.M., hours at which the earth's energy enhances human energy.
- **Purification:** This is used to remove "*ama*" (waste and impurity) from the body. Dr. Lonsdorf sees a parallel in the notion of removing *ama* and the effects of facilitating menstrual flow since iron, eliminated with the blood, is now being linked to heart disease when in excess in the body.[24] Dietary procedures to improve digestion and elimination include drinking plenty of warm to hot water and avoiding meat, cheese, caffeine, and alcohol. On the fourteenth or fifteenth day of the cycle, Dr. Lonsdorf suggests the use a laxative of four to five teaspoons of castor oil or senna tea followed by a light diet for the rest of the day.

Natural Hormone Therapy: The various symptoms women often experience for five to ten days before the onset of their menstrual periods—emotional ups and downs, headaches, depression, irritability, and weight gain—are typically caused by an insufficient production of progesterone,—due to stress and poor diet,—to balance the increased estrogen being produced, according to John R. Lee, M.D., of Sebastapol, California. "Unbalanced estrogen will cause cellular edema (watery swelling of cells), depression, loss of libido, irritability, and weight gain. Treatment with natural progesterone, given the ten days before menses, has been found to be very successful, as reported by Dr. Joel Hargrove of Vanderbilt University Medical School. Supplementation with modest doses of vitamin B_6, magnesium, and evening primrose oil may also be helpful.

"It is important that natural progesterone be used," cautions Dr. Lee. "Progestins, synthetic, or chemically altered progesterone, have a long list of side effects such as abnormal menstrual flow, fluid retention, nausea, insomnia, jaundice, fever, the development of masculine characteristics, and allergies. But with natural progesterone, side effects are extremely rare. In fact, we have only been able to find two minor problems related to its use. First, at higher dosages it may cause a feeling of euphoria. Second, in some individuals it might slightly alter the timing of their menstrual cycle.

"Although conditions other than premenstrual syndrome can cause nervousness, depression, and irritability, the diagnosis of PMS can be established by serial measurements of serum progesterone prior to therapy," adds Dr. Lee.

Craniosacral Therapy: "If migraines are part of the problem with premenstrual syndrome, craniosacral therapy can do wonders," says Dr. Frye. "I'm not sure that craniosacral therapy can provide long-term help with moods, but it is clearly helpful for some period of time when someone has the treatment. A patient typically will drift off and feel more relaxed than she's felt in years. How long that lasts depends on how many stressors she has."

Problems Related to Menopause

At the time of menopause, the hormonal output—instead of reducing gradually—alternately stops and starts. This general readjusting of the body's endocrine balance leads to many of menopause's symptoms. The estrogen supply eventually regulates itself and reaches a plateau, where it remains until around age seventy. Though doctors now know that the body still makes some estrogen, a common misconception is that menopause happens when a woman "runs out of estrogen." It was this generalization that led to the conclusion that simple estrogen replacement would remedy menopause, which was seen as a deficiency disease.

The symptoms of menopause are caused by estrogen dominance in the body as progesterone production declines in the years leading up to this change in a woman's body. Women may experience water retention, weight gain, memory loss, irritability, and depression. During menopause, decreased estrogen levels may cause bladder and vaginal atrophy, with the vaginal walls becoming drier and thinner, and a woman may have less interest in sex or slower arousal time. The hormonal changes also disrupt the delicate acid/alkaline balance of the vagina, which can lead to increased susceptibility to yeast and bacterial infections. Women may develop fibrocystic breasts, breast cancer, fibroids, or endometrial cancer. However, no symptom is inevitable. During this time many women also experience increased energy, greater focus on their life goals, and a renewed interest in sex since pregnancy cannot result. Further, many women in other cultures do not have the side effects of menopause that are common to American women: Japanese and Indonesian women report far fewer hot flashes than do women from Western societies, and Mayan women in Yucatan, Mexico, report no symptoms at menopause other than menstrual cycle irregularity.[25]

> *"I think that in all the lectures and workshops I give, the question that's asked of me most often is, 'What else can I take besides estrogen?'"*
> —Fredi Kronenberg, Ph.D.

A wide variety of alternative therapies are effective in treating menopause. Western science so far has provided women with little hard data on care strategies for menopause that would make personal health decisions easier. As a result, menopausal women may turn to other avenues of treatment, learning to take care of their health care in general. As Fredi Kronenberg, Ph.D., Director, Richard & Hinda Rosenthal Center for Alternative/Complementary Medicine, Columbia University College of Physicians and Surgeons in New York, notes, "I think that in all the lectures and workshops I have given, the question that's asked of me most often is, 'What else can I take besides estrogen?' We are seeing increasing interest in alternative approaches because women who are asking these questions are part of the generation that is outspoken about wanting things to change."

There are various approaches to treating the symptoms of menopause, some as simple as walking a half hour at the same time each day to stimulate the body's energies and to establish a calming regularity to life. Other approaches include dietary changes, herbs, homeopathy, and the disciplines of Chinese and Ayurvedic medicine. There are also treatments for specific problems of menopause—hot flashes, mood changes, vaginal atrophy—which are becoming word-of-mouth home remedies. A list of these treatments is provided for quick reference.

Symptoms of Menopause

Menopause can trigger a wide variety of symptoms, some commonly associated with the condition—such as hot flashes—and others that are more subtle and may seem like actual behavioral changes—such as anxiety and depression. Before a woman assumes that she is having a profound personality change, she should become familiar with all the symptoms of menopause and begin a plan to treat them.

Hot Flashes: According to Dr. Kronenberg, "hot flashes are defined subjectively as recurrent, transient periods of flushing, sweating, and a sensation of heat, often accompanied by palpitations and a feeling of anxiety, and sometimes followed by chills. There is no evidence that the physiology of nocturnal hot flashes (night sweats) is different from that of daytime hot flashes."[26] According to Dr. Lark, in the United States 85 percent of women have hot flashes, and 40 percent have symptoms severe enough to seek medical help.

Foods high in phytoestrogens (chemical compounds that the body can convert into usable estrogens) are thought to reduce the frequency of hot flashes. Japanese women have far fewer hot flashes than American women, and researchers have correlated this with the traditional Japanese diet that includes many soybean foods, which are high in natural phytoestrogens.[27] Dr. Lark emphasizes avoiding caffeine and alcohol, and taking nutritional supplements of vitamin E and the bioflavonoids.

"Herbs to treat hot flashes," says David Hoffmann, "include *dong quai*, ginseng, gotu kola, and motherwort to help with palpitations that accompany hot flashes."

Ayurveda recommends treating for a *pitta* imbalance. (See section on Premenstrual Syndrome, page 663.)

Homeopathy uses *Sepia*, *Lachesis*, and *Pulsatilla*, according to Dr. Jacobs, but she emphasizes that if hot flashes have become chronic, a woman should seek a more specific formula prescribed by a professional.

Traditional Chinese Medicine may use *dong quai* and ginseng but, again, according to Honora Wolfe, each patient needs a specific formula that only a doctor can give based on diagnosis.

"Estrogen has been found to be very effective in treating hot flashes, but considering the potential side effects of estrogen-replacement therapy, it is wise to attempt alternative treatment with vitamin E, a good diet, exercise, and simple perseverance, for they will eventually subside," says Dr. Lee. "If estrogen is chosen, however, it is especially important to include natural progesterone in the therapeutic plan."

Vaginal Dryness: According to Dr. O'Hanlan, "Low-dose estrogen vaginal cream is excellent. It works locally and it doesn't get absorbed systemically, being effective only in the immediate area." Dr. Lark also recommends estrogen replacement for vaginal dryness, but she also suggests vitamin E, taken orally and also applied directly to vaginal tissue.

According to Dr. Lee, the use of natural progesterone alone, used transdermally, is sufficient to treat vaginal atrophy. David Hoffmann suggests calendula flowers for vaginal dryness. There are also new lubricating jellies sold over the counter for this specific purpose.

Anxiety: According to David Hoffmann, skullcap eases anxiety associated with menopause. He recommends taking one-half teaspoon with chasteberry. Herbs such as passion flower and valerian root are often prescribed by Dr. Lark for their extraordinary calming properties. Other herbal remedies she recommends include chamomile, catnip, and peppermint teas.

Depression: For menopausal depression and its accompanying fatigue, stimulatory herbs such as oat straw, ginger, cayenne pepper, dandelion root, blessed thistle, and Siberian ginseng improve vitality, partly due to the high levels of essential nutrients contained in these herbs, notes Dr. Lark. "St. John's Wort can also lessen any depression that might occur," adds Hoffmann.

Perimenopause

During perimenopause, says Dr. Lark, "Estrogen levels swing between highly elevated and deficient with many side effects. The triumvirate of issues—PMS, bleeding, and fibroids—are very common. Often women who've had no PMS or very mild symptoms will begin noticing more irritability or touchiness, or classic PMS symptoms, food cravings, more tendency toward fluid retention, bloating, and breast tenderness. Combined with the more irregular menstrual cycle (the bleeding and even early onset of hot flashes) women can feel pretty awful during this transition time."

Dr. Lark notes, "The standard treatments are fairly draconian." These can include hormonal therapies, D&C's (in which a doctor dilates the cervix and inserts a small, spoon-shaped instrument, called a curette, which is used to remove pieces of the lining of the uterus), the use of medication to control the PMS symptoms, and even hysterectomy. "My goal is to get my patients through this vulnerable period with their uterus intact," continues Dr. Lark, "because once they've actually gone into menopause, these symptoms will subside and they will move into more of a simple estrogen-deficiency state; the fibroids will shrink, the PMS will go away, and the bleeding will stop."

Diet: Dr. Lark's outline for self-care includes a low-fat, high-fiber, vegetarian-based diet with whole grains, legumes, raw seeds and nuts, fruits, and vegetables making up the core of the diet. She advises avoiding salt, sugar, dairy products, alcohol, and caffeine in coffee, teas, colas, and chocolate.

Nutritional Supplements: Dr. Lark recommends the supplements vitamin B complex, vitamin B_6, vitamin E, vitamin C and bioflavonoids, magnesium, evening primrose oil, and borage oil.

Vitamin C and the bioflavonoids are recommended to be taken together. The combination has been shown to reduce heavy bleeding.[28] Bioflavonoids are available as supplements, but they are also prevalent in soy products, buckwheat, grape skins and cherry skins, and the inner peel and pulp of citrus fruit. The bioflavonoids are also weakly estrogenic and help even out estrogen levels when needed, reducing the body's own synthesis of estrogen or binding with estrogen receptor sites to increase the body's estrogen when low.[29] Dr. Lark points out, "Asian and African cultures, which feature bioflavonoid-containing foods, have lower rates of breast cancer, very few menopause symptoms, and do not tend to have these transition problems, either. The modulating effect of bioflavonoids also makes them beneficial for menopause."

Natural Hormone Therapy: Dr. Lee recommends supplementation with natural progesterone to correct any hormone imbalance during perimenopause if a woman is suffering from symptoms due to estrogen dominance such as water retention, loss of libido, weight gain, moodiness and irritability, depression, as well as fibrocystic breasts, breast cancer, or endometrial cancer.

General Recommendations for Menopause

The goal of any menopausal health program should be twofold: to eliminate the bother-somesymptoms of menopause and to prevent the degenerative ailments—osteoporosis and heart disease—that are associated with the post-menopausal period. Hormone-replacement therapy reduces the risk of these diseases, but not without potential side effects. "If a woman already has these diseases or is at unavoidable risk," says Dr. O'Hanlan, "these are reasons for taking hormones. In the case of osteoporosis, diet and exercise can also adequately prevent bone loss."[30]

Dr. Lark opposes an either/or approach to hormone-replacement therapy. "In an ideal world," she says, "one would make use of all the options available to women. You need to individualize a program for each woman, using a mix of lifestyle changes, hormonal therapy, or whatever else is needed."

Diet: Dr. Lark recommends the same type of diet prescribed for perimenopause, and notes, "These guidelines are also appropriate for the prevention of heart disease and osteoporosis."

In various societies, older women traditionally eat certain foods to remedy menopausal side effects. In the South Seas, for example, once a day women of menopausal age eat papaya, which contains phytoestrogens. Studies are beginning to show that these plant compounds can be helpful in menopause.[31] Traditional diets in Japan also are rich in phytoestrogens.[32] According to Dr. Kronenberg, "Studies of Japanese women with traditional Japanese diets show that these women's bodies contain levels of plant estrogens one hundred to one thousand times the level found in Western women. It may be that the reason these women don't have hot flashes is that they are eating a lot of weakly estrogenic substances all the time." She continues, "These women also have less incidence of breast cancer, and one of the reasons that is being suggested for this is that there are other things in the plant foods that are anticarcinogenic." In these studies, the higher estrogen levels were associated with intake of soybeans, soy products such as tofu, and miso and boiled beans.[33]

Dr. Lark points out, "As much as 50 percent of the Japanese diet contains phytoestrogen foods, whereas Westerners eat 10 percent or less. We really have very little dietary support as far as suppression of hot flashes and other menopausal symptoms."

Foods in the Western diet that do contain phytoestrogens are apples, carrots, yams, green beans, peas, potatoes, red beans, brown rice, whole wheat, rye, and sesame seeds. Though these foods may contain 1/400th or less estrogen than a single dose of hormone supplement, Dr. Jing-Nuan Wu, L.Ac., O.M.D., Director of the Taoist Center in Washington, D.C., suggests, "The thing that people have not really thought through is that the metabolism of a stronger dose of something may not be well incorporated into the body's system. If you have a steady drumbeat instead of a thunderclap, it may actually do much more for the body."

Legumes are excellent sources of minerals needed by postmenopausal women, containing calcium, magnesium, and potassium. They are also high in iron and in B complex, nutrients important for the health of the liver, which plays a role in the metabolism of estrogen.

Seeds and nuts are also good sources of calcium, magnesium, and potassium, and seeds such as flaxseed are mildly estrogenic. Seeds are also high in essential fatty acids. A deficiency of these oils may be responsible in part for the drying of the skin, hair, vaginal tissues, and other mucous membranes that occur with menopause; good sources are flaxseeds and pumpkin seeds. According to Dr. Lark, "The average healthy adult requires only four teaspoons per day of the essential oils in her diet, but menopausal women with extremely dry skin may need up to two to three tablespoons per day until the symptoms improve."[34]

Foods to avoid include most dairy products because of their high protein and fat content, caffeine because it can bring on hot flashes and mood swings, and alcohol because it can also lead to hot flashes.

Lifestyle: According to Dr. O'Hanlan, "When the data from the Framingham study of heart disease was first analyzed, it looked like women who worked had more heart disease. Then Suzanne G. Haynes, Ph.D., Chief of the NCI's Health Education Division, reanalyzed the data and found that actually it was the secretarial workers who had twice the rate of heart disease of housewives. The lowest risk was working women who were rewarded by their work. The stressor was jobs in which a woman had no autonomy or control of the environment, low recognition, accomplishment, and low pay."[35]

Nutritional Supplements: According to Dr. Lark, "Clinical studies have shown the remarkable ability of bioflavonoids to control hot flashes.[36] Unlike estrogen therapy, no harmful side effects have been noted with bioflavonoid therapy." She also recommends that women taking hormone therapy supplement with vitamin B_6 since they might become deficient in the vitamin. Dr. Lark also recommends vitamin E, calcium, magnesium, potassium, and aspartate. Evening primrose oil is a source of essential fatty acids.

Natural Hormone Therapy: "The most significant biologic consequence of menopause is the observed acceleration of osteoporosis. Due to anovulatory periods, poor diet, and lack of exercise, many women arrive at menopause with 25 to 30 percent loss of bone mass," reports Dr. Lee. "Any acceleration of osteoporosis at this time greatly increases their risk of fracture."

"Healthy bone tissue is continually being made, resorbed, and made anew," Dr. Lee continues. "This is accomplished by two sets of bone cells, osteoblasts and osteoclasts. New bone is made by osteoblasts and old bone is resorbed by osteoclasts. In this regard, the role of estrogen is to partially suppress osteoclast-mediated bone reabsorption, and the role of progesterone is to stimulate osteoblast-mediated new bone formation. Thus, the role of progesterone is of prime importance. Effective treatment of post-menopausal osteoporosis requires supplementation with progesterone. Various synthetic progestins have some positive bone-building effects, but none are as effective as natural progesterone which also is devoid of the adverse side effects of the progestins.

See Osteoporosis.

"There is no reason to assume that menopause signals the end of an active, healthy life," adds Dr. Lee. "Most women enjoy the absence of monthly menses. Most find to their surprise that their libido is unaffected. Their main concern is the aging they see in their female colleagues—the dryness and wrinkle lines that show in their face and body parts, the loss of fullness of their breasts, vaginal dryness, fracture proclivity, and the gray they see in their hair. Hormone replacement therapy promises many years of healthy life, though not the prevention of aging.

"Hormone replacement should consist of progesterone and, if hot flashes or vaginal dryness (signs of estrogen deficiency) occur, estrogen supplements. With progesterone, good diet, and exercise, their bones remain strong and their vigor for life also remains strong. Menopause is not the dreaded turning point of life as once was thought."

FEMALE RECONSTRUCTIVE SURGERY

Surgeon Vicki Hufnagel, M.D., of Beverly Hills, California, has developed a new approach to female surgery that is at once empowering and revolutionary in procedure, and which offers a new paradigm to other gynecological surgeons and the field of surgery as a whole.

"My work puts forth a philosophy that is the complete antithesis of conventional medicine," says Dr. Hufnagel, "a philosophy that views a woman's body as a whole organism that should be conserved and repaired at all times when possible." Dr. Hufnagel performs surgery for fibroids, endometriosis, and other conditions, and in the majority of cases is able to leave the reproductive organs intact. She believes that about 90 percent of all hysterectomies are unnecessary, and even conservative estimates of 16 percent to 27 percent are still high.[37]

From start to finish, her approach acknowledges that the patient has rights and deserves to be in control. "There is no reason to operate on someone who is frightened and uneducated," insists Dr. Hufnagel. Her preoperation education program requires the surgery candidate to talk with former patients and view twelve hours of video coverage on the anticipated procedure. "We provide pre-op care that may involve acupressure, naturopathy, and supplements of vitamins and amino acids," she says.

Dr. Hufnagel uses regional anesthetic for her major surgery, allowing the patient to watch the procedure and talk with the surgery team while the operation is in progress. Family is asked to be present in a neighboring room to watch the operation via camera and dialogue with the doctor. Dr. Hufnagel states, "This creates a completely different response post-op. The family becomes more involved and gives more assistance to the patient later."

During the procedure, Dr. Hufnagel bathes the exposed tissue in fluids to medicate and cleanse. She says, "In this way I can float a medication that can help prevent future endometriosis." Before closing the incision, she repairs muscle and ligaments so organs have good support and also removes any tissue stretched by a tumor that later would be unsightly. After surgery, Dr. Hufnagel often employs electromagnetic treatments and ultrasound to enhance healing, and she says her patients have better compliance in their post-op care because, as she notes, "A woman takes better care of herself when she doesn't see herself as a victim."

ESTROGEN-REPLACEMENT THERAPY

Perhaps the biggest debate today concerning women's health is the question of whether or not to supplement with hormones. Estrogen replacement therapy (ERT) is currently prescribed for osteoporosis and to relieve the symptoms of menopause. Some physicians recommend ERT when symptoms are "bothersome" while others use it only when symptoms become "disabling." Caution is used because estrogen has side effects, some highly debated. These include stroke, gallbladder disease, liver tumors and enlargement, fluid retention and weight gain, headaches, and endometrial cancer and fibroids. Estrogen is not recommended for patients with uterine or breast cancer, a strong family history of breast cancer, obesity, phlebitis, varicose veins, diabetes, hypertension, edema, fibroids, or fibrocystic breasts.

Herbal Medicine: David Hoffmann offers a simple formula, using chasteberry as the base, combined with a choice of other herbs used for specific symptoms. He recommends combining half a teaspoon of chasteberry with half a teaspoon of tincture of each herb added. Hoffmann states, "Chasteberry will ease the unfoldment of the natural process of menopause." The optional herbs include: St. John's Wort for depression, motherwort for palpitations accompanying hot flashes, and skullcap for anxiety.

Dr. Heron uses individualized formulas for her patients, but finds that a general formula works for most women. She prescribes herbs in liquid preparation, taken throughout the month, one teaspoon of tincture formula three times a day. As she states, "This is because menopause is not pathological (disease-causing) and these herbs are not drugs, just tonics to the female reproductive system." In developing an individual formula she selects from the following herbs: chasteberry, for its hormone-balancing effect; motherwort for its assistance in anxiety; false unicorn for hormonal and digestive benefit; *dong quai*, licorice, and alfalfa for estrogen enhancement; cramp bark or blackhaw bark because they both allay spasticity, which can promote hot flashes; and black cohosh as an antispasmodic and estrogen enhancer. The last herb was compared in a clinical study with estrogen replacement as a treatment for menopausal symptoms after hysterectomy (with intact ovaries). It was shown to be as effective as synthetic hormones.[38]

Dr. Hudson reports, "I have been using an herbal formula for eight years and it does relieve the symptoms of menopause in most women. It has two parts licorice, two parts burdock root, two parts *Dong quai*, one part wild yam, and one part motherwort. We powder the herbs and put them in capsules. The higher dose is two capsules three times a day, reducing it as needed."

Homeopathy: *Pulsatilla* is often suggested for a woman whose mood is changeable and is frequently weepy. When hot flushes extend all the way to the palms of the hands and soles of the feet, *Sulphur* is appropriate. *Bryonia* can help with a dry and thinning vagina."

Traditional Chinese Medicine: Traditional Chinese Medicine offers both herbs and acupuncture for the treatment of menopause, and assesses a woman's menopausal status in terms of various body organs and substances such as *qi* and blood in terms of *yin* and *yang*.

As Honora Lee Wolfe explains, "Symptoms of menopause result when hormonal fluctuations are causing *yin* and *yang* to come out of balance and be unstable for a time while the body readjusts its metabolism. The variations on this are quite complex. It is almost impossible to list herbs that work for menopause because the herbs are never given singly and because each person's diagnosis is very specific. However, there is one formula that is the most famous for menopause and this is the 'Two Immortals Decoction.'"

See Herbal Medicine, Traditional Chinese Medicine.

Traditional Chinese Medicine does, however, have a generalized diet recommended for menopause, which focuses on keeping the spleen and stomach strong. Wolfe says, "If the digestion is strong, then all the other symptoms are easier to treat or prevent. The diet is just a basic grounded, balanced diet that is easy to digest. It consists of cooked foods, a little bit of animal protein, which helps to keep the blood strong, some eggs, which are very good for the kidney energy, lots of fresh and lightly cooked vegetables, and fruits in season but not eaten cold or necessarily refrigerated. It's also important to go easy on the alcohol, caffeine, sugar, salt, and fat."

Wolfe also recommends as much moderate exercise as a woman has time for or feels comfortable with. She explains, "Exercise keeps the *qi* and blood from stagnating. As we age, more problems are due to stagnation, so movement of any kind is healthful. Stretching is good because it keeps ligaments and joints supple."

Ayurvedic Medicine: According to Dr. Lonsdorf, "Menopause is a natural transition time that shouldn't be creating disease if we are in balance. Basically, it is a *vata* imbalance."

Bladder Infections (Cystitis)

Cystitis refers to irritations or bacterial infections that occur anywhere from the lining of the vagina through the urethra (where the urine comes out from the bladder), to the lining of the bladder. These infections can occur in a single episode or recurrent episodes, or can exist as chronic conditions. Cystitis is common in sexually active women, and women in menopause have a tendency to develop cystitis because, as estrogen levels decline, bacteria is more prone to adhere to the bladder lining and vaginal tissue.

Symptoms include burning and pain on urination, increased urinary urgency and frequency, pain over the pubic area or lower back, and increased urination throughout the night. In women, as severity increases, blood may color the urine red. Signs that the kidneys have also become involved are fever, chills, nausea, vomiting, and severe high back and/or loin pain. For this a doctor must be seen.

Larrian Gillespie, M.D., Director of the Pelvic Pain Treatment Center and the Women's Clinic for Interstitial Cystitis, in Beverly Hills, California, specializes in the treatment of cystitis. She states, "A urinary tract infection is not a problem of bacteria getting into the bladder. It is a problem of bacteria not getting out. A study was done in which stool was placed directly into the bladder of medical students. By the second voiding, there was no more bacteria. So, an infection is directly the result of the bladder not efficiently evacuating the urine. It has nothing to do with the female anatomy being different from the male's, that is, 'too short'. If you can move 'dirt on the sidewalk' with your stream, instead of 'tinkling' drops out, you will not get a bladder infection."

There are a number of things a woman can do to avoid recurrent cystitis. First of all, do not urinate after intercourse until you feel the need to void, as squeezing out a few drops will not efficiently clean the bladder and the vagina. Second, an overly large fitted diaphragm will obstruct the bladder neck and prevent you from emptying your bladder after intercourse. The contraceptive sponge may also cause the same effect in women, so it is best to use either a cervical cap or have your diaphragm reduced in size, usually to a sixty-five millimeter or seventy millimeter size.

Some women, however, may develop symptoms of an infection when none exists. This hypersensitivity is often the result of changes in blood flow to the bladder. It can be caused by endometriosis, lower back problems, and hormone problems. The symptoms of pressure or burning relieved by urination are characteristic of the painful bladder syndrome, interstitial cystitis. New research by Dr. Gillespie now shows that the bladder is rarely the cause of this problem. "Hypersensitive bladder symptoms, such as those related to interstitial cystitis, can be caused by a stretch on the nerves which control blood flow into the bladder, bowel, and pelvic floor. By looking into the injury, we can switch the signals which are causing the bladder to lose oxygen and improve circulation. This can be done through back stabilization exercises and acupressure." In Dr. Gillespie's experience, many of the patients have unsuspected endometriosis, and it is necessary to perform microsurgery through a tiny incision in the belly button.

"It is important to first check your urine for the presence of nitrites," says Dr. Gillespie. These compounds are formed by actively-producing bacteria, and you can purchase a dip test from your pharmacy. If it is positive, you should contact your health practitioner for a single dose of antibiotics, according to Dr. Gillespie.

Diet: "If you have an infection, taking cranberry juice, which contains hippuronic acid, makes as much sense as putting out a fire with gasoline," states Dr. Gillespie. "It only adds *more* acid to the urine, which in turn, increases the burning sensation. Cranberry juice may be helpful if you want to prevent an infection, but if you already have one, it only makes matters worse. Rather, try one-quarter teaspoon of baking soda in water. You should feel the relief in twenty minutes." Corn silk tea contains silica which also acts as a soothing coating to inflamed bladder tissue.

Foods which are high in the amino acids phenylalanine, tryptophan, tyrosine, and tyramine can irritate the bladder of patients with hypersensitive symptoms, adds Dr. Gillespie. Try avoiding bananas, cranberries, pineapple, avocados, aspartame, figs, yogurt, chocolate, and the citrus fruits. Wines which do not undergo malolactic fermentation will not increase your pain, according to Dr. Gillespie.

Herbal Medicine: According to Hoffmann, herbs containing volatile oils that are excreted from the body via the kidneys produce good results in such infections. For an infection accompanied with pain and burning, he suggests combining tinctures of corn silk, bearberry, and buchu in equal parts and taking one teaspoonful of this mixture three times a day. Hot infusions often ease the symptoms. He also recommends combining equal parts of dried marshmallow leaf, corn silk, couch grass, and bearberry and drinking a cup of the infusion four to five times a day.

Vaginal Infections (Vaginitis)

Vaginal infections account for nearly 7 percent of all visits to gynecologists.[39] Hormonal vaginitis is primarily a problem of postmenopausal women, as the vaginal tissue becomes thin and susceptible to irritation. There may also be vaginal discharge. Infectious vaginitis may be sexually transmitted or may arise from a disturbance to the delicate ecology of the healthy vagina.

In the past twenty years, the yeast infection, *Candida albicans*, has increased two and one half times due to several factors, chief among them the increased use of antibiotics. The primary symptoms of candidal vaginitis are vulvar itching, which can be quite severe, and a thick, curdy discharge.[40]

"If a yeast infection is recurrent," advises Dr. Hudson, "it is important to go to a doctor to be diagnosed. Sometimes there are systemic health problems that cause it—diabetes, for instance—and more worrisome these days is that chronic yeast vaginitis is the primary presenting symptom of women who are HIV positive." Self-care for this condition includes diet and using suppositories for vaginal itching. One should also test for food, chemical, and environmental sensitivities.

Diet: A basic diet for vaginitis is low in fats, sugars, and refined foods.[41] For candidiasis, Dr. Hudson recommends that a woman follow a yeast-free diet, avoiding fermented foods and sugar, which feeds yeast growth, and increase her intake of acidophilus yogurt and garlic, both of which are antifungal.

Nutritional Supplements: Vaginal infections have been known to respond to vitamins A, B complex, C, E, and beta-carotene and the bioflavonoids. Zinc, lysine, lithium, acidophilus, and iodine as a topical douche, boric acid, and gentian violet are other options.[42]

Herbal Medicine: For vaginal infections, Dr. Heron recommends a douche of antiseptic herbs such as St. John's Wort, goldenseal, echinacea, fresh plantain, garlic, and calendula along with demulcent herbs like comfrey leaves and Self-heal to soothe the membranes. Calendula is both antiseptic and reparative. This douche is alternated with one of acidophilis. Sweet foods are to be avoided.

Suppositories: The suppository Dr. Hudson prescribes consists of powdered boric acid mixed with three herbs—berberis, hydrastis, and calendula, all antifungals—prepared in capsule form. "This works so well," says Dr. Hudson, "that I no longer prescribe douches for this condition."

Topical Treatment: Douches include apple cider vinegar (two tablespoons to one quart water), acidophilus (two opened capsules to one quart water), or a solution of water and garlic from capsules or fresh juice. Topical pau d'arco, black walnut, and tea tree oil are also options and vitamin E cream may relieve itching.

Problems with the Uterus

The uterus is an important female organ, and its health is an integral part of the health of the entire reproductive system. In recent years, problems with the uterus have been on the rise, because of lifestyle and environmental changes, according to Dr. Lark. Two common conditions affecting the uterus are fibroids and endometriosis.

Uterine Fibroids

A fibroid is a noncancerous tumor that arises from uterine muscle and connective tissue, almost all cases of which are benign. Since fibroids develop following the onset of menstruation, enlarge during pregnancy, and decrease after menopause, fibroids are thought to be estrogen dependent. One in five women in the United States has at least some evidence of fibroids, with most occurring in women in their thirties and forties.[43] Fibroids are much more common among black women than among white women, although the reason for this difference is not known.[44]

Fibroids are usually firm, spherical lumps that often occur in groups. They are of varying sizes, usually described in terms of vegetables and fruit—pea, lemon, apple, cantaloupe, etc. They can grow near the outer surface of the uterus, where they are easily detected during a pelvic examination, as well as near the inner lining of the uterus, where they may need ultrasound for detection. Fibroids normally shrink in size after menopause.

Most women have no symptoms at all, but there may be lower abdominal pain, a feeling of fullness and pressure in the lower abdomen, and frequent urination caused by tumor pressure on the bladder, plus heavy menstrual periods, bleeding between periods, and increased menstrual cramps. If a fibroid grows rapidly, it may outstrip its nutrition supply from nearby blood vessels, resulting in the degeneration and death of the oxygen-deprived tissue; severe abdominal pain may result. Rapid growth is common in pregnancy, when high estrogen levels stimulate tumor growth.

Birth control pills, with high levels of estrogen, and estrogen-replacement medication for menopause symptoms can also accelerate tumor growth. As Dr. Lark explains, "Fibroids are caused by periods of high estrogen production, and our strategy is to level these out so that the fibroids don't grow. We use a conservative approach, controlling estrogen production through nutrition and lifestyle and, if needed, reducing the bleeding in the same way. My issue with fibroids is that too many women have hysterectomies. A fibroid the size of a thirteen-week fetus (the size at which Western medicine begins discussing the need for a hysterectomy) and larger can be successfully treated by this approach. I've seen fibroid tumors shrink in women following a conservative approach."

In treatment, Dr. Lark uses anti-estrogenic substances, focusing on flavonoids. She explains, "The flavonoids have 1/400th to 1/50,000th the estrogenic effect that synthetic estrogen does and therefore these flavonoids contribute very little to the total body supply."

Diet: Dr. Lark recommends a whole foods diet with fresh vegetables and fruits, nuts, seeds, and whole grains. Foods to avoid include dairy products, red meat, fried fat, sugar, salt, caffeine, and alcohol.

Nutritional Supplements: Dr. Hudson suggests supplementing with vitamin C, beta-carotene, selenium, and zinc in treating fibroids.

Herbal Medicine: Hoffmann recommends a basic mixture of the tinctures of chasteberry, blue cohosh, wild yam, and cranesbill in equal amounts; one-half teaspoonful three times a day. If there is much cramping pain, he advises taking one-half a teaspoonful of cramp bark tincture in addition to the basic mixture.

Homeopathy: According to Joyce Frye, D.O., of Philadelphia, Pennsylvania, "Homeopathy may keep the fibroids from growing; it may change something about why this person got fibroids in the first place, but it's probably not going to get the fibroids to go away." And she continues, "There is often confusion about what the symptoms are, and if people have fibroids a lot of the other problems that they have get blamed on the fibroids—the back pain, a bleeding problem—and this isn't necessarily so. And homeopathy and craniosacral therapy can alleviate the symptoms."

Traditional Chinese Medicine: According to Honora Lee Wolfe, "Fibroids are an indication that something is not flowing—that is stagnation—but fibroids can also have an element of dampness and phlegm involvement, though each person's diagnosis may be somewhat different."

Ayurvedic Medicine: Dr. Lonsdorf recommends being more restful at the time of one's period because of incomplete elimination and buildup of toxins, and to avoid using tampons.

Endometriosis

In this condition, endometrial cells from the lining of the uterus migrate to locations where they are not normally found—in the uterine myometrium and outside the uterus on the ovaries, bladder, and gastrointestinal tract. It is estimated that 10 to 20 percent of all women in the United States have endometriosis. The probability of contracting the condition increases until age forty-four and then declines.[45] The condition is stimulated by excess estrogen production, but the exact cause is unknown. One theory is that the endometrial cells are carried upward through the fallopian tubes (called retrograde menstruation), enabling them to implant in the abdomen, where they grow to form endometriosis patches. Delayed first pregnancy and menstruation at an earlier age, both more common today than two or three generations ago, have also been linked to endometriosis in that the disease has become more common in the last few decades. In the past a woman might have had fewer than forty menstrual cycles before pregnancy, while now there might be twelve years of monthly periods before a woman decides to have a child.

The primary symptom of endometriosis is dysmenorrhea with dull, aching pain in the pelvis, lower abdomen, and back. Dr. Lee explains, "Once the endometrial cells are transplanted, they still respond to the monthly hormonal (estrogen) messages just as they would if remaining within the uterus; by filling with blood which is then released at the time of menses. The drops of blood, however, have nowhere to go and can become a focus of excruciating pain and inflammation. Despite their small size (some no larger than a pinhead), pelvic pain that results can be disabling. Symptoms tend to increase gradually over the years as the endometriosis areas slowly increase in size."

There are no specific laboratory tests that will detect endometriosis, but a biopsy can be performed in the office by a doctor.

For endometriosis, Dr. Lark follows the same protocol she does for fibroids—using weak estrogenic flavonoids to block the body's own production of estrogen—but she adds anti-inflammatory agents, since scarring and infection often accompany endometriosis. She advises, "The patient needs to include good sources of essential fatty acids because the body manufactures prostaglandins from these, which are anti-inflammatory agents. These EFA's are plentiful in fish such as salmon and in seeds and nuts. It is also equally important to reduce or eliminate meat, eggs, and especially dairy, because these foods are sources of arachidonic acid, which promotes inflammation."

Herbal Medicine: Many alternative therapies are also used to prevent and treat endome-

Ovarian cysts

The ovaries can develop various kinds of cysts, and of these, 75 to 85 percent are benign and do not require surgery. There are cysts that occur on the egg follicle and are the result of normal ovarian functions, follicular cysts that happen when a normal egg follicle ruptures as it releases an egg, and corpus luteum cysts, which can be a signal to check for ectopic or uterine pregnancy. A sign of a follicular cyst can be a sudden onset of pain on one side of the abdomen lasting a few hours and occurring halfway between monthly periods. The sign of a corpus luteum cyst can be abnormal or slight bleeding.

According to Tori Hudson, N.D., Academic Dean at National College of Naturopathic Medicine in Portland, Oregon, a diagnosis must encompass the patient's history, a physical exam, pelvic ultrasound, in some cases laparoscopy, and in even fewer cases, laparotomy (surgical opening of abdomen) to rule out malignancy. Acute problems from this condition can be pain and bleeding. In treating ovarian cysts, Dr. Hudson focuses on possible toxemia of the liver and designs treatments to maintain healthy liver function. She recommends a vegetarian diet using organic foods and nourishing the liver with beets, carrots, and lemons. Dr. Hudson advises, "There should be no fried foods, coffee, cigarettes, medications, alcohol, or sugar." She recommends as supplements vitamins A, E, C, beta-carotene, and zinc, as well as black currant oil and evening primrose oil.

Dr. Hudson suggests steps to be taken for self-care: Avoid chilling of the extremities, which can cause internal congestion; avoid wearing high heels, which can block pelvic circulation; heal past sexual or physical insults or abuses; and make an effort to express creativity.

triosis, and herbs are a good example. Dr. Heron treats endometriosis with a range of herbs meant to, as she explains, "increase circulation in the pelvis, thereby promoting drainage, discouraging adhesions, and facilitating removal of inflammatory substances. In addition, hormonal balance is reestablished, decreasing premenstrual syndrome." The herbs she chooses for treatment are intended to act as hormonal precursors and balancers, and also to improve liver function and digestion, all components of the disease. Dr. Heron states, "The result is usually symptom relief as a result of treating the underlying cause. Patients consistently report a marked decrease in dysmenorrhea, dyspareunia (pain with intercourse), digestive symptoms, menorrhagia, and ovulation pain, along with an improvement in mental outlook and decrease of lassitude."

Dr. Heron develops formulas of herbs fine-tuned for the individual. As she explains, "It's important not to use the catalogue of herbs like a cookbook, always prescribing the same herb for a given disease." She uses a polypharmacy approach, combining various herbs, because, as she says, "Most traditional systems combine herbs as the combination has an enhanced effect."

She uses three of her own formulas, one for each phase of the cycle: during menses itself, between menses and ovulation (approximately day fourteen or later), and from ovulation to the beginning of menses. Herbs that are included are: dandelion, Oregon grape root, pasque flower, chasteberry, false unicorn, cramp bark or blackhaw bark, black cohosh, motherwort, vervain, yarrow, hops, valerian, and borage.[46]

Nutritional Supplements: Dr. Hufnagel suggests supplementing the diet with vitamin C, vitamin B_6, folic acid, calcium, magnesium, essential fatty acids such linoleic acid, and evening primrose oil.[47]

Traditional Chinese Medicine: According to Honora Lee Wolfe, "This condition may be due to blood stasis, *qi* stagnation, phlegm and dampness, damp heat, or some combination of these, but in turn this can be based on some organs being empty or not strong enough. It's almost always a combination of patterns, a concurrent insufficiency, or vacuity."

Ayurvedic Medicine: "This condition is a *vata* imbalance," explains Dr. Lonsdorf. "We treat this as we would any *vata* imbalance (see section on Premenstrual Syndrome). For prevention we advise that a woman reduce her activities as much as possible for the first three days of her period each month, though this might be an unpopular suggestion to most busy women today. For exercise, we recommend a gentle walk rather than jarring aerobics classes at this time."

Endometrial Cancer

Endometrial cancer occurs most often in women between the ages of fifty-five and seventy. Cancer of the uterus accounts for 13 percent of all cancers in women, with 31,000 new cases in 1993.[48]

Spotting during menopause can be a sign of endometrial cancer, but, as Dr. O'Hanlan notes, "Ninety-five percent of all women who have spotting do not have cancer; however, it is important if there is irregular spotting to have a doctor do a biopsy of the uterine lining. This cancer is as much as 98 percent curable when it's found early,

MAMMOGRAMS AND BREAST CANCER

There is an information gap on the causes, monitoring, and prevention of breast cancer because so little conclusive research has been done on the subject. However, it is known that 75 percent of patients survive breast cancer, and most breast cancers are present for eight to ten years before they can be detected as a lump or on a mammogram, according to Susan M. Love, M.D., Associate Professor of Clinical Surgery at the University of California at Los Angeles, and Director of the Breast Center. The newly formed Women's Health Initiative will be launching some additional studies, and the National Breast Center Coalition in Washington, D.C., is lobbying for increased research funding, but women may have to wait five to ten years for solid answers. Dr. Love points out, "The problem of the prevention and treatment of breast cancer is the fact that 80 percent of women who get breast cancer don't have [the traditional] risk factors. A low-fat diet may be preventative, but we won't have the results from studies for a good five to ten years." Recent studies, however, have disputed the long-standing belief that the risk factor is greatly increased by a mother or sister's breast cancer, and state that although the risk of breast cancer is doubled among women whose mother had breast cancer before the age of forty or whose sister had breast cancer, the risk associated with a mother or sister history is much smaller than thought. The study indicated that within middle-aged women, only 2.5 percent of breast cancer cases were attributable to family history.[51]

Early detection is currently one of the primary strategies for prevention and successful treatment, which is why the self-breast examination is so important.

The benefits of mammography is still a subject of debate. Questions that are still present include whether low-level radiation used in the test can contribute to cancer, whether equivocal results lead to unnecessary surgery, and the accuracy rate of test results. According to the National Cancer Institute, in women ages forty to forty-nine, there is a high rate of "missed tumors," resulting in 40 percent false-negative test results. Breast tissue in younger women is denser, which makes it more difficult to detect tumors, and tumors grow more quickly in younger women, so tumors may develop between screenings. Because there is no reduction in mortality from breast cancer as a direct result of early mammograms, it is recommended that women under fifty avoid screening mammograms,[52] although the American Cancer Society is still recommending a mammogram every two years for women ages forty to forty-nine.

The Institute recommends that, after age thirty-five, women perform monthly breast self-exams. For women over fifty, most agree that mammograms are the best solution. As Dr. Love states, "We know that mammography works and will be a lifesaving tool for at least 30 percent."

and it usually is found early. The biopsy can be done in the office; it takes five minutes—it causes a major cramp that lasts two to three minutes at worst and then it goes away."

Estrogen-only therapy increases the risk of endometrial cancer, producing, according to Dr. O'Hanlan, "an eightfold increase in cancer risk of the uterine lining. However, when we give the progesterone with the estrogen, the cancer risk to the uterus is only one-half that of women who take no hormones at all." Dr. Lee takes this advice one step further, stating that, though synthetic progestin (commonly called progesterone) can be effective in the prevention of endometrial cancer,[49] natural progesterone provides even more protection. As he states, "With progestins, there can still be some hyperplasia, but with natural progesterone, the risk of endometrial cancer would approach zero."[50]

See Cancer.

Cervical Cancer

Cervical dysplasia is generally regarded as a precancerous lesion with risk factors similar to those of cervical cancer. Dr. Hudson states, "We have an excellent naturopathic protocol for treating this. Monitoring forty-three patients, we were able to completely cure thirty-eight of these, with three showing some improvement and the remaining two showing no change. Our protocol has three phases: herbal supplements, enzymes, and herbal paste applied locally to the cervix; systemic treatment using vitamin C, vitamin B, vitamin E, and beta-carotene; and dietary and lifestyle changes."

Ovarian Cancer

According to Patricia Cane, Ph.D., Research Associate in Ob. Gyn., Cedars Sinai Hospital, Los Angeles, symptoms of ovarian cancer can include bloating and abdominal discomfort. There are a wide variety of risk factors, but among the more predominant are age (over forty-five); family history of ovarian, breast, and gastrointestinal tumors; and personal history of breast cancer. Exposure to talc and asbestos, the number of children a woman has had, and obesity may also be factors, while oral contraceptives may actually be protective. According to Dr. Cane, "There is no good screening tool [for ovarian cancer], not a single one or a combination, and in early stages this cancer is asymptomatic. Consequently, the cancer is found at more advanced stages when it is more difficult to cure. Ultrasound is used to view any mass and to monitor color doplar flow, which indicates the flow characteristics of blood through tiny vessels associated with new growth. However, this test can create false negatives. Transvaginal ultrasound is preferred over abdominal ultrasound because the monitoring device can move closer to the area being investigated."

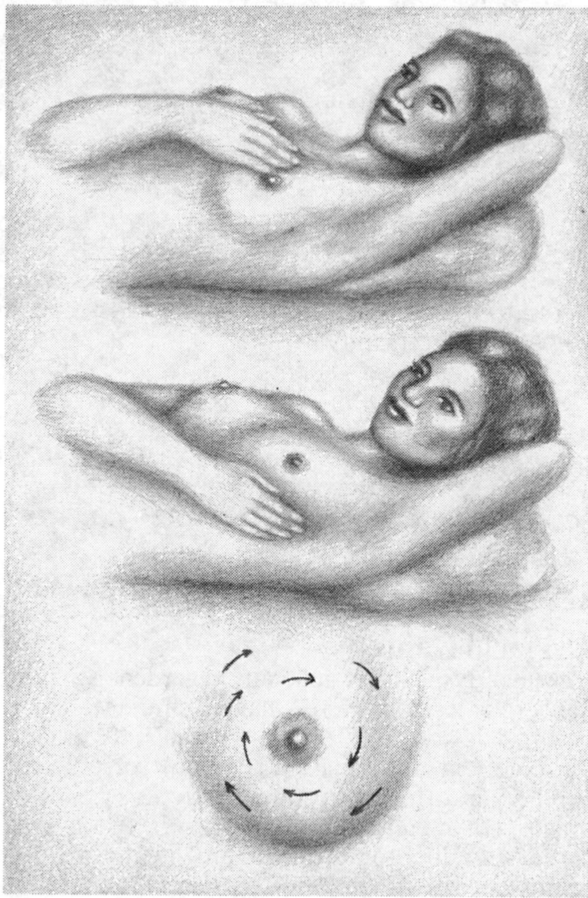

Breast self-examination.

Breast Problems

Breast disorders can be hereditary, and can also result from such environmental and lifestyle factors as diet, breast implants, and birth control pills. Since early detection of such problems—especially where cancer is concerned—is currently one of the primary strategies for prevention and successful treatment, it is important for women to examine their own breasts regularly. This must be done each month at the same time in a woman's cycle, in the same physical position, and using the same sequence of steps. Some lumps are easier to find when lying down, and others are more apparent when sitting or standing, so you may want to use a couple of positions. Using the flat part of the fingertips, feel each area of the breast, systematically moving around it and noting any changes. Some women draw a sketch each time to record what they feel.

"Since early detection of such problems—especially where cancer is concerned—is currently one of the primary strategies for prevention and successful treatment, it is important for women to examine their own breasts regularly."

Fibrocystic Breast Disease

"Fibrocystic breast disease occurs in 80 percent of premenopausal women," according to Susan M. Love, M.D., Associate Professor of Clinical Surgery at the University of California at Los Angeles, and Director of the Breast Center. Common symptoms of this condition include pain and tenderness, and the texture of the breast changing, with small lumps detectable to the touch. This is usually a component of premenstrual syndrome and is considered a low risk factor for breast cancer. Fibrocystic breasts are apparently caused by an increased estrogen-to-progesterone ratio.[53] Caroline M. Shreeve, M.D., says that benign disorders of the breast are common among women whose diets include a high proportion of saturated animal fat and rare among those who eat little saturated animal fat but take in a high proportion of essential fatty acids.[54]

Any breast lump that is painful is likely to be a cyst rather than a tumor, which usually is not tender. Diagnosis can be made by mammogram (see sidebar Mammograms and Breast Cancer) or by simple aspiration (a needle is inserted into the lump under local anesthetic and the cyst fluid is withdrawn). When fluid is withdrawn and the lump disappears, it is good evidence that the lump was not a tumor.

Jonathan Wright, M.D., Director of the Tahoma Clinic in Kent, Washington, reports success in eliminating breast cysts using a treatment of iodine (painted on intravaginally) and magnesium (administered intravenously) combined with a regimen of nutritional supplements including organic iodine tablets, chelated magnesium, B complex, vitamin E, vitamin B_6, and essential fatty acid capsules.

Diet: Dr. Wright recommends a primarily vegetarian, high-fiber, low-fat, dairy-free diet for patients with fibrocystic breast disease.

Nutritional Supplements: Dr. Hudson recommends vitamin E, beta-carotene, evening primrose oil, iodine, choline, flaxseed oil, vitamin B complex, and methionine.

Herbal Medicine: David Hoffmann says fibrocystic breasts can be treated with echinacea, goldenseal, herbal squaw vine, mullein, pau d'arco, poke root, and red clover. For long-term care, he recommends evening primrose oil and chasteberry. Dandelion is used for breast sores, tumors, and cysts, and parsley for swollen breasts.

Natural Hormone Therapy: Dr. Lee often recommends applying natural progesterone cream directly to the skin, allowing it to be absorbed transdermally. "Using this progesterone transdermally from day fifteen of the monthly cycle to day twenty-five will usually cause breast cysts to disappear," he states.

Self-Care

The following therapies can be undertaken at home under appropriate professional supervision:

Bladder Infections (Cystitis)

• Qigong

Aromatherapy: Massage or bath with bergamot, lavender, eucalyptus, sandalwood, camomile, juniper.

Ayurveda: Herbal mixture of *shatavari* 500 mg., *guduchi* 300 mg., *punarnava* 300 mg., and *kamadudha* 100 mg. Take one-quarter teaspoon of mixture twice daily after lunch and dinner with coriander tea.

Homeopathy: *Cantharis, Apis mel., Berberis.*

Hydrotherapy: Hot sitz baths two times a day for twenty minutes to relieve pain, with one cup of apple cider vinegar added to bath water. (The process is to pour half the apple cider vinegar in the water before getting in, and pouring the other half between the legs while sitting in the bath. Knees are up and apart so the solution can more readily enter the vagina).

Juice Therapy: • Equal parts carrot and apple juice • Cranberry juice • Watermelon juice • Garlic or onion juice may be added to carrot, beet, cucumber, or spinach juices. • Carrot, celery, spinach, and parsley

Topical Treatment: Half a teaspoon of yogurt around vaginal opening after intercourse.

Endometriosis

Aromatherapy: Cypress.

Hydrotherapy: Bleeding between periods: vaginal douches.

Menopause

• Meditation • Yoga

Aromatherapy: Clary sage.

Juice Therapy: Carrot, celery, parsley, and spinach.

Excessive Menstruation (Menorrhagia)

• Yoga

Ayurveda: Red raspberry or *manjistha.* Or try *shatavari* and *manjistha* in equal proportions.

Menstrual Cramps (Dysmenorrhea)

• Qigong • Yoga

Herbs: Mild diuretics may help remove some of the fluid retention.

Juice Therapy: One glass of blueberry and huckleberry juice daily.

Premenstrual Syndrome (PMS)

• Exercise • Meditation • Stress reduction • Relaxation • Yoga

Vaginal Infections

• Yoga

Homeopathy: *Cactus, Belladonna, Sepia.*

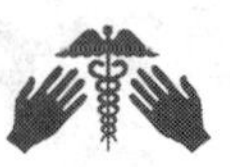

Professional Care

The following therapies can only be provided by a qualified health professional:

Bladder Infections (Cystitis)

• Acupuncture • Cell Therapy • Chiropractic • Environmental Medicine • Enzyme Therapy • Magnetic Field Therapy • Naturopathic Medicine • Osteopathy • Oxygen Therapy • Reflexology • Traditional Chinese Medicine

Endometriosis

• Chiropractic • Guided Imagery

Fibrocystic Breast Disease

• Biofeedback Training • Hypnotherapy • Relaxation Techniques

Menopause

• Acupressure

Menstrual Cramps (Dysmenorrhea)

Bodywork: Acupressure, massage.

Excessive Menstruation (Menorrhagia)

• Acupuncture • Biofeedback Training • Chiropractic • Craniosacral Therapy • Guided Imagery • Hypnotherapy • Light Therapy

Bodywork: Acupressure, reflexology, *shiatsu,* massage.

Premenstrual Syndrome (PMS)

• Acupuncture • Biofeedback Training • Guided Imagery • Hypnotherapy • Relaxation techniques • Yoga

Bodywork: Massage and hot baths relax the body and help release toxins. Acupressure, *shiatsu,* reflexology, Feldenkrais, Rolfing.

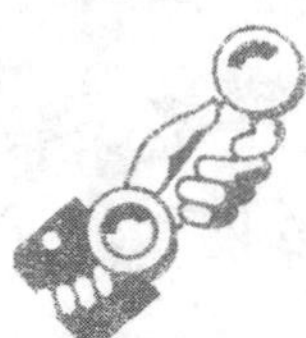

Where to Find Help

For information on female health conditions, or referrals to a qualified health care practitioner, contact the following organizations.

American Association of Acupuncture and Oriental Medicine
4101 Lake Boone Trail, Suite 201
Raleigh, North Carolina 27607
(919) 787-5181

The AAAOM is a national professional trade organization of acupuncturists who meet acceptable standards of minimum competency and can provide you the names and locations of local members. Referrals by written request only.

American Association of Naturopathic Physicians
2366 Eastlake Avenue, Suite 322
Seattle, Washington 98102
(206) 323-7610

Provides a directory of naturopathic physicians and offers referrals to a nationwide network of accredited or licensed practitioners. Publishes a quarterly newsletter for both professionals and the general public, sample copy free on request. Also offers a series of brochures and pamphlets on a variety of subjects.

American Foundation for Pain Research
120 S. Spalding Drive, Suite 210
Beverly Hills, California 90212

Provides information on cystitis, endometriosis, and other conditions leading to pelvic pain. Provides information on diet (including a complete list of foods to avoid for those suffering from cystitis) and self-help as well as a free video, "You Don't Have to Live with Pelvic Pain."

Foundation for New Options
2340 Sutter Street, Suite 205
San Francisco, California 94115
(415) 563-5502

A nonprofit organization dedicated to assisting people through the avenues of education and health promotion to make informed personal decisions. The foundation's primary objective is to provide individuals with an array of tools and a knowledge of individual options that can be used to take greater responsibility for personal actions and well-being.

International Foundation for Homeopathy
2366 Eastlake Avenue East, Suite 301
Seattle, Washington 98102
(206) 324-8230

Provides educational courses for professionals and the general public. Offers referrals to homeopathic health professionals.

Lifecycles for Women
101 1st Street, Suite 441
Los Altos, California 94022
(800) 862-9876

A clearinghouse for books by Dr. Susan Lark and for nutritional supplements for various women's health issues. Send or call for catalog.

Maharishi Ayur-Veda Medical Center
P.O. Box 282
Fairfield, Iowa 52556
(515) 472-5866

The center provides referrals to health centers, which offer treatment for prevention and the treatment of a broad range of illnesses. They also train practitioners and provide information to the lay public.

National Center for Homeopathy
801 North Fairfax, Suite 306
Alexandria, Virginia 22314
(703) 548-7790

Provides a referral list of practicing homeopaths and information. Gives courses for lay people and professionals, and organizes study groups around the country.

National Women's Health Network
1325 G Street, N.W.
Washington, D.C. 20005
(202) 347-1140
A clearinghouse of publications and information packets on all women's health issues.

WISE Essentials
716 Mount Curve Boulevard
St. Paul Minnesota 53116
(800) 705-9473
(612) 690-9626
A source for natural progesterone.

Women to Women
One Pleasant Street
Yarmouth, Maine 04096
(207) 846-6163
Publishes the Creating Health Guide, *a quarterly collection of articles written by the health care professionals at Women to Women. Focus is on creating wellness while enhancing the natural healing processes of the body regardless of one's starting point.*

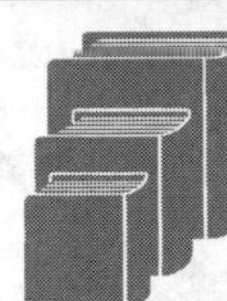

Recommended Reading

General Female Health

The New Our Bodies, Ourselves. The Boston Women's Health Collective. New York: Simon & Schuster, 1984, 1992.
With more than 3 million copies in print, this book continues to influence women and the health care industry around the world. Provides factual information about women's health care combined with women's own personal experiences and perspectives. Encourages women to challenge the medical establishment and take control of their own health.

Straight Talk with Your Gynecologist: How to Get Answers That Will Save Your Life. Sollie, Eddie C., M.D. Hillsborough, OR: Beyond Words Publishing, Inc., 1993.
Gives women the information and skills to form an equal partnership with their gynecologist. Provides frank talk on sexually transmitted diseases in simple language. Prevention and health maintenance receive in-depth coverage throughout the book.

Women's Health Alert. Wolfe, Sidney M., M.D., and the Public Citizen Health Research Group with Rhoda Donkin Jones. Reading, MA: Addison-Wesley Publishing Company, Inc., 1991.
This book provides up-to-date information on the practice of female medicine with data and statistics that can help a woman make wise decisions about her health. Hormone-replacement therapy and osteoporosis are detailed.

Fertility and Birth Control

Fertility: A Comprehensive Guide to Natural Family Planning. Clubb, Elizabeth; and Knight, Jone N. Ponfret, UT: David and Charles (U.K.), 1989.
Clear, accessible information for couples who want to take control of their own family planning without using chemicals or technology.

The Fertility Awareness Handbook. Kass-Annese, Barbara R.N., C.N.P.; and Danzer, Hal, M.D. Alameda, CA: Hunter House, Inc., Publishers, 1992.
Provides noninvasive and side effect-free natural family planning methods that teach you how to be more in touch with you body, more secure in your lovemaking, and more in control of your health and sexual well-being.

The New No Pill, No Risk Birth Control Guide. Aguilar, Nona. New York: McMillan, 1985.
The latest in natural family planning and contraception without drugs, chemicals, IUD's or barrier devices.

Your Fertility Signals. Winstein, Merryl. St. Louis, MO: Smooth Stone Press, 1991.
Naturally, cooperatively, and effectively achieve or prevent pregnancy, reduce or eliminate contraceptive use, enhance intimacy in your relationship, and possibly choose your baby's sex.

Menstruation and PMS

Exclusively Female: A Nutrition Guide for Better Menstrual Health. Ojeda, Linda, San Bernardino, CA: Borgo Press, 1985.

This book pioneered the nutritional approach to menstrual self-care. Menstrual problems are the result of hormonal imbalances which frequently are caused by nutritional deficiencies. Exclusively Female *was among the first books to give comprehensive guidelines on the use of diet and supplementation to alleviate these complaints.*

Premenstrual Syndrome Self-Help Book. Lark, Susan, M.D., Berkeley, CA: Celestial Arts, revised 1993.

Every month, 10 to 15 million women experience symptoms such as irritability, anxiety, mood swings, depression, weight gain, breast tenderness, bloating, and more. There are no magic cures. But there's a lot a woman can do for herself. Susan Lark, M.D., gives a complete step-by-step plan to help women cope with, and overcome PMS.

Menopause

Hormone Replacement Therapy, Yes or No: How to Make an Informed Decision. Kamen, Betty, Ph.D. Novato, CA: Nutrition Encounter, 1993

In the next twenty years approximately forty million women will enter menopause in the United States. Dr. Kamen presents the safe, non-toxic and medically valid alternatives to conventional hormone replacement treatment. This book shows how PMS, menopausal symptoms and osteoporosis can be avoided and reversed, along with the negative consequences caused by misdirected treatment.

Menopausal Years. Weed, Susan, S. New York: Ash Tree Publishing, 1992.

This book focuses on many aspects of women's health including osteoporosis, and reviews a wide range of remedies from massage and energy work to herbs, supplements, diet, and medications.

Menopause Naturally (updated): Preparing for the Second Half of Life. Greenwood, Sadja, M.D. Volcano, CA: Volcano Press, 1992.

This edition addresses the troubling questions women have about using postmenopausal hormones and the conflicting opinions they encounter. New information includes screening tests for osteoporosis, and nonhormonal treatments, new ways to deal with hot flashes, what natural progesterone is, testosterone therapy, exercise, diet, and maintaining postmenopausal health.

Menopause: A Second Spring. Wolfe, Honora Lee. Boulder, CO: Blue Poppy Press, 1992.

The first book-length description of the traditional Chinese medical view of menopause, menopausal syndrome, and postmenopausal disorders. Extensive sections on self-help, preventative therapies, and remedial treatment of specific problems, as well as a complete TCM explanation of menopausal symptoms.

The Menopause Self-Help Book. Lark, Susan, M., M.D. Berkeley, CA: Celestial Arts, 1990.

An easy-to-understand workbook on how to approach menopause. Dr. Lark explains what menopause is and its potential health problems. She explores the many natural treatments available and gives the pros and cons of estrogen replacement therapy. Resources are listed.

Menopause without Medicine (Second Edition). Ojeda, Linda, Ph.D., Alameda, CA: Hunter House Inc., Publishers, 1992.

Now, in a completely updated edition, the author presents the latest research on nutrition, exercise, and osteoporosis—including good news about the body's ability to rebuild bone later in life. Ojeda describes how women can best prepare their minds and bodies for the transition of menopause, and explains how women can prevent osteoporosis and control the disturbing symptoms of hot flashes, insomnia, fatigue, and weight gain.

Natural Menopause—Guide to a Woman's Most Misunderstood Passage. Perry, Susan; and O'Hanlan, Katherine, M.D. New York: Addison-Wesley, 1992.

Natural Menopause *dispels the common myths about menopause—the horror stories about raging hormones, violent mood swings, and the loss of femininity—by explaining to women what to expect during a time that, if approached as a natural phase rather that a crisis, can be a positive experience.*

150 Most-asked Questions about Menopause. Jacobwitz, Ruth S. New York: Hearst Books, 1993.

This book provides the plain facts on a host of topics including: the pros and cons of hormone replacement therapy; choosing the right doctor; how to de-stress your life; and twelve tips to make the most of a physician visit.

The Pause, Positive Approaches to Menopause. Barbach, Lonnie, Ph.D. New York: Dutton, 1993.

The Pause *gives a symptom-by-symptom breakdown of the physical changes that women experience as well as advice on how to choose the right treatment and make the right lifestyle adjustments. Barbach also offers the most up-to-date and practical ways to make the "third third" of a woman's life her healthiest and most productive.*

Startling New Facts About Osteoporosis: Why Calcium Alone Does Not Prevent Bone Disease. Kamen, Betty, Ph. D. Novato, CA: Nutrition Encounter, 1990

An up-dated edition of the best selling Osteoporosis, this book presents the latest medical evidence about calcium and other supplements in relation to osteoporosis. Dr. Kamen tells what women can do to prevent, control, and even reverse this debilitating and lethal disease. This booklet raises a multitude of fascinating new questions about osteoporosis, and anwers them with validating medical research.

What's Wrong with My Hormones? Gillian Ford. Newcastle, CA: Desmond Ford Publications, 1992.

This book discusses each of the major hormonal problems—PMS, postpartum depression, premenopause and menopause, and associated hypothyroidism. It describes the consequences of taking the pill, or having a tubal sterilization, ovarian surgery, or a hysterectomy. It also shows the connection between endometriosis and hormonal dysfunction. Also covers treatment, including information on both natural and hormonal remedies.

Newsletters

Breast Cancer Action
1280 Columbus Avenue, Suite 204
San Francisco, California 94133
(415) 922-8279

Holds monthly meetings and publishes a bi-monthly newsletter on topics related to breast cancer. Works closely with California Breast Cancer Organization, and the national Breast Cancer Coalition.

Menopause News
2074 Union Street
San Francisco, California 94123
(415) 567-2368

A bi-monthly publication featuring menopause basics and lively interviews and opinions on the most controversial midlife health issues for women.

Women's Health Forum
6113 Abbey Road
Aptos, California 95003

An interdisciplinary newsletter for physicians and medical students.

Gastrointestinal Disorders

Proper digestion is a requirement for optimum health. Disorders of the gastrointestinal tract are quite common and can lead to improper digestion, malabsorption, and nutritional deficiencies, all of which may contribute to the development of many other diseases. Alternative medicine treats these disorders with diet, nutritional supplements, herbal remedies, and stress reduction to restore proper digestion and enhance overall health.

The gastrointestinal (GI) tract is a tube twenty-five to thirty-two feet long, that begins at the mouth and ends at the anus. It comprises the mouth, pharynx, esophagus, stomach, small intestine (duodenum, jejunum, and ileum), large intestine (cecum, ascending colon, transverse colon, and descending colon), rectum, and anus. Accessory organs—the liver, pancreas, and gallbladder—all play an important role in digestion.

“The typical Western diet of high-fat, high-carbohydrate, highly processed foods with many additives and preservatives is the root cause of many digestive disorders.”

Digestion begins when food mixes with enzymes in saliva. The process is then carried on in the stomach by hydrochloric acid (HCl) and pepsin. Food is liquified in the stomach and passes into the small intestine, where it is further broken down by digestive enzymes from the pancreas (the enzyme protease digests proteins, the enzyme amylase digests carbohydrates, and the enzyme lipase digests fats). The gallbladder secretes bile, formed by the liver, to aid absorption of fats and fat-soluble vitamins.

Most food absorption takes place in the small intestine, while water, electrolytes (essential body chemicals), and some of the final products of digestion are absorbed in the large intestine.

Causes of Gastrointestinal Disorders

According to Patrick Donovan, N.D., of Seattle, Washington, there are many causes of GI disorders, including dietary and nutritional factors, food allergies, viral and bacterial infections, parasites, and stress. “They can also be secondary to problems with the pancreas, liver, or gallbladder, all of which are involved in the digestive process,” Dr. Donovan says. Many of these disorders involve inflammation of part of the digestive tract which may be secondary to any of the above causes. Disturbance of the digestive system can lead to malabsorption and nutritional deficiencies.

See Allergies, Diet, Enzyme Therapy, Nutritional Supplements, Parasitic Infections, Stress.

Poor Diet and Nutrition

The typical Western diet of high-fat, high-carbohydrate, highly processed foods with many additives and preservatives is the root cause of many digestive disorders.[1] Lack of fiber in such a diet makes the digestive system sluggish, and leads to improper elimination and constipation. This, in turn, leads to a buildup of toxins in the body and may lead to “leaky gut syndrome,” in which food particles cross the intestinal wall and enter the bloodstream, inducing an autoimmune reaction.

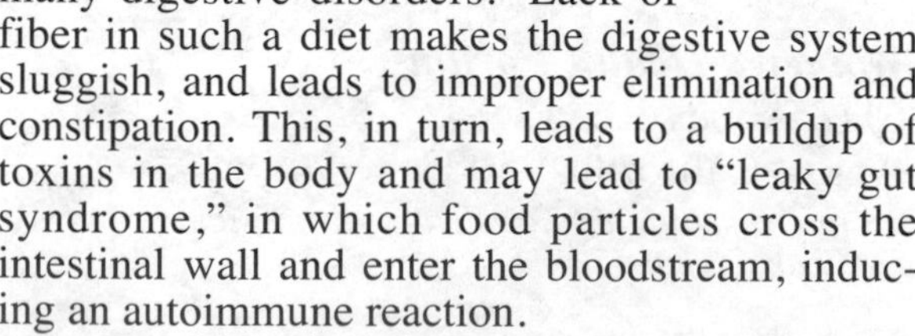

Nutritional deficiencies can also lead to poor digestion and malabsorption of food, as can deficiencies in digestive enzymes.

Food Allergies

Food allergies lie behind many disease processes and may be a factor in gastrointestinal disorders.[2] Common culprits are milk, dairy products, and wheat. Gluten intolerance can result in celiac disease (intestinal malabsorption due to gluten intolerance). Food allergies may also arise as a result of malabsorption syndrome, which occurs whenever there is injury to the surface layer of the digestive tract, according to Dr. Donovan. With poor digestion, large food particles cross the gut wall and enter the bloodstream, where they can cause food allergies.

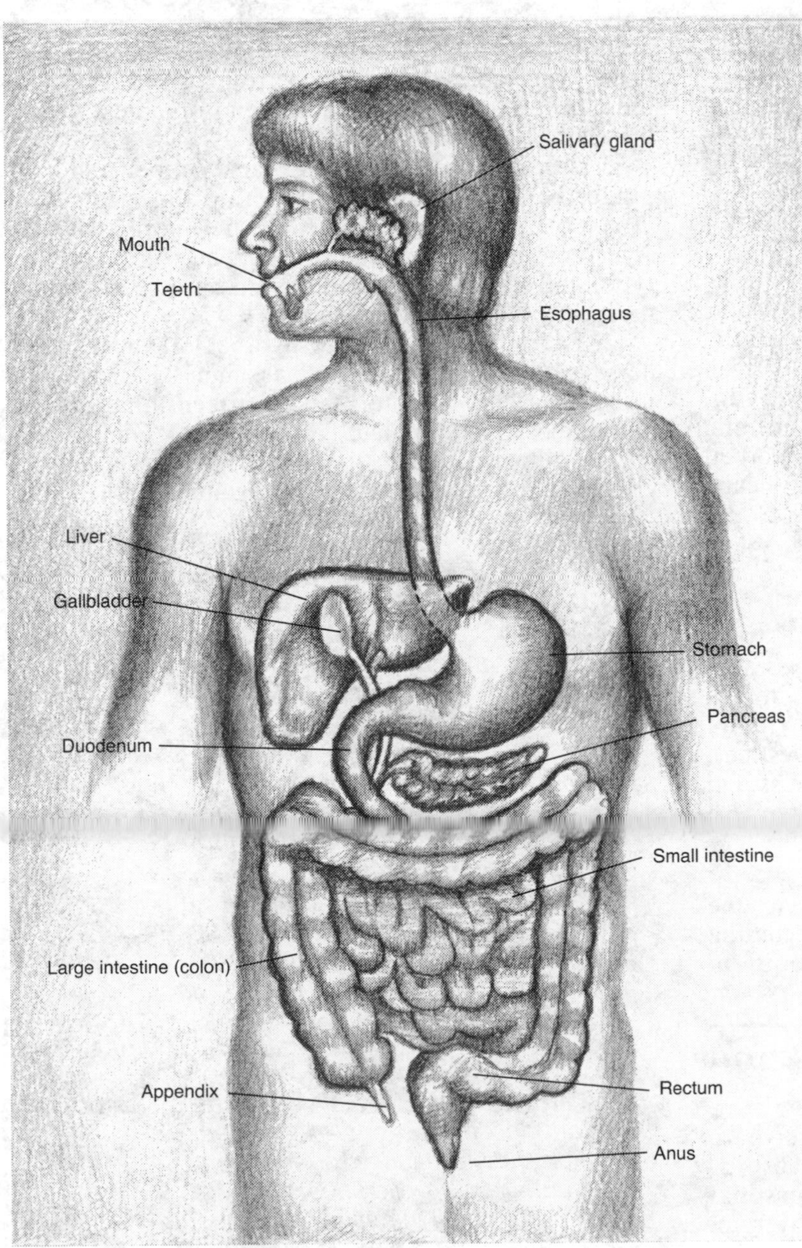

The digestive system.

Immunologic Factors

Several gastrointestinal disorders involve the immune system. People with deficient immune systems often suffer from malabsorption. If IgA, an antibody normally present in the intestine, is lacking or deficient, the patient suffers from an increased amount of gastrointestinal infections. Antibodies in the digestive tract which normally protect against infection and microbial toxins rid the body of parasitic worms, and help control the absorption of harmful antigens. Evidence suggests that immune mechanisms play a role in colitis (inflammation of the colon) and Crohn's disease (inflammation of the small intestine), since these patients have antibodies and white cells which react with cells that line their gastrointestinal tract.[3]

See Candidiasis.

Infections

Bacterial and viral infections, as well as parasitic infections, can also be harmful to the digestive system. Bacteria and viruses can cause gastroenteritis, an inflammation of the digestive system often called the stomach flu. They can also release toxins into the system which result in "leaky gut syndrome" and cause autoimmune reactions if they enter the circulation. Viruses and bacteria such as Epstein-Barr virus, cytomegalovirus, Pseudomonas, chlamydia, and Yersinia enterocolitica have, as well, all been associated with Crohn's disease.[4] Parasites also liberate toxins, and rob the body of essential nutrients.

An abnormal growth of organisms in the gut is known as *dysbiosis*. It occurs when you have pathogenic (disease-causing) organisms in the gut or the normal flora is imbalanced. Dysbiosis is a major factor in malabsorption, inflammatory bowel disease, and "leaky gut syndrome," according to Dr. Donovan.

High/Low Hydrochloric Acid Levels

Too much or too little hydrochloric acid secretion by the stomach is

Leaky gut syndrome

According to Patrick Donovan, N.D., of Seattle, Washington, the latest research shows that "leaky gut syndrome" has been associated with many disorders, and may be the focus from which autoimmune disorders originate. "Leaky gut syndrome" occurs when the intestinal mucosa is damaged and large food molecules, bacteria, and microorganisms pass across the intestinal wall to circulate through the body system. Antibodies are made against these molecules. If the molecules "look" like normal body components, the antibody cannot distinguish between the two, and may attack that body component (i.e., an autoimmune phenomenon occurs). This phenomenon can also occur with bacteria and certain drugs. "Bacterial antigens have been associated with rheumatoid arthritis, and ankylosing spondylitis (joint immobilization)," says Dr. Donovan.

another factor that can lead to digestive problems and malabsorption, according to Virender Sodhi, M.D. (Ayurveda), N.D., Director of the American School of Ayurvedic Sciences in Bellevue, Washington. "Too little acid can lead to anemia, as vitamin B_{12} and folic acid will not be absorbed effectively. And too much acid will give 'heartburn' and gas and may lead to ulcers," Dr. Sodhi explains.

Stress

There is little doubt that psychological stress affects the digestive system, causing excess acid production and poor digestive function. Crohn's disease, ulcerative colitis, as well as irritable bowel syndrome (irritation of the large intestine), are associated with, and aggravated by, stress, Dr. Donovan points out.

Insufficient Exercise

Insufficient exercise leads to a decrease in enzyme secretion and HCl needed for digestion, according to Dr. Sodhi. This will lead to malabsorption, nutritional deficiencies, and constipation.

Gastrointestinal Disorders and Their Treatment

Since a lot of gastrointestinal disorders share symptoms such as inflammation, poor absorption, bloating, gas, abdominal cramps, constipation, and diarrhea, the treatments often overlap. The alternative approach to such disorders includes dietary restrictions, nutritional supplementation, detection and elimination of food allergies, herbal remedies, and stress reduction.

Dr. Donovan recommends a whole foods diet to prevent gastrointestinal problems. "Get off all food additives and all prefabricated foods and junk foods," he says, "and eat a high-complex carbohydrate, high-fiber, moderate protein, extremely low-fat diet." He recommends staying away from red meat and nuts (unless they are fresh in their shells). Only high-quality, cold-pressed oils should be used, preferably flaxseed or olive oil. "Fats should make up only 10 to 15 percent of the daily calories," he adds. "I also recommend pastas, beans, vegetables, and protein from fish. If you must have meat, then I recommend organically grown, free-range lamb or poultry."

See Mental Health.

Dr. Sodhi recommends black pepper and ginger be sprinkled on foods to aid digestion. Olive oil and lemon may also be useful. In Ayurvedic medicine, treatment depends on body type, and different food dressings are recommended for different body types.

"Many people have low hydrochloric acid," he says. He recommends half a lemon squeezed into half a cup of water, ten to fifteen minutes before meals, to stimulate gastric juices. "Ginger tea, or ginger added to the lemon juice, is also effective," he says. "*Trikatu*, a mixture of Indian

Accessory organs of the digestive system

The pancreas, the liver, and the gallbladder facilitate digestion by acting as accessory organs to the gastrointestinal system.

The pancreas: *The pancreas produces digestive enzymes which act in the small intestine to digest protein, carbohydrate, and fat. If the pancreas does not produce sufficient enzymes, digestion will be incomplete and absorption of nutrients restricted.*

The liver: *The liver detoxifies toxins, produces proteins and cholesterol, stores the fat-soluble vitamins A, D, E, and K, and produces bile, which is essential for the absorption of fats and stimulates the small intestine. Any impairment of the liver will thus affect the digestive process.*

The gallbladder: *Although the gallbladder functions only as a storage vessel for bile, chemical disturbances in the body may result in the formation of gallstones, impeding the flow of bile to the small intestine, and thus the absorption of fats and fat-soluble vitamins.*

See Ayurvedic Medicine, Herbal Medicine.

long pepper, black pepper, and ginger, can be taken, as well, an effective dose being half a teaspoon before meals."

Dr. Sodhi had a patient suffering from an intestinal yeast infection for over a year. He found she had a low level of secretory IgA, an antibody which protects against infections. He put her on increasing doses of *trikatu* until her IgA levels returned to normal and the yeast infection cleared up completely.

Gastritis

Gastritis is an inflammation of the stomach. "The most common gastrointestinal disorder is a viral gastritis," says Dr. Donovan. "You often see it as a combination viral gastroenteritis, which means inflammation of the stomach and intestines—that's the name for the common stomach flu." Bacteria such as *Helicobacter pylori* can also cause gastritis, according to Dr. Donovan. "We find a correlation with the presence of *Helicobacter pylori* in about 93 percent of patients with gastritis and gastric ulcers," he says.

Gastritis can be induced chemically by medications such as aspirin, ibuprofen, Motrin, and Indocin, as well as steroids. It can also be due to an autoimmune reaction destroying the lining of the digestive tract. This often leads to pernicious anemia, an anemia due to interference of vitamin B_{12} absorption.

Alternative treatments for gastritis address the virus to restore balance within the system. These remedies include diet and nutritional supplementation, herbal medicine, and Ayurvedic medicine.

Food Combinations

Patrick Donovan, N.D., of Seattle, Washington, believes how people combine foods is important to prevent digestive problems. The general rule, he says, is that proteins are eaten alone or with green leafy vegetables. Fruits are eaten alone, and vegetables with grains and legumes. Starches and proteins should not be eaten together. Rice can be eaten with protein. "The rationale for this approach is the difference in digestion time for the various food groups," Dr. Donovan says. "Digestion is optimal if foods having roughly the same digestion time are eaten together."

A digestive stimulant prior to meals may also aid digestion. A couple of sips of green tea or alcohol, such as saki (rice wine) or white wine, over a ten-minute period, stimulates digestion. Herbal bitters or ginger tea are also helpful.

Diet and Nutrition: According to Dr. Donovan, shitake mushrooms activate the immune system and have a strong antiviral effect. He also recommends vitamin C to just below bowel tolerance (the highest dose which does not cause diarrhea), beta-carotene, zinc, and multivitamin-mineral supplements for the treatment of viral gastroenteritis. "The advantage of vitamin A, zinc, and beta-carotene is that they help the lining of the gastrointestinal tract repair and regenerate itself very well," he adds. He uses bismuth as an antibiotic and antiprotozoal agent against *Helicobacter pylori*, if it is present.

Herbal Medicine: Dr. Donovan recommends the use of herbs which stimulate the immune system while reducing inflammation and encouraging repair of the stomach lining, such as echinacea and goldenseal.

Ayurvedic Medicine: Dr. Sodhi uses meditation, the type varying with a person's body type. "*Vata* types need chanting or mantras," he states. "*Pitta* types are visually oriented and should meditate with visualization techniques. *Kapha* types are smell and taste oriented and should use incense or flowers."

Colitis and Crohn's Disease

Both these disorders involve inflammation and possible ulceration of the digestive tract. Symptoms include diarrhea, fever, anorexia, weight loss, gas, and abdominal tenderness. There may be bloody diarrhea if intestinal bleeding occurs. Colitis is confined to the colon, whereas Crohn's disease, though usually affecting the small intestine, can also affect the mouth, esophagus, and stomach. "The degeneration of the intestinal mucosa (surface layer of cells) often leads to poor absorption and nutritional deficiencies," says Dr. Donovan. "This is a major problem if the distal ileum is involved, since this is where vitamin B_{12} is absorbed.

"There may also be an autoimmune component to these diseases. The immune system may react to the cells as they break down, or may react to the food particles or bacteria which can cross the damaged intestinal walls."

Although colitis and Crohn's disease may result in similar symptoms, the causes are multifactorial and are often the result of autoimmune disorders or food allergies. Alternative treatments address these factors through diet, nutritional supplementation, herbal medicine, and Ayurvedic medicine.

Diet and Nutrition: Patients with colitis and Crohn's disease often have decreased food intake and suffer from nutritional deficiencies. Elimination diets are recommended to eliminate food allergies, which may be complicating the

DRUGS ASSOCIATED WITH A HIGHER INCIDENCE OF GASTROINTESTINAL REACTIONS

According to the Physicians Desk Reference *the following drugs are associated with side effects of gastrointestinal reactions. (Statistics refer to the percentage of individuals affected):*[5]

Accutane Capsules (Approximately 1 in 20)
Alka-Seltzer Effervescent Antacid and Pain Reliever (4.9% at doses of 1,000 milligrams daily)
Alka-Seltzer (Flavored) Effervescent Antacid and Pain Reliever (4.9% at doses of 1,000 milligrams daily)
Anturane Capsules, Tablets (Most frequent)
Genuine Bayer Aspirin Tablets and Caplets (4.9% at doses of 1,000 milligrams daily)
Bayer Plus Aspirin Tablets (4.9% of 4,500 people treated)
Regular Strength Bayer Enteric Aspirin Caplets (4.9% of 4,500 people tested)
Bufferin Analgesic Tablets and Caplets (4.8%)
Ceptaz (Most common)
Clinoril Tablets (3-9%)
Cuprimine Capsules (17%)
Ecotrin Enteric Coated Aspirin Maximum Strength Tablets and Caplets, Regular Strength Tablets and Caplets (4.9% at 1,000 milligrams daily)
Ecotrin Enteric Coated Aspirin (4.9% at 1,000 milligrams daily)
Eulexin Capsules (6% with LDRH Agonist)
Feldene Capsules (20%)
Fortaz (Most common)
Ilosone Liquid, Oral Suspensions, Pulvules, and Tablets (Most frequent)
Lamprene Capsules (40-50%)
Leukine for IV Infusion (37%)
Lopid Tablets (34.2%)
Lorabid Suspension and Pulvules (Most common)
Marplan Tablets (Among most frequent)
Meclomen Capsules (10%)
Norwich Enteric Safety Coated Aspirin-Maximum Strength (4.9%)
Novantrone for Injection Concentrate (58-88%)
Pancrease MT Capsules (Most frequent)
Paraplatin for Injection (17-21%)
Piroxicam Capsules USP (Approximately 20%)
Prepidil Gel (5.7%)
Prokine for I.V. Infusion (37%)
Retrovir Capsules, I.V. Infusion, Syrup (20%)
Rynatan Tablets (Among most common)
Rynatan-S Pediatric Suspension (Among most common)
Rynatuss Pediatric Suspension, Tablets (Among most common)
Supprelin Injection (3-10%)
Suprax Powder for Oral Suspension, Tablets (30%)
Tazicef for Injection (Most common)
Ticlid Tablets (30-40%)
Tolectin (200, 400, and 600 milligrams) (10%)
Toradol IM Injection, Oral (13%)
Trecator-SC Tablets (Among most common)
Trilisate Liquid, Tablets (Less than 20%)
Ultrase Capsules (Most frequent)
Vascor (200, 300, and 400 milligrams) Tablets (4.35-6.98%)
Voltaren Tablets (About 20%)

problem. According to Dr. Donovan, common allergenic foods are wheat, corn, dairy products, and carrageenan-containing foods (processed foods containing stabilizers and suspending agents). Supplements of magnesium, calcium, iron, potassium, and multivitamins are needed to counteract the decreased food intake and decreased absorption from the small intestine.

"One of the best factors to prevent colitis and Crohn's disease is a high-fiber diet," says Dr. Donovan, "but once active colitis is present you cannot use fiber since it is too harsh. As healing occurs, you can use soluble fibers." He suggests a liquid diet in the active phase, consisting of juices from cabbage and green leafy vegetables, because the chlorophyll has healing properties. A good source of chlorophyll is fresh water algae like chlorella.

Dr. Donovan also suggests vegetable broths and broths from the seaweeds *wakame, hijiki,* and *kombu,* as well as fish and meat broths in some patients. Vegetables are then gradually added back into the diet, then blended fruit juices. This is followed by the introduction of meat and fish broths, then solid fish. When patients are back to normal, they can add in animal proteins, grains, and beans.

A patient with a history of colitis for ten years and no relief from conventional therapy came to Dr. Donovan. He fasted the patient for four days and then put him on vegetable juices and lamb bone broth, after having determined which foods he was allergic to. His iron-deficiency anemia was treated with iron-containing herbs and foods such as spinach and kale. His symptoms began to resolve.

Over the next ten days he was put on raw and steamed vegetables and salads, and by the end of a month he was back on a whole foods vegetarian diet. Within thirty days he was able to return to work.

Herbal Medicine: Plant flavonoids such as quercetin are helpful in reducing the inflammatory response. According to David L. Hoffmann, B.Sc., M.N.I.M.H., of Sebastopol, California, past President of the American Herbalist Guild, chamomile and peppermint are beneficial for gas and colic, and for associated diarrhea. He recommends astringents such as bayberry, marshmallow root, or plantain and antispasmodics such as wild yam aid the healing process. He suggests a mixture of equal parts bayberry, agrimony, peppermint, wild yam, and valerian for a relaxing effect, one teaspoon taken three times a day. An infusion of chamomile or lemon balm should be drunk warm frequently.

Dr. Donovan recommends licorice root tea with marshmallow, slippery elm bark, geranium, yarrow, and goldenseal. He also uses Robert's Formula, which consists of a mixture of marshmallow root (a demulcent, to soften the tissues), wild indigo (for GI infections), echinacea (an antibacterial which promotes normalization of the immune system), *Geranium maculatum* (to prevent bleeding), goldenseal (to inhibit bacterial growth), poke root (for healing ulceration), comfrey (an anti-inflammatory and promoter of wound healing), and slippery elm (a demulcent).

Dr. Donovan recommends quercetin when food allergies are present. Butyric acid enemas are also part of his treatment. "They have an anti-inflammatory effect and help the mucosa of the intestine to heal and regenerate," he says. "Butyric acid comes from fiber in the diet, and patients with colitis and low butyric acid levels are prone to colon cancer."

Ayurvedic Medicine: "Treatment is mainly focused on relaxing the patient," says Dr. Sodhi. Meditation is recommended. He also believes there is a strong component of food allergies, so these are identified and eliminated. A complete stool analysis is done to see how well food is being digested, and if parasites or bacteria are present. Dr. Sodhi examined a patient with colitis and found she had allergies to milk, wheat, potatoes, and tomatoes. Once these were removed from her diet, all her symptoms went away.

Dr. Sodhi uses fish oils and flaxseed oil and the herb *boswellia* to reduce inflammation, and acidophilus to reconstitute the gut microflora. "Yogurt, cumin, and ginger are also helpful," he says. "But make sure the yogurt does not contain carrageenan, as this can cause bowel cancer."

Irritable Bowel Syndrome

Irritable bowel syndrome (IBS) is a condition in which the large intestine, or colon, fails to operate normally. It is a functional disorder, since there is no evidence of structural damage to the intestine. Symptoms include pain, constipation, diarrhea, gas, nausea, anorexia, and anxiety or depression.[6] The cause is unknown, but food allergies, excess dietary fats, and stress seem to be implicated in IBS.

Treatment of IBS aims to reduce the irritation to the digestive system and therefore relies heavily on dietary changes, herbal remedies, and stress reduction.

Diet and Nutrition: The usual treatment for IBS is to increase dietary fiber. To avoid food sensitivities (not allergies, since there does not seem to be an immune component in IBS[7]), fibers from a source other than grains are recommended, such as vegetables, fruits, oat bran, guar gum, psyllium, and legumes, such as beans and peas. According to James Braly, M.D., Medical Director of Immuno Labs, Inc., in Fort Lauderdale, Florida, nuts, seeds, and fruit with small seeds (such as raspberries) should be avoided, as should alcohol, caffeine, and spices. Dr. Braly also notes that supplements should include zinc, vitamin A, and evening primrose oil.

METHODS OF ACTION OF HERBAL REMEDIES

Herbs have many properties which can calm, heal, and rejuvenate the gastrointestinal tract.

- *Demulcents such as comfrey, marshmallow, and slippery elm, soothe the lining of the digestive system.*
- *Anti-inflammatories such as chamomile, meadowsweet, and marigold, reduce localized tissue inflammation.*
- *Astringents such as comfrey and meadowsweet, lessen local bleeding.*
- *Vulneraries such as comfrey, chamomile, and goldenseal, speed up local healing.*
- *Carminatives such as chamomile, peppermint, and valerian, relieve gas in the lower abdomen.*
- *Nervines such as chamomile, valerian, and hops, ease background stress.*
- *Bitters such as chamomile, yarrow, wormwood, and gentian, aid in the healing process in the latter stages but are contraindicated in early stages because they stimulate stomach acid and aggravate the problems.*

Herbal Medicine: Enteric-coated peppermint oil is used in Europe to treat IBS.[8] Without enteric coating, the peppermint oil is absorbed in the upper digestive tract, often causing heartburn and esophageal reflux (stomach acid regurgitating into the esophagus). Ginger has a long history of use to relieve digestive complaints.[9] Herbs such as chamomile, valerian, rosemary, and balm have antispasmodic effects on the intestines. David Hoffmann recommends a mixture of tinctures of bayberry, gentian, peppermint, and wild yam in equal parts, one teaspoon three times a day, and warm drinks of chamomile or lemon balm.

Stress Reduction: Stress reduction techniques such as biofeedback and hypnosis are often helpful in relieving IBS.[10]

Ulcers

Although traditionally ulcers have been associated with stress, there is evidence that food allergies and nutritional problems may also be responsible, according to Dr. Braly. Excessive dependency on aspirin and other anti-inflammatory medications, including steroids, can also cause ulcers. Symptoms of ulcers include stomach pain or upset, a burning sensation in the stomach, and feelings of acute hunger and pain after eating or lying down. Dr. Donovan has found a 93 percent correlation with the presence of *Helicobacter pylori* in the stomachs of patients with gastric ulcers.

Ulcers are another digestive disorder treated mainly with dietary changes, herbal remedies, and stress reduction.

Diet and Nutrition: Fats, alcohol, and caffeine should be avoided. Avoid aspirin and other anti-inflammatories. Linseed oil on a salad each day is recommended by Dr. Braly, who also suggests drinking three ounces of concentrated aloe vera juice twenty minutes before meals, and avoiding foods to which one is allergic. He also advises supplementation with zinc and vitamin A.

Dr. Donovan recommends bismuth for its antibacterial and antiprotozoal effects if *Helicobacter pylori* is present, and states that bananas and cabbage juice are both effective in treating ulcers in general.

Herbal Medicine: "By using plants that have demulcent, antacid, astringent, and vulnerary (speeding up natural wound healing) actions it is possible to bring about rapid and complete healing of most ulcers," says David Hoffmann. Some of these plants include marshmallow, calendula, meadowsweet, chamomile, and goldenseal. He suggests drinking an infusion made of one part chamomile and two parts marshmallow root, one teaspoon three times a day. An infusion of chamomile, linden flowers, or valerian may also help.

Dr. Donovan recommends licorice root or licorice root tea. It must be deglycerinated licorice or it will cause hypertension (high blood pressure) over the long term. Cayenne pepper also has a significant healing effect on ulcers, according to Dr. Donovan.

Ayurvedic Medicine: According to Dr. Sodhi, licorice is the best remedy. He recommends taking half a teaspoon of licorice powder three times a day. He also recommends bananas, coconut (the milk and the fruit), and the herb *ashwagandha*. "A mixture of cinnamon, cardamom, and cloves, ground into one quarter teaspoon of powder, can also prove helpful," Dr. Sodhi says. "This reduces acid secretion and relief should be seen immediately." Dr. Sodhi stresses the need to be under the care of a physician when treating GI disorders.

Stress Reduction: Stress reduction techniques such as yoga, meditation, biofeedback, and hypnosis may help reduce stress, which is a factor in most digestive system diseases.

Acupuncture: William Michael Cargile, B.S., D.C., F.I.A.C.A., Chairman of Research for the American Association of Acupuncture and Oriental Medicine, has had success treating ulcers with acupuncture. He reports on a case of an orthopedic surgeon who was taking Tagamet (a medication used in conventional medicine to treat ulcers) six times a day at two to three times the recommended dose and was getting worse. Dr. Cargile treated the patient twice in two days using the stomach meridian and he has not needed Tagamet since. In treating ulcer patients, Dr. Cargile uses the acupuncture points associated with stress, anxiety, and stomach/gastrointestinal problems.

See Acupuncture.

Diverticulosis and Diverticulitis

Diverticulosis is a condition in which the walls of the intestines balloon out forming pouches. A small percentage of these patients go on to develop diverticulitis, an inflammation of these pouches. Problems occur when undigested food particles and small seeds from fruits such as strawberries and raspberries lodge in these pouches. This causes irritation and can lead to inflammation.

"Diverticulosis and diverticulitis are much easier to prevent than to treat," says Dr. Donovan. "They are solely the result of the standard American diet. These diseases do not exist in cultures eating a whole foods, high-fiber diet." He also believes that a major cause of diverticulosis is constipation. "Regular bowel movements, two to three a day, will help prevent diverticulosis," he says.

Diet and Nutrition: A whole foods, high-fiber diet can prevent and relieve the symptoms of diverticulosis and diverticulitis. Dr. Donovan prefers soluble fibers such as flaxmeal, psyllium, and oat bran, but says a mixture of soluble and insoluble fibers can be used. Flaxmeal contains omega-3 fatty acids which are also beneficial. Foods with small seeds and foods difficult to digest should be avoided.

Food Allergies: Patients should be tested for food allergies, and any foods to which they are sensitive should be removed from the diet. An ELISA/ACT (enzyme-linked immunosorbent assay/advanced cell test) is the most sensitive way to determine delayed-type or hidden food allergies and can be used to screen for over 250 types of foods, according to Dr. Donovan.

Fasting: Dr. Donovan recommends a one- to three-day water or vegetable juice fast during acute attacks of diverticulitis. Nutrient-dense broths such as miso or lamb bone broth may also be used until the attack subsides.

Herbal Medicine: Dr. Donovan recommends Robert's Formula in combination with licorice root tea or deglycerinized licorice. For daily maintenance, he recommends Robert's Formula with liquid chlorophyll.

Homeopathy: Homeopathic remedies such as *Colosynthis, Brionia,* and *Belladonna* in low potencies are recommended by Dr. Donovan.

Diarrhea

Diarrhea is a common symptom of many disorders but should never be taken lightly and medical attention should be sought if it does not resolve in a few days. Diarrhea results in dehydration due to loss of fluids, and loss of electrolytes which can result in death if not replaced.

Many people suffer from a lactose (milk sugar) intolerance and will suffer from diarrhea if they eat dairy products. A bacterial, viral, or parasitic infection, often from drinking contaminated water, may injure the cells of the small intestine and result in diarrhea. Large amounts of some artificial sweeteners can cause diarrhea, as can megadoses of vitamin C.

See Constipation.

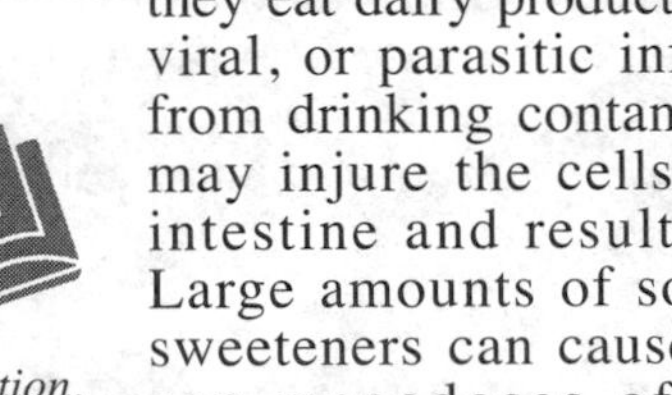

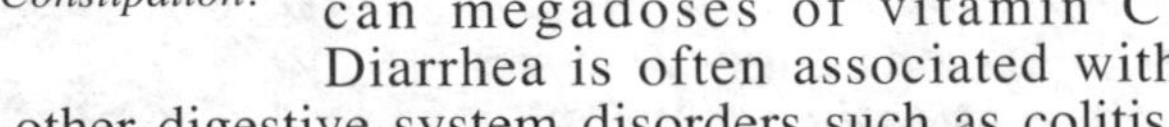

Diarrhea is often associated with other digestive system disorders such as colitis, Crohn's disease, and IBS.

Diarrhea is usually short-term and self-resolving, but steps can be taken to prevent or treat it. If it becomes chronic, professional advice should be sought.

Diet and Nutrition: According to Dr. Donovan, chronic diarrhea may be due to food allergies, so these need to be identified and eliminated. During the early stages, no food should be eaten. Fluids should be freely consumed and may include fruit and vegetable juices. This should be followed by soups, yogurt, and cooked fruits. Fats and fried foods should be avoided. Vitamin and mineral supplements may be necessary, as well, due to excessive loss.

Dr. Donovan treats pediatric diarrhea with barley water or rice water. A little sugar can be added to increase the absorption of minerals. In the case of a young patient, he had the mother cook a large pot of brown rice and barley, boil it up, and keep adding water. She then strained the water and gave it to the child. The diarrhea cleared within hours.

Pectin, found in the peel of citrus fruits, apples, carrots, potatoes, sugar beet, and tomatoes, helps relieve diarrhea. *Lactobacillus acidophilus* is needed after diarrhea to reconstitute the bowel flora.

Herbal Medicine: Goldenseal has proved beneficial in bacterial-induced diarrhea.[11] Robert's Formula also has a long history of use in relieving diarrhea, according to Dr. Donovan.

Ayurvedic Medicine: "*Triphala* can be taken as a treatment or a preventive medicine," Dr. Sodhi says. "Also, bael fruit cures many kinds of diarrhea. Bananas, too, are very effective, especially if blended to form a drink. The pectin in the banana absorbs toxins from the body. Goldenseal, Oregon grape, nutmeg, and cumin, however, can also be effective. Care should be taken with cumin, since it can be hallucinogenic, but it can be made into a paste and rubbed on the belly and forehead when treating children."

Hemorrhoids

Hemorrhoids are varicose veins appearing in the anal area. Symptoms are not usually evident until the patient is in his or her thirties. They are caused by a weakness of the veins, excessive venous blood pressure, pregnancy, straining at stool, standing or sitting for long periods, and heavy lifting.

While conventional medicine treats hemorrhoids with topical creams or surgery, there are natural remedies available, as well.

Diet and Nutrition: Hemorrhoids are rarely seen in parts of the world where high-fiber, unrefined diets are consumed. A high-fiber diet is the most important component in the prevention of hemorrhoids.[12] "A diet rich in vegetables, fruits, legumes, and grains promotes peristalsis and reduces straining during defecation," Dr. Donovan explains. Blackberries, cherries, and blueberries help strengthen the veins, and psyllium and guar gum are good sources of fiber. Dr. Donovan recommends vitamin C and flavonoids to strengthen the vascular walls of the colon, rectum, and anus.

Herbal Medicine: Butcher's broom and flavonoids are useful in enhancing the integrity of the veins, preventing hemorrhoids from developing.[13] David Hoffmann uses equal parts collinsonia, cranesbill, and *Ginkgo biloba*, in doses of one teaspoon taken three times a day for internal relief. For topical application, he recommends a mixture of ten milliliters of collinsonia with sixty milliliters of distilled witch hazel, applied after every bowel movement. He also recommends salves made of calendula, St. John's Wort, aloe, or plantain.

In addition, Dr. Donovan recommends herbal suppositories such as collinsonia, buckeye, and aesculus, which tighten the tissues and help get rid of hemorrhoids.

Hydrotherapy: A warm sitz bath (partial immersion of the pelvic region) at a temperature of 100 to 105 degrees Fahrenheit is an effective treatment for hemorrhoids.[14]

Exercise: Dr. Donovan has hemorrhoid patients do Kegel exercises, which are classic pelvic wall and rectal exercises. They are done by pulling up the lower pelvic wall and rectum, tightening up, and then relaxing. This increases the blood flow and circulation and pumps the blood back so that it doesn't pool in the area.

Self-Care

The following therapies can be undertaken at home under appropriate professional supervision:

Colitis

• Biofeedback Training • Fasting • Flower Remedies • Guided Imagery • Qigong • Yoga

Homeopathy: *Merc sol., Aloe, Allium sativa, Belladonna, Colchicum, Nux vomica, Arsen alb., Cantharis.*

Hydrotherapy: Sitz bath: contrast; apply daily when acute. Constitutional hydrotherapy: apply two to five times weekly.

Juice Therapy: • Cabbage, papaya, carrot juice • Wheatgrass juice • Drink juice of one-half lemon with warm water each morning, followed by: carrot and apple or carrot, beet, cucumber. • Aloe juice • Avoid citrus juices.

Reflexology: Colon, liver, adrenal, lower spine, diaphragm, gallbladder.

Crohn's Disease

• Flower Remedies • Meditation • Yoga

Aromatherapy: Basil.

Hydrotherapy: Constitutional hydrotherapy unless otherwise indicated: apply two to five times weekly.

Diarrhea

• Acupressure •Biofeedback Training • Fasting

Aromatherapy: • For stress-induced diarrhea: lavender, neroli. • Other antispasmodic oils include eucalyptus and cypress, chamomile.

Homeopathy: *Chamomilla, Colchicum, Sulfur, Arsen alb., Nux vomica, Argent nit., Ipecacuanha, Apis mel., Veratrum alb., Merc sol., Calc carb., Natrum Sulf.*

Hydrotherapy: Constitutional hydrotherapy: apply two to five times weekly.

Juice Therapy: • Carrot, apple juice • Carrot, celery, apple • Carrot, celery, spinach, parsley, garlic • Beets may speed up and worsen diarrhea in some cases.

Reflexology: Ascending colon, transverse colon, diaphragm, liver, adrenals.

Diverticulitis

• Flower Remedies

Aromatherapy: Rub abdomen with olive oil and a bit of essence of cinnamon.

Hydrotherapy: Constitutional hydrotherapy unless otherwise indicated: apply two to five times weekly.

Juice Therapy: • Carrot, celery, beet, cabbage juice • Green juices • Papaya, apple, lemon, pineapple

Irritable Bowel Syndrome

• Fasting • Guided Imagery • Meditation • Qigong • Yoga

Aromatherapy: Peppermint.

Homeopathy: *Merc sol., Aloe, Carbo veg., Nux vomica.*

Hydrotherapy: Constitutional hydrotherapy unless otherwise indicated: apply two to five times weekly.

Juice Therapy: Cabbage and family, carrot, celery, parsley

Ulcers

• Biofeedback Training • Guided Imagery • Meditation • Qigong • Yoga

Aromatherapy: Lemon oil, chamomile, geranium.

Homeopathy: *Silicea, Arsen alb., Lachesis, Acidum nit., Calendula, Hamamelis, Belladonna.*

Hydrotherapy: Constitutional hydrotherapy unless otherwise indicated: apply two to five times weekly.

Juice Therapy: • Drink fresh fruit and vegetable juices. • Wheatgrass juice. Duodenal ulcers: drink raw cabbage juice throughout the day (can be mixed with carrot or celery). Gastric or stomach ulcers: drink raw potato juice.

Reflexology: Diaphragm, stomach, duodenum, reflex pertaining to location of ulcer.

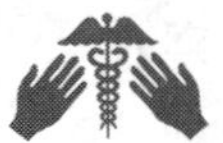

Professional Care

The following therapies should only be provided by a qualified health professional:

Colitis

• Cell Therapy • Chiropractic • Colon Therapy • Craniosacral Therapy • Magnetic Field Therapy • Naturopathic Medicine • Orthomolecular Medicine • Osteopathy • Traditional Chinese Medicine

Bodywork: Acupressure, *shiatsu*, Alexander technique, Feldenkrais, Therapeutic Touch.

Crohn's Disease

• Acupuncture • Biofeedback Training • Chiropractic • Colon Therapy • Hypnotherapy • Magnetic Field Therapy • Orthomolecular Medicine • Sound Therapy

Traditional Chinese Medicine: Barley soup or water.

Diarrhea

• Applied Kinesiology • Colon Therapy • Environmental Medicine • Enzyme Therapy • Magnetic Field Therapy • Naturopathic Medicine • Neural Therapy • Osteopathy • Traditional Chinese Medicine

Oxygen Therapy: • Hydrogen peroxide therapy • Hyperbaric oxygen therapy as adjunctive therapy to non-responding diarrhea

Diverticulitis

• Acupuncture • Biofeedback Training • Cell Therapy • Chiropractic • Colon Therapy • Magnetic Field Therapy • Osteopathy • Traditional Chinese Medicine

Irritable Bowel Syndrome

• Acupuncture • Biofeedback Training • Cell Therapy • Chiropractic • Colon Therapy • Environmental Medicine • Hypnotherapy • Magnetic Field Therapy • Naturopathic Medicine • Neural Therapy • Orthomolecular Medicine • Osteopathy • Reconstructive Therapy • Traditional Chinese Medicine

Detoxification Therapy: Indicated to assess the effects of diet, unless the person is depleted from diarrhea.

Oxygen Therapy: Hyperbaric oxygen therapy can be helpful.

Ulcers

• Craniosacral Therapy • Environmental Medicine • Enzyme Therapy • Fasting • Hypnotherapy • Naturopathic Medicine • Neural Therapy • Osteopathy • Traditional Chinese Medicine

Detoxification Therapy: Detoxification is usually helpful.

Oxygen Therapy: Ozone therapy.

Bodywork: Acupressure, Feldenkrais, Therapeutic Touch.

Where to Find Help

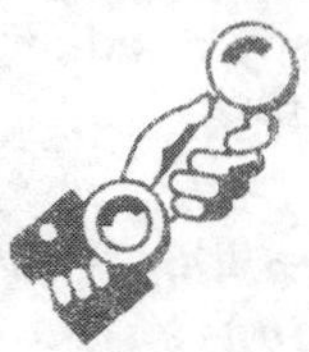

For more information on, and referrals for, treatment of gastrointestinal disorders, contact the following organizations.

American Association of Acupuncture and Oriental Medicine
4101 Lake Boone Trail, Suite 201
Raleigh, North Carolina 27607
(919) 787-5181

The AAAOM is a national professional trade organization of acupuncturists who meet acceptable standards of competency and can provide you with the names and locations of local members.

American Association of Naturopathic Physicians
2366 Eastlake Avenue, Suite 322
Seattle, Washington 98102
(206) 323-7610

Contact them for the location of a licensed naturopathic physician in your area.

International Foundation for Homeopathy
2366 Eastlake Avenue, East, Suite 301
Seattle, Washington 98102
(206) 324-8230

Provides educational courses for professionals and the general public. Offers referrals to homeopathic health professionals.

National Center for Homeopathy
801 North Fairfax, Suite 306
Alexandria, Virginia 22314
(703) 548-7790

Provides a referral list of practicing homeopaths and information. Gives courses for lay people and professionals, and organizes study groups around the country.

Recommended Reading

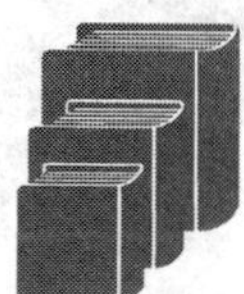

Dr. Braly's Food Allergy and Nutrition Revolution. Braly, James, M.D. New Canaan, CT: Keats Publishing, Inc., 1992.

A comprehensive investigation into food allergies and their link to other illnesses, including those of the gastrointestinal tract. Outlines the factors involved in GI disorders and how to treat them using diet, nutritional supplements, and exercise.

Eating Right for a Bad Gut. Scala, James. New York: Plume Books, 1992.

A guide to proper diet and nutrition for the treatment of gastrointestinal disorders.

Encyclopedia of Natural Medicine. Murray, Michael, N.D.; and Pizzorno, Joseph, N.D. Rocklin, CA: Prima Publishing, 1991.

An authoritative guide to naturopathic medicine outlining the basic principles of health and how they can be used to treat over sixty health conditions, including a full range of gastrointestinal disorders. Includes self-help approaches using diet, nutrition, and herbal medicine.

Gastrointestinal Health. Perkin, Steven, M.D. New York: Harper Perennial, 1992.

Comprehensive self-help guide for treating a full range of gastrointestinal disorders using diet and nutrition.

Irritable Bowel Syndrome and Diverticulosis. Trickett, Shirley. London, England: Thorson's/HarperCollins Publishers, 1992.

A comprehensive self-help approach for treating irritable bowel syndrome, diverticulosis, and other gastrointestinal tract conditions using diet, nutrition, bodywork, homeopathy, and exercise.

7 Weeks to a Healthy Stomach. Hoffman, Ronald, M.D. New York: Pocket Books, 1990.

A seven-week program to restore the gastrointestinal tract to optimal health, using diet, nutrition, and herbal medicine.

Headaches

Headaches affect almost everyone. Often, headaches are a sign of other underlying health conditions. While conventional medicine normally treats headaches by prescribing aspirin and other painkillers to deal with headache symptoms, alternative physicians treat both the headache and its cause to bring lasting relief from pain.

"Headaches are the most common health complaint," states Robert Milne, M.D., of Las Vegas, Nevada. Usually a headache is merely a symptom of another health problem in the body. "These occasional, or acute, headaches can be brought on by such conditions as eyestrain, a sinus infection, or the flu, for example," Dr. Milne says. Proper treatment of headaches first involves careful diagnosis to locate the disturbance actually causing headache pain. It is then essential to treat the root condition, rather than attempting to mask its symptomatic effects with temporary measures such as painkillers or tranquilizers.

Types of Headaches

Dr. Milne divides most headaches into two basic categories; those caused by muscle contraction, and those caused by vascular irregularities (the alternating constriction and expansion of the arteries). Certain conditions such as brain tumors, arterial inflammation, and irritation of the facial nerves also cause headaches but these are extremely rare.

Headaches Caused by Muscle Contraction

Dr. Milne has found that the most common type of headache is the tension headache, which begins in the back of the neck or head and spreads outward with dull, nonthrobbing pain. He estimates that 90 percent of all headaches involve excessive tension in the muscles of the face, head, and neck. "These headaches often feel like a tight band around the head, and the pain is usually constant," he says.

Dr. Milne attributes the pain to two mechanisms relating to muscle contraction: nerve compression within the muscle caused by poor posture, spinal misalignment, or physical and emotional stress; and nerve irritation caused by a buildup of metabolic wastes resulting from decreased blood and lymph circulation due to poor diet, constipation, or other digestive problems, and in women, pelvic irritation.

Headaches Caused by Vascular Irregularities

Headaches caused by vascular irregularities, including migraines, cluster headaches, and caffeine withdrawal headaches, account for less than 10 percent of all cases according to Dr. Milne. With vascular headaches, the alternating constriction and expansion of the arteries of the head exerts pressure on arterial nerves and causes sharp pain.

Migraine Headaches: Migraine headaches are surprisingly common, affecting 15 to 20 percent of men and 25 to 30 percent of women.[1] "This is probably because of the hormonal variations that occur due to the menstrual cycle," says Dr. Milne. "Many of my female patients report that they started getting migraines after some kind of hormonal shift, such as at the onset of puberty, while taking or stopping the birth control pills, or after a pregnancy. Migraines are also more likely to happen during certain times of a woman's cycle, usually at the beginning or the end of mense, and sometimes during ovulation." This indicates pelvic/ovarian weakness, inherited or acquired.

> *"Proper treatment of headaches first involves careful diagnosis to locate the disturbance actually causing headache pain."*

Migraine symptoms include lightheadedness, throbbing pain on one side of the head, nausea, vomiting, dizziness, blurred vision, hot and cold flashes, and hypersensitivity to light and sound. Migraine sufferers often experience warning symptoms or auras for a few minutes before experiencing pain. These auras consist of blurred vision, muddled thinking, exhaustion, worry, and numbness or tingling on one side of the body.

"Migraine pain is most often severe and localized on one side of the head, usually involving the temple and the eye," Dr. Milne explains. "In patients without preceding visual disturbances, there may or may not be any warning signs. Once the migraine occurs, the victim is forced to muddle through his day in pain, or else lie down in a quiet, darkened room."

Cluster Headaches: These are the most painful form of headache, with excruciating pain concentrated around the eye. They are often accompanied by tears, facial flushing, and nasal congestion. "Cluster headaches are much rarer than migraines and affect mostly men," says Dr. Milne. "As the name suggests, they occur in periodic clusters that can last anywhere from a few weeks to several months." During a cluster attack, sharp, intense pain afflicts the victim for a few hours, then subsides for a few hours more before returning again. "Due to the piercing and vicious nature of the pain involved, the victim can become highly agitated and unable to rest," Dr. Milne explains. "Sometimes sufferers might even bang their heads against the wall just to alter the sensation."

More so than for other types of headaches, sufferers of cluster headaches typically fit a certain profile. "The typical victim is normally a male between the ages of thirty and fifty," states David Bresler, Ph.D., founder and former Director of the UCLA Pain Control Unit. "Usually he is also a Type A personality, hard-driving and striving, who often also smokes or drinks. A lot of these people commit suicide because of the pain the clusters cause, although often their deaths are attributed to depression instead. But what is depression? It's psychological pain."

A genetic predisposition to cluster headaches also seems likely, according to Dr. Milne. "When this is the case, smoking and drinking alcohol only worsens the problem, particularly during the cluster periods," he says.

Caffeine Withdrawal Headaches: Headaches related to caffeine withdrawal involve a dull, throbbing pain on both sides of the head and are generally not as intense as migraines or cluster headaches, according to Dr. Milne. Such headaches occur as the body rids itself of the effects of caffeine addiction caused by consumption of coffee, soft drinks, certain teas, medications for weight control, colds and allergies, pain relief, and menstrual aids, among others. Normally, once the body rids itself of the caffeine's side effects, the headaches will disappear on their own. Such headache suffers, however, are often unaware that their problem is due to caffeine and so will not avoid it, causing the problem to reoccur.

Other Types of Headaches: Severe headache pain can also result from more serious conditions such as brain tumors or arterial inflammation. According to Dr. Milne, typical symptoms of these headaches include seizures, projectile vomiting, speech or personality changes, walking difficulty, and increasing pain. Temporal arteritis (an inflammation of the temporal arteries common among people over sixty) gives rise to burning, boring, or throbbing headache pain, often felt around the ear when chewing. A rare form of headache also cited by Dr. Milne is the short and stabbing pain from idiopathic cranial neuralgia (caused by an irritation of one of the nerves in the face) which occurs around the jaw or mouth and can last from several seconds to several minutes.

What Causes Headaches?

According to James Braly, M.D., Medical Director of Immuno Labs in Fort Lauderdale, Florida, determining the cause of headaches is a complicated matter, with, as yet, few established medical facts. Besides hidden food allergies and chemical sensitivities, he cites hormonal imbalances as one possible cause, which may explain the susceptibility of some teenagers to migraines that subsequently disappear when the sufferers enter adulthood. Other causes can also be be inherited.

"Because there are so many different types of headaches and headache patterns, identifying their underlying causes can be challenging," says Dr. Milne. "But since they are so hard to diagnose, all too often headaches are treated as an isolated problem, separate from the rest of the body. A chronic headache syndrome, however, is a sure sign that there is a systemic disturbance in the body that can be extremely complex and consisting of various conditions that interact and exacerbate one another." An example of such an interplay of conditions, Dr. Milne notes, is migraine headaches caused by hormonal imbalances occuring due to

"Among the causes of headaches are stress, allergies, blood clotting, smoking, poor posture, and dental factors."

yeast overgrowth, or candidiasis. The candidiasis, in turn, can also contribute to food allergies, which many alternative physicians now recognize as one of the primary causes of migraines. "Headaches, therefore, are extremely important and ought not to be ignored because they can direct attention to other health problems that might otherwise have gone undetected and untreated," Dr. Milne says.

Among the causes of headaches are stress, allergies, blood clotting, dental factors, smoking, poor posture, and pelvic irritation.

Stress

According to Dr. Milne, the most common cause of headaches is stress resulting from chemical, emotional, or physical factors. "Many of us carry stress in the muscles of the face, skull, neck, shoulders, and upper back, causing them to contract," he points out. "A person in whom these muscles are persistently contracted is likely to experience chronic tension headaches." Muscles that are constantly contracted can also become fatigued and suffer from a reduced supply of oxygen. In addition, the contractions can cause chemicals in the body, such as histamines, to accumulate, triggering neurons in the muscles to fire, creating pain. And once the headache occurs, the pain, coupled with the fear of the next headache attack, can result in additional stress and anxiety to perpetuate one of the vicious cycles associated with chronic headache complaints. Dr. Milne stresses that one must rule out toxic, metabolic stress in the liver and colon. These are the most common physical causes of these headaches.

"The most common cause of headaches is stress resulting from chemical, emotional, or physical factors."

Stress can also be due to mental or emotional factors related to the pressures of everyday life, regrets about the past, and worries about the future. Since the mind and body function as a whole, when such concerns are the present, the stress that they cause can often result in headache pain.

Leon Chaitow, N.D., D.O., of London, England, points out that another common source of stress that can lead to headaches is eye strain.

Children and Headaches

Contrary to popular belief, children can experience serious types of headaches, including migraines. Children of parents who suffer from migraines have an increased risk of developing such headaches, as well. According to Robert Milne, M.D., of Las Vegas, Nevada, "Sometimes these migraine conditions might take different forms in a child than they would in an adult. For example, headache pain might be 'vague' rather than localized. Or there may not be head pain at all. Instead, the child might experience spells of nausea, confusion, or dizziness." Children who are prone to motion sickness might also be susceptible to migraines as adults, Dr. Milne notes.

If you suspect your child is suffering from headache symptoms, be sensitive to the situation. "It's important not to focus so much on the problem that you worsen it by increasing your child's tension and fear," says Dr. Milne. "Address the experience in a loving manner and with sympathy, while at the same time gently allowing your child to develop his or her own individual coping mechanisms.

In addition, parents can help prevent the underlying conditions that can cause their children's headaches in the following ways:

- *Keep a record of your child's headaches in a diary. Note what he or she ate prior to the headache's occurrence. Also note any activities or stress your child experienced, as well as any chemicals or other environmental toxins he or she may have been exposed to. Such a record will provide you with clues to what triggers your child's headaches and enable you to avoid whatever factors are involved.*
- *By monitoring your child's diet, you will become aware of any food allergies or sensitivities he or she may have. Once you discover such foods, eliminate them from the diet. Also eliminate sugars in all of its forms, and try not to feed your child too much of the same type of food, such as corn or wheat, as repetition in the diet can also trigger headaches and other allergic reactions.*
- *Ensure that your child adopts regular sleep and eating patterns.*
- *Encourage your child to exercise and to spend time outdoors, breathing fresh air. Also help your child develop his or her ability to relax and enjoy quiet activities, such as reading and drawing.*
- *Finally, foster your child's ability to express whatever thoughts or emotions he or she may have, as repressing them can create additional stress and tension.*

As he explains, "There are many individuals whose chronic headaches disappear when they have their eyes checked. If there is a problem which is not corrected, it is common for the head to be held in a tilted manner to try to achieve focus." Dr. Chaitow states that eye glasses usually eliminate the need to tilt the head and frequently eliminate headaches as well. In addition, he suggests that eye exercises such as the Bates method may be helpful in curbing eye strain.

Dr. Chaitow also notes that eye strain and headaches can result from exposure to flickering neon or fluorescent overhead lighting, TV and video monitors, and computer screens.

Allergies

Based on his own clinical experience, Dr. Braly states that 90 percent of all migraine headaches are directly linked to food allergies or to reactions caused by additives, particularly certain preservatives and colorings, caffeine, and chocolate. A study reported in the British journal *The Lancet* confirms Dr. Braly's conviction. This study cited relief for 93 percent of the study's migraine sufferers when allergenic foods were eliminated from their diet. Most patients were allergic to more than one food, and surprisingly the offending allergens were often among the patients' favorite foods, with the most common offenders being cow's milk, eggs, wheat, cheese, and rye, along with benzoic acid (a preservative) and tartrazine (a popular food dye). A double-blind placebo test also proved that when these foods were reintroduced into the study group's diet, the migraine pain would reoccur.[2] According to Dr. Chaitow, aspartame (NutraSweet) has also been implicated in many headache cases, as has excessive salt intake.

Dr. Milne warns that other allergens may be "hidden" in complex foods. For example, he cites two common allergens, corn and brewer's yeast, which hide in many recipes and even in some vitamin pills. He recommends that treatment of headaches always start with a careful history of food and chemical intake to discover what role they may play in causing headache pain.

Are Painkillers Causing Your Headaches?

If painkillers are used too frequently, they may actually cause more pain than they relieve, according to Robert Milne, M.D., of Las Vegas, Nevada. "Excessive use of painkillers, especially of painkillers containing caffeine, can cause a rebound effect in which pain intensifies when the painkillers wear off," he says. For frequent users of these drugs, Dr. Milne recommends a gradual withdrawal over a one-week period. Afterward, several weeks may pass before the headaches caused by overused painkillers fully cease.

Posture and Headaches

Poor posture is a major cause of stress due to muscle strain, and the result can often be headache pain. But as Robert Milne, M.D., of Las Vegas, Nevada, points out, the classic depiction of bad posture with a person slouching, round-shouldered, with a protruding belly, is only one type of postural distortion, usually caused by poor diet and low energy. Holding oneself rigidly upright in a military-like posture can be just as hard on the body, because maintaining such a stance requires a great deal of muscular tension. In contrast, healthy posture features a spine with slight curvatures and well-toned muscles that maintain these curves.

"Good posture stems from having good energy and standing upright and tall, while still remaining relaxed," explains Dr. Milne. "Shoulders should drop, then be brought back slightly. The pelvis should be tucked in with the knees slightly bent. Shoulder and neck rolls can help relax tight muscles and rebalance posture."

Blood Clotting

Another common cause of headaches is blood clotting, also known as platelet aggregation.[3] Clotting creates constriction of the arteries, which results in inadequate blood supply to the brain. This is then followed by a rebound dilation of the blood vessels, leading to headaches. According to Julian Whitaker, M.D., of Newport Beach, California, the platelets of migraine patients release abnormal amounts of serotonin (a neurotransmitter), which enhances the arteries' constriction.

See Allergies, Candidiasis, Chronic Pain, Constipation, Gastrointestinal Disorders, Heart Disease, Hypertension, Stress, Vision Disorders.

James R. Privitera, M.D., Director of NutriScreen, Inc., in Covina, California, states that the evidence of clotting in headache sufferers is readily apparent when live blood cells are examined using a darkfield microscope. "Clinically, we have found that the majority of all headache sufferers not only have platelet aggregation, but that they also respond well to natural therapies such as diet, nutritional supplements, and herbal medicine," he says. In one study conducted by

Dr. Privitera, forty-one patients complaining of headaches were tested for clotting. "Thirty-nine people, or 95 percent of the group, showed significant clotting," he reports.

Dr. Privitera also points out that conventional practitioners normally do not test for clotting when they examine their patients, even though blood clots are known to contribute to heart attacks, strokes, arthritis, and other degenerative diseases.

Dental Factors

Dental stress can also contribute to headaches, according to Harold E. Ravins, D.D.S., of Los Angeles, who has been treating headaches in his dental practice for over twenty years. He estimates that more than half of his patients come to him because of headache problems that they have been unable to cure.

"Teeth that are under continuous stress affect other parts of the body," says Dr. Ravins. "Problems such as tooth decay, gum disease, muscle spasm, and low-grade infections from old fillings all cause stress in the lower jaw. The upper and lower jawbones move together at the temporomandibular joints, located just in front of each earlobe, to produce a pumping action. When the lower jaw hits the upper jaw in harmony, there is a natural flowing of energy whereupon the fluids of the brain, the electrolytes, can flow through the body properly. Dental stress factors can reduce this circulation in the brain area, because when the bones in the skull become more rigid, losing their flexibility and normal motion, they reduce blood flow. This causes the blood vessels to constrict, which can produce a headache."

See Biological Dentistry, Respiratory Conditions.

To rebalance the jaw, Dr. Ravins often has a headache patient use a removable appliance, usually worn at night. This treatment is in addition to healing the gums and teeth.

The following questions can help determine if dental stress is contributing to your headaches: Do you favor one side of your mouth when you chew? Do you grind your teeth? Do you have trouble swallowing three or four times in a row? Do you have a poor sense of balance? Do you feel tired after eating due to chewing? Do you have to strain to smile? Do your gums bleed? Do you make a clicking sound when you open or close your mouth? Answering yes to any of these questions can be an indication that you are experiencing some form of dental stress, which is most likely also contributing to headaches.

Dr. Ravins also recommends the following self-help technique that patients can do whenever they feel a migraine coming on: Put your thumb in your mouth on the side of the migraine pain; reach up with it and find the cheekbone, then press that bone up and out. Then do the same with the other side. Finally, place both thumbs inside on the upper palate and press the sides out. It may take several repetitions before the pain subsides.

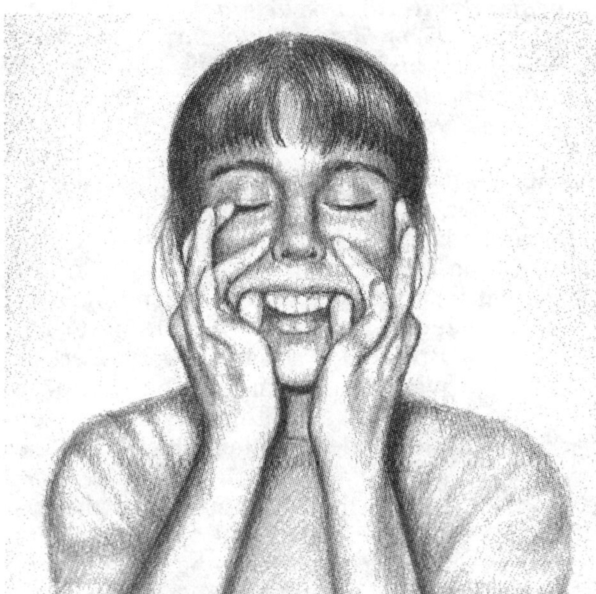

Self-help technique to prevent migraines.

Smoking

Smoking can also cause headaches, according to Dr. Milne. Nicotine constricts the blood vessels while inhaled carbon monoxide overly expands them, thus creating a condition which often triggers migraines and cluster headaches. Dr. Milne also points out that smoking cuts down the effectiveness of pain relievers, and may disrupt the nutritional balance of the body.

Treatment of Headaches

Although aspirin and other painkillers help alleviate headache pain, they usually provide only partial or temporary relief and fail to address the underlying conditions that headaches may be symptoms of. Some types of headaches have also proved resistant to even powerful drugs, which therefore can become easily abused by patients desperate for relief. Among the nondrug therapies which have proven most effective in treating headaches are diet, nutritional supplements, herbal medicine, bodywork, relaxation techniques, and hydrotherapy.

Caution: *When headaches are associated with fever, convulsions, head trauma, loss of consciousness, or localized pain in the ear, eye, or elsewhere, professional help should be sought* *immediately. Recurring headaches in children and the elderly, or headaches occurring suddenly with no prior history of headache, also require immediate medical attention.*

Diet

Because of the link between headaches and food allergies, Dr. Braly recommends that headache sufferers be laboratory tested for foods they may be allergic to. Another way to do this is to fast the patient for five days, during which time only distilled water is consumed. According to Dr. Braly, such a fast is a very effective way of allowing the body to free itself of symptoms as a first step toward determining which foods the patient is allergic to. He recommends that during the fast the patient be supervised by a competent physician, and that the patient avoid smoking and not use toothpaste, mouthwashes, and other personal hygiene products that contain chemicals. Once the fast is completed, the patient can then reintroduce individual foods one by one back into his or her diet. Those that cause a reaction should then be avoided. Keeping a food journal during this time can also be helpful, so that the patient can have a record of the offending foods and the symptoms they cause.

See Diet, Fasting, Nutritional Supplements, Orthomolecular Medicine.

After such foods are eliminated, Dr. Braly recommends a maintenance program that incorporates a rotation diet, with no food being eaten more frequently than once every four days. "Such a diet helps prevent the development of further allergies and reactions and also provides a more balanced diet which supplies a wider range of needed nutrients," Dr. Braly says.

The diet consists of eating foods high in nonallergenic complex carbohydrates and fiber, while avoiding simple and refined sugars, including dried fruit and fruit juices, chocolate, pastries, sodas, and candy; food additivies, colorings, and preservatives; alcohol; and caffeine. Margarine, shortenings, and other sources of partially hydrogenated oils are also avoided, and saturated fats from red meat, dairy products, eggs, and warm water fish are limited. These should be replaced with poultry, other types of fish, nongluten grains, and a variety of vegetables, fresh vegetable juices, and fresh fruit.

Dr. Braly reports that many of his headache patients have experienced substantial relief on this program. One of them was a teenage boy who came to him suffering from two to three migraines a week. He was also fifty pounds overweight, had previously seen a number of headache specialists without success, and was taking several drugs for his pain. He had also been diagnosed as being learning impaired and emotionally disabled. By use of the IgG Elisa lab test, Dr. Braly discovered that the boy was severely allergic to a number of foods, which were then eliminated from his diet. "After he gave up the offending foods and began following the rotation diet, he soon experienced complete relief from his headaches," Dr. Braly says. "He also was quickly able to shed forty-eight pounds and his learning and emotional difficulties improved. His mother told me I had given her son his life back, but all along the problem had simply been due to the foods he was eating."

Nutritional Supplements

Dr. Braly suggests that as a daily routine for health, the diet be supplemented with a multivitamin/mineral formula. For headache sufferers he recommends an increase of vitamin C (2 to 8 grams divided into three doses taken throughout the day), vitamin E (400 to 800 IU), niacinamide, a form of vitamin B_3, (500 milligrams), and calcium/magnesium (600 milligrams calcium/600 milligrams magnesium). [In addition, Dr. Braly has found that evening primrose oil (three to four capsules taken at breakfast and again at dinner); MaxEPA, a form of fish oil; and the amino acid DL-phenylalanine (one 275-milligram capsules taken two to three times daily between meals) should also be included.] "Evening primrose oil and MaxEPA are both sources of essential fatty acids which supply the body with anti-inflammatory agents and act to keep the blood vessels from constricting," Dr. Braly explains. "And DL-phenylalanine, when taken regularly, acts as a potent natural painkiller." Finally, Dr. Braly recommends the use of two herbs—standardized feverfew and querticin with bromelain—both often associated with relief of migraines.

A QUICK FIX FOR MIGRAINE HEADACHES

Robert Milne, M.D., of Las Vegas, Nevada, has found that the following simple procedure can often bring immediate relief for migraine headaches triggered by allergic reactions to food or chemical substances. As soon as the onset of migraine symptoms occur, take two tablets of AlkaSeltzer Gold in a glass of water. Let them dissolve, then drink. "The drink has the effect of creating an alkaline condition in the body," Dr. Milne explains. "This neutralizes the allergic mechanisms and prevents the migraine from fully taking hold."

According to Dr. Chaitow, a lack of potassium, which he describes as an excellent nerve tonic, can also contribute to various kinds of headaches. Potassium supplementation in the form of tablets or capsules is undersirable, however, according to Dr. Chaitow, since it can interfere with the functions of other nutrients. Instead, he recommends making a "potassium broth." "To make the broth," says Dr. Chaitow, "take an assortment of vegetables, or their skins (potatoes especially), and cover them with cold water. Boil the water, then allow the vegetables to simmer for ten minutes. Then strain the liquid from the pot. The broth will be very rich with potassium. Refrigerate and drink several cups of it throughout the day."

Herbal Medicine

There are a variety of herbs that offer relief to headache sufferers. Among them is feverfew, which has been shown to reduce the secretion of serotonin and the production of prostaglandin, an inflammatory agent which contributes to the onset of migraine headaches. In one study, 70 percent of 270 migraine patients tested reported that a daily dose of feverfew decreased the frequency and intensity of migraine attacks.[4]

For patients who do not respond to feverfew, Donald Brown, N.D., of Seattle, Washington, recommends *Ginkgo biloba*, which inhibits blood clotting, a condition related to the serotonin release which causes migraines in susceptible people. "Garlic and onion also inhibit blood clots and improve blood circulation," Dr. Brown says, "and can also bring relief when added to the diet."

Dr. Brown also recommends ginger, which reduces inflammation in the stomach and liver that can also contribute to migraine problems. "At the onset of a migraine attack, the patient can take 500 to 600 milligrams of powdered ginger," he says. "The dosage should then be repeated two more times during the day, with four hours between each dose. As an alternative, fresh ginger can be chewed or used in cooking."

Cayenne pepper is another useful herb for headache treatment. It is an excellent source of magnesium, which has been shown to be a migraine preventative, and, according to Dr. Milne, cayenne also reduces the likelihood of a migraine by stimulating digestion and increasing the body's metabolic rate.

Other useful herbs for treating headaches, according to Dr. Chaitow, include chamomile; tumeric, which is a natural anti-inflammatory agent; coriander, which reduces swelling and is an excellent source of potassium; bay leaves, which can be helpful for frontal headaches; skullcap, which can soothe headaches due to tension; valerian, a sedative and pain reliever; and willow bark, another pain reliever, which contains salicylic acid, the ingredient from which aspirin is derived. "Unlike aspirin, however, which is an isolated and concentrated chemical, willow bark acts gently and without aspirin's potential for irritating the stomach," Dr. Chaitow says.

Bodywork

Because of the relationship between headaches and muscle contraction, the field of bodywork has much to offer headache sufferers. "Many headaches occur due to tension spasms in the muscles that run between the base of the skull and along the top of the shoulders," explains William Cargile, B.S., D.C., L.Ac., F.I.A.C.A., Chairman of Research of the American Association of Acupuncture and Oriental Medicine. "A variety of bodywork therapies can address this problem by releasing muscle tension and normalizing the neurovascular system."

Bodywork methods that are appropriate for treating headaches include Rolfing, the Feldenkrais Method™, the Alexander technique, the Trager® approach, and polarity therapy. Such methods require the assistance of a trained professional, however. For a self-help approach, Dr. Cargile recommends acupressure. "One can achieve a great deal of relief using acupressure self-help techniques," he says.

Dr. Chaitow is another proponent of acupressure for headache relief. At the first sign of a headache, he suggests the following acupressure treatment, which stimulates the body's energy points: Hold your first finger and thumb straight and press them together. Their muscular effort forms a mound of flesh on the top of your hand (not the palm side). The highest point of this mound is a pressure point which should be pressed firmly, while keeping the hand muscles relaxed. To ease head and facial pain, press slightly toward the finger. "You should find that this area hurts when you press into it," Dr. Chaitow explains. "Maintain the pressure on the pain spot for up to a minute, and then repeat if necessary."

See Bodywork, Herbal Medicine.

The following acupressure points are also useful in treating headaches, according to Michael Reed Gach, Ph.D., Director of the Acupressure Institute in Berkeley, California:

GB20: With your thumbs, firmly press underneath the base of your skull into the hollow areas on either side. "These will be located two to three inches apart, depending on your head size," Dr. Gach says. "With your eyes closed, slowly tilt your head back and press up from underneath the

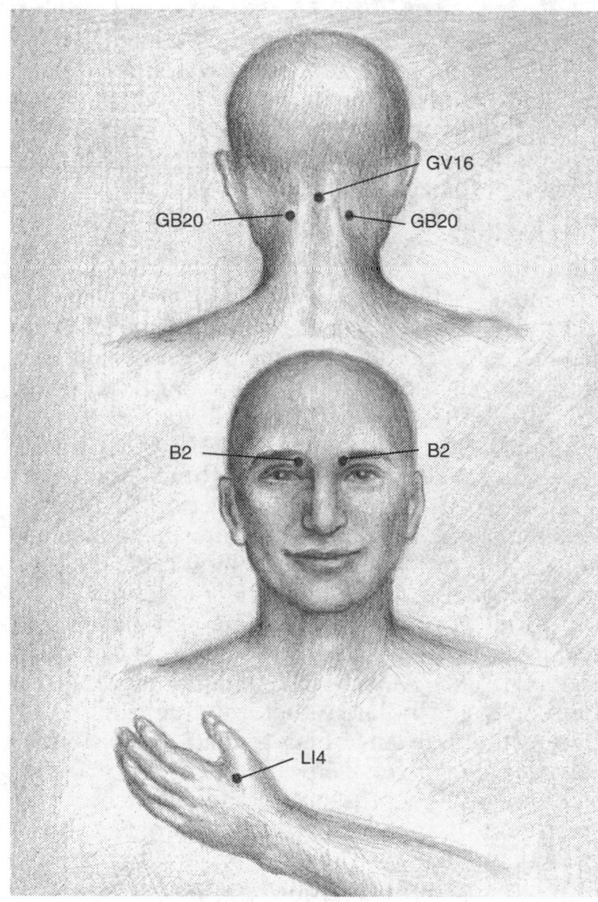

Acupressure headache points.

skull for one to two minutes. As you do so, take, long deep breaths through your diaphragm."

GV16 with B2: Using your right thumb, press the GV16 point located in the center hollow of the base of the skull. With your left thumb and index finger, simultaneously press point B_2 located in the upper hollows of your eye sockets, near the bridge of your nose. Once again, tilt your head back and breathe deeply for one to two minutes.

LI4: Place your right hand over the top of your left. With your right thumb, press the webbing between the thumb and index finger of your left hand, angling the pressure toward the bone that connects with the index finger. Hold for one minute, then reverse hands and press the point on your opposite hand for an equal length of time. "This point, which is known in acupressure as *ho-ku*, should not be used by pregnant women," Dr. Gach cautions, "because stimulating it can cause premature contractions of the uterus."

Relaxation Techniques

Relaxation is crucial to relieve the muscle tension and stress which cause many headaches. Some sufferers of severe headaches have to make radical lifestyle changes in order to alleviate their condition. A workaholic, male patient of Dr. Milne, for example, found relief from his throbbing, intensely painful headaches only when he began working fewer hours and spending more time relaxing with his family.

See Biofeedback Training, Guided Imagery, Meditation, Mind/Body Medicine, Yoga.

Many different techniques for relaxation exist for the headache sufferer. To promote vascular and muscle relaxation, Dr. Braly recommends the regular practice of meditation, deep relaxation, biofeedback, or yoga. He also advises patients to consider undertaking stress and behavior evaluation tests to identify possible emotional and lifestyle factors that might be triggering their headaches.

One of the easiest relaxation techniques suggested by Dr. Milne is slow, deep breathing for approximately five minutes. "Most people do not realize that they usually take short, shallow breaths, and that five minutes of slow deep breathing will trigger an involuntary relaxation response in muscles all over the body," he explains. Progressive muscle relaxation exercises can also help prevent nonvascular headaches. This is easily accomplished by tensing and then relaxing each of the muscle groups in the body.

Hydrotherapy

Hydrotherapy is another method of treating headaches without the use of drugs. "Hot baths, saunas, heat lamps, and steam baths all reduce

SELF-MASSAGE FOR HEADACHES

The following self-massage can provide effective relief from headache pain. Sit comfortably in a chair, taking care to breathe freely through the diaphragm. Cradle the back of your neck with your hand and squeeze gently, slowly rolling your head in a circle. Release for a few moments, then again squeeze your neck, slightly increasing the pressure. Repeat squeezing and releasing for twenty times.

Next, using your fingertips, press into any areas in your neck and shoulders that are sore or tender, moving your arms and shoulders in a gentle, rhythmic motion. Continue this for several minutes, until your headache fades.

Doing these exercises periodically throughout the day will often prevent your headaches from reoccurring. They can also be performed by a partner. As you seat yourself, have your partner stand behind you and follow the above instructions.

A PROGRESSIVE RELAXATION EXERCISE

The following exercise is a useful method that headache sufferers can use to learn how to relax and relieve the stress of muscle tension: Lie down, or lean back in a comfortable chair in a quiet room with subdued light. Take ten slow, deep breaths, taking a little longer to breathe out than you take to breathe in. The ideal timing is a two-second full inhalation followed by a slow, controlled four- or five-second exhalation. This starts the relaxation process.

Beginning with your feet, clench the muscles and toes tightly for a few seconds, then release. Then tighten the muscles of your leg, and relax. Repeat this process for the rest of your body: buttocks, back, abdomen, hands, arms, shoulders, neck, jaw, eyes, and finally the muscles of the face. Next, yawn several times, then squeeze your eyes open and shut, taking another ten deep breaths. Now notice how much more relaxed you are. Continue breathing, allowing that relaxation to grow stronger. Then resume your regular activities.

tension by increasing blood circulation," says Dr. Chaitow. "This, in turn, removes the metabolic wastes that are often the cause of headaches. A migraine headache, for instance, can sometimes be stopped dead in its tracks with the combination of a hot shower followed quickly with an ice-cold one." According to Dr. Chaitow, hot water may at first increase the migraine pain by temporarily dilating blood vessels, but this paves the way for fast relief when the vessels are constricted by the cold shower.

This "hot/cold" approach, however, can be too stressful for older people. They can get similar results by placing a piece of cracked ice in the back of the throat at the first sign of pain. "These techniques give the patient a measure of control," says Dr. Chaitow. "They also provide an opportunity to reduce and ultimately omit medication."

See Hydrotherapy.

For simple headache relief, Dr. Chaitow recommends cold applications of an ice pack to the head along with a simultaneous hot foot or hand bath. For the foot or hand bath, he advises mixing one teaspoon of dry mustard into two gallons of water. "But even a normal bath at body temperature can be therapeutic, especially at the onset of the headache," he notes.

Self Care

The following therapies can be undertaken at home under appropriate professional supervision:

• Biofeedback Training • Fasting • Guided Imagery • Meditation • Progressive Relaxation • Yoga

Aromatherapy: • Lavender, peppermint, rosemary, eucalyptus, chamomile • Rub a drop of lavender oil into temples to relieve pain. • Marjoram

Juice Therapy: • Carrot, celery • Carrot, beet, cucumber • Carrot, celery, spinach, parsley

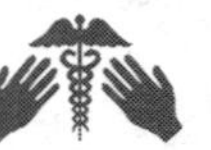

Professional Care

The following therapies should only be provided by a qualified health professional:

• Acupuncture • Chiropractic • Colon Therapy • Craniosacral Therapy • Environmental Medicine • Hypnotherapy • Magnetic Field Therapy • Osteopathy

Oxygen Therapy: • Hydrogen peroxide therapy • Hyperbaric oxygen therapy

Where to Find Help

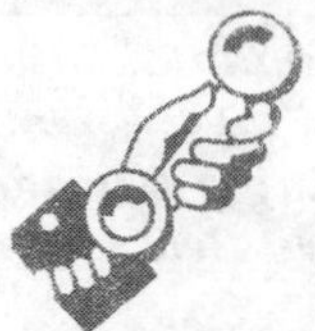

For information on headaches, or referrals to a qualified health care practitioner, contact the following organizations.

American Association of Naturopathic Physicians
2366 Eastlake Avenue, Suite 322
Seattle, Washington 98102
(206) 323-7610

Contact the association for the location of a licensed naturopathic physician in your area.

American Council for Headache Education
875 Kings Highway, Suite 200
West Deptford, New Jersey 08096
(800) 255-ACHE

Provides written information on causes of and treatment approaches to headaches. Also provides referrals to physicians nationwide who specialize in headache treatment, oversees local support groups, and publishes a newsletter. Call for further information.

The National Headache Foundation
5252 North Western Avenue
Chicago, Illinois 60625
(800) 843-2256

Supplies a state-by-state list of physicians who treat headaches, available by written request. Also provides free information on headaches. Membership available for annual fee.

Recommended Reading

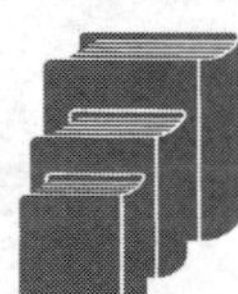

Dr. Braly's Food Allergy and Nutrition Revolution. Braly, James, M.D. New Canaan, CT: Keats Publishing, Inc., 1992.

An excellent overview of the role food allergies can play in a wide range of illnesses, including headaches and migraines. Includes a self-help approach to treatment based upon diet, nutrition, and exercise.

Freedom from Headaches. Saper, Joel, M.D.; and Magee, Kenneth, M.D. New York: Fireside Books, 1981.

A comprehensive, yet easy-to-read, discussion of the variety of headaches, their causes, and how to relieve them.

Migraine and the Allergy Connection. Mansfield, John, M.D. Rochester, NY: Healing Arts Press, 1990.

Explores the link between food and environmental allergies and migraine headaches, including how to safeguard yourself against exposure.

Migraine: Beating the Odds. Lipton, Richard, M.D.; Newman, Lawrence, M.D.; and MacLean, Helene. Reading, MA: Addison Wesley, 1992.

A self-help approach for avoiding and treating migraine headaches, using diet, nutrition, and a variety of mind/body medicine techniques.

Who Needs Headaches. Ingram, Cass, D.O. Cedar Rapids, IA: Literary Visions Publishing, 1991.

An overview on the various types of headaches, what causes them, and how to treat them, using diet, nutrition, herbal medicine, and bodywork. Available by calling (319) 366-5335.

Hearing and Ear Disorders

Disorders of the auditory system affect nearly 28 million Americans. Practitioners of alternative medicine believe that a large percentage of these disorders involve food and environmental allergies, as well as the overuse of antibiotics. Dietary changes, nutritional supplements, herbal therapy, and homeopathic remedies are often highly effective treatments, helping to eliminate the need for antibiotics or surgery.

The auditory system is responsible for the processing of sound and the regulation of balance, and is one of the body's most delicate and sensitive systems. When functioning properly, it enables a person to hear the faintest cry or maintain equilibrium in the most extreme circumstances. But the very complexity that allows for such precision also makes the ear susceptible to a wide range of ailments.

Ear disorders can affect people at any age, says Constantine A. Kotsanis, M.D., of Grapevine, Texas, and symptoms may include ear pain and stuffiness, inflammation, nerve damage, tinnitus (ringing in the ears), problems with balance, dizziness, vertigo, nerve damage, and hearing loss. "A slight loss in the ability to hear is not unusual with advancing age," adds Dr. Kotsanis, "but recently more and more young people are suffering from hearing loss equivalent to someone forty years his senior."

According to David Liscomb, M.D., of the University of Tennessee, more than 60 percent of incoming college students have impaired hearing in the high frequency range.[1]

Structure of the Ear

The ear comprises three distinct sections known as the inner, middle, and outer ear. The inner ear consists of two parts, the cochlea, which is responsible for hearing, and the vestibule and semicircular canals, which are responsible for equilibrium and balance. Lining the inner ear are tiny hair cells that act as sensory receptors to transmit balance and hearing signals to the nerves and the brain.

The middle ear houses the three hearing bones, or ossicles, and the auditory, or eustachian tube, which extends and opens to the back part of the nasal airway. Normally, the middle ear space is filled with air that enters through the nasal opening of the eustachian tube.

The external ear houses the external canal (where wax is produced), and the ear "drumhead." The physical external ear, the external canal, and the eardrum are separated from each other by thin, soft tissue walls.

Types of Ear Disorders

There are a wide variety of ear-related disorders, ranging from common ear infections to severe conditions such as chronic otitis media (ear infection), Meniere's disease, tinnitus, and hearing loss.

General Ear Pain

General ear pain is one of the most common patient complaints. According to Dr. Kotsanis, "The usual cause is a buildup of fluid in the middle ear, resulting in pressure that swells and closes the eustachian tube. When the tube closes fluid from the middle ear is prevented from flowing and begins to accumulate, and this stagnant fluid can lead to bacterial infection, causing acute pain, fever, and decreased hearing." General ear pain may also be attributed to wax buildup.

Otitis Media

Otitis media is an infection of the ear that is now the most common cause of hearing loss in chil-

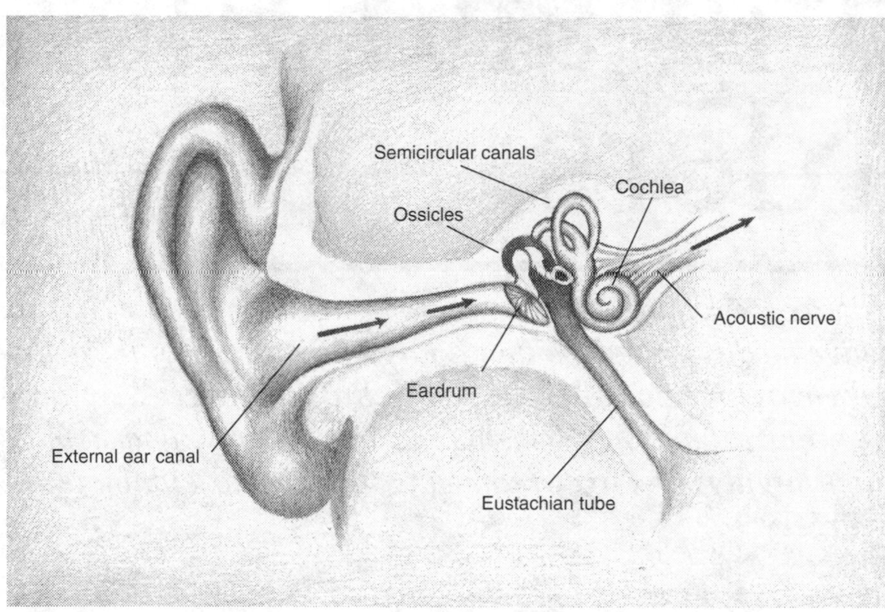

Diagram of the ear.

dren. Approximately $2 billion is spent annually on medical and surgical treatment of otitis media in the United States.[2] Its rise closely parallels the general rise of allergic diseases.[3]

There are two basic types of otitis media, acute and chronic. Acute otitis media is characterized by an infection of the middle ear (usually bacterial) and is often accompanied by an upper respiratory infection or allergy. Earache and irritability are common symptoms, as are fever, chills, and a red, swollen eardrum. Acute otitis media is most common in infants and children, though it may occur at any age. Recurrent acute otitis media is associated with early bottle feeding, while prolonged breastfeeding (minimum six months) has a prophylactic (preventative) effect due to antibodies contained in mother's milk.[4]

> *"Otitis media is now the most common cause of hearing loss in children, with approximately $2 billion spent annually on medical and surgical treatment of it in the United States."*

Chronic otitis media, also known as secretory or serous otitis media, refers to a constant swelling and blockage of the auditory tube, and is characterized by a dull, often throbbing pain. At some point it affects 20 to 40 percent of children under the age of six. "Chronic otitis media is usually accompanied by conductive hearing loss and can be caused by inflammation, swelling, or infection of the middle ear," says Dr. Kotsanis. He adds that, "Perforation of the membranes of the middle ear is usually present, and there may be a constant drainage from the ear." Dr. Kotsanis warns that any infection of the middle ear left untreated can lead to meningitis (inflammation of the membranes of the spinal cord or brain). Recurrent otitis media has also been linked to hyperactivity in children.[5]

Meniere's Disease

Meniere's disease is a serious dysfunction characterized by a buildup of fluid pressure of the inner ear which ultimately upsets the balance mechanism and can cause bouts of dizziness, nausea, and vomiting. Three common effects of Meniere's disease are vertigo, tinnitus, and sensory hearing loss.

The sudden, often violent attacks associated with Meniere's disease can last from ten minutes to several hours. Over time, as hearing loss becomes more profound, the number of attacks generally decrease, and often cease when hearing loss is total. Conventional treatment consists of diuretics to keep the fluid out of the ear canal, regular audiograms to monitor hearing loss and, as a last resort, surgery.

Tinnitus

Tinnitus is characterized by a continuous ringing or hissing in the ear, sometimes accompanied by pain. Causes can include excess ear wax, a blocked or impaired eustachian tube, and dysfunction of the auditory nerve. Dr. Kotsanis notes that the onset of tinnitus may also be linked to excessive drug use, aspirin, sustained exposure to loud noise, electrical stimulation, smoking, trauma, Meniere's disease, and temporomandibular joint syndrome (TMJ). Tinnitus in the elderly is often due to decreased circulation in and around the ear.

Caution: *People who suffer from tinnitus often complain of vertigo and dizziness, both of which can be symptoms related to problems of the inner ear, the heart, or the brain. These people should see a doctor to rule out anemia, atherosclerosis, labyrinthitis, and hypertension as possible causes of the tinnitus.*

Hearing Loss

Hearing loss can be sudden or gradual in onset. Problems that develop over a short period of time usually signify a blockage in either the outer or inner ear. Outer ear blockages are most often from wax buildup, while blockages of the inner ear are generally caused by fluid accumulation as a result of infection or allergy.

There are two basic types of hearing loss, conductive and sensory.

Conductive Hearing Loss: This type of hearing loss is associated with problems of either the external ear (wax or infection of the external canal) or the middle ear (eustachian tube dysfunction from infection or allergy, middle ear fluid, or fixation of one or all of the bones of the middle ear). Recurrent conductive hearing loss usually results from chronic ear infection or trauma.

Sensory Hearing Loss: Sensory hearing loss in adults is a common occurrence, usually resulting from a deterioration of the cochlea and from the loss of hair cells in the inner ear responsible for transmitting sound to the nerves. The most common causes of sensory hearing loss include aging, trauma, injury from high-frequency noise exposure, infection (mainly viral), and metabolic disorders such as diabetes, hypertension, and kidney problems. Dr. Kotsanis points out that toxins such as caffeine, tobacco, aspirin, certain diuretics, and chemotherapy can also cause sensory hearing loss, and adds that in some cases, vascular damage or benign tumors may be responsible. He recommends that hearing loss secondary to inner ear problems be investigated by an ear specialist. Dr. Kotsanis warns against purchasing a hearing aid without seeing an ear doctor first as some patients are not candidates for hearing aids even though they have a hearing loss.

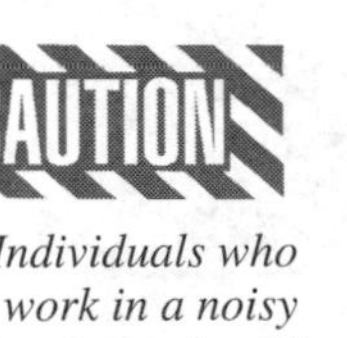

Individuals who work in a noisy environment should ask their employers for ear plugs and muffs. Federal regulations require employers to provide ear protection if the workplace is excessively noisy.

Causes of Ear Disorders

According to Dr. Kotsanis, "Many disorders of the ear can be traced to infection, loud noise, and a variety of food and environmental allergies. Other possible causes include drugs, smoking (as a result of its negative effects on circulation), trauma, sustained exposure to chlorine (swimmer's ear), and autoimmune and metabolic disorders. Medications such as aspirin, diuretics, and chemotherapy can also cause ear problems."

Excessive Wax Accumulation

The function of ear wax is to clean and moisten the ear canal. A healthy external ear canal produces a constant, small amount of wax, but a buildup can block the ear canal, causing a feeling of fullness in the ear, as well as earaches, deafness, and dizziness. Hearing loss due to wax buildup can be gradual or sudden, depending on whether one is predisposed to excessive wax production. According to Constantine A. Kotsanis, M.D., of Grapevine, Texas, excessive wax in the ears is seen mostly in the elderly and in patients with food or mold allergies. He notes that almost all children with excessive wax have allergies to cow's milk.

For wax buildup, Katie Data, N.D., of Fife, Washington, recommends a washing solution of lukewarm water with a few drops of vinegar or hydrogen peroxide. Virender Sodhi, M.D. (Ayurveda), N.D., Director of the American School of Ayurvedic Sciences in Bellevue, Washington, recommends warm herbal oils such as garlic or mullein in olive oil to remove ear wax.

Infection

Infection and inflammation often follow trauma to the ear. "A common cause is self-injury, usually from the overuse or misuse of cotton swabs and other objects placed in the ear for cleaning purposes," notes Dr. Kotsanis. "Infections are also commonly seen after swimming, especially in water that carries a heavy dose of either chlorine, bacteria, or fungi. Stubborn and repeated infections are usually fungal, and are commonly seen in patients with diabetes, allergies, cancer, and other chronic diseases."

Loud Noise

Twenty-eight million Americans suffer from some form of hearing and ear disorder, of which over one-third can be attributed to exposure to loud noise.[6] Depending on one's hearing sensitivity, sustained exposure to any sound over the 80 to 85 decibel level can cause permanent hearing damage. Potentially damaging sources of noise include jet planes (130 decibels at takeoff), jackhammers (110 decibels), personal stereos (110 decibels), and rock concerts (over 110 decibels). Sudden intense noise like a gunshot or dynamite blast can damage hearing instantly by tearing the tissue in the delicate inner ear.

Allergies

Researchers and physicians have drawn a link between repeated ear infections and allergic conditions such as hay fever, asthma, eczema, and hives.[7] Katie Data, N.D., of Fife, Washington, notes that an intolerance to particular foods such as wheat, and dairy products such as cow's milk, may encourage ear infections, inflammation, and hearing loss in some children. She notes that a large percentage of those who come to her with ear infections have ear problems related to the consumption of these foods. In such cases, young patients can often be successfully treated by the elimination of the offending foods from their diet.[8]

"Twenty-eight million Americans suffer from some form of hearing and ear disorder, of which over one-third can be attributed to exposure to loud noise."
—Gary Oberg, M.D.

According to Dr. Data, other factors to look for when treating infection or inflammation of the ear are environmental allergens such as dust, mold, and animal dander. She pays special attention to environmental allergens where a person sleeps.

Antibiotics

Otitis media is the most common reason parents bring their children to the doctor,[9] and accounts for 42 percent of all antibiotics prescribed to children.[10] According to Michael Schmidt, B.S., D.C., C.C.N., of Brookview Health Sciences in Anoka, Minnesota, while antibiotics are an important means of treating otitis media in some children, recent research has raised questions about their extensive use. One study from the University of Copenhagen in Denmark found that "eighty-eight percent of patients never need antibiotics, and that the frequency of recurrence of otitis media in the untreated group is low compared with those treated with antibiotics."[11] The study concluded that if a child is treated for an ear infection with an antibiotic within the first day or two of the onset of symptoms, the child is much more likely to get another ear infection within a month.

See Allergies, Antibiotics (in Appendix).

Another recent study raises doubts about the value of antibiotics in treating children with chronic, or longstanding earaches. In this study, children treated with the antibiotics amoxicillin, pediazole, and cefaclor fared no better than those given a placebo, and in fact, suffered recurrent middle ear fluid at a rate two to six times greater.[12] These findings are especially important when one considers that bacteria are only present in 50 to 70 percent of symptomatic ears. The remainder contain viruses, yeast, or inflammatory material which cannot be treated with antibiotics.[13]

According to William Crook, M.D., of Jackson, Tennessee, antibiotics used to treat ear infections upset the healthy balance of the normal intestinal flora, resulting in an overgrowth of the yeast, *Candida albicans*. Dr. Crook points out that this creates a cycle in which the immune system becomes suppressed, leading to recurrent ear infections.

Dr. Schmidt agrees, and cites a study in which children treated repeatedly with antibiotics for ear infections developed repeated yeast and fungal infections of the middle ear.[14] Lendon Smith, M.D., a pediatrician in Portland, Oregon, and author of many books on children's health, recommends that antibiotics only be used if the ear infection moves to the mastoid bone, found behind the ear, or the meninges (the three membranes covering the brain and spinal cord).

Treating Ear Disorders

Conventional medicine generally treats ear disorders with antibiotics and/or surgery. Every year, as treatment for otitis media, an estimated 1 million tympanotomy tubes (tubes inserted through the tympanic membrane, see ear diagram) are placed in the ears of American children to facilitate draining. Additionally, an equal number of children are given "prophylactic (preventative) antibiotics" in an effort to lessen the frequency of ear problems.[15]

These approaches, however, are often ineffective and can sometimes aggravate a condition. For instance, surgical implantation of ear tubes to promote drainage can lead to recurrent infections, while children who do not receive antibiotics for ear infections have fewer recurrences than those who do.[16]

When treating ear disorders, practitioners of alternative medicine first seek to identify the cause, be it diet, an intolerance to certain foods or environmental factors, infection, or trauma. Through the use of dietary changes, nutritional supplementation, allergy elimination, herbal remedies, homeopathy, Traditional Chinese Medicine, Ayurvedic medicine, craniosacral therapy, and auditory integration training, it is possible to alleviate conditions ranging from ear infections to tinnitus and hearing loss.

Dietary Changes

According to John Hibbs, N.D., of the Natural Health Clinic of Bastyr College in Seattle, Washington, making dietary changes such as cutting down on saturated fats and cholesterol, addressing intolerances to certain foods such as wheat and dairy products, and keeping sugar, sweets, and alcohol intake to a minimum (to limit yeast growth, especially if recurrent ear infections have been treated with antibiotics) are smart preventative steps that can have a profound effect on the health and well-being of the auditory system in both children and adults.

According to Katie Data, N.D., infants should not be bottle-fed while laying down, since this can lead to regurgitation into the middle ear, which can cause otitis media.

One diet-related study reveals a direct correlation between hearing and lipid (fat) levels. Several children with fluctuating sensorial hearing loss had their hearing return to near baseline when dietary controls were instituted.[24] In another study, over 1,400 patients with inner ear symptoms and increased lipoprotein (proteins that carry fat in the blood) levels were placed on individualized diets. In most patients, dizziness alleviated, the sensation of pressure in the ears dissipated, hearing improved and stabilized, and tinnitus often lessened in severity and sometimes disappeared.[25]

Nutritional Supplements

Dr. Hibbs points out that a deficiency of protein and iron in a child's diet can lead to ear infections, including otitis media. He recommends that, when necessary, a child's diet be supplemented with B vitamins as well as vitamins that contain iron to help prevent anemia, a condition that can lead to frequent ear infections. (Iron should not be given during an infection, and should only be given if an iron deficiency has been shown to exist. Excess iron can also lower immunity.)

When treating chronic otitis media, Dr. Data recommends supplements of beta-carotene and vitamin C, along with the use of N-acetyl cysteine, an amino acid, to remove the fluid. In

A NEW APPROACH TO TREATING OTITIS MEDIA

According to Michael Schmidt, B.S., D.C., C.C.N., of Brookview Health Sciences in Anoka, Minnesota, researchers are beginning to find important dietary, nutritional, and environmental correlations with otitis media. The middle ear fluid of children with repeated ear infections contains highly inflammatory substances that are, in part, related to dietary intake of essential fatty acids. These inflammatory substances can be reduced by modifying dietary fat intake and by taking antioxidant nutrients and certain trace elements such as zinc,[17] since children who suffer from repeated ear infections are more likely to be zinc deficient than their healthy counterparts.[18] Children exposed to heavy metals such as lead and mercury during their mothers' pregnancy are more likely to suffer from repeated infections of the ear, nose, and throat as well.[19]

Dr. Schmidt also points out that children who suffer viral infections, such as measles and chickenpox, commonly experience decreases in blood levels of vitamin A that may last for six to twelve months. This renders them more susceptible to secondary bacterial infections of the ears, nose, and throat.[20] Also, nutrient deficiencies that affect immune function have been found in various groups of children. For example, U.S. children had the lowest blood levels of vitamin E of any children in the industrialized world—one-half the level of Japanese children.[21]

A study of 104 children with chronic ear infections investigated the role that food may play. Of these, 81 were found to be allergic to one or more foods. When the offending foods were removed from the diet, 70 children experienced improvement of their middle ear condition. When the offending foods were reintroduced, most of the children experienced a worsening of their condition.[22] Another study found that 19 of 20 children with chronic earaches which had not responded to any other treatment, had their condition resolved after food allergy management.[23]

In conclusion, Dr. Schmidt points out that "the questions being raised about the safety and effectiveness of antibiotics and surgery (the placement of tympanotomy tubes), coupled with new discoveries about the role of diet, allergy, nutrition, environment, and other factors, should cause doctors and patients to take a new look at the problem of otitis media in children. At the very least, one should consider the role of food and food allergy. Perhaps we should not be asking, 'How can we kill this or that bacteria?', but, 'How can we optimize the immune defenses of all children?' Addressing the underlying reasons children become sick, while reserving antibiotics and surgery for those who truly need them, seems to be the most sensible solution to the nation's most common pediatric health problem."

cases where otitis media was treated with antibiotics, she stresses the importance of using acidophilus to reconstitute the normal digestive tract flora. Nutritional supplementation with vitamins A and C, bioflavinoids, and zinc may also be beneficial.[26] Additionally, thymus extract given orally has been shown to decrease children's food allergies, improve immune function, and may be of particular benefit in chronic otitis media.[27]

Allergy Elimination

In treating ear disorders, Dr. Hibbs gives high priority to identifying allergies. "I look for related problems such as allergies in the respiratory tract or any indication that other types of allergies might exist, including intolerance to certain foods, as these can create a type of immune weakness that leads not only to mechanical irritation but chronic ear infections as well. When there is an allergy to dairy products or wheat, congestion typically occurs in the middle ear."

When treating infants or children, Dr. Data explains that breast-feeding and the removal from the diet of any food to which the patient is allergic are the recommended preventative measures for otitis media, which occurs most frequently in infants and small children. Human milk provides immunologic protection for the child, and avoiding food allergens is important because a child's digestive tract is quite permeable to food antigens.[28]

Dr. Data cites the case of a fifteen-month-old baby suffering from chronic otitis media. The baby had not been breast-fed and had been given a milk-based formula from birth. After examination, she suggested the removal of all dairy and dairy-related products from the infant's diet (milk, cheese, and yogurt) and the use of herbal eardrops. The child's symptoms disappeared almost immediately.

Herbal Remedies

Herbal remedies have proven effective in treating a number of ear disorders, according to Dr. Hibbs. To treat ear infections, he uses a combination of goldenseal, mullein, and hypericum in a glycerine base to reduce ear pain and to help draw excess fluid out of the ear. Echinacea and goldenseal can also be used as antibacterials, adds Dr. Hibbs.

For otitis media, David L. Hoffmann, B.Sc., M.N.I.M.H., of Sebastopol, California, past President of the American Herbalist Guild, combines equal parts echinacea and cleavers tinctures and prescribes one teaspoonful three times a day (if this mixture is used for children, he recommends using the glycerates). Warm mullein flower oil introduced into the ear can be an effective anti-inflammatory, but he warns to avoid this treatment if there is any perforation of the ear drum.

Ginkgo biloba increases circulation in and around the ear area and is commonly used to treat tinnitus.[29] Hoffmann recommends combining the tinctures of black cohosh and *Ginkgo biloba* in equal parts and taking one teaspoon of this mixture three times a day.

See Herbal Medicine, Homeopathy.

Dr. Kotsanis reports one case of a teenage girl with severe tinnitus whom he successfully treated with *Ginkgo biloba*. Tests revealed an overall hearing level of twenty decibels, meaning the patient had trouble hearing sounds of a lower volume than twenty decibels. After six weeks of *Ginkgo biloba* treatments (Dr. Kotsanis' general recommendations are 50 to 200 milligrams three times a day for three months), the patient's tinnitus was relieved and, moreover, her hearing improved to the point that she could hear sounds in the one to five decibel range.

Homeopathy

Several homeopathic remedies are useful in the treatment of various stages of otitis media. Robert D. Milne, M.D., of Las Vegas, Nevada, recommends *Aconite* and *Ferrum phos.*, for the early stages of otitis media. For later stages or recurrent infections, he recommends *Belladonna, Chamomilla, Hepar sulf., Lycopodium, Merc sol., Pulsatilla,* and *Silicea*. Depending on the presenting symptoms, food sensitivities must be eliminated from the diet.

Dr. Milne points out that many patients who suffer from Meniere's disease have a history of migraines. Depending on the symptoms, he treats Meniere's with specific homeopathic remedies such as *Carboneum sulphuratum* and *Salicylicum acidum*, in addition to the herb *Ginkgo biloba* (to increase circulation), vitamin B_6 (to decrease fluid buildup) and restrictions on sodium, caffeine, and chocolate. The patient should also check for sensitivity to dental amalgams.

Several homeopathic remedies may help in the treatment of tinnitus as well, according to Dr. Milne. They include *Salicylicum acidum, Chenopodium,* and *Cinchona officinalis*. The appropriate remedy depends upon the type of noise heard by the patient.

Traditional Chinese Medicine

According to Traditional Chinese Medicine, ear problems are associated with kidney function. Thus, acupuncture points related to the kidney are used to treat a range of ear disorders. Roger Hirsh, O.M.D., of Santa Monica, California, treats ear disorders with a combination of acupuncture and Chinese herbs. He often uses an herbal preparation called *er long zuo gi wan*, a classical herbal remedy for kidney disturbances.

Dr. Hirsh cites the case of a thirty-five-year-old woman with nerve deafness in her left ear. After obtaining her medical history, acupuncture was recommended, and two acupuncture needles were placed in her ankles, two in her knees, two in her hand, and two near the ear. When the knee points were treated with moxa (herbs burned on the acupuncture needles), the hearing immediately returned to her left ear.

Dr. Hirsh also utilized acupuncture to treat a sixty-five-year-old woman with tinnitus. By increasing the circulation of *qi* (vital life energy) around the ear, the woman reported that, after six sessions, her tinnitus was 80 percent relieved.

Ayurvedic Medicine

Ayurvedic medicine uses a combination of oils, massage, herbs, and nutritional supplements to treat ear disorders. According to Virender Sodhi, M.D. (Ayurveda), N.D., Director of the American School of Ayurvedic Sciences in Bellevue, Washington, the most effective oil for treating ear infections is *neem*, which is both antibacterial and antifungal. Dr. Sodhi combines *neem* with warm *Adardica indica* oil, and places it in the ear.

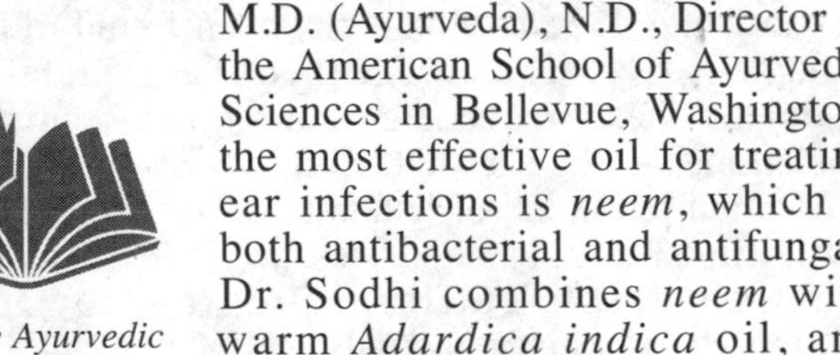

See Ayurvedic Medicine, Craniosacral Therapy, Sound Therapy, Traditional Chinese Medicine.

Dr. Sodhi also employs lymphatic massage outside the ears to open the eustachian tube and facilitate drainage. In addition, he uses the herb *amla*, which is not only antibacterial and antiviral, but a good source of vitamin C. It can be given in raw honey and helps stimulate the immune system.

Dr. Sodhi uses *albad* oil, herbs, and supplements to treat hearing loss. He recommends black pepper and Indian long pepper to improve digestion and elimination and to increase the circulation around the ear. Beneficial herbs include *ashwaganda*, *bala*, and *calamus*, all of which are known to increase circulation.

In treating Meniere's disease, Dr. Sodhi uses *albad* oil in the ear to draw out excess fluid. He also gives *albad* oil, sesame oil, and *ghee* (clarified butter) internally, and prescribes rest and lymphatic drainage massage. For tinnitus, Dr. Sodhi recommends warm *albad* oil in the ear.

Craniosacral Therapy

According to John Upledger, D.O., Medical Director of the Upledger Institute in Palm Beach Gardens, Florida, craniosacral therapy can be beneficial in treating hearing disorders caused by problems associated with the temporal bone (the bones on both sides of the skull at its base, one portion of which encloses the organ of hearing). "When the temporal bone is out of alignment with the rest of the bones of the cranium, hearing can be affected, and tinnitus may be the result," says Dr. Upledger. "This problem can be solved through craniosacral therapy by adjusting the temporal bone.

"The temporal bone can also be affected if the bite is off, and this can interfere with proper hearing," adds Dr. Upledger. "A problem with the bite can also prevent proper drainage of the eustachian tube, leading to a blockage which can result in hearing problems. Craniosacral therapy can successfully address both of these problems. It can also be used to relieve pressure on the temporal lobes of the brain which may be interfering with the hearing process," says Dr. Upledger. "Words may sound scrambled to the listener, and when the pressure is released, they can hear normally again."

Auditory Integration Training

Auditory integration training may be effective for patients who are hypersensitive to high-frequency sounds or suffer from loss of hearing in normal frequency ranges. The technique was developed by two French physicians, Alfred Tomatis, M.D., and Guy Berard, E.N.T. Both the Tomatis and the Berard methods provide auditory stimulation to the listener.

Dr. Tomatis theorizes that listening problems can begin at any time, even in utero, due to accident, illness, or physical or emotional trauma. Using a device called the Electronic Ear, Dr. Tomatis established a system of auditory training that emphasizes a connection between listening, language, and learning. Tomatis' method presents different types of sounds to the listener in an attempt to recreate critical periods of listening development. Specially prepared audiotapes containing music and voice are played into the Electronic Ear, which uses several controls, including filters, to simulate what Dr. Tomatis believes to be the developmental stages of listening. High- and low-frequency sounds are extracted from the sound source and then played to the listener. Low-frequency sounds are gradually eliminated in part of the program, leaving only the high frequencies which, according to Dr. Tomatis, "energize" the brain. In another part of the program, the person speaks into the Electronic

THE INVISIBLE DISABILITY—INFANTS AND HEARING LOSS

According to Katie Data, N.D., of Fife, Washington, although the incidence of pediatric hearing loss is thirteen per one thousand live births, the average age of identifying a child with significant hearing loss is two and a half years of age. This late identification has profound consequences in that it can leave a child unnecessarily handicapped for life. "A child is never too young to be evaluated for hearing loss," says Dr. Data.

Risk factors that can lead to hearing loss include premature birth, low birth weight, newborn jaundice, certain drugs (e.g. tobramycin, streptomycin, quinine, gentamycin, furosemide, ethacrynic acid), meningitis, and hereditary disorders such as otosclerosis (scarring of the membranes of the ear). Hearing loss may be present if a child does not respond to a spoken voice or ordinary household sounds. Delayed speech is also a significant sign.

Since the window for language acquisition is birth to four years of age, early identification of hearing loss is essential for normal language acquisition and development to occur. However, according to Dr. Data, most physicians and health care providers are not adequately trained to pick up hearing loss. Parents whose concerns are hastily dismissed should find a physician who will listen, says Dr. Data, emphasizing that "a child does not outgrow a hearing loss," and that "every minute of a child's development is precious."

There are many resources available once a hearing loss is detected, but early detection (before the first birthday) is critical to minimize the handicap in later years.

Ear microphone to listen to his or her own voice while repeating words and phrases, or reading, in order to establish good audio-vocal control.

A three-year-old girl who had been deaf for the first eighteen months of her life was treated with the Tomatis method. When she first began to hear at eighteen months, she was not able to process the sounds because they were so foreign to her, according to Billie Thompson, Ph.D., Director of the Sound, Listening and Learning Center in Phoenix, Arizona. Over the next year and a half she was unmanageable, displayed constant tantrums, and continually failed hearing tests. After sixty hours with the Electronic Ear, in conjunction with daily speech therapy, she began to speak, allowing her to enter nursery school where she is now fully functional.

Similar to the Tomatis method, Dr. Berard's method is based upon the belief that behavioral and cognitive problems can arise when certain frequencies are perceived in a distorted manner, and that this altered perception can then lead to difficulties in comprehension and behavior. By using a device called the Ears Education and Retraining System (EERS), Dr. Berard claims that distorted hearing and hypersensitivity to specific frequencies are reduced and that, ideally, all frequencies can be perceived equally well. The device takes music from a sound source (audio tape or compact disc) and filters out the frequencies to which the individual has been found to be hypersensitive. The EERS then electronically modulates these frequencies and returns them via headphones to the ears. Dr. Berard has found that after about ten hours of listening to the processed music (in twenty half-hour sessions), the listener usually makes significant progress toward hearing all frequencies equally well.

> *"A child is never too young to be evaluated for hearing loss."*
> —Katie Data, N.D.

One of Dr. Berard's patients was an eleven-year-old autistic girl who suffered from both a hypo- (low) and hyperacute (high) sense of hearing. Over the course of the twenty half-hour sessions using the EERS, Dr. Berard was able to decrease the hyperacute points of the girl's hearing while bringing the deficits up, thus creating a more normal hearing pattern. This also helped correct the girl's dyslexia, attention deficit, and hyperactivity. She is now a happily married college graduate, working on a University of Oregon research project to help autistic adults.

Professional Care

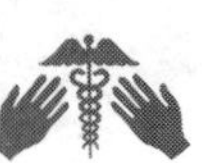

The following therapies should only be provided by a qualified health professional:

• Cell Therapy • Chiropractic • Environmental Medicine • Magnetic Field Therapy

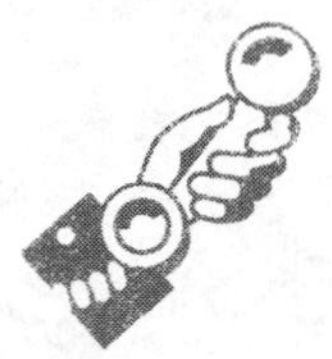

Where to Find Help

For more information on or referrals for the treatment of hearing and ear disorders, contact:

American Association of Acupuncture and Oriental Medicine (AAAOM)
4101 Lake Boone Trail, Suite 201
Raleigh, North Carolina 27607
(919) 787-5181
The AAAOM is a national professional trade organization of acupuncturists who meet acceptable standards of competency and can provide you with the names and locations of local members. Referrals by written request only.

American Academy of Environmental Medicine (AAEM)
P.O. Box 16106
Denver, Colorado 80216
(303) 622-9755
The academy offers extensive training for physicians interested in learning more about environmental medicine. For information on physicians practicing environmental medicine send a self-addressed, stamped envelope stating your request.

American Association of Naturopathic Physicians
2366 Eastlake Avenue, Suite 322
Seattle, Washington 98102
(206) 323-7610
Provides a directory of naturopathic physicians and offers referrals to a nationwide network of accredited or licensed practitioners. Publishes a quarterly newsletter for both professionals and the general public. Also offers a series of brochures and pamphlets on a variety of subjects.

American Holistic Medical Association
4101 Lake Boone Trail, Suite 201
Raleigh, North Carolina 27607
(919) 787-5181
A professional organization for holistic practitioners, the AHMA offers information and services for its members and lobbies for holistic issues. It also provides referrals for the public.

The Georgania Organization, Inc.
P.O. Box 2607
Westport, Connecticut 06880
(203) 454-1221
Provides education, workshops, consulting, and information on the Berard method.

International Foundation for Homeopathy
2366 Eastlake Avenue, East, Suite 301
Seattle, Washington 98102
(206) 324-8230
Provides educational courses for professionals and the general public. Offers referrals to homeopathic health professionals.

National Center for Homeopathy
801 North Fairfax, Suite 306
Alexandria, Virginia 22314
(703) 548-7790
Provides a referral list of practicing homeopaths and information. Gives courses for lay people and professionals, and organizes study groups around the country.

Sound, Listening & Learning Center
2701 East Camelback, Suite 205
Phoenix, Arizona 85016
(602) 381-0086
Provides education, workshops, consulting, therapeutic sessions, and information on the Tomatis method.

Recommended Reading

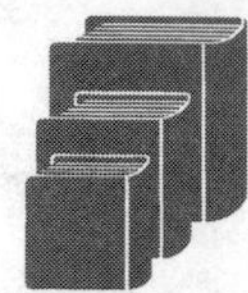

About the Tomatis Method. Gilmore, T.; Maudale, P.; and Thompson, B. Toronto: Listening Center Press, 1989.

Presents Alfred Tomatis' research on the ear, brain, and communication. Reveals the role of listening in human communication with specific attention to learning disabilities.

Beyond Antibiotics: Healthier Options for Families. Schmidt, Dr. Michael A.;, Smith, Dr. Lendon H.; and Sehnert, Dr. Keith W. Berkeley, CA: North Atlantic Books, 1992.

Contains an extensive discussion on the problems of antibiotic overuse. The focus of this book, however, is on practical alternatives in the area of diet, nutrition, lifestyle, environment, stress, and psychology with an emphasis on self care. It is written for the layperson, but contains an extensive list of references from the medical literature.

Childhood Ear Infections (What Every Parent and Physician Should Know). Schmidt, Michael, B.S., D.C., C.C.N., Berkeley, CA: North Atlantic Books, 1990.

This book details the story of Georgiana Stehli's recovery from autism, as well as Dr. Berard's auditory training technique.

The New Holistic Herbal. Hoffman, David. Shaftesbury, England: Ailment Books, 1990.

A comprehensive, introductory guide to the use of herbal medicine in holistic healing. It covers health and wellness as well as treatments for a range of different conditions and recipes for the preparation of herbal medicine.

Heart Disease

Although heart disease causes half of all deaths in the United States,[1] it is one of the most preventable chronic degenerative diseases. It now appears that the primary culprit in heart disease is not high cholesterol levels, but the presence of oxidized cholesterol in the bloodstream. Overwhelming evidence shows that the risk of heart attacks and strokes can be greatly decreased through dietary changes, exercise, stress reduction, and nutritional supplementation to help prevent excessive oxidation of cholesterol in the bloodstream.

The United States leads the world in death rates from heart disease, with over 60 million Americans currently suffering from the disease.[2] "The average American lifestyle, combining too little exercise, too much stress, and a diet of highly processed foods often deficient in essential nutrients, has rendered this nation's population especially vulnerable to the ravages of heart ailments," says William Lee Cowden, M.D., a cardiologist from Dallas, Texas.

> *"The average American lifestyle, combining too little exercise, too much stress, and a diet of highly processed foods often deficient in essential nutrients, has rendered this nation's population especially vulnerable to the ravages of heart ailments."*
> —William Lee Cowden, M.D.

Conventional medicine believes that the answer to fighting heart disease lies in treating symptoms such as high blood pressure or elevated cholesterol levels with medication. Expensive heart bypass surgeries and angioplasties (surgical alteration of blood vessels) are performed with increasing regularity, while cholesterol-lowering drugs further fuel the skyrocketing costs associated with heart disease. As a result, the medical cost of cardiovascular disease in the United States exceeds $56 billion a year.[3]

Some physicians choose to reduce a patient's risk factors for heart disease by considering preventive measures such as stress reduction, exercise, dietary improvement, weight control, and the elimination of smoking. "Although these methods have resulted in some leveling off of the rate of heart disease," says Garry F. Gordon, M.D., of Tempe, Arizona, co-founder of the American College of Advancement in Medicine, "the epidemic continues and conventional medicine continues to use drugs and surgery as the primary treatments for heart disease."

It is obvious that conventional medicine is largely failing in its battle against heart disease. Alternative medicine, by contrast, is providing exciting new options in treating the disease. In opposition to complicated, costly, and often dangerous surgery and drugs, many health care professionals who practice alternative medicine work to correct the nutritional and biochemical imbalances that can affect the functioning of the heart and deposition of plaque in the arteries. For example, raising blood or tissue levels of nutrients like vitamin B_6 and magnesium, as well as antioxidants such as vitamin E, vitamin C, coenzyme Q10, and selenium, has been shown to have a positive impact on heart disease.[4] Chelation therapy, acupuncture, and herbal remedies such as hawthorn berries, *Ginkgo biloba*, garlic, and cayenne[5] may also be effective in the treatment of heart disease.

See Hypertension.

Atherosclerosis: The Primary Cause of Cardiovascular Disease

A common precursor of heart disease is atherosclerosis, in which the inner arterial walls harden and thicken due to deposits of fatty substances. These substances form a plaque, which in turn causes a narrowing of the arteries.[6] Over time, plaque can block the arteries and interrupt blood flow to the organs they supply, including the heart and brain. Atherosclerosis of the coronary arteries (the arteries supplying the muscle of the heart), known as coronary heart disease, is one of the most common forms of heart disease in the United States today. Coronary heart disease can lead to angina and heart attack, while atherosclerosis of the cerebral arteries (the arteries that supply blood to the brain) can precipitate strokes.

Heart Attack

Atherosclerosis that occurs in the coronary arteries can deprive the heart of oxygen-rich blood until the affected area of the heart literally dies, causing a myocardial infarction (heart attack), sometimes leading to cardiac arrest or death. Heart attacks are responsible for over 550,000 deaths annually in the United States.[7]

Often, a diminished blood supply to the heart exhibits few symptoms until the blockage is so great that a heart attack results. But while a heart attack may appear to come on suddenly, it often begins with years of physical neglect, such as a poor diet and lack of exercise. Genetic predisposition can also be a crucial factor.

Angina

Angina, or discomfort, heaviness, or pressure in the chest or throat, may also be a symptom of coronary artery disease. Angina can result when there are lesions in either the coronary arteries, walls, or valves of the heart. These lesions diminish the supply of oxygenated blood to the heart muscle, causing discomfort to radiate from the throat or chest to the shoulder and down the left arm, in some cases. During exercise or increased effort, some people may suffer from chest discomfort as a result of a lack of oxygen in the heart muscle, while others experience angina without discomfort (silent angina). Angina is a warning sign that there are problems with the heart, but is not necessarily a precursor of a heart attack if appropriate treatment is initiated.

Stroke

Twenty-five percent of the blood pumped from the heart goes to the brain, and if the blood flow to a part of the brain is interrupted for any reason, the affected brain cells are deprived of oxygen and die, resulting in a stroke,[8] the third leading cause of death in the United States. Stroke can lead to loss of speech, physical movement, or eyesight, depending on the area of the brain affected. Of the 500,000 Americans who suffer a stroke every year, nearly two-thirds risk the possibility of becoming handicapped. There are currently over 2 million people in the United States disabled by stroke.[9]

Atherosclerosis of the cerebral arteries can affect blood flow to the brain and increase the risk of stroke. A stroke can also result from a blood clot that has formed in a narrowed cerebral artery, or as a result of a clot formed elsewhere in the body (an embolus), usually in the heart or arteries of the neck, and carried in the bloodstream to the head. Other causes include a blood vessel that ruptures or hemorrhages causing blood to spill into the brain, not only damaging the brain cells directly, but resulting in further damage to brain tissue due to lack of oxygen when the blood supply is interrupted. Strokes have also been associated with inherited disorders, birth defects, and certain rare blood diseases.[10]

How Plaque Forms in Arteries

Atherosclerosis may be well underway even at birth. In investigating the deaths of newborn babies in Scandinavia from a variety of causes, it was found that nearly 97 percent had some

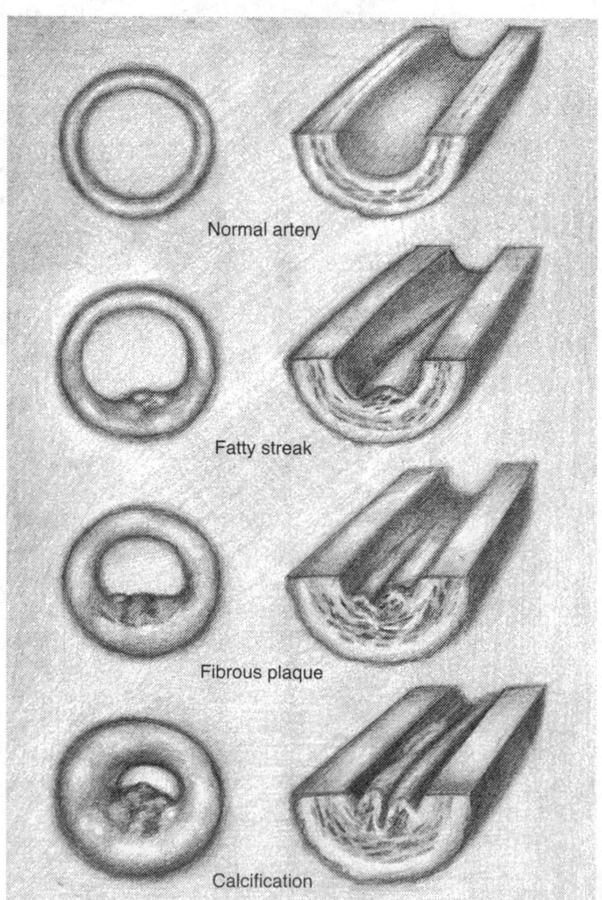

Advanced atherosclerotic plaque.

degree of arterial thickening, the first step in heart disease.[11] Plaque formation in arteries usually follows prior damage to the inner lining of the arteries. According to Dr. Cowden, deficiencies of nutrients such as vitamin C, vitamin E, and magnesium make this inner lining more susceptible to damage and plaque formation. "Small tears can occur in the lining of the arteries after a sudden very high blood pressure episode brought on by stress," explains Dr. Cowden, who adds that, "the vessels cannot always dilate rapidly enough to accommodate the sudden increase in pressure and tearing occurs." He explains how collagen (a protein of the connective tissue), clotting proteins, and other chemical substances are released into the bloodstream to repair the tear. These substances adhere at the site and attract platelets, special blood cells responsible for clotting. "Other cells are attracted to the repair site, including white blood cells laden with oxidized cholesterol which is deposited at the site and initiates soft plaque formation," says Dr. Cowden. "Calcium is then attracted to the site and solid plaques, which are more difficult to remove, are formed."

> *"In fact, in most people, less than 5 percent of the cholesterol in the bloodstream gets there through diet."*
> —William Lee Cowden, M.D.

Cholesterol, which has long been cast as the villain in heart disease, is a waxy, oily substance necessary for the maintenance of the body's cells. In fact, according to Dr. Cowden, the human liver synthesizes about three thousand milligrams of new cholesterol in any twenty-four hour period, a quantity equivalent to the amount contained in ten eggs. "This new cholesterol is used to repair cells," he says. "In fact, in most people less than 5 percent of the cholesterol in the bloodstream gets there through diet."

Cholesterol levels in the body are determined by measuring the levels of lipoproteins in the blood (proteins that carry fats in the bloodstream). This includes high density lipoprotein (HDL) and low density lipoprotein (LDL). Testing cholesterol levels allows physicians to determine how effectively the body is metabolizing cholesterol and how much remains in the bloodstream. LDL cho-

How Oxidized Cholesterol Is Formed

Oxidized cholesterol (known as oxysterols) enters the bloodstream either from processed foods, from the metabolism of ingested animal products, from environmental pollutants such as chlorine, fluoride, and chlorinated pesticides such as DDT, or from various stressors such as infections, traumas, and emotional stress.[12] According to researcher Joseph Hattersley, M.A., of Olympia, Washington, many oxysterols reach people through the air-dried powdered milk and eggs used in processed foods, as well as in fast food products.[13] Lard, kept hot and used repeatedly to cook French fries and potato chips, is loaded with oxysterols, as are gelatin preparations, says Hattersley.

"Scrambled eggs and hamburgers are big culprits in the production of oxysterols," according to James Privitera, M.D., of Covina, California. "Oxygen and intense heat from cooking quickly oxidizes unsaturated fats."

Another source of oxysterols is methionine, an essential amino acid found in red meat, milk, and milk products. Methionine is converted in the body to homocysteine, which is normally converted in the body to the harmless amino acid, cystathionine. But in individuals deficient in the enzyme necessary to convert homocysteine to cystathionine, homocysteine will be abnormally high. This excess homocysteine is capable of generating free radicals which are capable of producing oxysterols. It is reported that men with high homocysteine levels have three times more heart attacks than men with low levels.[14]

The conversion in the body of homocysteine to cystathionine requires sufficient levels of vitamin B_6, folic acid, and vitamin B_{12}.[15] Also, if sufficient antioxidants are present in the bloodstream (vitamin C, vitamin E, and beta-carotene for example), oxysterols can be neutralized and prevented from damaging the vessel walls. But stress depletes the body of vitamin B_6 and vitamin C, and this depletion can lead to a further buildup of homocysteine, which can in turn cause the generation of oxysterols.

Oxysterols can also be generated internally through exposure to environmental pollutants and pesticides. Chemicals that oxidize cholesterol include chlorine and fluoride, both of which are ingested from tap water.[16] Chlorine has been shown to have an effect on the arteries, and fluoride lowers thyroid function which in turn allows levels of cholesterol and homocysteine to rise.[17] Chlorine in drinking water also forms trihalomethanes (THM's—carcinogens formed when chlorine interacts with organic chemicals in water) which, according to Hattersley, create oxysterols.[18]

STRESS, HEART DISEASE, AND ATHEROSCLEROSIS

Stress can also contribute to the process of plaque buildup in the arteries. "When people are under stress, they form more free radicals, which cause a greater conversion of normal cholesterol into oxidized cholesterol (oxysterols)," says William Lee Cowden, M.D., a cardiologist in Dallas, Texas. "These oxysterols then build up in white blood cells and are carried to the site of damage in the arteries." He adds that stress also stimulates the release of adrenalin, which in turn has been shown to cause platelet aggregation (blood clotting) and increased blood viscosity (thickness).[23] *Increases in blood viscosity can result in spontaneous clot formation. These can either adhere to arterial walls, initiating further plaque formation, or become lodged in narrowed arteries or capillaries, initiating a heart attack or stroke.*

lesterol is often referred to as "bad" cholesterol because it appears to deposit fats on arterial walls and causes the most arterial damage.[19]

However, LDL cholesterol becomes harmful only after it has been oxidized (the process of a substance combining with oxygen) from exposure to free radical substances such as unstable oxygen molecules, homocysteine (an amino acid), or chlorine (from drinking chlorinated water), according to Dr. Cowden. Therefore, oxidized cholesterol should be considered the real culprit in atherosclerosis, as it can work to initiate plaque formation on arterial walls which can lead to atherosclerosis and ultimately to heart attacks and strokes.[20]

"We've been living on cholesterol phobia for twenty years," says Richard Passwater, Ph.D., of Berlin, Maryland, "but nothing matters unless you prevent the oxidation of cholesterol."

Preventing and Reversing Heart Disease

Through the use of a variety of natural therapies, the risk of heart disease may be greatly reduced. These same approaches may also benefit those already suffering from heart disease. They include dietary changes, nutritional supplementation, herbal medicine, chelation therapy, detoxification, oxygen therapy, exercise and stress reduction, Traditional Chinese Medicine, and Ayurvedic medicine.

During the teenage and young adult years when bad dietary and exercise habits can most easily be altered, much can be done to protect the body against heart disease. Although initial damage done to the arteries can cause the buildup of plaque, it can be corrected through diet and nutritional supplements.

Diet

Dietary management can be highly effective in reversing heart disease. Dean Ornish, M.D., Assistant Clinical Professor of Medicine at the University of California at San Francisco, used a vegetarian diet, exercise, and stress-reduction techniques to reverse arterial buildup of plaque.[21] His "reversal diet" is almost entirely free of cholesterol, animal fats, and oils. Dr. Ornish found that the condition of those patients who followed the diet improved, while the condition of those who continued eating a diet high in fat got worse.[22]

According to Dr. Cowden, however, the success of Dr. Ornish's diet is due, not primarily to low levels of cholesterol and fats, but to both low levels of methionine (an amino acid found in red meat, milk, and milk products, and a precursor to homocysteine, a free radical generator capable of oxidizing cholesterol), and to a high intake of vegetables and grains. These foods are rich in those vitamins (B_6, C, and E, and beta-carotene), which are necessary to act as co-factors for antioxidants and antiatherogenics (substances preventing atherosclerosis).

DRUGS ASSOCIATED WITH A HIGHER INCIDENCE OF CONGESTIVE HEART FAILURE

According to the Physicians Desk Reference *the following drugs are associated with side effects of congestive heart failure. (Statistics refer to the percentage of individuals affected.)*[24]

Emcyt Capsules (3%)
Ethmozine Tablets (1-5%)
Lupron Depot 3.75 milligrams (Among most frequent), Injection (5% or more)
Novantrone for Injection Concentrate (0-5%)
Rythmol tablets (0.8-3.7%)
Tambocor Tablets (Approximately 5%)
Tonocard Tablets (4%)
Zoladex (5%)

To reduce the level of oxidized cholesterol in the bloodstream, Dr. Passwater suggests combining a dietary regime (under 30 percent of daily calories from fat so as not to raise LDL cholesterol levels), with a personalized nutritional supplementation program. "What needs to be done," says Dr. Passwater, "is to first control the LDL cholesterol through diet, then raise the antioxidant level to prevent oxidized cholesterol from doing damage." Clearly, a healthy diet that limits sources of homocysteine-generating fat, such as red meat and fried food, can keep the body's systems operating more smoothly.

Supplementing the diet with essential fatty acids (EFA's) may also help to lower the level of homocysteine.[25] Omega-3 essential fatty acids are useful in reducing high LDL cholesterol levels and may prevent heart attacks by eliminating clotting and arterial damage.[26] Omega-6 EFA's have been shown to decrease the aggregation or stickiness of platelets, allowing them to pass through the arteries without danger of clotting.[27] Dr. Cowden notes that the best natural sources of omega-3 EFA's are flaxseed oil and cold saltwater fish such as Scandanavian salmon, orange roughy, and albacore tuna. Omega-6 EFA's are most abundantly found in borage oil, black currant oil, and evening primrose oil. These oils should not be rancid and should be cold-pressed so that no fatty acids are lost. Dr. Cowden recommends taking at least equal amounts of omega-3 whenever taking omega-6 fatty acids.

Dr. Cowden puts many of his heart patients through a detoxification regimen consisting of a vegetarian diet, vegetable juices mixed with garlic, and, in some cases, cayenne, as well as low temperature saunas. This program helps to cleanse the body of toxins which may be contributing to free radical damage to the artery walls and the buildup of arterial plaque. He also often uses homeopathic remedies to aid in the detoxification.

A NEW METHOD OF OBSERVING BLOOD CLOTTING ACTIVITY

James Privitera M.D., of Covina, California, has perfected a diagnostic technique to view patients' live blood cells as well as clotting activity through the use of a "darkfield" microscope, which illuminates the sample with specially angled halogen light. "Ninety percent of heart attacks are caused by blood clots at the site of an atherosclerotic lesion, and 90 percent of strokes are caused by platelet aggregation (blood clotting)," says Dr. Privitera, noting that dietary changes and nutritional supplements can be used to correct these problems. Dr. Privitera also suggests eating foods low in saturated fats and high in complex carbohydrates, and taking vitamins C, B_6, E, garlic and the essential fatty acids, EPA and DHA.

GENERAL DIETARY GUIDELINES

According to William Lee Cowden, M.D., a cardiologist from Dallas, Texas, the following dietary guidelines are helpful in preventing heart disease:

- *Eat minimally processed foods (avoid additives and preservatives or foods containing powdered eggs or powdered milk).*
- *Buy organic foods (free of pesticides, herbicides, steroids, and antibiotics) whenever possible.*
- *Avoid irradiated foods whenever possible.*
- *Increase fiber from sources like green leafy vegetables, fresh raw fruits, bran, whole grains, and psyllium.*
- *Reduce fat intake, especially fried foods, animal fats, and partially hydrogenated oils. Increase complex carbohydrates such as whole grains, beans, seeds, and potatoes.*
- *Use monounsaturated oils (such as cold-pressed olive oil and canola oil), omega-3 oils (flaxseed oil or oils from deep ocean fish) and omega-6 oils (borage, black currant oil, or evening primrose oil). Oils must be fresh and cold-pressed (rancid oils can be harmful).*
- *Reduce meat, sugar, tobacco, and alcohol consumption, which are all sources of free radicals. For example, sugar can cause damage to gallbladder and bowel function, which can in turn lead to reduced absorption of fat-soluble antioxidant nutrients like vitamin E and the increased absorption of free radicals produced by bacterial action in the stagnant colon.*

Nutritional Supplements

Because atherosclerosis and heart disease take many years to develop, a daily regimen of supplements may be helpful in preventing both. The amount of supplements needed varies from one individual to another depending on body weight and absorption levels, and it is best to consult with a nutritionally skilled physician or naturopathic physician before embarking on a routine of supplements.

Recent studies have shown that vitamins B_6, B_{12}, and folic acid can dramatically lower homocysteine, a free radical generator capable of oxidizing cholesterol, one of the major contributing factors in heart disease.[28]

Vitamin B_6: Researchers have found vitamin B_6 to be a safe and inexpensive supplement which may be helpful in preventing heart attacks and strokes.[29] Vitamin B_6 is needed for the conversion of homocysteine to the harmless chemical, cystathionine, thus preventing the homocysteine-induced oxidation of cholesterol.[30] It has also been suggested that vitamin B_6 inhibits the platelet aggregation which occurs in atherosclerosis.[31] The typical American diet, however, leaves many people significantly deficient in this vital nutrient.

In 1949, Moses M. Suzman, M.D., a South African neurologist and internist, gathered a group of pre-cardiac patients who showed signs of arterial damage and had them take one hundred milligrams of vitamin B_6 per day, while patients who had already had heart attacks or angina were given two hundred milligrams per day (half in a B complex including choline). In addition, the patients with the most serious conditions were given five milligrams of folic acid, one hundred to six hundred IU of vitamin E, magnesium, and zinc.[32]

Over the next twenty-three years, Dr. Suzman's patients recovered rapidly, as their angina and electrocardiographic irregularities diminished or disappeared. Those who dropped out of the vitamin and diet regimen, however, soon found their cardiac problems returning.[33]

Interest in vitamin B_6 deficiency and its relationship to heart disease revived in 1969, when Kilmer S. McCully, M.D., a Professor of Pathology at Harvard Medical School, found that heart patients had nearly 80 percent less of the vitamin than healthy individuals.[34] From this, Dr. McCully postulated that B_6 may help the body resist the arterial damage that precipitates heart disease. He also found that patients who had already suffered a heart attack or angina, and were then given two hundred milligrams of B_6 daily (half in a B complex including choline), combined with a low-fat, mostly vegetarian diet, recovered rapidly.[35]

Vitamin B_{12}: A deficiency in vitamin B_{12} is associated with elevated homocysteine levels.[36] When vitamin B_{12} is supplemented, homocysteine levels decrease.[37] This effect can be increased by also supplementing choline, folic acid, riboflavin, and B_6.[38]

Folic Acid: Folic acid is essential for the proper metabolism of homocysteine.[39]

Antioxidants such as vitamin E, vitamin C, selenium, and coenzyme Q10 have also proven in numerous studies to be effective in both the prevention and treatment of heart disease.[40]

Vitamin E: Vitamin E is a fat-soluble antioxidant which can help prevent abnormal blood clot formation. Dr. Passwater believes that any nutrient that prevents the oxidation of cholesterol, like vitamin E, beta-carotene, and coenzyme Q10, offers a protective factor. Supplementation of vitamin E may also inhibit platelet aggregation[41] and help repair lining cells of blood vessels.[42]

Two recent studies published in the *New England Journal of Medicine* suggest that vitamin E can contribute greatly to the prevention of heart disease in both men and women.[43] In one of the studies done at Harvard Medical School, involving a group of 87,245 female nurses, it was found that those who took one hundred IU of vitamin E daily for more than two years had a 46 percent lower risk of heart disease.[44] In the other study, also at Harvard, 39,910 male health professionals who took one hundred IU of vitamin E daily for an unspecified time period had a 37 percent lower risk of heart disease.[45] Groups who took higher doses of vitamin E for a longer time produced even greater results.

CAUTION

High dosages of vitamin E are not recommended for people with hypertension, rheumatic heart disease, or ischemic heart disease except under close medical supervision.[47] However, in hypertensive or ischemic heart disease patients, if the dose of vitamin E is raised gradually, the blood pressure will usually not rise significantly and there will not be a greater workload placed on the heart, according to Dr. Cowden.

In another study funded by the World Health Organization it was shown that among sixteen European study populations, those with low serum levels of vitamin E were at greater risk for heart disease than those with high blood pressure and high cholesterol levels.[46]

Vitamin C: The use of vitamin C (ascorbic acid) is believed to help prevent the formation of oxysterols.[47] By combining the amino acid lysine with vitamin C, it may be possible to dissolve clots in the bloodstream.[48] In a study conducted on guinea pigs, it was found that the equivalent of the U.S. Recommended Daily Allowance (U.S. RDA) of vitamin C offered virtually no protection against arterial damage. When the amount of vitamin C was increased to a dose equivalent to 2,800 milligrams for a 154 pound human, the researchers were able to reverse the damage.[49]

Studies also reveal that vitamin C is required for collagen synthesis, and is therefore necessary to maintain the integrity of the walls of arteries.[50] Nobel laureate Linus Pauling, Ph.D., believes that a deficiency of vitamin C may pre-

CAUTION

According to Dr. Cowden, high amounts of vitamin C taken over a prolonged period of time can leach calcium and other minerals out of the teeth, bones, and other tissues. He recommends that high amounts of vitamin C (ascorbic acid) be balanced by mineral ascorbates containing magnesium, potassium, zinc, and manganese.

cipitate arteriosclerosis because it causes defects in the arterial walls due to reduced collagen synthesis.[51] Dr. Pauling and Matthias Rath, M.D., Director of the Linus Pauling Institute of Science and Medicine, in Palo Alto, California, have shown in preliminary studies that vitamin C supplementation can reverse arteriosclerosis in humans.[52]

Research is needed into the role of nutritional supplements in preventing and reversing heart disease.

"Vitamin C reverses oxidation and prevents free radical formation," according to Dr. Cowden. "In a diet that involves reducing fats, vitamin C is an integral part of helping the body to repair itself." In patients with existing cardiovascular disease, Dr. Cowden recommends that vitamin C be taken to bowel tolerance (the maximum amount a person can take before causing loose stools or diarrhea). He suggests a minimum of three to four doses daily, increasing the amount until reaching bowel tolerance.

"For example," explains Dr. Cowden, "the first dose could be one thousand milligrams, the second dose two thousand milligrams, the third dose three thousand milligrams, and the fourth dose four thousand milligrams. Stay on bowel tolerance until cardiovascular disease is resolved, and then go on three thousand milligrams maintenance dose. For those who are well but want to prevent cardiovascular disease, three thousand to ten thousand milligrams daily is sufficient." Higher doses of vitamin C should be taken with adequate amounts of water, magnesium, and vitamin B_6, adds Dr. Cowden.

Coenzyme Q10: Over thirty years ago, Dr. Karl Folkers, a biomedical scientist at the University of Texas in Austin, discovered that coenzyme Q10 helps to strengthen the heart muscle and energize the cardiovascular system in many heart patients. Studies reveal that coenzyme Q10 may protect against atherosclerosis, and it has been shown to have antioxidant properties which may protect against the formation of oxysterols.[53]

Dr. Gordon reports success in helping infants avoid risky and unnecessary surgery using supplements of coenzyme Q10, amino acids, and herbs. "In one case, I went to see a newborn diagnosed with myocardiopathy (a disease of the heart muscle). I asked the attending doctor if he had tried coenzyme Q10 or carnitine [an amino acid]. He said that he had read about their effects, but would not use either. With the family's permission, I treated the baby with those supplements, as well as with magnesium, vitamin C, a multiple vitamin-mineral product, liquid garlic, and the herbal extract of hawthorn berry. The baby recovered without the heart transplant surgery that was being recommended by the university medical center."

Selenium: A positive relationship has been found between low serum selenium levels and cardiovascular disease, possibly related to selenium's antioxidant effects.[54] Selenium supplementation also reduces platelet aggregation,[55] and selenium is a co-factor for glutathione peroxidase, an important antioxidant enzyme.

The following minerals may also be effective in the treatment of heart disease:

Magnesium: It has been found that individuals who die suddenly of heart attacks have far lower levels of magnesium and potassium than control groups.[56] Magnesium helps to dilate arteries and ease the heart's pumping of blood, thus preventing arrhythmias (irregular heartbeats). Magnesium may also prevent calcification of the blood vessels, lower total cholesterol, raise HDL cholesterol, and inhibit platelet aggregation.[57] But simply taking magnesium supplements by mouth may not be sufficient. Dr. Cowden explains: "Most doctors don't use the best form for optimum absorption. It's more effective to use magnesium glycinate, taurate, or aspartate, or even herbal magnesium such as red raspberry, but some patients need intravenous or intramuscular magnesium to quickly raise their magnesium to ideal levels."

THE ROLE OF NIACIN IN HEART DISEASE

Niacin (vitamin B_3) helps to lower cholesterol levels and lessen the risk of heart disease.[57] It has also been shown to increase the longevity of patients who have suffered one heart attack. In one study, over eight thousand middle-aged men who had already had a heart attack were given supplements of either niacin, estrogen, thyroid hormone, or a placebo. Results showed that only niacin was beneficial in lowering the death rate and in increasing longevity.[59]

Abram Hoffer, M.D., Ph.D., of Victoria, British Columbia, saw a patient in 1992 who was a pilot and had not been able to fly since 1985 because of heart problems. Dr. Hoffer put him on three grams daily of niacin, and after one and a half years, he was given a clean bill of health and was able to fly again. Another of Dr. Hoffer's patients came to him twenty years ago with angina pectoris. This patient was also treated with niacin and, according to Dr. Hoffer, has had no signs of angina since.

Do cholesterol-lowering drugs work?

Since many people with heart disease also have elevated blood cholesterol levels, physicians have traditionally prescribed cholesterol-lowering drugs as part of their treatment program, although new research suggests that it is not the levels of cholesterol but the levels of oxidized cholesterol which represent high risk for heart disease.

There is also new information concerning the safety, side effects, and efficacy of cholesterol-lowering drugs. It has been found, for instance, that the drugs used to lower LDL (low density lipoprotein) cholesterol actually raise it in people who already have the highest levels.[68] In addition, these medications can lead to serious complications. A study conducted in Finland reported that deaths from heart attacks and strokes were 46 percent higher in those taking cholesterol-lowering drugs.[69] Newer drugs being touted as safer also have harmful side effects. Studies have shown that Mevacor (lovastatin) lowers the levels of coenzyme Q10 in the bloodstream, an antioxidant that helps the body resist heart damage.[70]

Alan R. Gaby, M.D., of Baltimore, Maryland, President-elect of the American Holistic Medical Association, has found that cases of congestive heart failure respond well to an intravenous injection of a "cocktail" composed of magnesium chloride hexahydrate, hydroxocobalamin, pyridoxine hydrochloride, dexpanthenol, B-complex vitamins, and vitamin C. (This is a modification of the nutrient cocktail popularized by John Myers, M.D.)

Calcium: Calcium supplementation may also decrease total cholesterol and inhibit platelet aggregation.[60]

Chromium: Chromium supplementation has been shown to lower total cholesterol and triglycerides and raise HDL cholesterol.[61] It is even more effective in lowering cholesterol when combined with niacin (vitamin B_3).[62] A chromium deficiency has been linked to coronary heart disease by several studies.[63]

Potassium: Hypertension (high blood pressure) is often present in heart disease. It has been found that supplements of potassium can help reduce a patient's reliance on blood pressure medication or diuretic drugs.[64]

Herbal Medicine

According to David L. Hoffman, B.Sc., M.N.I.M.H., of Sebastopol, California, past President of the American Herbalist Guild, "Some herbs have a potent and direct impact upon the heart itself, such as *Digitalis purpurea* (foxglove), and form the basis of drug therapy for heart failure."

One of the most promising herbs for the treatment of heart disease is the extract from the herb hawthorn berry, a commonly found shrub. Hawthorn berry has been found to help improve the circulation of blood to the heart by dilating the blood vessels and relieving spasms of the arterial walls.[65] According to Dr. Gordon, "Hawthorn berry may render unnecessary medications that decrease the rate and force of heart contraction in the treatment of heart disease as it performs a similar function to these drugs."

See Diet, Herbal Medicine, Nutritional Supplements.

Garlic and ginger also have many properties that make them valuable in treating heart disease. Garlic contains sulfur compounds, which work as antioxidants and also help dissolve clots.[66] Ginger has been shown to lower cholesterol levels and make the blood platelets less sticky.[67] While it's best to consult a skilled herbalist before taking herbs, the following is an example of a cardiac tonic that Hoffman recommends: an

Is fish oil as effective as aspirin in preventing heart attacks?

In the early 1980s physicians began prescribing aspirin as a preventative to those patients at risk for heart attacks and strokes. Many cited aspirin's anticoagulant effects, noting that aspirin prevents the blood from clotting in plaque-occluded arteries. William Lee Cowden, M.D., a cardiologist from Dallas, Texas, suggests that this approach may be misguided, since aspirin has been known to cause gastrointestinal bleeding and even perforated ulcers in some cases whereas eicosapentaenoic acid (EPA) from fish oils has no such risks and has also been shown to significantly reduce death from coronary heart disease.[71] In addition, EPA (especially when taken in conjunction with adequate antioxidant nutrients like vitamins E and C and beta-carotene) works on reducing stickiness of clotting cells in the blood by affecting prostoglandin ratios (like aspirin does). However, EPA also favorably alters blood lipid ratios and helps to lower blood pressure (which aspirin does not).[72]

ALTERNATIVE TREATMENTS FOR STROKE

In the same manner that coronary arteries can become blocked by plaque, causing a heart attack, so can arteries supplying the brain become blocked, leading to a stroke. The effects when the oxygen supply to a portion of the brain is blocked include loss of speech, movement, or eyesight.

Until now most stroke victims had little choice but to spend many months working with physical therapists, sometimes recovering only minimal bodily function. Researchers, particularly in Germany, have recognized that the loss of functioning of an arm or leg after a stroke was similar to the symptoms of the "bends," a sometimes fatal affliction deep sea divers can get from ascending too quickly to sea level. Restoring the balance of nitrogen and oxygen in the blood cured divers of the bends, and physicians suspected that victims of stroke or heart attack might be helped in a similar manner.

A hyperbaric oxygen chamber, which alters the atmospheric pressure, forces oxygen into the tissues so that it reaches the cells in its most easily utilized state. According to David Hughes, Ph.D., of the Hyperbaric Oxygen Institute, in San Bernardino, California, the treatment has been used quite successfully in West Germany. An infusion of highly diluted 35 percent hydrogen peroxide into the bloodstream may also have the same effect, and hydrogen peroxide has been shown to dissolve lipids from the arterial walls.[73]

William Lee Cowden, M.D., a cardiologist from Dallas, Texas, has noticed that if patients can be treated within the first twelve hours after a stroke with a combination of high antioxidant intake, essential fatty acids, and either hyperbaric oxygen therapy or ozone therapy (see Oxygen Therapy chapter), then a dramatic regression of symptoms of stroke can occur. Patients regain sensation, strength, and mental clarity, as well as motor and sensory skills and orientation. In his treatment he uses the antioxidants vitamin E, beta-carotene, ascorbyl palmitate (a fat-soluble form of vitamin C), and pycnogenol (a fat-soluble antioxidant found in pine needles and bark), as well as the essential fatty acid eicosapentaenoic acid (EPA) and docosahexaenoic acid (DHA) to help prevent damage to the fatty acid membranes in brain cells.

Harvey Bigelsen, M.D., Medical Director of the Center for Progressive Medicine in Scottsdale, Arizona, uses biological therapies developed by the late German bacteriologist, Gunther Enderlein, M.D., Ph.D., to help alleviate the symptoms of stroke. According to Dr. Bigelsen, Dr. Enderlein theorized that disease must be treated at the cellular level, and formulated his remedies accordingly. The remedies are extracts of plants and fungi which, once injected into the patient, work according to the principles of homeopathy. According to Dr. Enderlein, bacteria can take on both harmless and harmful forms. By injecting harmless forms of bacteria, those harmful entities in the body will revert to their harmless state, according to Dr. Enderlein.

Dr. Bigelsen uses these remedies intravenously to bring strokes-in-progress to a halt.[74] One such patient reportedly was treated intravenously, and within five minutes the crisis of the stroke was broken and the symptoms alleviated. The patient was then treated with cell therapy to stimulate the brain tissue and chelation therapy to help clear out the arteries. He was able to walk out of the hospital with no residual disability and resumed work a few days later.

Margaret A. Naeser, Ph.D., Associate Research Professor of Neurology at Boston University School of Medicine and a licensed acupuncturist in Massachusetts, has conducted research on the use of low-energy lasers (twenty milliwatt red to infrared laser beam light) in the treatment of paralysis in stroke. Five of her six subjects showed improvement, and patients with mild to moderate paralysis responded better than those with severe paralysis, according to Dr. Naeser. The improvements were observed even when treatments were begun three or four years after the stroke.

equal combination of the tinctures of hawthorn berries, *Ginkgo biloba*, and linden flowers (one-half teaspoonful three times a day). He also suggests the addition of tincture of motherwort to prevent palpitations, and garlic to help manage cholesterol.

Chelation Therapy

There is mounting evidence that chelation therapy offers an alternative to the hundreds of thousands of bypass surgeries and angioplasties performed each year. Chelation therapy is traditionally used to treat poisoning from toxic metals by removing them from the body with a chemical agent. Norman Clarke, Sr., M.D., Director of Research at Providence Hospital, Detroit, Michigan, hypothesized that since chelation with EDTA (ethylenediaminetetraacetic acid) removed calcium from pipes and boilers, it may be useful to remove calcium plaque in patients with arteriosclerosis. His experiments confirmed his theory, and angina patients treated by Dr. Clarke reported dramatic relief from chest pain.[75]

According to Dr. Gordon, in chelation therapy the chemical EDTA is given intravenously to remove plaque and calcium deposits from the arterial walls and then the unwanted material is excreted through the urine. The treatment is usually administered several times per week over a course of two or three months in order to restore complete circulation.

In a study completed in 1989, every patient suffering from a vascular disease who was treated with chelation therapy showed a measurable improvement midway through the course of treatment.[76] Another study showed that 88 percent of the patients receiving chelation therapy exhibited improved blood flow to the brain.[77] Charles Farr, M.D., Ph.D., of Oklahoma City, Oklahoma, cofounder of the American Board of Chelation Therapy, reports that during the past twenty-plus years, he has given more than five hundred thousand chelation treatments to over twenty thousand patients, 60 to 70 percent of which were for some form of cardiovascular disease or circulatory problems. He reports very positive results in 70 to 80 percent of the cases. "Many of our patients who were originally scheduled to have bypass surgery or angiograms continue to be healthy today, some ten to fifteen years past the time they were supposed to die if they did not have the surgery." According to Dr. Farr, chelation is remarkably effective in removing arterial plaque and dissolving clots, as well as softening up and dilating the blood vessels and allowing nutrients to get to damaged tissues.

See Biofeedback Training, Chelation Therapy, Guided Imagery, Meditation, Oxygen Therapies, Stress, Yoga.

Dr. Farr reports the case of a man who had several episodes of cardiovascular disease, and had been told by his doctor that he would die if he did not have immediate bypass surgery. Deciding against surgery, the man, who was unable to walk, went to Dr. Farr on referral and, despite the protests of his family, began chelation therapy. Within forty-five days of beginning chelation treatments, he had gone back to work running a construction company, and continued to work for many years.

Eliminating the Need for a Heart Transplant

While conventional medicine often relies on the high-risk procedure of heart transplant in treating heart disease, this radical method can often be avoided. William Lee Cowden, M.D., a cardiologist from Dallas, Texas, reports the case of a forty-five-year-old physician who was suffering from pneumonia and an enlarged heart. When given an ejection fraction test (measuring the percentage of the blood contained in the ventricle that is ejected on each heartbeat) his heart was only ejecting 16 percent of its contents (60 percent is normal), and his doctor told him his only hope was to receive a heart transplant. When he came into Dr. Cowden's office he could barely walk across the room without becoming out of breath.

Dr. Cowden immediately put him on a detoxification program that included a vegetarian diet and a three-day vegetable juice fast with garlic. He also had him follow a nutritional supplementation regimen including coenzyme Q10, vitamin C, magnesium, vitamin B complex, trace minerals, omega-3 fatty acids, lauric acid (an essential fatty acid), and carnitine, as well as the antiviral herbs, St. John's Wort, Pfaffia paniculata, *and* Lomantium dissectum.

Within three months, Dr Cowden reports, the patient could jog ten miles a day, and upon repeating the ejection fraction test, his score was up to 30 percent. Now he works sixty hours a week and continues to jog ten miles daily.

Oxygen Therapy

Studies at Baylor University twenty years ago found that an intravenous drip of hydrogen peroxide into leg arteries of atherosclerotic patients cleared arterial plaques.[78] In cardiac resuscitations hydrogen peroxide infusions often stopped ventricular fibrillation (rapid, ineffective contractions by ventricles of the heart), the heart's response to insufficient oxygen.[79] Dr. Farr reports success alternating treatments of intravenous diluted hydrogen peroxide and chelation therapy to bring patients out of high-output heart failure (where the heart fails even though it is pumping a high amount of blood).

Exercise and Stress Reduction

Stress-reduction techniques and exercise have been shown to be highly effective in reversing heart disease. In a study conducted by Dr. Ornish, an experimental group following a routine that combined a low-fat vegetarian diet, stress-management training, the elimination of smoking, and moderate exercise had a 91 percent decrease in the frequency of angina, as opposed to a control group which experienced a 165 percent increase in the frequency of angina.[80]

Dr. Cowden also includes stress-reduction exercises as part of his treatment. He believes that deep breathing and imaging techniques aimed at reducing stress should be conducted frequently throughout the day to reduce the output of adrenal hormones and lower the level of platelet aggregation. He encourages patients to do these techniques before meals and at bedtime, as they can not only reduce stress but can improve digestion. "Some of the nutrients we are giving have to be absorbed out of the gut [gastrointestinal tract]. If the gut is in a stressed state, it will not absorb those nutrients nearly as well as if it is in a relaxed state."

"Even ten minutes of extra exercise per day can significantly reduce the risk of heart disease."
—William Lee Cowden, M.D.

It is also important for people with heart disease to get plenty of exercise. "Even ten minutes of extra exercise per day can significantly reduce the risk of heart disease," adds Dr. Cowden.

Traditional Chinese Medicine

Traditional Chinese Medicine (TCM) views heart disease as a problem stemming from poor digestion, which causes the buildup of plaque in the arteries. Harvey Kaltsas, Ac. Phys. (FL.), D.Ac. (RI), Dip. Ac. (NCCA), President of the American Association of Acupuncture and Oriental Medicine, recommends herbs to strengthen the digestive functioning. "It has been understood in China for thousands of years that the circulation needs to flow unimpeded," states Dr. Kaltsas. An herbal extract made from a plant known as *mao-tung-ching* (*Ilex puibeceus*) is often used to dilate the blocked vessels. According to Dr. Kaltsas, a study was conducted in China in which *mao-tung-ching* was administered daily (four ounces orally, twenty milligrams intravenously) to 103 patients suffering from coronary heart disease. In 101 out of the 103 cases, there was significant improvement.[81]

Maoshing Ni, D.O.M., Ph.D., L.Ac., Vice-President of the Yo San University of Traditional Chinese Medicine in Santa Monica, California, views heart disease as either a weakness, or a block in the body's energy system. For acute problems such as pain or abnormal heart rates he uses acupuncture, but usually refers acute heart problem patients to a Western physician. He says that TCM is more suited to the treatment of chronic heart problems. For these, Dr. Ni uses a combination of acupuncture and herbs to dissolve plaque, lower cholesterol levels, raise blood flow rates, and relieve angina.

One patient came to Dr. Ni after having an angioplasty because of 70 percent blockage of the coronary arteries. After the angioplasty, he still had 55 percent blockage. Dr. Ni treated him with herbs and acupuncture and within three to four months, the blockage was reduced to 35 percent.

Ayurvedic Medicine

In treating heart disease, Ayurvedic physicians use several methods which result in the reduction of the generation of free radicals, which can contribute to the disease process in the arteries and heart. "Meat, cigarette smoke, alcohol, and environmental pollutants all generate free radicals," explains Hari Sharma, M.D., President of Maharishi Ayurveda Medical Association. By using specific herbal food supplements and *pancha karma* (detoxification and purification techniques), says Dr. Sharma, "free radicals and lipid peroxides are reduced." As it is especially important for those with heart disease to lower their level of stress, Dr. Sharma also recommends a program of Transcendental Meditation.

Virender Sodhi, M.D. (Ayurveda), N.D., Director of the American School of Ayurvedic Sciences in Bellevue, Washington, reports an interesting case of heart disease involving a fifty-five-year-old Asian male with chest pain so severe that he could not walk more than ten steps before having to sit down. He came to Dr. Sodhi's office after receiving word from the local hospital that he needed immediate bypass surgery. Refusing the surgery, doctors told him, would mean certain death.

Before beginning treatment, the man underwent a battery of tests, ordered by Dr. Sodhi. Angiographic studies showed that his patient's coronary arteries were blocked—the left main coronary artery was 90 percent narrowed, the anterior descending was 80 percent narrowed, and the right coronary was 30 percent blocked. Blood tests indicated elevated cholesterol levels at 278 and decreased HDL at 38. Dr. Sodhi determined his patient's metabolic type and started him on an appropriate cleansing program that included dietary changes and appropriate herbs. (See Ayurvedic Medicine chapter for discussion of metabolic type.)

See Ayurvedic Medicine, Traditional Chinese Medicine.

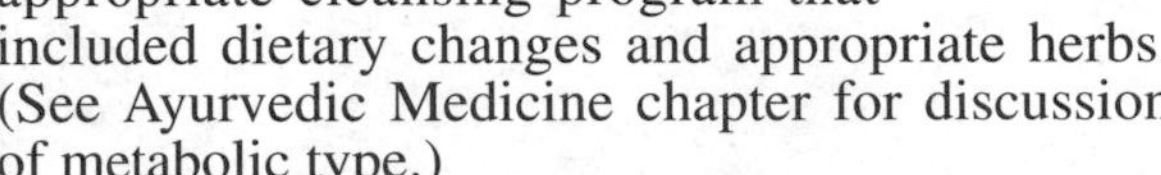

After three months, the man's cholesterol levels reportedly dropped more than 30 percent and his HDL's rose to 48. More importantly, though, his exercise tolerance had dramatically improved. "He was doing the treadmill exercise," reports Sodhi, "at the speed of five miles per hour for forty-five minutes without any angina." More than two years later, the patient is doing fine. He now jogs up and down hills with no symptoms, and his EKG has shown improvement. According to Dr. Sodhi, there is a hospital in Bombay, India, which has treated some 3,300 cases of coronary heart disease using this method, with about 99 percent success.

The Future of Heart Disease Treatment

Conventional treatments for heart disease tend to rely heavily on technological interventions such as bypass surgery, angiograms, angioplasty, and even the artificial heart. Coronary artery bypass surgery is often called an "overprescribed and unnecessary surgery" by many leading authorities.[82] Complications from such treatments are common and the expense to the health care system is extraordinarily high. For the most part, medicine is more equipped to treat heart disease only when it has reached its most serious and life-threatening stages.

A recent announcement by Mutual of Omaha Insurance Company, one of the nation's largest insurers providing coverage for about 10 million people, may help point the way for heart disease treatment in the future. The company will now offer insurance coverage for individuals participating in pilot programs testing Dr. Ornish's therapy, including a vegetarian diet, exercise, meditation, and support groups. According to Dr. Kenneth McDonough, Mutual of Omaha's Medical Director, "This isn't only a pilot program for coronary artery disease, it's a pilot for medicine in general."[83]

Clearly, much can be done in the early stages of heart disease. Maintaining a diet low in saturated fats to limit exposure to oxidized cholesterol, exercising regularly and using nutritional supplements such as vitamin B_6, vitamin B_{12}, folic acid, vitamin C, vitamin E, magnesium, and coenzyme Q10 can go a long way in preventing and treating heart disease.

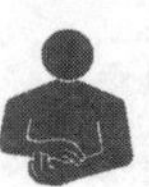

Self-Care

The following therapies can be undertaken at home under appropriate professional supervision:

• Fasting • Yoga

Aromatherapy: To strengthen heart muscle: garlic, lavender, peppermint, marjoram, rose, rosemary. For palpitations: lavender, melissa, neroli, ylang-ylang.

Hydrotherapy: Constitutional hydrotherapy: two to five times weekly.

Juice Therapy: • Carrot, celery, cucumber, beet (add a little garlic or hawthorn berries) • Blueberries, blackberies, black currant, red grapes

Professional Care

The following therapies can only be provided by a qualified health professional:

• Alexander Technique • Biofeedback Training • Cell Therapy • Environmental Medicine • Guided Imagery • Hypnotherapy • Magnetic Field Therapy • Meditation • Osteopathy

Biological Dentistry: Hal A. Huggins, D.D.S., reports the improvement or disappearance of many cardiovascular problems including angina, unidentified chest pains, and tachycardia (rapid heartbeat for no apparent reason) after removing toxic dental amalgams.

Body Therapy: Acupressure, reflexology, *shiatsu,* massage.

Chiropractic: To improve mid-back mobility and breathing.

Hydrotherapy: Leon Chaitow, N.D., D.O., reports that the neutral bath (patient immersed in water [35 degrees centigrade] for two hours) has been effective in treating mild heart failure problems which result in fluid retention.

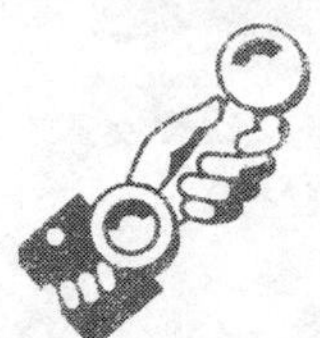

Where to Find Help

For additional information and referrals concerning treatment for heart disease, contact the following organizations.

American Association of Acupuncture and Oriental Medicine
4101 Lake Boone Trail, Suite 201
Raleigh, North Carolina 27607
(919) 787-5181

The AAAOM is a national professional trade organization of acupuncturists who meet acceptable standards of competency and can provide you with the names and locations of local members. Referrals by written request only.

American Association of Naturopathic Physicians
2366 Eastlake Avenue, Suite 322
Seattle, Washington 98102
(206) 323-7610

Provides a directory of naturopathic physicians and offers referrals to a nationwide network of accredited or licensed practitioners. Publishes a quarterly newsletter for both professionals and the general public. Also offers a series of brochures and pamphlets on a variety of subjects.

American College of Advancement in Medicine
P.O. Box 3427
Laguna Hills, California 92654
(714) 583-7666

This pioneer organization seeks to establish certification and standards of practice for chelation therapy. It provides training and education, and sponsors semiannual conferences for physicians and scientists. It provides referrals and informational material, including a directory listing of all physicians worldwide who have been trained in preventative medicine as well as in the ACAM protocol for chelation therapy. The directory is updated monthly. The organization also provides a copy of the ACAM protocol for chelation to the public.

American Holistic Medical Association
4101 Lake Boone Trail, Suite 201
Raleigh, North Carolina 27607
(919) 787-5181

A professional organization for holistic practitioners, the AHMA offers information and services for its members and lobbies for holistic issues. It also provides referrals for the public; requests must be in writing.

American School of Ayurvedic Sciences
10025 NE 4th Street
Bellevue, Washington 98004
(206) 453-8022

This college provides medical training for physicians and health care practitioners, as well as individual courses for lay people. Dr. Virender Sodhi's Ayurvedic, Naturopathic Medical Clinic is also located at this address.

Ayurvedic Institute
11311 Menaul NE, Suite A
Albuquerque, New Mexico 87112
(505) 291-9698

The institute, directed by Dr. Vasant Lad, trains people from all walks of life in most of the aspects of Ayurveda.

The College of Maharishi Ayur-Veda Medical Center
P.O. Box 282
Fairfield, Iowa 52556
(515) 472-5866

The center provides referrals to health centers, which offer methods of prevention and treatment of a broad range of illnesses. They also train practitioners and provide information to the lay public.

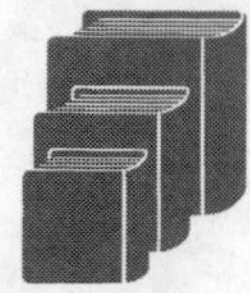

Recommended Reading

Bypassing Bypass. Cranton, Elmer. Troutdale, VA: Medex Publishers, 1992.

Dr. Cranton's book discusses metals, free radicals, and cross linking in relation to chelation therapy. His work on preventive medicine can enhance the benefits of surgery, as well as prevent surgery.

Coping with Angina. Wallace, Louise M. U.K.: Thorsons, 1990.

Practical advice on the management of angina, particularly stress and mental attitude, which are major factors in this condition.

Dr. Dean Ornish's Program for Reversing Heart Disease. Ornish, Dean, M.D. New York: Ballantine, 1990.

A step-by-step guide through Dr. Ornish's program of halting and even reversing heart disease through a change of lifestyle. Dr. Ornish goes beyond the physical aspects of health care to consider the psychological, emotional, and spiritual conditions that are vital to healing.

Encyclopedia of Natural Medicine. Murray, Michael, N.D.; and Pizzorno, Joseph, N.D. Rocklin, CA: Prima Publishing, 1991.

A definitive guide for the layperson on naturopathic medicine. Contains a chapter on atherosclerosis.

40 Something Forever. Brecker, Harold; and Brecker, Arlene. New York: Health Savers Press, 1992.

A consumer's guide to chelation and other recommendations for a healthy heart.

Good Cholesterol, Bad Cholesterol. Roth, Eli M., M.D.; and Streicher, Sandra L., R.N. Rocklin CA: Prima Publishers, 1993.

The first book written by a cardiovascular team teaches you the truth behind LDL (bad) cholesterol and HDL (good) choleserol and its cleansing ability. It also teaches you how to read labels to discover hidden cholesterol levels, how to eat out, and the benefits and side effects of available medications.

Heart Myths. Charash, Bruce D., M.D. New York: Viking Penguin, 1992.

A reevaluation of commonly held ideas about heart disease in light of current data and research.

The Johns Hopkins Complete Guide for Preventing and Reversing Heart Disease. Kwiterovich, Peter, M.D. Rocklin CA: Prima Publishers, 1993.

A winner of the prestigious Blakeslee Award from the American Heart Association, this is the most comprehensive and medically accurate book on preventing heart disease. Written by an internationally acclaimed expert from one of the world's great medical institutions, this book is information-packed with everything from types of heart disease to their prevention, from eating right to teaching children good health habits.

The New Supernutrition Book. Passwater, Richard A. New York: Pocket Books, 1991.

The celebrated nutritionist's book discusses the latest discoveries about, and solutions for, contemporary nutritional problems, including information on the relationship between diet and nutrition and supernutrients. Provides diet programs for specific problems.

Preventing Silent Heart Disease. Karpman, Harold L., M.D. New York: Henry Holt & Co., 1991.

How to diagnose and treat silent heart disease, which is the main cause of sudden death in America.

Reversing Heart Disease. Whitaker, Julian M., M.D. New York: Warner Books, 1985.

A complete cardiac care program that will help you prevent or cure heart disease the natural way.

Hypertension

Hypertension, or high blood pressure, affects nearly one out of four Americans. Alternative therapies can provide a natural and effective way of preventing or reducing hypertension, and can do so without the many side effects associated with orthodox high blood pressure medications.

Approximately 60 million Americans, two-thirds of whom are under sixty-five years of age, suffer from hypertension, indicating that this condition is not an inevitable result of aging but rather a condition affected by a number of risk factors, including smoking, obesity,[1] stress,[2] excessive alcohol consumption, and a diet high in fats and sodium chloride (table salt).[3] According to William Lee Cowden, M.D., a cardiologist from Dallas, Texas, "Individuals with diabetes are especially susceptible, as are those with a family history of hypertension. Stress and a sedentary lifestyle are other factors to consider when diagnosing and treating this condition."

Diagnosing Hypertension

Hypertension is the technical name for high blood pressure. It is measured by placing an inflatable cuff around the upper arm. As the cuff is inflated, the arm is squeezed tight. At this point the pulse cannot be heard through the stethoscope. As the cuff is slowly deflated, the pulse is heard again. This is the high number and measures the systolic pressure, when the heart is contracting to pump blood out into the body. A second reading is taken as the cuff is deflated even further and the pulse sound disappears again. This is the low number and measures the diastolic pressure, the pressure when the heart is relaxing to refill with blood.

A patient has hypertension if the high reading is over 140 and the low reading is over 90 when tested on two separate occasions.

Hypertension takes two forms: essential hypertension, when the cause is unknown, and secondary hypertension, when damage to the kidneys or endocrine dysfunction cause blood pressure to rise. Of the diagnosed cases of hypertension in the United States, over 90 percent are essential hypertension.[4]

The symptoms of hypertension appear throughout the body and may include dizziness, headache, fatigue, restlessness, difficulty breathing, insomnia, intestinal complaints, and emotional instability. In advanced stages, the hypertensive patient often experiences cardiovascular disease as well as damage to the heart, kidneys, and brain.

Causes of Hypertension

"High blood pressure often occurs due to a strain on the heart, which can arise from a variety of conditions, including diet, atherosclerosis [hardening of the arteries], high cholesterol, diabetes, environmental factors, as well as lifestyle choices," according to Dr. Cowden. When these factors combine with a genetic predisposition, hypertension can occur in two out of three individuals.[5]

Dietary Factors

"Although a combination of genetic and environmental factors such as behavior patterns and stress are believed to contribute to hypertension, the main cause appears to be a diet high in animal fat and sodium chloride, especially if high in relation to potassium and magnesium organic salts," says Dr. Cowden. Hypertension is closely associated with the Western diet and is found almost entirely in developed countries.[6] Recent studies of residents in remote areas of China, New Guinea, Panama, Brazil, and Africa show virtually no evidence of hypertension, even with advanced age. But individuals within these groups who moved to more industrialized areas showed increased incidences of hypertension in proportion not only to changes in diet, but with increased levels of body mass and fat. These studies concluded that changes in lifestyle, including dietary changes, significantly contributed to the higher levels of blood pressure.[7]

Nutritional deficiencies also play a major role in the development of hypertension. A diet high in sodium chloride and deficient in potassium has been associated with hypertension, and magnesium levels have been found to be consistently low in patients with high blood pressure.[8]

Lifestyle Factors

Lifestyle choices, including smoking and consumption of coffee and alcohol, have been shown to cause hypertension. A recent study conducted in Paris, France, showed higher systolic and diastolic levels in coffee drinkers compared to nondrinkers, with levels rising in direct correlation to the amount of coffee consumed each day.[9] Even moderate amounts of alcohol can produce hypertension in certain individuals, and chronic alcohol intake is one of the strongest predictors of high blood pressure.[10] Restricting alcohol and avoiding caffeine are recommended.

"Although a combination of genetic and environmental factors such as behavior patterns and stress are believed to contribute to hypertension, the main cause of hypertension appears to be a diet high in animal fat and sodium chloride."
—William Lee Cowden, M.D.

Smoking is a contributing factor to hypertension due to the fact that smokers are more prone to increased sugar, alcohol, and caffeine consumption.[11] Even smokeless tobacco (chewing tobacco, snuff, etc.) causes hypertension through its nicotine and sodium content.[12]

Environmental Factors

Environmental factors such as lead contamination from drinking water, as well as residues of heavy metals such as cadmium have also been shown to promote hypertension.[13] People whose hypertension has been left untreated have been shown to have blood cadmium levels three to four times higher than those with normal blood pressure.[14] It is important to rule out both lead and cadmium toxicity when treating hypertension.

See Chelation Therapy, Heart Disease.

ATHEROSCLEROSIS AND HYPERTENSION

Atherosclerosis involves the accumulation of plaque in the blood vessels which restricts blood flow and increases blood pressure. Consequently it is a common cause of hypertension as well as the main cause of coronary heart disease and strokes. According to Leon Chaitow, N.D., D.O., of London, England, "Blood pressure rises when the blood leaving the heart has to be pumped more vigorously due to a thicker consistency of the blood or to a greater resistance from the blood vessels themselves. The vessels may have become narrower, less elastic, or the muscles which surround them may be exerting more tension. The function of the muscles and breathing apparatus may also be inefficient in helping the heart to function properly. The relative health of the kidneys and liver (which filter the blood) also influences blood pressure."

Treating Hypertension

Conventional high blood pressure medications treat hypertension by reducing the heart output, lowering the blood pressure, or reducing the fluid retention through the use of diuretics. These medications may relieve the symptoms of hypertension but do little to address the cause. As many of these drugs have unwanted side effects, an alternative approach to reducing blood pressure may be preferable.

A careful evaluation of the factors[15] contributing to the patient's illness may reveal a need for dietary changes, nutritional supplementation, and lifestyle changes such as increased exercise, weight loss, and stress management. Other therapies include various forms of mind/body medicine, herbal medicine, detoxification therapies, Ayurvedic medicine, and Traditional Chinese Medicine.

Diet and Nutritional Supplementation

A diet low in fat, sugar, and salt, but rich in foods containing potassium, calcium, magnesium, and fiber, is highly recommended for hypertensives. Also, garlic and other members of the onion family should be included in any diet that aims to lower high blood pressure, as they significantly reduce systolic and diastolic pressure.[16]

Nutritional supplementation of the non-chloride salts of potassium, calcium, and magnesium can help reduce hypertension. Other beneficial supplements include vitamin A, vitamin C, vitamin E, niacin (vitamin B_3), bioflavinoids (particularly rutin) and the amino acid taurine.[17] To improve absorption of these and other essential nutrients, Dr. Cowden has his patients perform stress-reduction techniques before meals and at bedtime to reduce stress and improve digestion. Says Dr. Cowden, "The nutrients we recommend have to be absorbed out of the gastrointestinal tract. But if the gut is in a stressed state, it will not absorb those nutrients nearly as well as if it is in a relaxed state."

Eric R. Braverman, M.D., of Princeton Associates for Health (PATH) in Princeton, New Jersey, treats hypertension with a program centered around diet and nutritional supplementation. Dr. Braverman's dietary outline emphasizes low sodium, low saturated fat, and low refined carbohydrates combined with a high intake of vegetables from the starch group, with large amounts of fresh salad, and a high protein intake (particularly fish). Simple sugar, alcohol, caffeine, nicotine, and refined carbohydrates are reduced dramatically or eliminated. His nutritional program for a typical hypertensive patient includes fish oil (containing omega-3 fatty acids), garlic, Evening Primrose oil, magnesium, potassium, selenium, zinc, vitamin B_6, niacin, vitamin C, tryptophan, taurine, cysteine, and coenzyme Q10. One patient of Dr. Braverman had been treated with medication for high blood pressure for two years. His blood pressure on seeing Dr. Braverman was 150/90. He was started on multivitamins and supplements of B_6, folic acid, B_{12}, magnesium, taurine, garlic, and evening primrose oil, and within two weeks he was off medication and his blood pressure had dropped to 128/82.

Sodium and Potassium: In order to reduce blood pressure, sodium intake must be restricted while at the same time potassium intake increased.[18] Individuals with high blood pressure should be aware of "hidden" salt in processed foods.

Although their salt intake is comparable, vegetarians generally have less hypertension and cardiovascular disease than non-vegetarians because their diets contain more potassium, complex carbohydrates, polyunsaturated fat, fiber, calcium, magnesium, and vitamins A and C.[19]

According to Dr. Cowden, regular consumption of potassium-rich fruits such as avocados, bananas, cantaloupe, honeydew melon, grapefruit, nectarines, oranges, and vegetables such as asparagus, broccoli, cabbage, cauliflower, green peas, potatoes, and squash can lower high blood pressure. Steaming rather than boiling vegetables helps prevent vital nutrient loss.

Calcium: One thousand milligrams daily of calcium has been shown to lower blood pressure in hypertensives and young adults.[20]

Because many hypertensives have a lower daily calcium intake than people with normal blood pressure, calcium-rich foods, including nuts and leafy green vegetables, such as watercress and kale, should also supplement the diet.[21]

See Diet, Nutritional Supplements.

Magnesium: In one study, magnesium supplementation lowered blood pressure in nineteen of twenty hypertensives, compared to zero of four in the control group.[22] Dietary magnesium is found in nuts (almonds, cashews, pecans), rice, bananas, potatoes, wheat germ, kidney and lima beans, soy products, and molasses.

Caution: *High dosages of vitamin E are not recommended for people with hypertension, rheumatic heart disease, or ischemic heart disease except under close medical supervision.*[23]

DRUGS ASSOCIATED WITH A HIGHER INCIDENCE OF HYPERTENSION

According to the Physicians Desk Reference the following drugs are associated with side effects of hypertension. (Statistics refer to the percentage of individuals affected.)

- *Alfenta Injection (18%)*
- *Aredia for Injection (Up to 6%)*
- *Clozaril Tablets (4%)*
- *Dobutrex Solution Vials (Most patients)*
- *Epogen for Injection (0.75 to approximately 25%)*
- *Habitrol Nicotine Transdermal System (3-9% of patients)*
- *Lupron Depot 3.75 milligrams (Among most frequent), Injection (5% or more)*
- *Methergine Injection, Tablets (Most common)*
- *Orthoclone OKT3 Sterile Solution (8%)*
- *Polygam, Immune Globulin Intravenous (Human) (3-6%)*
- *Procrit for Injection (0.75-24%)*
- *Sandimmune I.V. Ampuls for Infusion, Oral Solution (13-53%)*
- *Sandimmune Soft Gelatin Capsules (13-53%)*
- *Stadol Injectable*
- *Sufenta Injection (3%)*
- *Tolectin (200, 400, and 600 milligrams) (3-9%)*
- *Velban Vials (Among most common)*
- *Ventolin Inhalation Aerosol and Refill (Fewer than 5 per 100 patients)*
- *Wellbutrin Tablets (4.3%)*

Lifestyle Changes

Lifestyle plays a major role in the development of hypertension, and any program to reduce blood pressure must take this into consideration. Dr. Cowden notes that any changes that are implemented must be maintained if blood pressure is to be controlled on a long-term basis. Smoking should be moderated, or preferably totally avoided, and alcohol intake should be kept to a minimum. Other factors for reducing and controlling hypertension include weight loss, increased exercise, and stress management.

"Meditation is so effective in reducing stress that in 1984 the National Institutes of Health recommended meditation over prescription drugs for mild hypertension."

Weight Loss: Weight loss reduces blood pressure in those with and without hypertension, and should be a primary goal for hypertensives who are obese or moderately overweight.

Exercise: Because exercise reduces both stress and blood pressure, it is highly recommended as a regular part of a person's lifestyle. Consistent aerobic exercise can prevent hypertension and help lower high blood pressure.[24] Before undertaking any exercise program, an individual with hypertension should consult a physician.

Stress Management: Stress-reduction techniques from the various disciplines of mind/body medicine such as biofeedback, yoga, meditation, *qigong*, relaxation exercises, and hypnotherapy have all proved successful in lowering blood pressure.[25] In fact, meditation is so effective in reducing stress that in 1984 the National Institutes of Health recommended meditation over prescription drugs for mild hypertension.[26]

See Biofeedback Training, Guided Imagery, Herbal Medicine, Meditation, Qigong, Stress, Yoga.

Biofeedback has proven particularly valuable in working to lower hypertension. Patients in one study were able to sustain lower blood pressure readings than those registered prior to treatment after three years of using biofeedback.[27] Combining biofeedback with other stress-reduction techniques can also help patients achieve optimum results. A study of mildly hypertensive males treated with either biofeedback, autogenic training, or breathing relaxation training showed a significant reduction in both systolic and diastolic blood pressure. The higher the pretreatment blood pressure, the greater the effects of relaxation training.[28]

Herbal Medicine

Many botanicals and herbs have hypotensive (blood pressure-lowering) properties. These include the garlic family, mistletoe, olive leaves, hawthorn berries, rauwolfia, and periwinkle.[29]

According to David Hoffmann, B.Sc., M.N.I.M.H., of Sebastopol, California, eating a clove of raw garlic daily will help considerably in preventing or reversing the effects of high blood pressure.

"An infusion of hawthorn berries drunk twice daily is a gentle and effective way of helping the body to normalize blood pressure," says Hoffmann. "The infusion can be strengthened by combining linden flowers or by adding chamomile or valerian if tension or headaches are present."

Detoxification

Detoxification is the body's natural process of eliminating internal toxins, and is accomplished through the various systems and organs of the body including the liver, kidneys, urine, feces, and perspiration. Everyone has a specific level of tolerance to toxicity that cannot be exceeded if good health is to be maintained; if the system becomes overwhelmed, various symptoms can occur, including hypertension.

Dr. Cowden puts hypertensive patients through a detoxification regimen consisting of daily saunas, homeopathic remedies, and a vegetarian diet supplemented with cayenne and garlic. "Cayenne (capsicum) mixed with vegetable juices or lemon juice is excellent for lowering blood pressure," says Dr. Cowden. He adds that after a few days of treatment, alternating cayenne/vegetable juice with cayenne/lemon juice, patients are often able to come off medication because this regime helps to cleanse the body of toxins which may be causing the high blood pressure.

"A clove of garlic a day will help considerably in preventing or reversing the effects of high blood pressure. For optimum results, garlic should be eaten raw."

—David L. Hoffmann, past President, American Herbalist Guild

Dr. Cowden notes that individuals with hypertension often suffer from a liver insufficiency, in which the liver does not properly clear steroid hormones (sex hormones and hormones of the adrenal gland as well as other toxic substances) from the blood. Saunas and a vegetarian diet can help to restore liver function and lower blood pressure. (Patients with more severe hypertension should have their saunas medically supervised.)

A toxic lymphatic system can also contribute to hypertension. Dr. Cowden suggests deep breathing exercises and ten minutes daily of dry brushing of the skin (vigorously brushing the entire body with a dry brush) for three weeks, in the direction of lymph flow (see illustration of lymphatic system in Detoxification Therapy chapter). Another way to stimulate the flow of lymph and to clear the lymph system of toxins is by using a small trampoline or rebounder for twenty minutes a day, says Dr. Cowden.

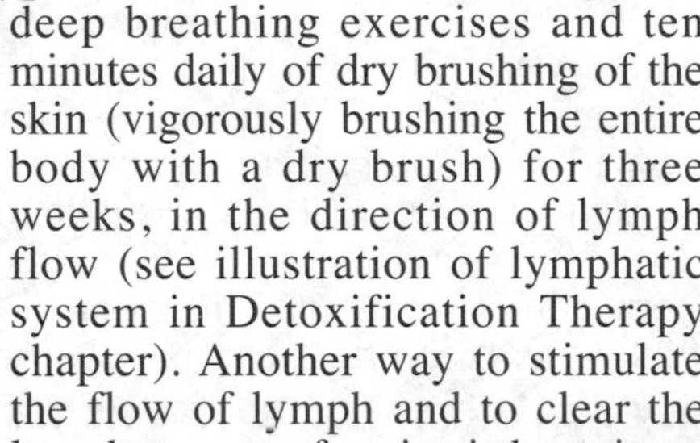

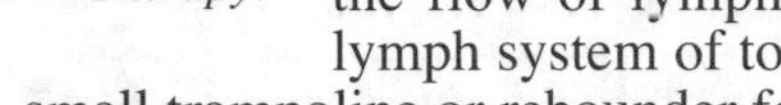

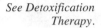

See Detoxification Therapy.

Dr. Cowden reports a case of a woman who was severely hypertensive, with blood pressure of 240/140, who had tried every prescription hypertensive drug and had adverse reactions to all of the medications. When she came to his office he found that, due to years of poor dietary habits and an unhealthy lifestyle, her system was highly toxic. He put her on a detoxification program that included a vegetarian diet, vegetable juice and lemon juice fasts with garlic and cayenne, supplements of oral magnesium, saunas, simple stress-reduction techniques, and cranial electrical stimulation. Within two weeks her blood pressure went down to 140/80, which according to Dr. Cowden, is ideal. She went off her hypertension medications, and her blood pressure continued to remain in that range during her follow-up visits over the next six months.

Ayurvedic Medicine

Ayurvedic medicine treats hypertension according to metabolic type. According to Virender Sodhi, M.D.(Ayurveda), N.D., Director of the American School of Ayurvedic Sciences in Bellevue, Washington, hypertension is found most often in *pitta* and *kapha* types and is usually due to a combination of genetics and lifestyle. Patients of Dr. Sodhi are put on a diet low in sodium, cholesterol, and triglycerides (the latter causes the blood to become very viscous and therefore raises blood pressure).

See the Three Metabolic Types in Ayurvedic Medicine.

Yogic breathing exercises help to relax the body and stimulate the cardiovascular system, effectively reducing hypertension, says Dr. Sodhi. "Breathing first with one nostril, then the other for ten to fifteen minutes, two to three times a day is highly effective in lowering blood pressure. I have patients try this in the office, and after ten minutes, their blood pressure drops considerably," he adds.

Herbs also play an important role in treating hypertension. Herbs are usually used in combinations, depending on the patient's individual needs, and are often combined with rose water and minerals such as calcium, magnesium, silicon, and zinc.

According to Dr. Sodhi, the following herbs are indicated for hypertension: *Convolvulus pluricaulis* has a calming effect, reduces anxiety and anger, and lowers serum cholesterol while increasing high-density lipoproteins (this helps to improve circulation and lower blood pressure). *Ashwaganda* also has a calming effect, and helps to reduce stress and thus blood pressure. Coral in rose water is an excellent tonic for the heart, as it contains calcium and magnesium, usually deficient in hypertensives.

HYPERTENSION AND HEAVY METAL TOXICITY

Jonathan Wright, M.D., of Kent, Washington, saw a patient with unexplained high blood pressure (156/100-80/110) for the duration of three years. Blood, urine, and kidney examinations were all normal. The patient was on a diet free from added salt, sugar, refined flour, and caffeine, high in vegetables, and fruits and supplemented with vitamins C and E. He exercised regularly and did not smoke.

The patient was an industrial painter, and Dr. Wright suspected that heavy metals in the paints such as lead and cadmium were the problem. Pubic hair analysis showed higher than usual amounts of lead, cobalt, and cadmium. He placed the patient on supplements of zinc to force the cadmium out of his system, and increased the vitamin C supplement to bowel tolerance. Dr. Wright recommended extra vitamin B_6 to prevent the increased vitamin C from causing kidney stones and he added selenium, which is known to protect against cadmium toxicity.

Dr. Wright also recommended linseed oil, which contains essential fatty acids known to reduce blood pressure. After six months, the patient's blood pressure had dropped to 154/96; after twelve months to 142/90; and after eighteen months to 134/80. At this time, the patient's supplements were cut back in dosage, but zinc and vitamin C were continued to prevent recurrence.

Rauwolfia, and its extract, reserpine, is particularly useful in helping to regulate blood pressure. Care must be taken when prescribing rauwolfia and reserpine, however, because they can cause central nervous system depression, and should not be given to patients suffering from depression.

Traditional Chinese Medicine

According to Traditional Chinese Medicine (TCM), essential hypertension is usually due to a problem in the circulation of energy (*qi*) in the body. Diet and long-term emotional distress such as chronic nervousness, anger, and depression can lead to this condition. "Treatment is aimed at bringing the energy flow of the body back into balance through a combination of acupuncture and herbs," says Harvey Kaltsas, Ac. Phys. (FL), D.Ac. (RI), Dip. Ac. (NCCA), of Sarasota, Florida, President of the American Association of Acupuncture and Oriental Medicine.

"Secondary hypertension often occurs when the energy reserves become exhausted (called "kidney *yin* deficiency" in Traditional Chinese Medicine), and can also be treated with a combination of acupuncture and herbs to build up and restore one's energy."

With early diagnosis and treatment, not only can hypertension be alleviated, but complications including damage to the heart, brain, kidney, and liver can be prevented. In addition to acupuncture and herbs, other important elements of treatment include exercises such as *qigong*, meditation, and a diet high in vegetables and low in fat, sugar, and alcohol.

Mark T. Holmes, O.M.D., L.Ac., Director of the Center for Regeneration in Beverly Hills, California, relates two cases in which TCM successfully controlled hypertension. The first case involved a forty-six-year-old, white, male attorney with essential hypertension, whose blood pressure was 160/90. Additional symptoms included impotence, insomnia, red eyes, nervousness, and a decreased desire to exercise. An inability to relax after work combined with a nightly habit of drinking two bottles of expensive wine were determined to be causative factors. Laboratory tests revealed elevated liver enzymes. In TCM this is referred to as a "flaring up of liver fire." After seven months of daily herbal intake combined with regular acupuncture treatments, the patient's hypertension was reversed. All other symptoms abated except the impotency, which significantly improved.

See Traditional Chinese Medicine.

Dr. Holmes also successfully treated an eighty-year-old woman suffering from secondary hypertension with a combination of Traditional Chinese Medicine and Western medication. Normally, her blood pressure remained high, between 210/90. This dropped moderately to 180/90 with the use of her prescribed medication. Using Chinese herbs combined with bimonthly acupuncture and homeopathic remedies, Dr. Holmes was able to stabilize her blood pressure at 130-140/85. A subsequent Western clinical examination revealed a 20 percent increase of carotid artery circulation.

Self-Care

The following therapies can be undertaken at home under appropriate professional supervision.

• Fasting • Yoga

Aromatherapy: Ylang ylang, marjoram, lavender.

Hydrotherapy: Constitutional hydrotherapy: apply two to five times weekly.

Juice Therapy: Celery, beet, and carrot or cucumber, spinach, and parsley. Add a little raw garlic to vegetable juices. Or, run a clove of garlic through juicer, followed by enough carrots to make eight ounces of juice. Drink once per day.

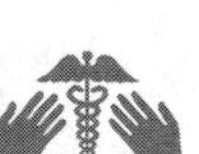

Professional Care

The following therapies should only be provided by a qualified health professional:

• Acupuncture • Chelation Therapy • Environmental Medicine • Hypnotherapy • Orthomolecular Medicine • Osteopathy

Bodywork: Acupressure, reflexology, *shiatsu,* massage, rolfing, Feldenkais, Alexander technique, Therapeutic Touch.

Magnetic Field Therapy: Recent studies from Russia show that magnetic treatments reduce blood pressure in certain patients with hypertension.[30]

Cranial Electrical Stimulation: William Lee Cowden, M.D., uses cranial electrical stimulation to treat hypertensive patients, reporting that it can lower blood pressure and can alleviate panic attacks within thirty to forty minutes of treatment.

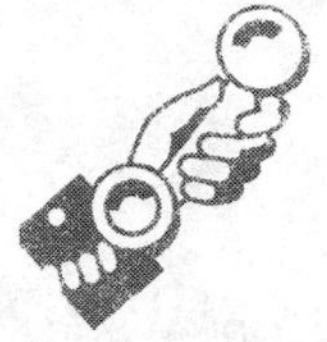

Where to Find Help

For additional information and referrals for hypertension treatment, contact the following organizations.

American Academy of Environmental Medicine
P.O. Box 16106
Denver, Colorado 80216
(303) 622-9755

The academy offers extensive training for physicians interested in learning more about environmental medicine. For information on physicians practicing environmental medicine send a self-addressed, stamped envelope stating your request.

American Association of Acupuncture and Oriental Medicine
4101 Lake Boone Trail, Suite 201
Raleigh, North Carolina 27607
(919) 787-5181

The AAAOM is a national professional trade organization of acupuncturists who meet acceptable standards of competency and can provide you with the names and locations of local members. Referrals by written request only.

American Association of Naturopathic Physicians
2366 Eastlake Avenue, Suite 322
Seattle, Washington 98102
(206) 323-7610

Provides a directory of naturopathic physicians and offers referrals to a nationwide network of accredited or licensed practitioners. Publishes a quarterly newsletter for both professionals and the general public. Also offers a series of brochures and pamphlets on a variety of subjects.

American Academy of Orthomolecular Medicine
The Huxley Institute for Biosocial Research
900 North Federal Highway
Boca Raton, Florida 33432
(800) 847-3802

This resource serves as a clearinghouse of information and as a referral service for physicians practicing orthomolecular medicine.

American College of Advancement in Medicine
P.O. Box 3427
Laguna Hills, California 92654
(714) 583-7666

This pioneer organization seeks to establish certification and standards of practice for chelation therapy. It provides training and education, and sponsors semi-annual conferences for physicians and scientists. It provides referrals and informational material, including a directory listing of all physicians worldwide who have been trained in preventative medicine as well as in the ACAM protocol for chelation therapy. The directory is updated monthly. The organization also provides a copy of the ACAM protocol for chelation to the public.

American Holistic Medical Association
4101 Lake Boone Trail, Suite 201
Raleigh, North Carolina 27607
(919) 787-5181

A professional organization for holistic practitioners, the AHMA offers information and services for its members and lobbies for holistic issues. It also provides referrals for the public; requests must be in writing.

American School of Ayurvedic Sciences
10025 NE 4th Street
Bellevue, Washington 98004
(206) 453-8022

This college provides medical training for physicians and health care practitioners, as well as individual courses for lay people. Dr. Virender Sodhi's Ayurvedic, Naturopathic Medical Clinic is also located at this address.

Ayurvedic Institute
11311 Menaul NE, Suite A
Albuquerque, New Mexico 87112
(505) 291-9698

The institute, directed by Dr. Vasant Lad, trains people from all walks of life in most of the aspects of Ayurveda.

Maharishi Ayur-Veda Medical Center
P.O. Box 282
Fairfield, Iowa 52556
(515) 472-5866

The center provides referrals to health centers, which offer treatment for prevention and the treatment of a broad range of illnesses. They also train practitioners and provide information to the lay public.

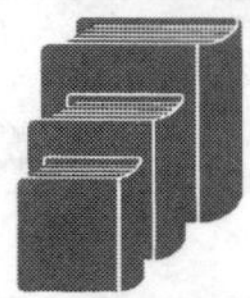

Recommended Reading

Choices for a Healthy Heart. Piscatelli, Joseph C. New York: Workman Publishing, 1987.

A guide to making the crucial choices about diet and lifestyle that can prevent coronary problems.

Controlling High Blood Pressure Without Drugs. Charles Bennett, M.D. New York: Doubleday Books, 1984.

A clear, practical plan for the management of diet, exercise, and stress that will increase health and decrease the need for expensive drugs.

Dr. Dean Ornish's Program for Reversing Heart Disease. Ornish, M.D., Dean. New York: Ballantine, 1990.

A step-by-step guide through Dr. Ornish's program of halting and even reversing heart disease through a change of lifestyle. Dr. Ornish goes beyond the physical aspects of health care to consider the psychological, emotional, and spiritual conditions that are vital to healing.

Encyclopedia of Natural Medicine. Murray, Michael, N.D.; and Pizzorno, Joseph, N.D. Rocklin, CA: Prima Publishing, 1991.

A definitive guide for the layperson on naturopathic medicine. Contains a chapter on hypertension.

High Blood Pressure. Chaitow, Leon. San Francisco, CA: Thorsons, 1988.

A clear, simple self-help guide that explains the causes of high blood pressure and describes ways to elevate it through diet, exercise, and other natural methods.

The High Blood Pressure Solution: Natural Prevention and Cure with the 'K' Factor. Moore, Richard, M.D., Ph.D. Rochester, VT: Healing Arts Press, 1993.

How to control high blood pressure by maintaining the proper ratio of potassium and sodium in the diet.

Hypertension and Your Diet. Carlson, Wade. New Canaan, CT: Keates Publishing, 1990.

The latest information on how to correct and avoid hypertension.

The New Supernutrition Book. Passwater, Richard A. New York: Pocket Books, 1991.

The celebrated nutritionist's book discusses the latest discoveries about, and solutions for, contemporary nutritional problems, including information on the relationships between diet and nutrition and supernutrients. Provides diet programs for specific problems.

Overcoming Hypertension. Cooper, Kenneth M.D., M.P.H. New York: Bantam, 1990.

The latest facts on coronary risks, a guide to hypertensive drugs, and complete fitness and diet programs.

The Relaxation Response. Benson, Herbert; and Klipper, Miriam Z. New York: Avon, 1976.

The relaxation response is a meditative technique derived from Transcendental Meditation, that can relieve stress, hypertension, anxiety, stress, and stress-related illnesses.

Stress Management. Gordon, James S., M.D. with introduction by C. Everett Koop, M.D., Sc.D. New York: Chelsea House Publishers, 1990.

Stress Management *traces the interaction between stress and bodily functions and describes a few of the many programs available to manage the condition before it becomes destructive. The book places special emphasis on holistic approaches such as wellness programs, which use biofeedback, massage, and body awareness techniques to promote relaxation and health.*

Male Health

Normal function of the male genitourinary tract is essential to the overall health of a man's body. Because this system is susceptible to a number of conditions and disorders, special attention must be paid to its health in order to maintain healthy sexual function, proper elimination, and general vitality.

Statistically, men experience higher rates of heart disease, cancer, chronic lung disorders, liver diseases, and diabetes than women, all of which contribute to an average life expectancy of seven years less than women. These conditions, however, are not unique to men. Therefore when a person thinks of male health the focus is primarily on disorders of their genitourinary organs.

Because the genitourinary tracts of men and women are distinct, each requires its own specific set of health requirements. Female health issues have been well publicized and discussed with relative openness. Men's health issues, on the other hand, are just beginning to be seen as equally important.

This is partly due to men in general, who traditionally have been less likely to seek medical attention than women, especially for minor problems which often serve as warning signs for more serious underlying illness. The result is higher morbidity and mortality rates resulting from the advanced state of the illness when it is eventually discovered. Social and economic pressures, as well as a lack of understanding of what constitutes normal function also contribute to men's ambivalence in issues of male health.

> *"It is estimated that about 10 million men in the United States are experiencing some form of impotency, of which only two hundred thousand per year seek medical help."*
>
> —Tom Kruzel, N.D.

Types of Male Health Disorders

The health of the genitourinary organs reflects a man's overall well-being, according to Dana Ullman, M.P.H., Director of Homeopathic Educational Services, in Berkeley, California. Individual sexual habits can also influence a person's state of health, just as the health of the body and the male reproductive system can be a determining factor for sexual habits and sexual drive. Some of the most common male health concerns include impotence, benign prostatic hypertrophy, prostatitis, and prostate cancer.

Impotence

Impotence is defined as the inability to sustain a satisfactory erection to perform intercourse and ejaculation. "It is estimated that about 10 million men in the United States are experiencing some form of impotence, of which only about two hundred thousand per year seek medical help," according to Tom Kruzel, N.D., of Gresham, Oregon. Although impotence has long been associated with aging, Dr. Kruzel points out that growing older is not necessarily an inevitable cause. "Rather, the amount and force of ejaculation decreases, while the recovery period between ejaculations becomes longer," he says. "This varies from person to person, depending on their overall health and vitality."

There are two forms of impotence—primary and secondary. "Primary impotence is rare and is almost always associated with severe psychopathology," says Dr. Kruzel. "This may include unreasonable fear of engaging in intercourse, fear of intimacy, or extreme feelings of guilt or anxiety about the act of intercourse. Low male sex hormone levels can also be a cause."

In cases of primary impotence, men are unable to engage in sexual intercourse.

Secondary impotence is the more common type of impotence and Dr. Kruzel estimates that it is related to psychological causes about 80 percent of the time. "Men who suffer from secondary impotence are only able to engage in intercourse 25 percent of the time," he says.

"This is most often situational in nature though, as the person may have become bored with the relationship, or the place and time may be less than optimal. Emotional factors such as low self-esteem, immaturity, performance anxiety, and depression can also play a role."

One way of evaluating the cause of any impotence is to evaluate whether or not an erection occurs while sleeping, which generally happens during REM (rapid eye movement) sleep. The usual method of doing this is called the "stamp test," which involves placing a ring of paper around the penis prior to bedtime. If the ring has been disrupted in the morning, the man has experienced an erection at some time during the night. This indicates that the cause of the impotence is most likely due to psychological factors rather than to physical causes.

Illness can also contribute to impotence, according to Dr. Kruzel, as can certain endocrine disorders such as hypothyroidism and hypopituitary function. Vascular diseases can also play a role due to their effects on the vessels of the penis. Neurological disorders from injury or brain disease have also been found to be causes, as have the various surgeries of the genitalia. Medications such as antihypertensives and psychotrophics are also a common reason for impotence, especially in elderly men taking multiple prescriptions.

THE PROSTATE GLAND'S RELATIONSHIP TO MALE HEALTH

The prostate gland lies at the base of the bladder, surrounding the urethra. It secretes a thin, milky white alkaline fluid during ejaculation to enhance delivery and fertility of the sperm. In addition, the prostate also acts as the genitourinary system's first line of defense against infection and disease.

Some of the more common problems associated with the prostate are benign prostatic hypertrophy, prostatitis, and prostatic cancer. All of these conditions are greatly influenced and accelerated by the aging process, and therefore need to be checked for regularly, especially as men move through middle age into older age.

Benign Prostatic Hypertrophy

According to Dr. Kruzel, by the age of fifty, about 30 percent of all men will start to experience difficulties with urination related to enlargement of the prostate gland or benign prostatic hypertrophy (BPH). Increases in the number of times a man has to visit the bathroom along with a frequent sensation of having to urinate—especially at night—are among some of the early signs. In addition, a reduction in the force and caliber of urination is also characteristic of prostatic enlargement. Instability of the detrusor muscle (the outer muscle layer of the bladder) can even result in urinary incontinence. "This occurs in 2 percent to 3 percent of patients with BPH," Dr. Kruzel says. "These symptoms often lead to an increased sense of frustration and embarrassment, as well as the disruption of normal activities, translating into several billion dollars a year in related health management costs."

"By the age of fifty, about 30 percent of all men will start to experience difficulties with urination related to enlargement of the prostate gland or benign prostatic hypertrophy."
—Tom Kruzel, N.D.

Enlargement of the prostate is usually caused by an abnormal overgrowth and/or swelling of the tissue of the prostate, which then blocks the urethra or opening from the bladder. Problems associated with this condition usually continue to worsen with age, increasing in incidence to about 50 percent of all males by the age of sixty, and up to almost 80 percent past age seventy.[1] Most physicians consider this to be a normal consequence of aging.

The growth of prostate tissue that results in BPH occurs due to the hormone testosterone which is produced by both the testicles and the adrenal glands, according to Dr. Kruzel. As a person ages the conversion of testosterone to its more active form of dihydrotestosterone (DHT) becomes greater. "The more active DHT results in a greater proliferation or growth of tissues in the prostate gland, which ultimately leads to the obstruction of the urethra which passes through it," Dr. Kruzel explains.

Chronic constipation has also been implicated as being a contributing factor to prostatic discomfort when there is an already enlarged gland. A correction of the constipation will bring some relief of symptoms since the rectum puts pressure on the prostate gland when it is enlarged. In addition, there is a buildup of waste products in the circulation with chronic constipation. This will indirectly have an effect on the function of the prostate.

Prostatitis

Prostatitis is an inflammation or infection of the prostate gland most often seen in men between

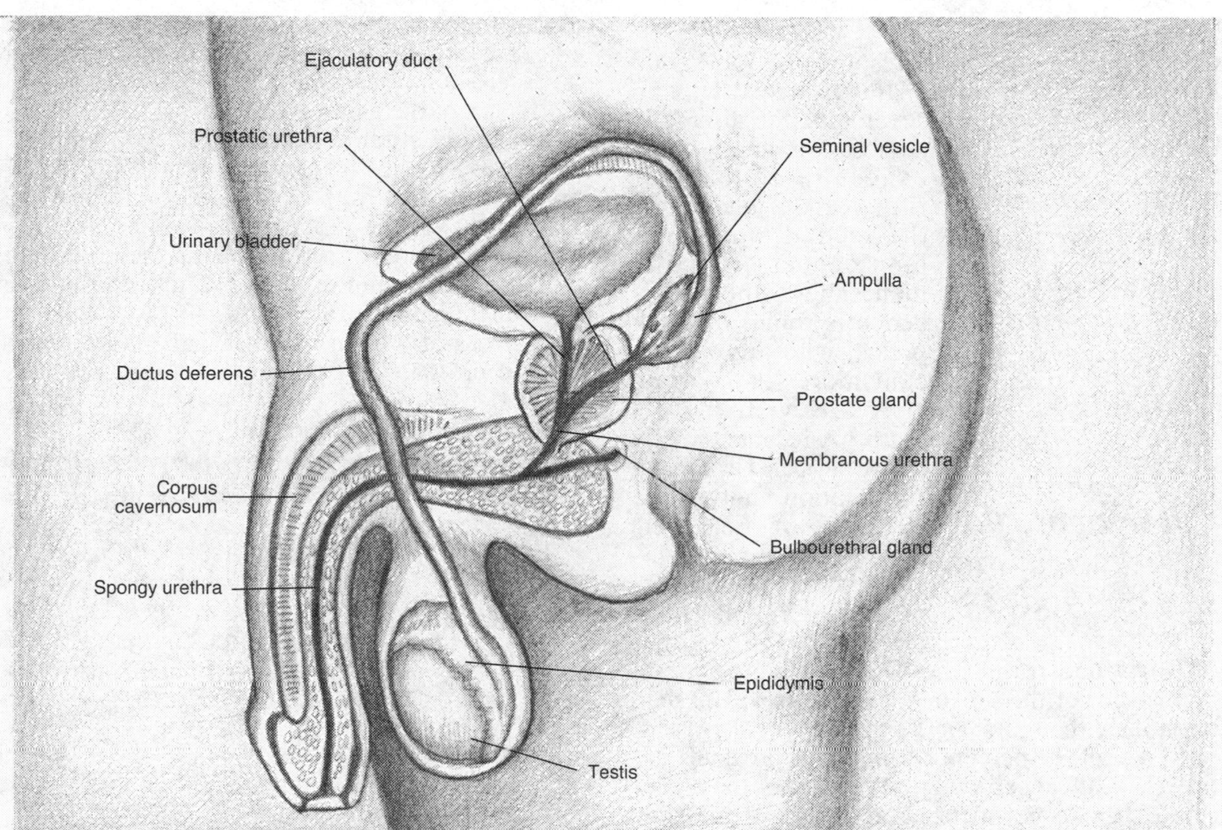

The prostate and the male genitourinary tract.

the ages of twenty to fifty. It is commonly viewed as being due to an infective agent such as a bacteria or chlamydia (an intracellular parasite transmitted through sexual contact). Bacteria in the urine, which passes through the urethra, can settle in the prostate which surrounds it. Noninfective forms of prostatitis are also recognized and may be associated with autoimmune disorders.[2] Several researchers have suggested that infective agents may not be the cause of the condition but are instead acting opportunistically upon a depleted glandular environment.[3]

Depletion of glandular elements such as zinc, ascorbic acid, and proteolytic enzymes (enzymes that break down complex proteins) make it easier for an infection to occur, states Dr. Kruzel. Prostatitis can also follow increased amounts of sexual activity, particularly with multiple partners, by depleting the prostate of enzymes and zinc which sterilize the urethra and protect the gland from infection, and introducing additional bacteriological factors. (It is advised that all sexual activity, including masturbation, be eliminated during infection in order to allow the prostate to renew itself, and to keep the infection from spreading further.) Excesses of caffeine, alcohol, and spicy foods also contribute to a lack of glandular nutrition which ultimately adds to depletion of the prostate and lowered immune function.[4]

Symptoms of prostatitis include difficulty, frequency, and urgency along with a burning sensation or pain during urination, and a discharge from the penis after bowel movements. These symptoms range from mild to severe, and come and go over time, with the prostate gland being susceptible to both acute and chronic infection or inflammation. According to Dr. Kruzel, an acute condition is often signaled by severe pain and tenderness in the region of the prostate, sometimes extending up into the genitals, pelvis, and back. Fever, chills, and overall fatigue can also follow.

Symptoms of a chronic condition are similar, but milder. More often than not these symptoms will be disregarded and treatment will be delayed or foregone completely. If the condition is caused by an infection which is untreated or unrecognized it may result in the infection of the sex partner as well, and can lead to more severe complications such as kidney infection, epididymitis (an inflammation of the epididymis, a tube along the backside of the testicles), and orchitis (a painful swelling of the testicles). Bladder outlet obstruction and prostate stones may also occur if chronic prostatitis is allowed to persist untreated.

Prostatic Cancer

Cancer of the prostate is responsible for 35,000 deaths every year in the United States, with an additional 165,000 men developing the disease in the same period.[5] It is the most commonly found cancer in males over fifty years of age and is the second most common cancer afflicting men. The highest incidence is found in black males, who are 40 percent more likely to be stricken with the disease.[6] A recent study by the American Urological Association showed the incidence of precancerous prostate gland lesions to range from 22 percent to 41 percent in males between the ages of thirty and forty-nine years.[7] "This suggests that cancer of the prostate is more prevalent than previously thought," Dr. Kruzel says.

"Cancer of the prostate is responsible for 35,000 deaths every year in the United States, with an additional 165,000 men developing the disease in the same period."

About 20 percent of enlarged prostates are the result of cancer. Fully 80 percent of these cancers either do not metastasize or are of the slow growing variety, often causing little if any problem.[8] The remaining forms spread more rapidly, primarily to the bones of the spine and lymph nodes of the pelvis. "One of the problems with cancer of the prostate lies in the fact that it may be present without any detectable symptoms, or with symptoms identical to those found in BPH," Dr. Kruzel explains. "Few of the classic cancer symptoms of weight loss, blood in the urine, urinary retention, pain, or the swelling of tissues due to the accumulation of lymph are present early on in the disease and may not show up at all until metastases has occurred. This can lead to its continued growth and subsequent spread throughout the body."

See Cancer.

As with other cancers, the precise cause of prostatic cancer is unknown. Genetic factors seem to play a role, and there are more occurrences in some families than in others, with black males showing a greater incidence than other ethnic groups. Hormonal factors may also affect the prostate as early on as puberty by delaying sexual development and maturity. Persons who enter puberty later also seem to have higher incidences of prostatic cancer, probably due to that late development, according to Dr. Kruzel.

Hormone levels certainly influence the course of cancer once it has become established. According to Dr. Kruzel, higher incidences of cancer found as the male population ages is related to the change in internal hormone levels, from testosterone to the more active DHT, that is normally part of the aging process.

Several studies indicate that men who undergo vasectomies have increased risks of developing prostate as well as testicular cancer.[9] This may be due to the production of allosperm antibodies which are formed following the procedure, which lower immune response and the body's subsequent inability to destroy cancerous cells.[10]

It has also been noted that there are higher rates of prostatic cancer, as well as other cancers, in males who are exposed to only chemical toxins. Workers in the petrochemical, rubber, and textile industries have among the highest cancer rates for industrial employees.[11] Urban areas have higher incidences as opposed to rural, which is thought to be due to air and other pollution.[12] Cadmium, a metallic element used in batteries, has also been implicated in cancer of the prostate, as evidenced by a demonstrably higher incidence of cancer found in men who work with batteries.[13]

DRUGS ASSOCIATED WITH A HIGHER INCIDENCE OF IMPOTENCE

According to the Physicians Desk Reference the following drugs are associated with side effects of impotence. (Statistics refer to the percentage of individuals affected.)[14]

- *Anafranil Capsules (Up to 20%)*
- *Eulexin Capsules (33% with LHRH agonist)*
- *Lupron Depot 3.75 milligrams (Among most frequent), 7.5 milligrams (5.4%)*
- *Lupron Injection (5% or more)*
- *Normodyne Injection, Tablets (1-4%)*
- *Paxil Tablets (1.9-10.0%)*
- *Proscar Tablets (3.7%)*
- *Roferon-A Injection (6%)*
- *Wellbutrin Tablets (3.4%)*

Treatment and Prevention of Male Disorders

Conventional Western medicine tends to view all genitourinary disorders as conditions that can be treated solely with medication, surgery, or medical devices. Alternative physicians, by contrast, look at the underlying causes as well, whether physical or mental, internal or external. This approach to health can result in a more pronounced and longer lasting improvement in overall health.

Some of the alternative modalities most often used in the treatment of male health issues include diet and nutrition, herbal medicine, homeopathy, acupuncture, Traditional Chinese Medicine, and Ayurvedic medicine.

Diet and Nutrition

"Poor nutrition is a primary cause of most conditions of the genitourinary tract," Dr. Kruzel states. "A good diet and nutritional program is a must for normal function. An avoidance of spicy foods, caffeine, alcohol, tobacco, and foods high in fat and carbohydrates is also imperative to the treatment of any disease of the prostate, as these factors can serve as irritants, negating the effects of essential nutrients such as vitamin C, vitamin E, and zinc." Supplementation of these nutrients is crucial for treating any prostate disorders as they are among the more prominent elements found in prostatic tissues. These nutrients are also necessary for the formation of seminal fluid.[15]

See Diet, Herbal Medicine, Homeopathy, Nutritional Supplements.

Vitamin C is a major component of the seminal vesicles and prostate gland, and high amounts are found in prostatic secretions. Vitamin E is also present and, due to its fat solubility, acts as an antioxidant and stabilizes membranes and lipids. Zinc has long been used in the treatment of prostatic disease, because of its prominent role in the metabolism of prostatic tissue as well as its sterilizing effect, which keeps the gland and urethra free of microorganisms.

> *"Poor nutrition is a primary cause of most conditions of the genitourinary tract."*
> Tom Kruzel, N.D.

A general vitamin and mineral supplementation routine is also beneficial, especially one high in B vitamins and magnesium. In numerous studies, magnesium has been shown to be an important nutrient which is deficient in most people. Garlic in its natural clove form can also help supply the body with vitamins and minerals and, most importantly, helps to prevent infection.

Essential fatty acids such as fish oils, olive oil, evening primrose oil, and eicosapentaenoic acid (EPA) are also needed in large amounts by the prostate gland. These become especially important if there is a high level of sexual activity, which can deplete the prostate gland of nutrients needed for normal function. They can also act to reduce blood clotting associated with prostate cancer, thus lowering the potential for the spreading of tumors.[16]

Glandular therapy has proven to be very effective in the treatment of disorders of the prostate gland. Extracts of bovine (cow) or porcine (pig) prostatic tissue taken orally or administered intramuscularly provides essential nutrients and growth factors to the gland. This is often coupled with other nutritional or herbal medicines.

Several researchers have also speculated that the prostate gland may be susceptible to autoimmune diseases. Glandular therapy may also provide a protective function against circulating autoantibodies or immune complexes due to the similarity of their cellular structures.[17]

NATURAL PROGESTERONE AND MALE HEALTH CONDITIONS

One doctor, who preferred not to be identified due to the current climate of medical politics, suggests that topical application of natural progesterone may prove beneficial in the treatment of prostate conditions. The doctor reports working with twelve men, all in their late seventies, who were suffering from osteoporosis. As it has been well established that natural progesterone, applied topically, can relieve osteoporosis, the physician suggested that the men systematically massage it into their skin on a daily basis. All of them began to experience relief from their condition, and later called to tell him that, after three months of daily massage, they were also experiencing an improved urine flow, with less pressure on their prostate glands and a noticeable decrease in nightly urination. Each patient was also suffering from enlarged prostates but had not mentioned it in the original exam as they had just attributed the condition to old age. Although the experience of the men is anecdotal, it suggests an area of research to determine exactly how natural progesterone can work to reverse prostatic disorders.

Herbal Medicine

Herbal medicine can offer many of the same therapeutic benefits for treatment of genitourinary tract disorders as drug therapy, without any of the potentially severe side effects. Herbal medications need to be specific to the individual condition in order for them to be most effective, according to Dr. Kruzel, and should always be taken under the guidance of a trained health practitioner to ensure maximum result.

Impotence: *Coryanthe yohimbe* and *Ginkgo biloba* are often used for the treatment of impotence due to their ability to stimulate vascular flow to the penis. *Coryanthe yohimbe* has also been shown to increase libido and decrease the latency period between ejaculations, as well as have a positive effect on impotence problems due to depression.[18] Several studies have confirmed the beneficial action of ginkgo, including one in which a *Ginkgo biloba* extract was found to increase penile blood flow in a group of patients who had not responded to traditional drug therapy. Half the group regained potency within six months.[19]

Aletrius farinosa, or true unicorn root, has been reported to be an excellent herbal medication for impotence in men, and has been used to promote fertility in both males and females.[20] Also, *Serenoa repens*, or saw palmetto, works well for impotence, especially if included with other medicines.

Strychnos Nux vomica is also used for the treatment of sexual dysfunction, especially if it is caused by an excess of alcohol, cigarettes, or dietary indiscretions. Since it contains small amounts of strychnine alkaloids, it can be very toxic if taken improperly and is only available through physicians trained in its use. It can also be used in the homeopathic dose with equal or better effect.[21]

Additionally, Siberian ginseng or *Panax ginseng* is widely believed to have aphrodisiac properties for which it has been prized over the centuries. Known as an adaptogen, it affects whichever system of the body may be in need of support. Its American counterpart, *Eleuthrococcus senticosus*, does not possess quite the stimulating properties, but is safer to use over the long term.[22]

Benign Prostatic Hypertrophy: Berries from the saw palmetto plant contain about 15 percent saturated and unsaturated fatty acids and sterols which have been found in studies to reduce prostatic swelling, stimulate immune function, and prevent the conversion of testosterone to its more potent DHT form. When used in clinical trials, saw palmetto has been shown to result in a significant decrease in prostate size and relief of symptoms.[23]

The powdered bark of the tree *Pygeum africanus* has also been used for centuries as a treatment for urinary disorders. Scientists in France who isolated its active compounds were able to conclude that the herbal preparation did in fact produce anti-inflammatory, antiedema, and cholesterol-lowering properties. Clinical trials on both animals and humans have clearly shown this herb to promote the regression of symptoms associated with BPH with no toxic side effects observed, even at large doses and with prolonged use.[24]

Another herb that has been indicated for problems associated with prostatic hypertrophy is *Aletrius farinosa*.[25]

A sixty-eight-year-old man complaining of blood in his urine, difficulty with urination, decreased urinary flow, slight urgency, frequently having to go to the bathroom, and a sensation of having a ball in his rectum was diagnosed as having an enlarged prostate gland and a bladder stone.

The patient was started on saw palmetto extract, prostate glandulars, and a combination of herbal medicines, which included *Pygeum africanus*, horsetail, and cornsilk, to reduce the size of the bladder stone.

Within ten days the patient reported a decrease in visible blood with urination, an increase in urinary flow and force of the stream, and a decrease in the ball sensation in his rectum. Microscopic examination of the urine three months later was normal and the patient was placed on a low dose of the saw palmetto extract to prevent further problems. According to Dr. Kruzel, this case is typical of patient response to treatment for an enlarged prostate gland and/or bladder or kidney stone.

Prostatitis: *Chimaphilia umbellata*, or pipsissewa, is an evergreen plant used in the treatment of urinary tract disorders. It is especially useful for the treatment of chronic prostatitis, as well as kidney and bladder stones. It contains arbutin, the active ingredient in uva ursi, a powerful urinary tract antiseptic, and also helps provide the urinary tract and prostate with increased blood flow and nutrition.[26]

Horsetail is also an excellent herbal medicine in the treatment of acute prostatic infection. It is also indicated for urinary loss due to inflammation of the bladder or prostate and can be used for the treatment of bladder and kidney stones as well.[27]

Echinacea angustifolia, or purple coneflower, is a powerful herbal antimicrobial agent which can be used against any infective process, including prostatitis.[28] The herbs *Delphinia staphysagria, Thuja occidentalis*, and *Anemone pulsatilla* are also indicated for inflammation of the prostate gland. These herbal agents act to decrease pain, vesicle irritation, swelling of the prostate, and impotence associated with prostatitis, according to Dr. Kruzel.

Prostate Cancer: Numerous herbal formulas are also available for the treatment of cancer of the prostate. In general herbal medicines are not specific for the different types of tumors encountered but rather act as an overall immune system stimulant. "Herbal medications perform a variety of functions when attacking cancerous tissue," Dr. Kruzel says. "They act to stimulate production and activation of both T and B cell systems of the lymphocytic variety of white blood cells. Additionally, herbal preparations will adhere to the tumor cell surface making it easier for the lymphocytes to attach and destroy the cell. Certain components of herbal medicines will also enter the tumor cell to disrupt its function, making it more vulnerable to destruction by the immune system. The herbs employed in such treatment also have built-in check and balance systems which make it less likely for them to become toxic and thus harmful to healthy tissues."

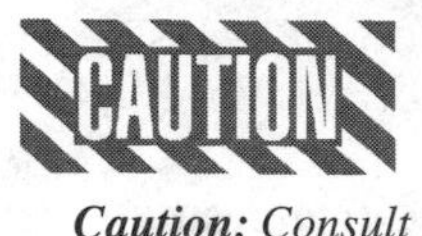

Caution: Consult your physician if you suspect you may have cancer.

Saw palmetto and *Pygeum africanus*, because of their ability to inhibit testosterone conversion, decrease swelling, and provide increased blood flow to the prostate, are essential parts of any herbal medicine program specifically for prostate cancer. Less specifically but equally important are the use of medicines such as *Phytolacca decandra*,[29] *Vinca rosa*,[30] *Viscum album*,[31] *Colchicum autumnale*,[32] *Conium maculatum*,[33] *Berberis aquifolium*,[34] *Echinacea angustifolia*,[35] *Digitalis purpuria*,[36] and *Arctium lappa*.[37] "These herbs have been found to effectively help treat cancer of the prostate and, when used along with a holistically oriented program, have as good as, or better, survival rates than conventional therapy," Dr. Kruzel states.

For a sixty-nine-year-old male diagnosed with prostate cancer, the immediate surgical removal of his testicles and prostate were recommended, as well as a course of chemotherapy. Dr. Kruzel placed him on saw palmetto extract, Hoxsey formula (an herbal formula developed by the late Harry Hoxsey, N.D., used to treat cancer), plus *Viscum album* (mistletoe), *Phytolacca decandra* (poke weed), and high doses of vitamins C and E. He was also begun on the homeopathic remedy *Lycopodium* and had already changed to a primarily vegetarian diet at the time of the first visit.

"Over the next six months the tumor size was monitored by the prostatic specific antigen test (PSA) and rectal ultrasound," Dr. Kruzel recounts. "Within the first sixty days the PSA dropped from a high reading of 4.5 (a normal reading is 0.5 to 4.0) to 3.0, but there was no change noted on ultrasound. By the end of the six month period, though, the tumor had decreased in size upon ultrasound examination and the PSA level had decreased to 2.6."

According to Dr. Kruzel, this patient will be kept on immune-stimulating herbal medication at low levels and saw palmetto extract until the tumor disappears completely on ultrasound or another biopsy shows that it is no longer present. It is his view that the patient has a very good prognosis as long as he continues to follow the dietary, herbal medicine, and vitamin recommendations. It is also recommended that the patient continue to take the saw palmetto extract indefinitely to keep the tumor from being acted upon by testosterone.

Homeopathy

By itself, homeopathy may work for a wide variety of urological conditions. It is also often combined with other treatments, such as herbal medicines and nutrition, to increase the healing action of the remedy and the degree of healing experienced.

Homeopathic remedies may work extremely well for problems of impotence, especially if the condition is due to psychological causes. Numerous homeopathic medications are also available for the treatment of benign prostatic hypertrophy and may be very effective in offering short- and long-term relief.

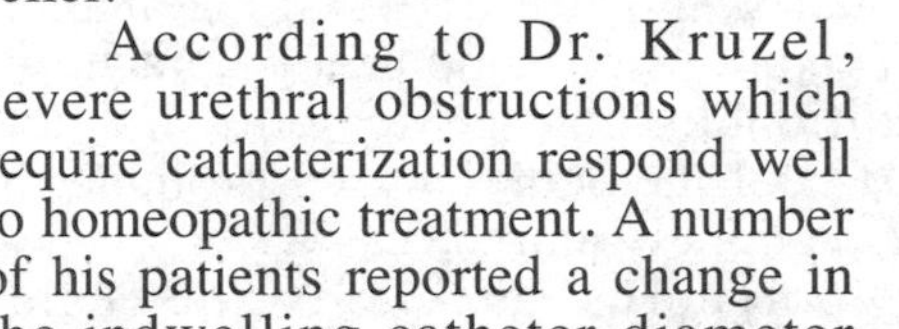

See Homeopathy.

According to Dr. Kruzel, severe urethral obstructions which require catheterization respond well to homeopathic treatment. A number of his patients reported a change in the indwelling catheter diameter during the course of homeopathic therapy as the prostate gland reduced in size. "Initial reduction in size occurred within the first week to ten days of therapy," he reports. "Ultimately the patients were able to urinate without them, as over the next six to eight weeks, normal urinary function returned."

Homeopathy has been used to treat all forms of prostatitis and works especially well with chronic prostatitis which has been unresponsive to conventional antibiotic treatment. "The patient may have experienced prolonged discomfort, sometimes lasting for years, because the condition was incompletely treated initially," says Dr. Kruzel.

Dr. Kruzel treated a thirty-eight-year-old male with severe aching pains in his hips, thighs, testicles, and prostate gland. His condition had been initially diagnosed twelve years earlier as gonococcal urethritis and was treated with antibiotics. Almost immediately after the disappearance of his discharge, the pains began in his hips and thighs. He received several courses of antibiotic therapy over a three-year period which did nothing to relieve his symptoms. He was later diagnosed by a rheumatologist as having arthritis and placed on nonsteroidal anti-inflammatory medication.

Dr. Kruzel reports he started him on homeopathic *Berberis* 30C and at his one-month follow-up the man reported that he was about 60 percent better. After three months on the homeopathic medication he was completely pain free and no longer taking the arthritis medicine.

Traditional Chinese Medicine

Disorders of the genitourinary tract are commonly regarded by practitioners of Traditional Chinese Medicine (TCM) and acupuncture as a combination of symptoms of the disease process itself and the effects of the patient's lifestyle. A patient is always evaluated for both his constitutional state, or *qi* (vital life energy), and his nutritional status. The condition is also viewed as to whether it is of an internal nature (psychological causes or an internal organ disharmony), or an external nature (physical causes such as spicy foods, alcohol, or drug use). From these the person is then diagnosed as being either *yin* or *yang*, hot or cold, possessing dampness or moisture, or whether he is hot and/or dry.

Prostatitis and urethritis are generally viewed as conditions of damp heat by practitioners of Traditional Chinese Medicine and acupuncture. Herbal medicines which promote the removal of dampness and excess water, such as polyporus, akebia, or the cephalanoplos, and Dianthus formulas with their potent herbal combinations, may be used to treat these conditions, according to Dr. Kruzel.

See Acupuncture, Ayurvedic Medicine, Traditional Chinese Medicine.

"Impotence, along with premature ejaculation, is seen primarily as a functional disorder by TCM with stress and nutritional indiscretions being the main contributors," Dr. Kruzel says. "Impotence due to low hormone output is considered a deficiency of kidney *yang*, while premature ejaculation is viewed as an inability to withhold the semen and is considered a deficiency of the kidney storage vessel."

Herbal medications such as *Eleutherococcus senticosus*, which enhances blood flow, is considered superior by many TCM physicians in the treatment of impotence.[38] This is not to be confused with its counterpart *Panax ginseng* which has long been prized as an aphrodisiac. "Many herbalists and physicians consider *Panax ginseng* too stimulating for long-term use as it tends to burn out the kidney fire," Dr. Kruzel says. "They prefer to substitute *Eleutherococcus senticosus* instead. Lyceum berries which are specific for enhancement of kidney and liver *qi* are also used as a *yin* tonic for sexual dysfunction." Herbals such as cascata and lotus seed have also been found to enhance sexual function and eliminate premature ejaculation.[39]

A number of acupuncture points along the Conception Vessel channel can also be used with certain spleen and bladder points to increase energy or *qi* flow to the sexual organs. Treatments are usually done over a period of weeks and tend to have a cumulative effect, gradually restoring normal function.

Nocturia, which is frequency of urination at night, is one the most common symptoms seen with benign prostatic hypertrophy and is treated with both acupuncture and herbal medicines. According to Rick Marinelli, N.D., M.Ac.O.M., of Beaverton, Oregon, benign prostatic hypertrophy responds very well to acupuncture and TCM. A person may remain on herbal medication for several months as the gland recovers, but Dr. Marinelli usually sees some improvement within the first three to six weeks of treatment, especially if coupled with acupuncture.

With chronic benign prostatic hypertrophy, Dr. Marinelli sometimes suspects a low-grade inflammation of the prostate as well, often finding signs and symptoms of burning, urgency, and fullness in the perineal area (the external region between the anus and the genitals). In these cases he suggests a more aggressive treatment plan until the symptoms have resolved.

Similar to the Western medicine view, cancer of the prostate gland is seen as a silent disease in that it may be present without signs or symptoms long before it is found. Yet, where conventional medicine tends to focus on the prostate tumor, Traditional Chinese Medicine tends to focus on the symptomology presented by the whole body.

A treatment plan is therefore designed to address the deficient immune system, based on the symptomology provided by the patient. The *Fu Zheng* treatment, which increases the body's energy flow, is used specifically to strengthen the body's immune function.

In China, most hospitals have departments of Western and Traditional Chinese Medicine which combine their efforts in the treatment of cancer. According to both Drs. Kruzel and Marinelli, patients undergoing conventional treatments such as chemotherapy or radiation often tolerate them better if they are combined with TCM.

Ayurvedic Medicine

According to Virender Sodhi, M.D. (Ayurveda), N.D., Director of the American School of Ayurvedic Sciences in Bellevue, Washington, Ayurvedic medicine can employ a number of herbal treatments to combat problems of the prostate, including *amla*, *triphala*, *neem*, and *shilajit*. Exercises such as the *ashiwin mudra*, which is the squeezing and relaxing of the anal sphincter, are also effective at helping relieve congestion and aiding circulation in the prostate gland, notes Dr. Sodhi.

Dr. Sodhi recalls treating a sixty-five-year-old man who had been diagnosed with BPH for five years, but had not wanted to go into surgery so had sought out alternative therapy. "When he came to me he was not able to urinate properly. A slow, feeble stream was all that was coming out," says Dr. Sodhi. "I had him practice the *ashiwin mudra* and gave him the herb *yashad bhasam*, as well as a preparation which was a combination of *shilajit* and zinc, plus other herbs such as *amla*, *triphala*, *ashwagandha*, and *bala*. We also did prostate massage. Within three months he was able to urinate properly and the prostate gland was softer and more gel-like, indicating significant improvement."

Prostatic Massage

Quite often a buildup of pressure in the prostate can also be due to lack of intercourse and ejaculation, according to Tom Kruzel, N.D., of Gresham, Oregon. "When this occurs, ejaculation through intercourse or masturbation is often recommended in order to relieve pressure," he notes. "In addition, prostatic massage has been shown to be an effective therapy for relieving pressure due to prostate enlargement." The massage is normally administered by a physician, who inserts a gloved finger in the patient's rectum to massage the prostate directly.

Done weekly for the first few weeks until symptoms begin to abate, periodic treatments follow as needed to relieve pressure. Prostatic massage does not affect the cause of the enlargement, but will only relieve symptoms. Excessive pressure by an overenthusiastic physician can also result in bleeding and soreness of the gland, Dr. Kruzel points out. "Prostatic massage is also contraindicated in cases of prostatitis, as it may cause the spread of the infection to other parts of the body, and in cancer, as it may disrupt the integrity of the tumor, causing the cancer to migrate," he says.

For prostatitis Dr. Sodhi recommends three things. First, changing sexual behavior if the infection is due in part to, or exacerbated by, sexual overstimulation. Secondly, increasing the diuresis (flow of urine) so that the patient will urinate more frequently, thereby helping to rid the body of the infection. This can be accomplished by drinking large amounts of water. The congestion can also be relieved with the help of the *ashiwin mudra* exercise and by soaking the testicles in cold water. Lastly, Dr. Sodhi recommends taking antibiotic type herbs such as *neem* to help stop the infection. *Amla* and *shilajit* can be taken as supportive herbs as well.

When a thirty-three-year-old male who had been treated unsuccessfully with antibiotics for his prostatitis came to see Dr. Sodhi, he immediately had the patient stop all sexual activity. "He was a little upset because his medical doctor had said he could have as much sexual activity as possible." Dr. Sodhi started him on berberine and *neem* as well as on zinc supplements. "I also had him soak his testicles and do the *ashiwin mudra* exercises," says Dr. Sodhi. "Within three months all symptoms of his prostatitis were gone."

Prostate cancer can be more difficult to treat according to Dr. Sodhi, "because sometimes by the time it is diagnosed it has already metastasized and spread to the spine or different organs of the body." Dr. Sodhi had one eighty-year-old man come to him who had been told he only had two months to live. "He didn't want to go through a lot of treatment because he felt he had lived a good life and if he only lived another couple months, that was okay." Dr. Sodhi prescribed just one supplement, an *amla* tonic, which is a preparation of *amla* and various extracts of different herbs. "I thought this was the best preparation for fighting the cancer and regenerating the body and the immune system," Dr. Sodhi explains. Dr. Sodhi then lost track of the man until two years later when he was lecturing in Phoenix, Arizona. "A man walked up to me and said, 'Dr. Sodhi, I don't know if you remember me or not, but I'm your patient who was diagnosed with prostate cancer and I'm still living and it's almost two years.'" The man had been reordering his prescription from Dr. Sodhi's office all this time. "I think the *amla* was very helpful to him," states Dr. Sodhi, "but I believe the man's mental attitude was equally as important, because he wasn't afraid of death, or of his cancer."

Prevention

Prevention is the best approach to maintaining the health of the male organs. "Considering the far-reaching effect problems of the genitourinary tract can have on the lives of sufferers in terms of discomfort, the side effects of standard treatments, and the enormous costs that are brought to bear, not to mention quality of life, prevention of these disorders should be undertaken by all men, of all ages," says Dr. Kruzel.

"Periodic examination coupled with a blood test for levels of prostatic specific antigen have been found to provide the best method of early detection for both BPH and cancer of the prostate. This should be coupled with a complete physical which includes a digital rectal examination (DRE)."

Caution: *It is recommended by the American Cancer Society that males over the age of forty receive yearly examinations for the presence of prostate enlargement and cancer. Reluctance to undergo examination on the part of many men often causes early treatment to be postponed, allowing the condition to become worse. It is only after symptoms become unbearable that many men seek treatment.*

Early detection has become much simpler and more refined with the introduction of a few relatively noninvasive diagnostic procedures such as blood testing, DRE, urinalysis, and ultrasound. Rectal ultrasound for visualization of the tumor is beneficial when used with these other tests. Because the procedure is relatively new, it is important that it be done by a physician experienced in the interpretation of ultrasound scans.

Along with frequent examinations should be changes in dietary habits. Several studies have found that decreasing the consumption of sugar leads to lower levels of prostate cancer, and decreased incidences of cancer in general are found in cultures which have lower intakes of refined sugar.[40]

See AIDS, Sexually Transmitted Diseases.

High-fat diets, especially diets high in animal fats, also contribute to higher rates of prostate cancer. Consumption of large amounts of red meat are associated with high fat intake due to the "fattening" process beef goes through just before marketing.[41] Cultures which consume high levels of red meat have higher levels of prostatic cancer.[42] A low-fat diet with a balance of proteins is the most beneficial to men over age thirty.

Lifestyle changes, especially those associated with sexual habits, are also important for prevention of genitourinary tract problems, as well as for a person's overall health, Dr. Kruzel notes. "Protected intercourse through the use of condoms not only helps to prevent unwanted pregnancy, but also contamination of the male urethra by normal vaginal flora," he says. "Likewise, it is the only defense, short of abstinence, a man can take against all forms of sexually transmitted disease, from herpes to AIDS."

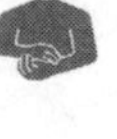

Self-Care

The following therapies can be undertaken at home under appropriate professional supervision:

Impotence

• ***Biofeedback Training*** • ***Meditation*** •***Yoga***

Aromatherapy: Sandalwood, jasmine, rose, clary sage, ylang ylang.

Hydrotherapy: Sitz bath: apply contrast two to five times weekly.

Juice Therapy: Red cabbage, celery, and lettuce juice twice daily.

Prostate Disorders

• ***Qigong*** •***Yoga***

Aromatherapy: Inflamed: lavender, cypress, thyme.

Juice Therapy: • Pumpkin juice • Carrot and celery with a little horseradish and watercress added • Carrot, cucumber, and beet, radish, garlic

Hydrotherapy: Sitz bath: apply contrast daily. Alternate hot and cold sitz baths, three minutes hot, thirty seconds cold. Repeat three times. Hot and cold sitz baths cause a flushing effect on the prostate, increasing blood flow to the gland, which results in an increase in metabolism as well as elevating the white blood cell population. Additionally, there is an effect upon the nerve flow to the pelvic organs allowing for better regulation and function.[43]

Practical Hints: Walk outdoors an hour daily.

Reflexology: Reproductive glands, bladder, lower spine, pituitary, adrenals, chronic prostate area.

Professional Care

The following therapies should only be provided by a qualified health professional:

Impotence

• ***Cell Therapy*** • ***Chiropractic*** • ***Feldenkrais*** • ***Hypnotherapy*** • ***Magnetic Field Therapy*** • ***Osteopathy*** • ***Traditional Chinese Medicine***

Bodywork: Acupressure, reflexology, *shiatsu.*

Chelation Therapy: Impotence: James Julian, M.D., estimates that over 60 percent of people with impotence also have a diminished blood supply. Chelation therapy may be indicated to improve both conditions.

Prostate Disorders

• ***Colon Therapy*** • ***Magnetic Field Therapy*** • ***Naturopathic Medicine*** • ***Osteopathy*** • ***Traditional Chinese Medicine***

Bodywork: Acupressure, reflexology, *shiatsu.*

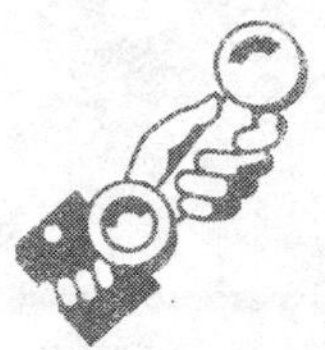

Where to Find Help

For information on male health and referrals to a qualified practitioner, contact the following organizations.

American Association of Acupuncture and Oriental Medicine
4101 Lake Boone Trail, Suite 201
Raleigh, North Carolina 27607
(919) 787-5181

The AAAOM is a national professional trade organization of acupuncturists who meet acceptable standards of minimum competency and can provide you with the names and locations of local members.

American Association of Naturopathic Physicians
2366 East Lake Avenue, Suite 322
Seattle, Washington 98102
(206) 323-7610

Provides referrals to a nationwide network of accredited or licensed practitioners. Publishes a quarterly newsletter for both professionals and the general public. Also offers a series of brochures and pamphlets on a variety of subjects.

Ayurvedic Institute
11311 Menaul NE, Suite A
Albuquerque, New Mexico 87112
(505) 291-9698

The institute, directed by Dr. Vasant Lad, trains people from all walks of life in most of the aspects of Ayurveda.

International Foundation for Homeopathy
2366 Eastlake Avenue East, Suite 301
Seattle, Washington 98102
(206) 324-8230

Provides referrals to homeopathic practitioners who have undergone training through the IFH. Also offered are classes for professionals and lay homeopaths.

National Center for Homeopathy
1500 Massachusetts Avenue NW, Suite 42
Washington, D.C. 20005
(703) 548-7790

Provides referrals to homeopathic practitioners who have undergone training through the National Center. Also offered are classes for professionals and lay homeopaths.

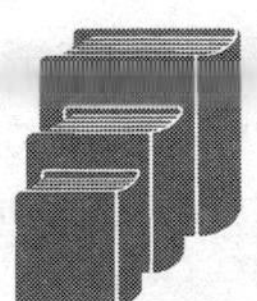

Recommended Reading

Encyclopedia of Natural Medicine. Murray, Michael, N.D.; and Pizzorno, Joseph, N.D. Rocklin, CA: Prima Publishing, 1991.

An authoritative guide to naturopathic medicine outlining the basic principles of health and how they can be used to treat over sixty health conditions, including prostate conditions. Includes self-help approaches using diet, nutrition, and herbal medicine.

Prostate Troubles. Chaitow, Leon, D.O., N.D. Wellingborough, England: Thorsons Publishers Ltd., 1988.

A comprehensive self-help guide for the prevention and treatment of prostate problems using diet, exercise, and other alternative therapies.

Mental Health

Any disturbance in behavior, emotion, or cognition can be considered a form of mental disorder. Recent evidence suggests that depression, anxiety, antisocial behavior, learning disorders, or schizophrenia can be caused by biochemical imbalances, toxins, allergies, food sensitivities, and other environmental factors. Advances in nutritional therapy, orthomolecular medicine, mind-body medicine, environmental medicine, and other alternative therapies now offer many solutions to the treatment of mental disorders.

According to the National Institute of Mental Health, over 28 percent of all Americans suffer from some type of mental disorder severe enough to require psychiatric treatment.[1] Incidences of depression and suicide are also rapidly increasing, especially among children and adolescents.

Types of Mental Disorders

Although there is no clear-cut way of defining mental disorders, they can be divided into several overlapping categories loosely defined as emotional, personality, and thought disorders.

Emotional Disorders

Two of the most common emotional disorders are depression and anxiety. Depression is characterized by feelings of persistent sadness, fear, unhappiness, pessimism, hopelessness, worthlessness, or despair. Serious depression, if not treated, can even lead to suicidal thoughts and feelings. Physiological symptoms may include a change in appetite (either increased or decreased), constipation, sleepiness, or sleeplessness.

Anxiety disorders, including phobias, affect roughly 10 million people,[2] with symptoms ranging from mild unease to intense fear and panic. These symptoms can often be manifested physically by a tightness in the chest, hyperventilation, heart palpitations, or gastrointestinal problems.

Personality Disorders

Personality disorders are characterized by a person's inability to effectively relate socially, for a variety of reasons. People suffering from paranoia, for instance, are overly suspicious, narcissistic people tend to be selfish and self-centered, and antisocial people fail to conform to societal rules and regulations. Other personality disorders can include overdependence, insecurity, obsessiveness, compulsiveness, passiveness, and aggression. Patients with borderline personality disorders often have difficulty maintaining stable relationships and are often socially inappropriate and moody. Addictions such as those to alcohol, drugs, and gambling are also considered forms of personality disorders.

Thought Disorders

Thought disorders include conditions such as behavioral problems, learning difficulties, schizophrenia, dementia (confused thinking), delusions, and brain dysfunction. Manic and depressive behaviors can also be considered forms of thought disorders.

Causes of Mental Disorders

Until recently, most mental disorders were considered either psychological in nature or genetically predisposed. Treatment options were generally limited to psychotherapy, or to medication, electroshock treatment, or surgical intervention. Today, however, many psychiatrists, psychologists, and researchers recognize that numerous factors can contribute to the onset of mental disorders, including social and cultural factors, age and gender, nutritional deficits, allergies and food sensitivities, alcohol and drug addictions, and even prescription drugs, including those prescribed to treat mental illness. Peter Breggin, M.D., a Harvard-trained psychiatrist, points out that drug therapy, while suppressing the symptoms of depression and other mental disorders, can also make a person chemically toxic, which will actually deepen the problem.[3]

Illness can also be a major contributor to mental illness, as well as stress, both physical and emotional, chronic and acute. Exposure to environmental stresses from chemicals, toxins, and electromagnetic fields can also play a major role in one's mental health.

Diet and Nutritional Factors

Diet and nutritional factors are probably the most significant determining factors, other than psychological or genetic causes, for predisposing mental disorder. Virtually any nutrient deficiency can result in depression. In fact, research shows that deficiencies in vitamin C, thiamine (B_1), vitamin B_6, vitamin B_{12}, niacin (B_3), and folic acid could be specifically linked to depression and other emotional disorders.[4]

In 1991, researchers found that babies deficient in iron, even though treated, scored lower on IQ and mental functioning tests than babies with normal iron levels, when checked at age five.[5] As far back as the 1950s, when the late Carl Pfeiffer, Ph.D., M.D., former Director of the Bio Brain Center in Princeton, New Jersey, discovered that trace metal imbalances could contribute to mental disorders; violent, criminal, and delinquent behaviors in both children and adults have been linked to these imbalances. "We've tested thousands of people in prisons, and many thousands more with behavior disorders," says William Walsh, Ph.D., a former research scientist at the Argonne National Laboratories and a colleague of Dr. Pfeiffer, "and we have found that 95 percent suffer from inborn chemical imbalances that predispose them to bad behavior."

"Diet and nutritional factors are probably the most significant determining factors, other than psychological or genetic causes, for predisposing mental disorders."

Dr. Walsh discovered that violent individuals often had elevated copper-zinc ratios and extremely low levels of sodium, potassium, and manganese. This group of people were considered underachievers and had numerous learning difficulties and attention deficit disorders. People with severe antisocial tendencies (lacking in remorse or conscience) showed a different biochemical pattern. They were low in copper, zinc, sodium, potassium, and manganese, but high in calcium and magnesium, often with toxic levels of lead. Another trace metal pattern involved people who were delinquent, impulsive, and irritable. Dr. Walsh found them to be low in all trace metals including calcium and magnesium. They also had low levels of most nutrients and amino acids, which may be caused by problems relating to nutritional absorption. "Many of these people have insufficient stomach acid," says Dr. Walsh. "When you correct the stomach acid, the body will often take over and treatment can be stopped."

Nutritional Therapy

Dr. Walsh classified a fourth type of individual who, though not violent or delinquent, did poorly in school and work, got irritable after eating sugar, and felt drowsy after meals. The basic problem, Dr. Walsh discovered, was hypoglycemia. Dr. Walsh's findings parallel a recent experiment conducted by the New York City public school system. Over a period of four years, they decreased the amount of sugar, food colorings, synthetic flavorings, and two commonly used preservatives in foods served at 803 schools. A dramatic 15.7 percent increase in academic performance was noted, compared to prior years in which no more than a 1 percent increase or decrease was reported.[7]

HISTAMINE LEVELS AND SCHIZOPHRENIA

In the 1950s, when the late Carl Pfeiffer, Ph.D., M.D., former Director of the Bio Brain Center in Princeton, New Jersey, found that trace metal imbalances (copper, zinc, lithium, cobalt) were linked to mental illness, he also found that nearly half of those suffering from schizophrenia had low levels of histamine, a chemical present in cells throughout the body that is in high concentration at the base of brain cells. He called these people histapenics. Histapenics are often classified as paranoid schizophrenics who suffer from severe depression, experience hallucinations, and become suicidal. Laboratory tests show that histapenics also have low blood basophils (white blood cells that store histamine), deficiencies in zinc and folic acid, along with unusually high levels of copper.[6]

Dr. Pfeiffer also found that nearly a third of the schizophrenics he analyzed had too much histamine in their systems. Histadelics, as Dr. Pfeiffer referred to them, are often obsessive-compulsive and delusional with severe impairment in their thinking, and high blood basophil levels. They are also suicidally depressed and may even become catatonic.

According to orthomolecular psychiatrist Harvey Ross, M.D., of Los Angeles, many patients who complain of depression also have hypoglycemia, which, in some cases, may even be the sole cause of the patient's depression. "Many times patients can feel depressed without being able to say why," says Dr. Ross. "They may also be experiencing low energy, feel irritable, or be having attacks of anxiety or fear, sometimes even to the point of developing phobias. Diabetes may also be part of their family history, but from a medical standpoint nothing seems wrong. Often they will be referred to a psychotherapist, usually without much success, when what they really need is to see a physician who treats hypoglycemia."

Leon Chaitow, N.D., D.O., of London, England, notes that another recently identified cause of depression is the excessive use of aspartame, the artificial sweetener widely used instead of sugar in diet colas and foods. "This is because aspartame is made up of amino acids, and when they are metabolized, they can cause an imbalance in brain chemistry because of their extreme concentration," Dr. Chaitow says. Depression that is otherwise unaccounted for can also be due to a specific food or chemical to which one is sensitive or allergic, Dr. Chaitow points out.

See Allergies, Diabetes, Diet, Environmental Medicine, Enzyme Therapy, Hypoglycemia, Nutritional Supplements.

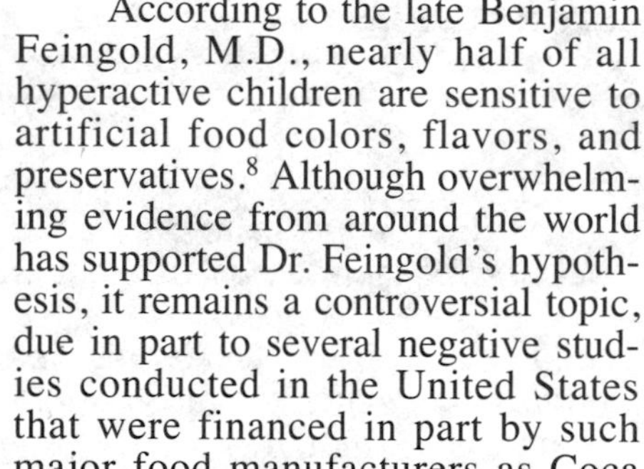

According to the late Benjamin Feingold, M.D., nearly half of all hyperactive children are sensitive to artificial food colors, flavors, and preservatives.[8] Although overwhelming evidence from around the world has supported Dr. Feingold's hypothesis, it remains a controversial topic, due in part to several negative studies conducted in the United States that were financed in part by such major food manufacturers as Coca Cola and General Foods.[9] Other countries have already restricted the use of artificial additives in foods because of their potential harmful effects. As a result, the National Institutes of Health has agreed to reconsider the issue.

Other studies have shown that food additives alone are sometimes not enough to provoke reactions in children, and that other food sensitivities are often involved. These include allergy reactions to milk, soy products, chocolate, grapes, oranges, apples, peanuts, wheat, corn, tomatoes, eggs, refined sugar, fish, and oats.[10] Doris Rapp, M.D., past President of the American Academy of Environmental Medicine, has demonstrated how just a few drops of allergenic substances can suddenly provoke anger, confusion, and hyperactivity in children.

Studies in Texas have also shown that when levels of the trace element lithium, commonly found in very small amounts in drinking water, are extremely low, the rate of suicide, homicide, and rape were significantly higher. When these levels are corrected by careful supplementation, aggressive behavior drops significantly.[11]

Addiction and Substance Abuse

According to Karl E. Humiston, M.D., of Albany, Oregon, when asked about their very first cigarette, most smokers will readily admit it made them pretty sick. "But after a bit of persistence, one gets used to it, builds up a tolerance for it, and, in fact, actually comes to like it and is uncomfortable only when going too long without smoking," Dr. Humiston says. "The same can basically be said about regular alcohol and drug users as well."

Orthodox physicians and psychiatrists usually give no thought to this phenomenon, however. "But for the human body to no longer be distressed by something as noxious as cigarette smoke, and perhaps even come to enjoy it, a profound change of some sort has had to occur in one's body chemistry," Dr. Humiston points out. "It is not just a psychological adaptation."

This phenomenon is called a "specific adaptation." This means that the body has adapted, at the chemical and energy levels, to a specific substance which is actually toxic or to which it is allergic. "This protects the body from instantly getting sick, but at the price of a heavy chronic stress that can grind away at one's immune system," says Dr. Humiston. "For example, most smokers don't get lung cancer, but all become much less healthy. Plus, in order to maintain the adaptive protection, you must maintain the exposure. In other words, you have to keep taking the stuff. If you go too long without it, then you get sick and can only be relieved by taking it again."

This is the physical basis for addiction. It is also the physical basis for a lot of mental and emotional illness. Adaptive/addictive reactions to toxic or allergic foods and chemicals account for much depression, confusion, irritability, anger, compulsive behaviors, and even psychosis, according to Dr. Humiston, as well as for obvious addictions such as to cigarettes, alcohol, and drugs. "Since symptoms mainly appear when you are not exposed to the substance, or occur in a chronic or erratic pattern, neither the patient nor the physician is likely to think of the connection unless trained in environmental medicine," he notes. "The person whose worst fits of anger occur on the days when he doesn't have toast for breakfast is not likely to think of this as reflecting a wheat allergy. Similarly, the person who knows that coffee works best to relieve his morning headache, is not likely to see this headache as a withdrawal symptom from an adaptive addiction to coffee, but that's what it is."

In a 1981 study, Stephen Perry, M.D., of Staffordshire, England, reported that people who lived near high-voltage lines had unusually high levels of depression and suicide.[12] A second study, conducted in 1988, showed that apartment-dwelling people who lived closest to the building's main power supplies and electrical cables showed as much as an 82 percent increase in depression.[13] A third study, conducted by David Dowson, M.D., of Southhampton, England, also showed an increase in depression from those who lived near power lines.[14]

See Addictions, Candidiasis, Light Therapy.

Numerous studies have shown that exposure to heavy metals, solvents, paints, and other toxic substances and fumes can also produce many psychological symptoms, including depression and fatigue,[15] as well as contributing to violent behavior. Post office slayer Patrick Sherril had extraordinarily high levels of lead and cadmium (in addition to a severe copper-zinc imbalance), which the University of Oklahoma attributed to his handling of ammunition. James Huberty, who shot twenty-four people at a McDonalds in San Ysidro, California, had an extremely high level of cadmium, which may have come from his seventeen years of work as a welder.[16] Scientific studies have also attributed many childhood learning disorders to high levels of mercury, cadmium, lead, copper, and manganese.[17]

The quality and quantity of light can also affect one's mental state, according to pioneering photobiologist John Nash Ott, Sc.D. (Hon.).[18] Dr. Ott discovered that artificial lighting (incandescent or fluorescent) not only interferes with the body's optimal absorption of nutrients, but contributes to a variety of mental and emotional disturbances, including fatigue, depression, hostility, alcoholism, drug abuse, a shortened lifespan, Alzheimer's disease, and cancer.[19] Damien Downing, O.D., Ph.D., Director of the Light Therapy Department at the Preventative Medical Center in San Rafael, California, confirmed these findings, stating that "by spending 90 percent of our lives indoors, in inadequate light conditions, we are causing, or worsening, a wide range of health problems, including depression, heart disease, hyperactivity in children, osteoporosis in the elderly, and lowered resistance to infection."[20]

Another form of this photobiological sensitivity is called seasonal affective disorder (SAD), a condition resulting from inadequate amounts of sunlight, usually during the winter months. According to Dr. Chaitow, between 5 and 10 percent of the population suffer from this disorder, which is often characterized by marked depression, extreme fatigue, and increased appetite.

Hugh Riordan, M.D., founder of the Center for the Improvement of Human Functioning International in Wichita, Kansas, adds that seasonal depression can also be triggered by mold and pollen allergies. Dr. Riordan notes that a monthly cycle of depression can also point to hormonal imbalances, especially in women.

According to Dr. Humiston, M.D., depression in women is often caused by toxicity from an overgrowth of yeast (*Candida albicans*) in the intestines, especially when the yeast organisms are stimulated by the artificial form of the hormone progesterone, which is commonly found in birth control pills.

Drugs Associated with a Higher Incidence of Mental Depression

According to the Physicians Desk Reference the following drugs are associated with side effects of mental depression. (Statistics refer to the percentage of individuals affected.)[35]

Depo-Provera Contraceptive Injection (1-5%)
Roferon-A Injection (16%)

Stress and Lowered Immune Function

While many physical conditions and disorders have been shown to cause psychological stress, studies have also found that psychological stress can likewise contribute to physical illness. According to the *Harvard Mental Health Letter*, the central nervous system, the endocrine system, and the immune system all respond to psychological stress. Depressed immune functioning is associated with many kinds of stress including bereavement, divorce, job loss, examinations, anxiety, depression, loneliness, and sleep deprivation.[21] Up to 80 percent of all American health problems are considered stress-related. In large-scale studies conducted in 1967, those who became seriously ill reported having more stressful life events than those who were well.[22]

Multiple daily stress has also been shown to undermine health.[23] British cardiologist Peter Nixon, M.D., suggests that when the body systems are overstimulated by stress, illness is likely to occur and cardiac disease may set in.[24]

Jeanne Achterberg, Ph.D., President of the Association for Transpersonal Psychology, adds that feelings of helplessness and hopelessness increase digestive problems and cancer growth. Fear, anxiety, and stress can also interfere with healing, compromise the immune system, and encourage cardiovascular disease.[25]

According to Carl Simonton, M.D., Director of the Simonton Cancer Center in Pacific Palisades, California, stress is the greatest single factor in cases of recurring cancer.[26] One study found that depressed men are more likely to develop cancer in the following twenty years and twice as likely to die of it, and, in another study, women who experienced stress are more likely to get breast cancer.[27]

“Stress is the greatest single factor in cases of recurring cancer. One study found that depressed men are more likely to develop cancer in the following twenty years and twice as likely to die of it.”

Grief and social isolation can also lead to weakened immune function, increased risk of cancer, and earlier death. One large nine-year study found that people with the lowest amount of social ties are two to three times more likely to die of all causes than those with the most social connectedness.[28]

Studies have also shown that psychotherapy helps to improve long-term health and immune function in cancer recovery patients. David Spiegel, M.D., of Stanford University, demonstrated that women with metastatic breast cancer who participate in a weekly support group live twice as long than those who do not.[29]

A recent experiment has also shown that the more stress a person is under, the greater the chance of viral infection. Four hundred and twenty people were evaluated for occurrences of stress during the prior year. These included such events as job loss, death in the family, moving, and divorce; feeling frightened, nervous, sad, angry, or irritated; or feeling unable to cope with current demands. They were then exposed to one of five cold viruses and then tested one month later for antibodies. Ninety percent of those who were under the greatest stress became infected, compared to 74 percent who experienced the least amount of stress.[30] In another study of one hundred subjects, the results indicated that people who experience stress (particularly tension and anger) are four times more likely to develop a cold or bacterial infection.[31]

See Cancer, Digestive Disorders, Heart Disease, Stress.

Researchers who have reviewed the influence of stress on immunity, have concluded that since the effect is not universal, with some people handling the stress well and showing no decline in immune efficiency, it is not the stress that is to blame, but the individual's means of handling it. “This has been called the ‘hardiness factor,’” says Dr. Chaitow. “It comprises a tendency to see problems as challenges not threats, having a commitment to involvement in society rather than having a sense of detachment from it, and having a feeling of control over life rather than a sense of being subject to the whims of fate.”

According to Dr. Chaitow, these three elements can be learned via appropriate counseling and therefore the absence of one or all of them from a person's personality profile is not necessarily a permanent feature. “People can learn to cope with stress so that it does not negatively affect

THE MIND/BODY CONNECTION

Research conducted in the fields of psychoneuroimmunology and mind/body medicine over the past two decades has established a definite and intimate relationship between the physiological and psychological processes of the body. Neurochemical substances known as neuropeptides, discovered by Candace Pert, Ph.D., a leading neuroscientist currently teaching at Rutgers University and a former Section Chief at the National Institute of Mental Health, were found to cause alterations in mood. Even more significant, perhaps, was the discovery that these substances can be found not only in the brain, but in the spinal cord, glands, organs, and other body tissues.[32] Among the most well-known of the neuropeptides are the endorphins, which can have a pain-relieving and pleasure-inducing effect when released. Dr. Pert looks at the neuropeptides as the “biochemical units of emotion,” and as “the bridge between the mental and the physical.”[33]

According to Leon Chaitow, N.D., D.O., of London, England, neuropeptides are the key to changes in emotion, because they increase or decrease the transmission of messages to and from the brain. Because these neuropeptides are found throughout the body, they can also affect the functioning of all the body's systems, including the immune system. “Viruses use the same receptors as a neuropeptide to enter into a cell,” explains Dr. Pert. “Depending on how much of the natural peptide for that receptor is around, the virus will have an easier or harder time getting into the cell. So our emotional state will affect whether we'll get sick from the same loading dose of a virus.”[34]

them," says Dr. Chaitow. This is also the basis of numerous healing modalities such as progressive relaxation, guided imagery, and biofeedback, which can be effectively used to treat both psychological and physiological disorders.

Treatment of Mental Disorders

A growing number of doctors and health practitioners have found that mental disorders, in many cases, can be successfully treated through means other than the traditional practices of psychotherapy, drug therapy, electroshock treatment, and surgery. These alternative methods include nutritional and herbal supplements, dietary changes, exercise, biofeedback, relaxation, guided imagery, and magnetic therapy.

Diet and Nutrition

According to Richard Kunin, M.D., of San Francisco, California, the most important dietary rules to follow for optimal psychological and physiological health are:

- **Variety:** Eat a little of a lot of different foods.
- **Moderation:** Don't overeat or binge.
- **Whole foods:** Eat natural foods (whole grains, fresh vegetables) rather than processed foods.
- **Purity:** Eat foods free of pesticides and additives, preferably organic.
- **Balance:** Eat a diet that is specifically suited to your own individual needs and body.

By following these basic guidelines, a person can go a long way in the prevention of mental disorders. Yet when certain conditions exist that contribute to the deterioration of one's mental state, more direct nutritional steps are often taken.

For treating hypoglycemia, Dr. Ross will have his patients begin an individualized program, which includes a strict diet and the use of nutritional supplements. He recommends a high-protein, low-carbohydrate diet, and in addition to three meals daily, the patient eats smaller snacks every two hours between meals until bedtime. After the first four months, patients are introduced to a maintenance diet that includes no more than three servings of fruit a day. Ideally, the patient will refrain from processed foods and sugars, but he or she may occasionally have a small amount of sugar. However, in times of increased stress, the patient may need to return to the stricter dietary program.

Raising serotonin (a chemical in the body that is important in sleep and sensory perception) levels in the body can also help reduce depressive symptoms, according to Dr. Riordan, who recommends the taking of walnut tea several times a day, which is high in serotonin. To make this tea, simply steep a broken half of an English walnut in boiling water, and drink it. Dr. Riordan adds that drinking plenty of water and breathing deeply are also effective ways to reduce depression. Studies conducted by Dr. Riordan showed that a nondepressed person breathes in six times the amount of air than does a person who is depressed.

Numerous herbs and botanicals also have antidepressive effects. For example, hypericum, commonly known as St. John's Wort, has been used historically as a mood elevator. A recent clinical study demonstrated that a standardized extract (two to four grams of dried herb, or two to four milliliters of fluid extract 1:1) led to significant improvement in symptoms of anxiety, depression, and sleep disorders in fifteen women.[36]

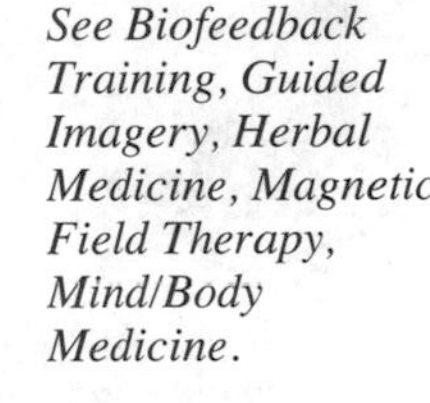

See Biofeedback Training, Guided Imagery, Herbal Medicine, Magnetic Field Therapy, Mind/Body Medicine.

One of the earliest and most important breakthroughs in alternative medicine was made in 1952, when Abram Hoffer, M.D., Ph.D., President of the Canadian Schizophrenia Foundation, and his colleague, Humphrey Osmond, M.R.C.P., F.R.C.P., of Tuscaloosa, Alabama, found that schizophrenia could be treated with megavitamins. Drs. Hoffer and Osmond demonstrated that vitamin B_3 (nicotinic acid or nicotinamide) can double the recovery rate of acute schizophrenics.[37] This discovery challenged some of psychiatry's basic concepts of schizophrenia and paved the way for orthomolecular medicine, which combines nutrition and the use of individualized supplements with other medical treatments.

These early studies, however, did not seem to help chronic patients, but progress was made when vitamin B_3 therapy was combined with other treatments. "Recently," says Dr. Hoffer, "I examined the outcome of treatment of twenty-six chronic patients who remained under my care for ten years and more. My survey showed that today eleven are working, two are married and looking after their families, two are single mothers caring for their children with no difficulty, and three are managing their own businesses. One patient received his B.Sc. from the local university, one was awarded her M.A., and another got a certificate from the community college. From this total group, eighteen are well, three are much improved, five are improved, and one has shown no improvement."[38] Compared to a recent study that showed only a 5 percent significant recovery from traditional psychiatric treatment,[39] orthomolecular treatment of medical disorders, Dr.

Hoffer believes, may soon become a standard medical practice.

In treating schizophrenia patients, Dr. Walsh has found that those with low histamine levels are much easier to treat with nutritional therapy than those with elevated histamine levels. To elevate histamine in histapenics, his medical staff prescribes folate and nutrients, basophil enhancement, and a specialized treatment that causes their bodies to get rid of excess copper. After several months of treatment, the nervousness, depression, and hallucinations often disappear. Paranoid symptoms, however, may take as long as a year to subside.[40]

With people whose histamine levels are high, treatment may begin with megadoses of calcium (for example, one thousand milligrams twice a day), which helps to release excess histamines from the body cells. Megadoses of the amino acid methylamine (one thousand to fifteen hundred milligrams), hastens the exit of histamine from the body. These people must also avoid multivitamins which contain histamine-elevating agents such as niacin and folic acid. "Unfortunately," adds Dr. Walsh, "these people may also have to stay away from many kinds of nutritious foods, like green leafy vegetables, or they will get worse." In each case, Dr. Walsh recommends individual nutritional counseling.

See Orthomolecular Medicine.

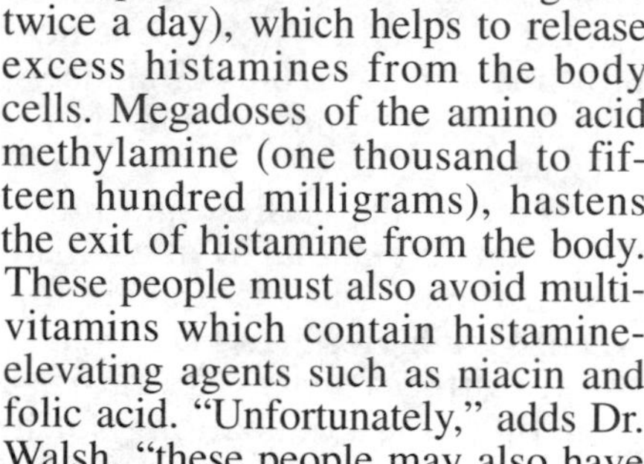

Dr. Walsh, along with the late Dr. Pfeiffer, has also treated children effectively with nutritional therapy, noting improvements in learning disability, hyperactivity, and attention deficit disorders. "After our first one thousand patients, we found we were getting major improvement with 70 percent of our behavior-disordered kids," says Dr. Walsh. "Twenty-two percent had improvement that was clear but not complete. Eight percent had little or no improvement. With learning disorders, 53 percent show great improvement, and 34 percent are better but still have a learning handicap. Approximately 13 percent showed no improvement at all."[41]

In one case, Dr. Walsh treated a ten-year-old boy who had explosive bouts of anger and hysteria, hitting people and destroying things. After four months of treatment, his parents reported that his behavior had significantly improved and was getting good grades in school. Another case involved a sixteen-year-old girl who was extremely emotional, with wild and erratic behavior, who lied, was sneaky, and was an underachiever in school. After four months of nutritional treatment, her fighting and emotional upheavals were gone. Unfortunately, she continued to do poorly in school.

In order to treat behavior and learning disorders, careful testing (blood, urine, hair chemistry analysis) must be carried out in order to identify each patient's biochemical individuality. Over 120 different determinations need to be made, which include testing for blood histamine, lead, copper, zinc; thyroid, kidney and liver function; protein levels; and electrolyte levels. "We also do a number of rather unusual tests," says Dr. Walsh.

"Many children who don't improve appear to have allergy problems in addition to biochemical imbalances," says Dr. Walsh. "For this particular group, diet is especially important." Some children, Dr. Walsh has found, are particularly sensitive to food dyes, particularly yellow and red, or sugar, while others may have a reaction to taking multivitamins and minerals. "Multivitamins are wonderful for most people, but if you happen to have the wrong biochemistry, it might make you dramatically worse.

ORTHOMOLECULAR MEDICINE

The term "orthomolecular" was first used by Nobel Prize-winning scientist Linus Pauling Ph.D., in 1968, to refer to the connection between nutrition and the mind. In 1991 Melvyn Werbach, M.D., published a 370-page volume which summarizes research studies supporting Dr. Pauling's original ideas about this connection. Dr. Werbach states, "It is clear that nutrition can powerfully influence cognition, emotion, and behavior. It is also clear that the effects of classical nutritional deficiency diseases upon mental function constitute only a small part of a rapidly expanding list of interfaces between nutrition and the mind."[42] He notes that patients in hospitals and nursing homes are often nutritionally deficient, adversely affecting their mental state.

Orthomolecular medicine has come a long way from the original discovery that large doses of B and C vitamins could improve the mental condition of schizophrenic persons. Yet, according to Joseph Beasley, M.D., Director of the Department of Medicine and Nutrition at the Brunswick Hospital Center in Amityville, New York, conventional medicine has largely ignored the overwhelming extent to which poor nutrition and toxic environments have damaged physical and mental health.[43] As further research is completed, though, it will become increasingly more difficult to ignore this important link between nutrition and mental health.

"This is particularly common for those with learning disabilities. One young man I saw had an extraordinary copper/zinc ratio. He was taking multiple vitamins which contain copper, and this was like poison to him."

Treatment in such cases is to avoid multiple vitamins and enriched foods containing copper, prescribing instead a supplement that will bring the copper and zinc levels back to normal. "We make sure that they don't drink water that may be copper-bearing, and suggest that they stay away from other possible sources of copper," adds Dr. Walsh. "Swimming pools, for example, are treated with antialgae agents which are loaded with copper, and patients ought to make sure they shower afterward and not drink any of the water."

Some children are sensitive to food dyes, particularly yellow and red, or sugar, while others may have a reaction to taking multivitamins and minerals.

A study involving fifteen autistic children and adults, ages six to twenty-two, indicated that autism can also be treated through the use of diet. According to the study, "These patients were socially isolated, resistant to learning, showed peculiar attachment to certain objects, had fear of unusual items and situations, and demonstrated both repetitive motor behavior and severe problems with emotional expression. Language problems and disturbed attention were also common."

Urine analysis samples showed that the patients with autistic syndromes have increased levels of peptides (simple proteins). Depending upon the specific urinary pattern, three types of diets were prescribed to reduce the overall peptide levels. Some patients received a gluten-free and milk-reduced diet, others received a milk-free and/or gluten-reduced diet, and a third group received a milk- and gluten-free diet.

Milk reduction was achieved by eliminating milk and cheese, and gluten reduction was achieved by giving only gluten-free bread and cakes. After one year, all the study subjects had changed toward the normal spectrum: they were less psychotic, were more communicative, and showed less bizarre behavior. Other statistically significant changes include improved attention and social integration, improved motor ability and skills, and a decrease in irrational emotional outbursts. Especially noteworthy is the decrease in resistance to learning demonstrated by all cases.[44]

Biofeedback and Relaxation Techniques

Several studies have found that children suffering from hyperactivity and attention deficits show improvements in academic performance when trained in biofeedback and relaxation techniques.[45] These findings provide further evidence that mental conditions can be improved through the use of exercises designed to reduce stress and promote physical awareness.

See Autism, Bodywork, Meditation, Yoga.

In many cases of extreme anxiety, according to Dr. Chaitow, hyperventilation patterns are pronounced, with breathing rapid and extremely shallow. This is something also seen frequently in people displaying phobic behavior, or who are subject to panic attacks. The person affected in this way will often report a sense of oppressive pressure on the chest and an inability to take a full breath.

Breathing retraining, coupled with expert bodywork to release the rib structures and breathing muscles, as well as with relaxation measures, will usually correct any habitual tendency toward hyperventilation. This nondrug approach is widely used in Europe for the treatment of chronic phobias and anxiety.[46]

USING WRITING AND GUIDED IMAGERY TO PREVENT NIGHTMARES

According to a recent study, nearly one out of ten people suffers from frequent nightmares. These people often also suffer from depression, hypochondria, and hysteria, and use more alcohol, tobacco, caffeine, and tranquilizers than others.[48] At the University of New Mexico, researchers found that two forms of behavior therapy could be used by patients at home to reduce the number of nightmares they experienced. The first technique, called desensitization, involves recalling the nightmare in detail while relaxing, and then writing it down on paper. The second technique, called rehearsal, is a form of guided imagery in which the person relaxes, and then, through visualization, changes the plot and the ending of his or her nightmare prior to writing it down. It took only one session to teach a group of twenty-eight people how to do these exercises. After seven months, twenty-three people reported having fewer nightmares (average reduction from 4.4 to 2.2) using either technique. In four cases, nightmares ceased entirely, and in one case a woman was able to eliminate her nightmares after three days of rehearsal practice. Previously, she had been plagued by nightmares four times a week for thirty years.[49]

Magnetic Field Therapy

William Philpott, M.D., of Choctaw, Oklahoma, a biomagnetic researcher, suggests that many psychological disorders are caused by electromagnetic imbalances in the body, and that these can be corrected through the application of magnetic therapy which uses specially designed magnetics placed on or above different parts of the body. "Anxieties, phobias, obsessions, compulsions, depression, psychosis, and seizures evoke an abnormal rise in the electrical activity of the central nervous system," says Dr. Philpott. Such conditions, according to Dr. Philpott, can be controlled through proper placement of negative magnetic energy devices, thus eliminating or reducing the severity of the mental disorder." Schizophrenics, he notes, have abnormally high electrical discharges deep within the brain, and through properly applied magnetic energy, a calming effect can be produced to alleviate their symptoms.[47]

Self-Care

The following therapies can be undertaken at home under appropriate professional supervision:

Depression

• ***Fasting*** • ***Flower Remedies*** • ***Meditation*** • ***Reflexology*** • ***Yoga***

Aromatherapy: • Sedative oils including chamomile, clary sage, lavender, ylang ylang and sandalwood may be helpful. • Neroli, jasmine, bergamot, melissa, rose, and geranium are antidepressants. • Propolis tincture

Hydrotherapy: Constitutional hydrotherapy, immersion bath, or wet sheet pack: apply two to five times weekly. Neutral application as needed for sedation.

Schizophrenia

Hydrotherapy: Constitutional hydrotherapy, immersion bath, or wet sheet pack: apply two to five times weekly. Neutral application as needed for sedation.

Juice Therapy: Seasonal fruit and vegetable juice. Short juice fasts (under medical guidance).

Professional Care

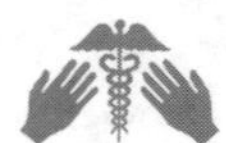

The following therapies should only be provided by a qualified health professional:

Depression

• ***Acupuncture*** • ***Applied Kinesiology*** • ***Chiropractic*** • ***Craniosacral Therapy*** • ***Environmental Medicine*** • ***Guided Imagery*** • ***Hypnotherapy*** • ***Magnetic Field Therapy*** • ***Osteopathy*** • ***Sound Therapy***

Dental Involvement: Hal A. Huggins, D.D.S., reports the improvement or disappearance of many emotional problems, such as depression, irritability, and suicidal tendencies after removing toxic dental amalgams. "Silver" fillings contain approximately 50 percent mercury and only 20 to 30 percent silver.

Bodywork: • massage • acupressure • *shiatsu* • Feldenkrais • Rolfing is very helpful if used in conjunction with psychotherapy.

Schizophrenia

• ***Acupuncture*** • ***Magnetic Field Therapy*** • ***Naturopathic Medicine*** • ***Sound Therapy*** • ***Traditional Chinese Medicine***

Bodywork: Rolfing.

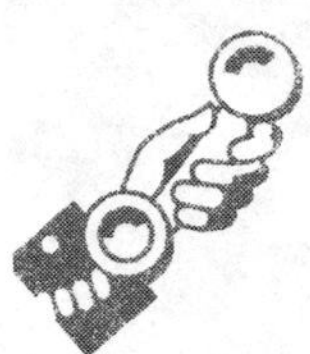

Where to Find Help

The following organizations can provide information on alternative approaches to treating mental illness, as well as referrals to alternative practitioners.

American Association of Naturopathic Physicians
P.O. Box 20386
Seattle, Washington 98102
(206) 323-7610

Refers to nationwide network of accredited or licensed practitioners. Publishes a quarterly newsletter for both professionals and the general public.

American Counseling Association
5999 Stevenson Avenue
Alexandria, Virignia 22304-3300
(703) 823-9800

The counseling profession grew out of education and therefore is largely based on principles of human development, of activating the power within, more than other mental health professions.

American Holistic Medical Association
4101 Lake Boone Trail, Suite 201
Raleigh, North Carolina 27607
(919) 787-4916

Large organization of physicians (M.D.'s and D.O.'s) who practice holistic medicine. Will provide referrals to holistic physicians in your area.

The Center for the Improvement of Human Function International
3100 North Hillside Avenue
Wichita, Kansas 67219-3904
(316) 682-3100

Medical, research, and educational facility specializing in the treatment of chronic illness. Is at the forefront of research in nutritional medicine. Treatments include counseling, stress reduction, biofeedback, acupuncture, hypnosis, pain control, and massage. The center also provides seminars and training programs for health care providers and publishes a monthly newsletter on contemporary health issues.

Foundation for the Advancement of Innovative Medicine
P.O. Box 338
Kinderhook, New York 12106

Organization of professionals and lay persons advocating for holistic and alternative practices. Best source of referrals in the New York City area.

Human Ecology Action League
P.O. Box 49126
Atlanta, Georgia 30359-1126
(404) 248-1898

A well-organized support organization for sufferers from environmental illness (sensitivity to foods, chemicals, etc.). They supply information regarding practitioners plus information about how to manage things yourself.

Well Mind Association of Greater Washington
11141 Georgia Avenue, Suite 326
Wheaton, Maryland
(301) 949-3484

Holistic mental health information and publications, public lectures in the Washington, D.C., area, and nationwide referrals.

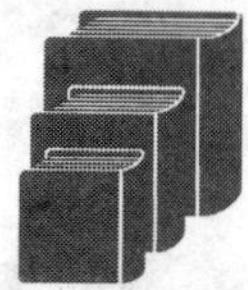

Recommended Reading

The Betrayal Of Health. Beasley, Joseph, M.D. New York: Times Books, 1991.
An investigation into the impact of nutrition, environment, and lifestyle choices on health, including mental illness.

The Healing Brain: A Scientific Reader. Ornstein, Robert; and David Sobel (Editors). New York: The Guilford Press, 1990.
An overview of scientific research into the role of the brain and the future of mental and physical health care, including the link of nutrients to behavior, stress, and emotion.

Brain Allergies: The Psychonutrient Connection. Philpott, William H., M.D.; and Kalita, Dwight, Ph.D. New Canaan, CT: Keats Publishing, Inc., 1980.
A comprehensive look at the role nutrition and orthomolecular medicine can play in treating brain allergies and the mental health conditions they can contribute to, including a self-help protocol and a special appendix for physicians.

"The competent physician, before he attempts to give medicine to the patient, makes himself acquainted not only with the disease, but also with the habits and constitution of the sick man"

—Cicero

Multiple Sclerosis

Nearly 350,000 Americans are affected by one of medicine's most misunderstood diseases, multiple sclerosis. Although there is no known cure, alternative medicine has recognized a number of contributing factors. Often, the early detection and identification of underlying causes combined with strict dietary and lifestyle guidelines can stabilize or reverse the symptoms.

Multiple sclerosis (MS) affects the central nervous system and usually occurs in early adult life. Normally, nerve fibers are surrounded by a layer of insulation called myelin. MS results when the nerve fibers of the central nervous system develop multiple patches of demyelination (removal of the myelin sheath). Nerve transmission is disrupted, leading to feelings of pins and needles in the hands and feet, numbness, loss of balance, clumsiness, sensitivity to heat and cold, blurred or double vision, and difficulty walking.

"Although the stereotype of an MS sufferer is that of a person in a wheelchair, many people are able to walk and continue working."
—Patrick Kingsley, M.D.

Patrick Kingsley, M.D., of Leicestershire, England, a specialist in nutrition and environmental medicine who has treated over two thousand multiple sclerosis patients, states that, "In advanced stages of MS, walking becomes more difficult, movements become more spastic, arms and hands may become weak, speech can become slurred, and chronic urinary urgency or incontinence may develop. Fatigue, one of the "silent" and most disabling symptoms of multiple sclerosis, may render even the smallest tasks difficult."

Dr. Kingsley adds, "Although the stereotype of an MS sufferer is that of a person in a wheelchair, many people with MS are able to walk and continue working. The disease can be benign, with a few minor attacks spread over many decades, or deterioration can be rapid. Most cases fall somewhere between these extremes."

Multiple sclerosis is often described as a relapsing/remitting disease, where attacks are followed by remission, leaving the MS sufferer worse off than he or she was before the exacerbation. Because no two cases of MS are identical, the severity of attacks and the state of health following a remission period differs from patient to patient. Unless steps are taken to slow or halt the disease, patients with chronic symptoms will probably become progressively worse.

Causes of Multiple Sclerosis

By the time multiple sclerosis is actually diagnosed—usually in a person's twenties or thirties—the disease is well established, having taken root in either adolescence or childhood. The medical establishment generally contends that there is "no known cause" for MS, yet billions of dollars have been spent researching potential causes and cures. Alternative medicine, however, regards MS as a complex, multifactorial disease involving several causes. When these causes are addressed, the symptoms may be alleviated or even reversed.

Dietary and Nutritional Deficiencies

People with multiple sclerosis typically have nutritional deficiencies. Studies show that essential fatty acids, the building blocks of the brain and nervous system, are lacking in many MS patients.[1] Multiple sclerosis is most common in Western countries where people consume large amounts of meats, dairy products, processed foods, and coconut and palm oils—all foods low in essential fatty acids, and is least common in countries where diets are high in unsaturated fats, including seed oils, olive oil, oily fish, fresh fruits, and vegetables—all foods high in essential fatty acids. The connection with saturated fat intake was first noted in 1950 by Roy Swank, M.D., of Oregon Health Sciences University in Portland, Oregon, and has been confirmed in more recent studies.[2]

See Allergies, Candidiasis.

Stephen Davies, B.M., B.Ch., who runs the Biolab Medical Unit in London, England, has found that even with a balanced diet, MS patients have difficulty absorbing essential nutrients. Although these differ from person to person, says Dr. Davies, the most common deficiencies are vitamin B_1, B_6, B_{12}, magnesium, zinc, folic acid, amino acids, manganese, selenium, as well essential fatty acids.

Food Sensitivities

Intolerances to certain foods are common in patients with multiple sclerosis. Among the most frequent are milk and dairy products, caffeine, tannin, yeast, sugar, fungi, wheat, gluten (found in wheat, barley, oats, and rye), corn, food additives, and fermented products such as ketchup, vinegar, and wine.

In a 1986 study it was found that of 135 MS patients, 65.9 percent had histories of sinusitis (inflammation of the sinuses), a classic symptom of an intolerance to milk and dairy products.[3]

Candidiasis

Candidiasis, an overgrowth of the yeast *Candida albicans,* is a major cause of food intolerances and, like nutritional deficiencies, can add to the stress on individuals with multiple sclerosis. William G. Crook, M.D., of Jackson, Tennessee, first made the connection between MS and the yeast *Candida albicans*, documenting several cases in which symptoms improved once the candida was treated.[4]

Environmental Toxins

Gary Oberg, M.D., past President of the American Academy of Environmental Medicine, notes several ways in which environmental toxins may contribute to multiple sclerosis. "Toxins may cause metabolic poisoning, interrupting the body's normal metabolic pathways and damaging the myelin sheath of nerves, which is the basic defect in MS. Certain substances, while not toxic to everyone, may initiate an autoimmune reaction in susceptible individuals. These individuals make antibodies to the foreign substance which cross-react with myelin, thus damaging the nerves and inducing symptoms characteristic of multiple sclerosis." According to Dr. Oberg, some of the substances that can produce or aggravate symptoms include chemicals in food and tap water, carbon monoxide, diesel fumes, fumes from domestic gas water heaters, solvents, aerosol sprays, and chipboard and foam in furniture and carpets. Dr. Oberg adds that MS symptoms may also be caused by internal toxins—toxins produced by bacteria and fungi in the gastrointestinal tract, including *Candida albicans*.

Toxicity from Mercury Dental Amalgams

Mercury is a highly toxic metal that, when used in dental amalgam fillings, can seep into body tissues where it accumulates and becomes capable of producing symptoms in the body that are indistinguishable from those of multiple sclerosis.[5]

According to Hal Huggins, D.D.S., of Colorado Springs, Colorado, mercury poisoning often remains undetected because patients' symptoms do not necessarily suggest mercury as the initiating cause, but the effects of mercury toxicity are potentially devastating. Mercury has been recognized as a poison since the 1500s, yet mercury amalgams have been used in dentistry since the 1820s. Mercury has been shown to bind to the DNA of cells and cell membranes, causing cell distortion and inhibited cell function.[6] When this happens the immune system no longer recognizes the cell as part of the body and initiates an autoimmune reaction, destroying myelin in the process. MS patients have been found to have over seven times higher levels of mercury in their cerebrospinal fluid (the fluid that surrounds the brain and spinal cord) as compared to neurologically healthy patients.[7]

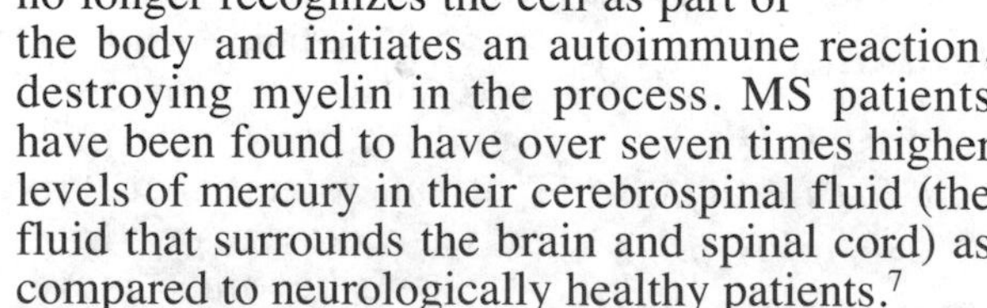

Research should be undertaken to explore the role of geopathic stress as a contributing factor to multiple sclerosis. See Geopathic Stress, page 563.

Stress and Trauma

Dr. Kingsley notes that a first episode of MS often follows a physical trauma or period of emotional stress, and that initial symptoms sometimes appear at the site of an injury (e.g., numbness in an arm or leg following a trauma in which that limb was injured).

The Viral Connection

Medical researchers have long suspected a viral involvement in MS. Recent research on patients infected with the Epstein-Barr virus (a form of herpes virus believed to be the causative agent in infectious mononucleosis) shows that levels of essential fatty acids are very low after the illness, similar to the low levels found in MS patients.[8] This virus interferes with the body's ability to metabolize essential fatty acids, causing a partial breakdown of the body's immune system. An acute episode of infection with the Epstein-Barr virus during adolescence could leave the door open to chronic illness such as MS some years later.

Genetic Predisposition

Although multiple sclerosis is not a hereditary disease, it is considered familial. First generation relatives of MS patients show a thirty to fifty times greater risk of developing the disease than the general population.[9]

Treating Multiple Sclerosis

An early diagnosis is an essential first step in treating multiple sclerosis. For the best rate of success, treatment of the disease should begin as soon as possible after diagnosis. Once the disability has gained a hold, it becomes harder to reverse the damage. "There is no question," says Dr. Swank, "at least in the minds of alternative physicians, that those MS patients who show the greatest improvement are the ones who start treatment earliest."

> *"There is no question that those MS patients who show the greatest improvement are the ones who start treatment earliest."*
> —Roy Swank, M.D.

Many health care professionals believe that if treatment begins soon enough and is adhered to it is possible to control multiple sclerosis in many, if not all, patients. Dr. Kingsley reasons that, "Cure is possible if the cause or causes can be found and then eliminated." He adds, "If mercury is eliminated from the body, and if the food and environmental sensitivities of the individual are pinpointed and sorted out, in addition to addressing any nutritional deficiencies, then I believe it is perfectly possible to cure people. But they must accept the fact that if they then return to their former diet and have mercury fillings put back in their teeth, they will probably get MS again because they have a predisposition toward it."

Because multiple sclerosis affects each patient differently, treatment programs are individualized. Dietary and nutritional needs are often addressed, as are food allergies and environmental toxins. Recommendations may be made for detoxification therapy, as well as for the removal of mercury amalgam dental fillings. Among practitioners of alternative medicine, there is a degree of consensus—not generally shared by conventional doctors—that multiple sclerosis can be controlled. This type of approach involves fundamental nutritional, environmental, and lifestyle changes. It is important that treatment be followed under the guidance of a qualified practitioner trained in these fields.

Diet

The best documented success with multiple sclerosis patients is Dr. Swank's work with a low-fat diet. He found that MS patients who ate the lowest amount of saturated fat realized the greatest improvement, and those who ate saturated fat in amounts larger than the prescribed maximum fared the worst.[10] Dr. Swank recommends that the maximum safe level of saturated fat for anyone with MS not exceed fifteen grams (about three teaspoons) a day. Patients need to be especially careful of hidden saturated fat found in processed and packaged foods. For best results, he advises the elimination of all saturated fat and a switch to the polyunsaturated type. Dr. Swank suggests oils such as sunflower, safflower, soya, and olive, which contain either polyunsaturated or monounsaturated fats (a minimum of four teaspoons of unsaturated oils a day, up to ten teaspoons for patients leading an active life).

While Dr. Swank's emphasis is on first reducing saturated fat intake, other doctors believe that the priority should be to increase an MS patient's intake of essential fatty acids found in poly- and monounsaturated oils. Either way, the result is a low-saturated fat/high polyunsaturated fat diet.

Thousands of patients can testify to the effectiveness of Dr. Swank's low-fat diet. Consider the case of one such patient, John. Before beginning Dr. Swank's diet, John exhibited typical MS symptoms: functional blindness, numbness of the left-side extremities, slurring of speech, difficulty walking, and lack of bladder control. After eliminating saturated fat from his diet, John began a nutritional supplement program outlined by Dr. Swank, and found that by maintaining a relatively stress-free lifestyle combined with a diet of fresh, pure produce, including fresh salads daily, his symptoms were relieved. John has had no real problems with multiple sclerosis for years, and can now work twelve to fourteen hours a day with no fatigue.[11]

Nutritional Supplements

For many health care practitioners, nutritional supplementation plays a vital role in treating multiple sclerosis. Important supplements include vitamins, minerals, amino acids, and essential fatty acids.

Essential Fatty Acids: The two families of essential fatty acids are omega-3 (linoleic acid), which is found mainly in seeds and seed oils, and omega-6 (alpha-linolenic acid), which is found mainly in fish, fish oils (cod liver oil), and green leafy vegetables such as spinach and kale.

Gamma linolenic acid (GLA), a vital member of the omega-6 family, is found in evening primrose oil, black currant oil, borage oil, and spirulina. Known primarily for its anti-inflammatory effect, GLA is necessary for the healthy functioning of the immune system, and helps to produce vital regulators called prostaglandins (biologically active unsaturated fatty acids) in the body.

Vitamins, Minerals, Trace Elements, and Amino Acids: Specific vitamins, minerals, trace elements, and amino acids may be recommended to make up for deficiencies as well as to act as "co-factors" for the efficient metabolism of essential fatty acids. These "co-factors" include vitamin C, vitamin B_3 (niacin), vitamin B_6, zinc, and magnesium. Other supplements frequently recommended are all the other B vitamins, including vitamin B_{12}, calcium, zinc, selenium, the amino acid glutathione, and the antioxidant beta-carotene.

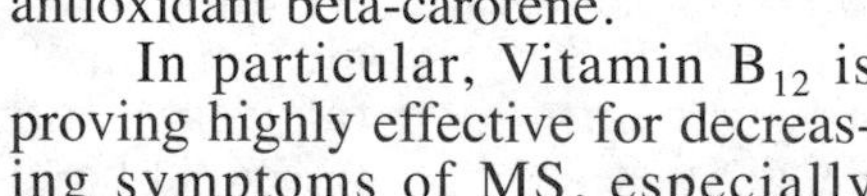

See Chelation Therapy, Environmental Medicine.

In particular, Vitamin B_{12} is proving highly effective for decreasing symptoms of MS, especially when associated with mercury poisoning. Dr. Kingsley sometimes prescribes doses, "as high as 12,000 micrograms once a week by intravenous infusion, usually with other essential nutrients. However, intramuscular doses are commonly between 4,000 and 8,000 micrograms once a week, and this can continue for many weeks until the person has become mercury negative." He says that in some cases he has been able to stem a relapse. "B_{12} is absolutely marvelous," says Dr. Kingsley. "We have been able to completely clear an MS relapse within half an hour of administering a suitably high dose of vitamin B_{12} intravenously."

Dr. Kingsley adds that textbooks on the subject of multiple sclerosis do not even mention the value of vitamin B_{12} or its use in MS.[12] "Many academics have been arguing that vitamin B_{12} is not necessary because they consider the condition to be a central nervous system disease. Yet they fail to recognize what the long-term effects of pernicious anemia (a severe blood disease marked by a progressive decrease in red blood cells, muscular weakness, as well as gastrointestinal and neural disturbances) are on the central nervous system. Their main reason for not recommending B_{12} to patients has been because the levels of B_{12} in the blood of MS patients are nearly always within the normal range. Now, however, studies are showing that the B_{12} levels in the cerebrospinal fluid of patients with MS are lower than those of control groups.[13]

One woman suffering from MS and experiencing numbness in her arms, legs, and hands, as well as pain in her arms, consulted with Dr. Kingsley. These symptoms had been occuring for approximately two years, and over that time she was eating a great deal of cheese and drinking six cups of tea and two cups of coffee daily. Dr. Kingsley identified milk and dairy products, tannin, caffeine, and yeast as the foods and substances to which she was sensitive. At his suggestion she made dramatic changes in her diet, eating plenty of fish, chicken, salads, fruit, and drinking herbal teas. Like all of Dr. Kingsley's patients, she had her amalgam fillings replaced and began chelation therapy. She also received regular injections of vitamin B_{12} in variable doses. "After about seven months she became symptom free for the first time, but then suffered periodic relapses, each one of which cleared with a suitable intravenous treatment of vitamin B_{12}. Apart from additional relapses in relation to a developing 'flu', or when under undue stress, the gap between each infusion of vitamin B_{12} has become longer and longer as time has gone by."

> *"Once environmental toxins are removed, it is entirely possible that remission can occur."*
> —Gary Oberg, M.D.

Magnesium is another important supplement. Dr. Davies stresses the importance of magnesium, as spasticity can often be traced to low levels of this mineral. One patient, a man who was diagnosed with MS at age forty, sought Dr. Davies' advice and was tested for nutrient levels and possible allergies. Very low levels of magnesium were found, so the patient was given weekly injections over two to three months. Allergies to wheat and all milk products were identified and it was recommended that the patient remove those foods from his diet. Also recommended were a multivitamin/mineral capsule, an evening primrose oil capsule, and cod liver oil. Dr. Davies notes that today, ten years later, the patient has multiple sclerosis under control, and is no longer plagued by bouts of double vision. He says that although the patient still has a limp, he is able to work full time.

Environmental Medicine

When treating MS patients, Dr. Oberg initially searches for the environmental or dietary factors that exacerbate multiple sclerosis symptoms. Dietary factors are examined by using an elimination diet—removing a particular substance from the diet and observing if the symptoms disappear. If they do, and reappear on reintroduction of the food into the diet, then that food must be avoided.

To diagnose dust, mold, pollen, food, or chemical sensitivities, Dr. Oberg also uses a diagnostic technique called maximum tolerated intradermal dose testing. By injecting the largest dose of an extract of the offending substance in an amount that does not cause a reaction (such as a skin wheal), the patient can be desensitized. "Once environmental or dietary substances to which the patient is individually sensitive are removed," says Dr. Oberg, "it is entirely possible that remission can occur."

Electroacupuncture biofeedback testing may also prove beneficial in determining toxins and allergens complicating MS.

Biological Dentistry

The removal of mercury-containing dental fillings is an intrinsic part of the treatment of multiple sclerosis. According to Dr. Huggins, mercury vapor escaping from dental fillings can interfere with the action of key enzymes, thus disturbing important enzymatic functions in the body. He adds that mercury vapor is implicated in chronic fatigue, a common MS symptom.

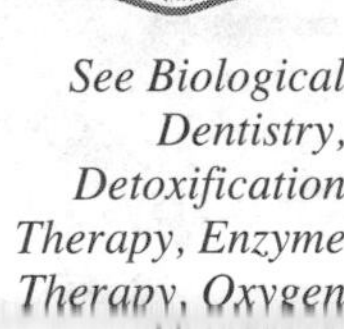

See Biological Dentistry, Detoxification Therapy, Enzyme Therapy, Oxygen Therapies.

Replacing mercury fillings with other kinds of material, however, is not as straightforward as it seems. Dr. Huggins warns that some plastic materials can contain aluminum and thereby create different problems for the patient. Before any work is begun, patients of Dr. Huggins first receive a "blood-serum bio-compatibility blood test" to determine which alternative material is biologically compatible. Dr. Huggins explains, "Patient blood serum is tested against multiple dental materials. Some dental materials cause immune reactions and others immune suppression. Neither are healthy conditions. An example of overreactivity is multiple sclerosis, and of immune suppression is AIDS. Since no material is 100 percent safe any more than no one prescription drug is safe for everyone, we do immunologic testing on each patient's blood to determine where reactivity is. After identifying the high and minimal reactivities, a computer matches dental materials with reactivity and suggests the safest materials for that particular patient."

Dr. Huggins's treatment is individualized and based on the results of extensive tests. After removal of the mercury fillings, a detoxification program is developed according to the requirements of each patient, and can include nutritional support, acupressure, and massage treatments. Chelating agents such as EDTA (ethylenediaminetetraacetic acid) and vitamin C can be used either intravenously or in tablet form. The program also has a psychological component, and Dr. Huggins warns that emotional release often occurs during detoxification. The program is then followed up with nutritional supplements to balance body chemistry, as well as individualized dietary and lifestyle guidelines. Recommendations are also made concerning the use of saunas and bodywork to enhance the detoxification process.

Dr. Huggins has seen approximately four hundred cases of MS at his center, 85 percent of which have improved. Positive changes include patients who have been able to walk again after having been confined to a wheelchair.

Hyperbaric Oxygen Therapy

In hyperbaric oxygen therapy (HBOT), a patient is placed in a oxygen chamber. Atmospheric pressure is then elevated in order to increase the amount of oxygen entering the body's tissues. As well as oxygenating the tissues, David Hughes, D.Sc., Director of the Hyperbaric Oxygen Institute in San Bernadino, California, notes that HBOT may also enhance the immune system, reduce inflammation via its effects on prostaglandins, help in the repair of damaged blood vessels, stimulate the circulation in the small blood vessels, and, in a variety of ways, assist in the production of myelin. Bladder and bowel dysfunction are two of the symptoms of multiple sclerosis which most improve with HBOT.[14]

Exactly how this procedure works for patients with MS is still a matter of conjecture and debate. While some medical literature refutes HBOT's effectiveness, in Britain, several thousand people with MS have received HBOT treatments. From 1983 to 1987, five hundred thousand individual sessions were provided, and nearly half of the four thousand people involved benefited in one or more ways.[15] HBOT seems to have been effective in keeping many people from getting worse, often improving their general condition and reversing many minor symptoms.

Enzyme Therapy

According to Hector H. Solorzano del Rio, M.D., D.Sc., Chairman of the Program for Studies of Alternative Medicine at the University of Guadalajara in Mexico, pancreatic enzymes can help patients with multiple sclerosis. He cites the case of a forty-year-old male patient confined to a wheelchair, who had not benefited from orthodox medical treatments. After a month of enzyme treatments he had gained sufficient strength to begin taking care of himself. Three months later he began to walk, and after six months he was leading a productive life.

Hundreds of MS patients in Mexico and Germany have sought out enzyme therapy. These same patients are also given unsaturated fatty acids and often supplements of selenium. Apparently, response to enzyme therapy is much faster if patients have not previously been given treatment that has suppressed the immune system.

Attitude and Lifestyle Changes

Dr. Kingsley advises that "taking an active role in treatment should be the first concern of a person diagnosed with multiple sclerosis. This includes positive cooperation with the practitioner, as well as possible fundamental lifestyle changes in work, relationships, and environmental conditions. Changes may be necessary to improve a person's condition; it may be inadvisable, even impossible, to carry on as if nothing has happened."

Dr. Swank finds stress to be the second most important cause of MS after high fat diets. "Continuing stress, such as from legal actions and family problems can cause MS," he says. Dr. Swank treats these patients with mild sedatives to help them sleep and be more relaxed during the day. For mild stress he suggests taking a short rest in the afternoon, and for more severe stress, he advises a rest mid-morning as well.

Self-Care

The following therapies can be undertaken at home under appropriate professional supervision:

• Fasting • Meditation • Yoga

Aromatherapy: Rub affected part with mixture of 95 percent olive oil and 5 percent essence of juniper or rosemary.

Ayurveda: The herb *ashwagandha* is recommended.

Exercise: Many people with MS are more disabled than they need be. Gentle exercise will help keep someone with MS toned, supple, and mobile. Any type of exercise will do, although yoga is particularly suited for helping patients regain lost movement.

Hydrotherapy: Constitutional hydrotherapy should be applied two to five times weekly.

Juice Therapy: Short fasts with fruit and vegetable juices.

Practical Hints: Avoid the use of electric heating pads, chlorinated water, as well as fluoridated water, toothpaste, and mouthwash.

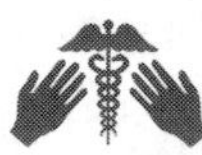

Professional Care

The following therapies should only be provided by a qualified health professional:

• Biofeedback Training • Cell Therapy • Chelation Therapy • Guided Imagery • Hypnotherapy •Traditional Chinese Medicine

Bodywork: Massage, Feldenkrais.

Osteopathy: To relieve symptoms.

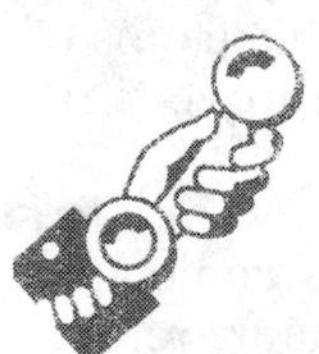

Where to Find Help

For additional information on, and referrals for, treatment of muiltiple sclerosis, contact the following organizations.

American Academy of Biological Dentistry
P.O. Box 856
Carmel Valley, California 93924
(408) 659-5385
(408) 659-2417 (Fax)

The purpose of the AABD is to promote biological dental medicine, which uses nontoxic diagnostic and therapeutic approaches in the field of clinical dentistry. The academy publishes a quarterly journal, Focus, *and holds regular seminars on biological diagnosis and therapy.*

American Association of Acupuncture and Oriental Medicine
4101 Lake Boone Trail, Suite 201
Raleigh, North Carolina 27607
(919) 787-5181

The AAAOM is a national professional trade organization of acupuncturists who meet acceptable standards of competency and can provide you with he names and locations of local members. Referrals by written request only.

American Holistic Medical Association
4101 Lake Boone Trail, Suite 201
Raleigh, North Carolina 27607
(919) 787-5181

A professional organization for holistic practitioners, the AHMA offers information and services for its members and lobbies for holistic issues. It also provides referrals for the public; requests must be in writing.

Environmental Dental Association
9974 Scripps Ranch Boulevard, Suite 36
San Diego, California 92131
(800) 388-8124

The EDA is an organization of alternative dentists who are concerned about potential toxic effects of various dental procedures and materials. Member dentists believe that the most important environment of all is the human body and that some dentistry can cause side effects to the body. The EDA provides a referral service for patients seeking alternative dentists in their area. It also offers books and products on alternative dentistry for the public. For a free packet of information call the EDA's toll-free number.

Foundation for Toxic-Free Dentistry
P.O. Box 608010
Orlando, Florida 32860-8010
(407) 299-4149

A nonprofit group whose main goal is to educate and refer the general public to biologic dentists all over the world. Send a self-addressed, stamped envelope with postage for two ounces and they will send you information and referrals.

Huggins Diagnostic Center
5080 List Drive
Colorado Springs, Colorado 80919
(719) 548-1600
(719) 522-0563 (Fax)

For information on removal of mercury fillings.

Swank Multiple Sclerosis Clinic
School of Medicine
Oregon Health Sciences University
3181 Sam Jackson Park Road
Portland, Oregon 97201
(503) 494-8370

Publishes Swank Multiple Sclerosis Newsletter.

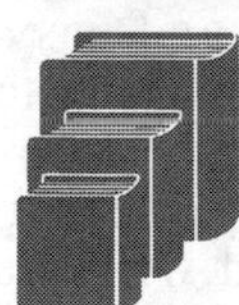

Recommended Reading

Enzyme Therapy. Wolf, Max, M.D., and Ransberger, Karl, Ph.D., New York: Biological Research Institute, 1972.

An in-depth study of enzymes and their therapeutic qualities in treating aging, cancer, virus diseases, and more.

It's All in Your Head. Huggins, Hal, D.D.S., Colorado Springs, CO: Life Science Press, 1986.

Dr. Huggins analyzes the diseases and symptoms associated with mercury poisoning, as well as providing diagnostics and a nutritional guide to recovery.

Multiple Sclerosis—A Self-Help Guide to Its Management. Graham, Judy. Rochester, VT: Healing Arts Press, 1989.

The author describes how she has controlled her own multiple sclerosis through exercises and a strict nutritional program that includes Evening Primrose oil, a dietary supplement shown to be an effective aid for those with MS.

The Multiple Sclerosis Diet Book. Swank, Roy L., M.D., Ph.D.; Duggan, Barbara Brewer. New York: Doubleday, 1987.

Supported by thirty-five years of clinical tests, Dr. Swank's diet can reduce the frequency and severity of multiple sclerosis attacks.

Obesity and Weight Management

Obesity clearly poses a danger to health, having been associated with numerous health problems including heart disease, high blood pressure, diabetes, and certain types of cancer. However, diets for weight loss have been shown to be ineffective and even damaging to health. A well-balanced diet which avoids fat-building foods, regular exercise, drinking adequate amounts of pure water, and stress reduction can help maintain a healthy weight compatible with one's body type.

Weight loss has become a national obsession in America. As many as 40 percent of women and 24 percent of men in the United States are trying to lose weight at any given time through such diverse methods as diets, exercise, behavior modification, and drugs.[1] While this obsession is often fueled by psychological needs (the urge to conform to an artificial standard of beauty fostered by media, fashion, and peer pressure) rather than physical needs, the underlying fact is that one-quarter to one-third of Americans are overweight.[2] Even more troubling, according to Joseph E. Pizzorno, N.D., President of Bastyr College in Seattle, Washington, is the fact that the number of severely obese children in the United States nearly doubled between 1965 and 1980. This trend, if it continues, will only lead to an even greater frequency of adult obesity as these children grow up.

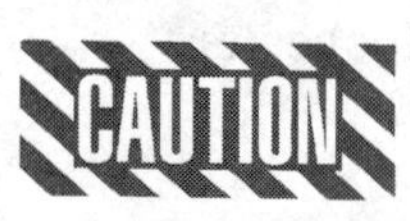

Professional help may be required if someone habitually eats for reasons other than hunger.

This is even more alarming because excess weight has been linked to a number of health problems, including high blood pressure, heart disease, diabetes, gallbladder disease, respiratory conditions, as well as breast and endometrial cancer in women, and cancer of the colon and rectum in men. Obesity has also been shown to result in a decreased lifespan for both women and men.[3] The answers to weight gain and weight loss though, are not always simple and easy. Under controlled settings, most people trying to lose weight are usually able to lose about 10 percent of their total body weight, but one-third to two-thirds of that weight is regained within a year, and almost all is regained within five years. Oftentimes, excessive dieting and weight loss regimens can actually lead to increased weight gain.

Causes of Obesity and Weight Gain

Obesity is indicated by an abnormally high proportion of body fat, but, according to Timothy Birdsall, N.D., of Sandpoint, Idaho, "Although it is commonly assumed that obesity is due to overeating, there is, in fact, a complex interaction between one's culture, environment, exercise habits, and eating styles, as well as one's genetic makeup, biochemical individuality, and physiological "set point."

The set point theory states that one's size and body fat are determined by genetics, eating patterns and calorie intake at certain key times in life such as early adolescence. "These patterns are relatively fixed," says Elson Haas, M.D., Director of the Preventive Medicine Center of Marin in San Rafael, California. "Attempting to arrive at a weight above or below one's set point range causes physiological mechanisms which ultimately force behavioral changes and a return to one's previous weight. A good example of this is the rapid weight gain that can happen after coming off a diet, especially a low-calorie starvation diet. The body reacts to what it perceives as a threat, quickly regaining the weight to once again reach its natural set point."

There are also cases where excess weight is gained because of conditions such as food allergies and nutritional deficiencies which are often treatable. Other times weight gain may be due to a sluggish metabolism, chemical toxicity, insulin imbalance, impaired thermogenesis (the mechanism by which fat is burned to produce heat), excessive dieting, or psychological factors. In rare cases obesity occurs as a signal that a more serious disease is present, such as hypothyroidism or Cushing's syndrome (hypersecretion of adrenal cortex, in which excessive glucocorticoids are produced, disrupting protein and carbohydrate metabolism).

Sluggish Metabolism

"Thin people have higher metabolic rates and burn calories at a much faster rate than their obese friends," says Majid Ali, M.D., Associate Professor of Pathology at Columbia University in New York. Metabolic rate can be understood as being the rate by which the body utilizes energy. The basal metabolic rate (BMR), which varies tremendously between individuals, is the minimum amount of energy needed to maintain normal body functions. Age, sex, body size, and fat to muscle ratio are all factors that influence how efficiently an individual burns calories. Even when individuals are matched for all of these factors, they can exhibit a 30 percent difference in BMR.[4] The types of food a person eats may also affect metabolic rate. According to Dr. Birdsall, carbohydrates are most effective in raising the metabolic rate. He points out that while fats can also increase the metabolic rate, they contain more calories per gram than carbohydrates and are therefore much less effective. "Fats have a negative net effect because, while they may increase the metabolic rate somewhat, they don't increase it enough to offset the added calories."

An inefficient thyroid gland (hypothyroidism) can be the cause of sluggish metabolic rate, according to Dr. Birdsall. And while it is possible that laboratory tests will not indicate the existence of hypothyroidism, other tests, such as basal body temperature, and symptoms, such as

Truths and Fallacies About Obesity

According to Gus Prosch, M.D., of Birmingham, Alabama, an obesity specialist who has treated tens of thousands of overweight patients since 1965, there are seven critical truths or facts relating to the problem of obesity, as well as seven fallacies.

"These truths and fallacies are accurate 99 percent of the time," says Dr. Prosch. "Understanding these before any entry into a weight control program will save an overweight person much time, effort, money, and disappointment."

The seven truths about obesity:

1. *If obese, you have a lifetime disease.*
2. *Your metabolic processes will always tend to be abnormal.*
3. *You cannot eat what others eat and stay thin.*
4. *Anyone can lose weight and stay slim provided the causes of weight gain are determined, addressed, and corrected.*
5. *Understanding insulin metabolism is the key to intelligently losing weight.*
6. *There is absolutely no physiological requirement for sugar or processed foods in your diet.*
7. *You cannot lose weight and keep it off successfully by strictly and solely following any special diet, or by taking a weight loss pill, or by following an exercise program. To succeed, you must address all the contributing factors causing obesity.*

The seven fallacies about obesity:

1. *Fad diets can successfully make you lose weight and keep the weight off.*
2. *Most physicians can successfully make you lose weight and keep the weight off.*
3. *Today's many and varied weight loss programs and weight clinics can successfully and permanently make you lose weight and keep the weight off.*
4. *Past experiences show that counting calories is a good way to help you lose weight and keep the weight off.*
5. *Your weight problem is caused from overeating and/or lack of exercise alone.*
6. *If you could only lose enough weight to get slim you could keep your weight off from then on.*
7. *There is no way that you can lose your weight successfully and keep the weight off.*

chronic constipation, fatigue, feeling cold, and a tendency to gain weight, may point to subclinical hypothyroidism. Correcting this problem can often lead to weight loss, adds Dr. Birdsall.

Impaired Thermogenesis

The body contains two types of fat tissue—white adipose tissue which stores fat, and brown adipose tissue (BAT), which burns up fat to produce heat in a process called thermogenesis. Evidence indicates that an impairment of the thermogenesis system in BAT may lead to obesity.[5] If fat from the diet is not burned up by BAT, it is stored as fat in white adipose tissue, thus contributing to excess body weight. Chronic dieting can alter BAT's responsiveness, lowering diet-induced thermogenesis and causing increased hunger, according to Dr. Birdsall.

Fat-Stored Chemical Toxins

For the past ten years, Zane R. Gard, M.D., of Beaverton, Oregon, and his partner and wife, Erma Brown, B.S.N., P.H.N., have been studying the effects of environmental toxins and detoxification on health. "Although humans adjust well to a changing environment, exposure to harmful chemicals is now occurring at a rate faster than the human body is able to adapt," says Dr. Gard. He notes that most environmental toxins are stored in fat tissue, and he refers to the accumulation and storage of these poisons in the body as "toxic bioaccumulation." He points out that one physical response to subtoxic chemical exposure is obesity and possibly a higher fat to muscle ratio.

Insulin Imbalance

"Many cases of obesity are due to an imbalance of the hormone insulin," says David K. Shefrin, N.D., of Beaverton, Oregon. Insulin allows the body to utilize glucose (sugar) and carbohydrates. Factors such as genetic predisposition, food allergies, eating habits, and stress may interfere with glucose and carbohydrate utilization, resulting in a condition known as glucose intolerance. Excessive sugar consumption (refined carbohydrates) may also contribute to glucose intolerance and obesity.[6]

> *“Research shows that overweight individuals burn up sugar less effectively than normal individuals, and that dieting only makes this problem worse.”*

"If insulin is not rapidly cleared from the bloodstream after a meal, it will cause an individual to feel hungry," says Dr. Shefrin. "Usually insulin will signal the body to stop eating, but if a person has chronically elevated glucose levels due to inefficient insulin, he may eat more." Thus, the more refined carbohydrates a person eats, the hungrier he or she may become.

Research also shows that overweight individuals burn up sugar less effectively than individuals of normal weight, and that dieting only makes this problem worse. The same research concludes that this trait is a part, not a consequence, of obesity.[7]

> *“The number of overweight and obese people in this country is constantly increasing, and the problem will continue to get even worse until our health leaders learn the truth and fulfill their responsibility to inform citizens of these facts.”*
>
> —Gus Prosch, M.D.

"When an overweight person becomes more obese, the insulin problem becomes worse as well, because the individual becomes more unresponsive to the action of insulin," says Gus Prosch, M.D., of Birmingham, Alabama, an obesity specialist. "In such a person, the simple carbohydrates are triggering the release of increasing amounts of insulin, but the body cannot use it efficiently. This is why we see high insulin levels in overweight people. Apparently the insulin receptors on their body cells are blocked from doing their function. This prevents insulin from stimulating the transfer of glucose to the cells to give them energy, which explains why so many overweight people feel tired so often. To make matters worse, since the insulin is not converting the glucose to energy, more glucose is then moved into the fat cells to create more fat."

See Diabetes, Hypoglycemia.

This imbalance in insulin hormone functioning can cause other dependent and related hormones to function abnormally and less efficiently as well, according to Dr. Prosch. "Ultimately, either the insulin receptors or the pancreas itself wears out or becomes exhausted, in which case diabetes can result," he says.

This excess insulin in overweight people can lead to other problems and complications, Dr. Prosch points out. These include:

- Increased salt and water retention
- Sleep disorders caused by insulin interference with neurotransmitters
- The production of more LDL, or bad cho-

lesterol, by the liver due to insulin stimulation
- Interference with the thyroid hormone thyroxine, thereby aggravating low metabolism
- Decreased cell wall permeability, which can cause an increase in cell size
- Hypoglycemia, hunger, and a further craving for simple carbohydrates

"These factors illustrate why simple carbohydrates are so detrimental to the health of America," says Dr. Prosch. "The number of overweight and obese people in this country is constantly increasing, and the problem will continue to get even worse until our health leaders learn the truth and fulfill their responsibility to inform citizens of these facts."

Dieting

Low-calorie diets and exercise have been the typical solution to losing weight. With thousands of diets and a multimillion dollar industry dedicated to weight control, shedding a few pounds should be easy. Unfortunately, the weight lost by dieters is almost always regained. As a result, many dieters fall into the "yo-yo trap"—a repetitive cycle of weight loss and gain.

Susan Kano, a national speaker and author on dieting and eating disorders, tells a story about a friend who had not only been trying to lose weight for years, but was also in the dieting business. Initially she struggled to get from 165 pounds down to 120. After a while, her weight returned to the 165 mark. Over the years, as she tried one diet after another, her weight yo-yoed up and down. Today she continues to diet and weighs over 200 pounds.

"Dieting leads to the emaciation of muscle cells, bloating of fat cells, accumulation of toxic fats in tissues, and fatigue. The more rapid the weight loss, the higher the risk of heart complications from muscle loss."
—Majid Ali, M.D.

There are several reasons why this happens and why food restriction for the purposes of weight loss should be avoided. "We have gotten fatter as a culture over the last few years," says Kano, "partly because of dieting." Whenever the body is deprived of food, whether from famine or dieting, it ensures survival by decreasing the metabolic rate in order to compensate for fewer calories. Energy is stored so efficiently in adipose (fat) tissues that someone of normal weight can survive for two months without eating. The desire to binge after food restriction, although disheartening to dieters, is another built-in survival mechanism intended to click on after a famine.[9] "Our innocent cellular metabolism has no way to tell the difference between self-imposed starvation and life-threatening famine," says Nancy Dunne, N.D., of Missoula, Montana.

How Weight Standards Are Determined

Traditionally, normal or ideal weight has been determined by weight and height charts first compiled by the Metropolitan Life Insurance Company (MLI) fifty years ago.[8] From these charts individuals were determined to either be overweight, obese (when weight is 20 percent or more above what is considered normal), or morbidly obese (when excessive weight interferes with normal activity and/or breathing). As obesity is more concerned with excessive fat, rather than excessive weight, there is some question among doctors now whether these standards are accurate.

Critics point out that when MLI first collected statistics for their charts, they used insurance clients as subjects for their information. Mortality rate, not health, was used to determine normal weight. Not only was this method flawed, but the population they used was not a representative sample. MLI charts also assume that being overweight means a person is overfat. Therefore, a muscular individual, who does not need to lose weight, may be considered obese on paper. Many experts now prefer using the body mass index (BMI). This type of system uses body fat, not body weight, as a guide.

Although there is no simple and precise means of assessing body composition, measuring a person's folds of fat or using charts such as the BMI, that more accurately correlate body fat and weight, are becoming common standards of weight measurement in doctor's offices. Despite this, most dieters still rely on old fashioned height-weight charts because they are easy to use.

"Dieting can be a cause of obesity, and not the way to lose weight," adds Dr. Ali. "Dieting not only slows down the metabolic enzymes, but leads to the emaciation of muscle cells, bloating of fat cells, accumulation of toxic fats in tissues, and fatigue. The more rapid the weight loss, the higher the risk of heart complications from muscle loss as well.

See Anorexia nervosa, Bulimia nervosa.

"An obese person needs to gain muscle mass and increase the amount of fat-burning tissue," continues Dr. Ali. "This usually means a slight initial weight gain, or at least absence of weight loss. This happens because muscle tissue is heavier than fat tissue. Only then can someone hope to increase the rate of burning, and losing, fat," says Dr. Ali.

Weight Loss Medications

Weight loss medications work in several ways, principally by either stimulating the nervous system or by suppressing appetite. All weight loss drugs have side effects though, according to Dr. Ali, and therefore he does not recommend anyone use them. Some of the more common problems associated with these drugs include adverse effects on the heart and blood pressure, an increased level of toxic fat in the tissues, as well as a variety of degenerative diseases.

Psychological Factors

Food is an intricate and tightly woven part of social activities, childhood memories, and psyches. Food is used to help celebrate almost all major holidays and events. In the United States, birthdays are marked by cakes and ice cream; Halloween is centered around candy and other treats; July 4th celebrates with picnics; and Thanksgiving, with its traditional feast of turkey, stuffing, and gravy, isn't complete without a thick slab of pumpkin pie and whipped cream. Even romantic dating centers around eating.

Dieting can make a person feel down, like he or she is actually depriving him- or herself of something, and eating can temporarily curb feelings of loneliness and depression. While many people eat "comfort foods" under stress, problems can emerge when unhappiness leads to chronic overeating. When someone eats for reasons other than hunger, especially if this is done frequently, professional help may be required.

The National Institutes of Health (NIH) has outlined a specific protocol for modifying unhealthy eating behavior brought on by psychological factors. First of all, each individual needs to identify the eating or related lifestyle behaviors to be changed, then one needs to set specific behavioral goals, modifying the psychological determinants of the behavior to be changed, and thus, reinforcing the desired behavior. According to the NIH, "The goal of behavior treatment is to modify eating and physical activity habits, typically focusing on gradual changes. Behavior modification can be undertaken through group or individual sessions under the guidance of professional or lay personnel, and alone or in conjunction with other approaches."[12]

HEALTH RISKS OF LIQUID PROTEIN DIETS

A severe example of dieting is the very low-calorie diet (VLCD) or liquid protein diet, supplying only four hundred to eight hundred calories per day. Like other restrictive diets, the VLCD reduces metabolic rate, but this only temporarily solves the problem of weight loss.

Although first popularized in the 1970s, the VLCD is regaining notoriety as celebrities promote several versions of this meal replacement plan. Twenty years ago, inadequate medical supervision and protein formulas lead to several deaths and medical problems among some VLCD users. Since that time, physicians have recognized the need for properly balanced protein supplements, as well as careful selection and monitoring of diet candidates. It is important to note that health risks for medically unsupervised individuals on a VLCD may include dehydration, disruption of the body's chemistry, low blood pressure, and increased uric acid levels. Even under the guidance of a doctor, patients can experience cold intolerance, headaches, fatigue, dizziness, stomach upset, and muscle cramping. If you binge after a VLCD, your heart, pancreas, or gallbladder may be affected.[10]

DRUGS ASSOCIATED WITH A HIGHER INCIDENCE OF WEIGHT GAIN

According to the Physicians Desk Reference *the following drugs are associated with side effects of weight gain (Statistics refer to percentage of individuals affected):*[11]

Anafranil Capsules (2-18%)
Clozaril Tablets (4%)
Hismanal Tablets (3%)
Hylorel Tablets (44.3%)
Proleukin for Injection (23%)
Supprelin Injection (3-10%)
Synarel Nasal Solution for Endometriosis (8% of patients)
Tolectin (200, 400, and 600 milligrams) (3-9%)
Wellbutrin Tablets (9.4-13.6%)

Treating Obesity

Dr. Birdsall believes that proper diet and exercise are the most effective ways to lose weight. However, he feels that it is not a matter of how much a person eats, but what the person eats that is important, and that one's diet must be high in complex carbohydrates. Other approaches to treating obesity include detoxification, stimulating thermogenesis, and correcting any underlying condition affecting one's weight such as insulin imbalance or hypothyroidism. Herbs and nutritional supplements may also prove beneficial in some cases.

Diet

The typical American diet includes more refined and processed foods than the diet of any other nation. When food is refined and processed, not only is fiber removed, but simple sugars often replace complex carbohydrates. A diet low in fiber and high in simple sugar can be a major contributing factor to excess weight gain. Fiber, on the other hand, can have a major impact on weight gain as evidenced by the almost complete lack of obesity in cultures that consume a diet high in fiber.[13] Fiber has been shown to not only reduce serum cholesterol, but to also pull dietary fat from the body into the feces. Other benefits of roughage include increasing chewing time, thus slowing down the eating process and inducing satiety, preventing constipation, and stabilizing blood glucose levels.[14]

A whole foods, whole grain, high-complex carbohydrate, low-fat (less than fifty milligrams daily), high-fiber diet is recommended by Dr. Birdsall. He suggests a maximum of 25 percent of the daily food intake be in the form of fat. In general, this amounts to forty-five to fifty grams per day, which represents about 450 calories. He believes lowering dietary fat and exercise are the two key factors to weight loss.

Dr. Haas points out that certain people will do better on different types of diets, with the one consistent factor being that the diets be low in fat. "For instance, some people will do better on a low-carbohydrate diet, instead of one that is high in carbohydrates," he says. "As long as the fat content of the diet remains low, the overweight person can have success." This was verified by a Cornell University study which showed that when women were allowed to eat as much as they wanted, with the only restriction being that they had to consume low-fat foods (only 20 to 25 percent of calories as fat), they lost weight.[15] This is due to the fact that fat contains more than twice as many calories per gram as protein or carbohydrates. A Swiss study also revealed that, unlike carbohydrates, approximately 90 percent of extra fat consumed during a meal is converted to body fat.[16] Very fatty foods may also encourage overeating because more needs to be consumed in order to maintain the body's natural storage of glucose.[17] Weight loss should therefore be directed toward a change in eating habits rather than dieting.

Alcohol should also be avoided or minimized, since it has been found to act like a fat in the body and promote weight gain. J. P. Flatt, Ph.D., from the University of Massachusetts Medical School, estimates that one ounce of alcohol represents one-half ounce of fat in the diet.[18] Cigarettes, which are used by many people to manage their weight, also appear to steer extra fat to the abdomen. In addition, both of these substances should be especially avoided by those who are prone to glucose intolerance.

Nutritional Supplements

Chromium plays an important role in sugar and fat metabolism. Over the years, research has demonstrated that chromium deficiency impairs glucose tolerance, increases circulating insulin levels, boosts blood sugar levels, allows sugar to spill into the urine, and elevates serum triglycerides and cholesterol.[19]

Zinc is needed for normal taste acuity and enhances the effectiveness of insulin. If a person overeats in part because food has no flavor, then zinc may be the answer.[20] A zinc taste test, performed by your physician, will determine if you have a zinc deficiency.

See Allergies, Diet, Nutritional Supplements.

According to James Braly, M.D., Medical Director of Immuno Labs, Inc., in Fort Lauderdale, Florida, other essential nutrients for weight loss and weight management include vitamin A, beta-carotene, vitamin B_3, vitamin B_6, biotin, vitamin C, and vitamin E.

Dr. Braly also recommends daily supplementation of essential fatty acids with evening primrose oil and MaxEPA (a fish oil), as well as two multiple amino acid capsules taken one half hour before each meal.

Detoxification

Obesity is almost always associated with toxicity, as many toxins are stored in fatty tissue, according to Dr. Haas. "When we lose weight we reduce our fat and thereby our toxic load. However, during weight loss we release more toxins and thus need protection through greater intake of water, fiber, and the antioxidant nutrients such as vitamins C and E, beta-carotene, selenium, and zinc." He adds that L-cysteine can also be used, as it helps liver and intestinal detoxification processes.

Michelle Pouliot, N.D., from Torrington, Connecticut, recalls a woman in her mid-forties who sought help for a weight problem. The woman had many surgeries and an extensive history of prescription drug use. Dr. Pouliot helped to stabilize the woman's health then put her on a detoxification program using a whole foods diet,

Specific Diets for Weight Loss and Weight Management

According to Elson Haas, M.D., Director of the Preventive Medicine Center of Marin in San Rafael, California, and author of Staying Healthy with Nutrition *(Celestial Arts), the following diets may prove effective for both weight loss and weight management as part of a general health maintenance program.*

***The Fish-Fowl-Green Vegetable Diet** includes fresh ocean fish, tuna, shrimp, and trout, plus organic poultry, and green vegetables, both raw and cooked. These can be eaten in any quantity desired, within reason. One piece of fresh fruit and one cooked egg are also suggested daily. Some bran and/or psyllium can be used to support bowel function. Salad dressing should be limited to one or two tablespoons daily of vegetable oil, such as olive, with some fresh lemon juice or vinegar. If no oils are used, an essential fatty acid supplement should be taken.*

Daily fluid intake should be eight to ten glasses (eight ounces) of spring or distilled water and/or herbal teas. Two glasses should be drunk first thing in the morning and then again thirty to sixty minutes before each meal. Some clear soup broths are also acceptable. "A general multivitamin should also be used daily for health insurance. Several pounds a week can be lost fairly easily with this diet even with only moderate activity, but the diet should go no longer than one or two months at the most," says Dr. Haas.

***The High-Fiber Starch Diet** can be a good weight-loss plan for overweight vegetarians, especially if they avoid excessive sweets, according to Dr. Haas. "Complex carbohydrates, such as whole grains, legumes, pasta, potatoes, and starchy vegetables are eaten at the beginning of a meal in order to provide bulk, thus decreasing the appetite and giving a feeling of fullness," he explains. "These foods are relatively low-calorie foods if they do not have sauces, gravies, butter, or oil added to them." Vegetables can also be consumed as desired, at least several cups daily. Dr. Haas also suggests a couple of pieces of fruit daily. "Dairy foods, red meats, and any fried, fatty, or refined foods should be avoided, as should sweets," he says.*

Water intake should be maintained at eight to ten glasses daily. A multivitamin can also be taken, along with some extra B_{12}. Care should also be taken that iron and calcium intake are adequate. These and other minerals might be supplemented, though most should be found in sufficient amounts in this diet.

***The Allergy-Rotation Diet** is becoming more popular for weight loss as well as for general health, especially when there are food allergies present. Any foods shown to be a possible problem should be eliminated from the diet for one to two months, depending on the degree of sensitivity. "If we seem to be addicted to any foods, that is, we crave them and eat them every day, sometimes even at every meal, those foods should be completely removed from the diet for at least several weeks before testing them, although avoiding them even for only four days will allow our body to be sensitive to their true effects," says Dr. Haas.*

To desensitize to other possible food allergies, a rotating diet means setting up a four-day rotation plan. "Any food eaten on one day must be excluded from the diet for the next three days," Dr. Haas explains. "For example, if apples, corn, or peas are eaten on Monday, we would not eat them again until Friday. Eliminating allergenic foods also reduces water retention through reduced immune reactions and secondary inflammation and may allow us to feel much better while we slim down."

***The Ideal Diet** is a well-balanced diet that incorporates aspects of all the previous diets. It is a rotation diet, good for food allergies; it has a high fiber content from the whole grains and vegetables; it is low in fat; and it contains good quality protein. The diet is as follows:*

- *Early morning: one or two pieces of fruit. Breakfast: starch, such as cereal grain or potatoes*
- *Midmorning:snack of fruit most days and occasionally nuts or seeds*
- *Lunch: protein and green and other vegeta bles*
- *Midafternoon: snack, vegetable, or fruit*
- *Dinner: starch or protein with vegetable*
- *Evening snack: vegetable or fruit, if needed*

Water should be consumed as usual, eight to ten glasses per day, mainly drunk about one hour before meals, and a basic multivitamin/mineral supplement can also be used. "Additional water and fiber and more filling low-calorie foods will help in decreasing the appetite," Dr. Haas says. "They will also support good colon function, which is helpful to detoxification and reducing food cravings."

an occasional two-day vegetable juice fast, mild exercise, and meditation.

To help the woman release toxins through her skin, Dr. Pouliot instructed her to soak in an Epsom salts bath and do dry brush massages three times per week. Drinking eight glasses of water per day supplemented with cranberry juice extract helped her kidneys flush out poisons. Fiber supplements moved waste out of her colon and milk thistle helped her liver detoxify substances more effectively. Finally, deep breathing exercised her lungs. After three weeks, she had lost seventeen pounds.

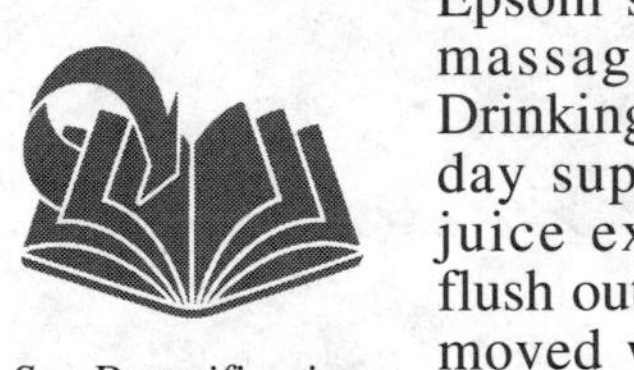

See Detoxification Therapy, Fasting.

Dr. Gard and Erma Brown have developed the BioToxic™ Reduction Program to detoxify individuals suffering from chemical toxicity. The program includes heat, physical therapy, nutritional supplements, and other treatments. Although people use the treatment program for detoxification, about 75 percent of the patients who are overweight end up losing weight. However, it is not wise to deliberately attempt to lose weight while going through a detoxification program since this makes it difficult to keep nutritional supplementation in proper balance.[21] Brown also cautions that such a program should only be undertaken with proper medical supervision.[22]

Important: *Fasting, a form of food restriction, is used by many health professionals for therapeutic reasons other than weight loss, particularly detoxification. While weight is invariably lost during any fast, the results are not usually permanent. Still, if you are considering a fast for any reason, do so only under the guidance of a trained health care provider.*

Correcting Insulin Imbalance

According to Dr. Pouliot, the insulin imbalance theory seems particularly applicable to women who have twenty pounds or less to lose. "A lot of women who are in this twenty pound range," says Dr. Pouliot, "have a history of yo-yo dieting and their bodies are very resistant to weight loss. With most women first I will try decreasing fat intake to thirty grams per day and increasing exercise. For some women that's enough to get them losing weight, and for others, not at all." For these women Dr. Pouliot uses a special plan that addresses insulin imbalance.

In one such case, a thirty-year-old fabric salesperson came to see Dr. Pouliot when she developed asthma after moving into a moldy basement apartment. Because the asthma, along with medications that were prescribed to treat it, restricted her activity, she also gained about thirty pounds. After Dr. Pouliot stabilized her health with various herbs and nutrients, and gave her ephedra and yohimbine, herbs which encourage the burning of fat (see Herbal Medicine section of this chapter). Dr. Pouliot also put her on a diet designed to rebalance her insulin and told her she could eat one meal a day containing unlimited amounts of carbohydrates, but the other two meals could not contain more than four grams of carbohydrates each. She also had her exercise every other day, when able. Not only did the woman lose the extra weight, but her asthma improved markedly.

Exercise

"Food fuels the furnace of metabolism; exercise stokes its fire," says Dr. Ali. Yet, almost as important as exercise, is what kind of exercise one does. Exercise that causes sweating and heavy breathing is sugar-burning exercise. Overweight people need fat-burning exercise, which requires slow, sustained activity. Dr. Birdsall recommends forty-five to sixty minutes of vigorous walking every day, if possible. Exercise such as walking possesses many health benefits including lowering the set point and increasing the metabolic rate.[23] The key is finding an activity one likes and then changing exercise plans periodically to alleviate boredom.

> *"Food fuels the furnace of metabolism; exercise stokes its fire."*
>
> —Majid Ali, M.D.

Herbal Medicine

For weight-loss programs, herbs are usually broken into two groups. The first group is taken to correct a condition that contributes to weight gain. For example, plantain for reducing absorption of fats and creating a feeling of fullness, fennel seed for digestion, burdock or dandelion root to enhance liver function, and kelp and bladderwrack to correct a sluggish thyroid gland. [24]

The second group of herbs is given to directly promote weight loss. *Ephedra sineca*, also known as *ma-huang,* has become a popular ingredient in natural weight-reducing formulas. Its effectiveness and ability to enhance the burning of fat, especially when taken with green tea or coffee, is due to the ephedrine in ephedra. Many people, particularly women who have a history of chronic dieting, can benefit from this herb as it helps to stabilize and enhance their metabolic rates.

Some people, however, will experience side effects like irritability, anxiety, insomnia, and hyperactivity. Used alone, ephedra can lead to rapid weight loss, but the pounds usually return once the herb is discontinued. For best results, ephedra should be part of a comprehensive program that includes permanent lifestyle changes, including diet and exercise.

Corynanthe johimbe, another herbal stimulant popular for weight loss, contains the fat-burning alkaloid, yohimbine. This herb works especially well for women with lower body fat, such as on the hips and thighs, by blocking fat-accumulating sites, called alpha-2 receptors, found predominantly on the breasts, buttocks, and thighs. These receptors become even more concentrated during pregnancy, low-calorie diets, and with normal aging. Like ephedra, yohimbine is useful for yo-yo dieters. These two herbs can also be used together.

Although both these herbs can have adverse side effects, Dr. Birdsall says they are rare and only short-term. In eight years of practice, he has only had three patients who had to discontinue ephedra. He finds both herbs to be highly effective, but cautions that they should only be used under professional supervision.

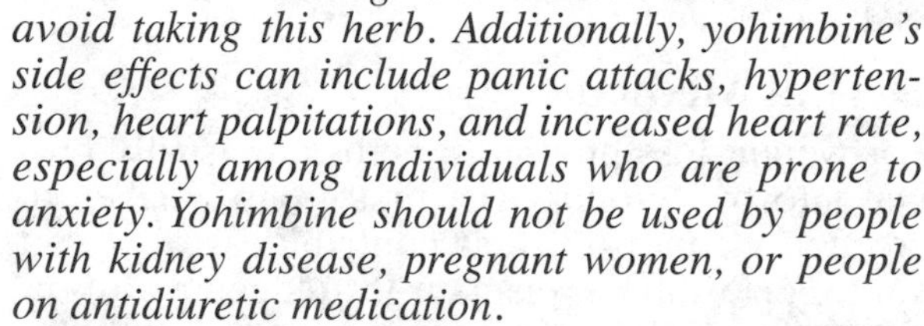

Caution: *Ephedra and yohimbine should be used only under medical supervision. Ephedra should not be used by anyone with heart disease, high blood pressure, thyroid disease, diabetes, or benign prostate hypertrophy. If using antidepressant drugs or medication for hypertension, avoid ephedra. Pregnant women should also avoid taking this herb. Additionally, yohimbine's side effects can include panic attacks, hypertension, heart palpitations, and increased heart rate, especially among individuals who are prone to anxiety. Yohimbine should not be used by people with kidney disease, pregnant women, or people on antidiuretic medication.*

Ayurvedic Medicine

According to Virender Sodhi, M.D. (Ayurveda), N.D., Director of the American School of Ayurvedic Sciences in Bellevue, Washington, the Ayurvedic approach to weight management includes both dietary considerations, such as watching the intake of sweets, dairy, and fats, and various herbal remedies. He recommends the herb *guggul* for lowering cholesterol and burning fat, *Garcinia cambozia* for suppressing appetite and aiding digestion, and the herbs boswellia, garlic, ginger, cayenne, black pepper, and fenugreek to help increase metabolism. To address carbohydrate indigestion (which can lead to the transformation of undigested carbohydrates into triglycerides), Dr. Sodhi recommends black pepper, long pepper, cayenne, ginger, and hot lemon juice before meals.

STIMULATING THERMOGENESIS

An over-the-counter preparation containing ephedrine can stimulate the brown adipose tissue (fat-burning tissue) to burn up fat, which produces heat that is dissipated by the body.[24] It also has a mild appetite suppressant action, according to Timothy Birdsall, N.D. The effects of ephedrine can be enhanced by caffeine, theophylline (a white, crystalline alkaloid derived from tea), and aspirin.[25] These preparations offer a way to burn up excess fat in patients with thermogenic deficiencies.

Caution: *These preparations should only be used under professional supervision and should not be used by persons with a history of cardiovascular disease, hypertension, or who are taking medications for these conditions. Diabetics, pregnant women, women trying to become pregnant, lactating mothers, and people sensitive to aspirin should not use these products.*

Psychological Counseling

Lauri Aesoph, N.D., from Sioux Falls, South Dakota, recalls a woman in her early forties who decided to investigate weight loss after her husband left her because he thought she was too fat. Over a series of visits, the woman was instructed in how to select foods that were healthy for her, and was encouraged to exercise regularly.

Midway through her program it was discovered that she had been sexually molested as a young woman. Eventually the woman came to understand that she may have gained weight to protect herself from sexual intimacy. To help her open the door to her feelings, she was given weekly guidance concerning the physical and emotional changes that were taking place in her life. The homeopathic remedy *Calcarea carbonica*, which fitted her constitutional symptoms, was prescribed. As the remedy began to work, her fears and apprehensions around sex and being thin surfaced, but as she continued to openly discuss her feelings and fears, her weight dropped until she reached her desired goal. At that point she felt that she no longer resisted feeling sexually attractive, and, according to Dr. Aesoph, she began to enjoy her new lifestyle and body.

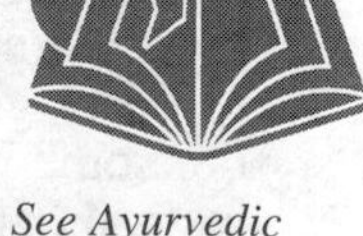

See Ayurvedic Medicine, Herbal Medicine.

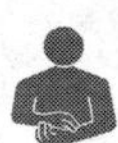

Self-Care

The following therapies can be undertaken at home under appropriate professional supervision:

Aromatherapy: Fennel, juniper, rosemary.

Juice Therapy: • Celery, watercress, parsley • Lemon, grapefruit, pineapple, grape • Carrot, celery • Carrot, spinach • Carrot, beet, cucumber • Cantaloupe/watermelon

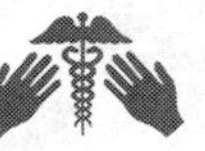

Professional Care

The following therapies should only be provided by a qualified health professional:

• Acupuncture • Cell Therapy • Environmental Medicine • Hypnotherapy • Magnetic Field Therapy • Naturopathic Medicine • Orthomolecular Medicine • Osteopathy • Oxygen Therapy

Where to Find Help

For more information on, and referrals for, treatment of obesity, contact the following organizations.

American Association of Naturopathic Physicians
2366 Eastlake Avenue, Suite 322
Seattle, Washington 98102
(206) 323-7610

Provides a directory of naturopathic physicians and offers referrals to a nationwide network of accredited or licensed practitioners. Publishes a quarterly newsletter for both professionals and the general public. Also offers a series of brochures and pamphlets on a variety of subjects.

American Society of Bariatric Physicians
5600 S. Quebec Street, Suite 160-D
Englewood, Colorado 80111
(303) 779-4833
(303) 850-0328 (Dial-a-tape)

Provides referrals for bariatric physicians (weight disorders specialists) to the general public and has a dial-a-tape phone line of prerecorded messages on nutrition, eating disorders, and weight loss.

National Association to Aid Fat Americans
P.O. Box 188620
Sacramento, California 95818
(916) 443-0303

A support, educational, and human rights group for overweight people. Newsletter available. Membership fee is nominal.

Overeaters Anonymous
World Services Office
P.O. Box 92870
Los Angeles, California 90009
(213) 936-4206

The aim of OA is to help people stop eating compulsively by offering support groups and a Twelve-Step method of healing. Call the World Services Office for the location of the nearest chapter.

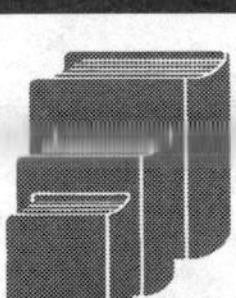

Recommended Reading

The Butterfly and Life Span Nutrition. Ali, Majid, M.D. Denville, NJ: Institute of Preventive Medicine, 1992.

Provides innovative and original solutions to the problems of nutrition, obesity, and health.

Dr. Braly's Food Allergy & Nutrition Revolution. James Braly, M.D. New Canaan, CT: Keats Publishing, Inc., 1992.

A valuable overview of food allergies and their link to health conditions, including an entire section devoted to losing weight effectively. Also includes a resource section of recipes.

Fat Is a Feminist Issue. Orbach, Susie. New York: Berkley Books, 1982.

One of the classics on self-acceptance of one's body, and how to lose weight without dieting.

Fat Is a Feminist Issue II. Orbach, Susie. New York: Berkley Books, 1987.

The anti-diet guide to permanent weight loss.

Feeding the Hungry Heart. Roth, Geneen. New York: New American Library, 1982.

This book discusses compulsive eating, why people do it, and how to overcome it.

Making Peace with Food. Kano, Susan. New York: Harper & Row, 1989.

An insightful book that discusses the myths behind being overweight. Also offers many useful exercises for redefining your own weight and how to adopt a healthier attitude and lifestyle.

No More Cravings. Hunt, Douglas, M.D. New York: Warner Books, 1987.

How to recognize and control food cravings.

What's Wrong with My Hormones? Ford, Gillian, M.D. Newcastle, CA: Desmond Ford Publications, 1992.

This book discusses each of the major hormonal problems—premenstrual syndrome, postpartum depression, premenopause and menopause, and associated hypothyroidism. It describes the consequences of taking the pill, or having a tubal sterilization, ovarian surgery, or a hysterectomy. It also shows the connection between endometriosis and hormonal dysfunction. This book also covers treatment, including information on both natural and hormonal remedies.

Staying Healthy with Nutrition. Elson Haas, M.D. Berkeley, CA: Celestial Arts, 1992.

Combining Eastern philosophies with his knowledge of Western medicine, Dr. Haas seeks to rejuvenate and cure using a mind/body approach to overall health. A comprehensive guide to diet and nutrition.

"Don't ask the doctor, ask the patient."

—Yiddish Proverb

Osteoporosis

Osteoporosis is a disabling disease affecting an estimated 20 million Americans.[1] Currently, one-third of postmenopausal women in the United States have osteoporosis, and the U.S. has the highest rate of osteoporotic fractures in the world.[2] However, the condition can be halted, and even reversed, using alternative treatments such as nutritional supplementation, diet, herbs, and natural hormonal therapy with progesterone cream.

Each year, in the United States, 1.3 million people over forty-five years of age experience bone fractures associated with osteoporosis (excessive bone mass reduction), mainly in the vertebral spinal column, wrist, and hip.[3] While these fractures can be painful, and vertebral fractures can lead to skeletal deformity, hip fractures are even more serious. Twelve to 20 percent of older people with hip fractures die within a year of the fracture.[4] The resulting immobility of hip fractures becomes debilitating in and of itself and causes a downward spiral with rapid loss of muscle, bone, endurance, strength, and appetite.

According to John R. Lee, M.D., of Sebastapol, California, "Osteoporosis affects women more than it does men because women have less bone mass than men and begin to lose bone far earlier. Up to age thirty-five, men and women have equal bone stability. For women, the most rapid rate of bone loss occurs in the first five years after menopause, beginning around age forty-five, when body hormone supplies undergo a dramatic change. Virtually all women lose 5 to 10 percent of bone mass during this period. The rate of bone loss then drops to about 1 percent per year. Men don't experience bone loss until after age seventy, but once they do contract osteoporosis, the condition can be severe."

Causes of Osteoporosis

Osteoporosis can be caused by decreased levels of estrogen and progesterone, hormones that play important roles in bone building. The disease can also result from a poor diet and insufficient exercise.[5]

Dietary Factors

The American diet of processed foods, carbonated soft drinks, caffeine, and high protein, sugar, and salt consumption can promote osteoporosis. According to Dr. Lee, "Processed foods lead directly to calcium loss because these foods are nutrient deficient. This in turn stimulates a need for protein, which, eaten in high amounts, can cause the body to lose calcium."

This relationship between protein intake and calcium loss has been known to researchers since 1920, but protein continues to be considered synonymous with being well fed.[6] The body cannot store protein, and the excess is metabolized and excreted in urine. Excess protein creates an excess of the waste products that result from the breakdown of protein, including ammonia and acids. Ammonia prevents calcium from being reabsorbed by the kidneys. The acids, which need to be buffered by calcium, also deplete bones of this mineral. Vegetarians seem to have a definite advantage in calcium balance. In one study involving 1,600 women, lacto-ovo vegetarians (vegetarians who eat milk and eggs) of twenty years had only 18 percent bone loss, as compared to omnivores (people who eat all types of food), who had lost 35 percent.[7]

> *"The American diet of processed foods, carbonated soft drinks, caffeine, and high protein, sugar, and salt consumption can promote osteoporosis."*

Another source of calcium loss is a high-sodium diet. Women eating 3,900 milligrams of sodium daily excreted 30 percent more calcium than those eating 1,600 milligrams daily.[8] Sugar has been linked to loss of calcium as well and can cause metabolic problems that eventually lead to mineral imbalances.[9]

Soft drinks and caffeine also put bones at risk, according to Dr. Lee. Consuming large amounts of soft drinks high in phosphorous can lead to high levels of phosphorus in the blood. Since the body needs to maintain blood levels of phosphorus and calcium in equal amounts, high phosphorus causes calcium to be drawn from the bones to meet the demand. Caffeine not only increases calcium excretion in the urine, but also allows more calcium to be secreted into the gastrointestinal tract.[10] One study found that individuals who drink more than three cups of coffee a day increase their risk of osteoporosis by 82 percent.[11]

“One study found that individuals who drink more than three cups of coffee a day increase their risk of osteoporosis by 82 percent.”

Alan R. Gaby, M.D., of Baltimore, Maryland, proposes that calcium is receiving more attention than it deserves, and that other nutrients may be equally critical to the prevention of osteoporosis. “Vitamin K, silicon, boron, folic acid, magnesium, and manganese all play a role in bone building and need to be consumed through diet or supplements,” he says.

Hormonal Factors

“A reduced supply of hormones is the primary cause of menopause-related osteoporosis, a condition that is generally attributed to a lack of estrogen, but the major hormone deficiency of concern in osteoporosis is progesterone,” says Dr. Lee. Progesterone is the hormone that stimulates monthly ovulation, but it also stimulates bone formation by stimulating osteoblast-mediated mineralization of bone.

“Before menopause actually begins, the body starts to decrease its output of progesterone,” points out Dr. Lee. “Because of the lack of progesterone, bones slowly begin to lose their mass even prior to menopause.”

“Menopause-related osteoporosis is generally attributed to a lack of estrogen, but the major hormone deficiency of concern is progesterone.”

—John. R. Lee, M.D.

With a combination of low progesterone and poor diet, osteoporosis may already be well underway as women approach menopause. Then, when menstruation ceases, osteoporosis accelerates because estrogen levels fall, and the already diminished bone mass is even more rapidly depleted.

HOW BONES GROW AND CHANGE SHAPE

Bones grow and develop throughout childhood and adolescence, and in a person's twenties bone mass increases by 15 percent. Every bone has a combination of compact tissue and spongy tissue, with the amount and proportion in constant flux. Some bones are so dense they appear solid, while others are primarily a complex webbing of bone tissue.

Two types of bone cells reshape bones. The “osteoclast” detects older or slightly damaged bone matter and slowly dissolves it, leaving behind a space. The “osteoblast” then moves into this space and spins out new bone matter to fill the space. With osteoclast/osteoblast equilibrium, bone mass remains stable. When the equilibrium shifts, bone mass is altered.

Bone, like all living tissue, requires adequate nutrition for proper growth. Bones need sufficient levels of minerals, especially calcium, phosphorous, magnesium, manganese, zinc, copper, and silicon, plus vitamins A, C, and K. Also, vitamin D is necessary to help ensure proper intestinal absorption and utilization of calcium. Physical stresses on a bone caused by gravitational pull and the contraction of muscle also stimulate it to increase in size. An arm placed in a cast for a week or two will lose bone mass, as will the bones of astronauts in the gravity-free atmosphere of space flight.

Hormones direct bone-building action. In females, estrogen exerts some control over the osteoclast after puberty, suppressing excessive bone loss, while progesterone stimulates the osteoblast to make new bone. In males, these functions are mediated by testosterone. For both sexes, the thyroid hormone calcitonin helps maintain proper levels of serum calcium while enhancing bone formation. Assuming a woman has no abnormalities in thyroid hormones, bone growth should continue normally as long as adequate levels of estrogen, progesterone, and nutrients are maintained.

Environmental Factors

Dr. Gaby points to the polluted world as another contributor to the widespread incidence of osteoporosis. He points out that heavy metals such as lead, cadmium, tin from tin cans, and aluminum, which is pervasive in products used daily, are all culprits. "Acid rain also leaches heavy metals out of the bedrock, moving them into our rivers and lakes, and eventually into the water we drink," says Dr. Gaby. "Acid rain has also caused our drinking water to become more acidic, which in turn challenges our body's buffering capacity, drawing calcium out of bones to provide alkalinity for balance. All this can lead to osteoporosis."

Other Osteoporosis Risk Factors

Dr. Lee cites a number of other risk factors for osteoporosis, including insufficient calcium absorption, the use of broad spectrum antibiotics and glucocorticoid medications (such as prednisone), fluoride, excess thyroxin (a hormone secreted by the thyroid gland), low body fat, and cigarette smoking.

Insufficient Calcium Absorption: Calcium is ingested in the form of relatively insoluble salts, whether the source is food or dietary supplements. According to Dr. Lee, for calcium to be absorbed, it requires not only vitamin D but adequate hydrochloric acid (HCl) in the stomach. With age, the amount of HCl secreted decreases. Since 50 percent of those seventy or older produce less HCl than is needed for calcium absorption, Dr. Lee recommends taking a supplement of either HCl, or calcium citrate (which is better absorbed under these conditions than other calcium compounds) with meals.

Broad Spectrum Antibiotics: Antibiotics used to treat a variety of diseases can often deplete normal intestinal flora that supply the body with vitamin K, which is needed in the building of bone. Yogurt and other nonpasteurized cultured milk products, or supplements of *Lactobacillus acidophilus* and *Bifidobacteria bifidum* can help replace this flora.

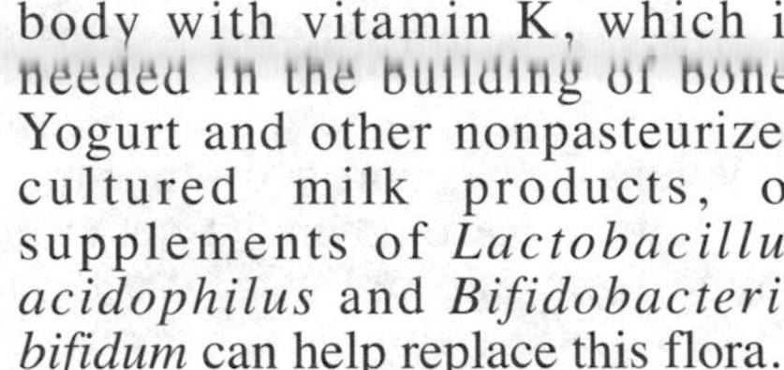

See Antibiotics (in Appendix), "Fluoridation", page 94.

Glucocorticoid Medications: Glucocorticoid medications, such as Prednisone, not only impair calcium absorption, but also inhibit osteoblast bone formation, which can lead to osteoporosis. Progesterone supplements taken with these medications can protect against this dangerous side effect, according to Dr. Lee.

Osteoporosis—A Modern Condition?

There is evidence that osteoporosis has not always been a consequence of aging and perhaps may be related to our modern diet and lifestyle. Recently, researchers were called in during a restoration program at a church in London to examine human skeletons discovered in a crypt. The bones, from the eighteenth and nineteenth centuries, were of women ages fifteen-to eighty-nine, all white (today, a high risk group for osteoporosis) and of Huguenot ancestry. Upon examination, these bones showed that in these earlier times there was no significant premenopausal loss of bone density, and that postmenopausal bone loss was less than would be expected today. This is in striking contrast to the incidence of bone loss of modern-day women.[12]

Fluoride: "Fluoride, once touted as an osteoporosis treatment, is, in fact, toxic to bone cells," says Dr. Lee. "When given in treatment doses, fluoride causes an apparent increase in bone mass, but the resulting bone is abnormal and lacks strength. Recent studies in the United States and England have shown that even smaller amounts of fluoride in common drinking water increases the risk of hip fracture.[13]

> *"Fluoride, once touted as an osteoporosis treatment, is, in fact, toxic to bone cells."*
>
> —John R. Lee, M.D.

High Levels of the Hormone Thyroxin: Thyroxin, the hormone secreted by the thyroid gland, stimulates minerals to be drawn out of the bones as part of the natural and ongoing process of bone remodeling. In hyperthyroidism, an excess of thyroxin causes excess bone depletion. Thyroid medication, which supplies thyroid hormone to the body, functions in the same way. People taking thyroid medication should have routine monitoring of their dose to check if it is in excess of what is needed.[14]

Low Body Fat: Being excessively lean, whether from weight loss or excessive exercise, such as training for marathon running, impairs hormone synthesis and eventually bone synthesis. Low body fat causes reduced progesterone, and if menstruation also ceases, both progesterone and estrogen are lowered. Under these circumstances, the consequences for bone mass are the same as

How to Test for Osteoporosis

The initial test for osteoporosis, according to Katherine O'Hanlan, M.D., of Stanford University, is measuring for a loss in height. "With osteoporosis, vertebrae shrink and this leads to height loss which can be observed," explains Dr. O'Hanlan. "This test, done carefully, should be performed routinely at regular office visits, as this is the earliest symptom of osteoporosis. A loss of one-half inch from what you've been all your life is significant." Once a loss of height is confirmed, bone density should also be measured.

"Bone density is best measured by DXA—dual x-ray absorptiometry—which has a 1 percent error rate," states Dr. O'Hanlan. "DPA—dual photon absorptiometry—is not the way to go, though it will be offered because a lot of people have the equipment, but it has an 8 percent error rate, so it may not pick up a 1 to 2 percent change in bone density." Regular x-rays can only detect osteoporosis after 25 percent of the bone mass has been lost. John R. Lee, M.D., of Sebastopol, California, also endorses DEXA (dual energy x-ray absorptiometry), which is 95 to 98 percent accurate and can detect a bone mass change of 3 to 5 percent.

In diagnosing osteoporosis, it is more effective to monitor certain bones according to Dr. Lee. He feels it is best to target a trabecular (spongy) area of bone, such as the spongy bone at the end of a long bone, a vertebra, or the heel bone, rather than a cortical bone, which is a denser bone of the limbs. The turnover rate of the spongy bone is more rapid and changes will show much earlier. He recommends using the lumbar spine since four vertebrae can be measured, reducing the chance of an erroneous reading of a single bone selected for testing. If a person elects to undergo treatment for osteoporosis, lumbar bone mineral density should be checked at six months and twelve months and the results compared.

they are from menopause. In fact, studies show that bones stressed by the weight of a large body are healthier than the bones of a small, thin person.[15] After menopause, estrogen levels are also higher in heavier women, as the hormone is synthesized in the adipose (fat) tissue.[16]

Cigarette Smoking: Studies indicate that cigarette smoking appears to promote osteoporosis by inhibiting estrogen's effect on osteoclast cells[17] and by lowering estrogen concentration in the blood stream. In addition, hampered breathing because of smoking prevents carbon dioxide from leaving the body as it normally does in an exhaled breath, and this too can affect bones. According to Dr. Lee, carbon dioxide retention leads to higher blood levels of carbonic acid which the body attempts to neutralize with calcium taken from bones.

Treatment of Osteoporosis

Alternative treatments for osteoporosis focus on supplementation with natural sources of calcium and hormones, balancing the body's own hormone production, as well as exercise and regulating diet. These approaches can be very effective without leading to side effects.

Diet and Nutritional Supplements

Nancy Appleton, Ph.D., a nutritional consultant in Santa Monica, California, believes that the standard American diet produces metabolic imbalances that reduce absorption and retention of minerals, including calcium. She adds that a diet of excess protein, dairy products, sugar, soft drinks, alcohol, caffeine, and fried foods has an acidifying effect on the body, causing calcium to be drawn from the bones to buffer this condition.

According to Dr. Lee, his recommended diet for treating osteoporosis is vegetarian-based, with whole grains, legumes, fruits, vegetables, nuts, and seeds, plus optional small amounts of animal meats and dairy. Leafy green vegetables, beans, and fish are used as primary calcium sources. If dairy products are used for calcium, yogurt is the preferred source since many older people are lactose intolerant and, in yogurt and other fermented dairy products, the lactose has been consumed by the fermenting culture and converted to lactic acid.

Calcium supplements are also recommended by some health practitioners. Michael T. Murray, N.D., of Bellevue, Washington, recommends the more soluble forms—calcium citrate, calcium lactate, and calcium aspartate. Combinations of calcium and other minerals are also prescribed. Recommended quantities of calcium range from approximately 800 milligrams per day to 1,500 milligrams per day, a significantly wide range that is still debated. Dr. Appleton also cautions about possible side effects associated with calcium supplementation. "Excess calcium can be redistributed in the body, and is often deposited in soft tissues, possibly causing arthritis, arteriosclerosis, glaucoma, kidney stones, and other problems," she says. Excess calcium can also imbalance stores of other minerals in the body."[18] Less calcium is needed if magnesium intake is adequate. Consult your health care professional in order to determine whether calcium supplementation is appropriate.

Dr. Murray also emphasizes other minerals, including the lesser known boron. "Boron can potentiate estrogen's role in building bones and it also helps in the conversion of vitamin D to its active form, which is necessary for the absorption of calcium," says Dr. Murray. He adds that though five milligrams per day is the optimum intake, the average American is only consuming one to three milligrams." Whole plant foods (whole grains, nuts, seeds, fruits, and vegetables) are good sources of boron.

See Diet, Female Health, Nutritional Supplements.

Honora Lee Wolfe, Dipl. Ac., of Boulder, Colorado, recommends supplements of natural microcrystalline hydroxyapatite (MCHC), a compound of calcium, phosphorus, magnesium, and fluoride, in amounts equal to the normal physiological proportions found in bone. MCHC has been found to not only halt bone loss but also to restore bone mass in cases of osteoporosis.[19] It can be used remedially and preventively without side effects.

Natural Hormonal Therapy

Natural progesterone, made from sterols (a group of substances related to fats) found in wild yams, is now drawing attention as a likely replacement for synthetic progesterone (progestin) which is used as a treatment for osteoporosis. "It is virtually the same molecule as the progesterone the body makes," explains Dr. Lee. By contrast, the synthetic progestin has additional chemical groups that change its shape. The danger is that cells that bind progesterone will receive this molecule, but once in place, the false proesterone cannot function properly, adds Dr. Lee. For example, with natural progesterone, sodium stays outside cells where it belongs. With progestin, sodium moves into the cells and brings water along with it. The result can be water retention and hypertension, and there are many other examples of similar dysfunction.[20]

Report any occurrence of unusual vaginal bleeding to your physician, as it may be a sign of hormonal imbalance.

The safety of natural progesterone has been confirmed by extensive testing at Vanderbilt University under Joel Hargrove, M.D., Department of Obstetrics and Gynecology.[21] Dr. Hargrove and his associates prescribe natural progesterone for premenstrual syndrome and menopausal hormone replacement therapy.

ARE CONVENTIONAL TREATMENTS EFFECTIVE?

In treating osteoporosis, conventional medical practice relies chiefly upon both hormone replacement (estrogen), and pharmaceutical drugs such as etidronate. Since estrogen has been shown in studies to slow bone resorption, it has become a standard prescription for women at menopause. But estrogen does nothing to maintain new bone formation. And with pharmaceutical drugs such as etidronate, the bone retained by treatment with this drug is increasingly made up of a larger percentage of old bone cells, which are inhibited from being absorbed into the blood. At the same time, new bone growth decreases. The resulting bone is more crystalline and brittle and may be more subject to fracture. In fact, the American College of Physicians says that the majority of women with hip fractures have a bone density that is within normal range.[22]

Further, since bone loss appears to resume at a pretreatment rate once the drug treatment is stopped,[23] therapy must be continued uninterrupted for twenty-plus years until bone loss abates around age seventy. Unfortunately, according to Dr. Lee, the longer estrogen is taken, the greater the risk of side effects and secondary diseases such as salt and water retention, increased fat synthesis, uterine fibroids, gallbladder and liver disease, heart disease, stroke, breast cancer, and endometrial (uterine) cancer. To offset the risk of endometrial cancer, a manufactured progesterone (progestin) is now added to prescriptions to help balance the estrogen. This also seems to slightly improve osteoporotic bones, but the introduction of progestin may in turn increase the chances for undesirable side effects of its own.[24]

Dr. Lee has used natural progesterone in his clinical practice since 1982 with positive results. In a clinical trial of one hundred patients, Dr. Lee reports a treatment program of diet, nutritional supplementation, and natural transdermal (absorbed through the skin) progesterone was virtually 100 percent successful in building bone mass. "The average increase in bone mass was 15 percent. The bone status of women with relatively good initial bone mass density (BMD) remained stable while the BMD of women with the lowest scores gained over 40 percent," states Dr. Lee. "Women with postmenopausal osteoporosis routinely showed true reversal of their disease,

A COMPREHENSIVE TREATMENT PLAN FOR OSTEOPOROSIS

According to John R. Lee, M.D., of Sebastopol, California, "A treatment plan for osteoporosis should recreate the conditions under which normal bone building occurs, including proper diet, nutritional supplements, hormone balance, exercise, and avoidance of known toxic factors such as fluoride and cigarette smoking."

Diet: *Emphasize leafy green vegetables and whole grains. Limit red meat to three or fewer times per week. Avoid excessive protein and all soft drinks. Also, limit alcohol consumption and restrict intake of fat, caffeine, and salt, which are implicated in excessive calcium loss.*

Nutritional supplements: *• Vitamin D: 350-400 IU daily. • Vitamin C: 2,000 milligrams daily in divided doses. • Beta-carotene: 15 milligrams daily (equiv. to 25,000 IU vitamin A). • Calcium: Goal of 800 milligrams daily by diet and/or supplement. Vitamins* B_6 *and K, magnesium, zinc, manganese, strontium, boron, silicon, and copper may be recommended. Add hydrochloric acid if needed.*

Hormonal supplements: *• Progesterone: One ounce of 3 percent cream per month; apply approximately one-quarter teaspoon at bedtime over a two-week to three-week time period each month. Alternate among different smooth skin sites. • Estrogen: If needed for hot flashes or vaginal dryness. Use 0.3-0.625 milligrams daily of conjugated estrogen for three weeks, timed to coincide with progesterone use. Do not use if contraindicated for any reason. (Check with physician.) Exercise: twenty minutes daily or half an hour three times a week.*

with significant improvement in bone mass and the virtual elimination of osteoporotic fractures."

Exercise

Regular exercise that delivers the force of impact to bones (dance versus swimming) builds bones, as does weight-bearing exercise.[25] Walkers can use weighted bracelets to add weight-bearing exercise to their aerobic activities. Thirty women increased their spinal bone mass by .5 percent in one year with fifty minutes of vigorous walking four times a week, irrespective of calcium intake, while non-exercisers lost 7 percent of spine bone mass.[26]

Herbal Medicine

Herbal therapy can be effective in treating osteoporosis, according to David L. Hoffmann, B.Sc., M.N.I.M.H., of Sebastopol, California, past President of the American Herbalist Guild. "Herbal and nutritional treatment cannot eliminate osteoporosis, but it can slow down the process," says Hoffmann. "There is a tradition in North America of using such herbs as horsetail, oat straw, and alfalfa for the long-term treatment of osteoporosis."

Some herbs are chosen for their calcium content, while other herbs are used for their ability to normalize hormones, says Hoffmann, who points out that, "These remedies can be useful if started early enough. Anti-rheumatic herbs will help with pain in the joints and muscles, and anti-inflammatory herbs will similarly reduce the discomfort associated with this problem."

See Herbal Medicine, Homeopathy, Traditional Chinese Medicine.

He recommends a tincture of two parts chasteberry, one part horsetail, one part black cohosh, one part oats, and one part alfalfa. Take one teaspoon (five millileters) of this mixture three times a day. Used as a dried herb, infuse two teaspoons to a cup of water and drink the mixture three times a day.

Homeopathy

In the homeopathic treatment of osteoporosis, Andrew H. Lockie, M.F. Hom., M.R.C.G.P., Dip. Obst., of Surrey, England, states, "Most authorities would agree that the best course of treatment is to treat the patient themselves, through homeopathic constitutional treatment, which takes into account any symptoms of imbalance that might be present as well as the osteoporosis. This would also include any remaining symptoms of menopause, for instance."

According to Dr. Lockie, the main homeopathic constitutional remedies would probably be *Calcarea carbonica* and *Calcarea phosphorica,* but *Calcarea fluorica*, *Carcinosin*, *Bufo*, *Silicea*, and a complex formula called vermiculate are also used.

Traditional Chinese Medicine

According to Traditional Chinese Medicine, the health of the bones is directly related to the health of the kidneys. Treatments for osteoporosis therefore focus on increasing the energy of the kidneys. As Wolfe states, "It is common for people in China, once they turn fifty to begin taking low-dose herbal formulas that boost kidney energy, and to continue this for years. Traditional Chinese Medicine views the aging of the kidneys as the aging of the body, and herbal therapy can slow down this process." According to Wolfe, two Chinese herbal formulas "Two Immortals Decoction, *er xian tang*" and "Eight Flavor Rehmannia, *shai di huang*" can be effective. However, she cautions specific recommendations for what a woman needs should be prescribed by a professional.

Maoshing Ni, D.O.M., Ph.D., L.Ac., Vice-President of Yo San University of Traditional Chinese Medicine in Santa Monica, California, provides the following anecdote. "A patient came to see me who was menopausal and complaining of back pain. According to x-rays, she had lost 30 percent of her bone density. The woman was Persian and because of certain beliefs did not want to take hormones which in Western medicine is the ideal therapy. We began to treat this using acupuncture and herbs, in particular eucommia, dipsaci, and *dong quai*. The acupuncture sessions were given twice a week for the first month and then tapered down after that. Happily, after six weeks of treatment, she was no longer experiencing the pains associated with the osteoporosis, and after x-rays, according to the radiologist, there was a 50 percent increase in bone density. Blood tests showed that there was also no question that her estrogen and progesterone levels had come back too, which goes hand in hand with the bone increase. There was not a complete reversal of the condition, but Traditional Chinese Medicine can indeed contribute to a healing."

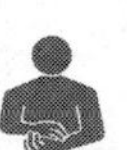

Self-Care

The following therapies can be undertaken at home under professional guidance:

• Fasting • Reflexology

Juice Therapy: • Green juice • Beet, carrot, and celery • Lemon, papaya, pineapple

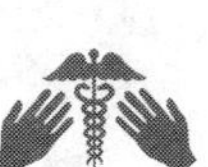

Professional Care

The following therapies can be provided by a qualified health professional:

• Acupuncture • Chelation Therapy • Chiropractic • Magnetic Field Therapy • Osteopathy

Ayurvedic Medicine: A traditional Ayurvedic formula for osteoporosis consists of one part sesame seeds (black seeds if possible), one-half part *shatavari* (the main Ayurvedic rejuvenative herb for the female), and one-half part ginger with raw sugar added to taste. Eat one ounce daily. The Ayurvedic herb *amla* is also recommended for osteoporosis.

Environmental Medicine: Excessive exposure to lead can cause a negative calcium balance, and cadmium can lead to a decrease in the mineral content of bone and contribute to osteoporosis.

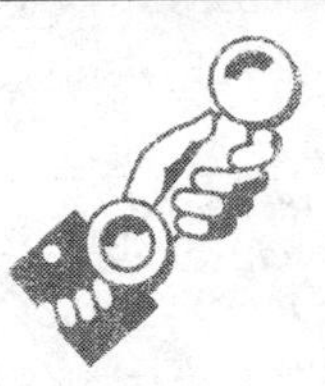

Where to Find Help

For more information on, or referrals for, the treatment of osteoporosis, contact the following organizations.

American Association of Acupuncture and Oriental Medicine
4101 Lake Boone Trail, Suite 201
Raleigh, North Carolina 27607
(919) 787-5181

The AAAOM is a national professional trade organization of acupuncturists who meet acceptable standards of competency and can provide you with the names and locations of local members.

American Association of Naturopathic Physicians
2366 Eastlake Avenue, Suite 322
Seattle, Washington 98102
(206) 323-7610

Provides a directory of naturopathic physicians and offers referrals to a nationwide network of accredited or licensed practitioners. Publishes a quarterly newsletter for both professionals and the general public. Also offers a series of brochures and pamphlets on a variety of subjects.

American Holistic Medical Association
4101 Lake Boone Trail, Suite 201
Raleigh, North Carolina 27607
(919) 787-5181

A professional organization for holistic practitioners, the AHMA offers information and services for its members and lobbies for holistic issues. It also provides referrals for the public.

Foundation for the Advancement of Innovative Medicine
2 Executive Boulevard, Suite 204
Suffern, New York. 10901
(914) 368-9797
A nonprofit organization that was founded to secure free choice in health-care by using alternative therapies.

Maharishi Ayur-Veda Medical Center
P.O. Box 282
Fairfield, Iowa 52556
(515) 472-5866
The medical center provides referrals to health centers which offer methods of prevention and treatment for a broad range of illnesses. They also train practitioners and provide information to the lay public.

National Center for Homeopathy
1500 Massachusetts Avenue NW, Suite 42
Washington, D.C. 20005
(703) 548-7790
Provides referrals to homeopathic practitioner who have undergone training through the National Center. Also offered are classes for professionals and lay homeopaths.

Professional and Technical Services, Inc.
3331 N.E. Sandy Boulevard
Portland, Oregon 97232
(800) 648-8211
This organization provides information concerning natural progesterone cream.

WISE Essentials
716 Mount Curve Boulevard
St. Paul Minnesota 53116
(800) 705-9473
(612) 690-9626
A source for natural progesterone.

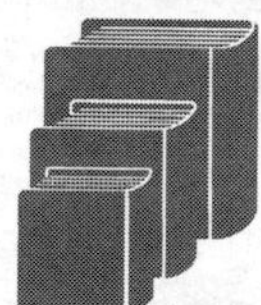

Recommended Reading

Healthy Bones. Appleton, Nancy, Ph.D. Garden City Park, NY: Avery Publishing Group Inc., 1991.
This book proposes that an imbalance in body chemistry is the fundamental cause of osteoporosis, rather than simply low calcium intake. A food plan is given, designed to keep bones strong.

Hormone Replacement Therapy, Yes or No: How to Make an Informed Decision. Kamen, Betty, Ph.D. Novato, CA: Nutrition Encounter, 1993
In the next twenty years approximately forty million women will enter menopause in the United States. Dr. Kamen presents the safe, non-toxic and medically valid alternatives to conventional hormone replacement treatment. This book shows how PMS, menopausal symptoms and osteoporosis can be avoided and reversed, along with the negative consequences caused by misdirected treatment.

Menopausal Years. Weed, Susan S. NY: Ash Tree Publishing, 1992.
The author addresses the goddess in each woman and offers this guide to health through the years of change. This book focuses on many aspects of women's health including osteoporosis, and reviews a wide range of remedies from massage and energy work to herbs, supplements, diet, and medications.

Menopause: A Second Spring. Wolfe, Lee Honora. Boulder, CO: Blue Poppy Press, 1992.
Using the perspective of Traditional Chinese Medicine, the author outlines various types of menopause and related symptoms. Recommendations are made for diet supplements, herbs, exercise, massage, and inner focus.

The Menopause Self-Help Book. Lark, Susan M., M.D. Berkeley, CA: Celestial Arts, 1990.
An easy-to-understand workbook on how to approach menopause. Dr. Lark explains what menopause is and its potential health problems. She explores the many natural treatments available and gives the pros and cons of estrogen replacement therapy. Resources are listed.

Natural Menopause: Guide to a Woman's Most Misunderstood Passage. Perry, S.; and O'Hanlan, K. A. NY: Addison-Wesley, 1992.
Natural Menopause *dispels the common myths about menopause—the horror stories about raging hormones, violent mood swings, and the loss of*

femininity—by explaining to women what to expect during a time that, if approached as a natural phase rather than a crisis, can be a positive experience.

150 Most-Asked Questions About Osteoporosis: What Women Really Want to Know. Jacobowitz, Ruth S., Emmaus, NY: Hearst Books, 1993.

This book answers the most common questions women have concerning osteoporosis.

Preventing and Reversing Osteoporosis. Gaby, Alan. Roseville, CA: Prima Publishing, 1993.

Gaby urges women to takes their fates into their own hands by treating and preventing osteoporosis through nutrition. Easy-to-read chapters explain what osteoporosis is, why it is so prevalent, what patients can do about bone loss, how diet affects this condition, plus news about vitamin K, food allergies and osteoporosis, and other nutritional issues.

Startling New Facts About Osteoporosis: Why Calcium Alone Does Not Prevent Bone Disease. Kamen, Betty, Ph. D. Novato, CA: Nutrition Encounter, 1990

An up-dated edition of the best selling Osteoporosis, this book presents the latest medical evidence about calcium and other supplements in relation to osteoporosis. Dr. Kamen tells what women can do to prevent, control, and even reverse this debilitating and lethal disease. This booklet raises a multitude of fascinating new questions about osteoporosis, and answers them with validating medical research.

What's Wrong with My Hormones? Ford, Gillian, M.D. Newcastle, CA: Desmond Ford Publications, 1992.

This book discusses each of the major hormonal problems—premenstrual syndrome, postpartum depression, premenopause and menopause, and associated hypothyroidism. It describes the consequences of taking birth control pills, or having a tubal sterilization, ovarian surgery, or a hysterectomy. It also shows the connection between endometriosis and hormonal dysfunction. This book also covers treatment, including information on both natural and hormonal remedies.

Women's Health Alert. Wolfe, Sidney, M., M.D. and the Public Citizen Health Research Group; with Rhoda Donkin Jones. Reading, MA: Addison-Wesley Publishing Company, Inc., 1991.

This book provides up-to-date information on the practice of female medicine with data and statistics that can help a woman make wise decisions about her health. Hormone replacement therapy and osteoporosis are detailed.

"Medicine absorbs the physician's whole being because it is concerned with the entire human organism."

—Johann Wolfgang von Goethe

Parasitic Infections

Recent medical research suggests that three out of five Americans will be infected by parasites at some point in their lives.[1] Living off the human body, these tiny organisms can contribute to a variety of acute and chronic illnesses, often going undetected, reproducing themselves year after year. Proper diagnosis and treatment is essential in order to maintain health and restore normal bodily functions.

Although technically any organism that lives off another host organism can be defined as "parasitic," according to Murray Susser, M.D., of Santa Monica, California, the term "parasite" refers specifically to those protozoa (single-cell organisms), arthropods (insects), and worms that invade and feed off host organisms, often causing harm. "Parasites have been co-evolving with man for millions of years," says Dr. Susser, "and, like viruses and fungi, their presence in the body serves no known purpose."

> *"Parasites have been co-evolving with man for millions of years and, like viruses and fungi, their presence in the body serves no known purpose."*
> —Murray Susser, M.D.

Illness can often result when disease-promoting parasites, which frequently contaminate food and water supplies, are ingested. Parasites can also infest the skin, as with scabies and lice, or can enter the bloodstream through insect bites, as with malaria and yellow fever parasites. They can also deplete the body of essential nutrients, taxing and overwhelming the immune system, which can lead to serious illness and even death.[2]

Medical researchers are beginning to recognize that parasitic infections contribute to a variety of major diseases, including Crohn's disease, ulcerative colitis, arthritis and rheumatoid symptoms, chronic fatigue syndrome (CFS), Epstein-Barr virus, and AIDS. In particular, a number of digestive complaints, such as diarrhea and irritable bowel syndrome, are now being linked to past or present parasitic infections.

What Are Parasites?

In the United States, the most common human parasites, apart from head lice, are of the microscopic protozoal variety, which can be transmitted by air, food, water, insects, animals, or other people. These tiny parasites include *Giardia lamblia,* a virulent form found in the contaminated waters of lakes, streams, and oceans, and a common cause of traveler's diarrhea; *Entamoeba histolytica,* which can cause dysentery and injure the liver and lungs; *Blastocystic hominis,* which is increasingly linked to acute and chronic illness;[3] and *Dientamoeba fragilis,* which is associated with diarrhea, abdominal pains, anal pruritus (intense itching sensation of the anus), and loose stools.[4] Another parasite, Cryptosporidium, poses a significant threat to those with immunologic diseases such as AIDS.[5]

Besides lice, the most common of arthropod parasites are mites, ticks, and fleas. These parasites, in turn, can carry other, smaller infectious organisms, such as *Borrelia burgdorferi,* a coiled spirochete-shaped parasite that causes Lyme disease, and *Yersinia pestis,* which causes the dreaded bubonic plague.[6]

The other type of parasites, commonly known as "worms," include pinworms, roundworms, tapeworms, *Trichinia spiralis* (worms usually acquired from eating tainted pork that inhabit the intestines and muscle tissue), hookworms, Guinea worms, and filaria (threadlike worms that inhabit the blood and tissues). Such worms can be contracted by those traveling in remote and underdeveloped regions of the world, as well as from contaminated water or from pets. Roundworms, for example, infect about 25 percent of the world's population and cause up to 1 million cases of disease annually.[7] Roundworms are particularly difficult to get rid of due to their high reinfection rate and the ability of their infective eggs to resist chemical treatment.[8] They are particularly prevalent in the Appalachian Mountains and adjacent regions to the east, south, and west,[9] and are the second most common intestinal worm in the United States. Pinworms, the most common type of intestinal worm, are especially found among children. Other common worms are the roundworm and the whipworm.

Leo Galland, M.D., of New York City, a specialist in parasitology, estimates that 10 percent of the American population may be infected by parasites. But even this estimate, he warns, may be too conservative. "For instance, in a recent study done at Johns Hopkins Hospital, 18 percent of a random selection of blood samples showed a past or present infection of the parasite Giardia lamblia," Dr. Galland points out. "And studies done in Arizona have shown a possible 50 percent rate of parasitic infection on Native American reservations."

Sources of Parasitic Infections

The most common mode of transmitting parasitic infections is through direct fecal-oral contamination.[10] For example, the global incidence of the disease giardiasis, caused by the Giardia lamblia protozoa, is estimated at 30 percent. Giardia lamblia is a highly contagious parasite and can be carried by virtually any species—wild animals, cats and dogs, as well as people. Giardiasis is particularly serious among those who live in institutions and overcrowded communities and can be spread by drinking or swimming in feces-contaminated water, and from person to person, or animal to person contact.

"Infection with protozoa parasites often follows drinking impure water," says Rita Bettenburg, N.D., of Portland, Oregon. "I have seen this in whole families who have been camping or waterskiing, or who have drunk from stream or river water. The signs in this case are usually diarrhea, cramps, and gastroenteritis." She adds that much of the ground water in North America has been infested with Giardia. A recent study also found 86 percent of the surveyed surface water source locations in Kansas to be contaminated with either Giardia, Cryptosporidium, or both.[11]

Day-care centers are now also recognized worldwide as breeding grounds for giardiasis, and other parasitic diseases. Dennis Juranek, of the Centers for Disease Control, Division of Parasitic Infection, in Atlanta, Georgia, reports that the current infection rates due to Giardia in day-care centers range from 21 percent to 44 percent in the United States.[12] A study of 900 children and 140 workers at Toronto, Canada, day-care centers showed an overall intestinal parasite infection rate of 19 percent for the children and 14 percent for the staff. Of those infections, the parasite Dientamoeba was in the largest number of people, with Giardia coming in a close second.[13]

Pediatric and dental clinics are another source for the spread of parasites, according to a 1983 University of California at Los Angeles study which found 38 percent of the attending children infected.[14] Again, the highest infection rate was found for Dientamoeba, followed closely by Giardia.

"Pinworms are also quite common in the United States," says Dr. Bettenburg. "They are often caught by children and then spread through the family." Some people may show symptoms of digestive upsets, but the usual sign is itching in the anal area, according to Dr. Bettenburg. The elderly are also particularly vulnerable to parasitic infection, and parasites can often be an unrecognized cause of much of the malnutrition, fatigue, and diarrhea found in the aged today.[15]

"The influx into this country of food grown around the world, as well as the popularity of ethnic foods such as sushi and sashimi, which are uncooked or undercooked, also contributes to the spread of parasites."

Dr. Bettenburg notes that people who travel may pick up worms in another country, as well, and it may be years before they are detected. "I have seen patients who have travelled in Africa and Asia, and it is sometimes five years before the parasites that they picked up are identified," she says. In some people the symptoms may be severe environmental sensitivity that develops for no known reason.

The influx into this country of food grown around the world, as well as the popularity of ethnic foods such as sushi and sashimi, which are uncooked or undercooked, also contributes to the spread of parasites.[16] Sometimes, simply poor digestion is a contributing cause of parasitic infection. "Someone who has a low acid level in his stomach won't digest food properly, so whatever parasites come through in the food won't get sterilized out," says Maoshing Ni, D.O.M., Ph.D., L.Ac., Vice-President of Yo San University in Santa Monica, California. "That's what the hydrochloric acid does, it sterilizes the food and kills off all the germs. When it's not effective at doing that, they get passed along into the intestines. That's why kids get a lot of parasites, because their digestive system is not yet as sophisticated as adults'."

Parasitic Infection and Disease

Large numbers of people throughout the world have parasitic infections compromising their health and contributing to illness, according to Dr. Galland, yet most who are infected don't even know it. Many parasites go undetected for years because they don't produce any serious symptoms, or only produce symptoms at one stage in their lives, which can easily be attributed to another cause.

"Many parasites go undetected for years because they don't produce any serious symptoms, or only produce symptoms at one stage of their life, which can easily be attributed to another cause."

Parasite longevity is another factor in their contribution to chronic diseases. In one recent study of chronic giardiasis, the mean duration was found to be 3.3 years,[17] with infection from *Strongyloides stercoralis*, an intestinal worm, often persisting for twenty to thirty years.[18]

Martin Lee, Ph.D., biochemist, microbiologist, and Director of Great Smokies Laboratory in North Carolina, conducted a study on the presence of parasites in chronically and acutely ill people. "In one group of lower-income immigrants who were acutely ill, 70 percent had parasites, with 20 percent of these parasites proving to be pathogenic (disease-producing)," Dr. Lee recounts. "In a second group, comprised of a broader and more affluent socioeconomic cross section of chronically ill people, 20 percent tested positive for the presence of parasites." Dr. Lee's results have subsequently been verified by the Centers for Disease Control.

Dr. Galland feels that major health problems can be caused by even mild parasitic infection. In his research, he reports that nearly half of the people diagnosed as suffering from irritable bowel syndrome had intestinal parasites, and that the majority were cured of their symptoms when treated for parasitic infection. Eighty-two percent of those who also suffered from chronic fatigue syndrome were relieved of these symptoms as well.

Dr. Galland's findings indicate that any person with chronic gastrointestinal complaints, such as bloating, diarrhea, abdominal pain, flatulence, chronic constipation, multiple allergies (especially to food), and patients with unexplained fatigue, should be screened for intestinal parasites.

Candidiasis, a condition that causes the overgrowth of yeasts such as *Candida albicans* in the intestinal tract, is reaching epidemic proportions in the United States and is often found as a complication of giardiasis. Candidiasis is an opportunistic infection (develops when the body is compromised by other infections) and has serious consequences since it increases gut permeability to undigested foods and bowel toxins, which then enter the bloodstream and induce an immune response, as well as promote intolerance or sensitivities to common foods.

See AIDS, Allergies, Candidiasis, Chronic Fatigue Syndrome, Constipation, Gastrointestinal Disorders.

Intestinal parasitic infections are also being linked to chronic fatigue syndrome. In one study, over one-third of the CFS patients tested were found to be infected with *Giardia lamblia*. Their complaints included depression, muscular pain and weakness, headache, and flulike symptoms present for an average of two to three years.[19]

Research has shown a connection between HIV (human immunodeficiency virus) and parasites. According to Leon Chaitow, N.D., D.O., of London, England, parasites are a common problem seen in people with AIDS. He finds AIDS patients often have treatment-resistant candidiasis due to "immunosuppressive factors" caused by many parasites. A recent study at the University of Virginia reports that a pathogenic species of amoeba (Entamoeba histolytica) produces a substance which attacks the immune defense cells that can inactivate the HIV virus. Because of this ability to actually disarm the body's own defense mechanism, amoeba parasites may play a role in the onset of AIDS.[20]

Symptoms of Parasitic Infections

Parasitic infection is usually evident within three to five days of exposure, sometimes beginning with explosive and watery diarrhea. Giardiasis has been found to be the number one cause of diarrhea in children and causes a variety of physical, behavioral, mental, and emotional problems.[21] Other symptoms may include intermittent diarrhea and constipation, indigestion, rashes, hives, gas, fatigue, and allergic reactions to food. If left untreated, rheumatoid and arthritic symptoms may emerge. Mucous in the stool, anorexia,

DIAGNOSIS OF PARASITIC INFECTIONS

One of the main problems related to the study of parasitic infections and their link to systemic illness, according to the Journal of Advancement in Medicine, *is due to the fact that "most parasitology laboratories fail to find the majority of intestinal parasites in stool specimens submitted to them."[22] David Casemore, M.D., of the Public Health Laboratories in Great Britain adds that parasitic infection "is almost certainly underdetected, possibly by a factor of ten or more."[23]*

Unfortunately, many afflicted individuals must struggle through prolonged pain and illness as a result of undiagnosed parasitic infection. Steven Bailey, N.D., of Portland, Oregon, reports of one patient with AIDS who required examination of twelve stool samples before giardiasis was diagnosed; and, at Children's Hospital in Orange, California, eight children with symptoms of chronic diarrhea, abdominal pain, cramping, and recurrent vomiting went undiagnosed despite multiple stool testing for parasites. Only after a rather invasive procedure called endoscopic brush cytology was used, was giardiasis finally detected.[24]

According to Martin Lee, Ph.D., Director of Great Smokies Laboratory in North Carolina, many doctors, hospitals, and laboratories fail to diagnose parasitic infection because they rarely allow the time for careful analysis or multiple procedures using stool specimens collected over several days. "Also, most tests are performed on single 'casual' stool specimens, rather than on multiple stool samples," he notes.

Dr. Lee suggests that if you suspect you may have an intestinal parasite, or just want to be tested as a preventative measure, make sure your physician, hospital, or lab follows the guidelines set up by the Centers for Disease Control and the Manual of Clinical Microbiology.

Some physicians also supplement conventional diagnostic testing for parasites with diagnostic tools such as electroacupuncture biofeedback to discover the type and degree of dysfunction going on within a particular organ that may be infested with parasites. Such methods can also be helpful for determining the body's tolerance of medications or remedies which may be prescribed.

Immunofluorescent staining is also proving a useful tool for detecting parasites. This technique uses antibodies against parasites tagged with fluorescent dyes which make them highly visible under the microscope. Because they specifically attack parasites, the antibodies will only show up where there is a parasitic presence.

cramping, constipation, nausea, vomiting, night sweats, and fever may also occur.

Acute cases can produce compromised immunity; malabsorption and malnutrition; deficiencies of vitamins A, B_6, and B_{12}, and potassium, calcium, and magnesium; electrolyte imbalance; and severe weight loss. The toxicity produced in extreme cases of parasite infestation can also cause blackouts, muscular and skeletal pain, wide swings in blood sugar levels, and menstrual irregularities.

Different parasites often infect different regions of the body, as well. While giardiasis mainly affects the functioning of the small intestine, amoebiasis (amoeba infestation) mainly involves the colon, and extreme cases can result in liver and lung abscesses. An amoebic infection can be hard to distinguish from ulcerative colitis (ulcer of the colon lining).

Treatment of Parasitic Infections

Although antibiotics and other drugs are often used to treat parasitic infections, such approaches can pose a threat to one's overall health by upsetting the natural balance of the body's own immunity, especially for those who are already immunosuppressed or chronically ill, according to Dr. Galland. Also, due to the toxicity of most of these drugs, they cannot be taken over an extended period of time, which can be a serious impediment in the treatment of Giardia and other long-standing, resistant protozoal infections. Because of this the cure rate for these drugs is considerably decreased, with the likelihood of recurrence greatly increased.

Many alternative physicians employ a multifaceted approach to treating parasitic infections. Among the options they make use of are diet and nutrition, herbal medicine, Traditional Chinese Medicine, and Ayurvedic medicine.

Diet and Nutrition

If an intestinal parasitic infection is suspected, it is advised that one eliminate all uncooked foods from the diet and cook all meats until well done; soak both organic and inorganic vegetables in salted water (one tablespoon per five cups) for a minimum of thirty minutes before cooking; eliminate coffee, all sugars, including fruits and honey; and eliminate all milk and dairy products from the diet, with the possible exception of raw goat's milk, which contains secretory IgA and IgG antibodies. According to Steven Bailey, N.D., of Portland, Oregon, these compounds have been found to be helpful in the treatment of parasites.

Since an intestinal parasitic infection may be only one element in the much larger issue of immunosuppression, nutritional supplementation is also important for the restoration of normal bowel and immune function. Nutritional supplements should include vitamin B_{12}, vitamin A, calcium, magnesium, and a probiotic culture, which can include *Lactobacillus acidophilus*, bifidobacteria, and *Lactobacillus bulgaricus*.

Dr. Chaitow recommends that any antiparasitic protocol begin by using high dosage probiotics to help rebuild intestinal flora ravaged by the parasitic infestation, as well as by other opportunistic infections, such as candidiasis. Probiotics are also imperative for fighting off any further infestation.

See Diet, Herbal Medicine, Nutritional Supplements.

Special nutritional support, including vitamins, and minerals, amino acids, and antioxidants are also given. Sweet or fermented foods, alcohol, tofu, and mushrooms are excluded from the diet, as are any other foods which might provoke an allergic or toxic reaction. Dr. Chaitow also encourages the eating of small meals during this regimen, with starch being consumed every four to six hours, and no food being taken within three hours of bedtime.

Dr. Chaitow has found that in cases of severe parasite infestation, coupled with yeast overgrowth, this nutritional protocol, combined with various herbal remedies such as artemisia and grapefruit seed extract, has had an excellent success rate returning patients to normal diet and function.

Herbal Medicine

The following herbal remedies have been found to be safe and effective for the treatment of parasitic infections. Any of these remedies can also be used as a preventative for parasitic infection when water or food conditions are questionable. According to Dr. Galland, it is also advisable to continue any treatment regimen until at least two parasitological tests, performed one month apart on "purged stool" specimens, are negative.

Citrus Seed Extract: Citrus seed extract is highly active against viruses, protozoa, bacteria, and yeast, and has been used for quite some time in other countries for the treatment of parasitic infections. It is not absorbed into the tissue, is nontoxic and generally hypoallergenic, and can be administered for up to several months, which may be required to eliminate Giardia and the candidiasis which often accompanies it.

The extract is available from several vitamin and supplement manufacturing companies and can be purchased through pharmacies and health food stores.

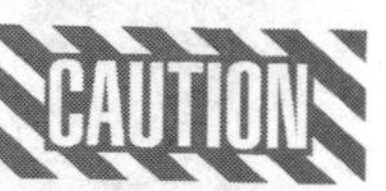

Before using any of the following herbal remedies, it is important that you first consult with a health professional who has been properly trained in their use. Both vermox and Artemisia annua should not be used during pregnancy due to the possibility that they might cause embryo toxicity. Vermox is also not recommended for children under the age of two.[25]

Artemisia Annua: This is an herbal remedy of Chinese origin. Its antiprotozoal activity is especially effective against Giardia, but some caution is advisable. It can initially cause a worsening of symptoms, allergic reactions, and some intestinal irritation. *Artemisia annua* is often prescribed by Dr. Galland, along with citrus seed extract. It may be used with additional herbs known for their antiparasitic activity with it, and it can also be used in conjunction with conventional drug therapy.

Artemisia Absinthium: According to Dr. Bailey, this is one of the oldest European medicinal plants. Known as "wormwood," it was highly prized by Hippocrates and used to expel worms similar to the *Artemisia annua* of Chinese herbal tradition. *Artemisia absinthium* taken alone can be toxic, though, and therefore should be used in combination with other herbs to nullify its toxicity.

Vermox: Although some protozoal infections can run their course and succumb to the body's defenses, with worm infestations this is rare, and intervention is almost always required. Dr. Galland has found vermox to be a very effective remedy for the elimination of worms, and has used it successfully against pinworm, whipworm, and hookworm, as well as giardia.

Traditional Chinese Medicine

With Traditional Chinese Medicine (TCM), the treatment of parasites depends upon where the infestation manifests itself, according to Dr. Ni. Incidents of parasites in the intestinal tract, the common bile duct, the blood, and the skin all require slightly different treatment protocols. Acupuncture, though not a primary treatment for ridding the body of parasites, is often used as an adjunct in acute cases where there is extreme pain, spasms, or obstructions of vital organs.

Intestinal Tract: Parasites in the intestinal tract are usually treated with purgative methods, according to Dr. Ni. Some of the safest and most common remedies used are pumpkin and quisqualis seeds. The pumpkin seeds are eaten raw, while the quisqualis seeds are usually roasted. Both are taken every morning on an empty stomach, approximately ten to twelve pieces of either, for about two weeks. "Quisqualis and pumpkin seeds are mild and safe enough for adults and children to take daily as a preventative measure as well," says Dr. Ni.

Meliae seeds are another remedy for parasites of the intestinal tract. They are much stronger than either the pumpkin or quisqualis, so should only be taken in more severe cases. The meliae seeds paralyze the parasites for approximately eight hours, allowing the body to eliminate them through the bowels. "It is very important to have proper bowel movements," Dr. Ni says, "otherwise when the parasites recover from their paralysis they'll go right back to clinging onto the intestinal wall. A couple of ways to do that would be to drink aloe vera juice, or to make a tea from rhubarb root and senna leaves to act as a laxative."

Betel nut is another common treatment for intestinal parasites. The nut is chewed raw like chewing tobacco. "It can give a certain sense of euphoria, too, because it is slightly toxic," says Dr. Ni. "This is negligible, though, meaning some people might get diarrhea."

For some patients, such as those with HIV, who have weak stomachs and weak intestines, taking these remedies orally can be difficult. "In cases like this, one would make a tea out of the these same herbs and then use them in a retention enema," says Dr. Ni. With a retention enema, the person lies on the stomach in such a way as to keep the fluid inside the rectal area for an hour to an hour and a half.

Common Bile Duct: Parasites in the common bile duct can cause tremendous amounts of pain and obstruction. Other than acupuncture for the immediate symptoms, Dr. Ni recommends using a tea made from the mume plum, which is also called the *umeboshi* plum by the Japanese, and the herbs listed above. Dr. Ni treated a case in which a man had been eating raw seafood and shellfish along the rural coast of China for years. "When the man got to me, he was having a severe attack of doubling over abdominal pain. We took an ultrasound and found all these shadows in the common bile duct area, and in the stool test, we confirmed parasites," says Dr. Ni.

"We used acupuncture to stabilize him so that he wasn't having doubling over pain and to get rid of his gallbladder spasms, which can be as painful as gallstones. Once we had stabilized the pain, we began to administer the herbs along with the laxatives. Within about three days we saw worms as long as eight or nine inches in his bowel movement. Two weeks later, after his symptoms had disappeared, we took another ultrasound, and the shadows had disappeared."

Blood: Depending on the type, parasites will be able to get through the intestinal walls and into the bloodstream. Others can enter through the air, or can get into the blood through insect bites. "In situations like this you have to use some very strong antibiotic-like herbs," says Dr. Ni. "Herbs such as goldenseal and coptidis are very strong antibiotic antiparasitic herbs."

How to Avoid Parasites

There are several precautions which will help you avoid parasites.

Food

- *Don't eat raw beef—it can be loaded with tapeworms and other parasites.*
- *Don't eat raw fish, sush—you are almost certain to get worms if you eat raw fish.*
- *Wash hands after handling raw meat or fish (including shrimp)—don't put your hands near your mouth without washing them first.*
- *Use a separate cutting board for meat and vegetables—spores from meat can seep into the board and contaminate vegetables or anything else you put on the board.*
- *Wash utensils thoroughly after cutting meat.*
- *Wash vegetables and fruit thoroughly—particularly salad items, as they often harbor parasites.Wash in one-half teaspoon Chlorox per one gallon of water. Soak for fifteen to twenty minutes. Then soak in fresh water for twenty minutes before refrigerating. Or substitute a few drops of grapefruit seed extract.*
- *Don't drink from streams and rivers.*

Pets

- *Don't sleep near your pets—they harbor many worms and other parasites.*
- *Deworm your pets regularly and keep their sleeping areas clean.*
- *Do not let pets lick your face.*
- *Do not let pets eat off your dishes.*
- *Don't walk barefoot around animals.*

General

- *Always wash your hands after using the bathroom.*
- *Wash your hands after working in the garden—the soil can be contaminated with spores and parasites.*

When traveling

- *Don't drink the water.*
- *Start taking Chinese herbs or other preventive medications two weeks before traveling, and continue them while you travel.*

Skin: Parasites can also manifest as skin lesions. "In these situations we would use the herbs externally, making a poultice or a concoction to wash," says Dr. Ni. "An herb that is quite effective for this is torryae seed. The seeds can be ground up and mixed with a little bit of aloe vera gel and then just smeared on." Fresh aloe vera is another good topical medicant for parasites.

The Immune System: According to Dr. Ni, "You can't really treat parasites without addressing the immune system at the same time. The immune system has to be strengthened in order to get at the underlying cause of much of parasitic infestations. There are various ways of doing this with nutrition and herbs such as ginseng, ligustri berries, and schisandra berries."

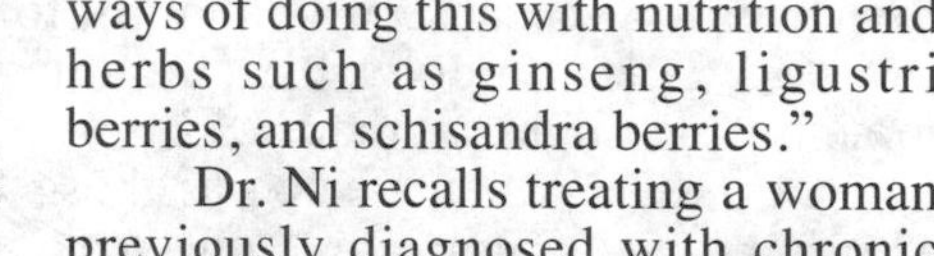

See Ayurvedic Medicine, Traditional Chinese Medicine.

Dr. Ni recalls treating a woman previously diagnosed with chronic fatigue syndrome, candidiasis, yeast problems, and severe stomach difficulties. "We did a stool test and found that she also had parasites. This woman was tremendously underweight. When she came to see me she weighed 86 pounds and was five feet, four inches tall. It took about three months for us to work on nourishing her body. Besides using herbs to kill off the parasites, I also used them to boost her immune system and to deal with the yeast problem and her digestive weakness. That's why she got the parasites in the first place. After the three months' treatment, her stool tests cleared up and remained clear, all her symptoms went away, and her weight went back up to 108 pounds."

Ayurvedic Medicine

Ayurvedic medicine has many natural remedies which address specific parasitic infections, according to Virender Sodhi, M.D. (Ayurveda), N.D., of Seattle, Washington. Although the following remedies are all safe and easy to self-administer, Dr. Sodhi still recommends that one should always consult with a doctor or qualified practitioner before beginning any treatment protocol in order to determine which of the various options will be best suited to one's individual needs and circumstances.

Pinworms: Bitter melon, a cucumber shaped vegetable found in Chinese, Japanese, and Korean markets, is especially effective against pinworms. It can be cut up and eaten in small pieces with other vegetables because of its bitter taste. Dr. Sodhi recommends eating one or two bitter melons a day for seven to ten days then repeating after one to three months to make sure the infestation has not returned. Dr. Sodhi adds that it is easy to tell if there is any recurrent infection, as thousands of little white bugs will show up in the stool the day after eating bitter melon if there is any pinworm presence. Bitter melon is very safe and has also been shown to be helpful for those suffering from AIDS and diabetes.

Roundworms: The herbs *embliaribes, vidang*, and *kamila* are most effective for roundworms, according to Dr. Sodhi. "Take one teaspoon of the herb powder extract twice a day with sweetened water or juice to attract the parasites. Do this for seven to ten days and then check your stool. If there is still evidence of infestation, repeat the cycle until you are parasite free."

Tapeworms: "*Kamila* is also effective for tapeworms," says Dr. Sodhi, "as well as betel nut, which can be chewed." The same kind of protocol as with pinworms and roundworms can be used. "Betel nut is also used quite a bit in veterinary medicine, as dog and cats get a lot of tapeworms, too," Dr. Sodhi adds.

Protozoal Parasites: For Giardia, amoebas, Cryptosporidium, and other protozoal parasites, the treatment is usually longer than for worms, taking up to several months, according to Dr. Sodhi. The herbs that are most effective for these microscopic intruders are *bilva, neem,* and berberine, which can be taken in combination. Dr. Sodhi also recommends bitter melon for protozoal infestations, as well as such nutritional supports as psyllium husk, tumeric, and acidophilus for the enhancement of the intestinal microflora.

Dr. Sodhi once had a patient come to him to be treated for a long-standing asthma condition. She had previously been treated with a variety of standard drugs which had not helped. "She was also having alternating constipation and diarrhea, and her white cell count was high," says Dr. Sodhi.

"I suggested that we do a stool test. We ran the tests on her and they came back positive for Giardia. When we started treating her for the Giardia with *bilva, neem*, and berberine, her asthma cleared up too. It's a well-known fact that whenever there are parasites, the white cell count gets higher, and you get more allergy prone, so there is some link there, although we don't know completely how it occurs."

Where to Find Help

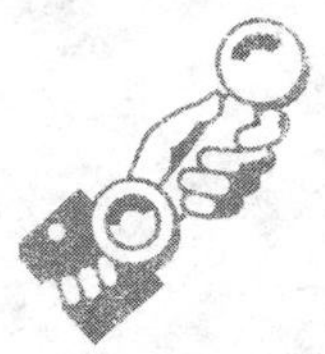

Dr. Lee recommends the use of laboratories of teaching institutions or universities where state-of-the-art equipment and procedures are available. The following laboratories may also be used or contacted for further information.

The Great Smokies Diagnostic Laboratory
18A Regent Park Boulevard
Asheville, North Carolina 28806
(800) 522-4762
Offers a comprehensive profile that includes the tests recommended in this article.

The Center for the Improvement of Human Functioning International, Inc.
3100 North Hillside Avenue
Wichita, Kansas 672191
(800) 447-7276
A complex medical, research, educational organization with four major divisions: Center for Healing Arts treats people who have not responded to standard medical care; Bio-Center Laboratory provides diagnostic services for physicians and hospitals throughout the United States; Bio-Medical Synergistics Education Institute provides learning opportunities for physicians, nurses, and health care personnel; and Bio-Communications Research Institute gathers clinical data about the effectiveness of treatment protocols and engages in clinical and basic research.

Medical Diagnostic Laboratory
3250 Westchester Avenue
Bronx, New York 10461
(212) 828-1500
Offers comprehensive parasitological testing.

Recommended Reading

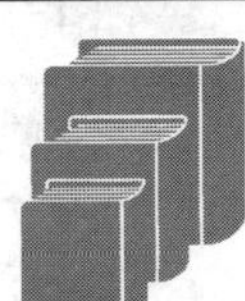

Solving the Puzzle of Chronic Fatigue Syndrome. Rosenbaum, Michael, M.D.; and Susser, Murray, M.D. Tacoma, WA: Life Sciences Press, 1992.
Although primarily about chronic fatigue syndrome, this book contains an informative chapter on parasites and includes a listing of recent published studies on the subject.

Super Immunity for Kids. Galland, Leo, M.D. New York: Dell Publishing, 1989.
Addresses the factors which can contribute to children's illnesses, including parasites. Includes precautions parents can take to protect their children, telltale signs to look for which can indicate parasite infestation, and types of treatment for dealing with them.

Pregnancy and Childbirth

The decisions a woman and her partner make during preconception, pregnancy, and childbirth will shape the life of their child. As alternative medicine increases in popularity, future parents and caregivers are looking toward natural therapies such as nutritional supplementation, homeopathy, herbology, massage, and aromatherapy in order to give birth to a healthier child.

This chapter explores the many available choices surrounding pregnancy and childbirth. A hospital birth is no longer seen as the only safe option for delivery. Many couples are opting to have their babies at home or in birth centers that offer the kind of care that is tailored to each couple's individual needs.

Currently, natural practitioners in the field of childbirth are addressing the need for dietary changes, abstinence from harmful substances, childbirth classes, and emotional support during the birth. Other options range from the modern technology of a hospital birth to water birth in the home; from obstetric care to midwifery; from medical drug intervention to labor-inducing herbs.

Preconception

"The idea of preconceptual preparation dates back to ancient times. Many cultures recognized the need to follow a balanced diet, exercise, and take proper relaxation for a period of time prior to conception, in order to cleanse and tonify the body to ensure optimum health for the child," according to Molly Linton, N.D., L.M., a naturopathic physician and licensed midwife from Seattle, Washington.

"A preconceptual checkup, including personal and family medical history, present lifestyle, and an assessment of both partner's health is an excellent beginning," says Helen Burst, R.N., M.Sc., Professor of Nurse Midwifery at Yale University. "Preconceptual care is a marvelous opportunity to screen for a wide range of factors which could be critical to not only the mother's health but the health of any child she brings into the world. This would include a complete head-to-toe physical examination and screening for breast and cervical cancer, sexually transmitted diseases, drug, alcohol, or tobacco abuse, as well as any history of sexual, physical, or verbal abuse."

> *"A preconceptual checkup, including personal and family medical history, present lifestyle, and an assessment of both partner's health is a good beginning."*

"The preparation for pregnancy begins six months to a year from the time of desired conception," according to Maoshing Ni, D.O.M., Ph.D., L.Ac., Vice-President of Yo San University of Traditional Chinese Medicine in Santa Monica, California. "This entails having the parents evaluate their diet and take herbs, so that the egg and sperm are fortified at the time of conception, and the health of their future child is maximized."

Diet and Nutritional Influences

According to the late Roger Williams, Ph.D., a pioneer of nutritional science, "Nature is so intent upon the continuance of the race that people will continue to propagate even when nutritional conditions are poor." A woman with very poor dietary habits, Dr. Williams explains, may not become impregnated at all. With a slightly improved, but still poor diet, she may conceive but then miscarry. And perhaps with yet a slightly better, albeit deficient nutritional intake, she may give birth to a baby with physical or mental anomalies.[1]

A vivid example of the effect of poor nutrition on the unborn child is the increase in congenital deformities that occurs during times of famine.[2]

In addition, Weston A. Price, D.D.S., discovered while studying people from traditional cultures, that it only takes one generation of eating a typically Western diet—one high in fats, salt, sugar, and low in complex carbohydrates—to compromise an offspring's health.[3]

A well-balanced diet is vital to ensure a healthy baby. Inadequate nutrition may also disrupt a woman's and man's reproductive system. Specific nutrients influence the production and maintenance of the egg and sperm, and thus affect the conception and subsequent health of the fetus," according to Dr. Linton. For example, studies on women suggest that folic acid and fatty acids play a role in fertility.[4] More specifically, health officials at the Centers for Disease Control now recommend that all women of child bearing age take 0.4 milligrams of folic acid to protect their future newborns from developing a neural tube defect, an anomaly of the spinal cord.[5]

Avoiding Drugs and Alcohol

The number one requirement for the good health of babies is the avoidance of harmful substances, such as caffeine, nicotine, recreational and some prescription drugs, and alcohol, according to Dr. Linton.

Caffeine: Studies on the effect of caffeine on the human reproductive cycle are mixed, however, one investigation indicated that women who consume a lot of caffeinated drinks are less fertile than those who drink caffeine occasionally or not at all.[6]

Nicotine: Approximately one-third of men and women in their reproductive years smoke cigarettes. Aside from the many diseases that smoking causes, male and female fertility are also negatively affected. Women who smoke may experience more ectopic pregnancies (ones in which the fertilized egg attaches to, and grows in, the fallopian tube). These women may also reach menopause earlier than their nonsmoking counterparts. They also risk compromising the health of their eggs, fallopian tubes, and cervix.[7]

Male smokers risk damage to their sperm from the carcinogenic substances found in cigarette smoke. Researchers claim that if a mutated sperm successfully fertilizes an egg, it may have adverse effects on the fetus.[8]

Recreational Drugs: The avoidance of recreational drugs is vital during preconception. Marijuana, for instance, once viewed as a fairly innocuous substance, carries a dual danger. The deep, extended inhalation, that is a typical practice among marijuana smokers, allows more tar and carbon monoxide to enter the lungs than regular cigarette smoking. Genetic material can be damaged by marijuana,[9] and in animals it has been linked to an increase in fetal deaths and malformations.[10]

Cocaine may be responsible for decreasing the concentration of sperm in semen. It is also thought to create deformities in the sperm's shape and to reduce the speed at which it swims after ejaculation.[11]

Tests have shown that men who use drugs increase their chances of producing abnormally developed offspring and the preconceptual use of cocaine has been linked to cases of neurological damage in children.[12]

Prescription Drugs: In the case of the effect of prescription drugs on fertility and conception, contact your physician for advice.

Alcohol: Alcohol consumption presents several threats to the health of potential parents and their future offspring. Alcohol depresses immune function and has a tremendous impact on the egg and sperm. Researchers studying the effects of alcohol consumption on rodents state that there may be a direct connection between moderate consumption by the parents and genetic damage to their offspring.[13] Miscarriage and mental and physical handicaps were also noted as possible results of alcohol consumption.

Adverse Environmental Effects

"Besides the poisons taken voluntarily, there is a myriad of unavoidable environmental hazards that can be detrimental to the health of future parents and, as a result, their offspring: toxins in the workplace, vehicle emissions, water and air pollution, to name but a few," says Dr. Linton. "It is important to be aware of these environmental hazards and to minimize exposure to them whenever possible."

See Environmental Medicine.

In an experimental investigation of two lamp factories, conducted in Italy, researchers tested the reproductive health of the women working in each factory—one group was exposed to mercury vapors on a daily basis, while the other was not. The mercury group experienced more menstrual difficulties, increased infertility, and a rise in vaginal bleeding during pregnancy. They also showed more miscarriages, preterm deliveries, and fetal malformations when compared to the nonexposed group.[14]

Emotional Factors

People are continually reminded that stress is detrimental to their health. Emotional and mental stressors have been linked to a host of illnesses ranging from fainting, nausea and weakness, heart disease, and dental cavities to the common cold.[15] "Stress can tear your health down faster than can inadequate nutrition," according to Dr. Linton. Therefore, during preconception, it is important that both partners try to maintain a positive state of mind. In terms of reproductive health, science provides an abundance of evidence showing that stress harms both men and women. Negative emotions can decrease sperm count and movement, as well as increase a woman's prolactin, the hormone responsible for milk production and breast growth during pregnancy.[16]

Most importantly for the future child, a couple must want to become parents—a twenty-two-year Czechoslovakian study found that children born to mothers who were denied abortions grew up with more emotional and psychological scars.[17]

Pregnancy

Fertilization usually takes place in the fallopian tube. Only one of the millions of sperm will pass through the membrane of the ovum (female egg) achieving conception.

Once the sperm has fertilized the ovum, enzymes in the egg alter the inner membrane and make it impossible for more sperm to enter. Once introduced, the nuclei of the sperm and the egg, each containing twenty-three chromosomes, unite to form one fertilized egg with the forty-six chromosomes needed for human development. The whole process of intermingling takes twenty-four hours. The fertilized egg then travels to the womb where it embeds itself like a seed in the lining of the uterus and begins to grow.

Physical Changes in the Mother During Pregnancy

During the first trimester, the uterus, a small, hard, pear-shaped organ becomes a soft, spherical sac through which the baby can be easily felt. By the end of the first trimester the uterus has expanded out from the pelvic cavity and touches the abdominal wall. It continues to grow and at term the uterus is between five hundred and one thousand times its prepregnant size. The actual growth of muscle fibers, not just the stretching of the uterus, is responsible for most of the increase in size. At the end of the ninth month the uterus almost touches the mother's liver just under the lower right rib.

The prepregnant cervix is firm and muscular. During pregnancy, from as early as the first trimester, the cervix begins to soften. This softening is caused by an increase in the number of blood vessels and mucous glands in the cervical lining. The cervix also becomes spongy in texture and creates a mucous plug that seals the cervical opening soon after fertilization takes place. This plug is released some time around the start of labor.

CAUTION

Maternal exposure to alcohol and cigarettes; the recreational drugs marijuana, cocaine, heroin, and LSD; medications such as lithium (to treat depression) and tetracycline (an antibiotic); pesticides; petroleum products; heavy metals such as lead and mercury; coffee; and even over-the-counter medicines such as aspirin can harm the fetus, and should be limited if not avoided altogether.

Soon after conception the vagina experiences an increase in blood flow and as a result it takes on a violet hue. Throughout pregnancy the vaginal wall thickens, elongates, and becomes looser and more elastic in order to prepare for the enormous amount of stretching that it will go through during the delivery. The opening to the vagina and the vulva become swollen and vaginal discharge becomes thick, white, and acidic, which helps guard against infection.

Within a couple of weeks after conception, the breasts can feel full, heavy, and sore. These sensations are due to the enlargement of ducts and milk glands—known as alveoli.

During the first trimester the breasts begin to increase in size. As time progresses, the areola, the pigmented area around the nipples, become wider and darker and the nipples themselves become larger and darker.

After the first trimester some women may notice a slight discharge of colostrum, a highly nutritious, yellowish liquid that the newborn suckles on until the milk comes in, around the third day after birth.

How to Have a Healthy Pregnancy

Although each individual responds to pregnancy differently, and there is no such thing as a perfect pregnancy, there are many ways to contribute to a healthy one. "Probably most important is that the woman realizes the physiological impact carrying a child has on her health and that she listen to her body's needs," says Dr. Linton. "Adequate rest, including naps, mental breaks, and sufficient

THE DEVELOPMENT OF THE FETUS DURING PREGNANCY

The first three months mark a period of intense development for the growing fetus. These early weeks of pregnancy are a critical time, because during this period the various organ systems are being fundamentally elaborated. It is at this stage that they are most sensitive to environmental chemicals, drugs, and viruses that can cause birth defects.[18] *During the second trimester developmental changes are less rapid and the baby's growth takes over. By the third trimester the baby's growth slows and the development of the senses as well as the brain and the sex organs is completed.*

The first trimester: *The first organs form around the* ***third week****, after the formation of a primitive spinal cord. Then the nervous system and the cardiovascular system begin to develop. The first blood cells are produced. Circulation of blood begins and by day twenty-one a primitive heart is functioning. Skeletal, nervous, and digestive systems are rapidly developing. Around this time the mother misses her period.*

During the ***fourth week,*** *small swellings that will eventually develop into arms and legs appear on the upper and lower sides of the body, as well as near the top of the head where the eyes will be. The liver is formed and the intestines, stomach, gallbladder, pancreas, and lungs begin to form.*

The ***fifth week*** *shows an increase in the size of the head and brain. The embryo's nervous system is beginning to function and it will display reflex movements in response to touch.*

At ***week six*** *arms and legs begin their primitive formations. The upper lip, throat, windpipe, and voice box form. The olfactory lobe, which deals with the sense of smell, and the pituitary gland begin formation in the brain. Around day forty, jaws, teeth, and facial muscles start to develop.*

The sexual organs are determined during ***week seven*** *and cartilage and some bone starts to form.*

During ***week eight,*** *the external genitalia are formed—the female clitoris and male scrotum develop around day fifty. By the end of this week the embryo is one and a quarter inches long. All of its organ systems are roughly formed, lower limbs have grown, and the embryo looks vaguely like a human infant.*

Week nine *marks the end of the embryonic stage. In this week the fetus undergoes a growth spurt and virtually doubles its size. Fingernails, toenails, and hair follicles appear. The skin thickens and becomes less transparent and baby teeth begin to form under the gumline. In the male fetus, the penis becomes distinguishable.*

By ***week ten*** *connections between the nervous system and the brain are mature enough to transmit sensory information. Consequently, the skin all over the body is now responsive and the fetus will move in response to touch. Fetal blood is now manufactured in the spleen and bone marrow.*

During ***week eleven*** *the vocal cords are formed. "Several of the digestive organs become functional: the liver begins to secrete bile; the pancreas begins to secrete insulin; and the intestines form into folds lined with villi and intestinal glands."*[19] *As the neural system matures, breathing, sucking and swallowing motions begin.*

Week twelve *marks the end of the first trimester. The fully formed baby is about three and a half inches from the top of the head to the rump and weighs only one ounce.*

The second trimester: *During the* ***fourth month*** *the fetus experiences an enormous growth spurt. This takes place largely in the body and limbs which brings its proportions close to those of a newborn. As the fetal movements become more pronounced and varied, the mother may feel them for the first time.*

In the ***fifth month*** *a fatty tissue called brown fat forms in the areas around the neck, chest, and crotch. This fat helps the fetus to maintain its body temperature. Vernix caseosa, a fatty substance now secreted from glands in the skin, forms a thick coating over the baby's skin to protect it during the long exposure to the amniotic fluid. A fine hair appears all over the body together with the formation of eyebrows and hair on the head.*

During the ***sixth month****, due to a lack of fat under the skin, the fetus appears lean and wrinkled. Its skin is a reddish color, a sign that the capillary system is developing. By the end of the month the lungs are developed to such an extent that it is now possible, for the first time, that the baby could survive outside the womb. Hearing and visual systems are now functioning primitively. The fetus has grown from eight to twelve inches.*

The third trimester: *By the* ***seventh month*** *the baby's senses are already fully developed. It can hear, see, smell, and taste. White fat forms in the innermost layer of the skin and smooths out wrinkles. In male babies, the testes descend into the scrotum. The brain increases in size and sophistication. It is just as advanced as that of a newborn. More refined movement and learning is now possible.*

During the ***eighth month*** *the baby's growth slows down and the new appearance of fat makes the body look more full and rounded.*

As the fetus begins its ***ninth month*** *in utero, its growth slows even more, but white fat is still produced and the baby becomes plumper. Most of the fine hair that covered the body has disappeared and the vernix now only covers the back. The baby receives antibodies from the mother's blood to protect and stimulate its immature immune system.*

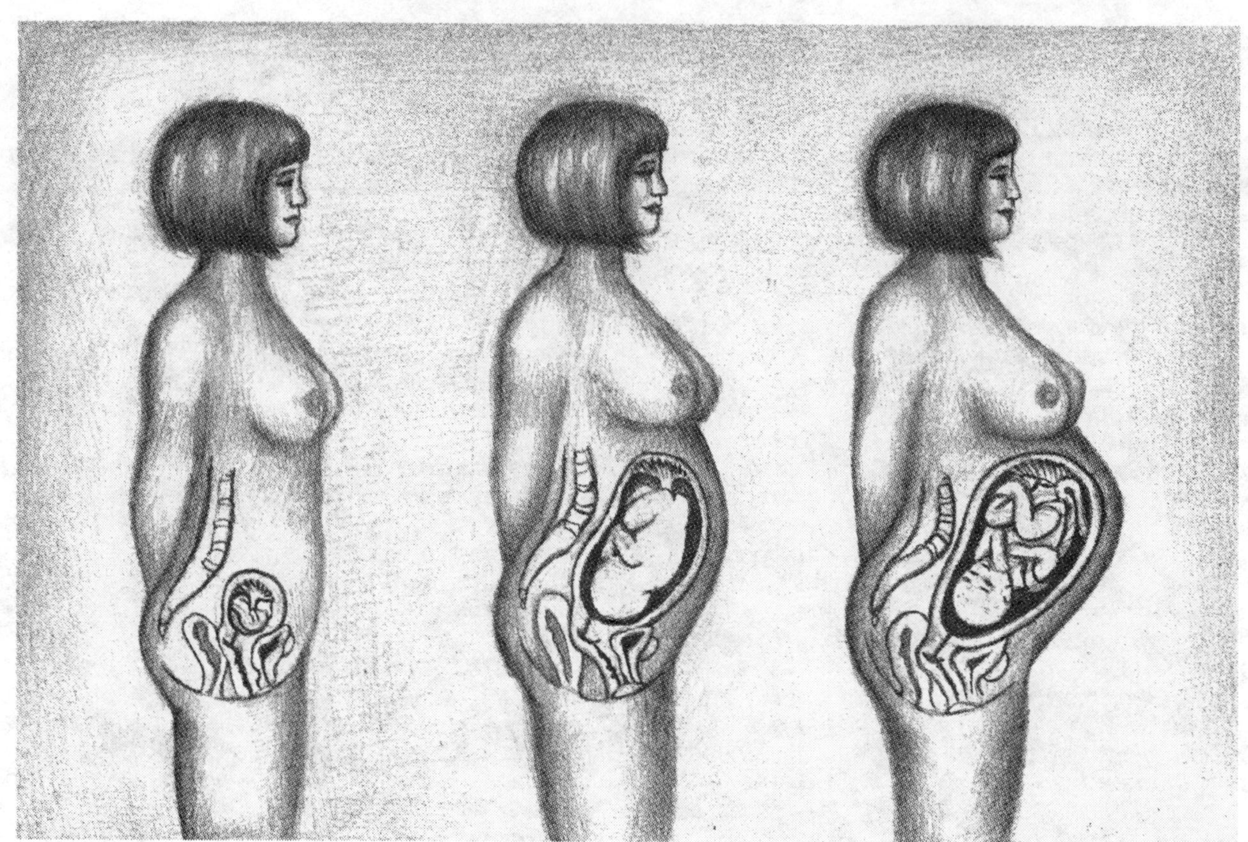

Development of the fetus in the three trimesters of pregnancy.

nighttime sleep is essential. Maintaining a positive outlook and keeping stress to a minimum are beneficial to both mother and baby. Comfortably paced, regular, non-jarring exercise, such as low-impact aerobics, walking, yoga, and swimming, can increase stamina for labor, strengthen muscles used during delivery, and may enhance the ability to cope better with labor."

Harmful Factors Affecting the Fetus: Maternal exposure to alcohol and cigarettes; the recreational drugs marijuana, cocaine, heroin, and LSD; medications such as lithium (to treat depression) and tetracycline (an antibiotic); pesticides; petroleum products; heavy metals such as lead and mercury[20]; coffee[21]; and even over-the-counter medicines such as aspirin, can harm the fetus, and should be limited if not avoided altogether.

There are two periods of pregnancy when the maternal consumption of alcohol is particularly threatening to the development of the fetus: from the twelfth to the eighteenth week and from the twenty-fourth to the thirty-sixth week. Experts at the U.S. National Institute of Alcohol Abuse and Alcoholism claim that three or four beers or glasses of wine a day can cause any one or more of the following defects: mental retardation, hyperactivity, a heart murmur, facial deformity such as a small head, or low-set ears.[22]

Cigarette smoking cuts the amount of oxygen available in the maternal blood which directly affects the growth of fetal tissue. According to recent studies, babies born to mothers who smoke thirteen or more high tar cigarettes a day are smaller and in poorer physical condition than those of nonsmoking mothers.[23]

Even over-the-counter drugs such as aspirin, when used during the first half of pregnancy, have been linked by researchers with lower than average IQ's in those babies.[24] Research into the effects of valium on chickens revealed an impairment of muscle cell development in their chicks, and suggests a possible risk in human pregnancy.[25]

Environmental factors such as pesticides, lead, and other chemicals brought home from a work environment on a parent's clothing can harm an unborn child.[26] X-ray exposure, to the mother, as well as preconception x-ray exposure to the father, is also harmful.[27]

Although most studies have not substantiated the claim that video display terminals (VDT's) adversely affect the fetus, many individuals are not convinced. In 1991, in response to this concern, San Francisco became the first American city to demand changes in this area. The city mandated that companies with fifteen or more employees protect their workers against potential adverse health effects from VDT's. They were required to provide wrist rests, antiglare shields, adjustable chairs, and regular breaks from sitting in front of a VDT screen. Louis Slesin, Publisher of *Microwave News* in New York, claims that the effect of using VDT's during pregnancy are unknown. He points out that studies concluding that VDT's are not harmful to the fetus do not assess the situation accurately. As so many people are now using video display terminals in their workplace, more reliable investigations need to be conducted.

Caution–Contraindicated Herbs, Vitamins, and Minerals: *Although many herbs are useful during pregnancy and childbirth, there are many that are discouraged. According to Tim Birdsall, N.D., birth attendant and the technical director of a national supplement company, herbs such as: autumn crocus, barberry, goldenseal, juniper, male fern, mandrake, pennyroyal, poke root, rue, sage, southernwood, tansy, thuja, and wormwood, may trigger a miscarriage. Use herbs with discretion and only under the guidance of a professional. "There are some herbs that are absolutely contraindicated in pregnancy." His list of herbs to avoid during this time includes some fairly common plants, such as the laxatives senna and cascara found in both herbal preparations and over-the-counter drugs. Cascara can cause abnormal development of the fetus. Senna has been listed as an herb that encourages menstruation and may promote miscarriage.*

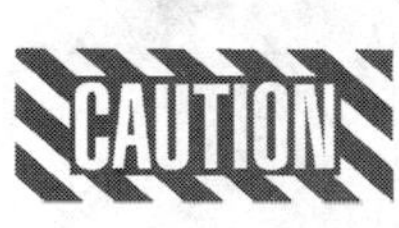

Herbs with high concentrations of the alkaloid berberine, found in goldenseal, barberry, and Oregon grape root, should not be used during pregnancy: "Historically," says Dr. Birdsall, "goldenseal was used to stop postpartum uterine hemorrhage. And it does that because it causes strong uterine contractions." Licorice contains estrogen-like substances and is to be avoided during pregnancy. Juniper can harm the fetus and possibly induce a miscarriage.

Pregnant women should use caution in taking vitamins and minerals. Doses of vitamin A as low as 15,000 IU have been associated with birth defects such as microcephaly (a congenital abnormal smallness of the head often seen in mental retardation).[28] *Beta-carotene, which is converted by the body into vitamin A, is relatively nontoxic and probably safe. However, Dr. Birdsall says, "I err on the side of caution in situations like that, and normally would not, at least early in pregnancy, use high doses of beta-carotene either." Regarding the use of supplementation during pregnancy, only take what is absolutely necessary.*

Nutrition During Pregnancy

It is important to the health of both mother and fetus that the mother eats a well-balanced and varied diet. Fresh fruits and vegetables, whole grains, legumes, beans, and fish are essential. Limit refined sugars, processed foods, and saturated fats. Organically grown produce, meats, and poultry are preferable. However, if produce is not organic, it should be washed to remove as much of the agricultural chemicals as possible.

Most physicians recommend eating plenty of dairy products during pregnancy, due to their calcium and protein content. Helen Burst suggests her patients use milk products. "If a woman is lactose intolerant," says Burst, "obviously you're going to find other ways of getting her the protein. If [she's] not lactose intolerant, I don't see any problems in using the milk and the dairy products." Other doctors are more wary about suggesting dairy as a mainstay of a pregnant woman's diet. Lendon Smith, M.D., a pediatrician and author of several books on children's nutrition, explains, "Many babies will develop a milk sensitivity before they are born because the mother followed the OB [obstetrician] dictum: 'Drink a quart of milk every day so the baby will get the calcium.' If a mother is already sensitive to dairy products and takes in milk, cheese, and ice cream, she may not be absorbing the calcium from those foods she is ingesting." Foods such as nuts, soybean products, such as tofu and soy milk, and goat milk products provide alternative sources of protein. Seaweed, green vegetables, and a mixture of sunflower, sesame, and pumpkin seeds are alternatives for calcium. No one food, including dairy, should be eaten on a daily basis, says Dr. Smith, as this practice increases an individual's chance of developing a food sensitivity.

Contrary to popular belief, a well-chosen vegetarian diet is healthy for a pregnant woman. On the other hand, vegetarians who consume no animal products at all, including dairy and eggs, should use a B_{12} supplement.

The idea that a pregnant woman needs to eat for two is a myth. A baby is not a parasite that depletes the mother of all her nutrition. Both undereating and overeating have their negative impacts, according to Dr. Linton. "The usual obstetric advice of increasing daily intake by three hundred calories is not supported by all, and some nutritionists feel that hunger, not calorie counting, is a more reliable guide to eating during pregnancy," says Dr. Linton.

Eating five to six small, nutrient-dense meals a day is a sensible idea. Restricting weight gain, which was very popular twenty years ago, was thought to ease a woman's labor. We now know that this is not necessarily so: "New guidelines, issued in June 1990 by the Institute of Medicine in Washington, D.C., recommend increased weight gains for healthy pregnant women. The range of optimal weight gains depends on the weight of the mother early in pregnancy: twenty-eight to forty pounds for 'underweight' women, fifteen to twenty-five pounds for 'overweight' women, and a minimum of fifteen pounds for 'obese' women."[29] These new guidelines "reflect current interests in preventing low-birth weight babies and thus reduce the incidence of infant mortality and mental and physical retardation."[30] Pregnancy is not the time to diet. Dr. Linton offers a simple formula. "If you are eating a whole foods diet, drinking plenty of water, and getting adequate exercise such as walking or swimming, then the weight you gain in your pregnancy is appropriate."

Opinions vary on the amount of protein that is needed during pregnancy. The U.S. Recommended Daily Allowance (U.S. RDA) indicates that a woman's requirements rise from forty-six to sixty grams per day. Some experts advocate consuming even more protein than the RDA: "I think that dietary protein," says Dr. Birdsall, "is probably the most common nutrient deficiency in pregnancy." Pregnant women need seventy to one hundred grams of protein daily, which most people will not get with a normal diet. These levels of protein, adds Birdsall, help feed increasing blood volume and guard against complications during pregnancy, such as preeclampsia, a potentially dangerous condition characterized by high blood pressure, swelling, and/or protein spilling into the urine.

Helen Burst agrees with Dr. Birdsall's sentiments. "I'm a big believer in the protein and calorie increase during pregnancy and certainly when breast-feeding too," she says. "To me the amounts given in the RDA are too low . . . I really and truly believe you can make a significant difference in the birth weights of babies born to women eating a good balance of protein and calories." Both Birdsall and Burst point out that a protein increase must be accompanied by more calories or else protein will be used for energy, rather than the construction of tissues, such as blood, the placenta, and an expanding uterus.

Salt Intake During Pregnancy: Sodium is needed to maintain fluid balance and blood volume. For this reason, salt restriction is one common nutritional advisement that does not apply during pregnancy. Restricting sodium and using diuretics, once routine treatments to prevent preeclampsia and swelling, are not only unnecessary, but potentially harmful.[31] It is best to use salt to taste.

Nutritional Supplements

If there is any concern that a mother's diet does not provide all the vitamins and minerals needed for a healthy pregnancy, she may want to add a prenatal supplement. Requirements for many nutrients do increase during this time and supplementing a poor diet results in a healthier pregnancy.[32] Dr. Linton notes that it is most important to have pregnant women eat well and then use supplements to optimize their health. Supplements of specific vitamins and minerals can also be used as safe treatments to certain problems during pregnancy. For example, vitamin B_6 may help alleviate morning sickness[33] and calcium can decrease hypertension.[34]

However, like any substance taken during this time discretion should be used. "Ideally, we all get our nutrients from foods," says Dr. Birdsall. "The unfortunate part is that none of us live in an ideal situation. We're all exposed to varying levels of toxins in our environment and in the food chain. Most of us are exposed to levels of stress in our lives that deplete us of nutrients. Many of the foods we consume are deficient in nutrients compared to what they were seventy-five or one hundred years ago." A prenatal supplement, he explains, acts as an insurance policy providing it contains reasonable amounts of vitamins and minerals.

See Diet, Nutritional Supplements.

Dr. Birdsall feels vitamin C is a nutrient that is chronically underdosed. He points out vitamin C's vital role in the formation of collagen—a major protein found in connective tissue, cartilage, and bone. Some doctors are concerned over a condition called rebound scurvy, thought to affect newborns whose mothers have ingested large amounts of vitamin C. In Dr. Birdsall's experience and research, this is a very rare phenomenon. "I have only been able to find two documented cases of rebound scurvy in the medical literature," he explains. If it does develop, he says, the infant recovers with no treatment in a relatively short period of time.

Folic acid, a B vitamin found in green leafy vegetables, nuts, and whole grains, can prevent neural tube defect in fetuses.[35] However, artificial supplementation of folic acid can decrease zinc absorption, a mineral required for proper fetal growth and immunity.[36] In unusually large doses (1,000 mcg.) folic acid is associated with maternal infection and abnormally slow fetal heart rate.[37] Extra iron may be warranted if the mother's hemoglobin tests suggest a deficiency. Yet routine supplementation of iron can block zinc absorption and has been linked with infection, cancer, and other conditions.[38] However, Dr. Birdsall states that iron is the only nutrient that the current dietary guidelines for pregnancy say should be supplemented and he sees adding this mineral to his pregnant patients' regimen as valuable.

Vitamin D should also be taken judiciously to avoid toxicity. The fetus can drain as much as three hundred milligrams daily of calcium from the mother during the third trimester, in order to facilitate bone development. However, absorption of vitamin D (a nutrient that aids in calcium uptake) and calcium are enhanced during pregnancy. Consequently, some experts are debating whether the current RDA of twelve hundred milligrams of calcium daily during pregnancy is perhaps too high. Excessive levels of this mineral in the body can result in its spillage into the urine. One in every fifteen hundred pregnant women who consumes high amounts of calcium may develop kidney stones, slightly higher than in nonpregnant women.[39] Dr. Birdsall agrees that physicians have tended to oversupplement pregnant women with calcium for two reasons. "We tend to ignore the relationship between calcium and the other minerals, particularly magnesium and zinc. And number two, most of the research done on calcium supplementation is done with relatively inefficient forms of calcium." Calcium citrate or citrate/malate are the most absorbable forms—the more efficiently the mineral is absorbed, the less you need to ingest.

While it is true that milk contains substantial amounts of this mineral, some experts question the availability of dairy's calcium," says Dr. Birdsall. "There is now some pretty good research to indicate that dairy consumption by the mom can in fact induce an allergic condition in the baby."

Using alternative calcium foods, such as dark green leafy vegetables, and avoiding calcium-robbing foods, such as coffee, sugar, and salt, will ensure adequate nourishment for a pregnant woman. With regard to salt, pregnancy is not a time to restrict salt intake, however it should be used in moderation as large amounts will decrease available calcium. Calcium supplementation can also help ease leg cramps during pregnancy.[40] Vitamins B_6, D, and K, and boron are examples of nutrients that are also involved in bone metabolism.

Preparing the Body for Childbirth

The stress, pain, and anxiety precipitating and accompanying childbirth can be eased by taking the proper steps to prepare one's body and mind. Exercises that strengthen the body are easy to do, but equally important are exercises that strengthen the intimacy between the expectant parents.

Kegel Exercises: The muscle that surrounds the vagina is called the PC muscle. It is usually in good tone, however, during pregnancy and childbirth it supports a lot of weight and can become slack. To keep the PC muscle toned it is important to practice Kegel exercises on a daily basis, both before and after the birth.

To find your PC muscle, sit on the toilet and spread your legs apart. As you start to urinate, see if you can control the flow of urine without moving your legs. The PC muscle is the one you use to turn the flow on and off.

- **Slow Kegels:** Tighten the PC muscle as if to stop the urine. Hold for a slow count of three, and then relax. Repeat ten times.
- **Quick Kegels:** Tighten and relax the PC muscle, as quickly as you can, five times. Relax and repeat ten times.
- **Pull in—push out:** Pull up the entire pelvic floor as though trying to suck water into the vagina. Then push out or bear down as if trying to push the imaginary water out. This exercise uses the stomach and abdominal muscles as well as the PC muscle. Do this four or five times in a row. Repeat ten times.

STRETCH MARK PREVENTION OINTMENT

Most women are concerned about stretch marks during pregnancy. Although many doctors feel stretch marks are hereditary, prevention is a good remedy. The consistent application of a mixture containing a blend of specific oils is your best protection. This should be applied once or twice a day and massaged onto the abdomen, breasts, and thighs. The best times to do this are in the morning when you wake up and before bed at night. You should start using your prevention routine as soon as your abdomen begins to swell as it is then that the skin begins to stretch.

All of the following ingredients can be found in most health food stores. Sweet almond oil can also be purchased where massage supplies are sold.

1 ounce vitamin E oil
5 tablespoons (2-1/2 fluid ounces) cocoa butter
4-1/2 ounces sweet almond oil

Carefully melt the cocoa butter in a double boiler—do not overheat it. Once the cocoa butter has turned to a liquid, add the vitamin E and sweet almond oils. Place the mixture in an eight-ounce plastic container. The ointment will solidify as it cools and may be stored at room temperature.

Ideally you should repeat each of these sets of exercises five times a day, beginning at the start of the pregnancy. After a few months you will notice an improvement in your performance and you can gradually increase the amount of times you practice each week. These exercises can be done anytime, anywhere. Practice while driving the car, watching television, washing dishes, or waiting in line. They will enhance vaginal elasticity and improve bladder control. It is also good to practice during sexual intercourse as this can help elevate sexual awareness and pleasure.

Perineal Massage: The perineum is the area between a woman's vagina and anus. During the last six weeks of pregnancy it should be massaged daily in order to prepare for the stretching it will do at birth. This technique can also help reduce the need for an episiotomy (a small surgical cut in the perineum, made by obstetricians to facilitate the emergence of the baby) and protect against tearing. This technique should be delayed if there are any vaginal problems, such as an active herpes sore or vaginitis. It can be resumed when the vagina has healed. Perineal massage can be performed by yourself or your partner.

Roy Dittman, O.M.D., of Santa Monica, California, offers these guidelines for a perineal massage:

- Wash your hands. Have a mirror handy, and find a warm private place to practice.
- Lubricate your perineum and your thumbs with vegetable oil, cocoa butter, KY jelly, or vitamin E oil. You can also use your own body secretions if you wish.
- Placing your thumbs about one to one and a half inches inside your vagina, press down and to the sides at the same time. Gently and firmly stretch the skin until you feel a slight tingling or burning sensation.
- Continue to hold this pressure for an additional two minutes until the perineum becomes more numb and the tingling is not as distinct.
- Take three to four minutes to massage the oil along the outside of the lower half of the vagina. Avoid moving upward toward the urethra.
- Pulling gently outward or forward, massage the lower part of your vagina with your thumbs. This massage motion helps to stretch the perineal skin, similar to the way your baby's head will stretch it during birth.

Intimacy During Pregnancy

A woman's physical and emotional comfort with her pregnancy determine her sexual attitudes and enjoyment at this time. Her feelings are often influenced by her partner's attitude to her appearance. This issue is complex and it is therefore vital that women and men discuss their feelings, fears, and beliefs about the changes that are shaping their lives, and consequently affecting their lovemaking.

During pregnancy, a woman's libido can oscillate from high to low. She may become anorgasmic for a period, or the symptoms of pregnancy may dampen her sexual drive. During the latter months, the awkwardness of her shape may inhibit her from lovemaking. Some couples are concerned that intercourse may harm the fetus and it is reassuring for them to learn that the penis rarely touches the cervix. The vagina lengthens during sexual excitement and the mucous plug covering the cervical opening to the uterus also provides protection. Semen is rich in prostaglandins, natural bodily chemicals that can help ripen and soften the cervix, and intercourse may initiate uterine contractions. However, these actions will not induce labor unless a woman is nearing the end of her pregnancy.

Helen Burst feels that sexual activity should depend on how the woman feels. "There are all sorts of things you can suggest in terms of alternatives to actual intercourse itself, if that is a problem for her," she explains. "The only time that I restrict sex is if she's having signs and symptoms of preterm labor." Other exceptions to sex or orgasm during pregnancy would be cases in which vaginal bleeding occurs, if the woman experiences continuing or painful cramps after intercourse, or if the woman has a new sexual partner with a sexually transmitted disease or AIDS. If there is a history of preterm labor, says Burst, she advises the use of condoms for sexual intercourse.

The father or birth coach should participate in the many decisions and educational opportunities during pregnancy. This includes touring the hospital (if this is the chosen location) and learning about the different stages of labor. The partner should discuss his or her concerns for the birth with both the pregnant woman and the birth attendant. He or she should feel free to disclose his or her feelings, positive or negative, surrounding the upcoming event[41] so that there are no uncertain feelings to hinder the support of the mother during labor.

Childbirth

All the planning, preparation, and events around pregnancy culminate with the birth of the child. Regarding childbirth, expectant parents must make some very important decisions including where the birth will take place, what type of practitioner will deliver the care, and what method will be used.

It is best to prepare for childbirth well in advance—preferably before conception. Good advice often comes by word of mouth from parents who have already gone through the birthing experience. There are also many great reading books on the subject. It is essential for couples to explore all the options available before deciding the type of birth they want.

Medical Intervention

Medical technology has its place in childbirth. However, the routine use of many standard interventions typically used in hospitals, such as pain medication, cesarean sections, and episiotomies, are being reevaluated. According to Susanne Houd, criticism of home births is unjustified especially when it is based on hospital knowledge. "It's like comparing oranges to apples."

A Canadian study discovered that the level of intervention increased when low-risk maternity patients delivered at facilities specializing in high-risk situations.[42] This situation has been referred to as the cascade effect. In an otherwise normal circumstance, one type of medical intervention can lead to complications and then more intervention. For example, a woman hooked up to a fetal heart monitor needs to remain inactive. As a result her labor slows down due to tension and inactivity. To hasten the labor, the physician may order a rupture of membranes which then enhances pain. Pain medications or anesthesia may follow, finally culminating in a cesarean section.[43]

Electronic Fetal Heart Rate Monitor (EFM): EFM is a machine used to determine the fetus's heart rate and mother's uterine contractions. EFM uses either ultrasound or electrodes attached to the baby, such as the scalp, and prints out a graph with the results. "I'm glad its there when we need it . . . because it can save lives," says Helen Burst. "And there are times where there are clear indications for fetal monitoring. To use it as a routine in perfectly normal pregnancy and childbirth, I think, is not the way management of care should be done." Risks involved, says Burst, include the fact that neither EFM readings nor their interpretations by practitioners are always totally accurate. When EFM was compared to auscultation (listening to the heartbeat with a stethoscope) in a series of studies at the University of Denver, there was no difference in fetal death and health between the two groups. The most glaring disparity was the 16.5 percent cesarean rate in the EFM group versus 6.8 percent in the non-EFM group.[44] Some experts have suggested that EFM has a positive influence on a child's neurological development later on. There has been no support for this theory.[45]

Pain Medication: Jack Pritchard, M.D., author of "Analgesia and Anesthesia" in *William's Obstetrics*,[46] says that medications are a risk for pain relief during childbirth. Part of that risk is the drugs the baby receives through the placenta. When pethidine, a type of pain medication, is given to laboring women it sedates newborns to the point of disturbing their early suckling pattern and possibly inhibiting successful breast-feeding.[47] Epidural analgesia, local pain medication injected in between the spine vertebrae, may diminish the bearing down reflex and perineal sensation. This can in turn delay the second stage of labor and lead to early surgical intervention, or use of forceps and a vacuum extractor.[48] Natalia Lopez speculates drug use during labor may be responsible for drug use among children and teens today.[49]

Episiotomy: The most common surgical procedure in childbirth and medicine overall is the episiotomy, an incision in the muscular wall surrounding the vagina intended to widen the opening and ease delivery. A recent Canadian study now recommends that routine episiotomies be

U. S. Hospitals with High Rates of Caesarean Sections

50 Percent or Greater Rate of a Caesarean Section

State	Facility Name	Total Births/Deliveries	Caesarean Rate
Louisiana	Abrom Kaplan Memorial Hospital	120	57.5%
Nevada	Humbolt Hospital	53	56.6%
Kentucky	Williamson Appalachian Regional Hospital	101	55.4%
Louisiana	Southern Baptist Hospital •	1,912	50.3%
Louisiana	Bunkie General Hospital	62	50.0%

• Indicates this facility has a neonatal intensive care unit (NICU).

Between 40 Percent and 50 Percent Rate of a Caesarean Section

State	Facility Name	Total Births/Deliveries	Caesarean Rate
Louisiana	Bogalusa Community Medical Center	251	49.8%
Pennsylvania	Tyrone Hospital	77	49.4%
Louisiana	Highland Hospital	395	48.4%
Florida	Hialeah Hospital	1,890	48.3%
Connecticut	University of Connecticut Health Center—John Dempsey	407	46.9%
Florida	Mt. Sinai Medical Center	1,244	46.6%
Louisiana	Lakeside Hospital •	2,899	46.5%
Louisiana	St. Anne Hospital	353	46.5%
Louisiana	St. Tammany Parish Hospital	285	46.3%
New Jersey	St. James Hospital	576	46.2%
New York	Carthage Area Hospital	266	45.9%
New York	Victory Memorial Hospital	924	45.6%
Louisiana	Abbeville General Hospital	347	44.7%
Mississippi	L.O. Crosby Memorial Hospital	399	44.4%
Louisiana	Thibodaux General Hospital	704	44.3%
Minnesota	Sleepy Eye Municipal Hospital	50	44.0%
Florida	HTI Plantation General Hospital	2,859	44.0%
Mississippi	Hancock General Hospital	150	44.0%
Tennessee	Perry Memorial Hospital	46	43.5%
Louisiana	Opelousas General Hospital	962	43.1%
Nevada	Humana Sunrise Hospital •	2,132	42.9%
Florida	Southeast Volusia Hospital	245	42.9%
Kentucky (1990)	Hazard Appalachia Regional Hospital	518	42.5%
New Jersey	Christ Hospital	1,188	42.5%
New York	Amsterdam Memorial Hospital	184	42.4%
West Virginia (1990)	Williamson Memorial Hospital	211	42.2%
Louisiana	St. Jude Medical Center (AMI) •	500	42.2%
West Virginia (1991)	Reynolds Memorial Hospital	211	42.2%
Maryland	Kent & Queen Anne's Hospital	228	42.1%
Louisiana	Physicians and Surgeons Hospital	150	42.0%
Illinois	Memorial Hospital Belleville	1,746	42.0%
California	Bakersfield Memorial Hospital •	2,172	41.9%
Kentucky (1990)	Caldwell County War Memorial Hospital	98	41.7%
Kentucky (1990)	Logan County Hospital	103	41.7%
Florida	Humana Hospital, Pembroke	709	41.6%
Louisiana	East Jefferson General Hospital •	1,321	41.5%
Florida	Humana Hospital, Bennett	249	41.4%
Georgia	Jenkins County Hospital	56	41.1%
Florida	AMI Palmetto General Hospital	595	41.0%
Kentucky (1990)	Highland Regional Medical Center	414	40.8%
Washington	Island Hospital	103	40.8%
Florida	AMI Palm Beach Gardens Medical Center •	809	40.7%
Nevada	Elko Hospital	344	40.7%
Florida	South Miami Hospital	3,082	40.6%
California	Circle City Hospital	838	40.5%
California	Nu Med. Regional Medical Center	520	40.4%
Mississippi	NW Mississippi Regional Medical Center	1,306	40.2%
New Jersey	Meadowlands Hospital Medical Center	2,036	40.1%
Ohio	Lawrence County General Hospital	60	40.0%
Pennsylvania	Suburban General Hospital, Norristown	380	40.0%
Kentucky (1990)	Paul B. Hall Regional Medical Center	355	40.0%
Washington	Island Hospital	103	40.8%
Florida	AMI Palm Beach Gardens Medical Center •	809	40.7%
Nevada	Elko Hospital	344	40.7%

State	Facility Name	Total Births/Deliveries	Caesarean Rate
Florida	South Miami Hospital	3,082	40.6%
California	Circle City Hospital	838	40.5%
California	Nu Med. Regional Medical Center	520	40.4%
Mississippi	NW Mississippi Regional Medical Center	1,306	40.2%
New Jersey	Meadowlands Hospital Medical Center	2,036	40.1%
Ohio	Lawrence County General Hospital	60	40.0%
Pennsylvania	Suburban General Hospital, Norristown	380	40.0%
Between 30 Percent and 40 Percent Rate of a Caesarean Section			
Nevada	Carson-Tahoe Hospital	386	39.9%
Pennsylvania	Springfield Hospital	83	39.8%
Tennessee	Jellico County Community Hospital	317	39.7%
New Jersey	Bayonne Hospital	480	39.6%
Ohio	Parma County General Hospital	1,027	39.6%
Florida	Mercy Hospital	1,272	39.6%
Florida	AMI Parkway Regional Medical Center	210	39.5%
Louisiana	St. Francis Cabrini Hospital	735	39.5%
California	Northridge Hospital Medical Center •	2,171	39.3%
Ohio	Doctors Hospital of Stark County	305	39.3%
New Hampshire	Parkland Medical Center	293	39.2%
Florida	St. Anthony's Hospital	296	39.2%
Florida	Humana Hospital, Lucerne	1,051	39.1%
North Carolina	Moore Regional Hospital	1,329	39.1%
Mississippi	Ocean Springs Hospital	538	39.0%
California	Mission Hospital Huntington Park	1,639	39.0%
Florida	HCA Northwest Regional Hospital	436	39.0%
Ohio	Deaconness Hospital of Cleveland	683	38.9%
Pennsylvania	Berwich Hospital Center	273	38.8%
Mississippi	North Sunflower County Hospital	62	38.7%
California	Wheeler Hospital	236	38.6%
Louisiana	Terrebonne Parish General Hospital	679	38.6%
Louisiana	Women's Hospital of Acadiana •	1,503	38.5%
Pennsylvania	Community General Osteopathic Hospital	73	38.4%
Tennessee	John W. Hartion Regional Medical Center	460	38.3%
New Hampshire	Androscoggin Hospital	94	38.3%
Ohio	Van Wert County Hospital	246	38.2%
Georgia	Gordon County Hospital	309	38.2%
Ohio	Fayette County Memorial Hospital	202	38.1%
Pennsylvania	Elk County General Hospital	202	38.1%
Nevada	Valley Hospital	571	38.0%
Tennessee	Smith County Memorial Hospital	58	37.9%
Nebraska	Cozad Community Hospital	58	37.9%
New York	Westchester County Medical Center •	1,048	37.8%
Tennessee	HCA Crockett General Hospital	421	37.8%
Missouri	Grim-Smith Hospital & Clinic	312	37.8%
California	El Centro Regional Medical Center	1,428	37.7%
Iowa	Stewart Memorial Community Hospital	106	37.7%
West Virginia (1990)	Thomas Memorial Hospital	313	37.7%
Mississippi	Methodist Medical Center	1,407	37.6%
California	Medical Center of Tarzana	1,952	37.6%
Indiana	Community Hospital of Munster	2,383	37.5%
California	San Clemente General Hospital	544	37.3%
Florida	St. Francis Hospital	282	37.1%
Kentucky (1990)	Tri-County Community Hospital	132	37.1%

• *Indicates this facility has a neonatal intensive care unit (nicu).*
Thanks to the Health Reasearch Group of The Public Citizen Foundation

abandoned. Instead, researchers suggest, this surgery should be reserved for cases of fetal distress or if a woman is unable to deliver her child without help. Episiotomies do not, as previously thought, prevent perineal tears or trauma, enhance later sexuality, or benefit the baby.[50] They are also not mandatory for all forcep or vacuum extraction use.[51] Burst says when she saw this study it angered her. The results, she says are "what we've been saying . . . for years. But it's not until the M.D.'s come out with an article that anybody pays attention to it."

Vacuum Extraction and Forceps: The use of forceps and vacuum extraction has recently been associated with decreased oxygen delivery and intracranial bleeding of the fetus during birth. Such instruments are used to forcibly pull the baby from the vagina and it is suggested that these methods are used more frequently on women who are less educated about childbirth. Forceps may later impair the baby's vision and cause foot problems. Vacuum extraction has resulted in leg problems.[52] One medical article entitled *Fatal Forceps* recounts a pathologist's findings that some infant deaths may be due to delivery by forceps.[53]

Caesarean Section (C-Section): Approximately 25 percent of all births in the United States are performed by c-section. One researcher claims that the high c-section rate is related in part to its financial compensation for the attending physician and hospital.[54] An English teaching hospital conducted an exercise to assess the need to perform c-sections in a number of birthing situations. Not only did auditors disagree with each other as to whether a c-section was indicated in each case, but when given identical information at different times, auditors were also inconsistent with their own decisions.[55]

Contrary to popular belief it is possible for a woman to have a vaginal birth after a cesarean. It is recommended by the American College of Obstetrics and Gynecology that appropriate patients try vaginal birth after previously having had a c-section.[56]

Vaginal births, statistically, create fewer complications. When a woman elects to have a c-section she is opting to undergo major surgery. It is a situation that may entail infection, bleeding, anesthesia complications, a longer recovery period, and less initial involvement with her newborn. Although it is estimated that 50 to 80 percent of VBAC's (Vaginal Birth After Caesarean) are successful, uterine rupture, the main concern of VBAC's, occurs in less than 0.5 percent of cases. VBAC's are not recommended for women with serious medical problems, such as diabetes, a multiple birth, a small pelvis, or a classical (vertical) c-section incision scar.[57]

Delivery

Originally, all women gave birth in their home environment. This first began to change in North America at the beginning of the twentieth century when childbirth gradually migrated from a female assisted experience in the home to a medical procedure based in a hospital.[58] Once the trend away from home birth had begun, the percentage of babies born in hospitals escalated and reached 90 percent in the 1950s.[59] In 1989 about 3.5 million births were performed in thirty-six hundred delivery rooms across the country.

Hospital Birth: An obstetrician (OB), a medical doctor specializing in the care of women during pregnancy and childbirth, will typically deliver babies in a hospital. A hospital environment is populated with modern technology, routine testing, and conventional medicines.

The rate of medical intervention (invasive medical procedures such as episiotomies, pain medications, and cesarean sections) is higher in a hospital than in a home environment, and according to Lewis Mehl of the Waisman Center at the University of Wisconsin, normal variations of childbirth can often be mistaken for complications by hospitals. This may be due to several reasons: the higher levels of tension in the hospital; the availability of consultants; modern tests and equipment; and the state of mind of hospital staff as they mediate between both high-risk situations and potentially normal births. It is also suggested that some physicians fear that the practice of minimum intervention could be translated by their colleagues as incompetence.[60]

However, the demand for a more natural approach to labor and delivery has motivated many hospitals to construct birth rooms or centers within their facilities. Such birthing rooms offer a more relaxed and personable atmosphere while maintaining contact with all the hospital benefits.

If a woman wants to have her baby in a hospital but still wants to have a natural birth it is important that she make her wishes clear to the obstetrician beforehand. Many women find it helpful to write up a birth plan, illustrating their wishes regarding medical intervention and the choice of birth position. These can be discussed with the woman's OB six to eight weeks before the due date. Usually a copy is sent to the hospital with the additional paperwork, and many women carry an extra copy with them.

Free-Standing Birth Centers: Free-standing birth centers (FSBC's) offer a happy compromise between a hospital and a home birth. They usually offer a homelike setting and are very casual about friends and relatives attending the birth. They are generally run by midwives who will follow the prenatal care and deliver the baby. Occasionally obstetricians will be called in to deliver.

In the 1970s, there were only thirty such centers in the United States; now there are around three hundred nationwide. In the case of an emergency or complication, they all have a written or verbal transfer agreement with a nearby hospital. Although most FSBC's offer technologies such as pain medication and fetal heart monitors, their care is less interventive, more personalized, and allows parents more active participation. Birthing in a FSBC is safe and can often be more economical. FSBC clients are carefully screened to confirm their low-risk status and so they can be assured a more natural childbirth. Some FSBC's also offer the use of warm water tubs for labor and birth.

Prenatal education, one-on-one care, and occasionally the use of natural remedies, such as homeopathic medicines and herbs, are part of a FSBC program.[61]

Home Birth: During the 1950s and until fairly recently, it was considered risky to give birth at home. Today, more people are considering home birth a viable option. Although hospital technology is not so readily at hand in home birthing situations, there are many advantages to birthing at home: familiarity and comfort; more control over the actual birth procedure; less chance of intervention; full-time supervision and care; and less expense.[62]

Recent investigations have determined that when low-risk women choose a home birth, it is as safe if not safer than a hospital birth in terms of interventions, birth injuries, and maternal hemorrhaging.[63] However, it is important that women are adequately screened for risk factors. High-risk complications include hypertension, heart disease, kidney disease, anemia, diabetes, epilepsy, multiple births, women who have had a cesarean section, and first-time mothers over the age of thirty-five. A home birth is generally not advisable if you fall into any of these categories.

Birth Attendants: "It's interesting that midwifery is the exception in the United States and not the norm," observes Susanne Houd, Program Director of the Department of Midwifery at The Michener Institute in Toronto, Ontario, Canada. Ms. Houd, a practicing midwife, former World Health Organization employee, and native of Denmark, offers a worldly view to the past and current state of midwifery. She notes that "sage femmes," Europe's female folk healers who also assisted in childbirth, were once trained by priests but gradually graduated to a medically-based education. The midwives act, a legislation ruling the practice of midwifery, went into effect around 150 years ago in most European countries. This did not happen in North America, she says. Instead the doctors just took over. "It was a new country," she explains. "The tradition may not have been that strong."

However, today the option of using a midwife is available to many women. A midwife [or in some states in the U.S., a naturopathic doctor (N.D.)], will usually be the one to attend a home birth. Certified nurse midwives (CNM's) are trained nurses with additional midwifery education and state certification. CNM's are permitted to attend hospital births and can also give sole care for women wanting a home birth. A midwife gives more personalized care than an OB, especially during labor and delivery. Most CNM's will have a backup doctor at a hospital, whom they use on a regular basis, in case of complications.

POINTS TO CONSIDER WHEN COMPOSING A PRELIMINARY BIRTH PLAN

The first point is to be aware. There are a wide variety of birth attendants available. Determine the extent of their training and experience. You need to know that their experience applies to your particular needs especially if you have a specific situation, such as hoping to have a vaginal birth after a cesarean section.

Ask for referrals from friends and childbirth educators. Make sure you talk to several people, as each person's idea of a good birth is different.

Establish how much control you will have over the birth and any additional procedures.

Ask about routine procedures such as an episiotomy, fetal heart monitoring, the use of forceps, vitamin K injections, and cutting the umbilical cord. Find out if you can decide for yourself whether you want these things or not.

Have an open, honest discussion with the attendant about your needs and wants. Be suspicious if a caregiver is not forthcoming with information or will not make time to discuss issues with you. Remember you are paying him or her for a service.

Even if you have a good idea of whom you want for an attendant, interview other caregivers as a comparison. It is important that you feel confident with your choice.

Midwives are more likely to have some knowledge of natural therapies such as herbology and homeopathy and may be able to suggest natural solutions to common health problems during pregnancy. Their philosophies usually support minimum intervention. Services generally include prenatal care, delivery, and postpartum checkups.

It is important for a woman to very carefully choose the professional who will deliver her baby. Prospective birth attendants should be interviewed thoroughly. It is essential that a woman feel completely comfortable and trusting of the person who is going to guide her through one of the most challenging and intimate moments of her life, and that this person's philosophies surrounding the birth mirror hers as much as possible, whether this person be an obstetrician or a midwife.

In order to prepare for the daunting task of choosing a birth attendant, it is helpful to write down any thoughts and questions about the birthing process. Whether considering a midwife or obstetrician, one can present this preliminary birth plan to him or her.

Water Birth: Pioneered by Dr. Michel Odent in France and Igor Tjarkovsky in Russia, birthing in water is increasing in popularity in the United States. It is a method of natural childbirth that is thought to ease the passing of the child from the dark and watery sanctuary of the womb to the outside world of air and gravity.

Dr. Michael Odent used hot tubs in his birth center as a means of relieving stress and pain during labor. He discovered that the allure of water often resulted in women delivering their babies underwater. This experience may lessen the length of labor and the difficulty of pushing.

Women who have experienced water births report that they felt relaxed during their labor. Some women maintain that the weightless feeling of the water eased their pain. Others feel that being in the water reduced the risk of perineal tearing. Advocates of water birth claim it is the least stressful way to give birth for both mother and baby.[64]

In Europe some of the more progressive hospitals now offer water birth. In the United States, however, it is a technique generally confined to free-standing birth centers or to women birthing at home. FSBC's usually provide large tubs rather like oversized baths for the process. A home water birth can be done in a portable inflatable tub—much like a portable spa tub—that can be rented specifically for water birth purposes.

During labor, the midwife or obstetrician will usually allow the mother to enter the pool when her cervix has dilated to between five and eight centimeters. Entering the pool before this can slow down or halt the labor. When it is time for the baby to emerge, the midwife simply guides the infant out into the water where it may float for a second before being lifted up out of the water by the midwife to be placed at the mother's breast. As the baby does not draw in breath until air hits its lungs, there is no risk of it drowning or breathing in water. The infant continues to get air through the umbilical cord until it stops pulsating some minutes after birth. Mother and baby remain happily in the water until it is time for the placenta to be delivered. This is usually done outside of the tub.

Preparing for Childbirth with Prenatal Classes

Although most expectant parents tend to participate in some form of prenatal preparation, expert opinions on the subject are divided. Elizabeth Noble, author of *Childbirth with Insight*, maintains that such prepared labor techniques are tiring and sometimes impossible to follow during labor. She explains that birth is of an "uncontrollable nature" and that control is not possible nor desirable. Noble recommends that a laboring woman should be supported with common sense and intuition to better serve her needs.[65]

For instance, it is important that she feels free to adopt whichever position is comfortable to her at the time and that she is encouraged to move around if she feels the urge to do so. Sometimes a woman will feel the need to vocalize, this is a natural instinct and can help tremendously during labor. Food and drink should be readily available to replenish her supply of energy, adds Dr. Lenton.

On the other hand, Penny Simkin, P.T., of Seattle, Washington, who has been intimately involved in childbirth for twenty-five years as an educator, labor support person, lecturer, consultant, and author, states, "For most women, this is the greatest physical challenge they will ever meet." She explains that most other physical and mental challenges such as mountain climbing, meditation, and playing a musical instrument are prepared for with training that includes specific breathing techniques, and she adds, "I can't see that childbirth should be an exception to that." Simkin maintains that when a person is in pain, gasping is often the result. There are, of course, exceptions and she explains that if a woman feels loved and cared for and is able to remain calm, she can, perhaps, rely on her instincts to guide her breathing. Very few women, however, allow themselves to follow their instincts during the birth process.

Most expectant parents take prenatal classes during the third trimester. According to Simkin, the earlier a woman can take a class, the better. The information offered in a prenatal course will help eliminate some of the doubt and fear that surrounds childbirth, as well as provide practical information such as prenatal nutrition. Classes will vary, so when researching those available, all prospective students should inquire about the class size, number of classes in the course, cost, philosophy, subjects covered, background, and training of the instructor. Couples should choose the class that fits comfortably with their own philosophy and needs. Techniques used in prenatal classes are varied, but all work toward preparing the couple for childbirth by teaching them how to reduce pain and anxiety.

Hypnosis: Hypnosis was used as early as 1837 for women giving birth. It was believed that having subjects focus on an idea rather than on the pain of labor would produce a state of anesthesia. These early ideas were taken further in Russia in the 1920s. The Russians developed their own theory of how hypnosis worked. They believed that hypnosis altered conditioned or learned reflexes, so that a negative reflex that was perceived as painful could be supplanted by a positive reflex that was perceived as a 'sensation'. By the 1960s, the Russians had used hypnosis in hundreds and thousands of births.

Today, in England, self-hypnosis is taught as a method of alleviating pain during labor. Gowri Motha, M.D., is an obstetrician who believes that preparing for birth by learning self-hypnosis techniques and using alternative therapies to clear the body of toxins and unnecessary tension will result in a stress-free and possibly pain-free labor. At her clinic in Northeast London she has developed a prenatal birth program that encompasses self-hypnosis, reflexology, massage, osteopathy, yoga, and other alternative healing methods in order that women may have a more pleasant birth experience. She delivers the majority of her babies in water and many of her women labor for under six hours.

The Grantly Dick-Read Method: An English obstetrician, Grantly Dick-Read, M.D., developed a theory that pain is not a necessary part of labor and childbirth. In delivering a baby to a woman who felt no pain during the process, he surmised that pain was essentially due to images of fear that women had learned from their society. He felt that these images could create muscle tension in the uterus, cervix, and abdomen, and cause real pain.

The Grantly Dick-Read method of prenatal classes employs three techniques. First it teaches women about the physiology and anatomy of childbirth. The classes are structured in a way that attempts to dispel the notion that childbirth must be painful. In fact the word pain is never used as it is thought that this alone would conjure up fear and, moreover, that the sensation felt during childbirth cannot be compared to any other known feeling of pain.

Second, mothers are taught relaxation, physical conditioning, and breathing exercises. They are encouraged to relax between contractions. Finally, the method stresses the importance of the relationship between the mother and her birth attendant. The woman must have absolute faith in her attendant to prevent fear, which ultimately creates tension within the body and thus pain.

Psychoprophylaxis: Similar to the Grantly Dick-Read method, psychoprophylaxis was developed in Russia in the 1940s and stemmed from the old technique of hypnosis. Doctors believed that pain is a learned reflex and that women can be reeducated not to focus on the pain during the birth process.

Like the Dick-Read method, mothers are taught anatomy in order to illustrate why birth does not have to be painful. They are also taught breathing techniques, relaxation, pushing methods, and positions to use during labor.

Lamaze: Lamaze was developed by a French obstetrician who adopted and changed the Russian method of psychoprophylaxis. He too taught anatomy and physiology but went into greater detail, adding instruction on how the fetus develops. Dr. Lamaze also showed how a woman, through conditioned reflexes, could learn to replace pain and fear with joyful expectation, and redefine contractions as sensations instead of birth pains. To the classes that taught breathing, relaxation, and delivery exercises, he added a pant-blow breathing technique to help with pushing in the second stage of labor. Today Lamaze is one of the most popular methods of prenatal preparation.

The Bradley Method: This program was developed from a combination of the Lamaze and Dick-Read methods, and incorporates the best elements of both with additional elements of its own. The key characteristic of the Bradley method is the emphasis on the father as the main labor coach.

The Birth

Emotional support during labor and delivery, whether from a partner, midwife, or birth assistant, is one of the most valuable forms of care a woman can receive. Women who feel their needs are being met emotionally, have fewer complications, less pain, a shorter labor, and less postpartum depression than those who don't.[66] Penny Simkin has reinforced this approach through her own research.

She wanted to assess women's long-term memory of their birth experience, and compared the birth stories of twenty female pupils who took her prenatal classes between the years 1968 and 1974 with information she gathered from in-depth interviews and questionnaires more than twenty years later. She relates: "I found that women don't forget . . . and the amount of detail that they recall is really very impressive." When she asked women to grade the satisfaction they felt during childbirth, a higher satisfaction and positive memories were associated with control and a sense of accomplishment. These birth experiences had enhanced the women's self-esteem. Simkin adds that these women had also "remembered positive words and actions from their doctors and their nurses." Those women that rated their satisfaction as lower felt entirely different. They held negative memories of a lack of control, fear, discomfort with doctors, and pain. The length of labor, however, did not influence satisfaction ratings.

A partner doesn't need to be experienced or trained in the birthing process to be effective. Sharing in the moment, being aware of the woman's needs, and ensuring her physical comfort are sufficient. Any friends or family who are also assisting should compliment the father's role without creating additional tension.[67]

Birthing Positions: "It has been found that standing and walking, activities that many women naturally gravitate toward during labor, can actually enhance the dilation of the cervix and aid the baby's descent," says Dr. Linton. "An active labor also reduces the need for medication as many women find it easier to cope with the pain when they can move around. Exclusive bed rest during labor can compress major blood vessels and compromise circulation. These two actions decrease maternal blood pressure, decrease uterine blood flow, and may result in fetal distress. The mother's breathing is also impaired when lying down."

"Some women find it helpful to squat with their partner supporting them," adds Dr. Linton. "It has been found that squatting increases the pelvic opening by half to a full centimeter, and when you are talking about a nine-and-a-half-centimeter head, that is significant." Others are more comfortable on their knees, supported in the front by a huge pile of cushions. Many women are also attracted to warm water during labor, such as a bath or jacuzzi. Yelling during labor is a common urge and a natural way of releasing tension and trapped emotions. It is extremely beneficial and ultimately helps relax the muscles in the uterus and the vagina.[68]

During the final phase of labor, many women automatically feel an urge to be upright or squatting, and grasping something, such the back of a chair, a partner's hands or a support bar. This is called the fetus ejection reflex. These instincts, as well as dilated pupils and the need to drink, are due to a rush of adrenaline. An advantage of this physiological process is that it enables a mother to be alert during the first few moments with her newborn.

Herbs: There are several botanicals and homeopathics useful during childbirth. Some commonly used herbs are blue cohosh, bethroot, and homeopathic *Calophyllum*. All are used to help stimulate uterine contractions to either initiate labor or to restart a stalled labor.

- Three to eight drops of blue cohosh tincture can be taken in a glass of warm water or herbal tea. Repeat every half an hour until contractions are regular.
- Bethroot tincture, widely used by Native Americans, starts and strengthens contractions. The dose is one-quarter to one-half teaspoon, in warm water or tea, every half an hour.
- A dose of homeopathic *Calophyllum* 200X can be taken every half an hour for two hours.

Caution: *It is always advisable to consult an herbalist, homeopath, naturopathic physician, midwife, or other expert before taking herbal or homeopathic preparations during pregnancy.*

Essential Oils During Labor: Essential oils are aromatic substances extracted from certain flowers, fruits, and leaves. Due to their high concentration and ability to penetrate the skin they have enormous healing potentials. During labor, certain essential oils can be used to relax and calm the mother. A few drops of an essential oil can be put into a base oil and massaged into the back and abdomen by the partner. Oils can also be put into a small amount of water and used on a diffuser or on a cotton wool ball on a warm radiator. Lavender, geranium, or neroli oils are excellent during labor.

- **Lavender** is calming and has a slight analgesic effect. It also stimulates circulation, which is great for both mother and baby, and has anti-inflammatory and antiseptic properties.
- **Geranium** is one of the best oils to stimulate circulation, which in turn facilitates easy breathing. It has a contractive effect

and helps pull together dilated tissues, so it is healing for the uterus and endometrium after the birth. Geranium is also an antidepressant and known for its uplifting effect.

- **Neroli** targets the nervous system where it too helps to make breathing easier. It has a great calming effect, increasing blood and oxygen to the brain. Use in low doses for relaxation. For instance, put one to two drops in water on a diffuser, as in higher doses it is a stimulant. Neroli is an antiseptic and an antidepressant.

After the Birth

Once the baby has been born, it is vital for the mother and her infant to bond. Placing the baby at the mother's breast will usually initiate suckling. This is very important to future breast-feeding. Most infants will imitate crawling motions toward the breast soon after delivery, and will be suckling in less than an hour if not drugged or disturbed.[69] Even though the mother's milk has not yet come in, the baby will suckle on the colostrum, or nutritious pre-milk fluid that is naturally present in the mother's breast.

The umbilical cord is often cut and the placenta discarded as soon as possible. Most physicians will wait for the cord to stop pulsating before severing it. However, many European doctors and natural childbirth attendants wait until the placenta is delivered or longer before cutting so the newborn can benefit from the oxygen-rich blood from the cord and placenta.[70] Likewise, Helen Burst adds that the placenta may be wrapped in a blanket and used as a warmer alongside the infant immediately after delivery.

Medications for the Infant: Check with local laws concerning procedures commonly performed on newborns at birth, such as silver nitrate, erythromycin, or tetracycline eye drops, and vitamin K shots (given during labor to prevent hemolytic disease in the newborn, characterized by anemia, jaundice, enlargement of the liver and spleen, and generalized edema) as they are required in most states and provinces.[71] Dr. Linton recommends allowing the baby to nurse before administering eye drops because it blurs the vision. She also prefers to check the mother's diet during pregnancy to see if she is deficient in vitamin K rather than automatically giving a shot. "If she is eating enough squash and dark green leafy vegetables such as spinach, chard, and kale, there is no reason to assume that the baby will be vitamin K deficient. If an expectant mother has not eaten these foods by the end of her pregnancy, we supplement with oral vitamin K during the last month of pregnancy. There is evidence that it crosses the placental barrier." There have been studies released linking intramuscular vitamin K shots with childhood cancer. On the other hand, no such ties were found when vitamin K was administered orally.[72]

Circumcision: This is a routine surgical procedure that is not required. It has been argued that this procedure is medically beneficial to prevent urinary tract infections and penile cancer. Scientific evidence now shows that the advantages of circumcision are insignificant when compared to the surgical risks.[73] "There is no medical reason to perform circumcision," says Dr. Linton. "It is totally a cosmetic decision on the part of the parents. In fact, most insurance companies no longer cover it because it is considered cosmetic surgery."

Postpartum Care

The care taken around pregnancy should not end with childbirth. After delivery both the mother and baby will have health concerns that can be addressed through alternative medicine.

Maternal Physical Changes After Birth

During the six- to eight-week period after the birth, the mother's body begins to return to its prepregnant self. Her reproductive organs shrink. She begins to lose her pregnancy weight. Pregnancy demarcations such as skin pigmentation and enhanced hair growth fade away. Estrogen and progesterone levels plummet and the vagina regains its original tone.

The uterus gradually begins to involute, or shrink, and returns to its normal size within five to six weeks. Nursing and uterine massage assist in this process and, during the first few days, prevent excessive blood loss. It is normal for a bloody vaginal discharge, called lochia, to flow from the uterus for four to eight weeks after the birth. At first lochia is heavy and red, but it gradually decreases in volume and changes to pale pink and finally to a white, yellowish, or brown color. Breast-feeding, body position, and activity may increase the flow of the lochia. Afterpains, caused by uterine contractions, may occur during the first week after birth especially while nursing or if the mother has given birth before. Resting and deep breathing will allay some of this discomfort.

The perineal area may be sore, particularly if an episiotomy was performed or if there is a perineal tear. The cervical opening decreases in size, however there remains a somewhat wider aperture than before. The labia shrinks, but remains larger, looser, and darker in color than its prepregnant state.

Besides the delivery of the baby and placenta, and the loss of a cup or more of blood, weight sheds gradually over the next few months to a year. At the beginning, frequent urination and increased perspiration expel up to five pounds of fluid during the first five days. Excess fat slowly recedes with exercise and a sensible diet. Lax abdominal muscles regain tone in about six weeks. There are mixed opinions and experiences on whether nursing aids in weight loss. Stretch marks will fade, but not completely unless precautions have been made during the pregnancy.

Maternal Emotional Changes

The emotional impact of new parenthood is one of the most difficult alterations to come to terms with. Some women experience much anxiety about caring for a new infant. Others experience mood swings from exhilaration to depression. Most mothers, both new and experienced, feel extremely tired. Unless the mother takes adequate and proper rest, chronic fatigue can intensify the physical and emotional challenge of adjusting to a new baby.

Breast-Feeding

Nursing mothers have an increased level of the hormones, prolactin, often called the mothering hormone, and oxytocin (pituitary hormone that stimulates release of milk from the mammary glands). These hormones, together with the baby's instinctive sucking motions, are essential to the cycle of milk production. For the first three to four days the infant will feed on colostrum, an easily digested liquid which is high in protein and antibodies, and low in fat and carbohydrates. The mother's milk ducts do not start producing mature milk until around the second to fourth day after birth.

Whether a woman nurses or not, the first lot of mature milk will still be produced and her breasts will pass through a stage of engorgement when they are hard, hot, and painful. Dr. Birdsall recommends vitamin B_6 and sage as natural remedies used to suppress lactation (the production of milk), if desired.

Cabbage leaves are wonderful for taking the heat out of engorged breasts. A couple of leaves can be torn off and placed under the bra. The leaves are removed and disguarded when they become warm and replaced with new ones.

If a woman is not nursing, menstruation resumes in one to two months. A breast-feeding mother can expect her period to begin in several months to a year or two after the birth, depending on how long she continues to nurse.

The Partner's Participation

The partner's response to the newborn will depend on how settled the partner is, his or her experience with infant care, medical and financial pressures, and the preconceived expectations

The Benefits of Breast-Feeding

Today there is more evidence than ever illustrating the positive health effects of nursing for both mother and child. Below are listed many of them.

For the infant, breast-feeding:

- *Enhances bonding between the mother and infant.[74]*
- *Provides optimum nutrition.[75]*
- *Provides disease-fighting constituents, such as lactoferrin, lysozyme, secretory immunoglobulins A,[76] T, and B lymphocytes,[77] and macrophages.[78]*
- *Encourages appropriate growth and development.[79]*
- *May increase survival rate for low birth weight newborns.[80]*
- *Decreases severity of gastrointestinal infections, such as diarrhea.[81]*
- *Supplies protection against necrotizing enterocolitis, a serious complication of the intestinal tract that occurs most often among premature or low birth weight babies.[82] Breast-feeding also protects against ear infections,[83] decreases the risk of colic,[84] decreases the risk of food allergies,[85] and may increase a child's intelligence.[86]*

For the mother, breast-feeding:

- *Stimulates contractions of the uterus and aids in controlling postpartum blood loss.[87]*
- *Increases mother's confidence in parenting skills.[88]*
- *Is convenient and economical.[89]*
- *If used with little or no supplementation, can help lengthen and space the birth of children by suppressing ovulation (although breast-feeding should not be relied on for birth control).[90]*
- *Is easier, especially at night, and less time-consuming than bottle feeding.[91] The milk is ready to serve, always at the perfect temperature, and there is no preparation "guess work" involved in the feeding process.*

he has of himself and the new mother. The introduction of a new family member, whether a first or additional child, often sets up a love triangle between mother, her partner, and baby. With the mother focusing her attention on her infant, together with disrupted sleep, a change in sexual patterns, and less freedom as a couple, it is normal for her partner to feel displaced and perhaps resentful of the new baby. However, with a little bit of planning, the partner can share in welcoming the new child to the world and enhance bonding time with the baby.

Before the birth, time with the child can be arranged by helping to prepare and freeze meals ahead of time, ensuring extra help during the first week or two after the birth from family, friends, or hired help, and learning about infant care. If possible, the partner should consider taking some time off from work after the baby's birth in order to spend precious moments with his new family.

Many partners are present during their child's birth and even assist in this process. Once the baby is delivered, this person can help in baby care such as changing, dressing, bathing, and bringing the baby to the mother for nursing. When the baby is old enough, the mother may consider pumping her milk so the partner can take over one nighttime feeding with a bottle. This will not only give the mother more uninterrupted sleep, but allows her partner to bond with the baby. This same strategy can be used when the mother wants to leave the house by herself or return to work.

For partners who feel left out of the natural mother-child bond during the first few months of life, it is reassuring to know that this will gradually change as the child gets older and grows more independent. If the partner develops a positive attitude toward the baby in the beginning, this will help foster a healthy, happy relationship within the entire family.

Postpartum Changes and Care

Pregnancy, labor, and delivery are taxing on a woman's body. It is important to recognize this. How the mother cares for herself after the baby comes depends on the nature of her delivery, for instance, whether the baby was born in the hospital, a birthing center, or at home, and whether or not there were any complications. If a woman is discharged early or her baby is born at home, she will need help with household tasks so she can devote her first postpartum week to bonding with her newborn and recovering from the birth. In fact, comments Helen Burst, "One of the nice things about home birth is that the couple assumes that responsibility (of caring for the baby) right from the beginning."

Women who have no complications can usually get up and move around shortly after birth. Not to do so, explains Burst, is physically and mentally unhealthy. A woman must take care of herself postpartum, "and part of taking care of yourself is getting up and around."

It is also important to do postpartum exercises which should include Kegels to strengthen the pelvic muscles. It is, of course, more difficult to adhere to this plan when other children are present. Women who are having their second or third child may take longer to recover than with their first. The mother should be guided by her own body and activities such as work, sex, housework, and exercise should be resumed when she feels ready. In a Western culture, people have demanding schedules and are used to instant results. It is therefore important for a woman to be aware of the stress her body has endured and the recovery it must make. Lack of sleep, nursing, and child care make extra demands on her body. Pacing oneself and taking slow steps are key in maintaining normal activities and optimum health.

Nutrition while nursing remains as important as during pregnancy. Eating a varied diet with plenty of whole foods and fluids still applies. Aggressive dieting during this time of healing and nurturing is detrimental to the health of both mother and baby.

Care of the Perineum: Correct perineal care is essential in order to prevent infection, particularly if an episiotomy was performed or a tear occurred and stitches were made. Douching and tampons should be avoided during this period. For the first twenty-four hours, half an hour of ice packs placed on the perineum with a cloth in between, followed by fifteen minutes of rest, helps reduce swelling. After the first day, heat as either a hot water bottle or heating lamp (not ultraviolet or sunlamp) should replace cold treatment. Twenty-minute, warm water sitz baths are also helpful. Witch hazel or essential oil of lavender applied to a sanitary napkin can also help with swelling.

Urination during the first week may be difficult and painful. Cleansing the perineum after urination will help. Warm water should be applied using a peri bottle available from the hospital or midwife. Women should always wash and wipe from the front to the back toward the rectum to avoid reinfection. Constipation may occur and/or bowel movements may be painful. To keep stools soft, drink a lot of fluids and eat plenty of fiber such as fresh fruits and vegetables.

Sleeping: Adjusting to a new sleeping schedule is probably the most important habit to get into. Exhaustion from the delivery and frequent awakenings for night feeding is inevitable. New mothers should nap when baby is sleeping and go to bed early.

Healing Remedies: In addition to rest and sound eating habits, overall recovery and healing can be enhanced by using Chinese medicines, homeopathic remedies, and nutrient supplementation, according to Dr. Dittman. He adds that acupuncture is effective in balancing hormones and strengthening the *qi* (the body's vital life energy) by retonifying the spleen, liver, kidneys, and uterus. In addition, Dr. Dittman recommends manipulating muscles, tendons, and ligaments using *cheng kua*, an ancient Chinese method.

Prenatal vitamins and minerals can be continued. Vitamin C, zinc, and beta-carotene during the first week will accelerate healing of perineal wounds. The homeopathic remedy, *Arnica,* is helpful during the first few days immediately following birth. It is indicated during injuries, shock, trauma, and bruising.[92]

Sex and Birth Control After the Birth

It is advisable to wait six to eight weeks before resuming sexual intercourse. Some health professionals believe that it is possible to get a uterine infection from early intercourse. However, a woman must determine for herself when she is ready.

Thirty years ago, when Helen Burst graduated from nursing school, episiotomies were regular procedure and left most women with stitches and a sore perineum. "Most women didn't much feel like having sexual intercourse for four to six weeks because of the healing of the episiotomy," recalls Burst. "I learned from the women years and years ago [that] many of them were having sex before I saw them at six weeks postpartum." Consequently, Burst decided that family planning discussions were necessary before the scheduled six-week checkup. She maintains that a woman should resume sexual relations when she feels ready.

Engorged breasts may also diminish a woman's sexual desire. Sexual drive, however, varies among new mothers from no or diminished libido to normal or enhanced drive. This is an area where communication between sexual partners is important. Many things can contribute to decreased libido including depression, anxiety, irritability, fatigue, pain, nursing, interruptions, and fear of pregnancy. Planning for intimacy can offset some of the frustrations of lovemaking. As with so many other areas of adjustment, sleep is one of the best aphrodisiacs. It softens the edges of irritability and feeds the libido. Sex for many new parents may get designated to bedtime when both partners are exhausted. A few hours of sleep before lovemaking may work. Hiring a babysitter away from home in the middle of the day when mother and father are more rested can also help partners resume sexual activity and intimacy.

A woman's natural vaginal lubrication may decrease during this time. Using an artificial lubricant, such as vegetable oil, or K-Y Jelly, can eliminate painful intercourse. Use positions that don't irritate the healing perineum or press on engorged breasts. Be aware that a slack vagina will tighten with time and the help of Kegel exercises.[93]

Probably the most important thing to feed a healthy sex life is a healthy relationship. Parents are often taught that children come first. But if a marriage or relationship is not attended to, there is no family. Partners should get out by themselves on a regular basis and find ways to attend to each other emotionally and not just sexually. Setting aside ten or fifteen minutes per day for discussing the events of the day is a pleasant way for partners to connect.

While breast-feeding appears to suppress ovulation somewhat and help in the spacing of children,[94] it is not a guaranteed form of birth control. The baby's frequent sucking while nursing initiates the release of hormones that appear to suspend menstruation and ovulation.[95] However, it is possible to ovulate and become fertile before menstruation returns. There are several effective and safe forms of birth control that can be used, for example, natural family planning which involves the daily charting of fertility signs, such as basal body temperature, consistency of the cervical mucous, as well as the positioning and the width of opening of the cervix; condoms; and barrier methods, such as the diaphragm used with spermicidal foam or jelly. Do not use oral contraceptives while nursing.

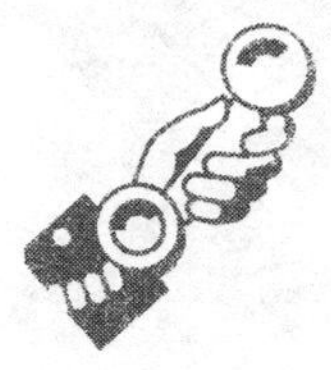

Where to Find Help

For more information and referrals to a qualified professional, contact the following organizations.

American Association of Naturopathic Physicians
2366 Eastlake Avenue, Suite 322
Seattle, Washington 98102
(206) 323-7610

Refers to a nationwide network of accredited or licensed practitioners. Publishes a quarterly newsletter for both professionals and the general public.

American College of Nurse Midwives
1522 K Street NW, Suite 1000
Washington, D.C. 20005
(202) 289-0171

Maintains a list of accredited nurse midwife programs. Will refer general public to midwives in their area.

Informed Birth and Parenting
P.O. Box 3675
Ann Arbor, Michigan 48106
(313) 662-6857

This program certifies childbirth educators and birth assistants. Books and videos on pregnancy, childbirth, and parenting are available for sale. Referral service for midwives throughout the United States and Canada.

International Association of Parents and Professionals for Safe Alternatives in Childbirth
Route 1, Box 646,
Marble Hill, Missouri 63764
(314) 238-2010

Educational organization encourages natural child birth in hospitals. Working to establish guidelines for safe home births. Provides parental education.

International Childbirth Education Association
P.O. Box 20048
Minneapolis, Minnesota 55420
(612) 854-8660

ICEA unites people who support family center maternity care and believe in freedom of choice based on knowledge of alternative medicine. They offer teaching certificates, seminars, continuing education workshops, and a mail order book center.

Read Natural Childbirth Foundation
P.O. Box 150956
San Rafael, California 94915
(415) 456-8462

A non-profit educational program preparing expectant parents for childbirth. Using the principles of Grantly Dick-Read, M.D., and the exercises developed by Mabel Lum Fitzhugh, R.P.T., the foundation certifies birthing teachers.

Recommended Reading

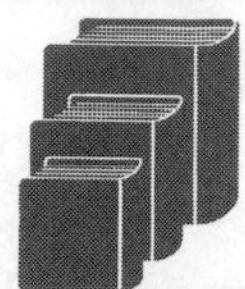

***A Child Is Born*.** Nilsson, L. New York: Dell Publishing, 1990.

A photographic journey from fertilization to birth, including advice and information for parents.

***Birth Without Violence*.** Leboyer, F. New York: Knopf, 1990.

Portrays the harsh experience of the conventional medical birth method as the beginning of the aggression displayed in society today. Maintains that natural child birth encourages the child to venture into the world gracefully based on the child's feelings of trust.

Evolution's End. Chilton Pearce, Joseph. New York: Harper Collins, 1992.

Points to five common practices which have caused rampant violence and deteriorated family and social structures; hospital childbirth, day-care, television, premature attempts at formal education, and synthetic growth hormones in food. Shows the route that needs to be followed to reach the next level of human evolution.

Nutrition in Pregnancy and Lactation. Worthington-Roberts, B.S.; Vermeersch, J.; and Williams, S.R. St. Louis, MO: Times/Mirror Mosby College Publishing, 1985.

A comprehensive book on the nutritional aspects of pregnancy and nursing—somewhat technical and well referenced.

***The Secret Life of The Unborn Child*.** Verny, M.D., Thomas; with Kelly, John. New York: Delacorte Publishing, 1981.

The ways in which you respond to and care for your unborn child may affect his or her physical and emotional well-being for life. The choices you make today about your child's birth may make a vital difference for years to come. This book shows you how you can prepare your unborn baby for a happy, healthy life.

***Spiritual Midwifery*.** Gaskin, I. M. Summertown, TN: The Book Publishing Co., 1980.

A collection of stories by women and midwives about their experience with pregnancy, miscarriage, and childbirth.

***Water Babies*.** Sidenbladh, Eric. New York: St. Martin's Press, 1982.

A book about Igor Ijarkovsky, the Russian researcher, and his innovative method of delivering and training children in water. Includes many photographs of his "swimming babies."

***The Well Pregnancy Book*.** Samuels, M.D. Mike: and Samuels, Nancy. New York: Fireside Books, 1986.

Comprehensive book on pregnancy, labor, and delivery. Covers all physical and emotional stages. Complete information on nutrition, exercise, sex, smoking, caffeine, drugs, and environmental substances.

Wise Woman Herbal for the Childbearing Year. Weed, Susan S. New York: Ash Tree Publishing, 1986.

Comprehensive guide with detailed instructions for sensible herbal use during pregnancy and childbirth.

Pregnancy, Childbirth and the Newborn. Simpkin, P.; Whalley, J.; Kepler, A. New York: Meadowbrook Press, 1991.

A comprehensive guide for parents beginning with gestation, going through childbirth and three months after. Covers everything from nutrition and exercise to medical care and birthing choices.

Respiratory Conditions

For the millions of people with respiratory difficulties, the simple act of breathing can be a constant struggle. Alternative medicine has much to offer such people, however, for many respiratory problems that have defied conventional medicine can be effectively treated through such methods as diet, nutritional supplements, herbal medicine, hydrotherapy, acupuncture, and Traditional Chinese Medicine.

Breathing is almost taken for granted. Yet, as John A. Sherman, N.D., of Portland, Oregon, states, "This constant motion has a profound effect on our overall health. The lungs relentlessly pump oxygen which helps rejuvenate blood vessels, digest food, stimulate the heart, and maximize brain function. The lungs also act as a major eliminative organ, where gaseous exchange can be accomplished."

According to Dr. Sherman, the respiratory system is a complex and sensitive network of organs which provides an immediate link with changes in the atmosphere. There are miles of air passages in the lungs, but by the time air reaches them, it has already been warmed and moistened by the nose, filtered through nose hairs and lymph tissue in the throat, and then constantly refiltered through millions of tiny cilia (hair-like projections along membranous cell tissue) to remove any particles which could damage the lungs.[1]

"We can fast, we can even restrict our fluids for long periods, but without a proper source of oxygen, we're gone in about six minutes," says Dr. Sherman. "This is why breathing properly is so important."

"We can fast, we can even restrict our fluids for long periods, but without a proper source of oxygen, we're gone in about six minutes. This is why breathing properly is so important."

—John A. Sherman, N.D.

Types of Respiratory Conditions and Their Causes

Respiratory problems can be caused by any number of factors, including viral and bacterial infections, pollen, environmental pollution, and smoking, as well as by a poor quality diet, food toxins and allergies, a stressful and inactive lifestyle, and the misuse of antibiotics. Respiratory problems also manifest in a variety of symptoms related to any one of a number of troublesome conditions. These include hay fever, bronchial asthma, bronchitis, pneumonia, sinusitis, emphysema, and lung cancer.

Hay Fever

Allergic rhinitis, or hay fever, affects as many as one out of every ten Americans.[1] It is an allergic condition commonly associated with pollen, but, says Dr. Sherman, "People allergic to pollen are only a subgroup of a larger group of sufferers who are sensitive to all kinds of environmental aggravations, including dust, cat and dog dander, mold spores, foods, medications, insect bites, even perfume. These allergens can affect a person all year round and cause a host of symptoms, including hives, eczema, digestive disorders, breathing difficulties, swelling, headaches, and even chronic fatigue syndrome."

According to Dr. Sherman, hay fever is a disorder of the immune system. "Just as the immune system is activated by a virus or bacteria, it also interprets a grain of pollen or dust particle as

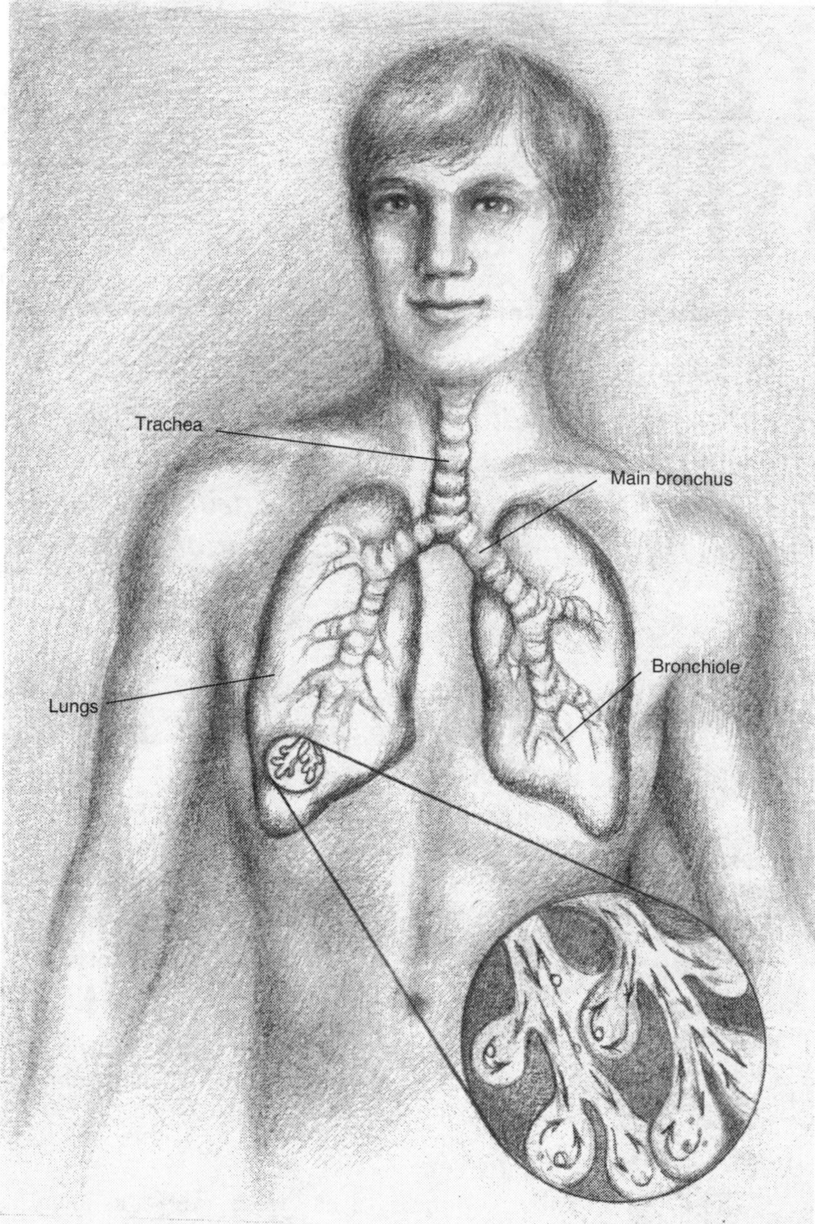

The respiratory system.

an intruder," he says. "Thus, whenever a person already has a weakened immune system from dealing with chronic food allergies or a vitamin deficiency such as for vitamin C, it tends to create a more severe reaction to the pollen."

The immune system can also be weakened by other sources of environmental pollution such as cigarette smoke, auto exhaust, or house dust. "People wondering if their runny noses and itchy eyes are caused by the common cold or by hay fever need to remember an allergic reaction will more often than not produce clear secretions, no fever, and bouts of multiple sneezes," Dr. Sherman adds.

Asthma

Asthma is the leading cause of disease and disability in children and teens ages two to seventeen years. It is also relatively common among all age groups, occurring in one out of forty people, with 65 percent of sufferers developing symptoms before the age of five.[3]

Asthma generally manifests itself in the form of an asthma attack. Between these attacks, an asthmatic will usually seem perfectly healthy. An attack is characterized by a narrowing of the bronchial passages, along with an excessive excretion of mucous, resulting in impaired breathing, with the severity of the symptoms often accelerating rapidly. "The greater the obstruction, the more difficult breathing will become," notes Dr. Sherman.

An attack will usually begin with an unproductive cough, followed by rapidly progressing difficulty in breathing. While the respiratory rate does not increase, expiration becomes prolonged and labored, resulting in wheezing that can often be heard from a distance.[4]

A number of allergic and environmental agents can bring on asthma attacks, including pollen, dust, mold, animal dander, feathers, textiles such as cotton and flax, detergents, petrochemicals, air pollution, and smoke. According to James Braly, M.D., Medical Director of the Immuno Labs in Fort Lauderdale, Florida, wheat, milk, and eggs are among the most likely foods that will trigger an asthma attack. He adds that chemical additives such as food coloring and food preservatives can also be at fault. Sensitivity to aspirin, exposure to cold air, and exercise can also prompt an asthmatic reaction.

See Allergies, Environmental Medicine.

Dr. Sherman points out that asthma that originates during infancy is generally due to food allergies; when it strikes between ages ten to thirty, it is usually due to inhalants; and when it occurs after age forty-five, it is commonly due to infections. "These factors can exist at any age and in any combination, however," he says.

He also notes that asthma attacks that occur only in the summer are normally caused by pollens or mold spores, while those that occur only in winter are usually due to infections. And attacks that occur at night tend to be emotionally related and may be due to suppressed anger.

In addition, up to 90 percent of asthmatics are or were mouth breathers (versus breathing through the nose), making it much easier for dust, pollution, organisms, and cold air to enter the lungs. Breath retraining can be of immense help in alleviating this additional cause of asthma.[5]

Bronchitis

Bronchitis refers to a severe inflammation of the bronchial tubes, with symptoms ranging from chills, fever, and coughing, to difficulty breathing and pain in the chest. Dr. Sherman identifies two types of bronchitis, acute and chronic. Acute bronchitis is a mild, short attack, sometimes accompanied by a secondary bacterial infection, while chronic bronchitis is characterized by constant inflammation, often accompanied by irritation of the bronchi, but without any infectious component.

> *"While antibiotics have greatly reduced fatality rates for pneumonia patients, their use has expanded the range of pathogens responsible for the disease."*

Bronchitis can be caused by infection, exposure to cold, or noxious agents. It is seen much more commonly in the winter as it usually follows some form of upper respiratory infection, such as a cold. In addition, notes Dr. Sherman, food or chemical allergies can provoke symptoms of bronchitis. Smokers or those exposed to excessive second-hand smoke may also be more vulnerable to chronic bronchitis.

Pneumonia

Pneumonia is defined as a severe inflammation of the lungs. It ranks as the fifth leading cause of death in the United States, leading all other infectious diseases in mortality.[6] It is particularly threatening for the elderly, according to Dr. Sherman.

"Like bronchitis, pneumonia is much more common during the winter months," Dr. Sherman says. "It is also a frequent complication of other serious illnesses, and is the most widespread of all fatal hospital-acquired infections. Symptoms include chest pain, coughing, difficulty in breathing, shortness of breath, fever, and single episodes of (but not persistent) shaking chills."

Joseph Pizzorno, N.D., co-founder and President of Bastyr College in Seattle, Washington, reports that pneumonia is usually seen in immune-compromised persons, including drug and alcohol abusers. People with HIV are especially vulnerable to the disease. Chronic lung diseases and debilitating illnesses can also cause pneumonia, as well as the use of immunosuppressive drugs or respiratory therapy.

Bacteria, fungi, and viruses can also be at fault, notes Dr. Sherman. The typical organisms which cause pneumonia are pneumococcus, staph, strep, klebsiella, *E. coli*, proteus, pseudomonas, hemophilus, and fungi. "Patients with bacterial pneumonia, though, are much more likely to have complications such as lung abscesses, pleurisy (inflammation of membrane enfolding the lungs),

FINDING THE ROOT CAUSE OF INFECTION

Conventional medicine usually considers bacterial or viral infection as the cause of congestion in the lungs. Many alternative physicians believe, however, that infection is instead the result of congestion in the lungs.

"Organisms only grow in the body when the 'soil' is right," explains John A. Sherman, N.D., of Portland, Oregon. "In the lungs, that means that congestion provides fruitful soil for the growth of infection. By only removing the infection, we do not solve the underlying problem."

David L. Hoffmann, B.Sc., M.N.I.M.H., past President of the American Herbalist Guild, adds, "One factor most often related to congestion is the quantity of mucous in the diet. If the body gets too much mucous-forming food, it increases secretion into the lungs as part of the natural cleansing process. Yet, if we inhibit the production of secretions with antibiotics, we can nurture congestion in the future and perhaps sow the seeds for chronic, degenerative diseases."

Respiratory difficulties that thrive on excessive mucous, such as asthma, suggest a diet low in mucous-forming foods. Dr. Sherman advises restricting the intake of dairy products (including goat's milk and yogurt), eggs, gluten-rich grains (wheat, oats, rye, and barley), sugar, potatoes, and other starchy root vegetables. Fresh fruits and their juices are good replacements.

and spread of infection through the bloodstream to other organs," Dr. Sherman says.

While antibiotics have greatly reduced fatality rates for pneumonia patients, their use has expanded the range of pathogens responsible for the disease, notes Dr. Sherman. This is especially true of hospitalized patients because the pathogens are more resistant to commonly used antibiotics.[7]

Sinusitis

Sinusitis is an unpleasant and often painful aggravation of the common cold or hay fever, resulting from the inflammation or infection of the air-filled bony cavities that surround the nasal passages. According to Richard Barrett, N.D., Associate Academic Dean of the National College of Naturopathic Medicine, in Portland, Oregon, negative pressure from trapped oxygen can build up inside the sinuses, causing extreme pain. If this swelling remains for any length of time, nature responds by filling the sinus cavity with a thin fluid excreted through the pores of the mucous membrane. This becomes an ideal medium for bacterial growth.

"The classic symptoms of a sinus infection are general malaise, fever, thick discharge from the nose, a nasal voice, and facial pain or headache that is aggravated by bending forward," states Dr. Barrett. He points out that only a small percentage of colds progress to sinusitis, however.

With chronic sinusitis, prolonged or repeated inflammation in the nasal passages can lead to a degeneration in the tissues that make up the sinus' mucous membrane, hampering the ability of the sinus to drain properly. The main symptoms of this condition are a dull pain over the involved sinus, persistent nasal congestion, thick discharge, chronic postnasal drip, and a diminished sense of smell. "Chronic sinusitis is rarely the result of an infectious process, although sufferers are at risk for acute infectious episodes," Dr. Barrett says.

Emphysema

Emphysema is characterized by a permanent enlargement of the air sacs and ducts in the lungs, along with destruction of the walls of these air spaces. In addition, there is a loss of the small blood vessels that supply these spaces, resulting in the lung tissue becoming inflamed and hardened.

According to Dr. Sherman, these changes are what produce the "barrel chest" effect common among emphysema sufferers, who are often referred to as "pink-puffers" because of the diffi-

THE HAZARDS OF SMOKING

It is no secret that smoking poses numerous health risks. The following is a brief list of some of the harmful effects associated with smoking.

- *Each cigarette steals away eight minutes of life.*
- *A pack a day equates to losing a month of life each year, and two packs a day means twelve to sixteen years off life expectancy for lifetime smokers.*
- *Just one cigarette can increase the heart rate twenty to twenty-five beats per minute and can increase blood pressure significantly.*
- *Cigarettes contain four thousand known toxic poisons.*
- *Smoking one pack of cigarettes a day depletes more vitamin C (five hundred milligrams) than most people ingest in a day.*
- *Cigarettes increase carbon monoxide levels in the blood, which compete with oxygen so thoroughly that it takes the circulatory system six hours to return to normal after smoking just one cigarette.*
- *Smoking is so immunosuppressive that it takes three months to reverse its damage to the immune system.*[8]

In addition, a direct link has been found between lung cancer and flue-dried tobacco, especially that to which sugar has been added, while no significant correlation between traditional sugar-free, air-dried tobacco and cancer has been found. Studies show that England and Wales, which have the highest male lung cancer rate in the world, also have the highest sugar content in cigarettes, about 17 percent. France, where tobacco is air-dried and contains only 2 percent sugar, has one-third less lung cancer. The United States, where sugar in tobacco averages 10 percent, has about half the male lung cancer death rate as Great Britain.[9]

Secondary cigarette smoke inhaled by nonsmokers can also pose health hazards. According to a recent report by the Environmental Protection Agency, it has been linked to 20 percent of all lung cancer in the United States not directly attributed to smoking. This equates to approximately 3,000 lung cancer deaths each year among nonsmokers. This risk is doubled for nonsmoking spouses married to people who smoke. Secondary smoking also causes 150,000 to 300,000 cases of respiratory illness, such as pneumonia, bronchitis, and asthma among infants and young children. Another study from the National Center for Health Statistics shows that babies are three times more likely to die if their mothers smoked during and after pregnancy.[10]

culty they have breathing. Symptoms of emphysema include wheezing, a hard and spasmodic cough, copious sputum (the substance produced by coughing or clearing the throat) production, as well as difficulty in breathing, varying from mild exertion to a marked lack of oxygen even while resting. Even the mere act of conversation by people with emphysema can initiate coughing attacks, Dr. Sherman notes.

The single major cause of emphysema is cigarette smoking,[11] with the risk running higher as the number of packs and years of smoking increase. Certain types of environmental pollutants are also linked with an increased incidence of emphysema, including cadmium fumes, which can be found in high concentrations in tobacco smoke as well. Emphysema has also been associated with gastric or duodenal ulcers (ulceration in the first part of the small intestine) caused by increased respiratory acidosis, an acidic condition caused by an insufficient supply of oxygen to the lungs that results in the retention of carbon dioxide.[12]

Lung Cancer

Lung cancer is the most common form of cancer in both men and women, and also the number one cause of death by cancer for either group, with the figures rapidly rising for women.[13]

The factors most responsible for causing lung cancer are cigarette smoking and air pollution, as well as exposure to toxic industrial materials such as asbestos, coal tars, and chemical pollutants.[14] Low levels of beta-carotene (a precursor to vitamin A in the body) has also been directly associated with the development of human lung cancer.[15]

Most patients with lung cancer acquire a cough as their first symptom, according to Dr. Sherman. "Those who already have a cough may note a change in its severity or character," he says. "Other symptoms can include feverishness, chills, sweating, weakness, loss of appetite, and weight loss, but in some 10 percent of cases, there may be no symptoms. Often a chest x-ray will be the only indication of a problem, and thus can provide the greatest likelihood of an early detection." Up to 70 percent of all cases can also be diagnosed from a sputum sample.[16]

See Cancer for a more in-depth discussion of lung cancer and alternative cancer treatments.

HAY FEVER "ADVANCE" PREVENTION

To lessen the effects of environmental allergens on hay fever victims, John A. Sherman, N.D., of Portland, Oregon, advises maintaining an active "advance" prevention program. This is done by determining what time of year to expect certain allergens and symptoms. "If you know when to expect allergens, you can start treating yourself for several weeks in advance of exposure," Dr. Sherman says.

"Test for specific allergens in your 'off season', while your immune system is at its peak," adds Dr. Sherman. Serum levels, applied kinesiology, and measuring changes in galvanic skin response are the testing methods he recommends using.

Leon Chaitow, N.D., D.O., of London, England, also reports that in Europe it is common for hay fever sufferers, sensitive to pollen, to start taking pollen extract supplements a few months before the season in which they are most likely to be troubled. This effectively desensitizes patients and usually reduces their symptoms dramatically, he says.

Treatment of Respiratory Conditions

A variety of alternative treatments exist for respiratory conditions, including diet and nutrition, herbal medicine, hydrotherapy, homeopathy, and acupuncture.

Hay Fever

An allergic reaction to airborne pollens, animal dander, dust, or foods, hay fever traditionally has been remedied with antihistamines, or other drugs given orally or as nose drops. The following treatments may offer relief for hay fever sufferers with fewer side effects.

Diet and Nutrition: A diet of high-fiber, whole foods including a generous amounts of fruits (non-citrus), vegetables, grains, nuts, and raw seeds may be helpful in combatting hay fever and reducing mucous production in the sinuses. It is also helpful to drink lots of fluids. Raw juices, in particular, are beneficial, particularly carrot, celery, beet, cucumber, spinach, and parsley.

Since hay fever is allergy-related, according to Dr. Sherman, it is best to avoid dairy products, wheat, eggs, citrus fruits, chocolate, peanuts, and shellfish, which are common allergens.

"Food coloring can also cause hay fever and sinus congestion," notes Dr. Braly. "These should also be avoided, as well as all preservatives, especially metasulfites, which are often used to keep food fresh in restaurants. Also eliminate caffeine, alcohol, tobacco, and sugar."

Dr. Braly also recommends nutrient supplementation for hay fever sufferers, particularly of

THE EFFECTIVENESS OF A "VEGAN" DIET FOR TREATING RESPIRATORY CONDITIONS

Joseph E. Pizzorno, N.D., President of Bastyr College in Seattle, Washington, has found that a vegan diet (elimination of all animal products, including dairy) can have a long-term positive effective on respiratory conditions, primarily asthma. In one study, Dr. Pizzorno noted significant improvement in 92 percent of twenty-five patients treated with a vegan diet.

The diet excluded all meat, fish, eggs, and dairy products, and drinking water was limited to spring water. Chlorinated tap water was specifically prohibited, as were coffee, tea, chocolate, sugar, and salt. Herbal spices and one and a half liters of herbal teas a day were allowed.

Vegetables used freely were lettuce, carrots, beets, onions, celery, cabbage, cauliflower, broccoli, cucumber, radishes, Jerusalem artichokes, and all beans except soy and green peas.

A number of fruits were allowed, including blueberries, strawberries, raspberries, cloudberries, black currants, gooseberries, plums, and pears. Apples and citrus fruits were not allowed. Grains were either eliminated or very restricted.

Additionally, Dr. Pizzorno says that 71 percent of the patients showed favorable results from the diet within just four months, and after one year a 92 percent success rate was reached.

vitamins A, C, and E, MaxEPA (an essential fatty acid), evening primrose oil, and vitamins B_5 (pantothenic acid) and B_6 (pyridoxine). He has used coenzyme Q10, raw thymus glandular, bee pollen, royal jelly, geranium, and zinc to good effect as well. Multivitamin/mineral tablets are also used as a simple supplement for children.

Dr. Braly recalls treating one hay fever patient who felt as though he were under attack from all sides. "He was sniffling, which he remarked was his permanent reaction to pollen, dust, cigarette smoke, and the sulfites in many foods. His hands were covered with a fiery rash, and he was having frightening bouts of lightheadedness. He'd been to several doctors already and was leery of adding even more medications to the several he was already taking."

Dr. Braly traced the man's light-headedness to petrochemicals in the drapes and rug of his new office. The man was also diagnosed with eleven food allergies. The allergic foods were eliminated from his diet, he began a program of aggressive supplementation to boost his immunity, and the offending drapes and rug were replaced with slatted blinds and tile.

"Eight months later, the patient's symptoms were so improved that for the first time in his life, he didn't have to carry around a packet of Kleenex like a 'security blanket,'" reports Dr. Braly.

Herbal Medicine: Dr. Sherman reports that the *Urtica* species of plants (nettle) has recently been reported as having the ability to clear the sinuses, and can greatly reduce the symptoms of hay fever. Tincture of licorice is also often recommended. One-half to one teaspoon should be taken in warm water twice daily, five days a week. This regimen is believed to be most effective if it's initiated a month before the season when symptoms usually appear.

A combination of the herbs black cohosh, skullcap, pleurisy, catnip, and red pepper have also proved effective for hay fever sufferers, according to Dr. Sherman. He also suggests a teaspoon of horseradish diluted in water and taken slowly over several hours to drain and help dry out the sinuses.

Comfrey tea and fenugreek tea taken daily can be beneficial to hay fever sufferers, as well, as can the fresh juice of coriander. Other herbs found to be effective include ginger root, angelica, astragalus, dandelion root, eyebright, goldenseal, ephedra, and mullein.

Hydrotherapy: Leon Chaitow, N.D., D.O., of London, England, recommends a variety of hydrotherapy methods that are useful in helping to decongest the sinuses. These include nasal lavage, in which a mixture of warm salt water is inhaled through the nostrils, alternating hot and cold compresses, hot foot baths, and steam inhalations.

Asthma

The advantages of using natural methods instead of conventional treatments for asthma are obvious, according to Dr. Sherman. The most common medications used by conventional medicine in the treatment of asthma include prednisone, a cortisone derivative, which can cause severe adverse reactions, including fluid and electrolyte disturbances, muscle weakness, peptic ulcers, impaired wound healing, headaches and dizziness, menstrual irregularities, and glaucoma. Prednisone may also help manifest latent diabetes.[17] Approaches such as diet and nutrition, herbal medicine, and hydrotherapy have shown positive results in the treatment of asthma, without the negative side effects associated with drug-based therapies.

Diet and Nutrition: "Strengthening the immune system is of primary concern in the treatment of asthma," states Dr. Braly. This can be accomplished by eliminating allergens in foods, correcting digestive problems, establishing the proper balance of essential fatty acids, such as those found in cold water fish, and supplying other nutrients important to the immune system.

In addition, good dietary management needs to be maintained in order to resist asthma. According to Dr. Braly, this can be accomplished by rotating the diet, and avoiding all artificial colorings (especially FD&C Yellow No. 5—tartrazine) and flavorings. He also advises avoiding caffeine, alcohol, tobacco, sugar, and all preservatives.

In addition to eliminating allergic foods, Alan Gaby, M.D., President-elect of the American Holistic Medical Association, suggests supplementing the diet with nutrients such as vitamins C, B_6, B_{12}, niacinamide, magnesium chloride, and calcium glycerophosphate. For acute asthma attacks, he recommends an intravenous injection of these same vitamins and minerals. Other nutrients of direct benefit to asthmatic patients include quercetin (a flavonoid found in onions), beta-carotene, selenium, and manganese.

Bee pollen has also proven helpful for some asthmatics affected by airborne allergens, according to Dr. Sherman. He points out that cases of asthma associated with low blood sugar also respond well to a hypoglycemic diet. This diet seems to especially help exercise-induced asthma.[18]

In addition, if asthma is due to a high-stress lifestyle, Dr. Sherman recommends adding half a teaspoon each of sea salt and baking soda to a sweet drink or juice for immediate relief. Research has also found that many patients are able to reduce their incidence of asthma attacks by taking one tablespoon of olive oil twice daily.[19]

Dr. Sherman reports that it may also be possible to remedy asthmatic patients' excess stomach acid with the use of hydrochloric acid or apple cider vinegar. This treatment eliminates the risk of exposing the patients to food allergies, which might weaken their immune systems and make them more vulnerable to asthma attacks.[20]

Herbal Medicine: Dr. Sherman recommends several herbal remedies for asthmatics which can be taken in the form of teas or tinctures. Among these are ephedra (in its natural rather than concentrated form), which he calls a very effective "bronchodilator," especially when combined with thyme, which acts as an antispasmodic.

Mullein tea soothes the mucous membranes and is especially good for night attacks. It can be combined with marshmallow and slippery elm tea for an additional mucous-secreting effect. Dr. Sherman also recommends passion flower tea or tincture for cases of asthma due to tension or nervous conditions.

TRADITIONAL CHINESE MEDICINE AND ASTHMA

Mark Cooper, N.D., L.Ac., of Portland, Oregon, recalls treating a woman suffering from a case of constant, acute asthma attacks. Using a variety of natural therapies including herbs, homeopathy, and spinal manipulation, he was able to alleviate only about half the symptoms. As a last resort, a cone of moxibustion (a Chinese herb) was placed over a specific acupuncture point on the woman's chest, on the lower part of the breast bone. The herb was then lit and burned until the patient could no longer stand the heat.

According to Traditional Chinese Medicine, this particular treatment is performed only once, but Dr. Cooper reports that the results in this case were dramatic and long lasting. The woman became free of her dependency on oxygen or any other medication, and gradually improved to the point where only mild wheezing was present. Dr. Cooper adds that this method can also be used in emergencies to alleviate difficult breathing in asthmatics.

According to Dr. Pizzorno, licorice root, Indian tobacco, capsaicin (cayenne pepper's major active component), skunk cabbage, gumweed, horse chestnut, jujube plum, green tea, onions, and garlic are also valuable aids for those suffering from asthma.

Hydrotherapy: For asthma sufferers, Dr. Sherman advises hot fomentations to the chest, especially for those suffering from acute attacks. He recommends combining these with hot foot baths, with the head kept cool with a fan or with cool water. The body should be covered up with wool or cotton blankets.

Dr. Sherman adds that Russian baths (a sauna with the head left outside the cabinet or steam bath) can also be very effective, but it is important the patient not get chilled afterward.

A twenty-minute hydrogen peroxide bath can help relieve asthma attacks as well, according to Dr. Sherman. Fill a bathtub with water at 98 to 100 degrees Fahrenheit. Add thirteen to sixteen ounces of hydrogen peroxide and soak while the release of oxygen relieves symptoms. Afterward, be sure to rest.

Bronchitis

In most cases of bronchitis it is important for mucous to be cleared from the lungs. Coughing can help this, notes Dr. Sherman, therefore cough suppressants should be avoided unless the patient is extremely weak from lack of sleep. Patients who cough once a minute for twenty minutes have shown a 41 percent clearance of mucous from the lungs in x-rays.[21] Deep breathing has also been shown to encourage mucous removal.

Diet and Nutrition: For bronchitis sufferers, Dr. Sherman first advises eating hot, spicy foods which open the air passages to bring relief. These foods include garlic, onion, chili peppers, horseradish, and mustard. Dairy products, starches, sugars, and eggs should be avoided in order to produce less mucous. In addition, a whole foods diet will strengthen the immune system, and drinking lots of fresh fluids is essential.

Dr. Sherman reports that vitamin A has been shown to be effective in relieving bronchitis, as have vitamins C and E. Zinc, proteolytic enzymes (taken between meals), garlic, thymus, selenium, and bioflavonoids are other very beneficial supplements.

Herbal Medicine: "Dry, irritating bronchitic coughing can be eased with a mixture of equal parts dried mullein, coltsfoot, and anise seed, drunk as a hot infusion several times a day," says David L. Hoffmann, B.Sc., M.N.I.M.H., of Sebastapol, California, past President of the American Herbalist Guild. Elecampane, horehound, goldenseal, echinacea, raw garlic, and ginseng are other medicinal herbs which have proven beneficial.

Dr. Sherman recommends a blend of poke root, licorice, echinacea, grindelia, and lobelia taken as a tea or tincture three to four times daily. This formula can be obtained from most naturopathic physicians or herbalists.

Hydrotherapy: Doug Lewis, N.D., Chair of Physical Medicine of Bastyr College in Seattle, Washington, recommends that bronchitis patients receive a cold friction rub or hyperthermia, applied every forty-eight hours. Walking (treading) in cold water for a few minutes daily to strengthen the body is also useful, as are full, hot baths taken for twenty to sixty minutes.

Pneumonia

According to Dr. Sherman, generally it takes a patient between two and three weeks to recover from pneumonia. Fever may come and go as well before any definitive treatment and recovery is completed.

Diet and Nutrition: For pneumonia, Dr. Sherman first advises patients to remove all known food allergens from the diet, and to drink plenty of fluids and fresh juices. "Diluted pear juice is especially effective at loosening up congestion in the lungs," he notes. "The juice of green and yellow vegetables and fruits is also beneficial, including lemon juice. Dairy products and processed food products should be avoided, though." He adds that fresh garlic, cayenne pepper, and chili peppers have proven effective against pneumonia, as well.

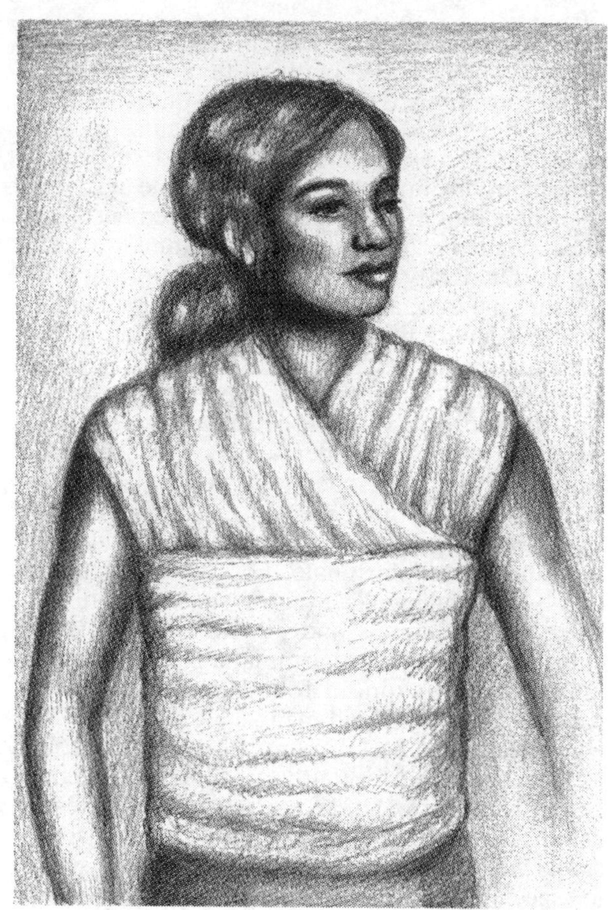

Pneumonia jacket.

Vitamins A and C, beta-carotene, zinc, proteolytic enzymes (taken between meals), acidophilus, bioflavonoids, thymus extract, and propolis are additional nutrients that have been found by Dr. Sherman to be of value in battling pneumonia.

Herbal Medicine: Dr. Sherman lists the following herbal remedies as being valuable for easing pneumonia symptoms: lobelia and sanguinaria used as expectorants, hydrastis as an infection fighter, plus the antiviral herbs arctostaphylos, uva ursi, *Cephaelis ipecacuanha*, *Hypericum perforatum*, *Juniperus communis*, and *Piper cubeba*.

Hydrotherapy: According to Dr. Sherman, pneumonia can be greatly relieved by using a "pneumonia jacket," applied by a professional. He recounts the case of one patient who "would almost beat the door down to get into the clinic to receive his daily treatment." It was the only thing that helped him feel human after three weeks of taking decongestants, antibiotics, and cough suppressants. Every treatment brought him closer and closer to health. By beating on his back with cupped hands after the jacket treatment I could loosen the mucous far more effectively for him than could any decongestant."

Dr. Sherman recommends that the jacket treatment be combined with a hot foot bath and a cold compress to the forehead. The feet should not be chilled. Patients with strong vitality should follow the jacket treatment with a cold mitten friction rub. This should be done after the chest is thoroughly reddened (about twenty minutes), and the feet are warmed.

Acupuncture: William Michael Cargile, L.Ac., D.C., F.I.A.C.A., Chairman of Research of the American Association of Acupuncture, has had dramatic success using acupuncture in the treatment of pneumonia. Dr. Cargile recalls a man who mistakenly took Chinese weight loss herbs designed for another person, who had a completely different constitution. The patient developed pneumonia almost immediately, and conventional medical treatment could not cure him, even after three weeks. "His condition was such that he could not lie down and had to sleep sitting up in a chair in order to breathe," Dr. Cargile says. "When he came to me, he had so much fluid in his lungs that his respiratory capacity was only about 40 percent."

After only one treatment session with Dr. Cargile, the patient was coughing up chunks of red, fleshy sputum, and within two days had returned to 80 percent of his normal breathing capacity.

Sinusitis

According to Dr. Barrett, dealing with sinusitis should begin with adequate treatment of hay fever and colds. "It is much easier to treat sinusitis in its early stages, before bacterial infections set in," he says. He attributes the prevalence of chronic sinusitis to the fact that Western medicine has been so unsuccessful in its treatment. As he states, "Conventional treatment is the province of ear, nose, and throat specialists. They employ a variety of antihistamines, decongestants, and antibiotics. If the condition persists, the last resort is surgery, cutting away the swollen mucous membrane and attempting to establish artificial drainage pathways."

Dr. Barrett recommends a different approach which addresses the root causes of the condition through diagnosis of allergies, regulation of diet, and other alternative methods. He advises that people prone to suffer from sinusitis first of all ensure that they get sufficient rest and a follow a simple diet which avoids sugar and any possible allergic foods.

Diet and Nutrition: At the onset of an acute sinusitis attack, Dr. Barrett often recommends a water fast, which frees the body to use its energy to fight the infection instead of digesting food. Otherwise, he advises a very light diet

Alleviating Environmental Stress

According to Richard Barrett, N.D., Associate Academic Dean of the National College of Naturopathic Medicine in Portland, Oregon, sinusitis can be caused or aggravated by environmental chemicals such as ozone, carbon monoxide, and nitrogen dioxide, which impact the immune system and make allergies more likely. Chronic sinusitis sufferers, therefore, should avoid living in cities which are extremely polluted. "If living in an urban area cannot be helped, avoid living near freeways, major roadways, and industrial parks," Dr. Barrett suggests.

Indoor air pollution can be as much of a problem for sinusitis, as well. "Whether you live in an existing home or plan to build, many choices in furnishings and building materials will affect your health," says Dr. Barrett. In general, he advises avoiding materials that are synthetic or plastic, as these tend to emit gas. Secondhand cigarette smoke, which is high in several toxic chemicals, including carbon monoxide and cadmium, is another all too common source of indoor air pollution.

Dust, which contains spores, animal dander, mites, pollen, plaster, bacteria, and viruses, is another major contributor to indoor air pollution. Dr. Barrett recommends the following in order to minimize the effects of dust:

- *Remove rugs and stuffed toys from bedrooms and damp dust twice a week.*
- *Change filters in heating systems regularly and have them cleaned professionally.*
- *Vacuum regularly with either a central system that vents dust away from the living areas, or use a water-trap vacuum which captures dust.*
- *Install air filters in heating systems or use free-standing ones to filter out dust from the air.*

Leon Chaitow, N.D., D.O., of London, England, points out that green plants with lots of foliage placed around the home act as extremely efficient agents for detoxifying the air due to their ability to absorb toxic chemicals such as formaldehyde.

which emphasizes fruits and vegetable broth. Concentrated sugars should be especially avoided since they slow down immune functions and encourage bacterial activity. "The basic rule is to follow your natural appetite," he explains. "If you don't feel hungry, don't eat."

Dr. Barrett also recommends the following regimen of nutritional supplementation for sufferers of sinusitis:

- **Vitamin A:** 50,000 IUs per day for one week only, or beta-carotene: 200,000 IUs per day.
- **Vitamin C:** One gram per hour to bowel tolerance.
- **Vitamin E:** 400 IUs per day.
- **Zinc:** Fifty milligrams per day.

For cases of chronic sinusitis, Dr. Barrett suggests also including selenium (two hundred micrograms per day), N-acetyl cysteine (five hundred milligrams per day), bioflavonoids (one to two grams per day), essential fatty acids in the form of evening primrose oil, black currant oil, or flaxseed oil, and vitamin B_5.

Chronic sinusitis sufferers should also avoid foods to which they have allergies or sensitivities. Proper digestion and elimination of stress are also crucial.

Herbal Medicine: Among the herbal remedies Dr. Barrett recommends are purple coneflower, ephedra, goldenseal, Oregon grape, horseradish, poke root, yarrow, garlic, wild indigo, and elder flowers.

According to Dr. Barrett, a good herbal formula for acute sinusitis is made using one part each of tinctures of eyebright, goldenseal, yarrow, horseradish, and ephedra. "Proper dosage is thirty drops every two hours for two days, then four times a day until symptoms are gone," he says.

Dr. Barrett also suggests an herbal formula for sinusitis attacks accompanied by infection: two parts of purple coneflower, two parts of wild indigo, and one part of poke root. Proper dosage is thirty drops every hour until the condition improves, then four times daily.

Other herbs Dr. Barrett recommends are stinging nettle, elder flowers, goldenrod (as a tincture), and eyebright compound.

Hydrotherapy: "Hydrotherapy is the most underrated of natural therapies," Dr. Barrett says, adding that hydrotherapy is invaluable for the treatment of sinusitis. In the early stages of sinusitis, he especially recommends nasal lavage using salt water and steam inhalations to loosen nasal secretions. This process cleanses the nasal passages and assists the sinuses in draining.

An alternative method for nasal lavage, according to Dr. Barrett, is to use one teaspoon of powdered goldenseal mixed in a cup of warm water. He also recommends hot foot baths with a cold compress placed over the affected sinuses. A hot compress can be applied over the sinuses for three minutes, followed by a cold compress for thirty seconds, as well. Repeat at least three times, being sure to finish with the cold application.

Inhaling steam is another treatment suggested by Dr. Barrett. Bend over a quart of boiling water and cover the head with a towel while inhaling the steam. Unless a homeopathic remedy is being used, small amounts of aromatic herbs like mint or eucalyptus can be added to the hot water. Cold water vaporizers are also useful.

Homeopathy: Sinusitis can also be treated with homeopathy, many times as a form of self-care. "A reasonable approach to home treatment would be to match the remedy with your symptoms, and then take two pellets of 30c potency taken every three to four hours, apart from food and other medicines, until symptoms abate," Dr. Barrett explains. "Afterward, repeat less frequently as needed. If none of these remedies seem to match the symptoms, seek out a homeopathic practitioner for treatment."

The following are some of the main homeopathic remedies for acute sinusitis:

- ***Arsenicum album:*** Use if the discharge is thin, watery, and burning as it comes out of the nose; the condition worsens with exposure to the open air; or there is a tendency to feel chilly, a desire for warm drinks and a sense of restlessness and anxiety.
- ***Kalium bichromium:*** Use if there is a feeling of pressure at the root of the nose and a foul smell or loss of smell; if the frontal sinuses are chronically stuffed up, with constant postnasal drip and nasal obstruction; or if the symptoms are relieved by warm applications, and worsen from exposure to cold damp air.
- ***Nux vomica:*** Use if passages are stuffed up, especially at night and outdoors; if frontal headaches are experienced, which ease with pressure placed against them; or if patients are chilly, irritable, and cannot bear noises or light.
- ***Mercurius iodatus:*** Use if nostrils are raw and ulcerated, if patients are worse at night, and suffer from extremes of temperature, either hot or cold; if the nasal discharge is yellow/green and tinged with blood; or if patients perspire easily which aggravates the condition.
- ***Silicea:*** Use if there are dry hard crusts in the nose which bleed easily, as well as pain experienced over the frontal and maxillary sinuses; if the nasal bones are

sensitive to touch; if the nose is obstructed with a loss of smell. *Silicea* types are also not very gritty or resilient, and they tend to be fair-skinned and very sensitive to the cold.

Acupuncture: According to Dr. Cargile, conditions of sinusitis are often linked to toxins in the bowel and intestines. "To effectively treat sinusitis, you want to stimulate the body to detoxify, so that it will raise its energy," he explains. "Once this happens, often the sinusitis will be better within minutes. And in some cases, the relief will last for weeks, and sometimes months, without the need for further treatments."

Dr. Cargile states that he has never had a patient with sinusitis who has not responded to acupuncture treatments. "And the irony is that in almost all of my sinusitis cases, I'm the last guy the patients came to, and everything else they tried, including the pharmaceutical treatments, failed," he says.

One of Dr. Cargile's patients was a female tennis player who was stricken with sinusitis in the midst of competing in a tournament. "She was trying to reach the finals, and was having severe difficulty because of how excruciating her symptoms were and the way her eyes were tearing," he says. She received one treatment from Dr. Cargile and gained immediate relief, remaining well throughout the rest of the tournament. After receiving an additional seven treatments spaced over three weeks, the woman's sinusitis completely cleared up and has not returned.

Emphysema

According to Dr. Sherman, the first and foremost thing that must be done in order to combat emphysema is to immediately stop smoking. Once that is accomplished, the alternative therapies outlined in this section will be much more effective.

Diet and Nutrition: "An increased quantity of raw foods in the diet will prove beneficial, as will hot and spicy foods such as garlic, onions, chili peppers, horseradish, and mustard," says Dr. Sherman. "Cold-pressed olive oil can be taken daily as well, and seaweed may also bring substantial relief."

Dr. Sherman advises avoiding mucous-forming foods such as dairy products, salt, eggs, meat, processed foods, "junk foods," and white flour products. He has found that grapes and raw grape juice provide beneficial aid, as do the raw juices from other fruits, including oranges, lemons, and black currants. "Raw vegetable juices such as carrot, spinach, celery, and watercress are strongly recommended, as well, and are even more beneficial when a small amount of garlic juice is added to them," he says. In crisis situations, Dr. Sherman suggests a three- to ten-day fast, drinking only vegetable juices.

Nutritional supplements recommended for the treatment of emphysema include zinc and vitamin B_6, to chelate cadmium; vitamin E, for decreasing the patient's dependence on oxygen tank therapy;[23] lethicin, to reduce the surface tension of fluids in the lungs, enabling easier elimination;[24] and vitamins A and C, protein, and folic acid, to help reestablish connective tissue elasticity. Chlorophyll, coenzyme Q10, L-cysteine, L-methionine, and vitamin B_{12} are also beneficial, according to Dr. Sherman.

Herbal Medicine: For emphysema sufferers, Dr. Sherman recommends a variety of herbal remedies. Coltsfoot tea is effective in helping raise and eliminate mucous. Anise oil mixed with

THREE THERAPIES TO HELP STOP SMOKING

John A. Sherman, N.D., of Portland, Oregon, suggests the combination of these three therapies to aid smokers in giving up their life-threatening addiction.

Aversion therapy: *Stop smoking except for one hour daily. Smoke constantly during that hour. Take fifteen drops of lobelia tincture a half-hour before the first cigarette and again at fifteen minutes before the last cigarette. Take this same quantity of lobelia tincture every fifteen minutes during the remainder of the smoking hour. This will produce nausea. Its association with smoking can eliminate the desire for cigarettes in just five to six days, according to Dr. Sherman.*

Hydrotherapy: *A simple Epsom salt bath, using a half a pound of salt per bath, helps pull nicotine and tar from the skin to prevent its introduction into the bloodstream. Shower or bathe normally after the Epsom salt bath to rinse them off. Dry with a white towel. The brownish residue of nicotine excreted by the skin visually enforces the desire and need to stop smoking. Exercise and colonic irrigations may also be useful in helping the body to eliminate toxins from smoking.*

Nutritional supplements: *The best withdrawal diet is a hypoglycemic diet which maintains constant blood sugar and avoids developing a flood of food cravings. This diet consists of six meals a day, largely consisting of fresh fruits, vegetables, proteins, and complex carbohydrates (whole grains and pasta). Sugar and baked flour products are to be avoided. This diet will help maintain a fairly even blood sugar through the day.*[22]

honey is very beneficial taken before each meal. The active ingredients of thyme help to break up lung secretions and speed their elimination. Ephedra tea quiets bronchospasms. And mullein helps prevent infections and aids in excreting fluid from the lungs.[24] Comfrey, fennel seed, fenugreek, licorice root, rosehips, and rosemary are other beneficial herbs which can be used.

"Relief from coughing may be expedited," adds David L. Hoffmann, "with a pleasant-tasting mixture of equal parts of coltsfoot, mullein, and licorice, taken three times a day. The flowers of these herbs, combined into an infusion, are not only effective but taste delicious. A blend of marshmallow, mallow, coltsfoot, violet, mullein, and red poppy flowers in equal parts, taken three times a day, is another very 'pleasant' medicine. White horehound is also highly effective in battling coughing, but its unpleasant taste needs to be masked by combining it with licorice or anise seed."

Hydrotherapy: According to Dr. Sherman, the "pneumonia jacket treatment" is also beneficial for emphysema sufferers with excessive or viscous mucous production. Once again, he cautions that it should only be administered under professional supervision.

Dr. Sherman also recommends long-term constitutional hydrotherapy. "This form of water treatment utilizes hot and cold water packs placed over the chest and abdomen at specific time intervals," he explains. "Sine wave electrical pads can also be employed to stimulate both the digestive tract and nervous system, helping to clear the lungs."

Fomentations, or hot compress applications, are also beneficial, states Dr. Sherman. A thick, folded flannel cloth is usually applied a number of times in succession at high temperatures to essentially produce a local vapor bath.

"This procedure is employed when it's necessary to reduce swelling, stimulate absorption of fluid, increase local blood supply, and awaken functional activity," Dr. Sherman says. "Full fomentations include a steam pack to the back, a hot foot bath, and cold compresses to the face, head, or neck."

Self-Care

The following therapies can be undertaken at home under appropriate professional supervision:

Asthma

• Biofeedback Training • Flower Remedies • Guided Imagery • Meditation • Qigong • Yoga

Acupressure: To relieve asthma place your thumbs on the outer portion of your upper chest, pressing on the muscles that run horizontally below your collarbone. Find a knot or sensitive spot on the chest muscles. Underneath that knot is LU1 (for an illustration of this point number please see the acupressure chart on page 874), an important acupressure point for relieving breathing difficulties. Let your head hang forward toward your chest, relaxing your neck, as you maintain firm pressure on those muscles with your thumbs. Continue to hold these points while breathing deeply for two minutes.

Aromatherapy: During an attack inhale bergamot, camphor, eucalyptus, lavender, hyssop, marjoram. Try frankincense for calming.

Ayurveda: • Make a tea from one-half teaspoon of licorice and ginger in one cup of water. • To relieve congestion and cough and alleviate breathlessness, try one-quarter cup of onion juice with a teaspoon of honey and one-eighth teaspoon black pepper. • Between attacks you may fortify the body with tonics such as *ashwagandha, shatavari,* gotu kola, licorice. • The Ayurvedic compound *triphala* is also recommended.

Homeopathy: *Antimonium tart., Nux vomica .*

***Juice Therapy*:** • Periodic fasting on juice or distilled water and lemon juice may be helpful. • Carrot and spinach • Carrot and celery • Carrot and radish • Radish, lemon, garlic, comfrey, horseradish mixed with carrots and beets • Lemon juice and water first thing in morning • Grapefruit

Bronchitis

• Acupressure • Fasting • Qigong • Yoga

Aromatherapy: Steam inhalation with benzoin, bergamot, camphor, eucalyptus, lavender, pine, sandalwood. Clear mucous with benzoin, bergamot, sandalwood, and thyme. In a hallmark study, a blend of clove, cinnamon, melissa, and lavender was as effective in treating bronchial conditions as were commercial antibiotics.

Ayurveda: An herbal mixture of: *sitopaladi* 500 mg., *punarnava* 300 mg., *trikatu* 100 mg., and *mahasudarshan* 300 mg., one-quarter teaspoon of this mixture generally taken twice a day after lunch and dinner with honey.

Homeopathy: • *Aconite, Bryonia, Phosphorus, Ferr phos., Sulfur, Arsen alb.* • *Lymphomyosot, Ferr. phos., Calc. sulph.*

Juice Therapy: • Carrot and radish juice • Wheatgrass juice • Carrot, beet, and cucumber • Carrot and spinach • Carrot and celery • Carrot, beet, and cucumber

Reflexology: Chest/lung, lymph system, pituitary.

Emphysema

• Acupressure • Biofeedback Training • Guided Imagery • Qigong • Reflexology • Yoga

Aromatherapy: Eucalyptus, pine.

Homeopathy: • *Aspidosperma* • *Carbo vegetabilis* when there is a feeling of being "hungry" for air and desire to be fanned

Juice Therapy: • Carrot, spinach, celery, wheatgrass, watercress, potatoes, barley juices. Add a little garlic to juices. • Grape, orange, lemon, black currant

Hay Fever

• Biofeedback Training • Guided Imagery • Yoga

Acupressure: To relieve hay fever place the thumb and index finger of one hand on the upper ridge of the eye socket B2 (for an illustration of this point number please see the acupressure chart on page 874), near the bridge of the nose. Press upward into the slight indentations in your eye socket. Spread the index and middle fingers of your other hand to press ST3 up underneath your cheekbones directly beneath your eyes. Hold these points for one minute with your eyes closed as you breathe deeply.

Aromatherapy: Lavender, eucalyptus, chamomile, melissa, rose.

Ayurveda: • Basil tea with honey (especially basil from India or Tulsi) • Calamus, gotu kola, ginger, cloves, ephedra, bayberry • Apply essential oils such as eucalyptus, menthol, or camphor (or ginger paste) to temple or root of nose.

Juice Therapy: • Carrot, celery juice • Carrot, beet, cucumber • Carrot, celery, spinach, parsley

Pneumonia

• Yoga

Aromatherapy: • Camphor, eucalyptus, teatree, pine, lavender, lemon.

Ayurveda: An herbal mixture of: *sitopaladi* 500 mg., *punarnava* 300 mg., *pippali* 200 mg., and *abhrak bhasma* 100 mg., one-quarter teaspoon taken with one teaspoon of *chyavanprash* three times a day or twice a day after lunch and dinner.

Juice Therapy: Carrot, spinach, parsley juice—add garlic, cumin.

Reflexology: Chest/lung, diaphragm, intestines, all glands, lymph system.

Professional Care

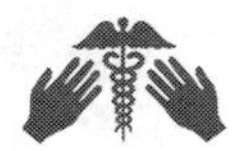

The following therapies should only be provided by a qualified health professional:

Asthma

• Acupuncture • Cell Therapy • Chelation Therapy • Chiropractic • Craniosacral Therapy • Environmental Medicine • Hypnotherapy • Light Therapy • Magnetic Field Therapy

Bodywork: • Alexander technique • Feldenkrais • Hellerwork • Massage • *Shiatsu* • Rolfing helps to free the rib cage and thereby promote better breathing, but cannot cure asthma.

Traditional Chinese Medicine: Ginseng is used in traditional formulas to treat asthma.

Oxygen Therapy: Ozone

Bronchitis

• Applied Kinesiology • Biofeedback Training • Cell Therapy • Colon Therapy • Environmental Medicine • Enzyme Therapy • Magnetic Field Therapy • Naturopathic Medicine • Osteopathy • Yoga

Detoxification Therapy: Often indicated if the person is strong enough and has other congestive conditions.

Oxygen Therapy: • Hydrogen peroxide therapy • Ozone therapy: extremely low concentrations of ozone/oxygen are anecdotally said to be helpful in healing. • Hyperbaric oxygen therapy

***Traditional Chinese Medicine*:** Treats bronchitis with fresh lotus root to strengthen the lungs, and pears help dry coughs.

Bodywork: Rolfing helps to free rib cage and promote better breathing but cannot cure bronchitis.

According to Leon Chaitow, N.D., D.O., many forms of massage are helpful in normalizing respiratory function.

Emphysema

• Acupuncture • Chiropractic • Magnetic Field Therapy • Osteopathy

Bodywork: • Rolfing helps free the rib cage and promotes better breathing but cannot cure emphysema. • *Shiatsu* • Reflexology

Hay Fever

• Acupuncture • Applied Kinesiology • Chelation Therapy • Chiropractic • Craniosacral Therapy • Hypnotherapy • Osteopathy

Bodywork: Acupressure, reflexology, Rolfing.

Pneumonia

• ***Acupuncture • Magnetic Field Therapy***
• ***Naturopathic Medicine • Osteopathy***

Bodywork: Osteopathy and Rolfing both help to free up the rib cage, thereby promoting better breathing, but do not cure pneumonia.

Fasting: According to Dr. Chaitow, fasting is useful in the early stages if patient is not too frail.

He has fasted elderly patients with pneumonia for forty-eight hours with excellent results. He uses repetitive soft tissue manipulation methods to help breathing function, along with herbal

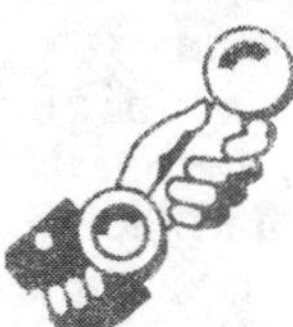

Where to Find Help

For information on respiratory conditions or referrals to a qualified health care practitioner, contact the following organizations.

American Association of Naturopathic Physicians
2366 Eastlake Avenue, Suite 322
Seattle, Washington 98102
(206) 323-7610
Contact for the location of a licensed naturopathic physician in your area.

American Association of Acupuncture and Oriental Medicine
4101 Lake Boone Trail, Suite 201
Raleigh, North Carolina 27607
(919) 787-5181
The AAAOM is a national professional trade organization of acupuncturists who meet acceptable standards of competency and can provide you with the names and locations of local members.

International Foundation for Homeopathy
2366 Eastlake Avenue, East, Suite 301
Seattle, Washington 98102
(206) 324-8230
Provides educational courses for professionals and the general public. Offers referrals to homeopathic health professionals.

National Center for Homeopathy
801 North Fairfax, Suite 306
Alexandria, Virginia 22314
(703) 548-7790
Provides a referral list of practicing homeopaths and information. Gives courses for lay people and professionals, and organizes study groups around the country.

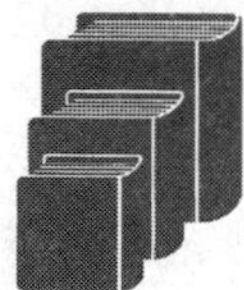

Recommended Reading

Sinus Survival. Ivker, Robert, M.D. Los Angeles: Jeremy P. Tarcher, Inc., 1992.
A self-help guide for treating bronchitis, sinusitis, colds, and allergies.

Breathe Free. Gagnon, David; and Morningstar, Amadea. Wilimot, WI: Lotus Press, 1990.
A nutritional and herbal self-help guide to treating a full range of respiratory conditions.

Encyclopedia of Natural Medicine. Murray, Michael, N.D.; and Pizzorno, Joseph, N.D. Rocklin, CA: Prima Publishing, 1991.
An authoritative guide to naturopathic medicine outlining the basic principles of health and how they can be used to treat over sixty health conditions, including a full range of respiratory conditions. Includes self-help approaches using diet, nutrition, and herbal medicine.

Dr. Braly's Food Allergy and Nutrition Revolution. Braly, James, M.D. New Canaan, CT: Keats Publishing, Inc., 1992.
A comprehensive investigation into food allergies and their link to other illnesses, including asthma. Outlines the factors involved in asthma and how to treat them using diet, nutritional supplements, and exercise.

Sexually Transmitted Diseases

Sexually transmitted diseases (STD's) are more varied and prevalent than ever before, with traditionally common STD's, such as gonorrhea and syphilis, being joined by chlamydia and the deadliest newcomer, AIDS. While prevention is the ideal way to deal with STDs, many natural treatments such as herbs, homeopathy, and nutritional supplements are effective depending on the specific condition and its severity.

Venereal diseases, or what is now called sexually transmitted diseases (STD's), can affect anyone. It is possible to have only one sexual partner and still acquire an STD. Even newborn babies are susceptible if the mother is infected.

"Most sexually transmitted diseases are caused by either a bacteria or a virus," says Tori Hudson, N.D., Director of the Portland Naturopathic Clinic in Oregon. "For example, diseases such as chlamydia, gonorrhea, and syphilis are caused by bacteria while viruses cause herpes simplex, hepatitis B, and HIV (human immunodeficiency virus).

Because of the many variables and potential problems associated with an STD, a trained health professional should be consulted if infection is suspected.

As the name suggests, STD's are usually transmitted through intimate sexual contact involving a variety of body parts, such as the genitals, mouth, and anus, but they can also be transmitted nonsexually. For example, hepatitis B, often spread sexually, can be transmitted by sharing a hypodermic needle or through a human bite.

Because of the many variables and potential problems associated with an STD, a trained health professional should be consulted if infection is suspected. The potential for contracting an STD depends on the disease type, the gender of both the carrier and the receiver, and the nature of the sexual contact. A person may experience no symptoms or only very mild symptoms for a short or extended period of time. During this phase, serious complications may result and the STD can be passed to a sexual partner or, in the case of a pregnant woman, her unborn child.

See AIDS, Female Health, Male Health.

Because of the many variables and potential problems associated with an STD, a trained health professional should be consulted if infection is suspected.

Prevention

To avoid STD's, Dr. Hudson offers the following precautions:

- **Take care when selecting a sex partner.** Find out about your partner's health and sexual history before pursuing a sexual relationship. Have sex only if the person has no apparent signs of infection and is willing to assure your protection during sexual intimacy. Be prepared to talk and inquire about past experiences. Be direct and persistent. Make conversations about health a natural part of the sexual relationship.

- **Limit your number of sex partners.** The more sexual partners a person has, the more vulnerable he or she is to STD's. Although "safer sex" (there is no such thing as safe sex) is an essential form of protection for many STD's, open lesions can occur on parts of the body that cannot be covered by a condom or other latex barrier.
- **Use latex barriers.** Except for people in long-term, monogamous relationships, a barrier-style contraceptive should always be used. Latex condoms give the best protection against STD's. Condoms made from natural products such as sheepskin are not as reliable as latex, and no condom can guarantee 100 percent protection. A latex dental dam—a device that, when inserted in the mouth, prevents secretions from being swallowed—is suitable for partners with genital warts or genital herpes. The recently developed female condom may help prevent the spread of STD's to and from the external genitals.
- **Stay healthy.** If you have sex with more than one person or if your partner does, have a checkup for STD's at least once a year. Pap smears should be considered an important part of a woman's exam. It is also important that both women and men urinate after intercourse to help clear the urethra, thus preventing infection.
- **If you think you have been exposed to an STD, act responsibly.** See your physician or clinician immediately. Urge your partner to be examined and treated as well. Follow the treatment regimen exactly and do not have sex until you and your partner have been tested again or until you know how to ensure each other's protection.

Common STD's and Their Treatment

From an alternative approach, the key to treating any disease is stimulating the immune system. In the case of STD's, this can be done by eliminating fatty foods, sugar, white flour, salt, and coffee from the diet, according to Dr. Hudson. The diet should be high in complex carbohydrates and contain a low to moderate amount of protein. The immune system can be protected by drinking pure water and eliminating alcohol, tobacco, and mood-altering drugs. Several nutrients including vitamins A, C, and E and zinc are necessary for optimal immune function, while herbs such as echinacea and goldenseal fight off the offending organism while bolstering the immune system.

In the case of any STD, it is important to consult a physician who can evaluate the condition and determine whether antibiotics or other pharmaceutical drugs are necessary, or whether natural remedies alone will be effective. Even where conventional medicine seems the best choice, one can always add natural therapies under the supervision of an alternative physician. For instance, with conditions for which antibiotics are required, the patient may take acidophilus to counteract yeast overgrowth brought on by the drug and may also benefit greatly by utilizing liver herbs to help clear the prescription drugs from the system.

See Diet, Herbal Medicine, Nutritional Supplements.

Chlamydia

Chlamydia are a group of microorganisms which cause primary lesions on the genitals and inflammation of the regional lymph nodes. Chlamydia is the most prevalent STD in the United States, costing billions of dollars in medical care each year. Only about half of state governments require medical personnel to report cases of chlamydia, but it is estimated that 4 million individuals are infected annually.[1]

Chlamydia is a dangerous disease because it is often symptom free. This poses a particular threat for women and the children they bear. If chlamydia goes untreated or is not treated appropriately, it can cause tubal pregnancies and infertility in women, and prematurity or death in newborns. Chlamydia has also been known to cause pneumonia as well as ear and eye infections in infants.

In women, chlamydia can infect the cervix, urethra, eyes, and throat. Most commonly, though, chlamydia strikes the upper genital tract, including the fallopian tubes, endometrium (lining of the uterus), and pelvic peritoneum (lining of the pelvis), in a condition known as pelvic inflammatory disease (PID). In fact, chlamydia is responsible for half of the 1 million cases of PID that occur yearly. Symptoms, which can range from mild to intense, typically include vaginal discharge and/or bleeding, pelvic pain, pain with intercourse, changes in urination, and fever.[2]

Because acute pelvic inflammatory disease (PID) can be severe or even life-threatening, proper diagnosis and medical care is essential. It is unwise to diagnose and treat PID from a self-care point of view without consultation with a licensed health care practitioner.

Although the consequences are not as dire, men are also susceptible to chlamydia, especially in the urethra and epididymis part of the excretory duct of the testes. In fact, urethritis, the most common STD seen in men, is frequently caused by chlamydia. In these cases it is called nongonococcal urethritis. As in women, this infection often has no symptoms and is thus difficult to prevent and treat. However, when detectable complaints include discharge from the penis, urethral itching, or changes in urination, medical care should be sought.

An infection of the epididymis on the other hand, is characterized by one-sided pain in the scrotum, as well as swelling and/or pain in that same region. Providing pain relief is an important part of the treatment of epididymitis.

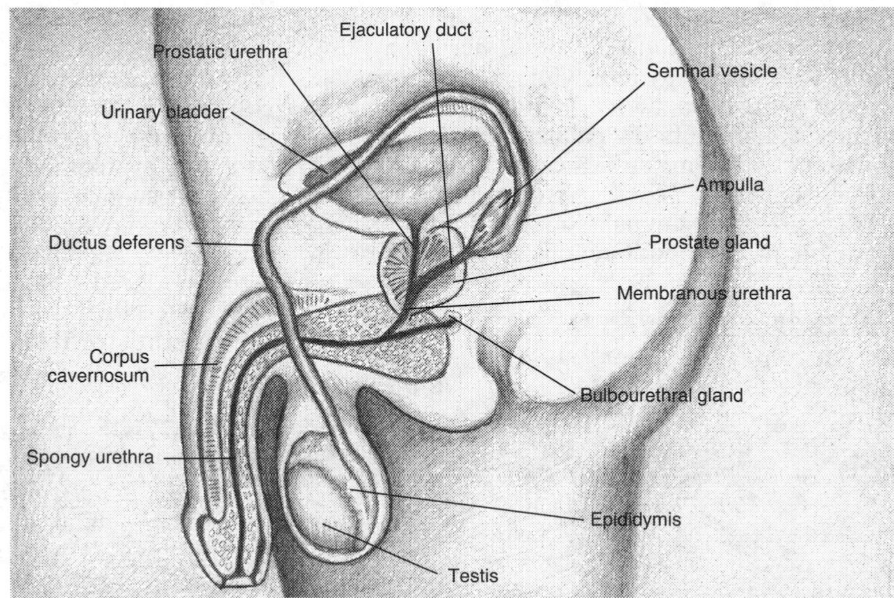

Male reproductive system.

Treatment: According to Dr. Hudson, when using natural therapies for PID, urethritis, or any other genital chlamydial infection, the purpose is to increase circulation to the affected area. When this occurs, inflammation is reduced, healing quickens, the infection subsides, and the body's immunity is stimulated. There are several ways this can be accomplished.

If the infection is acute, such as PID, or pain is severe, as in epididymitis, a three-day water fast is beneficial in minimizing the pain, says Dr. Hudson. Digesting as few nutrients as possible allows the body's healing mechanisms to work more effectively. If a patient cannot tolerate a water fast for either medical or nonmedical reasons, a fast using fruit and vegetable juices is an alternative. If the person infected is unable to undergo such a fast, or the condition is chronic, then a light diet of fresh fruits and vegetables for three to five days is another option.

Whether fasting or not, fluids should be increased. In addition to water, utilize the therapeutic effects of juices from watermelons, apples, nectarines, grapes, carrots, and green vegetables. Carrot juice, for example, is very high in beta-carotene, the nontoxic precursor to vitamin A. According to Dr. Hudson, other juices, such as pomegranate, cranberry, celery, parsley, and cucumber, have been used for decades to treat urethritis. These foods are considered therapeutic because they promote urination.

When herbal preparations are used to treat epididymitis, it is best to consult a trained practitioner, says Dr. Hudson. Many old botanical texts recommend pulsatilla and podophyllum specifically for epididymal infections. However, both of these plants are potentially toxic and therefore must be administered by a knowledgeable professional in

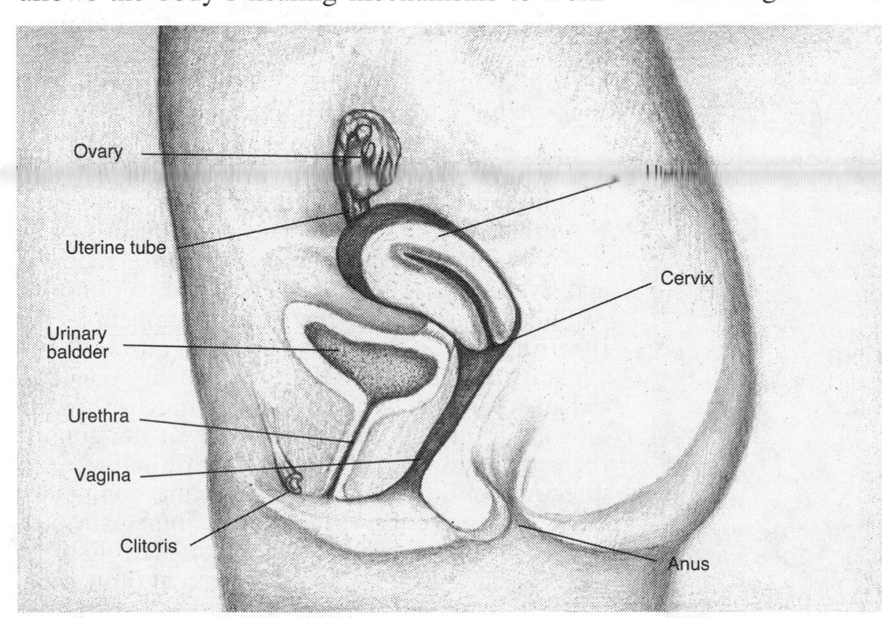

Female reproductive system.

order to ensure a safe dose. "Given in medicinal doses," says Dr. Hudson, "these herbs have the ability to treat epididymitis with results comparable to conventional medicine." Other herbs such as echinacea, horsetail, saw palmetto berries, cranberry extract, and chimaphilla are also recommended.

Tom Kruzel, N.D., Associate Professor of Medicine at the National College of Naturopathic Medicine in Portland, Oregon, who specializes in the treatment of male genital and urological infections, finds that saw palmetto is the most important herb in treating men for these infections. Berberine, an active constituent of goldenseal, has been shown to stimulate some parts of the immune system.[3] In India, berberine drops are used on patients with chlamydial eye infections. When this treatment was compared to the standard drug, sulphacetamide, it was found that the drug produced better initial results, but that only berberine killed the chlamydial parasite and only berberine-treated patients suffered no recurrences.[4]

A CASE OF EPIDIDYMITIS

Tom Kruzel, N.D., Associate Professor of Medicine at the National College of Naturopathic Medicine in Portland, Oregon, specializes in the treatment of male genital and urological infections. One of his cases involved a forty-five-year-old man who visited his office following treatment for an itchy, red rash on his penis and scrotum. His previous doctor had given him cortisone cream, which cleared up the rash, but three weeks later the patient developed a right-sided epididymitis. When Dr. Kruzel examined the man, the infection had progressed from a dull aching to a sharp pain accompanied by slight swelling.

Although Dr. Kruzel suspected the infection may have been due to chlamydia, he did not confirm it with a culture because, he explains, "I rarely do a culture for chlamydia, partially because it doesn't really alter my treatment plan that much and I'm not using antibiotics." Dr. Kruzel adds that it is often difficult, particularly with chlamydia, to gather an adequate sample on a male, and when it is done, it is very painful for the patient. "What is most important to me is to have the symptoms delineated because that way I can choose the botanical or homeopathic medicine that will work."

For this case, Dr. Kruzel chose saw palmetto and horsetail, both specific for the epididymis; pulsatilla, a good herb for swelling and pain seen in male genitourinary diseases; and Staphysagria, *previously given to this patient in homeopathic form for mental and emotional issues. A homeopathic constitutional remedy of* Lycopodium *was also prescribed for the rash.*

At his three-week follow-up visit, the patient reported an 85 percent improvement of the pain, but the rash had returned, although with no itching. Without adjusting his patient's medications, Dr. Kruzel told him to return in one month. "On the return visit, he was completely painfree and the skin rash was just about gone." The pain and rash completely disappeared within four months and there has been no recurrence.

Gonorrhea

Gonorrhea is caused by the bacterium *Gonococcus neisseria*, and causes an inflammation of the genital mucous membranes. It may also affect the oral mucosa, conjunctiva of the eye, the rectum, or the joints. Gonorrhea's presence has been overshadowed by more common STD's, such as chlamydia and genital warts, as well as AIDS, but in the United States, gonorrhea is still a significant problem, with approximately 2.5 million or more cases per year. Of the sexually transmitted diseases that American physicians are required to report to public health officials, gonorrhea is the most prevalent.[5]

"Of the sexually transmitted diseases that American physicians are required to report to public health officials, gonorrhea is the most prevalent."

In women, gonorrhea can infect the vagina, cervix, urethra, rectum, and throat, or can travel up to the uterus, ovaries, or fallopian tubes and cause pelvic inflammatory disease. Men's reproductive organs, such as the penis and epididymis, are similarly infected by gonorrhea, as are the rectum and throat. When urethritis is caused by gonorrhea, it is called gonococcal urethritis.

A gonorrheal infection can cause redness and swelling in the affected area. The painful urination and pus-like discharge from the penis seen in nongonococcal urethritis (caused by Chlamydia trachomatis), are similar in gonococcal urethritis. Frequency of urination or an urgency to urinate may also occur. If the gonorrhea organism escapes from its original site of infection and enters the bloodstream, complications such as fever, skin rash, or joint pain can occur. While about 95 percent of men display some symptoms, only 50 to 75 percent of women do.[6] However, Dr. Hudson notes, "Follow-up testing is critical in order to ascertain if there is a need for antibiotics."

Treatment: Natural therapies for gonorrhea, especially urethritis, epididymitis, and PID, are similar to those used for chlamydia.

Syphilis

Syphilis is caused by a bacterial microorganism and causes lesions which may involve any organ or tissue. It usually causes skin lesions in the early stages, but may not present any symptoms for many years. Syphilis should not be treated with natural therapies. According to Dr. Hudson, "Syphilis is a serious and potentially debilitating and life-threatening illness, and requires conventional treatment with penicillin or other antibiotics such as tetracycline. You would be putting yourself out on a limb to treat syphilis any other way."

> *"Syphilis is a serious and potentially debilitating and life-threatening illness, and requires conventional treatment with penicillin or other antibiotics such as tetracycline. You would be putting yourself out on a limb to treat syphilis any other way."*
> —Tori Hudson, N.D.

However, Dr. Hudson says homeopaths may use *Syphilinum* to stimulate the immune response and avoid long-term, more subtle problems from the disease. "Even though the organism is killed by penicillin, homeopaths believe there are alterations of the patient's vital force as a result of the disease. The disease leaves an imprint that is long lasting, which a parent can even pass along to a child," says Dr. Hudson. "Homeopathic remedies used in conjunction with other medicines can avert that process and help avoid long term consequences."

Herpes

There are two main kinds of herpes. The first type, also known as a cold sore, is caused by herpes simplex virus type 1 (HSV1). Genital herpes, the most common type of genital ulceration, is brought about by herpes simplex virus type 2 (HSV2). The first signs of an HSV2 infection can occur four to seven days after sexual contact with an infected partner. Tingling, burning, or a persistent itch usually herald a herpes outbreak. A day or two later, small, pimple-like bumps appear over reddened skin. As the itching and tingling continue, the herpes pimples transform into painful blisters, which burst and exude blood and a yellowish pus. Five to seven days after the first tingling sensation, scabs form and healing begins.

In women, blisters tend to accumulate on the external genital region, cervix, and around the anus. In men, lesions may occur on the glans penis (the bulbous end of the penis), the prepuce (the foreskin or fold of skin over the glans penis), and shaft of the penis, as well as around the anus and rectum. Herpes simplex virus can also cause nongonococcal urethritis infections in men.

Treatment: Treating herpes with natural medicines can significantly reduce the frequency and number of eruptions. Dr. Hudson reports that some patients suffering from chronic herpes are able to reduce their outbreaks from monthly to once or twice a year.

Recurrent herpes is clearly a stress-related illness. Anxiety is the greatest predictor of a herpes eruption, and thus stress reduction can help prevent herpes attacks.[7] A specific diet may also help. Many HSV2 sufferers have decreased their herpes outbreaks by eating foods high in the amino acid lysine, such as fish, seafood, chicken, turkey, eggs, dairy products, potatoes, and brewer's yeast, reports Dr. Hudson. Supplemental lysine can be taken as well.

A diet containing large amounts of arginine, another amino acid, appears to aggravate herpes. Foods to avoid include chocolate, nuts (specifically peanuts, almonds, cashews, walnuts), seeds (sunflower and sesame), and coconut. Foods containing a moderate amount of arginine should be eaten with discretion. These include wheat, soy, lentils, oats, corn, rice, barley, tomato, and squash. Those suffering from an outbreak should avoid these foods until the blisters have disappeared. Immunosuppressants such as drugs, alcohol, and tobacco should also be eliminated from the diet.

Aromatherapy uses essential oils that have been proven to be very effective in treating herpes simplex due to their strong antiviral properties. Combinations of oils such as lemon and geranium or eucalyptus and bergamot applied topically at the first sign of outbreak can lessen or prevent a full flare-up. Other essential oils that can be used are true rose oil or true melissa oil, both of which, according to Dr. (rer. nat.) Dietrich Wabner, a professor at the Technical University of Munich, have contributed, in some cases, to complete remission of herpes simplex lesions after a one-time application.

See Aromatherapy, Fasting, Homeopathy, Juice Therapy.

Herbal remedies can also be used to treat herpes. "Herbs that strengthen the immune system and help the body to resist infection can be taken internally. Tinctures of echinacea, Siberian ginseng, nettle, and goldenseal should be combined in equal parts, and one-half teaspoon taken three times a day," says David Hoffmann, B.Sc., M.N.I.M.H., an herbalist from Sebastopol, California, and past President of the American Herbalist Guild.

When preventive measures do not stop herpes sores from appearing, there are several ways to diminish the discomfort and/or hasten recovery. Ice applied to the sores at the very beginning of an eruption can help. Cool compresses or baking soda compresses also soothe lesions. Aloe, goldenseal, lavender, and lycopodium can be applied directly to the herpes lesions in a salve. A popular topical ointment among naturopathic physicians contains licorice root. Italian researchers discovered that glycyrrhizic acid, a constituent of licorice, inactivates HSV1-infected cell cultures.[8]

“Anxiety is the greatest predictor of a herpes eruption, and thus stress reduction can help prevent herpes attacks.”

As with other STD's, herpes is most effectively controlled by halting its spread between partners. Herpes is potentially contagious from the first signs of tingling until the skin is healed. During an attack, the following precautions should be taken:

- Underwear should be worn to bed.
- Hands should be washed before and after touching any part of the body.
- No clothing, utensils, or other objects should be shared.
- Sexual contact should be avoided if lesions are on genitals, as condoms will not guarantee safety.
- Kissing should be avoided if blisters are on the lips or in the mouth. If lesions are on an area that can be covered with a dressing, then intimate contact may be allowed.
- When being treated or examined by a health-care worker, notify that person if you have an active case so precautions can be taken.

Trichomonas

Although less well known than some STD's, trichomonas vaginalis, a protozoa (a single-cell parasite), is nonetheless a relatively frequent venereal condition. It is the third most common cause of vaginitis in women. Symptoms include a copious, odorous discharge from the vagina, intense itching, and burning and redness of the genital region. Although the fact is debated by some clinicians, trichomonas vaginalis is also thought to infect men, leading to urethritis, prostatitis, epididymitis, and perhaps infertility.

Treatment: Trichomonas can be difficult to treat with natural medicines. "As in other acute infections, it is always beneficial to decrease sweets and refined carbohydrates," says Dr. Hudson. "Increase fresh fruits and vegetables, whole grains like brown rice, whole wheat flour, and oatmeal, and avoid coffee, rich foods, and junk foods." Dr. Hudson has also found that nutritional supplements are helpful, including vitamins A, C, and E, and zinc. She relates the case of a New Zealand research team from Auckland Hospital who discovered the effectiveness of zinc while treating a young woman with trichomoniasis. The woman was initially put on several different drugs, such as metronidazole and amoxycillin, with no success. Finally, the medical team measured zinc levels in her blood and urine and found them to be abnormally low. High dosages of zinc cleared up her infection in three weeks.[9]

It is vital that both sexual partners be treated at the same time if trichomonas is diagnosed, even if it is found in only one partner.

When treating trichomonas, Jill E. Stansbury, N.D., of Battle Ground, Washington, mixes various herbs such as calendula, goldenseal, and echinacea, and prescribes them as a douche. She has her patients douche with this formula once or twice a day or use the herbal douche in the morning and a plain yogurt douche at night.

Genital Warts

It is estimated that between 40 and 80 percent of the U.S. population is infected with the human papilloma virus (HPV), the organism that causes genital warts. The reason this condition is so prevalent and the estimated infection rate is so wide is partly because HPV is difficult to detect.

Not only are one-quarter of HPV infections in regression and thus undetectable, but the virus' life cycle is unpredictable. HPV can be transmitted from person to person in several ways. Any sexual contact, genital or oral, can spread HPV. This virus can also be picked up from inanimate objects that have been recently exposed to HPV and not properly cleaned, for example, medical equipment (such as gloves or a speculum), underwear, tanning salon beds, and sexual aids or devices.

Most infected individuals exhibit no lesions or warts. A scant 2 to 3 percent have visible warts, while another 2 to 3 percent have flat warts which are not visible to the naked eye. Many times there are no symptoms associated with either the flat or visible warts. In other cases, burning, itching, and general irritation are felt and the affected skin may be red. This is especially true of flat warts. If a doctor suspects flat warts because of exposure or symptoms, he or she can verify this by applying white vinegar and then inspecting the area with a magnifying glass. Spots that turn white are often a positive indicator of warts.

> *"It is estimated that between 40 and 80 percent of the U.S. population is infected with the human papilloma virus (HPV), the organism that causes genital warts."*

Visible warts are usually small, raised, soft, moist bumps that are pink or red. They often resemble a tiny cauliflower. These cauliflower warts are easily spotted on a man's penis, at the opening to the urethra, or on his scrotum. Less detectable, although visible to the eye when found, are warts around a man's anus and in his rectum. Because a woman's genitals are less accessible, a closer inspection must be performed to locate warts on her vulva, vaginal wall, cervix, or anus.

The flat wart is the most dangerous for women. The HPV virus can cause changes in the cervical cells, progressing to more severe cell abnormalities (called dysplasia), and finally cancer. Typically, there are no symptoms to alert the woman of a problem. This is why an annual Pap smear, the most effective screening tool for detecting abnormalities, is vital.

Treatment: Conventional office procedures for treating raised warts include local removal using electrocautery (burning the wart off), freezing the wart with liquid nitrogen, or applying acid or podophyllin, a prescription drug. Many natural methods can be used alone or in addition to conventional treatment.

Dr. Hudson has developed an ointment of vitamin A and the herbs thuja and lomatium. When applied directly to the wart, this antiviral and immune-supportive mixture inhibits HPV. Lomatium and thuja can also be taken orally as a botanical. *Thuja* is a common homeopathic remedy for warts as well.

Deficiencies in vitamins A and C and folic acid can aggravate HPV infections, and may be risk factors in cervical dysplasia and cancer. Smoking, which robs the body of vitamin C, is another risk factor.

Yeast Infection

Many women are familiar with the itching, irritation, and odorous discharge associated with a yeast or candida infection. What has been debated in medical circles, and may be unknown to many women, is that yeast infections can be sexually transmitted. This may be one reason why a woman suffers from chronic yeast infections.[11]

RESEARCH ON CERVICAL CANCER

Tori Hudson, N.D., Director of the Portland Naturopathic Clinic in Oregon, spends much of her time conducting research on natural therapies for women's health conditions, including cervical cancer. Cervical dysplasia (abnormal changes in the tissues covering the cervix uteri) and cervical cancer are caused by the human papilloma virus,[10] a sexually transmitted virus, but, according to Dr. Hudson, there are other significant factors in the development of the disease, including smoking, and deficiencies of vitamins A and C, folic acid, and birth control pills.

One of Dr. Hudson's studies examined the effect of a naturopathic protocol on various stages of dysplasia and cervical cancer in forty-three women. Besides instructing her subjects to follow a healthy diet, take an herbal formula, and take various vitamins such as beta-carotene, vitamin C, and folic acid, Dr. Hudson recommended that herbs and enzymes be applied locally and topically to the cervix.

After six months, thirty-eight patients following this protocol became disease free, three patients partially improved, and two patients showed no improvement. None of the forty-three patients' condition worsened during the naturopathic treatment.

While seeking proper medical evaluation and either conventional or alternative treatment, the following aspects of Dr. Hudson's treatment can be applied:

Self-treatment:

- *Beta-carotene: 150,000 IU/daily.*
- *Vitamin C: 2,000 milligrams daily. (Decrease this dosage if diarrhea occurs and consult a physician first if you have a history of kidney stones.)*
- *Folic acid: 10 milligrams daily.*
- *A diet of fresh fruit, fresh vegetables, and whole grains, along with the elimination of dairy products, meats, sugar, refined grains, junk food, coffee, and alcohol.*

Methods of prevention:

- *Use condoms during intercourse and avoid unprotected sexual contact with anyone who has genital warts.*
- *Women should avoid smoking, which is the most significant co-factor in the development of cervical dysplasia and cervical cancer.*

The incidence of this fungal condition, topping the list as the most common cause of vaginal infections, has increased dramatically over the past twenty-five years.

There is also evidence that vaginal candida infections suppress immunity.[12] Mary Miles, M.D., and her colleagues found that all women they tested who harbored yeast in their vaginas also had yeast in their stools.[13] This suggests that when a woman is infected with vaginal candida, she should also be checked for gastrointestinal candida and her overall health and immunity should be addressed.

See Candidiasis, Gastrointestinal Disorders.

Treatment: Once a vaginal yeast infection has been confirmed, many of the therapies used to treat gastrointestinal candida apply including a special diet. Items that encourage yeast growth should be avoided, including fermented foods such as soy sauce, tofu, cheese, and pickles; sweets of all kinds, including sweet fruits; fungi such as mushrooms; and prepared foods containing baking or brewer's yeast.

For years, women have eaten yogurt and used it in douches for self-treatment of yeast vaginitis. Up until recently, the research on this therapy has been inconclusive. However, new studies are now demonstrating the successful use of unsweetened yogurt containing *Lactobacillus acidophilus* in curing vaginal yeast infections.[14] Herbs such as calendula, usnea, echinacea, yarrow, marshmallow, and goldenseal are also effective as douches. They can be made into a strong tea with one pint used as a douche twice a day for one to two weeks. Garlic, either as an herb, or in foods, should also be consumed.

Dr. Hudson reports that the most consistently successful home treatment for yeast vaginitis is boric acid powder capsules. Cornell University investigators compared boric acid capsules with the leading prescription and over-the-counter drugs for vaginal yeast infections. Boric acid capsule suppositories were successful 98 percent of the time.[15] Do not use boric acid crystals, however, as they are not the same remedy.

Faizi Medeiros, N.D., a partner of the Upper Valley Naturopathic Clinic in Norwich, Vermont, recalls a thirty-seven-year-old woman who came to her office complaining of vaginal discharge and itching. "In the past," says Dr. Medeiros, "she had been treated quite often with Nystatin (an antifungal medication) and she kept getting recurrent yeast infections, so I decided to do an elimination diet with her using only rice and vegetables for ten days." In addition to this, Dr. Medeiros gave her nutrients targeted at her bowel, liver, and immune system—important body systems to consider when treating chronic health problems.

About one month after being on this regimen, the woman came back. She said that the infection had returned, although it was not as bad as usual. Medeiros augmented her treatment plan by instructing her patient to use tea tree oil suppositories for four nights, along with alternating hot and cold sitz baths. The patient, says Dr. Medeiros, has not returned with any complaints since that time.

SPECIAL CONSIDERATIONS FOR MEN

Men with untreated STD's, says Tom Kruzel, N.D., run the risk of infertility or impotence. Unfortunately, sometimes the only indications that an STD is present are mild symptoms, such as an aching in the hip or lower back or a mild pain in the testicles or scrotum. If it is a low-grade infection, the STD may persist for a long time, causing only fatigue, minimal fever, or malaise. Unaware of the consequences, many men will ignore these warning signs. A man also must remember to seek treatment if his partner is infected, even if he has no symptoms.

SPECIAL CONSIDERATIONS FOR WOMEN

STD's often affect each sex differently. Chlamydia, for example, may cause pelvic inflammatory disease in women, which can result in infertility. Natural health care methods may not be enough for a woman in cases such as this, especially if she is considering getting pregnant in the future. She should always talk to her health care practitioner about the possible use of antibiotics, along with natural remedies, because, when a woman has a STD and does become pregnant, she always runs the risk of passing the infection along to her baby.

It is now standard procedure among most obstetricians and midwives to screen women for STD's, often including HIV, during prenatal care. If you are pregnant and have an STD, check with a health-care provider before taking any medications, including herbal preparations or nutritional supplements. Boric acid, for example, should not be used during pregnancy, though most herbal douches and suppositories are safe.

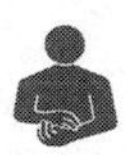

Self-Care

The following therapies can be undertaken at home under appropriate professional supervision:

Syphilis

Herbs: Add two tablespoons each of sarsaparilla and yellowdock root in one quart boiling water. Simmer five minutes and add three and a half teaspoons dried thyme. Steep covered for one hour. Drink one to three cups per day. Women should also use often as a douche.

Hydrotherapy: Contrast sitz bath applied daily.

Herpes

• Enzyme Therapy • Biofeedback Training

Aromatherapy: • Tea tree, bergamot, eucalyptus, lavender, camomile, palmarosa • True rose oil or true melissa oil

Ayurveda: An herbal mixture can be made of: 500 mg. *shatavari*, 200 mg. *guwel sattva*, 200 mg. *kamadudha*, and 300 mg. *neem*. Take two teaspoons of this mixture twice a day after lunch and dinner. Also *tikta ghee* can be applied locally, or one teaspoon can be taken on an empty stomach.

Homeopathy: *Rhus tox., Sepia, Nartum mur., Hepar sulph., Arsen alb., Caladium, Acidum nit.*

Hydrotherapy: Hyperthermia (heat aggravates herpes infection but may accelerate the healing process if tolerated) applied daily or every other day, followed by short cold bath, or sitz bath. Apply contrast daily.

Juice Therapy: • Carrot, beet, celery juice • Avoid citrus, pineapple.

Topical Treatment: • Glycyrrhizic acid (licorice) applied to the skin lesions[16] • Squeeze vitamin E capsule onto cotton roll. • Zinc sulfate ointment • Calendula cream • Tea tree oil (one teaspoon to one quart water).

Professional Care

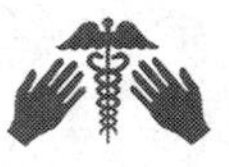

The following therapies should only be provided by a qualified health professional:

Syphilis

• Magnetic Field Therapy • Naturopathic Medicine

Herpes

• Cell Therapy • Environmental Medicine • Fasting • Magnetic Field Therapy • Naturopathic Medicine • Orthomolecular Medicine

Detoxification Therapy: May be indicated, depending on the condition of the person.

Energy Medicine: Electro-Acuscope.

Oxygen Therapy: • Hydrogen peroxide therapy (IV) • Ozone inactivates the genital herpes virus. Treatment is autohemotherapy.

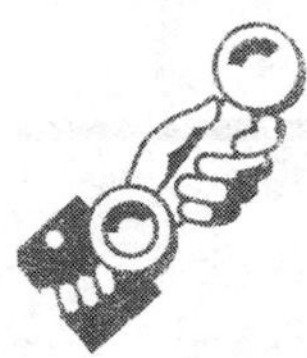

Where to Find Help

For referrals and more information on, and treatment for, sexually transmitted diseases, contact:

American Association of Naturopathic Physicians
2366 Eastlake Avenue, Suite 322
Seattle, Washington 98102
(206) 323-7610

Provides a directory of naturopathic physicians and offers referrals to a nationwide network of accredited or licensed practitioners. Publishes a quarterly newsletter for both professionals and the general public. Also offers a series of brochures and pamphlets on a variety of subjects.

American Foundation for the Prevention of Venereal Disease
799 Broadway, Suite 638
New York, New York 10003
(212) 759-2069

The foundation provides educational material for the prevention of STD's and encourages responsible sexual relations.

American Holistic Medical Association
4101 Lake Boone Trail, Suite 201
Raleigh, North Carolina 27607
(919) 787-5181

A professional organization for holistic practitioners, the AHMA offers information and services for its members and lobbies for holistic issues. It also provides referrals for the public; requests must be in writing.

American Social Health Association
P.O. Box 13827
Research Triangle Park, North Carolina 27709
(919) 361-8400

A voluntary health agency dedicated to eliminating STD's as a social health problem.

American Venereal Disease Association
P.O. Box 1753
Baltimore, Maryland 21203-1753
(301) 955-3150
An association of professionals and lay people interested in understanding and controlling STD's.

Citizens Alliance for VD Awareness
P.O. Box 1073
Chicago, Illinois 60648
The Citizens Alliance provides information to the public, especially high-risk groups, on symptoms, treatment, and prevention of STD's, including AIDS.

Herpes Resource Center
P.O. Box 13827
Research Triangle Park, North Carolina 27709
(919) 361-8488
The Herpes Resource Center provides emotional support and information to individuals with recurrent genital herpes infections.

International Women's Health Coalition
24 East 21st Street
New York, New York 10010
(212) 979-8500
An organization which provides information to women, particularly, about sexually transmitted diseases and other health concerns. Free pamphlets available upon request.

Portland Naturopathic Clinic
The Teaching Clinic of National College of Naturopathic Medicine
11231 S.E. Market Street
Portland, Oregon 97216
(503) 255-7355
A full-service outpatient clinic in naturopathic medicine with diagnostic services, a full scope of naturopathic treatments and a large natural pharmacy.

The following will provide a list of clinics, pamphlets, and other educational information, as well as free condoms and a counseling hotline:

Long Beach Department of Health and Human Services
2525 Grand Avenue
Long Beach, California 90815
STD Clinic Information Line (ask for a counselor): (310) 570-4315

Los Angeles County Department of Health Services
Public Health Programs and Services
Sexually Transmitted Disease Program
12838 Erickson Avenue
Downey, California 90242
(310) 940-8011

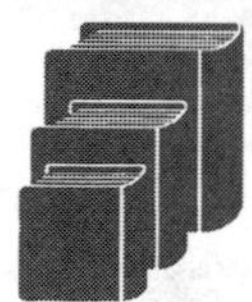

Recommended Reading

Color Atlas and Synopsis of Sexually Transmitted Diseases. Handsfield, H. Hunter, M.D. New York: McGraw Hill, 1991.
The rising incidence of sexually transmitted disease in the general patient population has necessitated a working knowledge of the diagnosis and management of these disorders by the primary care physician. Color Atlas and Synopsis of Sexually Transmitted Diseases *gives you that knowledge base in 138 full-color photographs and succinct clinical summaries that emphasize recognition and diagnosis of each condition.*

The Culture of Silence. Published by the International Women's Health Coalition, 24 East 21st Street, New York, New York 10010. (212) 979-8500.
This booklet offers an in-depth discussion of the causes and consequences of reproductive tract infections.

Encyclopedia of Natural Medicine. Murray, Michael, N.D.; and Pizzorno, Joseph, N.D. Rocklin, CA: Prima Publishing, 1991.
Naturopathic approach to treating sexually transmitted diseases.

The Sex Encyclopedia. Bechtel, Stephen, et. al. New York: Fireside, 1993.
An A to Z guide to the latest information on sexual health, safety, and technique from the nation's top sex experts.

Sexual Disease and Its Treatment. Banerjee, Prosad, M.D. West Bengal, India: Shiva and Company Medical Publishers, 1991.
A list of sexual diseases and their homeopathic cures.

Sexual Ills and Diseases. Anshultz, E. P. M.D., New Delhi: B. Jain Publishers Pvt. Ltd., 1992.
Sexual diseases and cures based on homeopathic practice and textbooks.

Sexually Transmitted Diseases (Second Edition). Eds. Holmes, King K., et al. New York: McGraw Hill, 1990.
The new, second edition of Sexually Transmitted Diseases *has been thoroughly updated and substantially revised to reflect the epidemiologic trends and diagnostic and therapeutic advances that have occurred since the appearance of the first edition nearly five years ago. Like its critically acclaimed predecessor, the second edition provides practicing clinicians, specialists, and public health professionals with the most comprehensive and readily accessible coverage available of the signs, symptoms, and management of the ever-increasing numbers of STD's.*

What Doctors Can't Heal. Jackson, Bernard. Inglewood, CA: Strictly Honest, 1993.
The unflattering truth about sexual diseases and individual responsibility.

"He's the best physician who know the worthlessness of most medicines."

—Benjamin Franklin

Sleep Disorders

Over 50 million Americans suffer from sleep disorders, including insomnia, excessive drowsiness, and restless movement during sleep. According to many practitioners of alternative medicine, these disorders often are related to nutritional or behavioral factors, and may be remedied by addressing the various causes and symptoms underlying the condition.

Sleep is a restorative process that serves to replenish both physiologically and psychologically. As an essential part of the daily human cycle, sleep is a determining factor in the state of a person's health.

"The quantity and quality of sleep vary from person to person, but how well and how long one sleeps is ultimately the result of varying physical and psychological influences," says John Zimmerman, Ph.D., Laboratory Director of the Washoe Sleep Disorders Center in Reno, Nevada. Not only can stress, illness, and anxiety contribute to sleep disorders, but so can external circumstances such as a noisy sleeping room, as well as disturbed biological rhythms such as those occurring due to night-shift work, and jet lag, adds Dr. Zimmerman. A shortened attention span, the loss of physical strength, and difficulty in responding to unfamiliar situations are all common symptoms of sleep disorders.

THE CYCLES OF SLEEP

The phenomenon of sleep can be seen as a cycle consisting of two distinct states: rapid eye movement (REM), also known as dream sleep because almost all dreaming occurs in this state, and non-REM (NREM). Four stages of sleep take place during NREM, beginning when the person falling asleep passes from relaxed wakefulness (stage I) to an early stage of light sleep (stage II), and then to increasing degrees of deep sleep (stages III and IV, also referred to as "delta" sleep). Most stage IV sleep (the deepest) occurs in the first several hours of sleep. A period of REM sleep normally follows each period of NREM sleep.

Types of Sleep Disorders

Sleep disorders are a particularly troublesome health concern. Not only can they be the result of other, often undetected ailments, but they also generate their own health complications. Insomnia, sleep apnea, and periodic leg movement syndrome (PLMS)/restless leg syndrome are common sleep disorders.

Insomnia

Insomnia, characterized by an inability either to fall asleep or to remain asleep during the course of the night, can be traced to a number of physical, mental, behavioral, and situational factors.

Insomnia has been classified in terms of the time of night that it effects. According to Dr. Zimmerman, there are three main types of insomnia: sleep-onset insomnia, sleep-maintenance insomnia, and early-morning-awakening insomnia. People who take hours to fall asleep but sleep relatively well throughout the remainder of the night have sleep-onset insomnia. Those who wake up several times in the middle of the night and have trouble falling back to sleep suffer from sleep-maintenance insomnia. Individuals who awaken too early have what is called early-morning-awakening insomnia.

Psychophysiological insomnia, notes Dr. Zimmerman, is an official diagnostic category the symptoms of which often include sleep onset insomnia. In psychophysiological insomnia a person's normal presleep rituals, behavior, or sleeping environment trigger insomnia. In this case, the more the sufferer worries about falling asleep, the worse it becomes.

Sleep Apnea

Sleep apnea refers to a serious condition in which there is intermittent cessation of breathing during sleep which forces the individual to repeatedly wake up to take breaths of air. This disturbs the continuity of sleep and is a primary cause of the excessive daytime sleepiness associated with this disorder.

There are three types of sleep apnea, according to Dr. Zimmerman: central sleep apnea, obstructive sleep apnea, and a combination of the first two types called mixed-type sleep apnea.

Central sleep apnea refers to a defect in the central nervous system which affects the diaphragm. It can result in poor quality sleep, frequent awakening during the night, and excessive fatigue throughout the day. Obstructive sleep apnea occurs when a blockage develops in the upper airway, preventing normal air flow. Individuals who have obstructive sleep apnea usually snore and are often excessively tired and sleepy throughout the day.

Periodic Leg Movement Syndrome and Restless Leg Syndrome

Periodic leg movement syndrome causes repeated leg movements during the onset of sleep or during sleep itself. These occur as a series of stereotyped, repetitive movements throughout the night. A related disorder called restless leg syndrome is characterized by periodic leg movements and uncomfortable leg sensations.

Causes of Sleep Disorders

Sleep disorders occur for many reasons: psychological, such as anxiety, biochemical (such as the inappropriate use of sleeping pills or other drugs), or medical (such as the physiological problems often associated with sleep apnea, PLMS, or restless leg syndrome), as well as daily living activities (such as poor diet and lack of exercise).

Diet

Diet is a primary factor when considering sleep disorders. Intolerance to certain foods, eating excessively, the consumption of caffeine, and the intake of drugs and alcohol are important concerns.

> *"Even a few cups of coffee in the morning can interfere with the quality and quantity of sleep at night."*
> —Konrad Kail, N.D.

Caffeine: Konrad Kail, N.D., past President of the American Association of Naturopathic Physicians, notes that caffeine can have a pronounced effect on sleeping habits. "Even a few cups of coffee in the morning can interfere with the quality and quantity of sleep at night," says Dr. Kail, adding that, "Caffeine consumption has been associated with insomnia, periodic leg movements syndrome, and restless leg syndrome." He points out that many over-the-counter medications such as cold and cough preparations that contain caffeine, or caffeine-related substances, can also increase sleep disorders.

Drugs and Alcohol: The sleeping process can be significantly disturbed by drug and alcohol intake. Drugs which may lead to insomnia include thyroid preparations, oral contraceptives, beta-blockers, and marijuana.[1] Heavy drinking can reduce overall sleep time, including both REM and non-REM sleep.[2]

Food Intolerance: Katie Data, N.D., of Fife, Washington, first looks for intolerances to certain foods when treating patients with sleep disorders. She finds the most common foods that people are sensitive to are dairy products, wheat, corn, and chocolate.

Herbert Rinkel, M.D., former Associate Instructor in Medicine at the University of Oklahoma School of Medicine, is considered one of the first to bring to light the issue of food sen-

NARCOLEPSY

Narcolepsy is a condition that causes sufferers to suddenly fall asleep. This can happen at any time, and is often accompanied by a loss of muscle tone or partial paralysis, a condition called cataplexy that is triggered by the experience of a strong emotion, usually laughter or anger. These cataplexy episodes occur during the day, sometimes many times a day. Then, at night, people with narcolepsy may suffer from sleep paralysis, a condition of being unable to speak or move even though fully aware of external events. Richard Wilkinson, M.D., of the Yakima Allergy Clinic in Yakima, Washington, recalls a patient—a high school principal—suffering from narcolepsy. The onset of narcolepsy in meetings with teachers and students caused him great embarrassment, so he sought the help of Dr. Wilkinson who prescribed a single-food diet (eating only one food per meal) as a diagnostic measure. Almost immediately, the patient's narcolepsy disappeared, and several days later, when a meal of potatoes caused the patient to fall instantly asleep, Dr. Wilkinson determined that the patient had an allergy to potatoes. In the future, the patient could avoid narcolepsy completely by simply avoiding the consumption of potatoes.

DRUGS ASSOCIATED WITH A HIGHER INCIDENCE OF SLEEPLESSNESS

According to the Physicians Desk Reference the following drugs are associated with side effects of sleeplessness. (Statistics refer to the percentage of indivuals affected.)[4]

Anafranil capsules (11-25%)
Atrofen Tablets (2-7%)
Benadryl capsules, Kapseals (Among most frequent)
BuSpar (3%)
Cylert Chewable Tablets, Tablets (Most frequent)
Depo-Provera Contraceptive Injection (1-5%)
Desyrel and Desyrel Dividose (6.4-9.9%)
Emcyt Capsules (3%)
Floxin I.V., Tablets (3-7%)
Habitrol Nicotine Transdermal System (3-9% of patients)
Intron A (Up to 5%)
Kerlone Tablets (1.2-5%)
Lioresal Tablets (2-7%)
Lupron Injection (5% or more)
Marplan Tablets (Among most frequent)
Mazicon for Injection (3-9%)
Mepron Tablets (10-19%)
Nicoderm Nicotine Transdermal System (23%)
Nipent for Injection (3-10%)
Orudis Capsules (Greater than 3%)
Paxil Tablets (13.3%)
Permax Tablets (7.9%)
Prostep (nicotine transdermal system) (3-9% of patients)
Prozac Pulvules and Liquid, Oral Solution (13.8%)
Retrovir Capsules, Syrup (2.4-5%), I.V. Infusion (5%)
Ritalin Tablets (One of the two most common), SR Tablets (Among most common)
Sanorex Tablets (Among most common)
Sectral Capsules (3%)
Seldane-D Extended-Release Tablets (25.9%)
Stadol Injectable, NS Nasal Spray (11%)
Supprelin Injection (3-10%)
Symmetrel Capsules and Syrup (5-10%)
Synarel Nasal Solution for Endometriosis (8% of patients)
Tenex Tablets (Less than 3-5%)
Theo-X Extended-Release Tablets (Among most consistent)
Toradol IM Ijection, Oral (14%)
Ventolin Inhalation Solution (3.1%)
Videx Tablets, Powder for Oral Solution, and Pediatric Powder for Oral Solution (2-25%)
Visken Tablets (10%)
Wellbutrin Tablets (18.6%)
Xanax Tablets (29.4%)
Zoladex (5%)
Zoloft Tablets (16.4%)

sitivities. While still a medical student, he discovered his own intolerance to eggs, and began to research the field. Dr. Rinkel found that symptoms of tension and jitteriness, common to food-sensitive individuals, are apt to manifest in restlessness and inattentiveness by day, and insomnia by night. He concluded that insomnia, as well as tossing about or crying out at night, are very frequent manifestations of food intolerance.

Dr. Rinkel says that fatigue is often one of the first symptoms of food intolerance, and is most troublesome early in the morning upon rising. This is particularly noticeable in children with food intolerances. People suffering from food intolerances are often irritable during the morning hours and may need a nap in the late afternoon. They frequently suffer from insomnia as well, according to Dr. Rinkel.[3]

According to Dr. Kail, intolerance to certain foods can cause histamine (a substance produced by the body during an allergic reaction) to be released in the brain, which in turn can disturb a person's biochemistry, and can, in some cases, lead to sleep disturbance. He explains that in the brain, histamine replaces neurotransmitters, but because it does not function like other neurotransmitters, it creates a dysfunction in the biochemical pathways of the brain (which are responsible for thinking, mood, and behavior). When these pathways are disrupted, the consequence is exhibited as symptoms, one of which is insomnia.

See Allergies, Environmental Medicine, Mind/Body Medicine.

Environmental Factors

"Items that interfere with the body's electromagnetic field and create electromagnetic fields of their own can disrupt sleep," states Anthony Scott-Morley, D.S.C., Ph.D., M.D. (alt. med.), B.A., from Dorset, England. "These include electric blankets, electrically heated waterbeds, electric clocks (at the head of the bed), and 60 cycle frequencies (household electric current), as well as power lines and generators. Also sleeping near or over geopathic stress zones (areas of harmful earth radiation) seriously affect the sleep habits of sensitive individuals."

Dr. Zimmerman adds that sleep problems can sometimes be attributed to factors like ventilation, humidity, noise, or an uncomfortable mattress.

Mental/Emotional Factors

Numerous mental and emotional factors can precipitate sleep disorders, especially insomnia, according to Dr. Zimmerman. These include grief, depression, anxiety, fear, and excitement. Dr. Kail agrees. "Anxiety and depression are two common causes of insomnia. If the insomnia is simply due to a short-term reaction to a situation in one's life, the insomnia will normally disappear as soon as the situation changes. It is rare to see a patient who has a severe case of insomnia due to purely emotional factors, however," he adds. "It is normally a biochemical problem, and biochemical breakdown can take place in many ways. For example, if your digestive system is stressed and unable to digest protein, the amino acids which affect neurotransmission will not be available to your brain and you can become ill emotionally without having anything emotionally stressful going on in your life."

Physiological Factors

John Hibbs, N.D., of the Natural Health Clinic of Bastyr College in Seattle, Washington, points out that adrenal function can have a significant effect on sleep patterns. In particular, he notes that high nighttime levels of cortisone are associated with many sleep disorders. Cortisone is a hormone secreted by the adrenal glands in the morning, or during periods of wakefulness and activity.

Dr. Hibbs also points out that insomnia can result from any number of conditions that interrupt the sleeping process, including stomach problems or bladder ailments. Concerning periodic leg movement syndrome, Dr. Hibbs notes that it is sometimes triggered by a rheumatic disorder or nervous system illness, while sleep apnea may be linked to obesity, particularly if the obese patient also has lung problems from chronic smoking or heart disease.

Treating Sleep Disorders

Treatments for sleep disorders vary, but effective cures include simple dietary changes, nutritional supplements, hormone therapy, behavioral treatment, bedtime and nocturnal respiratory therapy, herbal and homeopathic remedies, Traditional Chinese Medicine, and Ayurvedic medicine.

Insomnia

Insomnia is the most common sleep disorder, and there are several approaches which may prove useful, including diet alteration, nutritional supplementation, herbs, homeopathy, Traditional Chinese Medicine, Ayurvedic medicine, and behavioral treatments.

Diet: Diet is especially important when treating sleep disorders, and it is essential to rule out food intolerances as a cause. In one study of infants, sleeplessness was eliminated by removing cow's milk from the diet and then reproduced by its reintroduction.[8] Leon Chaitow, N.D., D.O., of London, England, recommends a combination of nutritional adjustments to aid sleep, including:

- A marked reduction in alcohol consumption
- Avoiding caffeine in all forms (tea, coffee, cola, chocolate)
- Taking a protein-rich snack at bedtime (yogurt is one example)
- Taking one gram of niacinamide (vitamin B_3) at bedtime (for the type that sleeps easily but wakes and cannot get back to sleep)

ARE CONVENTIONAL TREATMENTS EFFECTIVE?

Each year 4 to 6 million Americans receive prescriptions for sedative hypnotics (sleeping pills).[5] But many medications prescribed by conventional medical practitioners can often hide the root cause of a sleep disorder and can lead to even more dangerous health risks and dependencies. According to Konrad Kail, N.D., past President of the American Association of Naturopathic Physicians, over-the-counter or prescription sleeping pills can alter the brainwave patterns of sleep, thereby preventing a normal cycle of sleep stages. He adds that although they may work initially, sleeping pills lose their effectiveness after a few weeks.

The prescription of hypnotics, such as benzodiazepines, to combat sleep disorders can cause a number of side effects including tolerance, dependence, withdrawal symptoms, a hangover effect, alteration of the memory process, and may potentiate the effects of alcohol.[6] Another serious side effect that can occur is rebound insomnia; upon discontinuation of the drug, sleep can actually worsen compared to pretreatment levels.[7]

- Taking a half of gram of chlorella or other green or blue algae product at bedtime (as a source of tryptophan)

Dr. Chaitow points out that it is beneficial to follow the same sleep ritual patterns (bath, shower, reading), and stress reduction tactics (relaxation, deep breathing).

Nutritional Supplements: The following information, provided by Dr. Hibbs, highlights specific nutritional supplements known to aid sleep:

- **Calcium**, especially when contained in food, has a sedative effect on the body, says Dr. Hibbs, who notes that, for adults, doses of approximately 600 milligrams of liquid calcium have been shown to have a relaxing effect.
- **Magnesium**, in doses of approximately 250 milligrams, can also help induce sleep, according to Dr. Hibbs. Magnesium-rich foods include kelp, wheat bran, almonds, cashews, blackstrap molasses, and brewer's yeast.
- **The B vitamins** are known to have a sedative effect on the nerves, and vitamin B_6 supplements of 50 to 100 milligrams daily can help to prevent insomnia. Dr. Hibbs notes that a tablespoon or two of nutritional yeast is an excellent source of B_6 and can be stirred into a glass of juice. Fifty milligrams of activated vitamin B_6 is often more efficiently used by the body than B_6 in tablet form.
- **Vitamin B_{12}** is another important supplement to consider when treating insomnia, notes Dr. Hibbs, who adds that 25 milligrams of vitamin B_{12}, supplemented with 100 milligrams of pantothenic acid (B_5), can serve as an effective anti-insomnia vitamin regimen. The best food sources of the B vitamins are liver, whole grains, wheat germ, tuna, walnuts, peanuts, bananas, sunflower seeds, and blackstrap molasses.
- **Chromium**, available in liquid or capsule form, is often effective for someone with a blood sugar problem that is keeping them awake at nights. Dr. Hibbs recommends brewer's yeast as a source or, alternatively, taking 250 to 500 micrograms twice a day.
- **L-tryptophan**, found in foods such as milk and turkey, was banned in the United States by the FDA (Food and Drug Administration) after a contaminated batch from a Japanese manufacturer was suspected of causing a serious blood disease in several people. It is considered the best amino acid for sleeping problems, according to Dr. Hibbs.
- **Phosphatidylserine**, an amino acid which helps the hypothalamus regulate the amount of cortisone produced by the adrenals, is helpful for those who cannot sleep because of high cortisone levels, usually induced by stress. Cortisone is usually at high levels in the morning, for wakefulness, but in stressed individuals it may be high at night and prevent sleeping.

Jonathan Wright, M.D., Director of the Tahoma Clinic in Kent, Washington, has had success in treating insomnia using supplements of essential amino acids. He reports the case of a man who had been suffering from insomnia most of his adult life. Over the previous eighteen years, doctors had prescribed fourteen different drugs, starting with sleeping pills and progressing to antidepressants. The sleeping pills left him feeling groggy while the antidepressants resulted in nightmares and, in the case of two drugs, heartbeat trouble. He had also tried supplements of the amino acid L-tryptophan, but his insomnia did not improve.

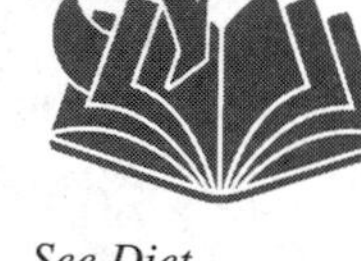

See Diet, Nutritional Supplements.

A blood test determined that the patient was deficient in five of the eight essential amino acids (his tryptophan levels were normal). Using a computer to calculate the proper proportions, Dr. Wright prescribed an amino acid blend to be taken, stirred into applesauce, twice a day. After three weeks, the patient's condition had improved markedly, and within three months, his insomnia had cleared up completely.

Natural Hormone Therapy: John R. Lee, M.D., of Sebastopol, California, treats women who are having trouble sleeping with natural progesterone. Estrogen tends to cause brain cells to swell and causes the irritability and sleep disturbances associated with premenstrual syndrome and menopause, according to Dr. Lee. Progesterone restores hormonal balance, and its calming effect promotes sleep. He cites one woman who came to him with hot flashes which kept her awake at night. After only six weeks of natural progesterone supplements, she was able to sleep peacefully again.

Behavioral Treatments: There are many behavioral self-help techniques that can be used for treating insomnia. Dr. Zimmerman offers the following suggestions for a better night's sleep:

1. Don't look at the clock during the sleep period: Few people realize this, but the awareness of how long you have been trying to fall asleep can be a major contributing cause of insomnia. Worrying about how late it is, or how much time is left before you have to get up in the morning, can only contribute to anxiety.

2. Do not spend too much time in bed trying to fall asleep: If you cannot fall asleep in a comfortable period of time, get out of bed and out of the bedroom. Sit or lie down comfortably in another area of the house and engage in some quiet, relaxing activity such as reading, watching television, or listening to music. When you start to feel sleepy, then, and only then, go back to bed. Do not fall asleep on the sofa or in a chair as it is important to reserve the sleepy feeling only for the bed. This will strengthen the association of being sleepy and being in bed. Repeat this process as often as necessary during the night and eventually you will break the psychological association of being in bed yet not feeling sleepy enough to fall asleep. By the second or third night you will be so sleepy from getting out of bed so often that you will be able to fall asleep quickly the next time you try to do so.

MELATONIN—RESETTING THE BIOLOGICAL CLOCK

William Lee Cowden, M.D., of Dallas, Texas, has had excellent success using melatonin (pineal gland extract), a powerful antioxidant, in treating insomnia. He suggests giving melatonin capsules nightly, between 10:00 P.M. and midnight, for one to two weeks to reset the biological clock, then every other night for several months to normalize sleep habits.

Dr. Cowden reports one man from Florida who came to see him who had suffered from insomnia for ten years, sleeping only three hours a night. He had visited numerous sleep disorders centers, as well as dozens of sleep specialists, and had tried virtually every prescription drug for insomnia, to no avail. Because of his condition, he had become extremely irritable and hard to live with. Dr. Cowden instructed him to avoid sugar and caffeine, sleep in a totally darkened room, remove all electrical devices such as clocks, radios, and televisions, and to take melatonin nightly for two weeks and then every other night for two months. He also gave him supplements of vitamin C and omega-3 oils. After a few days he was sleeping seven to eight hours a night, and after two months he said he was sleeping like he had slept as a child.

In addition, avoid most non-sleeping behaviors in bed. Eliminate reading or watching television in bed and note the results.

3. Try sleep restriction therapy: This behavioral self-help measure is based on the observation that many insomniacs spend a great deal of time in bed when they are not actually sleeping. In order to get a good idea if you are spending too much time in bed without sleeping, compute your sleep efficiency index: Divide the estimated total amount of sleep you get on a given night by the total amount of time you spend in bed from the time you turned out the lights until you get up in the morning. If your total sleep time is only six hours and your total time in bed is eight hours, your sleep efficiency index is only 75 percent—a figure indicating that you could benefit from sleep restriction therapy. A normal sleep efficiency index is usually 85 percent or higher, preferably in the 90 percent range.

In order to do sleep restriction therapy, compute your sleep efficiency index for one week. If it averages less than 90 percent, deliberately go to bed later and/or wake up earlier in the morning. By restricting your time in bed to be about equal to your typical total sleep time, you will increase your sleep efficiency. If you begin to feel sleepy during the day, reward yourself by going to bed earlier or waking up a little later until you have reached a total in-bed time that is not substantially longer than your total sleep time.

“Studies have shown that exercise in the late afternoon or early evening increases the amount of deep sleep that a person gets at night.”

4. Exercise: Studies have shown that exercise in the late afternoon or early evening increases the amount of deep sleep that a person gets at night. Evening is a good time for light exercise such as walking. Most physicians recommend a program which elevates the heart rate by 50 to 75 percent for at least twenty minutes each day.[9] Be warned, however, that the timing of the exercise is important. Exercise done too close to bedtime has a counterproductive effect, since it raises the heart rate and gets the adrenalin going.

5. Spend some time in bright sunlight during the morning hours: Dr. Zimmerman states that few people realize what a powerful influence the bright early morning sunlight has upon circadian rhythms, or biological clocks. Studies have shown that exposure to bright, early morning sunlight (between about 7:00 A.M. and 9:00 A.M.) for at least fifteen minutes is perhaps the most powerful signal that "sets" the biological clocks each morning and entrains them to the twenty-four-hour light/dark cycle. Humans naturally have a 24.8 hour circadian rhythm, and would naturally go to bed about an hour later each night and wake up about that much later each morning. Studies of people living in caves or specially designed "chronobiology" laboratories have confirmed this fact. Bright sunlight each morning coaxes the biological clock to conform to the twenty-four-hour day.

> *"If one is prone to insomnia caused by worrying, evenings are definitely not the time to balance a checkbook or to worry about the next day's business activities."*

Depression is one of the most common causes of early-morning-awakening insomnia, and depressed individuals frequently wake up too early and cannot go back to sleep. Bright light in the morning has a beneficial effect upon depression and what is often known as "winter depression" or seasonal affective disorder (SAD).

Bedtime Rituals—Exercise, Meditation, Baths, Massage, Breathing Exercises: Meditating before bed may help to ease worry about falling asleep. If one is prone to insomnia caused by worrying, evenings are definitely not the time to balance a checkbook or to worry about the next day's business.

Dr. Zimmerman recommends a warm bath before retiring to help increase circulation to the skin and relax the muscles, and adds that baking soda in bath water will soothe the nerves on the surface of the skin. A few drops of pine needle essence, oil of eucalyptus, or mustard powder can also help to relax an individual.

Massage is one of the best ways to relieve muscular tension before sleep. Also, breathing techniques can calm the body and promote sleep. Controlled breathing, such as yogic breathing can help people fall asleep more quickly.

See Bodywork, Herbal Medicine, Homeopathy, Meditation, Yoga.

The following breathing exercise is recommended to bring on drowsiness: Lie on your back or side, eyes closed, and begin with a few very deep inhalations, filling your lungs as much as possible. Then exhale fully, drawing in your abdomen to expel as much air as possible. Repeat this three times, and at the end of the third exhalation hold your breath as long as you can. Repeat this procedure two or three times, or until you feel drowsy.

Herbal Medicine: Certain herbs have long been known to induce a peaceful and restful sleep. Chamomile tea and lime blossom tea with a pinch of skullcap are both soothing remedies. Valerian can also bring on a restful sleep. Studies have shown that valerian has an extremely beneficial effect among poor or irregular sleepers (particularly women), and people with difficulty falling asleep.[10] These herbs should be taken about forty-five minutes before bedtime.[11]

For insomnia, David Hoffmann, B.Sc., M.N.I.M.H., of Sebastopol, California, past President of the American Herbalist Guild, recommends linden flowers, which are especially effective for people with blood pressure problems. Stronger remedies such as passion flower or hops can be very relaxing. Hoffman also suggests an herb bath before going to bed. Fill a muslin bag with chamomile, linden flowers, or lavender, and hang it from the faucet so that the hot water runs through it. He also recommends herbs such as Siberian ginseng and licorice, nutrients such as pantothenic acid (vitamin B_5), and exercise, all of which can help return the adrenal glands to normal functioning.

Biofeedback Treatment for Insomnia

Steven L. Fahrion, Ph.D., Director of the Center for Applied Psychophysiology at the Menninger Clinic in Topeka, Kansas, reports on the successful treatment of a patient with insomnia using biofeedback techniques. The patient had undergone psychotherapy and was on sleeping medication, neither of which helped her problem. She was a very stressed person, and lay awake thinking through the problems of the day. Her sleep ritual included watching television and reading for about an hour before she could fall asleep. Dr. Fahrion found out what kind of relaxation exercises would work for her by monitoring muscle relaxation and hand skin temperature.

Because she wanted to get off the medication, Dr. Fahrion first sent her home with a relaxation tape, and as she used this she was gradually able to taper off her medication, until after three months she could go to sleep without any medication whatsoever. She also cut out reading and by the time Dr. Fahrion stopped seeing her (after about nine months) it only took her about thirty minutes to get to sleep.

Homeopathy: The homeopathic approach to sleep disorders seeks to identify the specific physical or emotional cause of the problem as well as the general nature of the patient. According to Robert Milne, M.D., of Las Vegas, Nevada, a host of factors or confirming symptoms must be taken into account in order to prescribe the appropriate homeopathic remedy. Since many cases of insomnia are related to digestive disturbances and pelvic problems (especially in women), these conditions should be ruled out and/or treated.

Dr. Milne traces many cases of insomnia to grief. For grieving individuals whose confirming factors include irritability, sobbing, and muscle spasms, *Ignatia amara* is often used as a treatment. Another remedy, *Muriaticum acidum*, is recommended for grief-stricken insomnia patients who are marked by extreme emotional sensitivity (another symptom may be an intolerance of sunlight).

Anxiety is also commonly regarded in homeopathic medicine as a cause of insomnia, and it is often treated with *Nux vomica*. Confirming symptoms for people with anxiety-induced insomnia, include sensitivity to cold and irritability toward anything that slows them down.

Dr. Milne points out that in order for homeopathic remedies to be effective, substances such as coffee, marijuana, and cocaine must be avoided.

Traditional Chinese Medicine: Traditional Chinese Medicine views almost all sleep disorders as stemming from kidney problems or weakness. According to Roger Hirsh, O.M.D., of Santa Monica, California, the kidneys, like all the body's organs, store energy. When the kidney's ability to store energy is compromised, sleep disorders can result.

Dr. Hirsh cites the example of people who get a surge of energy at eleven o'clock at night, preventing them from falling asleep. "The energy should go deep in the body," says Dr. Hirsh, "but because there is kidney energy deficiency, the kidney is unable to hold the energy in and, instead, it ascends and disturbs the heart (spirit) which in turn, keeps the person awake."

Though the energy reserves of the kidney are depleted during the aging process, a person can help preserve or restore energy vital to the sleep process by tonifying the kidneys. This is done primarily with herbal remedies, such as a commonly available six-herb formula known as *er long zuo gi wan*. In addition, *qigong* postures and exercises are beneficial to the kidneys, and can thus help the sleep process.

Studies show that some insomnia may be due to a deficiency of endorphins (the body's own natural painkillers), and thus acupuncture is often a useful therapy. During acupuncture, patients tend to become drowsy or even fall asleep, possibly because of increased levels of central nervous system endorphins.[12]

Traditional Chinese Medicine also stresses the need to observe the body's natural daily cycle. Dr. Hirsh notes that the "organ time clock" specifies certain times for restoring the energy of certain organs: 11:00 P.M. to 1:00 A.M. for the gallbladder, 1:00 A.M. to 3:00 A.M. for the liver, 3:00 A.M. to 5:00 A.M. for the lungs, and 5:00 A.M. to 7:00 A.M. for the large intestine. "By going to bed at 9:00 P.M., you put money in the bank," says Hirsh. "A 10:00 P.M. bedtime means that you are spending what you have earned, and an 11:00 P.M. bedtime translates into living on credit."

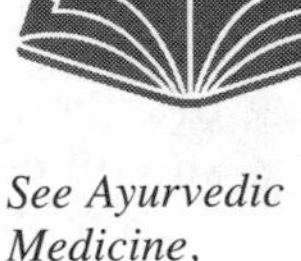

See Ayurvedic Medicine, Traditional Chinese Medicine.

Ayurvedic Medicine: The Ayurvedic approach to sleep disorders focuses on *vata*, the constitutional unit of the body that regulates breathing and circulation. According to Virender Sodhi, M.D. (Ayurveda), N.D., founder of the American School of Ayurvedic Sciences in Bellevue, Washington, people with a *vata* imbalance frequently exhibit irritability, anxiety, and fear, making it difficult for them to rest or relax. "Our aim," says Dr. Sodhi, "is to calm down, relax, and pacify the excessive *vata* system."

A primary treatment for sleep disorders is the topical application of oil to the head and feet. Depending on an individual's body type, different kinds of oil are used at varying temperatures to relax the nervous system. These include coconut oil (*pitta* type, used at room temperature), sesame oil (*vata* type, applied warm), and mustard oil (*kapha* type, applied warm).

A MULTIFACTORIAL APPROACH TO INSOMNIA

John Hibbs, N.D., of the Natural Health Clinic of Bastyr College in Seattle, Washington, cites the case of a forty-year-old patient with chronic insomnia. The patient was slightly overweight, did not exercise, and was tired and depressed. A regimen was devised that combined the amino acid phosphatidylserine, supplements of calcium, magnesium, and the B vitamins, especially B_6 and B_{12}, as well as a constitutional homeopathic remedy, acupuncture, relaxation exercises, and dietary changes. Within a few weeks, the patient had begun to dream again, and after several months, the insomnia had been reduced to approximately one night a week.

Meditation is another form of treatment. Dr. Sodhi explains that by repeating soothing mantras, such as "I sleep properly," in the morning and evening, it is possible to alleviate the anxiety and fear that can interfere with normal sleeping habits. Other forms of meditation, including the use of visualization and aromas (sandalwood, chamomile, jasmine, rose), can also be effective.

Addressing Electromagnetic Pollution and Geopathic Stress: To minimize the effects of electromagnetic pollution on sleep, Dr. Scott-Morley recommends "that all electrical appliances such as radios, alarm clocks, televisions, and computers should be at least six feet from the bed. Electric blankets should not be used. All appliances should be unplugged at the socket before sleeping. The bed frame should be made of wood with no metal parts, and the mattress should not contain metal coils. Water beds should be avoided. Do not sleep directly over garages, fuel tanks, or steel girders.

"Because geopathic stresses are usually confined to a small area, moving the bed to another location may be sufficient to avoid these stresses. The best way to detect geopathic disturbance is with instruments such as the magnetometer despite some limitations. If dowsing is employed, then at least two dowsers should independently survey the property to see if both obtain the same results.

Sleep Apnea

Sleep apnea is not well understood, and can be a difficult condition to treat, but practitioners of alternative medicine are having some success with behavioral treatments, homeopathy, and exercise and weight loss programs.

"Because many of those who suffer from sleep apnea are either overweight or obese, weight loss and exercise can be an effective form of treatment."

Exercise and Weight Loss: Because many of those who suffer from sleep apnea are either overweight or obese, weight loss and exercise can be an effective form of treatment, says Dr. Hibbs, who notes that sleep apnea is generally, though not always, thought to occur because of structural problems. This means that the breathing airways become obstructed while a person is sleeping.

Homeopathy: In treating sleep apnea, *Lachesis* and homeopathic opium are useful, depending on the personality type. Dr. Milne recommends *Lachesis* for extroverted, charismatic, angry individuals while homeopathic opium is prescribed for more temperate people with a history of emotional or physical pain. He points out that sleep apnea relates to loss of energy. Therefore, diet must be carefully chosen, eliminating sugar and other allergic foods.

Avoiding Drugs and Alcohol: One should avoid alcohol and sleeping pills, because they slow down the respiratory drive needed during sleep and cause further relaxation of the throat muscles, which makes obstructive sleep apnea more likely to occur. Sleep laboratory tests reveal that eliminating alcohol dramatically reduces the number of sleep apnea episodes, increases the oxygen saturation levels of the blood, and leads to deeper, more restful sleep.

Behavioral Treatments: Sleeping on one's back may allow the tongue to fall back into the airway and cause an obstruction, leading to sleep apnea. To avoid this position, Dr. Zimmerman recommends cutting a tennis ball in half and sewing each part onto the inside seam of a pajama top—one near the neck and one about mid-back level. This should stop you from rolling over onto your back at night, by making the supine position uncomfortable.

Many people panic when they wake up unable to breathe and try to inhale vigorously. This only worsens the problem and the fear. If this happens, forcefully breathe out, then breathe in again slowly.

Continuous Positive Airway Pressure (CPAP): The most common treatment for sleep apnea used today is a form of respiratory therapy administrated at night called continuous positive airway pressure. CPAP is nothing more than a blower unit, tube, over-the-nose mask, and head gear to keep the mask sealed around the nose to allow the person to breath air under pressure. CPAP involves blowing a soft stream of slightly pressurized air into the nose. The positive pressure in the upper airway counteracts the negative pressure which causes the snoring, the airway narrowing (hypoanea) or the airway collapse (apnea).

Dr. Zimmerman finds that this treatment is highly successful with his patients, who report better quality sleep and increased energy levels. Patients and their spouses are equally pleased with the cessation of snoring, and patients are less likely to awaken to go to the bathroom in the middle of the night.

Dental Treatments: Dental treatments may help alleviate mild and moderate conditions of sleep apnea. But medication and surgery, which have been used in severe cases, are potentially dangerous and costly. Surgery, for example, can sometimes stop the snoring but have no beneficial effect on the sleep apnea, according to Dr. Zimmerman. In some cases, the number of apneic episodes or degree of oxygen desaturation is worse after surgery than before.

Periodic Leg Movement Syndrome and Restless Leg Syndrome

Like sleep apnea, periodic leg movement syndrome and restless leg syndrome can be difficult to treat. Weight reduction (if necessary) and regular exercise are recommended, as are the avoidance of alcohol and the alleviation of any stress-related situations.[13]

Diet and Nutritional Supplements: Dr. Hibbs has had success in treating restless leg syndrome, which he believes is caused by decreased circulation to the legs. He has found vitamin E supplements of 400 IU two or three times a day to be extremely effective in alleviating this condition (he cautions that vitamin E can elevate the blood pressure slightly). In one study concerning vitamin E and restless leg syndrome, a seventy-eight-year-old female with a history of restless and "jumpy" legs found that after two months of 300 IU daily, she was completely cured.[14] In another study, a thirty-seven-year-old female with a ten-year history of severe nightly "restless legs" was placed on 300 IU daily for six weeks and 200 IU daily for the following four weeks with complete relief.[15]

Further information comes from Dr. Chaitow, who recommends avoidance of caffeine in all forms, the elimination of food allergies and sensitivities, and a supplement of blue or green algae (as a substitute for L-tryptophan, and especially for those people whose symptoms can be resolved by massage or movement of the limbs). He also recommends two to three grams of folic acid daily, to be given under strict supervision to avoid toxicity.

Homeopathy: According to Dr. Milne, restless leg syndrome and PLMS are treated with *Rhus tox.* (for rheumatism-related conditions) or *Causticum* (for nervous system-related conditions). Pelvic or prostate problems should also be treated.

Self-Care

The following therapies can be undertaken at home under appropriate professional supervision:

• Biofeedback Training • Guided Imagery • Qigong

Hydrotherapy: Immersion bath or wet sheet pack: neutral application as needed for sedation.

Juice Therapy: Carrot, spinach, lettuce, celery juice.

Light Therapy: Full-spectrum and bright-light therapies have been effective in treating a wide range of depressive and affective disorders including sleep disorders, seasonal affective disorder and premenstrual syndrome.

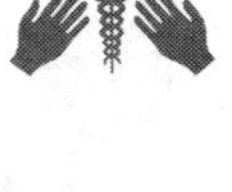

Professional Care

The following therapies should only be provided by a qualified health professional:

• Acupuncture • Chiropractic • Craniosacral Therapy • Magnetic Field Therapy • Osteopathy • Naturopathic Medicine

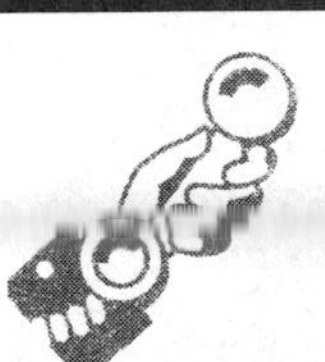

Where to Find Help

For more information on sleep disorders, or referrals to a qualified health care practitioner, contact the following organizations:

American Association of Acupuncture and Oriental Medicine
4101 Lake Boone Trail, Suite 201
Raleigh, North Carolina 27607
(919) 787-5181

The AAAOM is a national professional trade organization of acupuncturists who meet acceptable standards of competency and can provide you with the names and locations of local members.

American Association of Naturopathic Physicians
2366 Eastlake Avenue, Suite 322
Seattle, Washington 98102
(206) 323-7610

Provides referrals to a nationwide network of accredited or licensed practitioners. Publishes a quarterly newsletter for both professionals and the general public. Also offers a series of brochures and pamphlets on a variety of subjects.

American Holistic Medical Association
4101 Lake Boone Trail, Suite 201
Raleigh, North Carolina 27607
(919) 787-5181

A professional organization for holistic practitioners, the AHMA offers information and services for its members and lobbies for holistic issues. It also provides referrals for the public; requests must be in writing.

American Sleep Disorders Association
1610 14th Street, N.W., Suite 300
Rochester, Minnesota 55901
(507) 287-6006

The ASDA can refer you to a sleep disorders center near you where your sleep or wakefulness problem can receive the expert and professional attention it deserves.

American School of Ayurvedic Sciences
10025 NE 4th Street
Bellevue, Washington 98004
(206) 453-8022

This college provides medical training for physicians and health care practitioners, as well as individual courses for lay people. Dr. Virender Sodhi's Ayurvedic, Naturopathic Medical Clinic is also located at this address.

Ayurvedic Institute
11311 Menaul NE, Suite A
Albuquerque, New Mexico 87112
(505) 291-9698

The institute, directed by Dr. Vasant Lad, trains people from all walks of life in most of the aspects of Ayurveda.

The College of Maharishi Ayur-Veda Medical Center
P.O. Box 282
Fairfield, Iowa 52556
(515) 472-5866

The center provides referrals to health centers, which offer methods of prevention and treatment of a broad range of illnesses. They also train practitioners and provide information to the lay public.

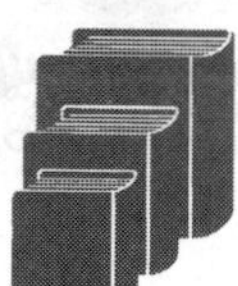

Recommended Reading

Everybody's Guide to Natural Sleep. Kaufman, Daniel.; Goldberg, Philip; Los Angeles: Jeremy P. Tarcher, 1990.

This book allows the reader to assess his or her individual sleep problems and then presents a multitude of techniques to permanently conquer insomnia.

Losing Sleep. Dotto, Lydia. New York: Quill, 1990.

What sleep is, what it means when you don't get enough, and what can be done about insomnia and other sleep disorders.

No More Sleepless Nights. Hauri, P., Ph.D.; Linde, Shirley, Ph.D., New York: Wiley Press.

Offers a comprehensive look at insomnia, and outlines the steps necessary to overcome this problem by helping patients to identify the cause of sleeplessness rather than simply covering it up with sleeping pills.

Solve Your Child's Sleep Problems. Ferber, Richard, M.D. New York: Simon & Schuster, Inc., 1985.

A valuable book on the common sleep problems of children, from babies to teens, that offers clear explanations and common sense solutions. This book is backed by six years of research offering ideas to help you with your child's sleep problems.

Stress Management. Gordon, James S. New York: Chelsea House, 1990.

Stress Management *traces the interaction between stress and bodily functions and describes a few of the many programs available to manage the condition before it becomes destructive. The book places special emphasis on holistic approaches such as wellness programs, which use biofeedback, massage, and body-awareness techniques to promote relaxation and health.*

Stress

Current estimates show that between 70 and 80 percent of all visits to physicians are for stress-related disorders.[1] Chronic stress directly affects the immune system, and if not effectively dealt with, can seriously compromise health. Alternative medicine offers many beneficial strategies for reducing stress and its effects, including acupuncture, biofeedback, meditation, guided imagery, and lifestyle counseling, as well as diet and nutritional programs.

Stress can be defined as a reaction to any stimulus or interference that upsets normal functioning and disturbs mental or physical health. It can be brought on by internal conditions such as illness, pain, or emotional conflict, or by external circumstances such as a death in the family, or financial problems. Even a positive experience—a new marriage, a job promotion, or financial gain—can be a stress-provoking event.

"Stress can also be caused by allergic reactions, poor diet, nutritional deficiencies, substance abuse, or biochemical imbalances in the body," according to Konrad Kail, N.D., past President of the American Association of Naturopathic Physicians. "These internal imbalances are a major contributing factor to stress. They help to set up a cycle in which a stressor causes a biochemical imbalance in the body. This, in turn, depletes the immune system, causing illness, which creates more stress for the person, and the cycle continues."

> *"Although a certain amount of stress is a normal part of our lives, prolonged bouts of stress can lead to exhaustion and illness, along with more serious health problems."*

Although a certain amount of stress is a normal part of our lives, prolonged bouts of stress can lead to exhaustion and minor illness, along with more serious health problems. Eric Peper, Ph.D, Associate Director of the Institute of Holistic Healing Studies at San Francisco State University, states that up to 80 percent of the health problems in America today are considered stress-related. According to Dr. Kail, "Repeated incidences of stress can interfere with digestion, alter brain chemistry, increase heart rate and blood pressure, and affect metabolic and immune functioning."

He cites studies that show depressed immune functioning to be associated with many stress-inducing experiences and conditions, including bereavement, divorce, job loss, school or professional examinations, depression, loneliness, and sleep deprivation.[2]

Fortunately, stress and its effects can be reduced through exercise, relaxation, biofeedback, guided imagery, counseling, involvement in social groups and support groups, meditation, acupuncture, massage, yoga, deep breathing, and other lifestyle changes. These therapeutic approaches can help restore normal function to the internal biochemical processes and help to reverse chronic stress.

How Stress Affects Health

Everyone experiences stress on a daily basis. "Although stress itself is not a disease, it can aggravate numerous conditions, including allergies, arthritis, asthma, atherosclerosis, cancer, colitis, diabetes, emphysema, gastritis, hypertension, hypoglycemia, neuromuscular syndromes, speech problems, and ulcers," according to Dr. Kail. "Whatever the source or cause of the stress, human beings respond biochemically to stress in a very predictable manner," he adds. "Stress begets illness which increases stress, thereby aggravating the illness."

Dr. Kail's review of the available research reveals the following recurrent themes associated with stress:

- High levels of emotional stress increase susceptibility to illness.[3]
- Chronic stress results in a suppression of

the immune system, which in turn creates increased susceptibility to illness—especially to immune-related disorders and cancer.[4]

- Emotional stress also leads to hormonal imbalances (adrenal, pituitary, thyroid, thymus, and others) that further interfere with immune function.[5]

Pioneering stress researcher Hans Selye, M.D., a Canadian physiologist, noted a consistent pattern of response to stress in his studies and termed these the general adaptation syndrome (GAS). Outlined in three stages, they consist of the alarm reaction, the stage of resistance, and the stage of exhaustion.[6]

Initially, the body's biochemistry tends to react to stress in an orderly fashion.[7] Stimulation of the sympathetic nervous system (part of the autonomic nervous system consisting of ganglia, nerves, and plexuses that supply the involuntary muscles) activates the secretion of hormones from endocrine glands, and constricts both the blood vessels and the involuntary muscles of the body. When the endocrine glands are stimulated, heart rate, glucose metabolism, and oxygen consumption increase. The parasympathetic nervous system (the craniosacral division of the autonomic nervous system) is also stimulated, which begins a process of relaxation. The pituitary gland responds by releasing a variety of hormones throughout the body which influence the defensive and adaptive mechanisms. Endorphins, the body's own natural painkillers, are also released.[8]

> *"Although stress itself is not a disease, it can aggravate numerous conditions, including allergies, arthritis, asthma, atherosclerosis, cancer, colitis, diabetes, emphysema, gastritis, hypertension, hypoglycemia, neuromuscular syndromes, speech problems, and ulcers."*
> —Konrad Kail, N.D.

Dr. Selye points out, however, that eventually chronic stress depletes the body's resources and its ability to adapt. If stress continues and remains unattended for a long period, coping functions will be compromised and illness will result.

British cardiologist Peter Nixon, M.D., notes that excessive or chronic stress inhibits immune function, protein synthesis, and cardiac functioning. Dr. Nixon adds that chronic stress can deplete not only the body's reserves, but can exhaust other physiological functions. This process can lead to cancer and heart disease.[9]

William Lee Cowden, M.D., a Dallas, Texas-based cardiologist, confirms that stress may precipitate heart disease. He believes that it may be significant that most heart attacks occur on Monday mornings. "In response to stress the arterial wall may spasm, causing heartbeat irregularities which lead to cardiac arrest," says Dr. Cowden. He explains that this is often not a sudden response, but one brought on by years of not dealing properly with stress.

Stress-Related Anxiety

Stress is not always an unhealthy experience, and some people even seem to thrive on it. Dr. Kail explains, for example, that stress can help top-level executives control anxiety. Middle-management employees, by contrast, are far more susceptible to uncontrollable situations, and, as it turns out, are at higher risk for cancer. According to Frederick Levenson, Ph.D., who teaches at Hofstra University and the Center for Modern Psychoanalytic Studies in New York, "Any stress that allows an individual to defend against anxiety . . . is anticancer. Any stress that places the individual in high performance anxiety situations in which the variables cannot be manipulated will produce high levels of internal carcinogens."[10]

See Cancer, Colds and Flu, Heart Disease, Hypertension.

Everyone reacts differently to stress, and the amount of emotional stress a person experiences depends on the individual's coping functions. Likewise, the degree of anxiety that a person experiences often indicates how well he or she is coping.

Some common symptoms of anxiety include excessive or unwarranted worrying, a rising sense of panic, restlessness, insomnia, trembling or feeling shaky, muscle tension, fatigue, shortness of breath, heart palpitations, sweaty or clammy hands, hot flashes or chills, dizziness, irritability, and difficulty concentrating.

Increased Susceptibility to Colds and Viral Infections

In an experiment on the relationship between stress and the probability of viral infection, 420 people were evaluated for occurrences of stress during the course of a year. These included such events as job loss, death in the family, moving, divorce, or feeling frightened, nervous, sad, angry, irritated, or unable to cope with current demands. They were then exposed to one of five cold viruses and tested one month later for antibodies. Ninety percent of those who were under the greatest stress became infected, compared to 74 percent of those who experienced the least amount of stress.[11]

In another study of 100 subjects, those who experienced stress (particularly the type of stress associated with tension and anger) were four times more likely to develop a cold or bacterial infection.[12]

Allergies

Dr. Kail reports that physicians are seeing increasing numbers of patients complaining of stress-related disorders such as allergies, candida overgrowth, and chronic fatigue syndrome. He explains that an allergic reaction is a stressor which can trigger a variety of symptoms, including irritability, aggressive behavior, depression, and anxiety.

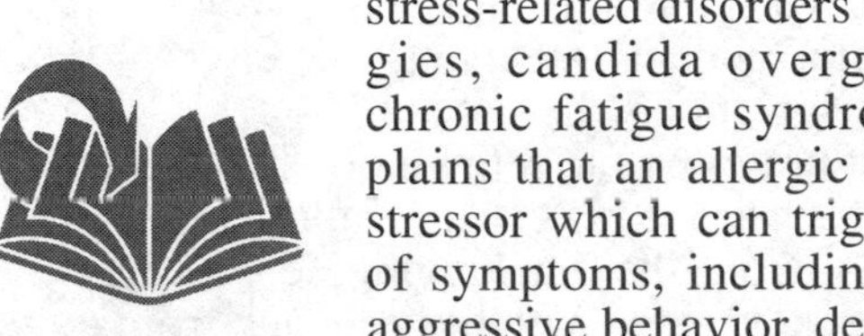

See Allergies, Environmental Medicine.

During an allergic reaction, the body releases histamine, a chemical that is present in cells throughout the body. Histamine causes inflammation, excess stomach acid, a narrowing of the air pathways in the lungs, and increased stress on other organs and glands. Dr. Kail also notes that because stress affects the immune and endocrine systems, leaving them in a weakened, susceptible state, chronic stress may actually precipitate the allergic reaction in the first place. "Allergies are significant stressors," says Dr. Kail. "Their proper diagnosis and treatment should be included in any medical checkup."

Treating and Reducing Stress

If stress contributes to illness, then stress reduction should promote healing. This theory for alleviating stress is the basis of numerous approaches such as meditation, progressive relaxation, guided imagery, biofeedback, yoga, and *qigong*. Other methods include dietary changes, herbal medicine, Ayurvedic medicine, and Traditional Chinese Medicine techniques such as acupuncture and acupressure.

"More important than the stressors themselves is the person's ability to cope with them."

Life experiences, beginning with infancy and childhood, shape behavior in significant ways. How these experiences are handled often affects our ability to deal with stress in the future. Therefore, it is important for both children and adults to learn effective coping skills when dealing with stressful stimuli and events. Failure to do so, says Dr. Kail, can result in emotional imbalance, which in turn affects the biochemistry of the body, and can lead to serious psychological and physiological problems.

Relaxation Therapies

Meditation, biofeedback, guided imagery, yoga, and *qigong* all have one thing in common, they facilitate deep relaxation and reduce stress. Herbert Benson, M.D., of Harvard Medical School, called this physiological mechanism "the relaxation response" and has applied its principles to the treatment of cardiac disease, using it to lower blood pressure and decrease gastric acid secretion.[13] Dean Ornish, M.D., Assistant Clinical Professor of Medicine at the University of California at San Francisco, has been able to reverse coronary heart disease by employing a

MIND/BODY MEDICINE: THE PSYCHOLOGY OF STRESS

A basic premise in mind/body medicine is that chronic stress can contribute to illness, and that relaxation, positive ways of coping with stress, and restoration of integral physical and mental/emotional functioning will improve one's health. More important than the stressors themselves is the person's ability to cope with them.

If there is a psychological process that is conducive to the development of chronic disease, as the science of psychoneuroimmunology suggests, then there is a corresponding psychological process for recovery. This process may include counseling, involvement in a therapeutic support group, and/or the conscious decision to alter one's lifestyle and behavior. Feelings of hope and renewed optimism not only improve one's psychological state, but also promote better immune functioning of the body.

In a recent research review, Jeanne Achterberg, Ph.D., President of the Association for Transpersonal Psychology, cited numerous studies demonstrating that feelings of security, coupled with the ability to cope, counter negative emotions that can interfere with healing, compromise the immune system, and encourage cardiovascular disease.[15] Pioneering stress researcher Hans Selye, M.D., pointed out that overambitious goals and personal objectives which exceed one's experience and skill are a common stressor. He suggested that a person measure the benefit of performing a stressful task to determine if it is worth the involvement. He also recommended that people avoid unnecessary stress and try to limit stress or stressful situations to more manageable scheduled times whenever possible.

combination of meditation, stress-reduction exercises, psychotherapy, and a vegetarian diet.[14] Stress-reduction techniques often employ deep breathing and visualization in order to enhance the relaxation process.

Meditation: At the University of Massachusetts Medical School, Jon Kabat-Zinn, Ph.D., founded the Stress Reduction Clinic in 1979 to help people suffering from chronic pain, chronic diseases such as cancer and heart disease, as well as stress-related disorders such as abdominal pain, chronic diarrhea, and ulcers. According to Dr. Kabat-Zinn, these conditions are often the most difficult to treat, and the patients have frequently tried other, more conventional forms of medicine without complete success.

"Meditation is so effective in reducing stress and tension that, in 1984, the National Institutes of Health recommended meditation over prescription drugs as the first treatment for mild hypertension."

Dr. Kabat-Zinn's stress-reduction program was originally designed to test the value of using mindfulness meditation to help patients develop effective coping strategies for stress, and to see whether meditation would have any effect on their chronic medical conditions. According to Dr. Kabat-Zinn, it turned out that it did, and that the majority of people improved in a number of different ways.[16]

Meditation is so effective in reducing stress and tension that in 1984, the National Institutes of Health recommended meditation over prescription drugs as the first treatment for mild hypertension.[17] In addition, Dr. Benson has documented that meditation has the beneficial physiological effect of slowing the breathing rate, increasing oxygen consumption, creating a more relaxed brain wave rhythm, and increasing blood flow.[18] Meditation has also been shown to have a positive effect on immune functions and in strengthening the body's defenses against infectious disease.[19]

Biofeedback Training: Biofeedback training is another method for learning how to regulate a person's body functions to reduce physical and psychological stress, and is often used in conjunction with other relaxation and stress-reduction techniques. Through the use of visual or auditory signals from a machine that records a person's physiological responses, one can learn to voluntarily relax specific muscles, alter the brain's electrical activity, reduce heart rate and blood pressure, increase body warmth, and improve gastrointestinal functioning.[20]

Steven Fahrion, Ph.D., Director of the Center for Applied Psychophysiology at the Menninger Clinic in Topeka, Kansas, reports on a forty-six-year-old male who was having problems with dizziness and vertigo. When he stood up he would have an excessively high heart rate and inefficient blood pumping so that the brain was getting an inadequate blood supply. He had been treated unsuccessfully with medications and psychotherapy over a period of several months and was referred for biofeedback treatment.

See Biofeedback Training, Guided Imagery, Light Therapy, Meditation, Qigong, Yoga.

Dr. Fahrion found the patient's hand temperature to be far below normal and that he was breathing from his chest (shallow breathing) instead of from the diaphragm. He was also breathing at a rapid rate. With biofeedback from a thermometer, he was taught to increase the temperature in his hands and to slow diaphragmatic breathing. Within three weeks his symptoms had greatly improved and he was off medication.

Guided Imagery: Guided imagery is a very common relaxation technique. Many people find guided imagery to be an easy way to learn to relax, as the active nature of this practice makes it comfortable and enjoyable.

A typical application, as described by Martin L. Rossman, M.D., Co-director of the Academy of Guided Imagery in Mill Valley, California, is to close your eyes, take a few deep, easy breaths, and recall a time and place when you felt relaxed and peaceful. You should then imagine being there, noticing in detail the sights, sounds, and smells of this place, focusing especially on the specific feelings of peacefulness and relaxation. This simple practice can be used in combination with other relaxation techniques or alone as a quick stress reducer.

Guided imagery can also be used to accomplish specific objectives besides relaxation and stress reduction, such as increasing immune response, reducing susceptibility to disease, controlling pain, losing weight, or dealing with anxiety or depression. The relaxation-imagery process can also serve as a method of evaluating current belief systems and altering those beliefs. Alterations in the symbols and pictures that one uses can dramatically change beliefs to those more compatible with optimizing health.

Yoga: Yoga has long been associated with reducing stress. The physical postures, meditation, and breathing exercises that are part of the practice of yoga can have a healing and relaxing effect on both body and mind. In fact, the concept behind the study of yoga is the integration of mind and body, explained by the observation that when the mind is restless and agitated, the health of the body will be adversely affected, and that when the body is ill, mental functioning will be compromised.

Since the early 1970s, more than one thousand studies of yoga and meditation have demonstrated their effectiveness in reducing stress and anxiety, lowering blood pressure and heart rate, alleviating pain, providing relief from addictions, heightening visual and auditory perceptions, and improving memory, intelligence, and motor skills, as well as metabolic and respiratory functioning.[21] Yoga has also been shown to markedly reduce blood pressure in adults suffering from hypertension thereby decreasing the need for drug therapy.[22]

PROGRESSIVE RELAXATION EXERCISE

- *Find a quiet place with soft lighting. Sit in a comfortable chair, feet flat on the floor, eyes closed.*
- *Become aware of your breathing.*
- *Take in a few deep breaths, and mentally say, as you let out each breath, "Relax."*
- *Concentrate on your face, feeling any tension in your face and eyes. Make a mental picture of this tension—such as a rope tied in a knot or a clenched fist—and then mentally picture it relaxing or being untied and becoming comfortable, lying limp, like a relaxed rubberband.*
- *Experience your face and eyes becoming relaxed. As they relax, feel a wave of relaxation spreading throughout your body.*
- *Tense your eyes and face, squeezing tightly, then relax and feel the relaxation spreading throughout your body.*
- *Apply the previous instructions to other parts of your body. Move slowly down your body—jaw, neck, shoulders, back, upper and lower arms, hands, chest, abdomen, thighs, calves, ankles, feet, toes—until every part of your body is relaxed. Mentally picture the tension in each part of the body, then picture the tension melting away; tense the area and then relax.*
- *When you have relaxed each part of your body, rest quietly in this comfortable state for two to five minutes.*
- *Now let the muscles in your eyelids lighten up and prepare to open your eyes and become aware of the room.*
- *Finally, let your eyes open. You are ready to continue with the day's activities, refreshed and relaxed.*

Qigong: According to recent medical studies in both China and the United States, *qigong* (pronounced "chi-kung") can also reduce stress. This ancient Chinese exercise combines graceful movements and rhythmic breathing, and if practiced regularly can improve muscular strength and flexibility and reverse damage caused by prior injuries and disease. Research has shown that *qigong* also initiates the "relaxation response," leading to decreased heart rate, lowered blood pressure, stress reduction, and increased energy and tissue regeneration.[23]

Diet and Nutritional Supplements

According to Dr. Kail, "Often, symptoms of stress such as anxiety, depression, allergic-like reactions, food and chemical intolerances, and hyperactivity can be explained by a careful examination of diet, as well as vitamin, mineral, enzyme, and other nutrient levels." He suggests that those suffering from stress avoid caffeine and food additives, and stick to a fresh, whole foods diet that is high in complex carbohydrates, moderate in protein, and low in fat. Less than 2 percent of the diet should consist of simple sugars, and those should come from fruit, not fruit juice.

Stress also tends to increase the likelihood of maldigestion and malabsorption, and because of this, many individuals may have vitamin deficiencies, says Dr. Kail. For example, he notes that vitamin B_6 is rapidly depleted during times of stress and needs to be replenished on a regular basis. His nutritional program includes supplements of multivitamins and minerals, particularly B-complex vitamins and vitamins A, C, and E, as well as calcium and trace elements. He finds these deficient in most people. Dr. Kail also strongly encourages his patients to use stress-reduction techniques and plenty of exercise in conjunction with his nutritional program.

See Diabetes, Diet, Hypoglycemia, Nutritional Supplements.

Hypoglycemia is one stress-related disorder that can be directly addressed by diet. Harvey Ross, M.D., an orthomolecular psychiatrist from Los Angeles, notes that people with hypoglycemia (low blood sugar) are particularly vulnerable to stress because they have low energy and often their thinking and concentration are impaired. "Their mood is usually depressed. When life's little stresses—or big stresses—come up they just don't have the tools to deal with them." He believes a person is genetically predisposed to hypoglycemia, and a poor diet—usually high in refined carbohydrates—and stress set off the symptoms. "If a person has poor energy and depression not directly related to life's events, and he is anxious and irritable, yet his doctor tells him everything is normal, he should start thinking about a nutritional cause for these problems—particularly hypoglycemia."

In treating hypoglycemia, Dr. Ross uses an individualized program that includes a strict diet and the addition of nutritional supplementation with multivitamins, chromium (100 to 200 milligrams daily), and glutamine (1,000 milligrams, three times a day half an hour before meals). He recommends a high-protein, low-carbohydrate diet, and instead of three meals daily, the patient eats smaller meals five times a day, with frequent high-protein snacks. After the first four months, patients are introduced to a maintenance diet that includes no more than three servings of fruit a day. Ideally, patients will refrain from processed foods and sugars, but they may occasionally have a small amount of sugar. However, in times of increased stress, they may need to return to the stricter dietary program, cautions Dr. Ross.

Exercise

Physical exercise is commonly regarded as an effective means of reducing stress. But while a good workout can have beneficial effects, over-exercising can wear on the body's resources and contribute to stress. It is important, therefore, to devise an exercise routine appropriate to the needs of the individual.

> *"I don't think there's a single thing in life that's as therapeutic as the right kind of exercise program applied over time. But misapplied, it can be just another stressor."*
> —John Hibbs, N.D.

"I don't think there's a single thing in life that's as therapeutic as the right kind of exercise program applied over time," says John Hibbs, N.D., of Bastyr College in Seattle, Washington. "But misapplied, it can be just another stressor." Dr. Hibbs cites the example of Type A individuals, whose lives are defined by a constant drive to achieve. "Turn them loose in the gym and what are they inclined to do? The same thing. Work really hard, pump, pump, pump. There are studies now showing that such exercise does not decrease your chance of heart disease and stroke, it might even increase it."

Instead, Dr. Hibbs recommends what he calls tissue aerobic exercise: relaxing exercise that allows blood flow to continue to the tissues. "The heart rate should increase and you should wind up sweating, but many doctors are switching over to a lower heart rate now. You don't need to go up to 140," says Dr. Hibbs.

Virender Sodhi, M.D. (Ayurveda), N.D., Director of the American School of Ayurvedic Sciences in Bellevue, Washington, emphasizes exercise geared to the specific nature of the individual. For *vata* (thin, restless, nervous) types, nonstrenuous exercise such as walking is recommended. *Pitta* (moderate build) types, says Dr. Sodhi, should engage in moderate forms of exercise. For *kapha* (large body frame) types, Dr. Sodhi suggests heavy exercise, including running or weightlifting.

Herbal Medicine

One of the most universal methods of relaxing is drinking a hot cup of tea. Many herbalists suggest brewing certain herbs known for their stress-relieving properties.

Daniel O. Gagnon, a medical herbalist affiliated with the Botanical Research and Educational Institute in Santa Fe, New Mexico, recommends chamomile to help promote relaxation. Chamomile tea is used daily by millions of people worldwide to decrease their stress level. Gagnon has found it to be one of the best herbal remedies for treating acute and chronic gastritis and gastric ulcers, which are often caused by an inability to deal effectively with stress. Among its many properties (anti-inflammatory, relaxing, antispasmodic), chamomile works to strengthen the stomach. Another effective herbal treatment is passion flower. It may be used safely during the day as it

See Flower Remedies, Herbal Medicine, Naturopathic Medicine.

Flower Remedies for Stress

Many people who have difficulty coping with stress find flower remedies to be helpful. Flower remedies were originally developed earlier this century by Edward Bach, M.B., B.S., D.P.H., a British physician interested in the link between emotions and physical illness. He began to investigate the healing potential of the wildflowers native to the English countryside and found that the essences distilled from thirty-eight flowering plants and trees had a profound effect on the underlying psychological and emotional states that influence physical illness. These thirty-eight remedies became known as the Bach flower remedies. Today, there are numerous flower remedies available to address the specific psychological and emotional factors involved in many minor stress-related conditions.[24]

will not cause drowsiness. Gagnon recommends it for the chronic worrier and for the overly busy mind.

To keep the central nervous system from being overwhelmed, Gagnon suggests valerian, which is especially useful when dealing with high emotional stress. He also recommends American ginseng (*Panax quinquefolius*) to help support the entire body during stressful times, noting that it is underutilized for this purpose. American ginseng can help protect against the effects of emotional, mental and physical stress because of its ability to work as an adaptogen, a substance described by Gagnon as one which "helps the body be more prepared and more resistant to everyday stresses."[25]

Traditional Chinese Medicine

According to Traditional Chinese Medicine (TCM), stress may be a factor in the development of many diseases. Treatment of stress in TCM includes acupuncture and herbs to help balance the body's energies and relieve the tension that constricts the functioning of a particular part of the body.

Maoshing Ni, D.O.M., Ph.D, L.Ac.,Vice-President of Yo San University of Traditional Chinese Medicine in Santa Monica, California, says that stress is a nervous response of the body to external or internal irritants. According to TCM, the liver is affected first, and continued stress then impacts other organs.

Dr. Ni treats stress with a combination of acupuncture and herbs such as astragalus, ligus-

A NATUROPATHIC PHYSICIAN'S APPROACH TO STRESS

Konrad Kail, N.D., past President of the American Association of Naturopathic Physicians, recalls a thirty-year-old sales representative and mother of two who came to him with a two-year history of stress-related disorders. "Her symptoms included recurrent episodes of fatigue, difficulty concentrating, confusion, dizziness, emotional swings, body aches, gastrointestinal upset, night sweats, recurrent low-grade fevers, swollen glands, and severe premenstrual symptoms," says Dr. Kail. "To her advantage, she did not smoke or drink, and tried to eat a wholesome diet, but she consumed two cups of coffee and three glasses of black tea daily. Recently, she had become more susceptible to minor illnesses such as colds and flus. Her past history included mononucleosis and frequent childhood ear infections.

"A symptom survey showed findings compatible with digestive disturbance, liver-gallbladder dysfunction, and multi-endocrine deficit (inadequately functioning hormonal glands). The physical examination was fairly normal except for findings of rhinitis (inflammation of nasal mucosa) and other signs of allergy, and a few tender lymph nodes in the neck. Her spleen and thyroid were marginally enlarged and her neck and shoulder muscles were tight. Also, anxiety and depression scores were in the mild to moderate range."

Laboratory tests ordered by Dr. Kail suggested poor protein digestion, mild bowel toxicity, possible hydrochloric acid deficiency, adrenal fatigue, and a severe vitamin C deficiency. Further lab work revealed allergy/sensitivity, candida overgrowth, and chronic Epstein-Barr virus infection. According to Dr. Kail, "These stressors had caused malabsorption, adrenal fatigue, hypoglycemia, and hypothyroidism, and were interfering with her body's ability to defend against minor illness. Also, her average body temperature was very low, suggesting thyroid dysfunction, and transit time of foodstuff in her digestive system was thirty-two hours, indicating constipation."

Dr. Kail reported his findings, explaining that her biochemical systems were having trouble maintaining a state of balance, most likely caused by a combination of physical and mental/emotional stressors. For treatment, he prescribed digestive aids in the form of plant enzymes to take before meals. Dr. Kail prefers plant enzymes to animal enzymes since they work over a broader pH (acid-base balance) range. Adrenal and thyroid supplements were also recommended, as were the herbs black radish and dandelion to stimulate liver function and to regulate her hormones. Additionally, she was given a therapeutic dose multivitamin-mineral to replace any nutritional deficiencies. Dr. Kail used acupressure to treat her allergies, and an herbal preparation of Urtica dioica *which inhibits histamine, the chemical mediator of allergic reactions, to treat chronic fatigue syndrome. The candida was treated with grapefruit seed extract.*

Finally, Dr. Kail asked his patient to exercise strenuously and to spend thirty minutes a day practicing a variety of relaxation and visualization techniques. According to Dr. Kail, over the course of a year she was able to attain 90 percent of her previous energy and strength capabilities and her symptoms were reduced greatly.

INCREASING YOUR ABILITY TO COPE WITH STRESS

Although stress and stressful situations are unavoidable, increasing one's coping functions is recommended so that stress will not damage health and contribute to the development of a chronic disease. The following guidelines are suggested by Dr. Kail:

- *In addition to practicing relaxation and stress-management techniques, plan regular diversions and cultivate outside interests.*
- *Get enough sleep and rest. Set up a ritual that establishes a regular hour of bedtime. Avoid sleeping pills.*
- *Get regular vigorous exercise. Relaxed muscles mean relaxed nerves. Choose whatever exercise you enjoy that is appropriate for your age and physical condition, but do it on a daily basis.*
- *Avoid hurry and avoid worry. These far too common behaviors alter your patterns of eating, sleeping, working, and recreation. They are learned behaviors and can be unlearned.*
- *Don't be afraid of compromise. In a stressful situation you can either fight back, back off, or compromise. Seldom is the ideal situation available.*
- *Love more. Learn to use things and love people, instead of using people and loving things.*
- *Identify your fears, even list them. Fear adds to paralysis. To break this cycle, make a decision, right or wrong, and then act on it. Anxiety results when you sit in the middle and let your fears tug at you from opposite directions.*
- *Laugh more. Laughter is a good tension breaker.*
- *Try to maintain calm in the face of stressful situations. Reestablish calm after unavoidable upsets.*
- *Avoid self-pity.*
- *Avoid loneliness. Reach out and take the initiative in friendship. Treat people as though they were already your friends. Seek out people with common interests.*
- *Avoid coping solutions that involve alcohol or drugs. Using a chemical means of escaping from your problems soon leads to addiction and increases your problems. This also applies to stimulants such as tobacco, caffeine, and sugar.*
- *Consider meditation, yoga,* tai chi chuan, *autogenic training, biofeedback, prayer, self-hypnosis, or other techniques used to increase coping functions, alleviate stress, and achieve a state of relaxed awareness.*

tra, and ginseng. He also prescribes visualization and breathing exercises through the practice of *qigong* and *tai chi*.

One of Dr. Ni's patients, a fifty-two year-old lawyer who worked eighty hours a week, came to him complaining of headaches, neck pain, low back pain, insomnia, high blood pressure, and impotence of six months' duration. Dr. Ni treated the patient with acupuncture and herbs, and gave him some *qigong* exercises which he could do at work. After weekly treatment for one and a half months, his pain became minimal, his blood pressure returned to normal, he no longer was impotent, and he only occasionally suffered from insomnia. Dr. Ni points out that such patients need to be treated at least once a month on a continuing basis to maintain the effects.

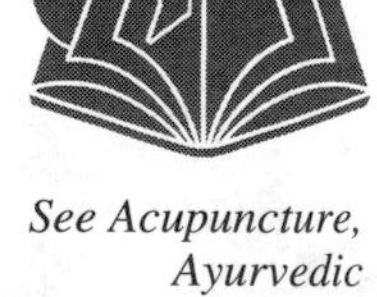

See Acupuncture, Ayurvedic Medicine, Traditional Chinese Medicine.

Ayurvedic Medicine

"In treating stress through Maharishi Ayurveda, we look at four areas: consciousness, physiology, behavior, and environment," says Hari Sharma, M.D., President of the Maharishi Ayurveda Medical Association. Exact treatment varies according to body type, Dr. Sharma says, but the same four areas are addressed. Mental stress is relieved by Transcendental Meditation. Physiology is addressed by dietary changes that include avoiding stimulants and eating a whole foods diet and daily massages with sesame oil. Behavior modification involves adhering to a daily routine, with regular hours of work, sleep, and meals, and an organized lifestyle. The patient's environment is improved through music and aromatherapy, and a cleaner, more restful living space (i.e., one should keep the bedroom a soothing and pleasing place to rest, devoid of work materials and clutter).

If these four areas of life are attended to, stress should be relieved within a few days, according to Dr. Sharma. The most important factor, he says, is to keep the regular daily schedule as stress free as possible.

Self-Care

The following therapies can be undertaken at home under appropriate professional supervision:

Acupressure: To relieve anxiety place your fingertips on CV17 in the indentation of your breastbone at the level of your heart. Hold firmly for two minutes while you take long slow deep breaths. (See acupressure chart on page 874)

Aromatherapy: For anxiety: benzoin, bergamot, chamomile, camphor, cedarwood, clary sage, cypress, frankincense, geranium, hyssop, jasmine, juniper, lavender, lemon, marjoram, melissa, neroli, rose, sandalwood, ylang ylang.

Hydrotherapy: Constitutional hydrotherapy, immersion bath or wet sheet pack: apply two to five times weekly, neutral application as needed for sedation. • Leon Chaitow, N.D., D.O., of London, England, reports that the neutral bath where one is immersed in 35 degrees centigrade water for two hours has a sedative effect and can be helpful in achieving complete relaxation in anyone who is suffering from severe anxiety, agitation, irritability, exhaustion, chronic pain, or insomnia.

Juice Therapy: To reduce anxiety: equal parts lettuce and carrot juice two times a day.

Professional Care

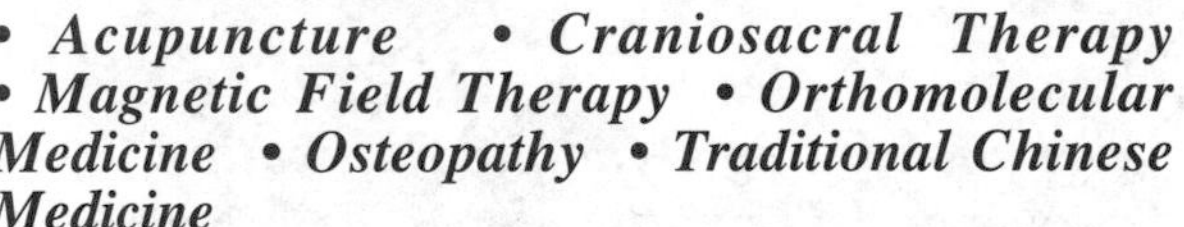

The following therapies should only be provided by a qualified health professional:

• Acupuncture • Craniosacral Therapy • Magnetic Field Therapy • Orthomolecular Medicine • Osteopathy • Traditional Chinese Medicine

Bodywork: • Massage with essential oils. • Acupressure, reflexology, *shiatsu*, Alexander Technique, Feldenkrais • Rolfing can be very helpful in conjunction with psychotherapy.

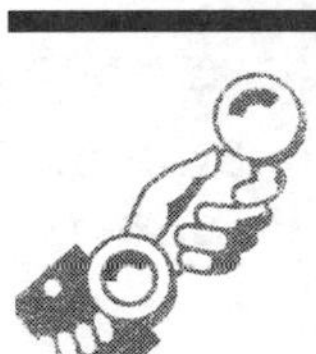

Where to Find Help

For additional information and referrals for treatment of stress, contact the following organizations:

American Association of Acupuncture and Oriental Medicine
4101 Lake Boone Trail, Suite 201
Raleigh, North Carolina 27607
(919) 787-5181

The AAAOM is a national professional trade organization of acupuncturists who meet acceptable standards and can provide you with the names and locations of local members. Referrals by written request only.

American Association of Naturopathic Physicians
2366 Eastlake Avenue, Suite 322
Seattle, Washington 98102
(206) 323-7610

Provides a directory of naturopathic physicians and offers referrals to a nationwide network of accredited or licensed practitioners. Publishes a quarterly newsletter for both professionals and the general public, sample copy free on request. Also offers a series of brochures and pamphlets on a variety of subjects.

American Holistic Medical Association
4101 Lake Boone Trail, Suite 201
Raleigh, North Carolina 27607
(919) 787-5181

A professional organization for holistic practitioners, the AHMA offers information and services for its members and lobbies for holistic issues. It also provides referrals for the public; requests must be in writing.

Maharishi Ayur-Veda Medical Center
P.O. Box 282
Fairfield, Iowa 52556
(515) 472-5866

The center provides referrals to health centers which offer prevention and treatment for a broad range of illnesses. They also train practitioners and provide information to the public.

Mind-Body Clinic
New Deaconess Hospital
Harvard Medical School
185 Pilgram Road
Cambridge, Massachusetts 02215
(617) 632-9530

A treatment program at a medical center where the Relaxation Response can be learned. The clinic uses yoga, meditation, and stress reduction as part of its program.

Stress Reduction and Relaxation Program
University of Massachusetts Medical Center
55 Lake Avenue
North Worcester, Massachusetts 01655
(508) 856-2656

The Stress Reduction and Relaxation Program is a training program to teach meditative-type awareness.

Recommended Reading

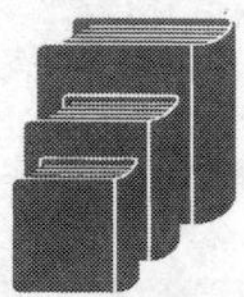

Creating Wholeness: A Self-Healing Workbook Using Dynamic Relaxation, Images and Thoughts. Peper, Erik; and Holt, Catherine. New York: Plenum, 1993.

A simple and accessible self-help program that teaches physical, cognitive, and imagery-based techniques to reduce stress and promote health.

Full Catastrophe Living. Kabat-Zinn, Jon, Ph.D. New York: Dell Publishing, 1990.

A practical guide to stress-reduction and healing based on meditation techniques taught by Dr. Kabat-Zinn. This book explains how to develop a meditation schedule in order to reduce stress and enhance wellness.

Mind/Body Medicine: How to Use Your Mind for Better Health. Goleman, D.; and Gurin, J. New York: Consumer Reports Books, 1993.

A comprehensive and informative book on the power of the mind. A well-researched collection of essays and case histories by more than twenty-four researchers and doctors.

Minding the Body/Mending the Mind. Borysenko, Joan. New York: Bantam Books, 1989.

Based on ground-breaking work at the Mind-Body Clinic at New Deaconess Hospital, this book tells of dramatic success with conditions ranging from allergies to cancer. A unique blend of physical and mental exercises are explained, which show how to elicit the mind's relaxation response, boost the immune system, overcome chronic pain, and alleviate stress-related illnesses.

The Relaxation Response. Benson, Herbert; and Klipper, Miriam Z. New York: Avon, 1976.

The relaxation response is a meditative technique derived from Transcendental Meditation, that can relieve stress, hypertension, anxiety, stress, and stress-related illnesses.

Stress Management. Gordon, James S., M.D. with introduction by C. Everett Koop, M.D., Sc.D. N.Y.: Chelsea House Publishers, 1990.

Stress Management *traces the interaction between stress and bodily functions and describes a few of the many programs available to manage the condition before it becomes destructive. The book places special emphasis on holistic approaches such as wellness programs, which use biofeedback, massage, and body-awareness techniques to promote relaxation and health.*

Stress Without Distress. Selye, Hans, M.D. New York: Signet, 1975.

Pioneering stress researcher Hans Selye explains the psychological mechanisms of stress, and gives specific advise for avoiding harmful levels and amounts of stress.

Vision Disorders

Nearly 60 percent of all Americans require vision correction by the time they reach adulthood, but standard treatments such as corrective lenses or surgery may in fact contribute to further visual impairment. Fortunately, many vision problems can be prevented or treated through the use of nutrition, eye exercises, behavioral optometry, biofeedback, Ayurvedic medicine, and Traditional Chinese Medicine.

Many people grow accustomed to their vision problems, assuming that their eyes are deteriorating as a result of aging. However, poor diet and nutrition, physical, mental, and emotional stress, poor visual skills, and side effects of pharmaceutical drugs are the cause of many vision problems, which are often unrelated to eye disease or to error in the functioning of the visual system.

"The proper functioning of our visual system has far-reaching effects on our general health, beyond an ability to see clearly," says Glen Swartwout, O.D., of Hilo, Hawaii. "Information processed by the eyes helps to regulate functions such as biological rhythms, as well as the nervous, endocrine, and immune systems. It also provides the dominant source of information for human perception, thinking, and coordination of movement."

The ability to process visual information depends upon a highly refined eye/brain communication. As light strikes the retina (the innermost layer of the eye, which receives images), chemical changes convert the light energy to a visual impulse, which is then processed by the brain. According to Dr. Swartwout, when eye/brain communication is disrupted, related problems include blurred vision, altered depth perception, loss of central or peripheral vision, double vision, sensitivity to light, and changes in color perception. If not treated, impaired vision can lead to any number of physiological or psychological problems, including lack of coordination, spatial disorientation, or reading, writing, and learning difficulties.

Types of Vision Disorders

Conditions that can impair vision range from relatively minor problems such as myopia (nearsightedness), to more serious illnesses like glaucoma (increased pressure in the eye), and cataracts. The following are some of the more common vision disorders.

Poor Eyesight

Poor eyesight, including nearsightedness, farsightedness, and astigmatism, is a condition that usually results from a refractive error (deflection of a light ray from a straight path as it moves through the eye).

Nearsightedness: Nearsightedness occurs when the visual image falls in front of the retina, preventing proper focusing on distant objects. Causes stem from a longer than normal eye, a steeply curved cornea, or the inability of the lens of the eye to sufficiently relax.

Farsightedness: Farsightedness (hyperopia) occurs when the visual image falls behind the retina, preventing proper focusing on nearby objects. Causes stem from the eye being shorter than normal, the cornea too flat, lack of muscle tone in the ciliary muscle that controls the lens, or from a combination of these.

Astigmatism: Astigmatism is a condition in which the shape of the cornea is more oval than round, causing the eye to focus on two points instead of one. Blurring, fatigue, and/or headaches are often the result.

Cataracts

Defined as a partial or complete clouding of the clear lens of the eye, cataracts is the leading cause of impaired vision and blindness in the United States.[1] Though one can develop cataracts at any age, it occurs most frequently in the older adult. Dr. Swartwout notes that in addition to the aging process, risk factors include extensive exposure to radiation or infrared light, certain

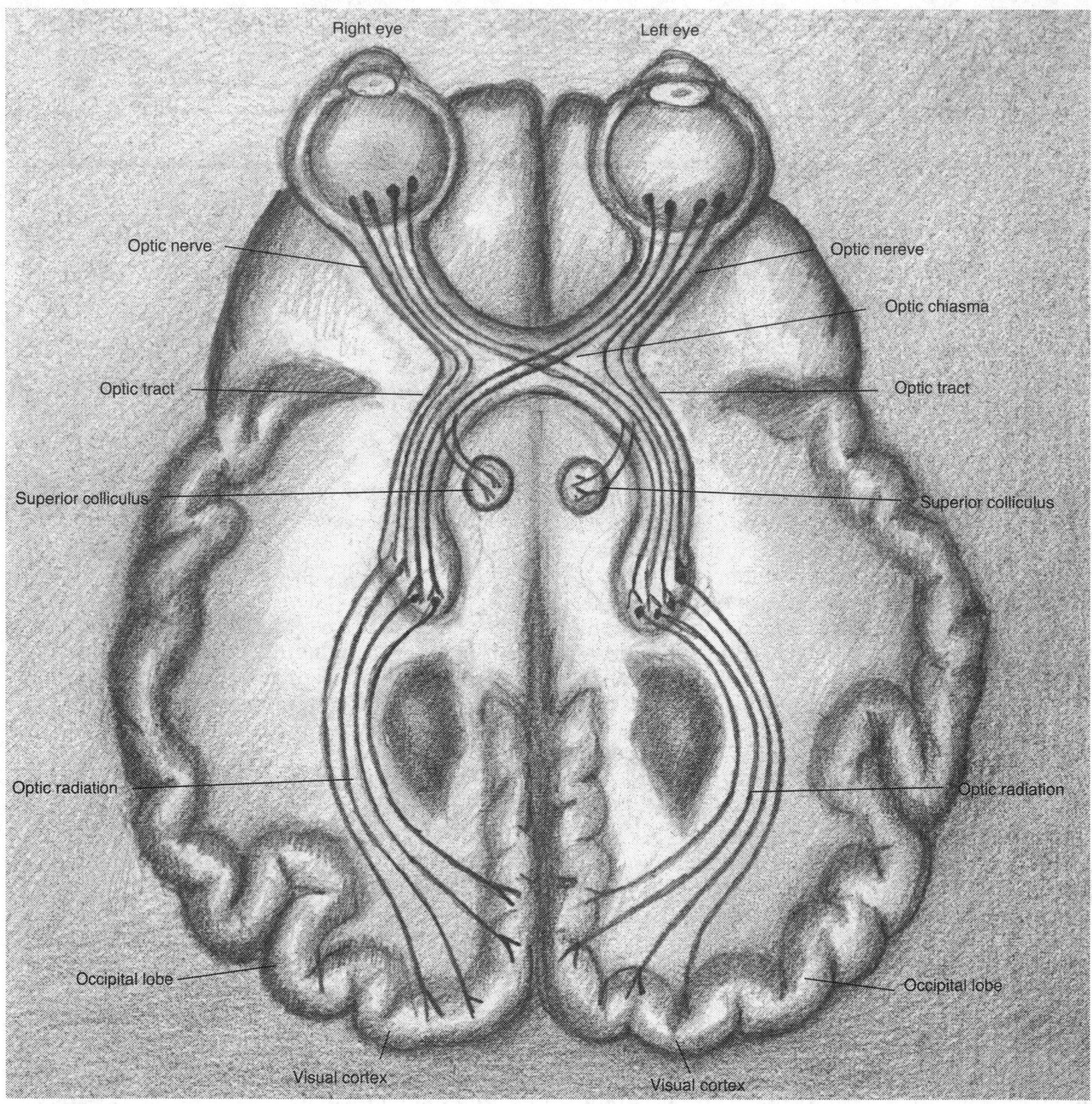

Diagram of the eye and connections to the brain.

medications such as steroids, various injuries, and diseases. He adds that cataracts has also been linked to vitamin, mineral, and protein imbalances.

Conjunctivitis

Also known as pink eye, conjunctivitis is an irritating inflammation of the conjunctiva, the mucous membrane that lines the eye and eyelid. Symptoms include discharge from the eye (often containing pus), pain, swelling, and redness, as well as itching and discomfort with bright lights. Eyelids may stick together upon awakening. Causes of conjunctivitis include infections, allergies, stress, and poor nutrient levels.

Glaucoma

Glaucoma is a group of several diseases generally characterized by loss of peripheral vision which is accompanied in many cases by an increase in pressure of the fluid within the eyeball. It is frequently asymptomatic in the early stages and often goes undetected. Today, there are 2 million known cases of glaucoma in the United States, making it a leading cause of blindness among the older adult.[2] And although the aging process is a factor, other causes include serious eye injuries, eye surgery, certain medications including steroids, and eye tumors. Glaucoma may also be linked to nutritional deficiency in the retina and optic nerve, and to excess toxins and metabolic wastes.

Lazy Eye

Usually beginning in childhood, lazy eye, or amblyopia, results when one eye begins to function below capacity. It occurs when the brain receives dissimilar information from the eyes (for example, if one eye is myopic and the other astigmatic) and favors one eye in order to focus on a single image. The affected eye then becomes accustomed to being ignored, and the result is diminished overall vision.

Macular Degeneration

Macular degeneration is a condition in which the macula, the central area of the retina, deteriorates, resulting in the loss of sharp vision. It is the leading cause of severe visual loss in both the United States and Europe for those fifty-five years or older, and is the third leading cause of impaired vision among those over sixty-five.[3] In addition to aging, risk factors include atherosclerosis and hypertension. Macular degeneration may also be linked to nutritional deficiencies.

See Diabetes.

Night Blindness

Night blindness is often a symptom of retinitis pigmentosa, a disease that causes deterioration of the rods (cells which distinguish light and dark) in the retina and progressive loss of sight. Vitamin A and zinc deficiencies can also lead to night blindness.

Retinal Detachment

Retinal detachment, a peeling away of the retina from the back of the eye, can result in blindness. It occurs when a hole or tear in the retina permits fluid to collect between it and the back of the eye. Injuries to the eyes are the leading, but not exclusive, cause of retinal detachment.

Retinopathy

Retinopathy is a serious visual disorder characterized by hemorrhages of the retinal blood vessels. It is usually associated with either hypertension or diabetes, and is a major cause of blindness among diabetics.

Causes of Vision Disorders

Dr. Swartwout notes that a great many factors can contribute to visual problems, including nutritional deficiency, alcohol, drugs, physical strain, dental problems, poor posture, environmental pollution, harmful lighting, and emotional stress. If these problems go untreated, vision disorders and eye disease can occur. He adds that, "Drugs and surgery do not correct or eliminate the causes of [eye] disease, which are often individual and multifactorial."

Poor Diet and Nutrition

Many eye ailments can be traced in part to poor dietary and nutritional habits. According to Dr. Swartwout, cataracts, glaucoma, and macular degeneration have been linked to vitamin and mineral deficiencies, while the muscles that control eye movement (and thus visual performance) are affected by nutritional imbalances and deficiencies. In his experience, specific foods that often contribute to eye disease and vision impairment include sugar, eggs, dairy products, fats, fried and processed foods, wheat, alcohol, tobacco, and coffee.

> *"Drugs and surgery do not correct or eliminate the causes of [eye] disease, which are often individual and multifactorial."*
> —Glen Swartwout, O.D.

Dr. Swartwout also notes that imbalances in the metabolic system also interfere with vision. "If the blood pH (acid-base balance) becomes too acidic, muscle tone increases, turning the eyes inward, while an alkaline pH will interfere with normal muscle tone, leaving the eyes posturing outward and generally fatigued. Blindness and cataracts are linked to diabetes, a metabolic disorder, and reduced night vision is often linked to impaired liver functioning. Gastrointestinal disorders such as candida overgrowth and parasites contribute to vision problems because they interfere with the normal assimilation of proteins, vitamins, and nutrients."

Pharmaceutical Drugs

According to Leonard Levine, Ph.D., certain prescription drugs can "impair the biological health of the visual system."[4] For example, the *Physicians Desk Reference* lists ninety-four medications that can cause glaucoma, including antihypertensives, steroids, and antidepressants. A partial list of drugs that adversely affect the eyes includes the following:

- **Antihistamines** (antiallergic drugs that increase pressure in the eye)
- **Chlorothiazide and furosemide** (diuretics that can cause blurred vision and dryness in the eyes)
- **Chlorpromazine** (a drug used to treat mental disorders that can cause blurred vision)

- **Digoxin** (a heart medication that can cause distorted or blurred vision)
- **Ethambutol** (a drug used to treat tuberculosis that can cause severe loss of vision and altered color perception)
- **Gold** (a drug used to treat arthritis and lupus that can cause corneal inflammation and blurred vision)
- **Haloperidol** (a drug used to treat mental disorders that can temporarily paralyze the eye muscles and cause blurred vision)
- **Hydroxychloroquine sulfate** (a drug used to treat arthritis, lupus erythematosus, and malaria that can reduce the ability to see red and distort central vision)
- **Oral contraceptives** (birth control drugs that can cause blurred vision and a variety of other problems)
- **Steroids** (anti-inflammatory drugs that can cause cataracts, glaucoma, and other problems)
- **Tetracycline** (an antibiotic that can reduce visual acuity and alter color vision)[5]

Dr. Levine adds that of the ten most frequently prescribed drugs, many "hamper the optometric examination or cause erroneous findings such as cataracts and decreased accommodation (the inability of the eye to properly adjust to various distances) and may result in misdiagnosis or inappropriate treatment."

The Physicians Desk Reference *lists ninety-four medications that can cause glaucoma, including antihypertensives, steroids, and anti-depressants.*

Environmental Factors

"Fluorescent lighting, electromagnetic stress, computer monitors, lack of sunlight, and poorly lit work and school environments are all potential hazards for the eyes," says Dr. Swartwout. In one major study involving 160,000 Texas schoolchildren, 98 percent of the students entered kindergarten without major eye disorders, but at the close of sixth grade over 50 percent had developed vision problems. When researchers redesigned the classrooms to allow for optimal visual performance, incidences of chronic disorders decreased significantly.[6]

Mental/Emotional Factors

According to Dr. Swartwout, when the eyes are not functioning properly, psychological capacities can be significantly impaired. Conversely, mental disorders can cause vision problems. For example, emotional disturbances in a child's life, such as divorce or other severe stress and abuse, can lead to eye turns (an eye that turns inward, or wanders outward) and lazy eye, while school-related stress often triggers nearsightedness and astigmatism.

Dr. Swartwout also points out, "Each time there is a change in the cognitive demand of our visual activity or a change in our emotional state, our focus changes. Stress heightens the demand on the near focusing response, requiring increased precision and muscular response."

Physical Factors

Any tension in the neck, shoulders, or face interferes with the flexibility a person needs to smoothly and accurately track objects and judge distance and depth. The performance of many skills depends on vision, especially driving and sports-related activities. Excess physical tension also promotes fatigue, which interferes with information processing, such as reading.

Treating Vision Disorders

A new generation of optometrists is investing postgraduate years mastering programs designed to prevent and eliminate vision impairment and improve visual performance. People with poor vision can reduce their dependency on prescription lenses, and in some cases eliminate the need altogether. A combination of approaches including diet/nutrition, behavioral optometry, syntonic optometry, biofeedback training, light therapy, the Bates method, herbal remedies, Traditional Chinese Medicine, and Ayurvedic medicine can not only enhance visual performance, but can play an important role in improving movement, coordination, and learning abilities.

Diet and Nutritional Supplements

Diet and nutrition play a central role in the proper functioning of the eyes. Vision disorders, including cataracts, glaucoma, and macular degeneration, can be traced in part to nutritional deficiencies, and a number of physicians have developed nutritional therapy programs to treat and prevent specific vision ailments.

See Diet, Nutritional Supplements.

Dr. Swartwout reports that cataracts can result from a nutritional disorder, and are further aggravated by smoking, drinking alcohol, and the use of some prescription drugs (especially cortisone and other steroids). In a study conducted by Dr. Swartwout, two-thirds of his patients showed improved vision beginning within four weeks of making changes in diet, health habits, and nutritional supplementation.[8] These findings are supported by the indi-

ARE CONVENTIONAL TREATMENTS FOR VISION DISORDERS EFFECTIVE?

It is often thought that once vision is impaired, it can only be restored through corrective lenses, drugs, or surgery. Glen Swartwout, O.D., of Hilo, Hawaii, points out that not only is this untrue, these remedies may even contribute to further visual impairment.

Corrective lenses: *As a person's eyes grow progressively weaker, doctors often prescribe stronger and stronger corrective lenses. But prescription eyeglasses can contribute to the progression of nearsightedness and astigmatism because they make the image smaller, leading to insufficient movement of the extraocular eye muscles (muscles that control eye movement and coordination). Corrective lenses also contribute to the progressive worsening of farsightedness by forcing the ciliary muscle (muscle that facilitates near vision) to relax its tone, thus losing its ability to compensate for the farsightedness without glasses.*

Long-term dependency on corrective lenses can lead to reduced flexibility of the eye muscles, sensitivity to artificial light, and a loss of depth perception, according to Dr. Swartwout. He points out that some optometrists now recommend using progressively weaker lenses to help strengthen the eyes. In the case of myopia—often triggered by a spasm of the ciliary muscle—which is usually corrected with negative, or concave lenses, Dr. Swartwout uses a positive, or convex, lens which helps the ciliary muscles relax, and thus vision is improved.

Contact lenses may pose their own problems. For instance, a recent article in The Lancet *revealed a 65 percent higher incidence of microbial keratitis (inflammation of the cornea due to infection) in contact lens wearers.*[7] *Extended-wear soft contacts carry the highest risk, but any foreign object worn in the eye is a potential danger, says Dr. Swartwout. He adds that, not only can contact lens wearers suffer from "dry eye" problems and become dependent on pharmacological eye drops, but medicated eye drops that "get the red out" often have a rebound effect, leaving the eye even redder when they wear off. He recommends eye drops with ingredients like vitamin A and the herb eyebright.*

Prescription drugs: *Drugs are commonly used in the treatment of glaucoma and certain retinal disorders. But while medications may prove effective in halting the progress of a vision disorder, they can also prevent its cure. For instance, Dr. Swartwout notes that eye drops are widely prescribed to reduce pressure in the eyes due to glaucoma. This elevated pressure, however, is generally a response to some imbalance, and drugs can complicate the body's effort to eliminate this imbalance.*

"It is essential to be able to identify and remove the cause of a problem," says Dr. Swartwout. "The danger of drugs is that they only partially control the symptoms of a disease, and very often their effectiveness wanes, requiring stronger doses, new medications, or more radical measures. Side effects of drugs pose yet another hazard."

Surgery: *Surgery is used for a wide variety of eye ailments, from nearsightedness and crossed eyes to cataracts, glaucoma, and retinal detachments. But because the visual mechanism is extraordinarily delicate, complications from surgical treatment for chronic eye problems are common, and even a "successful" operation can disrupt the subtle functions of the eyes. Depending on the nature of the procedure and the circumstances of the case, the hazards range from various vision distortions to partial or total loss of eyesight.*

Dr. Swartwout believes that surgery to correct refractive errors (nearsightedness, farsightedness, astigmatism) is generally unwarranted. He points out that radial keratotomy, a common operation used to remedy myopia, requires the surgeon to cut 90 percent of the way through the cornea. In some cases, the cornea has been completely penetrated resulting in blindness. And because of scar tissue, the eye is weak and cannot withstand the pressures generated by subsequent injury. This can result in a complete loss of vision, even following a perfect surgical result.

Radial keratotomy can also lead to less severe problems, such as vision distortion and fluctuation, and nighttime glare. Dr. Swartwout notes that because of these complications, the Federal Aviation Administration has adopted a policy forbidding any pilot to fly who has had radial keratotomy. A more natural alternative for treating myopia is a process called orthokeratology which safely reshapes the cornea using special gas-permeable contact lenses.

Eye muscle surgery, used to treat such conditions as crossed eyes and wall eye (an eye that wanders outward), also carries significant risks and for the most part can be avoided in favor of nonsurgical techniques. In the case of severe disorders such as cataracts and glaucoma, the dangers of the condition sometimes outweigh those of the surgery. Yet as Dr. Swartwout says, "If we can treat them preventively at an earlier stage, then we can prevent the need for most eye surgeries."

vidual research of other doctors, including Gary Todd, M.D., an ophthalmologist from North Carolina, and Stuart Kemeny, M.D., an ophthalmologist from California. In a two-year study of fifty patients, Dr. Todd found that nutritional supplementation eliminated the need for cataract surgery in over 50 percent of his patients. In addition, 88 percent showed improved vision. In two studies conducted by Dr. Kemeny at the International Cataract Clinic in Mexico, subjects were prescribed nutritional supplements, ultraviolet light-absorbing glasses, and special eye drops. Vision improved in 54 percent of his patients in the first study and 85 percent in the second.[9]

When treating cataracts and glaucoma, Dr. Swartwout stresses the relationship between nutrition and vision. For prevention of both disorders, he recommends a diet consisting of unrefined, natural foods, in addition to vitamin and nutritional supplements. Conversely, refined, processed, and junk foods may contribute to the development of cataracts and glaucoma, along with stress, alcohol, caffeine, sugar, and smoking—all of which deplete essential nutrients.

> *"It is often thought that once vision is impaired, it can only be restored through corrective lenses, drugs, or surgery. Not only is this untrue, but these remedies may even contribute to further visual impairment."*

Like cataracts and glaucoma, macular degeneration can also be linked to nutritional deficiencies, especially among older individuals. Jonathan Wright, M.D., Director of the Tahoma Clinic in Kent, Washington, and Alan Gaby, M.D., of Baltimore, Maryland, point out that there is a large body of clinical evidence suggesting that nutrient supplementation, particularly with antioxidants, may retard the aging process. According to Drs. Gaby and Wright, "With advancing age nutritional status tends to decline because of reduced gastrointestinal absorption and impaired cellular uptake of nutrients. The sensory organs involved in vision, hearing, smell, and taste appear to be especially vulnerable to the effects of nutritional deficiency, and the purposes of supplementation are to delay the inevitable process of cellular degeneration and to enhance the function of those cells which are living."[10]

Drs. Gaby and Wright recently reviewed the role of nutritional factors in cataract and macular degeneration, and found the following nutrients to be beneficial:[11]

- **Zinc:** Necessary for normal visual function and adaptation to the dark. Zinc deficiency may lead to cataracts, and supplementation reduces visual loss in macular degeneration.
- **Selenium:** Is an antioxidant, and may help prevent cataracts. Visual acuity improved in patients with macular degeneration when supplemented with selenium and vitamin E.
- **Taurine:** May protect cells from harmful effects of ultraviolet light.
- **Vitamin C (Ascorbic acid):** One of the most important antioxidants in the eye. Supplementation can improve vision in those with cataracts.
- **Vitamin E:** A deficiency of this important antioxidant may lead to cataracts. Vitamin E in large doses can prevent macular degeneration.
- **Vitamin A:** Necessary for maintenance of healthy rods and cones (the visual cells of the eye) in the retina.
- **Riboflavin:** Necessary co-factor for the antioxidant enzyme glutathione reductase. Riboflavin deficiency in animals leads to cataracts.
- **N-acetylcysteine:** Has antioxidant activity and may prevent cataracts and other degenerative changes in the eye.
- ***Ginkgo biloba* extract:** Has antioxidant activity, improves arterial blood flow and enhances cellular metabolism. Is known for its antiaging properties, which may prevent degenerative changes in the eye.
- **Flavonoids:** A group of compounds found in plants. Flavonoids have antioxidant and anti-inflammatory effects. Found in high concentrations in blueberries and grapes. Improves night vision and adaptation to the dark. Improves visual acuity and improves capillary integrity to reduce hemorrhage in diabetic retinopathy.

One patient of Dr. Wright's, a woman in her early seventies, came to him with rapidly deteriorating central vision in both eyes (20/100 in the right eye, 20/80 in the left). He recommended a program combining zinc, selenium, vitamin E, and taurine, an amino acid. To ensure proper absorption, the zinc and selenium were administered intravenously; the vitamin E and taurine were taken orally, along with additional supplements of zinc and selenium.

According to Dr. Wright, the patient responded well to the treatment, with significant improvement in both her eyes (20/40 in the right eye, 20/30 in the left). She was able to discontinue the IV's after thirteen months, but found it necessary to maintain the oral supplements. Since she had low stomach acidity, she also added supplements of hydrochloric acid with every meal to enhance mineral absorption.

Behavioral Optometry

Defined as "the art and science of developing visual abilities to achieve optimal visual performance and comfort,"[12] behavioral optometry is based on the work of the late A. M. Skeffington, O.D., D.O.S., who believed that vision is learned and can be enhanced through education, training, and corrective lenses. Behavioral optometry helps patients recognize old behaviors which interfere with vision-related activities and teaches them new, more efficient behaviors by developing the following skills:

- Eye movement (ocular motility)
- Eye focus (accommodation)
- Eye teaming (binocularity)
- Peripheral vision
- Eye-hand coordination
- Visual memory
- Visual perception
- Information processing
- Visualization

Problems in visual tracking and acuity contribute to reading, speaking, and writing difficulties.[13] Therefore, when visual skills are improved, learning becomes easier. According to Harold Solan, O.D., Director of the Learning Disabilities Unit at State University of New York, the proper development of visual perception skills is essential for the formation of reading comprehension and arithmetic skills in the elementary grades. Through the use of appropriate visual testing and training, behavioral optometrists can help children whose problems in reading and math relate to poor visual functioning.[14]

Ray Gottlieb, O.D., Ph.D., a behavioral optometrist in Madison, New Jersey, cites the case of a first-grader named Eric. When Eric began working with Dr. Gottlieb he was lagging far behind his classmates in all subjects. He suffered from poor memory, a short attention span, and a lack of athletic ability. He spent much of the time daydreaming aimlessly with his head flopped backward, his eyes upturned, and his mouth gaping open.

Dr. Gottlieb's visual examination of Eric revealed poor eye movement skills, faulty eye posturing, and inadequate focusing. After six weeks of working with Dr. Gottlieb, Eric's vision problems began improving. His teachers reported significant progress in both his learning skills and physical appearance, and his athletic ability improved to the point that in six months he was playing on both the soccer and basketball teams.

> *"The proper development of visual perception skills is essential for the formation of reading comprehension and arithmetic skills in the elementary grades."*
>
> —Harold Sloan, O.D.

Behavioral optometrists address learning-related visual problems, and problems with motor coordination, sensory integration, environmental sensitivity, and educational dysfunctions as they relate to perception. The effects of emotional and psychological factors upon vision are also considered, and with proper training, significant changes in academic, athletic, and social/emotional behavior can occur.

Syntonic Optometry

In recent years, researchers have found that full-spectrum light (sunlight, or an artificial light source containing sunlight's full spectrum) improves the functioning of the nervous, endocrine, and immune systems. Syntonic optometry, or colored light therapy, selects specific bands of frequencies (seen as colored lights) within this full-spectrum, to improve visual ability and to treat some eye ailments, including peripheral vision problems, color and night blindness, crossed eyes, and lazy eye. Many optometrists are also discouraging the use of standard incandescent and fluorescent lights, which do not contain the full spectrum of light found in natural sunlight and therefore can contribute to vision problems.

An instrument called the Lumatron Light Stimulator® is utilized by syntonic optometrists to help alleviate peripheral vision problems, night blindness, light sensitivity, and color blindness. Developed by John Downing, O.D., Ph.D., Director of the Light Therapy Department at the Preventive Medical Center in San Rafael, California, the Lumatron emits eleven wave bands of color, ranging from red through violet, at a rate of anywhere from zero to sixty cycles a second. Patients sit underneath a hood at the front of the instrument and look at the light, which restimulates the neural/visual system.

See Light Therapy.

According to Dr. Downing, "The visual field significantly expands after stimulation, which is an indication that more photocurrent is traveling from the eye to the visual cortex." A typical treatment consists of twenty-five to thirty sessions over four to six weeks. The Lumatron is currently being used in some twenty countries by hundreds of physicians.

Biofeedback Training

Biofeedback is used to measure and regulate various bodily functions, and can be used to treat refractive errors, lazy eye, crossed eyes, macular degeneration, and glaucoma.

Joseph Trachtman, O.D., Ph.D., a New York-based optometric physician, is the inventor of the Accommotrac Vision Trainer®, an instrument that measures the retina for clarity of image. As the patient's focusing changes, the Accommotrac converts the visual image into sound so that very small changes can be detected and then controlled. The treatment consists of weekly, hour-long sessions in which patients learn how to refine control over the eye muscle thus allowing both nearsighted and farsighted individuals to significantly improve their vision.

See Biofeedback Testing, Herbal Medicine.

According to Dr. Trachtman, "We're able to take people who have extremely poor vision and either eliminate or reduce the need for their eyeglasses." He recalls one patient who, after six months of treatment, showed an improvement in vision from 20/400 to about 20/30. When Dr. Trachtman saw the patient a couple of years after the treatment, he found that the patient had maintained most of the improvement.

The Accommotrac is also sensitive to eye position, and can be used to treat crossed eyes, lazy eye, and a condition called nystagmus, characterized by oscillating eye movement. Dr. Trachtman has also helped patients suffering from macular degeneration by training them to use a part of the eye other than the deteriorating macula.

Steve Fahrion, Ph.D., Director of the Center for Applied Psychophysiology at the Menninger Clinic in Topeka, Kansas, says that, based on several studies, the use of biofeedback to relax the forehead muscles can reduce the pressure in the eyeball, based on several studies in the literature, and therefore can be used to treat glaucoma. This technique involves placing electrodes on the forehead in order to get an auditory tone that indicates the level of stress. By increasing relaxation, the pressure in the eye area can be reduced. According to Dr. Fahrion, one of his colleagues at the clinic has used this approach successfully to control his glaucoma for the past several years.

The Bates Method

Pioneering New York ophthalmologist William Bates, M.D. (1860-1931), was the first to discover that chronic eye problems were frequently stress-related. He demonstrated the correlation between various vision disorders and tension unconsciously placed on the muscles that control the eyes. From this, Dr. Bates developed a set of eye exercises to reduce eye stress and correct eye and vision-related disorders.

Dr. Bates further explained that "perfect sight is a product of perfectly relaxed organs, unconsciously controlled," and that vision improves naturally when people stop interfering with it.[15] Under relaxed conditions, refractive errors tend to be self-correcting.

> *"Perfect sight is a product of perfectly relaxed organs, unconsciously controlled."*
>
> —William Bates, M.D.

Paul Anderson, a Bates method practitioner in Kirkland, Washington, succeeded in correcting his own vision from 20/300 to 20/20, and advocates natural vision-improvement techniques be included in schools and workplaces. "Putting on glasses to correct an image distorted by mental strain will not, in the long run, prove beneficial to the child or to society," he says.[16]

Herbal Remedies

David Hoffmann, B.Sc., M.N.I.M.H., of Sebastopol, California, past President of the American Herbalist Guild, treats cataracts with an eye wash of an infusion of eyebright. A stronger mix can be made with equal parts eyebright and goldenseal.

In treating macular degeneration, European research shows that *Ginkgo biloba* and bilberry can be very beneficial.[17] In addition to *Ginkgo biloba*, David Hoffman recommends taking one 100-milligram tablet of milk thistle and one 100-milligram tablet of bilberry three times a day. Hoffman also notes that Siberian ginseng may be helpful in treating some forms of color blindness.[18]

For conjunctivitis, a simple home remedy suggested by Joseph Pizzorno, N.D., President of Bastyr College in Seattle, Washington, is made by adding one tablespoon goldenseal root powder, one teaspoon salt, and 250 milligrams of vitamin C, to a quart of water. After letting the solution settle, the clear liquid is used to thoroughly wash out the eye several times a day.

Traditional Chinese Medicine

The Chinese approach traces most vision ailments to liver function. Treatment often combines acupuncture, herbs, and dietary changes.

According to Maoshing Ni, D.O.M., Ph.D., L.Ac, Vice-President of Yo San University of Traditional Chinese Medicine in Santa Monica, California, acupuncture is very effective in balancing and readjusting the tension in the eye muscles, thereby improving the shape of the eye and its ability to function properly. For nearsightedness and farsightedness, a typical course of treatment involves ten acupuncture sessions. Eye exercises are often recommended to help maintain the improvements.

With more serious disorders such as cataracts and glaucoma, treatment involves the use of herbs and dietary changes. For glaucoma, this regimen can significantly decrease interocular pressure, allowing a patient to reduce or forego medication and postpone surgery. Dr. Ni cites the example of one man who underwent treatment for glaucoma for three months, which included weekly acupuncture sessions, herbal treatments, and dietary changes. By the end of the course, the patient's eye pressure had returned to normal, allowing him to discontinue his medication and postpone surgery indefinitely. Upon discharge, Dr. Ni provided stress-management techniques and instructed the man to maintain his modified diet. A similar approach can sometimes stop or even reverse the growth of a cataract, according to Dr. Ni.

In a much simpler case, Dr. Ni used acupuncture, herbs, and herbal cream to treat a thirteen-year-old girl with conjunctivitis. Within a week, the condition had cleared up completely.

Ayurvedic Medicine

Ayurvedic medicine generally considers vision disorders to be caused by digestive problems. Ayurvedic techniques attempt to improve metabolic function, and eye exercises are used to strengthen ailing vision and prevent healthy eyes from deteriorating.

Herbal remedies and nutritional supplements are the basis of Ayurvedic treatment for vision problems. Herbs such as *amla*, *triphala*, and licorice, along with beta-carotene-rich substances like carrots and spinach, are prescribed to stimulate the digestive system and strengthen the eyes.

See Ayurvedic Medicine, Traditional Chinese Medicine.

Virender Sodhi, M.D. (Ayurveda), N.D., Director of the American School of Ayurvedic Sciences in Bellevue, Washington,

Eye Exercises

One of the easiest treatments for improving visual fitness and efficiency is to allow your eyes frequent breaks throughout the day. Here are a few exercises for relaxing the eyes:

- *Every thirty to sixty minutes, give your eyes a five-minute rest from concentrated work. Look up from your work, relax your gaze, and let your eyes wander across the room, or simply stare off into space.*
- *The eyes need oxygen and will function better when the body is rested and circulation is improved. Breathe deeply for several minutes, then stretch your neck and shoulders. Roll your head around in a circle, side to side and up and down. Touch your ear to your shoulder and repeat for the other side. Yawn and stretch the muscles of your face, which often hold a lot of tension.*
- *Blink regularly to reduce eye strain. Blinking also increases the amount of concentrated work your eyes can accomplish comfortably.*
- *"Palming" is easy to practice and offers effective eye relief. Sit comfortably in a relaxed position, and breathe deeply as you gently cover your eyes with your palms. Yogis suggest that you first rub your hands together vigorously to create some penetrating warmth and energy that will provide additional comfort to your eyes.*

The process of "accommodation"—which means switching one's focus between near and distant objects without losing clarity—becomes more difficult as the lenses of the eyes grow less flexible with age. To enhance flexibility, try each of these procedures daily for fifteen to twenty seconds, with prescription lenses removed:

- *Perform rapid switches from a close-up to a long-range focus in a smooth and effortless manner by pretending to follow an imaginary ping-pong game.*
- *Tack some reading material to the wall and read it from a comfortable distance, then increase the distance a little bit each day. Eventually, you'll be able to read the material from across the room. Near vision can also be improved by getting closer to the material each day.*

recalls treating his mother who was suffering from retinal hemorrhages and had been declared legally blind. A previous physician had prescribed heavy doses of cortisone, which had no effect on her vision but caused her to gain nearly sixty pounds and develop high blood pressure. Dr. Sodhi treated her using *amla* tablets combined with a series of eye exercises. As a result her vision improved substantially, allowing her to regain the ability to read and write.

Any effective prevention-oriented regimen includes annual visits to an optometrist. If you are feeling a persistent irritation in your eyes, however, or if objects begin to look markedly different to you, don't wait to consult a professional. Early detection of potentially serious conditions greatly increases the likelihood that only minimal treatment will be required to restore your eyes to their natural state.

In another case, Dr. Sodhi treated a nine-year-old girl suffering from severe corneal ulcers in one eye. The patient's ophthalmologist, observing that the eye was badly scarred, recommended corneal transplant surgery, which has a 50 percent chance of failure. But when Dr. Sodhi discovered an allergy to chocolate was causing blurred vision and severe headaches, he instituted a three-month dietary treatment combined with herbal treatment. To strengthen the musculature of the eye and increase the pliability of the cornea, eye exercises were prescribed, as were eye rinses with the water of *triphala*. At the end of treatment, the ulcers were gone and there was no trace of scarring.

Craniosacral Therapy

According to John Upledger, D.O., Medical Director of the Upledger Institute in Palm Beach Gardens, Florida, visual motor disturbances can occur if the membranes attached to the temporal bone puts pressure on the nerves to the eye. He uses Craniosacral therapy to relieve the pressure and help restore motor control of the eyes.

See Craniosacral Therapy.

Other structural problems can also interfere with vision according to Dr. Upledger. He recalls one patient whose vision improved from 20/200 to 20/40 within a matter of minutes after treating her cervical vertebrae (spinal neck vertebrae). "In addition, manipulation of the bones of the occipital region (base of the skull) can release pressure on the occipital lobes of the brain and improve vision by allowing the correct messages to get through to these areas," says Dr. Upledger.

Self-Care

The following therapies can be undertaken at home under appropriate professional supervision:

• Qigong • Yoga

Juice Therapy Fresh carrot juice, or combine carrot with celery, parsley, spinach, or cucumber.

***Topical Treatment*:** Eye strain, pressure on eyeball: raw-potato eye pack. Grate organic, unsprayed white potatoes (peel and pulp) and place a small spoonful on the eyelid and over entire eye. Cover with a piece of gauze and leave on for one or two hours.

Eye infections or irritations: wash hands thoroughly. Cut off chunk of cucumber, peel, and grate. Put grated cucumber in large sterile gauze pad or boiled cheesecloth. Squeeze a few drops of cucumber juice directly into eye. Use fresh cucumber and gauze each time.

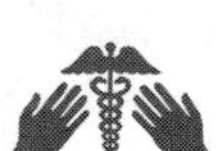

Professional Care

The following therapies should only be provided by a qualified health professional:

• Chelation Therapy • Chiropractic • Colon Therapy • Magnetic Field Therapy • Naturopathic Medicine • Osteopathy

Bodywork: Acupressure, reflexology, *shiatsu* massage to relieve accompanying muscular tension. Rolfing, Feldenkrais, and Alexander technique can help reduce vision-affecting physical and emotional stress.

Environmental Medicine: Environmental medicine takes into consideration chemical or food sensitivities, electro-magnetic pollution, and geopathic stress, environmental hazards to which the retina is particularly sensitive.[20]

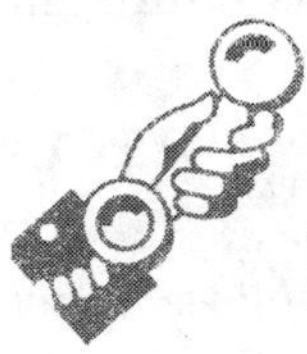

Where to Find Help

Vision-improvement practitioners may be listed in the phone book under the category "Eyesight Training." They may or may not be licensed. A licensed eye doctor can also help you find alternative care, or you can contact the following organizations:

Behavioral Optometry

College of Optometrists in Vision Development (COVD)
353 H. Street, Suite C
Chula Vista, California 92010
or
Box 285
Chula Vista, California 91912
(619) 425-6191
(619) 420-3010

The College of Optometrists in Vision Development is an international certifying organization for optometrists who specialize in vision therapy.

Optometric Extension Program Foundation, Inc.
2912 South Daimler Street
Santa Ana, California 92705
(714) 250-8070

Offers continuing education in behavioral optometry for consumers and optometrists.

Syntonic Optometry

College of Syntonic Optometry
1200 Robeson
Fall River, Massachusetts 02720
(508) 673-1251

A society of optometrists who practice phototherapy. They offer courses on the optometric application of phototherapy.

Other Resources

American Association of Acupuncture and Oriental Medicine
4101 Lake Boone Trail, Suite 201
Raleigh, North Carolina 27607
(919) 787-5181

The AAAOM is a national professional trade organization of acupuncturists who meet acceptable standards of competency and can provide you with names and locations of local members. Referrals by written request only.

The College of Maharishi Ayur-Veda Medical Center
P.O. Box 282
Fairfield, Iowa 52556
(515) 472-5866

The center provides referrals to health centers, which offer methods of prevention and treatment for a broad range of illnesses. They also train practitioners and provide information to the lay public.

National Eye Research Foundation
910 Skokie Boulevard, Suite 207A
Northbrook, Illinois 60062
800 621-2258

Has history with contact lens safety and advocacy. They use color fields to uncover systemic diseases and alternatives to surgical intervention for crossed eyes.

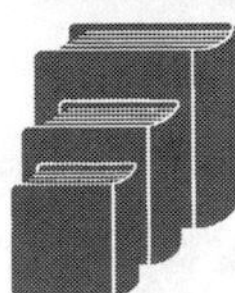

Recommended Reading

The Bates Method for Better Eyesight Without Glasses. Bates, W.H. New York: Henry Holt & Co./Owl Books, 1981.

Bates' revolutionary, commonsensible theory of self-taught improved eyesight is outlined here. Originally published in 1940, this text has become a classic in its field. Includes an eye chart.

The Eyes Have It: A Self-Help Manual for Better Vision. Cheney, E. York Beach, ME: Samuel Weiser, Inc., 1987.

Includes step-by-step instructions and exercises using the Bates method, plus holistic, herbal, folk, spiritual, and yogic techniques. Latest medical breakthroughs are included, as well as a discussion on the many daily things one can do to save your eyes.

Light, Medicine of the Future: How We Can Use It To Heal Ourselves NOW. Liberman, Jacob, O.D., Ph.D. Santa Fe, NM: Bear & Company Publishing, 1991.
Dr. Liberman challenges the myth that sunlight is dangerous and argues that technological advancements and indoor lifestyles have been more harmful than helpful. He also discusses the use of light in treating a variety of conditions.

Seeing Beyond 20/20: Improve the Quality of Your Vision and Your Life. Kaplan, Michael, R., M.D. Hillsboro, OR: Beyond Words Publishing, 1987.
Gives readers a practical, solidly researched twenty-one-day program for self-help toward clearer vision. Topics include nutrition, aerobics for the eyes, the eyes as a biofeedback device, and the relationship of inner vision with outer sight.

"Only freedom from prejudice and tireless zeal avail for the most holy of the endeavours of mankind, the practice of the true art of healing."

—Samuel Hahnemann, Founder of Homeopathy (1755-1843)

Quick Reference Guide to Additional Health Conditions

An Important Message

This book is intended as an educational tool to acquaint the reader with alternative methods for the maintenance of good health and the treatment of illness. The publisher hopes the book will enable the reader to improve his or her well-being and to better understand, assess, and choose the appropriate course of treatment for an illness or health condition. Because the methods described in this book are, by definition, **alternative** methods, many of them have not been investigated and/or approved by any government or regulatory agency. National, state, and local laws vary regarding the use and application of many of the treatments that are discussed. Accordingly, this book should not be substituted for the advice and treatment of a physician or other licensed health professional, but rather should be used in conjunction with professional care. Pregnant women in particular are especially urged to consult with their physician before using any therapy.

Your health is important. Use this book wisely. Discuss the alternative treatment options described herein with your doctor. Ultimately, you, the reader, must take full responsibility for your health and how you use this book. The publisher expressly disclaims responsibility for any adverse effects resulting from your use of the information contained herein.

How to Use This Section

This Quick Reference Guide covers 106 health conditions. Each condition is briefly described, and information is supplied concerning its causes and symptoms. A self-care/professional care section cross references each condition with the alternative therapies most appropriate for its treatment.

Self-care refers to treatments that can be undertaken in the privacy of your own home, under the guidance of your physician. Professional care means you must see a qualified practitioner of this therapy for this condition. (Each of the thirty-three health condition chapters in Part Three also contains a self-care/professional care section at the end of the main text that follows the same guidelines.)

Self-care modalities are not only cost-effective, but help you begin to take your health and welfare into your own hands. Self-care therapies include diet, nutritional supplementation, juice therapy, flower remedies, meditation, yoga and *qigong*, self-acupressure, and reflexology, and in some cases, herbs, hydrotherapy, aromatherapy, and fasting. Ayurvedic medicine, naturopathic medicine, herbal medicine, homeopathy, detoxification therapies, acupressure, reflexology, guided imagery, and biofeedback all have self-care practices that can be practiced at home under the guidance of a physician, as well as more sophisticated applications for which you will need to see a professional.

Therapies requiring direct professional care include the following:

- Acupuncture
- Applied Kinesiology
- Biological Dentistry
- Bodywork (Acupressure, Alexander Technique, Aston-Patterning, Feldenkrais, Hellerwork, massage, myotherapy, reflexology, Rolfing, *shiatsu*, Therapeutic Touch, Trager)
- Cell Therapy
- Chelation Therapy
- Chiropractic
- Colon Therapy
- Craniosacral Therapy
- Environmental Medicine
- Enzyme Therapy
- Fasting
- Flower Remedies
- Guided Imagery
- Herbal Medicine
- Hyperthermia
- Hypnotherapy
- Light Therapy
- Magnetic Field Therapy
- Mind/Body Medicine
- Naturopathic Medicine
- Neural Therapy
- Neuro-Linguistic Programming
- Orthomolecular Medicine
- Osteopathy
- Oxygen Therapy (hydrogen peroxide therapy, ozone therapy)
- Reconstructive Therapy
- Traditional Chinese Medicine

Regardless of whether you choose primarily self-care approaches or those involving professional services, it is recommended that you find an open-minded physician or health professional you trust and respect who can help you create an effective health-maintenance program.

Choosing Alternative Therapies for Health Conditions

Look up the health condition you are interested in under its alphabetical listing. Choose the alternative therapies listed for the health condition you want to investigate. In order to read about a particular therapy in greater detail, refer back to its chapter in Part Two. If you have further questions about the therapies, contact the professional organizations listed there for more information, as well as for referrals to physicians or other health professionals in your area who offer this service.

The possible contributing factors discussed under special notes give you and your physician more information (particularly if he or she is a specialist) concerning what underlying factors may be contributing to your health condition.

One crucial concept to keep in mind is that no one treatment method is effective for a particular condition in people. Healing is complex because individuals are biochemically unique. What works for someone else may not work for you. It is important to find a therapy that works for you and has the least long-lasting negative effects on your body, while at the same time building the longest term positive effects on your overall lifestyle. The intention of this book is not to promote one therapy over another, but to help inform you about all of the therapies available so that you can decide which therapy best suits you.

By making use of the information this book provides, you will be able to make intelligent, informed choices and take charge of your own health, in cooperation with your primary health practitioner.

The Alternative Therapies

When examining the alternative therapies listed in the A-Z section, remember the following facts:

- Self-care is indicated by the icon.
- Professional care is indicated by the icon.
- These sections are intended to expose you to these alternatives. If you have questions, or if you have symptoms that do not respond as they should, ask a qualified practitioner for guidance and answers. See the Where to Find Help section in the Alternative Therapies chapters in Part Two.
- Diet and nutritional supplements are recommended for virtually every condition. Be sure to check with your physician before undertaking a dietary or nutritional program.

Instructions for Self-Care

Acupressure

Refer to the following acupressure charts to locate points referred to in the Quick Reference Guide and self-care sections of health condition chapters.

Aromatherapy

See the How to Use Aromatherapy section in the Aromatherapy chapter for instructions on how to use the essential oils listed under each condition. You may also want to read Some Essential Oils and Their Applications and Purchasing Oils sections in the same chapter. (See the Where to Find Help section at the end of the Aromatherapy chapter for organizations that can refer you to a qualified aromatherapist.)

Ayurveda

Simple dietary, herbal, and topical treatments are provided that you can employ in the privacy of your own home. You may want to read the chapter on Ayurvedic Medicine to see if you would like to consult an Ayurvedic physician. (See Where to Find Help section at the end of the Ayurvedic Medicine chapter for organizations that can refer you to a qualified Ayurvedic physician.)

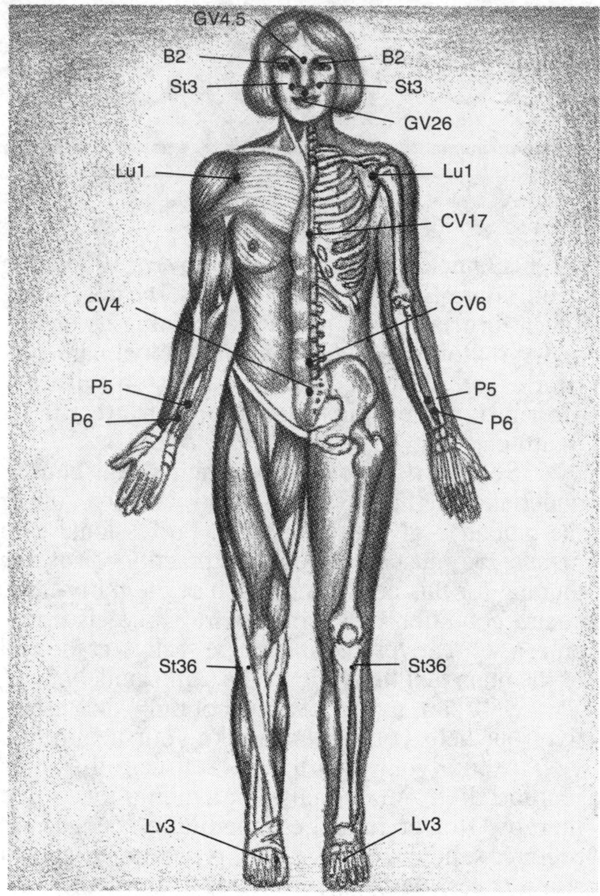

Acupressure points. Front view.

Diet

Diet plays an enormous role in health. General dietary guidelines are normally provided for each condition, such as a whole foods diet, vegetarian diet, low-fat diet, or raw foods diet. Pay particular attention to the foods which are beneficial to the condition and those which should be avoided. If you are ill or are considering a major dietary change please consult a health professional trained in nutritional medicine. (See Where to Find Help section in Diet chapter for organizations that can provide referrals for nutritional counseling.)

Herbs

Many herbs can be prepared as teas, although in some cases it is suggested to make a decoction, infusion, or other preparation. Certain herbs may be used in baths, steam inhalations, and in compresses to be applied topically to the body. In all cases please refer to the chapter on Herbal Medicine, particularly The Herbal Medicine Chest section which describes twenty-five herbs, their therapeutic action, recommended uses, and sup-

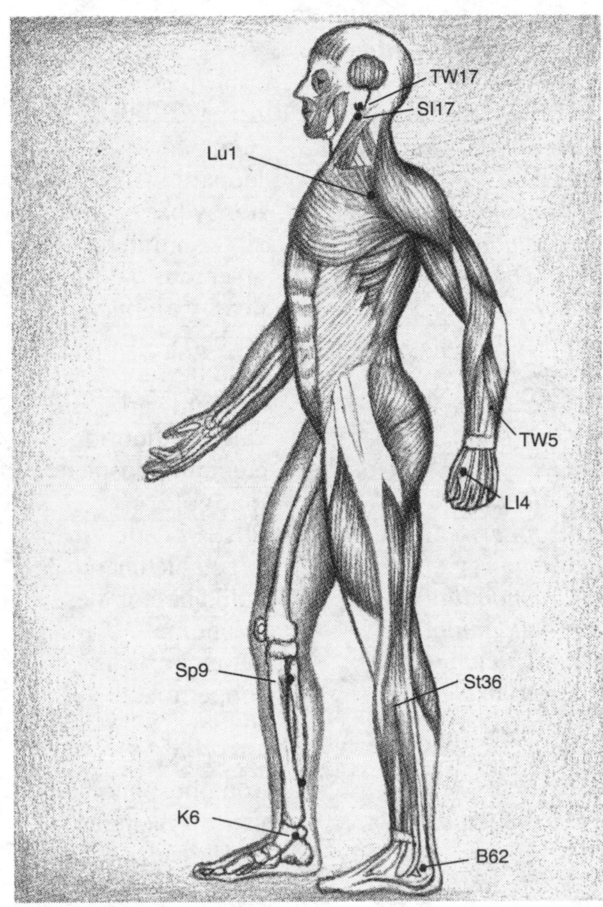

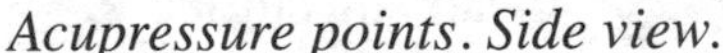
Acupressure points. Side view.

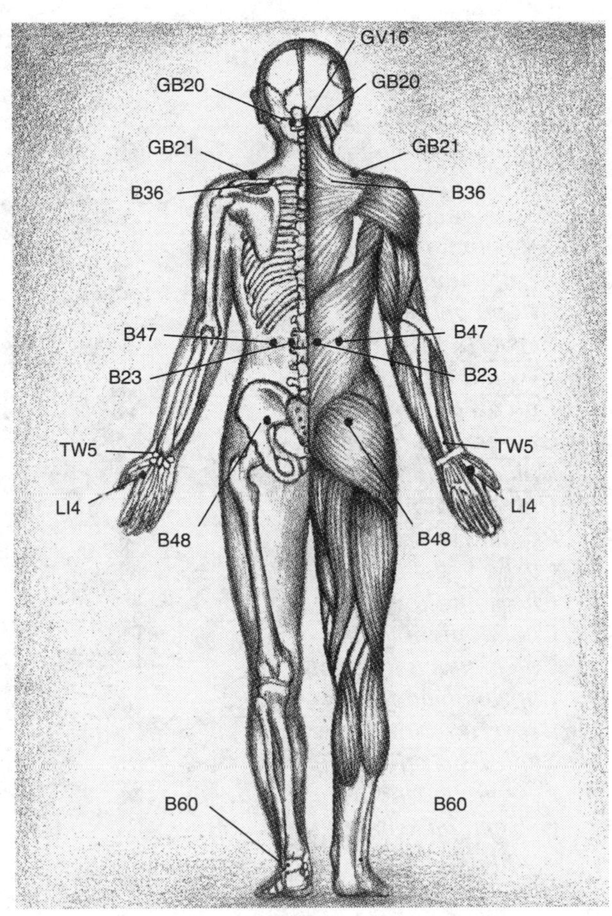

Acupressure points. Back view.

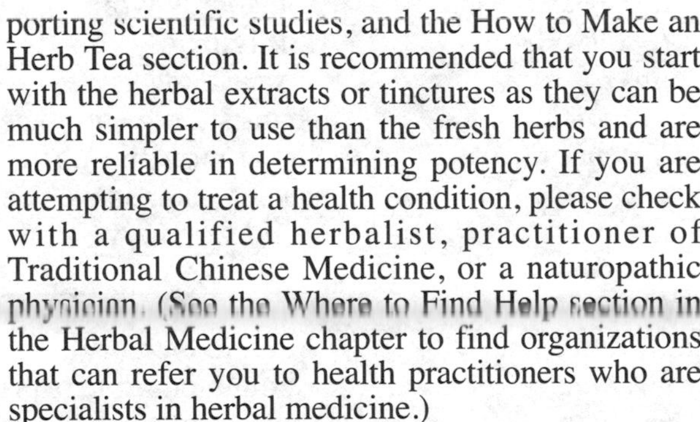
porting scientific studies, and the How to Make an Herb Tea section. It is recommended that you start with the herbal extracts or tinctures as they can be much simpler to use than the fresh herbs and are more reliable in determining potency. If you are attempting to treat a health condition, please check with a qualified herbalist, practitioner of Traditional Chinese Medicine, or a naturopathic physician. (See the Where to Find Help section in the Herbal Medicine chapter to find organizations that can refer you to health practitioners who are specialists in herbal medicine.)

Homeopathy

Remedies listed in the chart on the following page may be used individually or in combination with other remedies. Trevor Cook, Ph.D., D.I. Hom., President of the United Kingdom Homeopathic Medical Association, has created a simple system to make your own combination homeopathic remedies from the single remedies associated with particular symptoms of a health condition. According to Dr. Cook, nearly every combination prescription can be made from these forty-eight individual remedies. These remedies may be purchased separately or as a special combination kit consisting of each of the remedies in their liquid or pellet form.

How to Prepare the Homeopathic Remedies: The kit may also include a number of empty dropper bottles for combining the remedies. All potencies in kits are normally 12X potency (a low potency which is considered safe for most people).

To prepare a combination treatment, add ten drops of each remedy indicated for a particular condition to an empty bottle. Mix well, lightly tapping a firm, resilient surface about ten times and label the dropper bottle clearly. The standard dose for a combination remedy is ten drops taken in a clean mouth under the tongue. For a more in-depth discussion of homeopathy, refer to the Homeopathy chapter. (See the Where to Find Help section in the Homeopathy chapter to find organizations that can refer you to a qualified Homeopathic physician.)

Hydrotherapy

There are many water therapy treatments which you can easily do in the privacy of your own

Homeopathic Remedies Used in Quick Reference Guide

Full Name	Source	Abbreviation	Common Name
Aconitum napellus	P	*Aconite*	monkshood
Arnica montana	P	*Amica*	leopard's bane
Apis mellefica	A	*Apis mel.*	honey bee
Argentum nitricum	M	*Argen nit.*	silver nitrate
Arsenicum album	M	*Arsen alb.*	arsenious oxide
Atropa belladonna	P	*Belladonna*	deadly nightshade
Berberis vulgaris	P	*Berberis*	barberry
Bryonia alba	P	*Bryonia*	wild bryony
Calcarea carbonica	M	*Calc carb.*	calcium carbonate
Calcarea fluorica	M	*Calc fluor.*	calcium fluoride
Calcarea phosphorica	M	*Calc phos.*	calcium phosphate
Calendula officinalis	P	*Calendula*	marigold
Cantharis vesicatoria	A	*Cantharis*	blister beetle
Carbo vegetabilis	M	*Carbo veg.*	vegetable charcoal
Chamomilla	P	*Chamomilla*	wild chamomile
Chelidonium majus	P	*Chelidonium*	celandine
Colchicum autumnale	P	*Colchicum*	autumn crocus
Cuprum metallicum	M	*Cuprum met.*	copper metal
Drosera rotundifolia	P	*Drosera*	sundew
Euphrasia officinalis	P	*Euphrasia*	eyebright
Ferrum phosphoricum	M	*Ferrum phos.*	iron phosphate
Gelsemium sempervirens	P	*Gelsemium*	yellow yasmine
Graphites	M	*Graphites*	black lead
Hamamelis virginiana	P	*Hamainelis*	witch hazel
Hepar sulfuris	M	*Hepar sulf.*	calcium sulfide
Hydrastis canadensis	P	*Hydrastis*	goldenseal
Hypericum perforatum	P	*Hypericum*	St. John's Wort
Ignatia amara	P	*Ignada*	St. Ignatius bean
Ipecacuanha	P	*Ipecac*	ipecacuanha
Kalium bichromicum	M	*Kali bich.*	potassium bichromate
Kalium phosphoricum	M	*Kali phos.*	potassium phosphate
Lachesis mutus	A	*Lachesis*	bushmaster snake venom
Ledum palustre	P	*Ledum*	wild rosemary
Lycopodium clavatum	P	*Lycopodium*	club moss
Magnesium phosphorica	M	*Mag phos.*	magnesium phosphate
Mercurius solubilis	M	*Merc sol.*	soluble mercury
Natrum muriaticum	M	*Nat mur.*	sodium chloride (salt)
Nux vomica	P	*Nux vom.*	poison nut
Phosphorus	M	*Phosphorus*	
Pulsatilla nigricans	P	*Pulsatifla*	windflower
Rhus toxicodendron	P	*Rhus tox.*	poison ivy
Ruta graveolens	P	*Ruta grav.*	bitterwort
Sepia officinalis	A	*Sepia*	juice of cuttlefish
Silicea	M	*Silicea*	
Sulfur	M	*Sulfur*	
Symphytum officinalis	P	*Symphytum*	comfrey
Thuja occidentalis	P	*Thuja*	tree of life
Urtica urens	P	*Urtica*	stinging nettle

Source: P: Plant M: Mineral A: Animal

home for little or no cost. Please consult the Hydrotherapy chapter for complete instructions on how to perform the following hydrotherapy procedures:

- Cold compress
- Cold friction rub
- Constitutional hydrotherapy
- Contrast applications
- Enema/colon irrigation
- Hot packs
- Heating compress
- Hyperthermia
- Hot blanket pack
- Ice packs
- Immersion baths
- Sitz bath
- Sprays/showers
- Steam/sauna
- Wet sheet pack

See the Where to Find Help section in Hydrotherapy chapter for organizations that can refer you to a physical therapist or naturopathic physician who is knowledgeable of hydrotherapy procedures.

Juice Therapy

Unless otherwise indicated, the raw juices in this section can be either used for a short three-day juice fast or incorporated into your daily diet. Check with your physician before undertaking a fast.

Nutritional Supplements

This section gives you the most important nutritional supplements (vitamins, minerals, amino acids, enzymes, glandulars, and antioxidants) for helping to deal with each health condition.

Before going on a new regime of supplementation it is important to consult with a qualified health professional or call an organization listed in the Where to Find Help section in the Nutritional Supplements chapter that can refer you to a physician specializing in nutritional medicine.

Qigong

Qigong exercises that may be helpful for the various health conditions are described and illustrated in the *Qigong* chapter in Part Two. Although *qigong* can be practiced at home, it is advised that you first receive proper instruction from a qualified instructor. (See the Where to Find Help section in *Qigong* chapter for organizations that can refer you to a qualified teacher or therapist.)

Reflexology

Use the chart below to locate the reflex areas described in the Quick Reference Guide and the self-care section of the health condition chapters.

Yoga

The yoga postures described and illustrated in the Yoga chapter may be beneficial for a variety of health conditions. Although yoga can be practiced at home, it is advised that you first receive proper instruction from a qualified yoga instructor or yoga therapist. (See the Where to Find Help section in Yoga chapter for organizations that can refer you to a qualified teacher or therapist.)

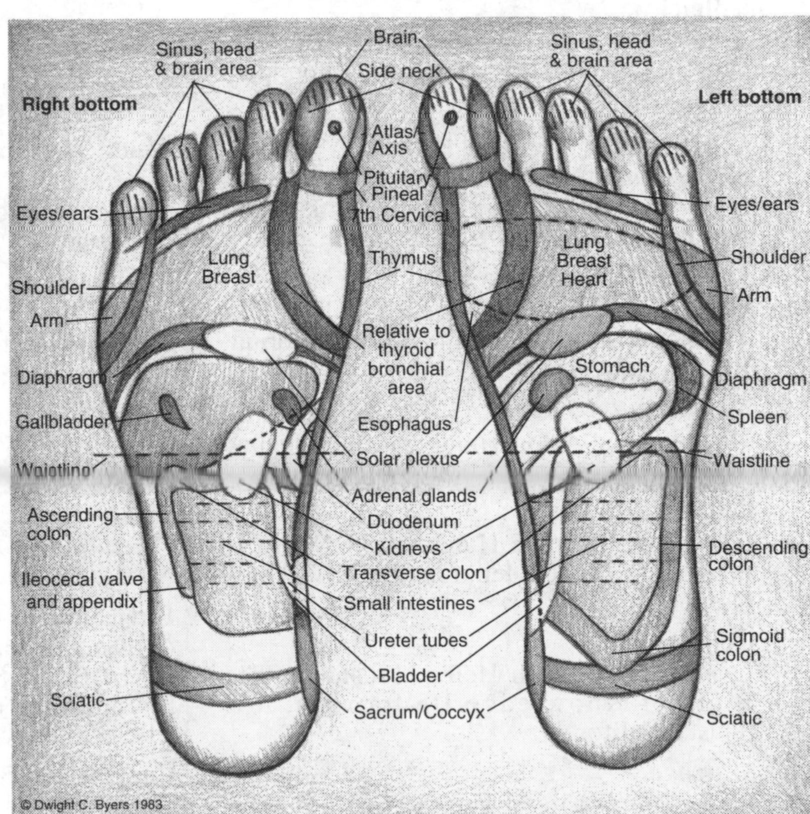

Foot reflexology chart.

Consultants for Quick Reference Section

Senior Editor Quick Reference Section
D. Lindsey Berkson, D.C., M.A., Nutritionist and Educator, Santa Fe, New Mexico

Acupuncture
Consultant: Maoshing Ni, D.O.M., Ph.D., L.Ac., Vice-President, Yo San University of Traditional Chinese Medicine, Santa Monica, California

Applied Kinesiology
Consultant: George Goodheart, D.C., F.I.C.C., D.I.B.A.K., Research Director, International College of Applied Kinesiology, Grosse Pointe Woods, Michigan

Aromatherapy
Consultant: Ann Berwick, founder and President, National Association of Holistic Aromatherapy, Boulder, Colorado

Ayurveda
Consultant: Dr. Vasant Lad, Director, Ayurvedic Institute, Albuquerque, New Mexico

Biofeedback
Consultant: Marjorie Toomim, Ph.D., Director, Biofeedback Institute, Los Angeles, California

Bodywork

- **Acupressure**
  Consultant: Michael Reed Gach, Ph.D., Director, The Acupressure Institute, Berkeley, California
- **Alexander Technique**
  Consultant: Frank Ottowell, Alexander Training Institute, San Francisco, California
- **Aston-Patterning**
  Consultant: Judith Aston, founder and Director, The Aston Training Center, Incline Village, Nevada
- **Feldenkrais**
  Consultant: Bonnie Humiston, R.N., M.S., President, The Feldenkrais Guild, Albany, Oregon
- **Hellerwork**
  Consultant: Joseph Heller, President, The Body of Knowledge/Hellerwork, Mt. Shasta, California
- **Massage**
  Consultant: Eileen Henry, C.A., C.M.T, Director, Institute of Psycho-Structural Balancing, Santa Monica, California
- **Myotherapy**
  Consultant: Bonnie Prudden, founder and Director, Bonnie Prudden, Inc., Stockbridge, Massachusetts
- **Reflexology**
  Consultant: Dwight Byers, President, International Institute of Reflexology, St. Petersburg, Florida
- **Rolfing**
  Consultant: Jeff Maitland, Faculty Chair, The Rolf Institute, Boulder, Colorado
- **Therapeutic Touch**
  Consultant: Dolores Krieger, R.N., Ph.D., founder, Therapeutic Touch, Port Chester, New York
- **Trager**
  Consultant: Deane Juhan, Trager instructor,, Mill Valley, California

Cell Therapy
Consultant: Peter Stephan, M.D., Director, The Stephan Clinic, London, England

Chelation Therapy
Elmer Cranton, M.D., past President, American College of Advancement in Medicine, Troutdale, Virginia

Chiropractic
Consultant: Stuart Garber, D.C., Director, Westside Health Clinic, Los Angeles, California

Colon Therapy
Consultant: Connie Allred, President, American Colon Therapy Association, Los Angeles, California

Craniosacral Therapy
Consultant: Robert Norett, D.C., Director, Stillpoint Health Center, Venice, California

Detoxification Therapy
Consultant: Elson Haas, M.D., Director, Marin Clinic of Preventive Medicine and Health, San Rafael, California

Diet
Consultant: D. Lindsey Berkson, D.C., M.A., Nutritionist and Educator, Santa Fe, New Mexico

Environmental Medicine
Consultant: Marshall Mandell, M.D., F.A.C.A.I., F.A.A.E.M., Medical Director, New England Foundation for Allergic and Environmental Diseases, Norwalk, Connecticut

Enzyme Therapy
Consultant: Hector Solorzano, M.D., D.Sc., Coordinator, Program for Studies of Alternative Medicine, Professor of Pharmacology, University of Guadalajara, Guadalajara, Mexico

Fasting
Consultant: Steven Bailey, N.D., Graduate Assistant Professor, National College of Naturopathic Medicine; Director, Northwest Naturopathic Clinic, Portland, Oregon

Flower Remedies
Consultant: Julian Barnard, author, *Guide to the Bach Flower Remedies* and *The Healing Herbs of Edward Bach,* Hereford, England

Guided Imagery
Consultant: Martin L. Rossman, M.D., founder and Co-director, Academy of Guided Imagery, Mill Valley, California

Herbs
Consultant: David L. Hoffmann, B.Sc., M.N.I.M.H., past President, American Herbalists Guild, Sebastopol, California

Homeopathy
Consultant: Trevor Cook, Ph.D., D.I.Hom., President, United Kingdom Homeopathic Medical Association; Director, British Institute of Homeopathy, London, England

Hydrotherapy
Consultant: Douglas Lewis, N.D., Chairperson, Department of Physical Medicine, Bastyr College, Seattle, Washington

Hypnotherapy
Consultant: A. M. Krassner, Ph.D., founder and Director, American Institute of Hypnotherapy, Santa Ana, California

Juice Therapy
Consultant: Steven Bailey, N.D., Graduate Assistant Professor, National College of Naturopathic Medicine; Director, Northwest Naturopathic Clinic, Portland, Oregon

Light Therapy
Consultant: Glen Swartwout, O.D., founder, Achievement of Excellence Research Academy International, Hilo, Hawaii

Magnetic Field Therapy
Consultant: William H. Philpott, M.D. Chairman, Bio-Electro-Magnetic Institute Institutional Review Board, Choctaw, Oklahoma

Naturopathic Medicine
Consultant: Joseph Pizzorno, N.D., President, Bastyr College, Seattle, Washington

Neural Therapy
Consultant: James Carlson, D.O., past President, American Association of Orthopedic Medicine, Knoxville, Tennessee

Nutritional Supplements
Consultant: D. Lindsey Berkson, D.C., M.A., Nutritionist and Educator, Santa Fe, New Mexico

Orthomolecular Medicine
Consultant: Abram Hoffer, M.D., Ph.D., Editor-in-Chief, *Journal of Orthomolecular Medicine*; President, Canadian Schizophrenia Foundation, Victoria, British Columbia, Canada

Osteopathy
Consultant: Leon Chaitow, N.D., D.O., Editor, *Journal of Alternative and Complementary Medicine*; Director, Nutrition and Health Research Associates, London, England

Oxygen Therapy

• Hydrogen Peroxlde Therapy
Consultant: Charles Farr, M.D., Ph.D., President, International Bio-Oxidative Medicine Association; Medical Director, Genesis Medical Center, Oklahoma City, Oklahoma

• Hyperbaric Oxygen Therapy
Consultant: David Hughes, D.Sc., Director, Hyperbaric Oxygen Institute, San Bernardino, California

• Ozone Therapy
Consultant: Gerald Sunnen, M.D., Associate Professor of Psychiatry, New York University-Bellevue Hospital Medical Center, New York City, New York

Qigong
Consultant: Roger Jankhe, O.M.D., L.Ac., Dipl. (NCCA), Director, Health Action, Santa Barbara, California

Reconstructive Therapy
Consultant: William Faber, D.O., Milwaukee Pain Clinic, Milwaukee, Wisconsin

Traditional Chinese Medicine
Consultant: Roger Hirsh, O.M.D., Director, Metamedical Group, Santa Monica, California

Yoga
Consultant: Rudolph Ballentine, M.D., author; Board of Trustees, Medical Staff, Himalyan Institute, New York City, New York

"To wish to be well is part of becoming well."

—Seneca

Abscess

Accumulation of pus, usually caused by bacterial infection (or viral, parasitic, fungal), in almost any body part (most common: face, armpit, extremities, rectum, and female breast during lactation).

Symptoms: Heat, swelling, tenderness, or redness over the infected area. These increase with severity. A severe abscess may cause fever, cellulitis (inflammation of cellular tissue, usually with associated pus formation), fatigue, weight loss, chills, abnormal functioning depending on the area affected or, at worst, blood infection and rupture.

Consider: Boils, allergic infections, poor immune response, poor diet, and nutrient deficiencies. Chronic or recurrent abscesses may suggest food, environmental, or chemical allergies.

Special Notes: *Mild:* External abscesses may respond to gentle heat from warm water soaks and to improved nutrition. Most abscesses, however, need to be treated with antibiotics or herbs. This requires acidophilus, B vitamins, and an increase in fluids. Need for specific treatment such as drainage, compression bandage, or surgery should be assessed by a doctor. *Moderate to severe:* May require bed rest, increased fluids, local ice packs, or hot baths. Incomplete drainage may result in fibrous wall with calcium accumulation resulting in a hardened mass. May be caused or worsened by decreased immune functioning.

An abscess should start to clear up in several days. A failure to clear up or bouts of reoccurrences may indicate problems with immune functioning and overall health and require professional care. Assess lifestyle to reduce stress or problems that may be contributing to decreased general health and immune functioning, and get plenty of rest.

Alternative Treatments

Refer to alternative therapy chapters for more information before evaluating or applying any treatment. Some conditions, including yours, may require a physician's care.

Diet: Increase liquids such as filtered water, fresh vegetable and fruit juices, and immune enhancer herbal teas like astragalus or nettle (eight to ten glasses per day). Avoid all stressor foods, especially refined sugars, and alcohol for at least two weeks. Avoid cow's milk dairy products and processed foods. Drink water and juice of one fresh lemon on rising and before bed. If chronic, eat plenty of berries (fresh or frozen) or drink berry leaf teas.

Nutritional Therapy: • Vitamin A (50,000 IU for two weeks) • Beta-carotene (100,000 IU for two weeks) • Zinc (60 mg. daily for two weeks) • Vitamin C (5-10 grams daily) • Liquid chlorophyll • Acidophilus • Bifidobacteria culture (several times per day) • Proteolytic enzymes (on empty stomach) • B complex vitamins • Pantothenic acid • Garlic capsules • If recurrent, consider an imbalance in the system and need for bowel cleanse and rejuvenation.

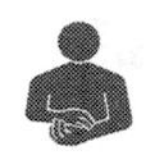

Self-Care

The following therapies can be undertaken at home under appropriate professional supervision.

Aromatherapy: • Lavender • Hot compress of bergamot, tea tree, lavender, chamomile, garlic

Fasting: Leon Chaitow N.D., D.O., suggests a short (forty-eight-hour) water or juice fast to encourage more rapid detoxification and healing.

Herbs: Burdock root, cayenne, dandelion root, echinacea, goldenseal, red clover, yarrow, and yellowdock root.

Homeopathy: *Belladonna, Merc sol., Hepar sulph., Silica, Bryonia.*

Hydrotherapy: Contrast application: apply daily.

Juice Therapy: • Carrot, beet, and celery juice • Cucumber • Wheat grass • Spinach • Also can add a small amount of yellowdock leaf juice (5 percent of total juice).

Naturopathic Medicine: Use a paste of goldenseal root powder and calendula succus (the juice of the marigold flower). Place the paste over the abscess and leave it on twelve to twenty-four hours. It will often draw out the infection, while stimulating regeneration of the damaged tissues.

Topical Treatment: • Calendula ointment • Apply mixture of the following: zinc oxide cream plus squeeze vitamin A capsule (10,000 IU) and liquid chlorophyll, locally on external abscess, three times daily. If all three are not available use whichever you can obtain. • Apply raw, unprocessed honey to infected area.

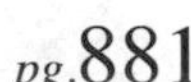

Professional Care

The following therapies should only be provided by a qualified health professional.

• Craniosacral Therapy • Detoxification Therapy • Environmental Medicine • Guided Imagery • Light Therapy • Naturopathic Medicine • Osteopathy • Traditional Chinese Medicine

Oxygen Therapy: • Hydrogen peroxide therapy (IV) • Hyperbaric oxygen therapy

Acne

Inflammation of skin because a sebaceous gland, located at the bottom of each hair follicle, becomes trapped with natural oils, causing bacterial buildup and inflammation. This condition may be worsened at adolescence, premenstrually, or mid-menstrual cycle due to hormonal action, and when under stress, eating a poor diet, or on contraceptives.

Symptoms: Inflamed spots or elevations either on or under the skin. Blackheads form when the oil combines with skin pigments and gets trapped. Blackheads may suggest the need for better hygiene, or magnesium and vitamin A. Chronic, numerous whiteheads may suggest B_1 deficiency or absorption problems. Consistent raised spots on the outside of the arms and sometimes even the thighs, resembling "chicken skin," may suggest need for magnesium, vitamin A, or essential fatty acids or the need to avoid foods that inhibit the absorption of these, such as trans-fatty acids found in margarine and hydrogenated oils, such as cottonseed oil and palm kernel oil.

Consider: Food allergies, allergies to facial creams, soaps, shampoos, makeup, excess intake of refined sugars. Certain foods may aggravate (chocolate, fruit juices, carbonated beverages, caffeinated beverages, milk products). Excessive long-term seafood or other high iodine foods may also bring on acne bouts in some people.

Special Notes: Vitamin B_6 may help for premenstrual or mid-menstrual cycle acne. Coexisting gum problems suggest the need for folic acid.

A separate acne condition may occur in women thirty to forty years old due to physical exercising or working all day with face makeup, lowered resistance due to stress, or hyper-response to bacteria or hormone problems. Another acne problem, acne rosacea (reddish spots in a pattern over nose and cheeks), may be sign of low B vitamins or low hydrochloric acid in the stomach.

It may take up to one year to eliminate skin problems. They are some of the slowest conditions to respond to natural therapies, but the response is often more complete than with drugs.

Alternative Treatments

Refer to alternative therapy chapters for more information before applying any treatment. Some conditions, including yours, may require a physician's care.

Diet: Whole foods diet with special emphasis on vegetables (four to five servings per day, try to eat half of servings raw) and whole fruits (one to three times per day). The more severe the acne the more you should reduce fats. Reduce especially animal fats (saturated) and also cut down on vegetable fats. Some people get acne in response to stressor foods such as caffeine, refined sugars, and alcohol. Processed foods such as colas, candies, and frozen and preprepared foods may also be a problem.

Increase fiber. Mono-cleansing diets for one to two days per week for several months may be helpful in people who are not hypoglycemic (low blood sugar, debilitated, or require food to keep up strength for working). Examples are: steamed vegetables and brown rice without any animal products. Fasting one day a week is helpful for some: fresh vegetable juices, filtered water, lemon and honey, or water from wheatberries soaked for twelve hours.

Nutritional Therapy: • Vitamin A (50,000 IU for two weeks. Some orthomolecular physicians recommend higher initial doses.) • Beta-carotene (50,000 IU for one month then reduce to 25,000 IU) • Zinc (80 mg. daily unless it causes nausea; if so, reduce by 20 mg.) • Vitamin B complex (two to three times daily) • Vitamin B_6 • Thiamine (vitamin B_1) • Essential fatty acids (One to two daily for one year. Acne may be a symptom of an omega-3 fatty acid deficiency.) • Brewer's yeast • Chlorophyll • Pancreatin with meals (three times daily) • Vitamin C • See Female Health chapter if this is hormonally related.

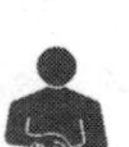

Self-Care

The following therapies can be undertaken at home under appropriate professional supervision.

• Fasting • Guided Imagery • Hypnotherapy • Meditation • Yoga

Aromatherapy: • Bergamot, lavender, rosemary, rosewood, thyme-linalol, tea tree oil • Massage with bergamot, camphor, geranium, juniper, lavender, neroli.

Ayurveda: • Apply tumeric and sandalwood paste externally (one-half teaspoon of each and enough water to make a paste). • Drink one-half cup aloe vera juice twice daily until acne clears.

Bodywork: • Massage, acupressure, *shiatsu*,

and reflexology are often recommended for skin problems. • Lymphatic drainage massage

Herbs: When used with appropriate nutritional support, herbs may be helpful in the treatment of acne. Combine the tinctures of sarsaparilla, burdock, and cleavers in equal parts and take one-half teaspoonful of this mixture three times a day. An infusion of nettle can also be drunk two or three times a day. An infusion of calendula mixed with equal parts of distilled witch hazel may be applied topically as a cleansing wash. • Try a steam sauna for face with red clover, lavender, and strawberry leaves.

Homeopathy: *Pulsatilla, Silicea, Berberis, Ledum, Sulfur, Arsen alb., Belladonna, Carbo veg.*

Hydrotherapy: • Contrast application: apply daily. • Or, try hot Epsom salts baths two to three times a week.

Juice Therapy: • Two glasses raw juice daily • Carrot, beet, and celery juice • Any combination of carrot, cucumber, lettuce (not iceberg), spinach, with carrot predominating

Naturopathic Medicine: While long-term improvement for acne requires treating the lifestyle and metabolic causes, improvement may be hastened by a proper facial hygiene. Washing the face three times a day with a soap made with the herb *Calendula officinalis* (marigold flowers) can be very effective in keeping the face clean and the cyst-forming infections minimized.

Practical Health Hints: Expose whole body to sun and air but take caution not to sunburn. Fresh air and daily exercise are very important. Be sure to get sufficient relaxation and sleep. Do not squeeze pimples or whiteheads, as this may lead to infection. Use non-oil-based makeup and wash off thoroughly each night. Avoid cosmetic products containing lanolin, isopropyl myristate, sodium laurel sulfate, laureth-4, and D and C red dyes, as they may be too rich for the skin and cause blackheads. Drink eight glasses of water a day. Use 100 percent cotton clothing and bed linen.

Reflexology: Liver, adrenals, all glands, kidneys, intestines, thyroid, diaphragm.

Stress Reduction: A study of teenagers taught methods of relaxation, including biofeedback, showed a marked reduction in acne outbreaks in severely affected individuals. Those who continued to practice at home maintained the progress they had made.[1]

Topical: Wipe face in the morning and evening with vitamin A-E emulsion, liquid chlorophyll, and aloe vera gel, or with cider vinegar and dash of cayenne pepper. Wipe three times daily with tea made from alfalfa, burdock root, echinacea, with a teaspoon of apple cider vinegar and a dash of cayenne pepper. Apply tea tree oil.

Facial cleansing: Gently wash face with mild soap and water two to four times daily. Alternatives to soap are milk, diluted lemon juice, or a solution of one part rubbing alcohol to ten parts water. Rinse face with warm water and pat dry. Try to keep skin free of oil and use water-based products. Eric Jones, N.D., instructor of pediatrics and dermatology at John Bastyr College of Naturopathic Medicine in Seattle, Washington, and Chief Medical Officer of the college's Natural Health Clinic, recommends the use of soaps containing the herb calendula, to help clean the pores without irritating the skin.

Facial masks: The following foods may be applied to the cleansed skin as a masque for thirty minutes before rinsing off with warm water: cooked and mashed carrots (let cool first), grated cucumber or sliced cucumber soaked in rum, whisked egg yolk, oatmeal, cooked in milk until thick and then cooled. Or apply baking soda and water mixture to face, rinse immediately with water, and then rinse or spray with apple cider vinegar, plus do a final rinse with filtered water. • A bentonite clay mask, left on the skin for fifteen to twenty minutes to help draw out inflammatory by-products of acne. • Rub oil from a vitamin E capsule over freshly washed and dried skin. Let remain for thirty minutes. Then apply a coating of whisked egg whites over the vitamin E and leave for another thirty minutes. Rinse with filtered water. • Apply poultice made from chaparral, dandelion, and yellowdock root to affected area. • Or try a compress of goldenseal tea. • Overnight mask for drying the skin: diluted liquid hand soap or shampoo patted on a cleansed and dried face.

Professional Care

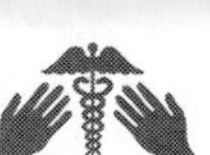

The following therapies should only be provided by a qualified health professional.

• Colon Therapy • Environmental Medicine • Enzyme Therapy • Magnetic Field Therapy • Naturopathic Medicine • Orthomolecular Medicine • Osteopathy • Traditional Chinese Medicine

Detoxification Therapy: Detoxification may be indicated, especially of the colon.

Oxygen Therapy: • Hydrogen peroxide therapy (IV)

Addictions

See Addictions chapter, page 485.

AIDS

See AIDS chapter, page 494.

Alcoholism

See Addictions chapter, page 492.

Allergies

See Allergies chapter, page 510.

Alzheimer's Disease

See Alzheimer's Disease chapter, page 521.

Amenorrhea

See Female Health chapter, page 661.

Angina

See Heart Disease chapter, page 712.

Ankylosing Spondylitis

A rare rheumatologic condition that causes stiffness and inflammation of the spine and sacroiliac joints. Characterized by "bent forward" posture. May have genetic risk.

Symptoms: *Mild and early:* Recurrent low back pain, pain along sciatic nerve that can go from buttocks to down the leg and foot, and stiffness on rising in the morning. *Progresses:* Pain spreads from low back up to middle and/or higher in the neck. Pain in arms and legs. Fatigue, muscle rigidity and more stiffness, anemia, weight loss.

Occurrence: Ninety percent occurs in males from age twenty to forty.

Consider: Test for identifying gut problems, stool sample and scraping to identify amoebic, bacteriaL, fungal, or other parasitic problems. Test for food allergies and assess need for digestive enzymes.

Alternative Treatments

Refer to alternative therapy chapters for more information before evaluating or applying any treatment. Some conditions, including yours, may require a physician's care.

Diet: Whole foods diet with emphasis on variety and ruling out food allergies. Alan R. Gaby, M.D., has treated ankylosing spondylitis successfully by identifying allergic foods and recommending avoidance and food allergy nutrients. Gut health may be related and bowel program may be useful. Two cups of vegetable broth daily. Researchers at King College Hospital in London have found a link between ankylosing spondylitis and bowel dysbiosis (incursion or overgrowth by undesirable bacteria, in this case klebsiella). They discovered that the majority of patients placed on a low-starch diet had the disease process halted.[2]

Leon Chaitow, N.D., D.O., of London, England, feels that an overgrowth of *Candida albicans* (a naturally occuring fungus in the body) is also involved in creating the damage to the gastrointestinal tract which allows the klebsiella bacteria to enter the bloodstream. He recommends further measures, including the use of friendly bacteria such as acidophilus and bulgaricus to reestablish a normal bowel flora, and an anti-candida approach, which includes a low-fat diet. He believes that the results of the low-fat diet in the King College Hospital study may have been due to controlling both the klebsiella bacteria and the candida.

Nutritional Therapy: Vitamin C to bowel tolerance. (See Orthomolecular Medicine chapter, page 402.)

Self-Care

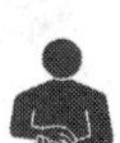

The following therapies can be undertaken at home under appropriate professional supervision.

• Fasting • Yoga

Herbs: Many anti-inflammatory and alternative herbs have been used to alleviate the symptoms of this condition. The following mixture has been used over long periods of time: a combination of the tinctures of meadowsweet, willow bark, black cohosh, prickly ash, celery seed, and nettle in equal parts, one-half teaspoonful of this mixture taken three times a day. In cases of rheumatoid arthritis add wild yam and valerian to the mixture and take one teaspoonful of this mixture three times a day.

Hydrotherapy: Constitutional hydrotherapy: apply two to five times weekly. Or contrast application: apply daily as needed for relief of inflammation.

Juice Therapy: Carrot, beet celery, parsley, potato, alfalfa.

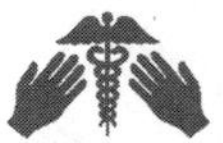

Professional Care

The following therapies should only be provided by a qualified health professional.

• Applied Kinesiology • Cell Therapy • Chelation Therapy • Chiropractic • Craniosacral Therapy • Environmental Medicine • Magnetic Field Therapy • Naturopathic Medicine • Neural Therapy • Osteopathy • Pancreatic Enzyme Therapy • Reconstructive Therapy

Acupuncture: For chronic condition: moxa stick used up and down the spine for five to ten minutes a day along with herbs.

Bodywork: • Feldenkrais • Rolfing can sometimes ease the pain and stiffness associated with ankylosing spondylitis, but cannot cure.

Oxygen Therapy: Hydrogen peroxide therapy (IV).

Anorexia Nervosa

An eating disorder where weight loss becomes an obsession and starvation begins to affect thinking patterns and personality.

Symptoms: Physical symptoms include wasting of the body, including the muscle tissue, arrest of sexual development and cessation of menstruation, drying and yellowing of the skin, loss of texture of the hair, pain to the touch, lowered blood pressure and metabolic weight, anemia, and severe sleep disturbances.

Mentally, the patient still sees herself as fat, may have a preoccupation with death, and often exercises frantically to keep physically fit. She often is manipulative, trying always to be the center of attention, and may become socially isolated.

Occurrence: Predominantly in teenage females and is a problem only in developed countries.

Special Notes: In both anorexia nervosa and bulimia nervosa, the underlying causative factors were believed to be solely due to an obsession with body fat, a fear of being (or becoming) fat, or overconcern with perfectionism. Although all of these factors are important, recent studies also show that in most cases, an underlying zinc deficiency may contribute to the maintenance of the disorder.

Alternative Treatments

Refer to alternative therapy chapters for more information before evaluating or applying any treatment. Some conditions, including yours, may require a physician's care.

Diet: A well-balanced diet, high in fiber, should be followed when a regular eating pattern is being established. Avoid sugar and white flour products.

Nutritional Therapy: Ten years of study indicate that a liquid form of a zinc sulfate heptahydrate supplement (Zinc Talley, Zinc Drink) is beneficial in the diagnosis and treatment of anorexia nervosa. According to Alexander Schauss, Ph.D., a Certified Eating Disorder Specialist, the inability to taste a tablespoon of this supplement in the mouth may be indicative of inadequate zinc status. He recommends 100-120 ml./day of the zinc solution until symptoms improve, which may take two weeks to experience.

Vitamin B_{12}, D, and E levels in the blood are often low in anorexia nervosa.

Intravenous feeding may be necessary in acute cases to replace lost calories and reverse protein deficiency. Psychological counseling by trained specialists, combined with nutritional therapy, is highly recommended.

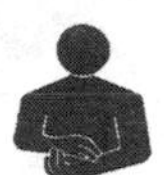

Self-Care

The following therapies can be undertaken at home under appropriate professional supervision.

• Biofeedback Training • Yoga

Aromatherapy: As anti-depressants—bergamot, basil, chamomile, clary sage, lavender, neroli, ylang ylang.

Ayurveda: Cardamom, fennel, and fresh ginger to help regulate digestion and stop vomiting. Follow a bland diet and avoid coffee, tea, and other stimulants. For calming effect, valerian, nutmeg, *ashwagandha*, and sandalwood. Massage head and feet with sesame oil.

Herbs: To stimulate appetite: ginger root, ginseng, gotu kola, peppermint.

Hydrotherapy: Constitutional hydrotherapy: apply two to five times weekly.

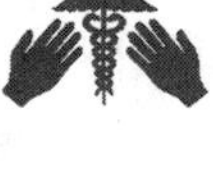

Professional Care

The following therapies should only be provided by a qualified health professional.

• Hypnotherapy • Magnetic Field Therapy • Traditional Chinese Medicine

Arthritis

See Arthritis chapter, page 530.

Asthma

See Respiratory Conditions chapter, page 814.

Astigmatism

See Vision Disorders chapter, page 859.

Autism

See Autism chapter, page 540.

Back Pain

See Back Pain chapter, page 546.

Bad Breath

Bad breath, or halitosis, is an unpleasant odor emanating from the mouth, usually caused by some health problem in the mouth, teeth, gums, throat, or gastrointestinal tract. Other problems may be smoking, liver disease, and poor protein digestion. The mouth is one window into the body. If there is a bad odor it is a general sign that there is some underlying cause and imbalance that needs to be treated.

Symptoms: Bad odor coming from the mouth that is usually not detectable by the person him- or herself. Astute health practitioners smell the breath and examine carefully the tongue and mouth of all patients.

Special Notes: Certain smells are associated with specific disease, for example a metallic smell may represent diabetes or an active metabolism undergoing rapid weight loss. Sour smells may represent stomach problems or tumors. Orthodox physicians do not agree that halitosis may represent intestinal problems, but anecdotal evidence by many alternative practitioners finds differently.

Bad breath may also be caused by chronically infected sinuses, tonsils, or lungs.

Alternative Treatments

Refer to alternative therapy chapters for more information before evaluating or applying any treatment. Some conditions, including yours, may require a physician's care.

Diet: Whole foods diet with plenty of raw foods. Water with juice of fresh lemon and/or one teaspoon chlorophyll on rising and before bed. Include fiber in diet: oat bran, rice bran. Chew food well, don't overeat, and drink lots of liquids.

See Diet chapter for information on the role antioxidants play in relieving bad breath.

Nutritional Therapy: • If needed, bowel cleanse and rejuvenation • Proteolytic enzymes (two between meals, three times daily, and two with each meal) • Vitamin B complex (100 mg. two times daily) • Vitamin C • Chlorophyll • Thiamine (vitamin B_1) • Niacin (vitamin B_3) • Vitamin B_6 • Alfalfa tablets • Garlic capsules • PABA (para-aminobenzoic acid) • Vitamin A • Beta-carotene • Acidophilus • Digestive enzymes • Magnesium • Zinc • Charcoal

Self-Care

The following therapies can be undertaken at home under appropriate professional supervision.

• Fasting • Yoga

Aromatherapy: Peppermint, lavender, cardamom.

Ayurveda: *Triphala*, one-half teaspoon with warm water, half an hour before bed at night. Chew roasted cumin, fennel, and coriander seeds after each meal.

Herbs: • Chewing seeds of fennel or anise as needed will mask the odor and have a mild local antimicrobial effect. Alternatively chew parsley leaves. Attention must be given to underlying causes, such as tooth and gum disease or digestive illness. • Peppermint tea

Homeopathy: *Arnica, Merc sol., Nux vom., Kali phos., Chelidonium.*

Hydrotherapy: Constitutional hydrotherapy: apply two to five times weekly.

Juice Therapy: • Carrot and celery with parsley, spinach, watercress, alfalfa, comfrey, or beet tops • Wheat grass juice • Green juice • Carrot, spinach, and cucumber • Half a lemon in warm water each morning

Naturopathic Medicine: According to Joseph Pizzorno, N.D., bad breath is far more often due to maldigestion and a toxic bowel than to poor oral hygiene. People who experience bad breath, abdominal bloating and gas, and tiredness after meals may be deficient in stomach acid.

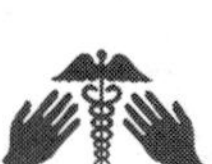

Professional Care

The following therapies should only be provided by a qualified health professional.

• Applied Kinesiology • Colon Therapy • Environmental Medicine • Naturopathic Medicine

Detoxification Therapy: Bad breath is often related to gastrointestinal toxicity, suggesting a need for intestinal detox with diet change.

Oxygen Therapy: Use of ozonated water gargle may be effective.

Traditional Chinese Medicine: As this is considered a symptom of "stomach heat" it is most important to address the deeper cause of the digestive problem.

Bed Sores

Ulcers of the skin formed by prolonged bed rest, which causes sustained pressure over bony areas of the body, such as the buttocks, hips, sacrum, and shoulder blades.

Symptoms: Areas of redness, deep ulceration, and painful.

Special Notes: Patients need to be moved frequently, and also require fresh air and light bed clothes. Daily baths with gentle soaps containing vitamin E and aloe vera, and sufficient natural light may be helpful.

Occurrence: In physically restricted patients such as the disabled, comatose, and bedridden elderly.

Time: Should start to heal within one week and may take up to six, depending on severity of situation.

Alternative Treatments

Refer to alternative therapy chapters for more information before evaluating or applying any treatment. Some conditions, including yours, may require a physician's care.

Diet: Drink plenty of liquids (distilled water, herbal teas, fresh juices). Include plenty of fiber in diet to keep colon clean. Oat bran, guar gum are both excellent. (If bowels do not move, use an enema.) Five to seven vegetables and fruits a day is optimal.

Nutritional Therapy: • Oral vitamin E • Zinc • Vitamin A • Beta-carotene • Vitamin C • Vitamin B complex • Zinc with copper • Vitamin D • Protein supplement (free-form amino acids) • Garlic capsules • If not responding to the above, pancreatic enzymes in between meals (six to twelve per day for one week along with bioflavonoid and vitamin C may be helpful). Vitamin C to bowel tolerance. (See Orthomolecular Medicine chapter, page 402.)

Self-Care

The following therapies can be undertaken at home under appropriate professional supervision.

• Guided Imagery

Herbs: Comfrey root powder, echinacea powder, goldenseal, myrrh gum, pau d'arco, slippery elm powder, suma.

Homeopathy: *Calendula, Hypericum, Merc sol., Chamomilla, Phosphorus, Hamamelis, Silicea, Belladonna.*

Hydrotherapy: • Contrast application: apply several times daily to promote healing. • Periodic cold compresses to stimulate sore areas

Juice Therapy: Carrot, beet, cantaloupe, currant, red grapes.

Naturopathic Medicine: A standard naturopathic approach is to wash the open wound with *Calendula succus* (juice of the marigold flower) and then cover it with zinc oxide.

Topical Treatment: Application of a paste of goldenseal powder, vitamin E squeezed from capsule, along with zinc oxide applied topically. Also enzyme cream, vitamin E cream, aloe vera gel, comfrey ointment, calendula cream.

Leon Chaitow, N.D., D.O., suggests the "safest and oldest approach—application of raw honey or granulated sugar paste to open ulcers from bed/pressure sores—which have now been well researched medically and shown to be at least as effective as medicated creams."

Professional Care

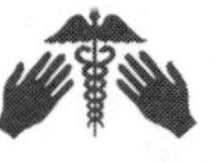

The following therapies should only be provided by a qualified health professional.

• Acupuncture • Chelation Training • Magnetic Field Therapy • Naturopathic Medicine

Oxygen Therapy: • Ozone therapy is useful applied externally in a fitted plastic bag. • Hyperbaric oxygen therapy

Bedwetting

Involuntary wetting of the bed in the middle of night during childhood. Usually spontaneously stops by teenage years. Often a general sign that there is some underlying problem.

Consider: Hypoglycemia, diabetes, food allergies, and urinary tract infections.

Special Notes: Cause of bedwetting is unknown and controversial. Low blood sugar is one nutritional theory. Others are emotional stress, small and weak bladders that cannot hold the urine all night long, excessive consumption of liquid beverages, sleeping too soundly, food allergies, heredity, and behavioral problems.

Time: Improvement may take up to several months but some improvement may be seen within the first two weeks.

Alternative Treatments

Refer to alternative therapy chapters for more information before evaluating or applying any treatment. Some conditions, including yours, may require a physician's care.

Diet: Eat more frequent and smaller meals throughout the day, up to five or six. Consume slow release complex carbohydrates such as potatoes, yams, whole grains, breads, and beans. Avoid liquids around bedtime. Avoid drinking very sweet beverages such as fruit juice or cola more than one time per day. Take two teaspoons of raw honey at bedtime. Take small piece of protein from chicken, fish, soy, goat cheese, or nut butter, before bed.

Nutritional Therapy: • Mixed amino acid supplements (two, two or three times daily ten minutes before meals) • Magnesium (100 mg. two times daily) • Calcium (250 mg. with dinner and before bed) • Vitamin B complex (one with breakfast and lunch) • Multivitamin (two to three daily)

Self-Care

The following therapies can be undertaken at home under appropriate professional supervision.

Aromatherapy: Before bedtime a rub of the child's abdomen with olive oil and 3 to 5 percent cypress essence.

Flower Remedies: For emotional states as appropriate.

Herbs: If bedwetting occurs because of lack of nervous control of the bladder, use of an infusion of one part each of horsetail, St. John's Wort, cornsilk, and lemon balm. Half a cup given three times a day, with the last dose well over an hour before bedtime.

Homeopathy: *Berberis.*

Hydrotherapy: A cool sitz bath for five minutes.

Naturopathic Medicine: According to Joseph Pizzorno, N.D., supplemental magnesium has helped several children with this problem.

Reflexology: Kidneys, diaphragm, ureters, adrenals, lower spine.

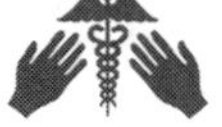

Professional Care

The following therapies should only be provided by a qualified health professional.

• Acupuncture • Biofeedback Training • Chiropractic • Hypnotherapy • Magnetic Field Therapy

Bodywork: *Shiatsu.*

Environmental Medicine: Allergies can be a major cause of bedwetting. Allergic reactions to food or environmental factors can cause sudden and violent contractions in the muscles of the bladder.

Bee and Insect Stings

See Insect Bites.

Benign Prostatic Hypertrophy

See Male Health chapter, page 734.

Beriberi

A deficiency of thiamine (vitamin B_1) causing neurologic, mental, and cardiovascular problems.

Symptoms: *Mild:* fatigue, irritation, slow learning and confusion, poor cold tolerance, nausea, vomiting, whiteheads on face or upper torso. *Severe:* memory loss, heart pain, weight loss, abdominal and heart discomfort, poor digestion, gas, diarrhea, constipation, extreme fatigue, mood swings, mental confusion, tachycardia (rapid heart rate), heart failure, death.

Consider: Parasites, gastrointestinal or liver disease, food allergies, severe stress syndrome.

Special Notes: *Primary beriberi:* Occurs due to inadequate intake of vitamin B_1 through food. This is found especially in people eating highly refined diets, as B_1 is lost in the milling process. Especially prevalent in people subsisting on polished (white) rice. However, boiling before milling disperses the B_1 from the husk throughout the kernel and tends to make less B_1 lost through this processing.

Secondary beriberi: Occurs due to loss by poor utilization, such as in liver disease, gastrointestinal problems, or alcoholism and drug addiction, through increased requirements, such as pregnancy, hyperthyroidism (overactive thyroid), breast-feeding, fever, stress (emotional and physical), genetic need for more than the average individual, and impaired absorption, such as with diarrhea, parasites, gastrointestinal loss of friendly bacteria, damage to the lining of the gastrointestinal tract by drugs, alcohol, stress, amoeba, food allergies, celiac or borderline celiac disease (wheat intolerance), or other gut problems.

Time: Response should start within a few days to one week depending on severity of deficiency and symptoms.

Alternative Treatments

Refer to alternative therapy chapters for more information before evaluating or applying any treatment. Some conditions, including yours, may require a physician's care.

Diet: Eat foods rich in thiamine and other B

vitamins such as brown rice, whole grains, raw fruits and vegetables, especially green leafy vegetables, legumes, seeds, nuts, and yogurt. Drinking excessive liquids (more than one glass) with meals may wash out thiamine and other B vitamins. Avoid raw fish.

Nutritional Therapy: *Mild deficiency:* • Thiamine (vitamin B_1), (30 mg. a day in divided dosages) *Severe:* Thiamine (30-100 mg. day in divided dosages) • Vitamin B complex • Multivitamin and mineral complex • Vitamin C

With severe cardiac and mental symptoms such as in cardiovascular beriberi or Wernicke-Korsakoff syndrome (marked reduction of blood flow to the head with dramatic symptoms) B_1 needs to be given 50-100 mg. by injection two times daily.

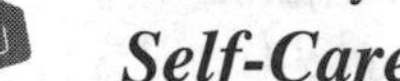

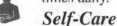

Self-Care

The following therapies can be undertaken at home under appropriate professional supervision.

Homeopathy: *Sulfur.*

Professional Care

The following therapies should only be provided by a qualified health professional.

• Naturopathic Medicine • Orthomolecular Medicine • Traditional Chinese Medicine

Bladder Infections (Cystitis)

See Female Health chapter, page 669.

Blood Clots

Clots (thrombi) of blood formed inside major blood vessels which are the major cause of many heart attacks, strokes, and other cardiovascular disorders.

Symptoms: Usually silent.

Special Notes: Blood solidification, clotting, usually occurs as a healthy response, within minutes, after the skin is cut or there is trauma that causes bleeding. A clot helps seal the damage. However, blood clotting can be dangerous if it is inside healthy blood vessels. Unhealthy clotting can occur from platelets that get "activated" to clump together (get sticky). This occurs when platelets come in contact with damaged arterial walls (see Heart Disease chapter), or due to nutrient deficiencies, poor dietary habits, or genetics. Once platelets get sticky their shape changes and they easily mesh or clump together, causing a clot. Another factor is the production of fibrin that helps bind the clump of platelets together. Fibrin is the end product of a cascade of coagulation (clumping) factors that occurs with just the activation of one molecule that can lead to the explosion of up to thirty thousand molecules of fibrin at the site of injury at the arterial wall.

Factors that may cause a buildup of platelet stickiness and fibrin are: birth control pills, late stages of pregnancy, nutrient deficiencies, smoking, free radical pathology (inadequate antioxidant nutrients), a high cholesterol diet, low essential fatty acids, nutrient deficiencies, genetics, a diet high in saturated fat and low in vegetables and fish, and liver disease.

Some doctors and medical researchers have found that prolonged sitting on long airline flights, especially in cramped conditions, puts a person at risk for developing pulmonary thrombosis.[3] Blood clots forming in the legs or another part of the body break loose and then block one of the arteries to the lungs. Some practical preventive measures include: getting up and walking the aisle every hour, wearing loose, comfortable clothing, periodically stretching the legs and tightening and loosening the muscles of the abdomen and buttocks, and taking some slow, deep breaths.

In studies done at Duke University, Salvatore V. Pizzo, M.D., showed that moderate exercise may help protect against heart attacks and strokes by enhancing the body's natural mechanism for dissolving blood clots. In addition, Dr. Pizzo found that the higher risk of blood clotting in women taking oral contraceptives can be significantly reduced by exercise.[4]

Alternative Treatments

Refer to alternative therapy chapters for more information before evaluating or applying any treatment. Some conditions, including yours, may require a physician's care.

Diet: Foods that act to decrease platelet stickiness and fibrin formation are garlic, ginger, onions, and hot peppers (capsicum) which protect against heart attack and stroke. Use granulated garlic on food as a regular spice. Fish oils help to reduce clotting of blood. Increase consumption of cold water fish at least three times per week.

Decrease sucrose consumption as sugar intake increases platelet stickiness.[5]

Nutritional Therapy: • Vitamin B_6 • Garlic capsules • Niacin (vitamin B_3) • Lipotrophic factors (combination useful for liver metabolism of fat, produced by many vitamin companies) • Omega-3 and omega-6 fatty acids • Bromelain • Vitamin E may be useful in helping to dissolve blood clots. • Vitamin C • Zinc • Magnesium • Manganese

If you are on aspirin as daily preventive therapy, you may want to begin a gut rejuvenation program to stimulate healing and proper gastrointestinal wall functioning, in order to offset aspirin's traumatization of the gut wall when taken on daily basis. It is a good idea to do bowel cleanse and rejuvenation several times a year when on daily aspirin. (Consult your physician for guidance.)

Self-Care

The following therapies can be undertaken at home under appropriate professional supervision.

• Fasting

Herbs: Hawthorne berry.

Homeopathy: *Hamamelis.*

Hydrotherapy: Contrast application: apply several times daily.

Juice Therapy: Garlic, carrot, parsley, spinach, celery, beet.

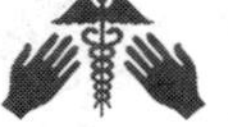

Professional Care

The following therapies should only be provided by a qualified health professional.

• Environmental Medicine • Osteopathy • Naturopathic Medicine

Oxygen Therapy: Hydrogen peroxide therapy (IV).

Body Odor

The most common cause of unpleasant smells coming off the body is poor hygiene and uncleanliness. Sweat has no odor, but if left on the skin for a few hours, bacteria decompose the sweat and can cause odor. The next most common cause is sweat containing a high level of garlic, curry, or other spicy food. However, when a person is very healthy, usually the foods can be eaten without lasting odor effects.

The other causes for body odor that are not often appreciated are nutrient deficiencies (usually zinc), underlying health problems (usually liver disease or diabetes), or gastrointestinal problems (such as parasites or chronic constipation).

Consider: Recommendation is to wash effectively once a day. Feet are areas most affected due to warm, airless environment, so check condition of feet and shoes. Consider excessive caffeine consumption or emotional stress which can influence body odors.

Special Notes: The more wholesome the diet and the balance of nutrient biochemistry in the body, the less there are unpleasant odors emanating from the body even under high risk situations.

Alternative Treatments

Refer to alternative therapy chapters for more information before evaluating or applying any treatment. Some conditions, including yours, may require a physician's care.

Diet: Whole foods diet with at least one-third to one-half raw foods. Increase fluids, quality water seven to eight glasses per day. On rising and before bed, one glass of water with juice of fresh lemon and one teaspoon of chlorophyll.

Nutritional Therapy: • Bowel cleanse and rejuvenation program several times a year • Vitamin B_1 (50 mg. two times daily while problem exists and then 20-30 mg. one time daily several times a week for one year) • Vitamin B complex • If not on a gut rejuvenation program, take Vitamin A (25,000 IU daily for a few weeks). • Vitamin C (increase amount and frequency under periods of stress). • Vitamin B_6 (pyridoxine) • Chlorophyll • Magnesium • Zinc • PABA (para-aminobenzoic acid) • Liver glandulars and liver program may be helpful.

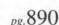

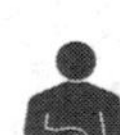

Self-Care

The following therapies can be undertaken at home under appropriate professional supervision.

• Fasting

Aromatherapy: Sage.

Juice Therapy: Fresh vegetable juices.

Homeopathy: *Hepar sulph., Sulfur.*

Hydrotherapy: One of the following: immersion bath, wet sheet pack, or steam/sauna. Apply daily to produce sweating and elimination.

Naturopathic Medicine: Leon Chaitow, N.D., D.O., suggests skin brushing daily—in which a natural bristle brush is gently used to scrub the skin of the entire body in gentle circular motions to encourage removal of dead skin, improved local circulation, elimination through the skin, and enhanced skin function generally. This should ideally be followed by a bath in which essential oils are used.

Topical Treatment: Apply baking soda under arms and between toes. Avoid aluminum-based antiperspirants.

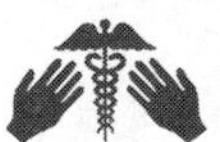

Professional Care

The following therapies should only be provided by a qualified health professional.

• Applied Kinesiology • Colon Therapy • Environmental Medicine • Naturopathic Medicine • Traditional Chinese Medicine

Detoxification Therapy: Detoxification may be indicated, depending on the person's condition.

Boils

A pus-filled, inflamed area of the skin, that can occur anywhere on the body, usually at an infected hair follicle. Most common sites are low back, thighs, buttocks, back of neck, and armpits. The infection is usually due to the bacteria Staphylococcus aureus.

Symptoms: Starts as a very painful slightly red bump. It then becomes more swollen, more painful, redder, filled with pus, gets a yellowish-white tip, and will keep draining or causing pain until the very "core," a slight sac surrounding the pus, is expelled.

Special Notes: Recurrent boils may occur in people with decreased immune function, diabetes, chronic gastrointestinal problems, underactive thyroid, or lowered resistance due to borderline nutrient deficiencies and chronic emotional stress. Bursting a boil can spread it, leaves scars, and does no good until the "core" is expelled.

Alternative Treatments

Refer to alternative therapy chapters for more information before evaluating or applying any treatment. Some conditions, including yours, may require a physician's care.

Diet: Lots of green, orange, and yellow vegetables which are cleansing (try to have at least four different types of green vegetables a day, keep this up for at least six months as much as possible). Increase fluids, drink water throughout the day, and drink water with juice of fresh lemon and one teaspoon of chlorophyll on rising and before bed. A cleansing fast may be helpful in some people but not others, especially if the immune system is not built up afterward. Check for nutritional deficiencies, particularly overconsumption of white sugar and white flour products.

A drink made by mixing greens (parsley, spinach, celery) in blender with pineapple juice may be used to help purify the blood. According to Leon Chaitow, N.D., D.O., fresh or bottled beet root juice is traditionally used in Europe as a blood purifying drink.

Nutritional Therapy: • Garlic capsules • Chlorophyll • Proteolytic (pancreatic) enzymes (taken on empty stomach two to three times daily away from meals) • Vitamin E emulsion • Coenzyme Q10 • Raw thymus glandular • Kelp • Zinc • Beta-carotene • Vitamin A

Emphasize the role of building up the immune system and liver functioning, and in reducing chronic emotional stress, in the case of chronic boils. Thus, consider thymus glandular, 1 gram of B_5 four times daily, vitamin C, 1 gram every hour, adrenal glandulars, blueberry leaf tea, liver programs, and bowel programs.

Direct application of mixture of honey, oil from vitamins E and A capsules, and some zinc oxide, several times a day up to one time an hour, may be helpful.

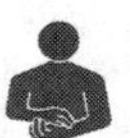

Self-Care

The following therapies can be undertaken at home under appropriate professional supervision.

• Fasting • Guided Imagery

Aromatherapy: Draw out the boil with bergamot, lavender, chamomile, clary sage.

Ayurveda: To bring boil to a head: application of a poultice of cooked onions. Wrap in cloth and do not apply onion directly to boils. Application of a paste of one-half teaspoon each of tumeric and ginger powder directly to boil.

Bodywork: Acupressure, reflexology, *Shiatsu.*

Herbs: A blend of the tinctures of echinacea, cleavers, and yellowdock in equal parts, taken one teaspoonful three times a day. Additionally, drink a cup of an infusion of nettle, preferably fresh herb, twice a day.

Homeopathy: *Bellis, Belladonna, Hepar sulph., Arnica, Silicea, Apis mel., Arsen alb., Lachesis* • *Phytolacca* must be taken alone, not in combination with other remedies.

Hydrotherapy: • Contrast application: apply daily. • Warm Epsom salts baths

Juice Therapy: • Wheat grass juice • Carrot, beet, and celery juice • Carrot, beet, and cucumber • Carrot, spinach • Carrot, lettuce, spinach and yellowdock (5 percent)

Topical Treatment: • Poultice of goldenseal root powder paste • Hot Epsom salts pack (two tablespoons in one cup water) • Tea tree oil applied to boils • One part sesame oil and one part lime juice mixed and applied externally

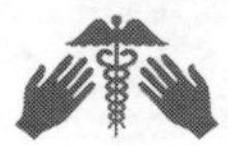

Professional Care

The following therapies should only be provided by a qualified health professional.

• Environmental Medicine • Magnetic Field Therapy • Naturopathic Medicin • Osteopathy • Traditional Chinese Medicine

Detoxification Therapy: Detoxification is indicated after controlling the infection.

Oxygen Therapy: Hydrogen peroxide therapy (IV)

Breast Cancer

See Female Health chapter, page 673.

Bronchitis

See Respiratory Conditions chapter, page 815.

Bruises

A darkish black and blue mark on the skin, formed usually without a cut, due to blood that leaks out of capillaries, usually after an injury, and collects just beneath the surface of the skin.

Symptoms: First discolorations are black and blue. Then, when the hemoglobin of the blood breaks down the color turns to yellow. Often associated with some swelling and surrounding redness of the tissues.

Occurrence: More common in children from accidents. More frequently in women than men, may be due to estrogen demands of vitamin C on the body.

Special Notes: Bruises that do not fade after a week, or are recurrent without cause, may be signs of bleeding disorders or vitamin C and bioflavonoid deficiencies, or signs of underlying stresses on the body that continually deplete the vitamin C stores. See a physician.

Alternative Treatments

Refer to alternative therapy chapters for more information before evaluating or applying any treatment. Some conditions, including yours, may require a physician's care.

Diet: Whole foods diet with emphasis on foods rich in vitamin C and bioflavonoids such as fresh fruits, green leafy vegetables, and buckwheat.

Nutritional Therapy: • Vitamin C with bioflavonoids and rutin • Alfalfa tablets • Vitamin B_6 • Folic acid • Vitamin E • Iron

Nutritional biochemist Jeffrey Bland, Ph.D., reports that higher doses of some bioflavonoids (especially rutin) increase blood vessel elasticity and so help to prevent rupturing of small blood vessels and easy bruising.

When the bruises are not responsive to high dosages of vitamin C, increase the bioflavonoids to 2 grams several times a day along with adrenal support: pantothenic acid up to 3-4 grams per day, adrenal glandulars, blueberry leaf tea.

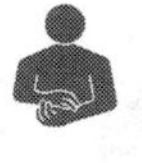

Self-Care

The following therapies can be undertaken at home under appropriate professional supervision.

• Fasting • Guided Imagery

Aromatherapy: • Camphor, fennel, hyssop, lavender • Put a few drops of lavender oil on gauze compress and place on bruise.

Herbs: • Liberal applications of arnica salve on the effected area. Alternatively application of a compress made with oil of hyssop or a mixture of tumeric and honey to bruise. • See Herbal chapter for the use of St. John's Wort for bruises.

Homeopathy: • *Arnica, Ruta grav., Hypericum, Hamamelis, Symphytum.* Do not apply *Arnica* cream to open wounds.

Hydrotherapy: Contrast application: apply several times daily as needed.

Juice Therapy: Carrot, beet, high bioflavonoid sources.

Topical Treatment: *Herbal poultices:* • Mashed yerba santa leaves soaked in hot water, applied to the bruise and covered with a clean cloth. • Compress of chilled infusion of comfrey or sage. Remove when dry and apply comfrey ointment or calendula ointment. • Apply slice of raw onion to bruise. • *Witch hazel:* Soak one ounce of witch hazel leaves and twigs in two cups of 151 proof alcohol for two weeks. Shake the mixture daily. Strain and use directly on bruise. (Or use commercial witch hazel solution.)

Leon Chaitow, N.D., D.O., suggests hot and cold applications (ring out towels in appropriate temperature water) applied locally in a sequence of twenty seconds hot, ten seconds cold, for several minutes every hour will help reduce the congestion of bruising. The sooner after the blow this is done the better.

Professional Care

The following therapies should only be provided by a qualified health professional.

• Applied Kinesiology • Environmental Medicine • Naturopathic Medicine • Traditional Chinese Medicine • Orthomolecular Medicine • Osteopathy

Oxygen Therapy: Hyperbaric oxygen therapy may be useful for extensive bruising (crash injuries).

Bulimia

An eating disorder characterized by bouts of extreme overeating (bingeing) followed by self-induced vomiting. Often, but not always, associated with anorexia, in which bingeing and dieting are both carried out to extremes.

Symptoms: Bulimics may be thin, normal, or slightly underweight. If anorexia is part of the eating disorder, there will be extreme loss of body weight. Bingeing and vomiting may occur several times a day, after most meals, or less frequently. Gastric symptoms, loss of menstruation, swollen face and neck especially after coming out of bathroom after eating meals, fatigue, dizziness, irritability, poor cold tolerance, severe food cravings, excessive exercise habits, poor stress coping skills, depression, and even suicidal tendencies may manifest. Vomiting exposes the teeth to gastric juice and there may be dental erosion. Using the hand to force vomiting may cause callouses on the back of the hands where the skin hits the teeth during the procedure.

Occurrence: This disorder is often performed in "secret," so that the rate of occurrence is not fully established. However, it is much more prevalent in women between the ages of twelve and thirty.

Consider: Nutrient deficiencies, especially zinc, food allergies, amino acid imbalances.

Special Notes: In both anorexia nervosa and bulimia nervosa, the underlying causative factors were believed to be solely due to an obsession with body fat, a fear of being (or becoming) fat, or overconcern with perfectionism. Although all of these factors are important, recent studies also show that in most cases, an underlying zinc deficiency may contribute to the maintenance of the disorder.

Alternative Treatments

Refer to alternative therapy chapters for more information before evaluating or applying any treatment. Some conditions, including yours, may require a physician's care.

Diet: A whole foods diet with regular eating patterns is paramount. Avoid all sugar and white flour products. Identification and avoidance of allergic foods. Sufficient protein sources to adequately nourish the body.

Nutritional Therapy: Ten years of study indicate that a liquid form of a zinc sulfate heptahydrate supplement (Zinc Talley, Zinc Drink) is beneficial in the diagnosis and treatment of anorexia nervosa. According to Alexander Schauss, Ph.D., a Certified Eating Disorder Specialist, the inability to taste a tablespoon of this supplement in the mouth may be indicative of inadequate zinc status. He recommends 100-120 ml./day of the zinc solution until symptoms improve, which may take two weeks to experience.

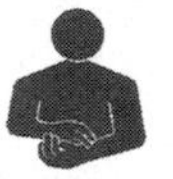

Self-Care

The following therapies can be undertaken at home under appropriate professional supervision.

• ***Qigong***

Homeopathy: *Calc carb., Ipecac., Graphites.*

Hydrotherapy: Constitutional hydrotherapy: apply two to five times weekly.

Naturopathic Medicine: When associated with anorexia, it seems to respond well to supplemental zinc.

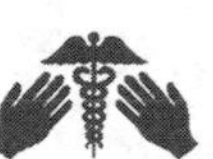

Professional Care

The following therapies should only be provided by a qualified health professional.

• ***Biofeedback Training*** • ***Hypnotherapy*** • ***Light Therapy*** • ***Naturopathic Medicine*** • ***Traditional Chinese Medicine***

Bunions

Enlarged area of the inner part of the big toe associated with a fluid-filled pad (bursae) underneath the often hardened outer skin. This is caused by a swelling of the bursa of the metatarsophalangeal joint (joining toe to foot) of the big toe which forces the toe to point inward as the joint itself protrudes outward.

Symptoms: Large toe moves inward. Can become inflamed and create mild to extreme pain.

Occurrence: More frequently in women from wearing pointed and tight-fitting shoes. According to Jonathan Wright, M.D., bunions are often hereditary.

Special Notes: Bunions need to be treated or will get worse. Mild bunions can be treated mechanically though larger ones may require surgery.

Alternative Treatments

Refer to alternative therapy chapters for more information before evaluating or applying any treatment. Some conditions, including yours, may require a physician's care.

Nutritional Therapy: • This is palliative, may improve symptoms of pain and inflammation, but is not curative, will not get rid of the symptoms. Thus, these need to be taken on a regular basis several times per day to keep blood levels up and improvement usually takes up to one month and will go away a short time after these are no longer taken. • DL-phenylalanine or D-phenylalanine • Niacinamide • Magnesium

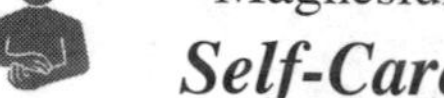

Self-Care

The following therapies can be undertaken at home under appropriate professional supervision.

Herbs: Aloe vera juice, parsley tea, calendula.

Hints: Walk barefoot whenever possible. Exercise foot, rolling back and forth, from heel to toe, over a bottle.

Homeopathy: • *Ruta grav., Silicea, Arnica* • *Benz ac.* must be taken alone, not in combination with other remedies.

Hydrotherapy: • Contrast application: apply daily. • Hot Epsom salts foot baths; to aid circulation use a whirlpool bath.

Reflexology: Work around and directly on bunion.

Topical Treatment: Apply aloe vera gel.

Professional Care

The following therapies should only be provided by a qualified health professional.

• Acupuncture • Chiropractic • Magnetic Field Therapy • Naturopathic Medicine • Osteopathy • Reconstructive Therapy

Bodywork: • Alexander technique • Foot massage • Manipulation of joint of big toe

According to Leon Chaitow, N.D., D.O., to correct or improve a bunion, structural and functional correction is needed of the postural and mechanical (weight-bearing) factors which led to its development. Fallen arches, postural muscle imbalance in the legs and pelvic area, problems involving low back and pelvic joint mechanics, as well as habits of use (running, walking, and standing postures relating to work, sport, and general function) all need attention from skilled practitioners using manipulation and rehabilitation methods, including physical therapists, chiropractors, and osteopaths.

Burns

Heating of the skin, anything over 120 degrees Fahrenheit, so that damage occurs.

Symptoms: *First degree burns:* Skin reddens, as only the top layer of the skin is affected (epidermis). Skin may peel away in several days and heals quickly. *Second degree burns:* Blisters are created due to damage to the deeper layer of the skin. Usually heal without scarring. *Third degree burns:* The full thickness of the skin is damaged by the heat. Area looks charred or white, and tissues below bones and muscles may be exposed. Requires burn specialist to treat properly.

Special Notes: Immediately run cold water over the burn. According to Leon Chaitow, N.D., D.O., if possible and practical, run cold water over the area for as long as possible (hours if necessary). This will also help prevent blisters. Cover.

On second degree burns place mixture of baking soda mixed with olive oil, zinc ointment, and pure vitamin E to promote healing and prevent scarring. Do not break blisters. Elevate area of burn higher than heart if possible to alleviate swelling. To remove substances melted on skin such as plastic or tar, use ice-cold water.

Copper and zinc are lost through wound seepage. Loss of these minerals may significantly increases the need for supplementation during burns.

Alternative Treatments

Refer to alternative therapy chapters for more information before evaluating or applying any treatment. Some conditions, including yours, may require a physician's care.

Diet: High protein diet for second and third degree burns to promote repair of damaged tissue. Increase intake of fluids. Increase high zinc foods such as pumpkin seeds and oysters.

Nutritional Therapy: • Vitamin E • Vitamin C with bioflavonoids • Zinc • Protein supplement (free-form amino acids) • Vitamin A • Vitamin B complex • Pantothenic acid (B_5) • Spray burned area with vitamin C solution. • Vitamin E can have a dramatic effect on burns of all kinds: fire, chemical, electrical, and sunburn. • Apply 100 percent solution of dimethyl sulfoxide (DMSO) to minimize scarring and prevent loss of skin.

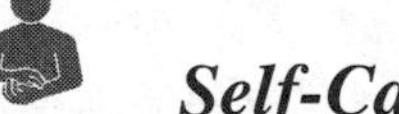

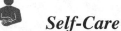

Self-Care

The following therapies can be undertaken at home under appropriate professional supervision.

• Fasting • Guided Imagery

Aromatherapy: • Lavender, geranium, camphor • Prevent blistering: apply two to three drops of lavender oil. The discovery of the healing properties of lavender oil on burns was actually the basis for research into and development of the field of aromatherapy by French chemist René-Maurice Gattefossé. (See Aromatherapy chapter, page 56.)

Ayurveda: Application of a paste made of fresh aloe vera gel or plain *ghee*, coconut oil, licorice *ghee*, or *tikta ghee*.

Herbs: If a mild burn, application of a poultice, salve, or juice of plantain to the burn. Cool aloe vera gel may also be applied. Severe burns require immediate professional attention. For sunburn cool aloe vera gel applied liberally to the burnt area may be helpful. If badly burned a salve made with St. John's Wort and calendula flowers may be helpful.

Homeopathy: *First degree: Calendula, Hypericum, Arnica* (for shock), *Urtica Urens, Belladonna. Second degree: Arnica* (for shock), *Cantharis, Belladonna. Third degree:* consult a physician. *Sunburn: Nat mur.* (as preventative), *Urtica urens, Rhus tox.*

Hydrotherapy: Cold compress: apply immediately and as needed to control pain.

Juice Therapy: Carrot, cantaloupe, currants (add garlic to juice).

Naturopathic Medicine: Gel from the freshly cut aloe vera leaf.

Topical Treatment: Ice and vinegar.

Professional Care

The following therapies should only be provided by a qualified health professional.

• Cell Therapy • Light Therapy • Naturopathic Medicine • Orthomolecular Medicine

Special Notes: Studies indicate up to 95 percent of burned tissue can be healed with minimal scarring with negative ion therapy. This method is also greatly helpful for pain reduction.[6]

Magnetic Field Therapy: Magnetic treatments pioneered in the former Soviet Union have been demonstrated to be effective in the healing of burns.[7]

Oxygen Therapy: • Hydrogen peroxide therapy (IV) • Hyperbaric oxygen therapy • Ozone therapy: In infected burns, especially if not too extensive and relatively dry, ozone therapy has healing value. In wet burns, too much ozone may be absorbed.

Traditional Chinese Medicine: A salve made with Lithospermum root *(zi cao)* and black sesame oil has been used for burns. Ginger juice has been applied fresh topically in Traditional Chinese Medicine.

Bursitis

Inflammation of bursa, which are sac-like cavities filled with lubricating fluid (synovial), at areas where friction is likely to occur, such as where muscles or tendons pass over bony places. Inflammation may be acute or chronic.

Symptoms: Acute and chronic: Localized pain and tenderness, sometimes swelling and redness, may be associated with loss of normal range of motion of that joint, and sometimes becomes reddish colored and warm.

Consider: Trauma, malposition of specific joint or joints above and below, chronic overuse, acute or chronic infection, calcium deposits secondary to calcium malabsorption, magnesium deficiency or localized trauma, allergies especially airborne or food, vitamin B_{12} malabsorption, inflammatory arthritis, gout, rheumatoid arthritis, infective organisms (especially *Staphylococcus aureus*), and, rarely, tuberculosis organisms.

Special Notes: Most commonly affected joints are shoulder, elbow, and hip which are often referred to as "frozen" due to the loss of normal range of motion.

Time: Improvement should start within first ten days and not take longer than two months if appropriate. Splinting and rest are helpful for acute bouts but much less for chronic.

Alternative Treatments

Refer to alternative therapy chapters for more information before evaluating or applying any treatment. Some conditions, including yours, may require a physician's care.

Diet: Identify and avoid food allergies. Eat foods high in magnesium: dark leafy green and many different green and yellow vegetables. Drink filtered water, apple cider vinegar, and honey on rising, before bed and several times throughout the day. Avoid foods from the nightshade family: tomatoes, potatoes, eggplant. Take one tablespoon cod liver oil one to two hours before meals.

Nutritional Therapy: • Vitamin B_{12} (intramuscular injection) repeated on a daily basis • Calcium • Magnesium • Proteolytic enzymes between meals • Vitamin C and bioflavonoids

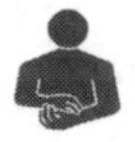

Self-Care

The following therapies can be undertaken at home under appropriate professional supervision.

• Fasting • Guided Imagery

Aromatherapy: Juniper, chamomile, cypress.

Herbs: Combine the tinctures of meadowsweet, horsetail, and willow bark in equal parts and take one teaspoonful three times a day. Topically either gently rub into the affected area a mixture of equal parts tincture of lobelia and cramp bark to the effected muscles. Drink strong chamomile tea, particularly at bedtime to help relieve pain. Aloe vera gel may be helpful.

Homeopathy: *Belladonna, Arnica, Ruta grav., Silicea.*

Hydrotherapy: Contrast application: apply one to three times daily. If acute; ice pack: apply twenty minutes out of each hour for the first twenty-four to thirty-six hours.

According to Leon Chaitow, N.D., D.O., any hot treatment (or bath) should finish with the area being chilled by a compress or spray (shower).

• Epsom salts baths. A pound or more of Epsom salts per bath. Soak for twenty-five to thirty minutes. Rinse and rub down with hot olive oil. Do once a week. • Also try rosemary soaks for hands and feet or a bath for the whole body. Soak for ten to fifteen minutes, two to three times a day. • Ice packs: Place one above joint and one below for twenty minutes three times a day for one month (six ice cubes to a quart of cold water, or mix two-thirds water and one-third alcohol and freeze until slushy).

Juice Therapy: Equal parts carrot, celery, cucumber, beet.

Lifestyle: At the onset of inflammation rest the affected area for a few days. Otherwise the problem may last for weeks.

Reflexology: Reflex to affected area, adrenals, referral area to affected area.

Topical Treatment: Mullein hot packs: boil three to four fresh mullein leaves in water for three minutes. Place over joint. Wrap with hot moist towel, then dry towel. Leave for twenty minutes three times a day.

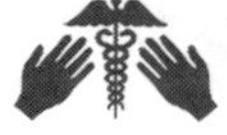

Professional Care

The following therapies should only be provided by a qualified health professional.

• Acupuncture • Applied Kinesiology • Chiropractic • Craniosacral Therapy • Environmental Medicine • Magnetic Field Therapy • Naturopathic Medicine • Neural Therapy • Osteopathy • Reconstructive Therapy • Traditional Chinese Medicine

Bodywork: Reflexology, acupressure, Feldenkrais, Rolfing.

Detoxification Therapy: Detoxification may be indicated, depending on the condition of the person.

Oxygen Therapy: • Hydrogen peroxide therapy (IV) • Hyperbaric oxygen therapy is in regular use internationally but not in the United States.

Ultrasound: To break up calcium deposits and adhesions.

Energy Medicine: Electro-Acuscope, Light Beam Generator.

Light Therapy: Cold (soft) laser photo stimulation therapy.

Cadmium Toxicity

A trace metal, that is toxic to the body in any amount, and may accumulate in body tissues.

Symptoms: Mild symptoms; fatigue, irritability, dulled sense of taste and/or smell. Cadmium toxicity may be associated with high blood pressure, prostate enlargement of a benign nature, hair loss, weight loss, bone loss, pain in the joints and muscles, poor immune response, learning disabilities, dry and scaling skin, and in severe conditions, kidney and liver damage.

Occurrence: High in cigarette smokers as it is found in high concentrations in tobacco.

Special Notes: Risk and severity of cadmium toxicity increases with zinc deficiency. Cadmium binds to tissue sites where zinc would normally bind, so it lowers tissue levels of zinc and worsens zinc deficiencies.

Alternative Treatments

Refer to alternative therapy chapters for more information before evaluating or applying any treatment. Some conditions, including yours, may require a physician's care.

Diet: • High fiber diet • Pumpkin seeds • Apple pectin in form of apples or apple sauce • Beans at least four times a week • Eight glasses of filtered water a day

William L. Cowden, M.D., recommends a diet of organic vegetables, fruits, seeds, grains, and nuts. He adds that a small percentage of the population whose ancestors lived in the very Northern latitudes cannot tolerate this diet. Symptoms of intolerance would be fatigue, sometimes muscle weakness, difficulty with memory and concentration, and feeling low-grade flulike symptoms If these symptoms occur as a result of the dietary changes, test for urine pH (acid-base balance). If urine is too alkaline, add some organic meats and/or dairy products if no allergies to dairy are present.

Nutritional Therapy: • Vitamin C • Zinc • Garlic capsules • Two weeks of a diet high in vegetables (five to seven servings daily; emphasis on green vegetables) and no meat, along with one-quarter teaspoon of baking soda in water three times daily between meals with 2 grams of vitamin C which helps reduce cellular toxicity from tobacco and especially helps reduce smoking craving and helps eliminate smoking addiction.

According to Leon Chaitow, N.D., D.O., the amino acids taurine, glutathione, and cysteine have all been shown to protect human cells against toxicity resulting from tobacco usage.

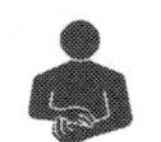

Self-Care

The following therapies can be undertaken at home under appropriate professional supervision.

• ***Fasting***

Herbs: See Chemical Poisoning.

Hydrotherapy: Hazel Parcells, N.D., D.C., Ph.D., reports excellent success with the following bath for heavy metal poisoning: Put one cup household bleach in a full bath of water as hot as you comfortably can stand it. Stay in until it cools to body temperature. The therapeutic value is in the exchange of fluids between tissues. The heat brings the toxins to the surface. As it cools the toxins are drawn out of the body and into the water.

Juice Therapy: • Carrot, celery, parsley, cucumber • Steven Bailey, N.D., of Portland, Oregon, reports a patient with elevated levels of cadmium via hair and serum (blood) tests. Employing increased juices, flaxseed oil, and zinc, within four weeks of niacin/sweat program (see Detoxification chapter, page 156) serum levels went from 6 to nondetectable.

Professional Care

The following therapies should only be provided by a qualified health professional.

• ***Acupuncture*** • ***Magnetic Field Therapy*** • ***Naturopathic Medicine***

Chelation Therapy: According to Leon Chaitow, N.D., D.O., chelation should be considered as the first form of treatment.

Cancer

See Cancer chapter, page 556.

Candidiasis

See Candidiasis chapter, page 587.

Canker Sores

Painful ulcers on the movable mucous membrane surface of the mouth, cheek, or tongue that occur singly or in groups.

Symptoms: *Mild:* Less than one centimeter, last ten days to two weeks and heal without scarring. *Severe:* More than one centimeter, last several weeks to several months, leave scarring. Recurring attacks are common with anywhere from several to many ulcers. Ulcers have whitish centers surrounded by redness.

Occurrence: Women more than men.

Consider: Bowel flora imbalances in people with parasites, poor digestion, food sensitivities, chronic constipation or diarrhea, Crohn's disease.

Special Notes: Stress, extreme heat such as associated with physical exertion, hot weather, extreme fatigue, fever, localized trauma such as after dental work, and with nutrient deficiencies such as lysine, iron, vitamin B_{12}, and folic acid. These may be contagious if resulting from infectious agent.

Alternative Treatments

Refer to alternative therapy chapters for more information before evaluating or applying any treatment. Some conditions, including yours, may require a physician's care.

Diet: • Vary grains and add a variety of beans, seeds, and nuts. Mono-wheat diets contribute to canker sores. Avoid foods that may irritate the ulcers such as coffee, alcohol, refined sugar, citrus fruits, spicy foods, mouthwashes, and smoking.

Severe: Cut down on acid-forming foods such as animal products, grains, beans, and seeds, in ratio to amount of vegetables and fruits.

According to Leon Chaitow, N.D., D.O., some cases develop from food sensitivity, with the most common culprits being milk, cheese, wheat, tomato, vinegar, lemon, pineapple, and mustard.

Nutritional Therapy: • Vitamin C • Lysine (4 grams for first four days, then 500 mg. three times daily, on empty stomach and away from meals) • Vitamin B complex lozenges or vitamin B complex (two to three daily with meals with folic acid and B_{12}) • Iron • Zinc gluconate lozenges • Acidophilus • Pantothenic acid

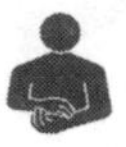

Self-Care

The following therapies can be undertaken at home under appropriate professional supervision.

• Fasting • Guided Imagery

Herbs: For symptomatic relief use a mouthwash made with sage and chamomile. Combine equal amounts and then infuse. Use as a gargle as often as needed. Internally take a combination of equal parts tincture of echinacea and cleavers, one-half teaspoonful three times a day.

Juice Therapy: Carrot, celery, cantaloupe. Avoid high acids (pineapple, citrus).

Naturopathic Medicine: While many local therapies exist, naturopathic physicians believe the basic cause is most likely an allergy to wheat and possibly other grains. Local relief of pain can be achieved using a paste made up of echinacea tincture and myrrh gum.

Topical Treatment: Using a cotton swab, dab each sore with an 8 percent solution of zinc chloride (from your pharmacist).

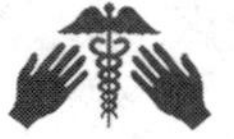

Professional Care

The following therapies should only be provided by a qualified health professional.

• Colon Therapy • Environmental Medicine • Magnetic Field Therapy • Naturopathic Medicine

Traditional Chinese Medicine: Watermelon frost powder.

Detoxification Therapy: Detoxification may be indicated, depending on the condition of the person.

Oxygen Therapy: • Hydrogen peroxide therapy (IV) • Ozone therapy

Carbuncles

A cluster of interconnecting boils with the infection spreading underneath the skin. Great amount of pus, slow healing, and often associated with scarring. (See Boils.) Infective organism is usually Staphyloccus aureus.

Symptoms: These develop more slowly than boils, are localized over a larger area, are extremely painful, swollen, and red, and may be accompanied by general feelings of fatigue, debilitation, and fever.

Occurrence: More frequently in men, at the nape of the neck, buttocks, or thighs. Even though they can occur in very healthy people, they are often associated with diseases that are very debilitating, associated with diabetes mellitus, and found in the elderly. These are very contagious and often are spread to family and friends.

Special Notes: Carbuncles should be cultured to identify the infective organism and antibiotics used if needed. Carbuncles or boils in the nose require antibiotics as the infection can easily spread to the brain.

Alternative Treatments

Refer to alternative therapy chapters for more information before evaluating or applying any treatment. Some conditions, including yours, may require a physician's care.

Diet: (See Boils.) Drink plenty of filtered water. Whole foods with lots of green, leafy vegetables, and grains such as buckwheat.

Nutritional Therapy: (See Boils.) • Vitamin A • Vitamin C • Chlorophyll • Garlic • Proteolytic enzymes (empty stomach away from meals) • Acidophilus

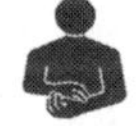

Self-Care

The following therapies can be undertaken at home under appropriate professional supervision.

• Fasting • Guided Imagery

Herbs: Please refer to Boils.

Homeopathy: *Ledum, Belladonna, Arsen alb., Lachesis.*

Hydrotherapy: Contrast application: apply daily.

Juice Therapy: • Carrot, beet, and celery juice, garlic • Wheat grass juice • Cucumber

Topical Treatment: Please refer to boils.

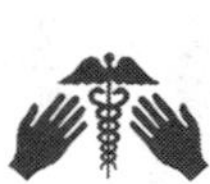

Professional Care

The following therapies should only be provided by a qualified health professional.

• Magnetic Field Therapy • Naturopathic Medicine • Osteopathy • Traditional Chinese Medicine

Detoxification Therapy: May be indicated, depending on the condition of the person.

Oxygen Therapy: Hydrogen peroxide therapy (IV)

Carpal Tunnel Syndrome

Compression of a nerve in the wrist (median) that produces numbness, tingling, and sometimes pain. Weakness and tingling of the first three fingers and thumb may also occur. Symptoms:

tingling of palm surface of hands, first three fingers, often worse at night or with driving. Can also be associated with tingling, burning, and pain of entire arm, neck and hip, and thigh. May be one or two sided.

Occurrence: More common in women after the age of thirty-five.

Consider: Conditions that can create swelling or fluid shifts (to contribute to pressure on nerve) such as pregnancy, low thyroid, occupations which require forceful or repetitive wrist movements, vitamin B_6 deficiencies, nerve disorders, or compression of the nerve root of the sixth cervical vertebrae due to misalignment of the neck, muscular spasm, osteoarthritis, disk disease, or tumor. May be secondary to other wrist conditions.

Special Notes: Treatment varies, symptoms may improve in one week or take several months. Often carpal tunnel can be successfully treated without the need for surgery, although sometimes surgery is necessary.

According to Steven Bailey, N.D., of Portland, Oregon, carpal tunnel is often a misdiagnosis of thoracic outlet compression syndrome (a syndrome in which pressure to lower cervical and upper thoracic nerves results in dysfunction of the tissues and nerves associated with the brachial nerves).

Alternative Treatments

Refer to alternative therapy chapters for more information before evaluating or applying any treatment. Some conditions, including yours, may require a physician's care.

Diet: Whole foods diet. Limit protein intake. Eliminate foods high in yellow dyes. Good foods to focus on: whole grains, seeds, and nuts, soybeans, fresh salmon, brewer's yeast, molasses, liver, wheat bran and germ, and cod. Avoid stressor foods that deplete the body's level of B_6 such as excessive consumption of sugars, caffeine, and processed grains and corn.

Nutritional Therapy: • Vitamin B_6 • Vitamin B complex • Magnesium • Essential fatty acids • Folic acid • Thyroid hormone

People with carpal tunnel syndrome often have a large deficiency of vitamin B_6, or have lifestyle factors that inhibit B_6 metabolism such as stress, or ingesting Yellow Dye No. 5, and tartrazine derivatives. It may also be that a deficiency of vitamin B_6 (pyridoxine) may cause a pyridoxine-responsive neuropathy (nerve disorder). Treatment with B_6 may relieve the symptoms in many cases, eliminating need for surgery. Daily dosage ranges from 25-300 mg., depending on the person's biochemistry.

Caution: *Pyridoxine supplementation may create a nerve disorder (sensory neuropathy) in dosages as low as 300 mg. if taken daily for long periods. Most of the cases of vitamin B_6 toxicity have been reported with dosages from 2-5 grams per day.*

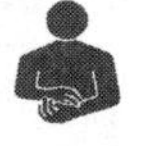

Self-Care

The following therapies can be undertaken at home under appropriate professional supervision.

• Biofeedback Training • Fasting • Qigong

Acupressure: To relieve carpal tunnel wrist pain firmly press P6 and TW5 (for an illustration of these point numbers please see the acupressure chart on pages 874-875) on the affected hand for two minutes. Position the fingertips between the bones of the forearm two finger widths below the wrist crease. Grasp these points firmly to strengthen the wrist joint and relieve the carpal tunnel pain. Repeat three times daily for a month.

Aromatherapy: Marjoram, lavender, eucalyptus.

Herbs: Anti-inflammatory herbs effectively support the broader treatment. A simple approach involves combining equal parts of meadowsweet and willow bark tinctures and taking one teaspoonful of this mixture three times a day.

Homeopathy: • *Aconite, Arsen alb., Ignatia, Nat mur., Chamomilla, Colchicum.* Homeopathic treatment tends to be constitutional in nature and is therefore normally long-term, but usually successful.

Hydrotherapy: Contrast application: apply one to three times daily.

Lifestyle: Avoid repetitive wrist movement. Monoamine oxidase inhibitor anti-depressant drugs can create a deficiency in vitamin B_6 and should therefore be avoided if possible.

Naturopathic Medicine: Vitamin B_6 is believed to be highly effective, but patience is necessary—most people don't respond for at least six weeks.

Professional Care

The following therapies should only be provided by a qualified health professional.

• Applied Kinesiology • Chiropractic • Craniosacral Therapy • Light Therapy • Naturopathic Medicine • Orthomolecular Medicine • Osteopathy • Reconstructive Therapy

Acupuncture: Acupuncture treatments have proved effective in giving substantial relief in pain and discomfort.

Bodywork: Acupressure, Feldenkrais, Hellerwork, Rolfing.

Detoxification Therapy: May be indicated, depending on the condition of the person.

Energy Medicine: Electro-Acuscope.

Neural Therapy: According to Deitrich Klinghardt, M.D., many cases can be traced to interference fields in the arm, shoulders, or neck, often caused by vaccination scars. Dr. Klinghardt reports great success using neural therapy to alleviate the problem.

Oxygen Therapy: Hyperbaric oxygen therapy.

Cataracts

See Vision Disorders chapter, page 859.

Cellulite

This is really not a condition, but a lay term for unsightly looking dimples in various parts of the body, especially the thighs, knees, buttocks, stomach, and arms.

Symptoms: Loose, dimpled skin.

Occurrence: More frequently in women.

Special Notes: In general, this condition is considered to be due to an increased ratio of fat cells to lean body mass. Based on this assumption, reducing body fat content and building up muscle mass is imperative. Spot reducing, aimed at fat reduction at specific body sites, is extremely difficult. Most experts say that it is not possible.

However, notes Dennis Pies, B.A., M.A., P.T., of Santa Fe, New Mexico, cellulite is formed by fibroid masses of protein that have accumulated in the spaces between the cells due to faulty elimination through the lymph system. He has achieved a 100 percent success rate in the elimination of this condition using lymphatic therapy.

Pies suggests that since gravity is the primary force that creates cellulite, the following exercise is beneficial: First, gently jump on a trampoline (if available) to create pumping action in the lymph system. Then, using gravity to drain the lymph system, place your legs up against a wall or over a chair and massage, very lightly, the crease formed by the legs and the abdomen in order to open the deep inguinal lymph nodes which is where all of the accumulation that forms the cellulite must pass to be eliminated from the body.

Alternative Treatments

Refer to alternative therapy chapters for more information before evaluating or applying any treatment. Some conditions, including yours, may require a physician's care.

Diet: Whole foods diet with less complex carbohydrates and sugars than is usually recommended for the average person. Large amounts of filtered water. Decrease fats to below 20 percent of the total diet and avoid as much as possible animal fats and processed fats.

Pies recommends not eating protein at night as unused protein in the body puts a greater load on the lymph system.

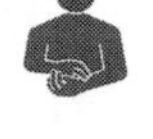

Self-Care

The following therapies can be undertaken at home under appropriate professional supervision.

• Fasting • Hydrotherapy

Aromatherapy: Juniper, rosemary, lavender, lemon, geranium.

Bodywork: Self-massage: massage affected area regularly.

Herbs: Combine equal parts of horse chestnut bark and gotu kola tinctures and take one-half teaspoonful three times a day. Topically apply a compress made with white birch oil morning and evening or apply an ointment or lotion made from horse chestnut twice a day.

Juice Therapy: Beet, carrot.

Topical Treatment: Aloe vera extract.

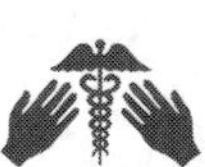

Professional Care

The following therapies should only be provided by a qualified health professional.

• Cell Therapy • Magnetic Field Therapy • Naturopathic Medicine

Detoxification Therapy: May be indicated, depending on the condition of the person.

Energy Medicine: Light Beam Generator.

Cerebral Palsy

A general classification for a number of congenital (occurs at birth) conditions that are lifelong and are characterized by impairments in voluntary muscular movements (motor handicaps). Cerebral palsy is incurable, but much can be done to optimize patients' capabilities, through lifelong and complex therapies and a variety of interventions.

Symptoms: Seventy percent of cases are spastic (abnormal stiffness of muscles). The spasticity may be mild or severe. Hemiplegia characterizes both limbs involved on one side, such as one arm and leg. The arm is usually more severe. Paraplegia means both legs are involved and the arms may not be or may be very mildly involved. Quadriplegia means that all four limbs are involved to some degree. Affected limbs are usually poorly developed, sometimes rigid due to excessive muscle tone, weakness, with a tendency to spasm and contracture (severe spasm that may lead to bone deformity unless there is some intervention). Sometimes the first symptoms are "floppy baby syndrome" where the baby's muscles have too little tone and the baby flops around when held. The parents may recognize that something "seems wrong," but are not sure exactly what it is.

Special Notes: Diagnosis may take up to the second year due to moving through certain developmental patterns.

The Peto Institute in Hungary and the United Kingdom provides an intensive physical therapy and exercise program called conductive education, which has for some forty years treated children with cerebral palsy with sometimes dramatic success in terms of improved function and speech.

Alternative Treatments

Refer to alternative therapy chapters for more information before evaluating or applying any treatment. Some conditions, including yours, may require a physician's care.

Diet: Marshall Mandell, M.D., of Norwalk, Connecticut, reports that his studies show that victims of cerebral palsy may have sensitivities or allergies to certain foods or elements they breathe in or come in contact with that may cause an increased reaction or intensified symptoms. He refers to this as a sort of hay fever of the brain, and explains how food is passed through the digestive track into the bloodstream and eventually to the brain where the allergy triggers exaggerated symptoms.

In some patients he has identified intermittent, unpredictable flare-ups of allergies, aggravating what he calls "biological weak spots," areas that may have healed up to degree but are still supersensitive to outside irritation.

Nutritional Therapy: Identification and avoidance of food allergies may improve muscle tone or decrease the higher percentage of health problems associated with this condition usually due to the decreased immune system functioning because of loss of normal range of movement and muscle tone. Certain nutrients may help muscle tone: magnesium, vitamin B_1, vitamin B_6, vitamin C, and bioflavonoids.

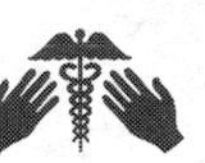

Professional Care

The following therapies should only be provided by a qualified health professional.

• Acupuncture • Biofeedback Training • Craniosacral Therapy • Fasting • Magnetic Field Therapy • Naturopathic Medicine • Traditional Chinese Medicine

Bodywork: Reflexology, Feldenkrais, Rolfing can be helpful with less severe cases.

Environmental Medicine: Dr. Mandell has found that many cases of cerebral palsy are exacerbated by brain allergies. He has found that treating the brain allergies can often stabilize and improve cerebral palsy.

Osteopathy: According to Leon Chaitow, N.D., D.O., osteopathy is the first choice, but only if cranial osteopathy (craniosacral therapy) is used.

Cranial osteopathy, if provided by a fully qualified practitioner within hours or days of birth can prevent much of the subsequent damage caused by a difficult labor or forceps delivery, which may have caused the cranial distortion which is impeding normal function of the brain and nervous system. In older infants results will often be less dramatic, but nevertheless substantial. (See Craniosacral Therapy chapter, page 149 and Pregnancy and Childbirth chapter, page 802.)

Oxygen Therapy: • Hydrogen peroxide therapy (IV) • Hyperbaric oxygen therapy

Vision Therapy: Vision therapy may improve cerebral palsy with prism therapy. The prisms manipulate posture and perception to awaken and alter brain function.

Cervical Cancer

See Female Health chapter, page 673.

Chemical Poisoning

(See Detoxification chapter, page 156.)

Overexposure to chemicals that have harmful effects on the body such as damage to the liver.

Symptoms: Can be anything from skin conditions such as rashes and boils, to organ damage such as kidney or liver failure.

Occurrence: Most often occurs in the home from household chemicals or in people who are exposed to chemicals on the job.

Special Notes: Poisons may enter from topical exposure to skin, breathing poison in, chronic poisoning from gradual exposure such as from a job, accidental poisoning in the home most often from young children who swallow prescription drugs or household chemicals, or by a suicide attempt.

Leon Chaitow, N.D., D.O., states that anyone living in an industrial or urban or even rural setting is likely to be somewhat affected long-term by toxicity from chemicals. He adds that there is now evidence that everyone on the planet carries in his or her fatty tissues residues of dioxin and DDT, and that lead burdens are now two hundred times that present in skeletal remains of people living one thousand years ago—and rising. Everyone can benefit from reducing this load.

In severe, acute cases, seek emergency help.

Alternative Treatments

Refer to alternative therapy chapters for more information before evaluating or applying any treatment. Some conditions, including yours, may require a physician's care.

Diet: Eat organically grown foods as much as possible. Short, periodic fasts are recommended to reduce toxicity. Eat a high-fiber diet to help cleanse the system. Recommended foods include: brown rice, beans, barley, lentils, oatmeal, beets, carrots, spinach, garlic, onions, almonds, brazil nuts, bananas, lemons, grapes, dates, yogurt, fish.

Nutritional Therapy: • According to Jonathan Wright, M.D., in emergency situations, a very high dose of vitamin C and glutathione given intravenously can be very helpful. • Vitamin B complex with choline and inositol • Vitamin C with bioflavonoids • Vitamin E • Superoxide dismutase (SOD) • Raw liver extract • Protein supplements (free-form amino acids) • Selenium • L-cysteine and L-methionine • Garlic capsules • Co-enzyme Q10

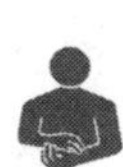

Self-Care

The following therapies can be undertaken at home under appropriate professional supervision.

• ***Fasting***

Herbs: Herbs that help the regeneration of liver cells are helpful, combined with ones that facilitate elimination of waste from the body. Specific details depend upon the chemicals involved, but one general practice is to combine the tinctures of milk thistle, licorice, and dandelion leaf in equal parts and take one teaspoonful of this mixture three times a day.

Hydrotherapy: Hazel Parcells, N.D., D.C., Ph.D., reports excellent success with the following bath for pesticide and carbon monoxide poisoning. *Pesticides:* one cup household bleach in a full bath of water as hot as you comfortably can stand it. Stay in until it cools to body temperature. The therapeutic value is in the exchange of fluids between tissues. The heat brings the toxins to the surface. As it cools the toxins are drawn out of the body and into the water. *Carbon monoxide poisoning:* Add five drops of household bleach to a glass of water. Saunas may also be effective in helping chemical poisoning.

Dr. Chaitow suggests regular Epsom salts baths, and skin brushing to encourage skin function.

William L Cowden, M.D., recommends the following protocol (under a physician's care): essential fatty acids like flaxseed, canola, safflower, or sunflower oil (two to three tablespoons to as much as one-eighth cup); co-enzymated B complex; vitamin C plus lecithin, all immediately before a light exercise session or a light, dry sauna. Immediately after exercise or sauna take a cool shower with a good quality soap.

Dr. Cowden suggests that people who are very ill from the toxins should take homeopathic detoxification remedies and work into the exercise and sauna program very slowly.

Naturopathic Medicine: In addition to the appropriate specific therapy to neutralize the chemical poison, the liver is treated to help it detoxify the chemical and minimize the damage to the liver cells. Considerable research and clinical experience has shown that the herb *Silybum marianum* (milk thistle) is very effective in assisting the liver when exposed to chemical toxins.

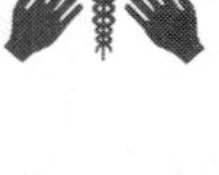

Professional Care

The following therapies should only be provided by a qualified health professional.

• ***Homeopathy*** • ***Naturopathic Medicine***

Oxygen Therapy: • Hydrogen peroxide therapy (IV) • Hyperbaric oxygen therapy may be useful for cyanide, carbon monoxide, smoke inhalation.

Chest Pain

See Heart Disease chapter, page 711.

Chicken Pox

See Children's Health chapter, page 608.

Childbirth

See Pregnancy and Childbirth chapter, page 799.

Children's Health

See Children's Health chapter, page 595.

Chills

An attack of feeling very cold, that results in shivering, chattering of teeth, and paleness.

Consider: Poor cold tolerance which means that one gets cold very easily and has difficulty getting and staying warm. This can be a sign of decreased health due to many conditions. Most common: thyroid disorder, adrenal disorder, poor digestion, and chronic respiratory disorders.

The most common first sign of nutrient deficiencies (especially the B vitamins) or borderline nutrient deficiencies is poor cold tolerance.

According to Leon Chaitow, N.D., D.O., evidence from the United Kingdom and Germany shows that people who are easily chilled can have their circulatory and temperature regulatory mechanisms normalized by a slow progressive exposure to cold over a period of six months. During this time the individual should on a daily basis start the day in a warm bathroom standing feet only (moving the feet up and down as if marching on the spot) in cold water for ten to twenty seconds. Week by week this increases to the point where after a month the individual is standing up to the mid-calf for a minute or so in cold water. At this point he or she should end the process by sitting in the water (up to the waist) for ten seconds. Progressively he or she should reach a point where he or she can, after some months, lie in the bath for several minutes each morning. By this time the circulatory and heat control mechanisms will be trained and hardened and chills will be a thing of the past, says Dr. Chaitow.

Special Notes: This is frequently associated with a fever, especially one associated with an infection.

Alternative Treatments

Refer to alternative therapy chapters for more information before evaluating or applying any treatment. Some conditions, including yours, may require a physician's care.

Nutritional Therapy: • Vitamin B complex (two to three times daily with meals) • Vitamin C • Niacin (B_3—some people this helps and some it makes worse) • Vitamin B_{12}, mixed amino acids (two, ten minutes before meals, three times daily) • Thyroid support

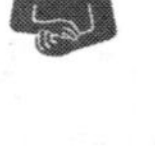

Self-Care

The following therapies can be undertaken at home under appropriate professional supervision.

• Fasting • Yoga

Herbs: Teas of chamomile, boneset, ginger, pennyroyal, or yarrow.

Homeopathy: *Aconite* (sudden onset), *Euphrasia, Nat mur., Arsen alb., Sulfur, Pulsatilla.*

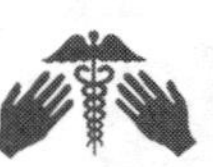

Professional Care

The following therapies should only be provided by a qualified health professional.

• Acupuncture • Applied Kinesiology • Colon Therapy • Environmental Medicine • Naturopathic Medicine

Oxygen Therapy: Hydrogen peroxide therapy (IV)

Chlamydia

See Sexually Transmitted Diseases chapter, page 828.

Chronic Fatigue Syndrome

See Chronic Fatigue Syndrome chapter, page 616.

Chronic Pain

See Chronic Pain chapter, page 625.

Cirrhosis

A group of chronic liver diseases associated with abnormal changes in the normal microscopic architecture (interstitial cells) of the liver which cause hardening and inflammation of the liver itself. (Sometimes the term cirrhosis is used to refer to any organ that has chronic interstitial inflammation.) The liver becomes damaged and cannot perform its many functions: storage and filtering of blood, production of bile (which helps digest fat and fat-soluble vitamins), production of bilirubin (which gives stool its color) and many metabolic actions like the production of sugar into glycogen (form in which carbohydrates are stored in the body); stored energy for the body (thus, another classic symptom of liver disease is extreme fatigue).

Symptoms: Cirrhosis of the liver usually has a very long period of latency, meaning no overt symptoms. Some signs of mild liver disease may be fatigue, itching, rashes of unknown causes, constipation or diarrhea, alternating color of the stools, fever, and indigestion. Suddenly there is abdominal swelling, pain, vomiting of blood, swelling of the body in general and jaundice (yellowing of the skin). Advanced stages lead to very severe symptoms which may lead to coma and death.

Special Notes: Biliary cirrhosis first affects the bile ducts, then moves into the liver and is a disease of unknown causes. It is most frequent in women thirty-five to sixty years of age. Thirty percent have no symptoms but are discovered through abnormal blood tests. Fifty percent have itching, rash, and fatigue as the initial signs that may occur months or even years before the actual disease is identified. Fifty percent of people, at time of diagnosis, have enlarged excessively firm but nontender livers and enlarged spleens. Ten percent of people have patches of darkness on skin and less then 10 percent have jaundice. Other possible signs are: clubbing of nails, yellow stools, kidney, bone, and nerve disease.

Alternative Treatments

Refer to alternative therapy chapters for more information before evaluating or applying any treatment. Some conditions, including yours, may require a physician's care.

Diet: Whole foods diet including seeds, nuts, whole grains, beans, and milks from soy, nuts, rice, and goat. According to Jonathan Wright, M.D., the current and best diet recommendations for cirrhosis are for a low-protein diet. Avoid processed fats such as margarine, hydrogenated oils, processed foods with these oils added, rancid oils, and hardened vegetable fats.

Use cold-processed oils. Use nitrogen-packed nuts. Increase consumption of foods high in good amino acids and potassium such as nuts, seeds, bananas, raisins, rice, wheat bran, kelp, dulse, brewer's yeast, and molasses. Drink plenty of filtered water. Avoid animal protein as well as raw or undercooked fish. Limit intake of fish. Strictly avoid alcohol.

Stressors on the liver: overeating, drugs of any kind, a highly processed diet, especially with processed fats, powders, additives, and foods high in animal protein, and accumulation of toxins from chemicals that have to be processed by the liver such as alcohol, drugs, the new aspirin substitute acetaminophen, insecticides, chemicals from rancid and processed oils, possibly toxins given off from colonies of candida organisms within the body, possibly contraceptives, and preservatives.

Nutritional Therapy: • Lipotrophic factors • Vitamin B complex • Vitamin B_{12} • Folic acid • Niacin (B_3—in small doses such as 10-30 mg. three times) • Liver glandulars • Vitamin C • Multidigestive enzymes with HCl and ox bile extract • Amino acids: L-methionine, L-carnitine, L-cysteine, L-glutathione, L-arginine

According to Jonathan Wright, M.D., anything that helps support the remaining liver function is very important. These include: vitamin C, vitamin E, silymarin, phylanthrus, lipoic acid, raw liver tablets.

With liver disease, do not use more than 10,000 IU of vitamin A daily and avoid cod liver oil entirely.

The liver is further stressed by a toxic bowel. Bowel cleanse and rejuvenation techniques may be very important. Eat whole foods diet for two weeks, then do bowel cleanse and follow with bowel rejuvenation. Repeat bowel cleanse once a month as needed and stay on bowel nutrients for up to one year depending on severity of condition and response to treatment.

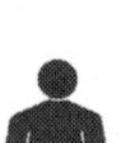

Self-Care

The following therapies can be undertaken at home under appropriate professional supervision.

• Fasting • Flower Remedies • Qigong

Aromatherapy: Juniper, rosemary, rose.

Ayurveda: An herbal mixture of: *kutki* 200 mg., *shanka pushpi* 500 mg., and *guduchi* 300 mg., one-quarter teaspoon of this mixture generally taken twice a day after lunch and dinner with aloe vera juice.

Herbs: Milk thistle may contribute to the treatment of cirrhosis as it helps liver cells regenerate. It may be taken in the form of tablets or the nonalcohol extract called a glycerate. The dose is based upon the content of silymarin (the active ingredient of milk thistle) and so standardized extracts are preferable. The dosage range is 70-200 mg. of silymarin daily. The actual dosage of tablet of extract this translates to will appear on the manufacturer's label. Another important herb is licorice.

Hydrotherapy: Constitutional hydrotherapy: if severe illness, apply two to seven times weekly. Contrast application or cold friction to stimulate liver function: apply daily.

Leon Chaitow, N.D., D.O., reports that the neutral bath (patient immersed in water of body temperature for two hours) has been effective in reducing excessive fluid retention in a patient suffering from cirrhosis of the liver.

Juice Therapy: • Beet and carrot juice • Wheat grass juice • Add raw flaxseed oil and garlic as tolerated.

Reflexology: Liver, pancreas, all glands.

Professional Care

The following therapies should only be provided by a qualified health professional.

• Cell Therapy • Colon Therapy • Magnetic Field Therapy • Naturopathic Medicine

Detoxification Therapy: Detoxification may be indicated, depending on the condition of the person. Stay off alcohol, chemicals, and fats.

Traditional Chinese Medicine: The Chinese herb bupleurum *(chai-hu)* may be helpful.

Cold Sores (Herpes Simplex)

Small fever blisters, often recurrent, found anywhere around the mouth, caused by the virus herpes simplex 1 (HSV1). Groupings of these blisters are called a cluster.

Symptoms: The first bout may be accompanied by flulike symptoms, with fever, neck ache, neck lymph node enlargement, and fatigue, or it may go unnoticed. After the first attack, the virus remains dormant in nerve cells, but can be reactivated by stress, colds, hot weather, anxiety, nutrient deficiencies, or other illnesses, especially ones with accompanying fever. Prolonged bouts may occur in people with immune suppression or in healthy people under large amounts of stress. Recurrent attacks start with a burning sensation that soon is followed by blisters that can be very sore and itch. Within a few days to several weeks they burst, dry, encrust, and disappear.

Occurrence: Ninety percent of people have this infection at least one time during their lives.

Consider: Herpes zoster, coxsackie virus, low thyroid, health problems depressing immune function.

Special Notes: These sores are very contagious. Oral sex can spread HSV1 from the mouth to the genitalia.

The drug acyclovir is prescribed orally and topically. However, it may cause an increase in symptoms on cessation of the drug. Also, antiviral drugs are very strong to be able to penetrate the well-protected viruses, so they are very hard on the body and especially the liver.

Alternative Treatments

Refer to alternative therapy chapters for more information before evaluating or applying any treatment. Some conditions, including yours, may require a physician's care.

Diet: Whole foods diet with more raw vegetables and cultured products such as yogurt and sauerkraut.

Nutritional Therapy: • L-lysine cream applied directly on blisters • Lysine (4 grams daily for first four days, then 500 mg. three times daily for two weeks): do not take daily on maintenance basis as it may create an imbalance among other amino acids, unless you have had your amino acid screen run and are working with a qualified practitioner. If continual daily lysine is the only way for you to prevent recurrent attacks, then decrease wheat and add other grains to diet and take lysine in small dosages with backup amino acid blends and consider amino acid testing. • Vitamin B complex • Zinc gluconate lozenges • Vitamin C with bioflavonoids • Thymus extract • Acidophilus • Vitamin E

According to Jonathan Wright, M.D., the two amino acids that appear to be important in herpes infections are lysine and arginine. Arginine induces the growth and reproduction of the herpes simplex virus, while lysine inhibits the virus. What's important is the ratio of arginine to lysine. The higher the arginine to lysine ratio, the more herpes virus is likely to grow. Conversely, if lysine is high with respect to arginine, the growth is inhibited. Chocolate, peanuts, most cereal grains, nuts, and seeds have more arginine than lysine.

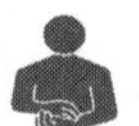

Self-Care

The following therapies can be undertaken at home under appropriate professional supervision.

• Biofeedback Training • Fasting • Guided Imagery

Aromatherapy: Geranium, lemon, chamomile, tea tree, lavender.

Herbs: Herbs that boost resistance and strengthen the immune response should be taken internally. Combine the tinctures of echinacea, Siberian ginseng, nettle, and goldenseal in equal parts and take one-half teaspoonful of this mixture three times a day. Externally apply dilute tincture of myrrh or calendula.

Hydrotherapy: Early stages: ice application. On ten minutes, off five minutes.

Juice Therapy: Avoid citrus, pineapple.

Topical Treatment: Vitamin E ointment or saturate gauze with vitamin E oil and hold on for fifteen minutes. A mixture of butylated hydroxytoluene (BHT) and alcohol applied topically can also be helpful.

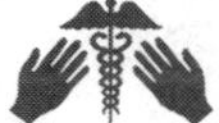

Professional Care

The following therapies should only be provided by a qualified health professional.

• Cell Therapy • Environmental Medicine • Homeopathy • Magnetic Field Therapy • Naturopathic Medicine • Orthomolecular Medicine • Traditional Chinese Medicine

Oxygen Therapy: • Hydrogen peroxide therapy (IV) • Ozone therapy inactivates herpes I and promotes skin healing.

Colds and Flu

See Colds and Flu chapter, page 632.

Colic

See Children's Health chapter, page 601.

Colitis

See Gastrointestinal Disorders chapter, page 684.

Conjunctivitis

See Vision Disorders chapter, page 860.

Constipation

See Constipation chapter, page 640.

Convulsions

(Seek medical attention promptly. See Epilepsy.)

A variety of nonvoluntary contractions (single or series) of the voluntary muscles, from mild to severe, due to sudden uncontrolled changes in the electrical activity of the brain.

Symptoms: May be mild, only slight muscle twitches and tingling, all the way to violent, jerking whole body movements, sometimes associated with intense feelings of fear, familiarity, possible hallucinations, and sometimes a lapse of consciousness, which is then called grand mal seizure. Seizures that reoccur are called epilepsy.

Special Notes: Convulsions or seizures may be caused by many medical problems such as: stroke, brain tumor, withdrawal from alcohol and drugs, metabolic disturbances, neurological disorders, and trauma from head injury. A febrile seizure or twitching, jerking convulsion associated with loss of consciousness in a child with a rapidly rising fever (often due to infections such as middle ear or tonsillitis), are common in children between six months and five years old, and tend to run in the same families. They are usually not serious, even though they are frightening, and occur in one out of twenty children.

Alternative Treatments

Refer to alternative therapy chapters for more information before evaluating or applying any treatment. Some conditions, including yours, may require a physician's care.

Diet: According to Melvyn Werbach, M.D., epileptics should have normal, well-balanced meals at regular intervals and children should not be allowed to take large meals as these predispose toward seizures.

Alcohol is totally contraindicated as is caffeine (cola drinks, coffee, tea, chocolate).

Aspartame (NutraSweet) has been implicated in some cases of seizure.

Nutritional Therapy: • Taurine • Magnesium • Vitamin B_6 • Manganese • Have an amino acid blood screen. Working with a qualified practitioner is important.

Supplementation with amino acids taurine, dimethyl glycine, and/or DL-glutamic acid have been shown to beneficial.

There are multiple nutritional deficiencies associated with seizures, including folic acid, niacin (vitamin B_3), thiamine (vitamin B_1), vitamin B_6, vitamin D, copper, magnesium, manganese, and selenium. Some of these deficiencies may relate to anticonvulsant medication, while others may be related to the cause of the seizures.

Any supplementation should be with the awareness of the medical practitioner responsible for the care of the individual.

Omega-6 fatty acid supplementation may trigger or exacerbate temporal lobe epilepsy.

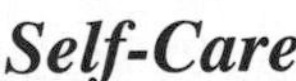

Self-Care

The following therapies can be undertaken at home under appropriate professional supervision.

• Guided Imagery

Acupressure: A hospital study in Germany[8] found that when a seizure (fit) occurred, and while nurses were preparing medication for injection, in almost all cases (over one hundred were evaluated) very firm stimulation of the center of the nasal philtrum (the depression above the upper lip below the center of the nose) using the nail of the thumb, caused consciousness to be restored in an average of under thirty seconds. This was long before the medication was ready for use (and therefore making its use unnecessary).

This point is governor vessel point 26 in Traditional Chinese Medicine. The only cases in which it failed to work were where the child was still partially conscious and the stimulation was therefore unacceptable causing the child to wriggle thus preventing sustained contact on the point. The only side effect noted was slight bruising of the lip area. No comparable study has been done on adults.

Aromatherapy: Chamomile, clary sage, lavender, neroli.

Herbs: Asafetida, mugwort, skullcap, valerian root.

Hydrotherapy: Constitutional hydrotherapy: apply two to five times weekly.

Homeopathy: *Cuprum met., Belladonna, Cicuta.*

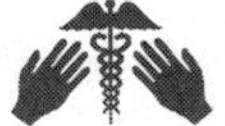

Professional Care

The following therapies should only be provided by a qualified health professional.

• Chiropractic • Environmental Medicine • Fasting • Light Therapy • Magnetic Field Therapy • Naturopathic Medicine • Osteopathy • Traditional Chinese Medicine

Detoxification Therapy: *Not* indicated unless the condition is due to specific toxicity.

Corns

A painful, hardened, cone-shaped area of increased growth of the corneous layer of the skin, found mainly over the toe joints and between the toes on the foot.

Symptoms: Mostly pea-sized or slightly larger hardened areas on the feet, occurring where bony protuberances occur. Corns may only hurt in response to pressure or may hurt spontaneously.

Consider: Calluses, warts, localized injury and inflammation, infection, or poor circulation. Corns, when pared away with a sharp instrument, have a clearly outlined translucent core.

Special Notes: The harder corns are called "hard" corns and occur mainly on the toes, while the "soft" corns occur mainly between the toes.

Prevention is the most important cure, and this is accomplished by eliminating undue pressure at certain sites of the foot. Thus, assessment by a podiatrist, osteopath, or chiropractor who can evaluate foot gait, the role of other joints such as pelvis in foot pressure problems, shoes, and need for orthotics, pad, mole-skins, etc., is very important in prevention as well as treatment.

Treatment also involves better fitting shoes. Corns do disappear when the inappropriate pressure is eliminated. Podiatrists can "pare" the corn away but the cause still needs to be assessed. Patients with recurring corns and calluses need ongoing treatment by a podiatrist.

Patients with poor circulation from serious diseases such as diabetes mellitus require special and regular care.

Alternative Treatments

Refer to alternative therapy chapters for more information before evaluating or applying any treatment. Some conditions, including yours, may require a physician's care.

Diet: A whole foods diet is recommended.

Nutritional Therapy: • Vitamin A and Vitamin E topically and orally • Essential fatty acids

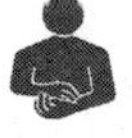

Self-Care

The following therapies can be undertaken at home under appropriate professional supervision.

Aromatherapy: Lemon, verucas.

Herbs: Apply a salve made from calendula petals two to three times a day. This will soon soften the tissue and acts as an anti-inflammatory.

Homeopathy: *Graphites, Silicea, Antim crud.*

Hydrotherapy: • Contrast application: apply daily. • Hot Epsom salts foot bath • Hot foot bath and then rub corns with fresh lemon juice

Reflexology: Around and directly on them.

Topical Treatment: • Aloe vera gel • Rub castor oil on corn twice daily.

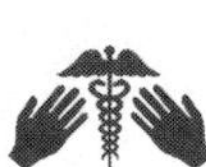

Professional Care

The following therapies should only be provided by a qualified health professional.

• Magnetic Field Therapy • Naturopathic Medicine

Coughs

Sudden, explosive expulsion of air from the lungs, usually in order to expel something from the air passages. Usually accompanied by a sound.

Productive coughing brings up mucous (referred to as sputum or phlegm) and an unproductive, dry cough does not.

Symptoms: Different cough sound characteristics may signal different problems. (A qualified practitioner should be able to evaluate.)

Examples: Constant, severe coughing with thick mucous production may signal chronic bronchitis (bronchitis often associated with smoking or passive smoke exposure). A very dry cough with profound symptoms of fever and fatigue may signal an approaching severe bout of acute bronchitis. Viral bronchitis usually has a persistent cough that disturbs sleep. Dry coughs that are usually worse at night may signal bronchospasm (temporary narrowing of the bronchi, larger tubes of airways) that can be associated with asthma, infection, or allergies. Allergic coughs may occur along with running nose, wheezing, or begin after certain foods are consumed or at different times of the year. Coughing associated with changes of posture suggest lung abscess or other severe diseases. Coughs associated with eating may suggest serious swallowing or trachea problems. Coughs due to exercise or cold air may signal asthma. In young children with inflammation of the respiratory tract, the airways can narrow so much that the cough sound produces a huge noise called the croup. Persistent short, mild, dry coughs in the spring may signal hay fever. Rattles of secretions associated with a dry, barking cough may signal an infection of the trachea. Pneumonia (lung inflammation secondary to infection) usually has painful coughing associated with flecks of blood. Cancers of the airways may produce a mild cough at first that gets worse and then produces mucous that is blood flecked. Some coughing is a nervous manifestation, especially in children.

Sputum (expectorated matter) produced with the cough signals the following: changes (white to yellowish, green, or brown) mean that an infection is involved; blood streaking means infection is getting worse, must definitely see a doctor; gritty material in sputum may mean a serious condition of the lungs called broncholithiasis—inflammation or obstruction caused by calculi (stone, usually formed by mineral salts) in the bronchi. Cough sputum up for observation by a practitioner.

Consider: Coughing may be due to a simple illness like upper respiratory illness or the common cold, or may signal a more serious illness, such as cancer. May also be due to irritation from environment (smoke, dust, pollens), mucous dripping in back of the throat, a sign of nervousness, or a symptom of an underlying health disorder.

Special Notes: Important questions about coughing: How long? Did it come on suddenly? Has it changed recently? What factors make it worse? What time of day? Is the cough associated with production of mucous? What color is the mucous? Are there any other pains or symptoms? Is the cough association with work or exercise?

Treatment of the cough depends entirely on the underlying cause.

Coughing up blood (hemoptysis): Blood comes up in sputum due to rupturing of blood vessels in airways, lungs, nose, or throat secondary to causes that may be mild or serious and need to be evaluated. May appear as bright red or rusty-brown streaks, pinkish froth, or bright red pure blood. Need chest x-ray. If x-rays show abnormalities, if person is over forty, a smoker, or has coughed up blood before, may need bronchoscopy, a procedure that allows direct viewing of the lungs by insertion of a soft, flexible tube. One-third of people undergoing this procedure are found to have no underlying serious problem.

Alternative Treatments

Refer to alternative therapy chapters for more information before evaluating or applying any treatment. Some conditions, including yours, may require a physician's care.

Diet: • Eat whole foods including lots of raw fruits and vegetables. • With mucous: avoid sugar, salty foods, dairy products, starches. • Dry cough: *umeiboshi* plum paste

According to George Sarantakos, Ph.D., a cough syrup can be made from eight ounces of warm pineapple juice and two teaspoons honey. The bromelain in the pineapple juice is activated by the honey.

Cough medicine to keep on hand: Mix juice of one lemon with two tablespoons glycerine, then add twelve teaspoons honey and stir. Stir before each use. Take one teaspoon every half hour, reducing as needed. (Do not refrigerate.)

Nutritional Therapy: • Zinc lozenges

• Vitamin A • Folic acid • Vitamin C and bioflavonoids • Vitamin E

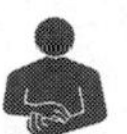

Self-Care

The following therapies can be undertaken at home under appropriate professional supervision.

• Fasting • Guided Imagery • Yoga

Aromatherapy: Steam with thyme, benzoin, eucalyptus, frankincense, peppermint, sandalwood, chamomile, juniper. Also try myrrh.

Ayurveda: • Take equal parts lemon juice and honey in teaspoon doses. • *Cough with mucous:* make a tea of one-half teaspoon ginger powder, a pinch of clove, and a pinch of cinnamon powder in one cup of water. • *Gargle:* add one pinch of salt and two pinches of tumeric powder to glass of water.

For chronic coughs: a confection of one part sesame seeds (black seeds if possible), one-half part *shatavari*. Add ginger and raw sugar to taste and take one ounce daily. • An herbal mixture of: *sitopaladi* 500 mg., *yasti madhu* 300 mg., *punarnava* 300 mg., *kant kari* 200 mg., and *vasaka* 300 mg., one-quarter teaspoon of this mixture generally taken twice a day after lunch and dinner.

Herbs: A cough is an important diagnostic signal from the body, and should not be simply suppressed. Any long-standing or intransigent coughing should receive professional attention. Home treatment is safe and effective for minor coughs of short duration or associated with mild infections, but if in doubt seek skilled advice. Coltsfoot and mullein have been found to be safe and effective for children and adults. Use as an infusion at least three times a day while the symptoms remain. For a dry irritating cough use an infusion of marshmallow leaves. Mullein and horehound are appropriate for adult coughs. There are many effective kitchen remedies for coughs. Slice an onion into a deep bowl and cover in honey, let stand overnight. Strain the mixture of juice and honey. This makes a simple cough elixir. Take a dessertspoonful four or five times a day.

Homeopathy: *For dry coughs:* • *Belladonna, Aconite, Drosera, Bryonia, Phosphorus.* • *Hyoscyamus, rumex*, and *spongia* must be taken alone, not in combination with other remedies. *For loose coughs: Ipecac, Merc sol., Pulsatilla, Kali bich., Kali carb.*

Hydrotherapy: • Hot pack: apply to chest as needed to aid in expectoration. • Benzoin steam inhalation

Juice Therapy: • Fresh fruit and vegetable juices • Hot pear juice with cinnamon stick, can add cardamon, cumin to juices.

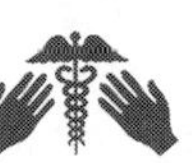

Professional Care

The following therapies should only be provided by a qualified health professional.

• Applied Kinesiology • Chiropractic • Colon Therapy • Environmental Medicine • Magnetic Field Therapy • Naturopathic Medicine • Neural Therapy • Osteopathy • Traditional Chinese Medicine

Bodywork: Acupressure, reflexology, *shiatsu*.

Detoxification Therapy: Detoxification may be helpful, depending on the condition of the person. (If due to infection—maybe; if due to allergies—yes.)

Oxygen Therapy: Hydrogen peroxide therapy (IV)

Cuts

Breaking of skin that causes bleeding and may be mild or severe. The more severe it is, the more underlying tissues may be involved, the longer it may take to heal, and may require therapeutic stitching to assist in the healing.

Alternative Treatments

Refer to alternative therapy chapters for more information before evaluating or applying any treatment. Some conditions, including yours, may require a physician's care.

Nutritional Therapy: • *If mild:* after cleaning, cover with mixture of zinc oxide cream and vitamin E oil. When healing has begun, and signs of inflammation, infection, and redness are gone, use topical aloe vera. • *If the laceration is severe, and thus referred to as a wound:* apply pressure until the bleeding stops. Keep covered with a bandage that creates some pressure. Ascertain if stitches are necessary (outside help such as sutures will be needed to stop bleeding and keep structures together for healing). If stitches are necessary, go immediately to an emergency room. If stitches are not necessary, may treat as mentioned above. • Vitamin C • Zinc • Vitamin A • Pantothenic acid

Problems with healing: increase vitamin C (three to six times daily), add proteolytic enzymes (three to four times daily, on empty stomach, until healing gets well underway).

The amino acid arginine improves both the speed and quality of wound healing (it stimulates production by the body of growth hormone which is involved in any new tissue growth).

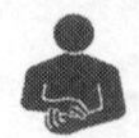

Self-Care

The following therapies can be undertaken at home under appropriate professional supervision.

• *Guided Imagery*

Ayurveda: For minor cuts: aloe vera gel with tumeric applied locally, or *tikta ghee.*

Fasting: If infection is a component, fasting may be beneficial.

Herbs: Clean the cut and then apply comfrey leaf as an ointment or compress. Do not use comfrey for puncture wounds as the skin will heal before the deeper tissue. An alternative is calendula.

Homeopathy: *Calendula, Hepar sulph., Ledum, Hypericum, Arnica* ointment.

Hydrotherapy: Ice pack: apply to the arterial trunk that supplies the area.

Topical Treatment: Green clay, found in health food stores, is very effective for healing when made into a paste and applied topically to cuts.

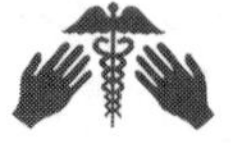

Professional Care

The following therapies should only be provided by a qualified health professional.

• *Acupuncture* • *Naturopathic Medicine*

Oxygen Therapy: Hyperbaric oxygen therapy for accelerated wound healing.

Cystitis (Bladder Infection)

See Female Health chapter, page 669.

Dandruff

A common scalp condition in which the dead skin is shed producing irritating white flakes. Dandruff frequently accompanies scalp disease and is a primary cause of baldness and general hair loss. Its character is that of a unspecified seborrheal dermatitis, a mild scalp inflammation with excessive fatty secretions, and is frequently due to digestive disturbances. It is highly dependent on the general health of the whole body.

Symptoms: White flakes appear on the hair and fall onto the shoulders and clothes. There may be itching, scaling, and redness of the scalp, and may also occur on other skin surfaces such as the face, chest, and back. Yellow crusting may appear. It does not cause the hair to fall out.

Special Notes: The most common cause of dandruff is seborrheic dermatitis. This is a skin condition that usually starts as dry or greasy scaling of the skin but may progress to yellow-red scaling bumps along hairline, behind the ears, in the ear canals, on the eyebrows, on the bridge of the nose, in the folds around the nose or on the breastbone. Don't pick or scratch scalp.

When infants get this it is called cradle cap. According to Leon Chaitow, N.D., D.O., cradle cap is a yeast problem and many skin experts in Europe find that dandruff in adults is also a yeast problem. The problem should then be treated as for candidiasis.

Alternative Treatments

Refer to alternative therapy chapters for more information before evaluating or applying any treatment. Some conditions, including yours, may require a physician's care.

Diet: Increase raw foods within whole foods diet. Eat more salads and green vegetables. Avoid fried foods. Reduce intake of fats, sugar, dairy products, chocolate, seafood, nuts.

Nutritional Therapy: • Vitamin B_6 • Vitamin A • Vitamin B complex • Essential fatty acids (omega-6) • Vitamin C • Vitamin E • Beta-carotene • Kelp tablets • Zinc

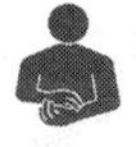

Self-Care

The following therapies can be undertaken at home under appropriate professional supervision.

• *Fasting*

Aromatherapy: Patchouli, rosemary, tea tree.

Herbs: Rinse the hair and scalp with a strong infusion of nettle, sage, and rosemary. Drink a cup of nettle tea and take three oil of Evening Primrose capsules daily.

Homeopathy: *Arsen alb., Graphites, Lycopodium, Thuja, Sepia, Sulfur, Cantharis.*

Hydrotherapy: Contrast application: apply daily to scalp (contrast shower).

Topical Treatment: • Pour warm apple cider vinegar over head and wrap head in a towel. After one hour, wash hair. • Apply vitamin E oil to scalp nightly for three weeks.

According to Dr. Chaitow, selenium-based shampoos are effective because the selenium acts as an antifungal agent. Massage cold-pressed linseed oil into the scalp at night and wash it off in the morning. (Use an old pillowcase.) This is often successful in restoring scalp health.

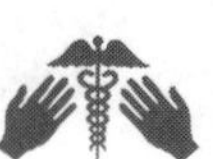

Professional Care

The following therapies should only be provided by a qualified health professional.

• *Environmental Medicine* • *Magnetic Field Therapy* • *Naturopathic Medicine* • *Traditional Chinese Medicine*

Detoxification Therapy: May be indicated, depending on the condition of the person.

Dermatitis

A variety of inflammations of the most superficial portion of the skin, most frequently caused by allergies (food allergies, contact allergies: from substances such as makeup, metal from jewelry [especially nickel], perfumes, creams, or toxic plant allergies such as poison ivy or poison oak). (Many medical sources use the terms dermatitis and eczema interchangeably.)

Symptoms: Itching, flaking, color oozing, crusting, scaling, and thickening of the skin.

Special Notes: If allergic cause is not removed, and/or there is much scratching, the dermatitis may spread and become very severe.

There are many types of dermatitis:

Contact dermatitis: Inflammation produced by substances that touch the skin from direct irritants, to allergic substances, to exposure to light.

Atopic dermatitis: A severe, chronic, itching and inflammation of the skin in individuals with a family history of allergic disorders such as asthma, hay fever, and milk allergies.

Seborrheic dermatitis: Inflammation of skin usually on scalp, face, and, rarely, on sternum (breastbone).

Nummular dermatitis: Coin-shaped red bumps that severely itch seen in middle-age people under stress and more often in the winter.

There can also be chronic dermatitis of the hands and feet, and a generalized dermatitis that affects wide areas of the skin with extreme scaling.

Alternative Treatments

Refer to alternative therapy chapters for more information before evaluating or applying any treatment. Some conditions, including yours, may require a physician's care.

Diet: Identify and avoid food allergies and other allergic substances. Try a gluten-free diet. No wheat, oats, rye, barley.

According to Leon Chaitow, N.D., D.O., in Europe the most likely allergy would be dairy foods, especially cow's milk as many studies have shown this to be the likeliest culprit food, followed by wheat.

Lots of yogurt, sauerkraut, and naturally fermented foods.

Nutritional Therapy: • Vitamin B_6 • Vitamin B complex • Evening Primrose oil or omega-6 fatty acids from other sources • Acidophilus • Zinc • Magnesium • Assess need for digestive enzymes or gastrointestinal problems such as parasites.

Self-Care

The following therapies can be undertaken at home under appropriate professional supervision.

• *Fasting* • *Flower Remedies* • *Hypnotherapy* • *Reflexology* • *Relaxation* • *Yoga*

Aromatherapy: Benzoin, chamomile, lavender, bergamot, geranium.

Herbs: Combine the tinctures of nettle, red clover, and cleavers in equal parts and take one-half teaspoonful of this mixture three times a day. Drink an infusion of fresh nettle or cleavers twice a day. To alleviate itching bathe the area with lukewarm or cold chickweed infusion. For cracked, dry, or painful skin use a salve made from calendula flowers and St. John's Wort leaves.

Homeopathy: *Pulsatilla, Arsen alb., Lycopodium, Graphites, Petroleum, Sulfur, Thuja, Sepia.*

Hydrotherapy: Cold compress: apply as needed to control pain and/or itching.

Juice Therapy: • Carrot, beet, cucumber, celery • Carrot, celery, apple • Cantaloupe

Topical Treatment: • Aloe vera gel • Pyridoxine ointment • For itching: mix vitamin E, vitamin A, unflavored yogurt, a little honey and zinc oxide, and place onto skin. • Evening Primrose oil applied directly to cracks and sore areas of the skin (folds such as elbows and behind the knee for example) can be very helpful in promoting healing.

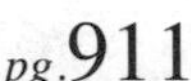

Professional Care

The following therapies should only be provided by a qualified health professional.

• *Acupuncture* • *Cell Therapy* • *Environmental Medicine* • *Magnetic Field Therapy* • *Naturopathic Medicine* • *Osteopathy*

Detoxification Therapy: May be indicated, depending on the condition of the person.

Oxygen Therapy: Hydrogen peroxide therapy (IV)

Diabetes

See Diabetes chapter, page 647.

Diarrhea

See Gastrointestinal Disorders chapter, page 687.

Diverticulitis

See Gastrointestinal Disorders chapter, page 686.

Dizziness

Can be very mild: defined as dizziness, a short-lived sensation of faintness, unsteadiness with lightheadedness. May be more severe: defined as vertigo, either as subjective vertigo (individual has impression he or she is spinning in the room) or objective vertigo (impression that objects are spinning around the individual). True vertigo has to do with a problem somewhere within the equilibratory system: middle ear, eighth (acoustic nerve) cranial nerve, the brain (brain stem), or the eyes. Unlike dizziness, vertigo is usually associated with nausea, vomiting, and severe sweating.

Consider: True vertigo is never a sign of anxiety, but lightheadedness, giddiness, and fear of losing one's balance; may be a sign of depression or anxiety.

Special Notes: True "dizziness" is usually caused by a sudden drop of blood pressure in the brain from standing up too quickly from lying or sitting down (postural hypotension), fatigue, stress, low blood sugar (hypoglycemia), temporary blockage of blood to the brain as in a transient ischemic attack, low blood oxygenation (anemia), low blood iron, and certain drugs. Vertigo is mainly caused by labyrinthitis (usually viral infection of fluid filled canals of inner ear) and Meniere's disease, a disease characterized by bouts of severe nausea, vomiting, ringing in the ears (tinnitus), hearing loss, and vertigo that can persist for days and weeks.

With any dizziness, first take a few deep breaths and sit down to rest. Severe or prolonged dizziness needs to be evaluated by an exam and blood tests.

According to Leon Chaitow, N.D., D.O., when dizziness comes on when standing up after sitting or lying it can be an indication of adrenal exhaustion. The individual should take action to restore adrenal health by stopping use of stimulants (caffeine, tobacco, alcohol) and via rest and normalization of lifestyle and nutritional balance. When you feel this sensation upon standing it helps if you can immediately squat down or cross your legs strongly pressing them against each other, as this forces circulation back up from the lower body/limbs to the trunk and head.

Alternative Treatments

Refer to alternative therapy chapters for more information before evaluating or applying any treatment. Some conditions, including yours, may require a physician's care.

Diet: Whole foods diet. *If hypoglycemic:* eat smaller meals throughout the day and restrict refined sugars, caffeinated beverages, and alcohol. *If anemic:* consume green drinks, more chicken, and dark green vegetables, and raw seeds.

Nutritional Therapy: • Vitamin B complex • Niacin (B_3) • Vitamin E • Iron

Specific nutritional support (adrenal exhaustion) involves supplementation with vitamin C (3-5 grams daily) and vitamin B_5 (500-1000 mg. daily of pantothenic acid/calcium pantothenate).

Self-Care

The following therapies can be undertaken at home under appropriate professional supervision.

• Fasting • Guided Imagery

Acupressure: To relieve dizziness, firmly press GV26 (for an illustration of this point number please see the acupressure chart on page 874) two-thirds of the way up from the upper lip to the nose using your index fingertip. Press deeply, applying firm pressure into the center of your upper gum for one minute.

Bodywork: Acupressure, *shiatsu*, massage, Alexander technique.

Herbs: Ginger, ginkgo leaf extract.

Homeopathy: *Gelsemium, Phosphorus, Cocculus, Convallaria, Granatum.*

Hydrotherapy: Hot foot bath.

Reflexology: Side of neck, ear reflex, cervicals.

Professional Care

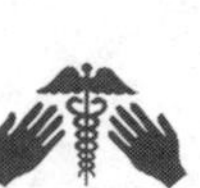

The following therapies should only be provided by a qualified health professional.

• Cell Therapy • Chiropractic • Craniosacral Therapy • Environmental Medicine • Hypnotherapy • Magnetic Field Therapy • Naturopathic Medicine • Osteopathy

• ***Traditional Chinese Medicine***

Biological Dentistry: Check for mercury toxicity from amalgams.

Detoxification Therapy: If allergies are present, detoxification is possibly helpful.

Oxygen Therapy: Hydrogen peroxide therapy (IV)

Dysentery

(Amoebiasis—See Parasites.)

An infection of the intestines, caused by either a group of bacteria called shigella (thus, dysentery is called shigellosis) or by protozoan (single-celled) parasites called Entamoeba (this dysentery is called amebic dysentery).

Symptoms: *Shigellosis:* Sudden diarrhea that is very watery, and sometimes bacterial contamination of the blood (toxemia) occurs. In severe cases, shigellosis may lead to bacteremic shock or cardiovascular collapse. *Amebic dysentery:* More gradual development of diarrhea. Diarrhea can become mixed with blood, pus, and mucous, and much straining and sitting on toilet may result in very little blood-stained watery mucous. Dehydration may occur and fluids must be replenished in the body. Possible complications of amebic dysentery include amebic cysts in liver brain and other important organs.

Special Notes: If you are suffering from shigella or *Entamoeba histolytica* you should seek medical help. Antibiotics may be necessary.

Alternative Treatments

Refer to alternative therapy chapters for more information before evaluating or applying any treatment. Some conditions, including yours, may require a physician's care.

Diet: Clove of garlic morning and evening followed by hot tea with lemon (unsugared). Lots of unflavored yogurt. Avoid refined sugars and alcohol during and for week after episode.

Nutritional Therapy: During and several weeks after episode: • Acidophilus • Bifidobacteria and *Lactobacillus bulgaricus* • Vitamin A • Citrus seed extract

Self-Care

The following therapies can be undertaken at home under appropriate professional supervision.

• ***Fasting*** • ***Yoga***

Aromatherapy: Chamomile, black pepper, cypress, eucalyptus, lemon, melissa.

Herbs: Use a decoction of oak bark to reduce the diarrhea and fluid loss. Drink an infusion of meadowsweet and chamomile to ease abdominal discomfort. Eat a clove of raw garlic morning and evening. Take electrolyte replacement if needed, made by dissolving one teaspoon of salt and four teaspoon of sugar (which helps intestines absorb both) in one quart of water. Be accurate with salt or may create more dehydration.

Hydrotherapy: Constitutional hydrotherapy unless otherwise indicated: apply two to five times weekly.

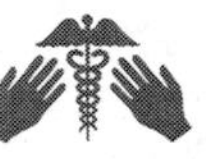

Professional Care

The following therapies should only be provided by a qualified health professional.

• ***Applied Kinesiology*** • ***Colon Therapy*** • ***Magnetic Field Therapy*** • ***Naturopathic Medicine*** • ***Osteopathy (Except Amebic Dysentery)*** • ***Traditional Chinese Medicine***

Dysmenorrhea (Menstrual Cramps)

See Female Health chapter, page 660.

Ear Pain, Ear Infections (Otitis Media)

See Hearing and Ear Disorders chapter, page 701.

Eczema

Inflammation of the skin, usually associated with blisters, red bumps, swelling, oozing, scaling, crusting, and itching. Eczema is often called dermatitis.

Consider: There are different types of eczema depending on their causes and where they occur on the body. Eczema can be due to allergies, allergies secondary to digestive disorders such as hydrochloric acid deficiency, rashes secondary to immune diseases, genetic metabolic disorders, or nutritional deficiencies such as vitamin B [especially niacin (vitamin B_3) and B_6].

Special Notes: There are various types of eczema. *Contact eczema or dermatitis:* Sharp demarcations where substance contact skin and create rash (may be direct irritants, allergic substances, from exposure to light or certain chemicals or perfumes). *Atopic dermatitis or eczema:* Occurs in people with family histories of allergy, vitamin B_{12} problems, asthma, and allergic respiratory problems such as hay fever. Infants, two to eighteen months: weeping, crusty, red spots on face, scalp, and extremities or in older children and adults it may be more localized and chronic. May subside by three to four years and may reoccur in adolescence or adulthood.

Seborrheic dermatitis or eczema: Of scalp, face, and chest.

Nummular dermatitis or eczema: Coin-shaped chronic red spots with crusting and scaling. Normally occurs after thirty-five years of age and often associated with emotional stress and in winter with dry skin.

Chronic eczema: Of hands or feet which can get very severe.

Generalized eczema: That is widespread over much of the skin.

Stasis eczema: In lower legs associated with poor venous return of the blood and tendency toward skin to turn brownish.

Localized scratch dermatitis or eczema: Occurring in specific patches often with whitish areas well demarcated by areas of increased pigmentation or color, such as arms, legs, ankles, around the genitals, and made worse by stress and scratching. Much more frequent in women between twenty and fifty years.

Avoid irritating substances, wear natural nonirritating materials, use soothing ointments, and assess if diet, nutrients, and allergic components need to be considered.

Alternative Treatments

Refer to alternative therapy chapters for more information before evaluating or applying any treatment. Some conditions, including yours, may require a physician's care.

Diet: Whole foods diet with identification and avoidance of allergic foods especially wheat and cow's milk products. Lemon juice mixed with equal part olive or almond oil applied externally and taken internally. Excess consumption of fruit, especially citrus and sour, may aggravate symptoms.

Eczema may be a symptom of an omega-3 fatty acid deficiency.

If there is a family history of asthma, hay fever, and food allergies, it may be helpful to delay solid food introduction to infants as preventative measure. A ten-year study in New Zealand involving 1,265 children showed that children who were introduced to four or more types of solid foods before the age of four months were 2.9 times more likely to develop recurrent eczema than children not exposed to early solid feeding.[9]

Nutritional Therapy: • Zinc • Essential fatty acids (sometimes containing GLA) • Vitamin E • Vitamin A • Vitamin B complex • Vitamin B_6 • Magnesium

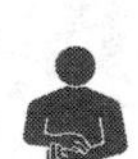

Self-Care

The following therapies can be undertaken at home under appropriate professional supervision.

• Fasting • Flower Remedies • Yoga

Aromatherapy: Bergamot, chamomile, lavender, melissa, neroli, eucalyptus, geranium, juniper.

Ayurveda: An herbal mixture of: *kutki* 200 mg., *manjista* 300 mg., *tumeric* 200 mg. and *neem* 200 mg., one teaspoon of this mixture generally taken twice a day after lunch and dinner. Externally apply *neem* oil. Do not eat salt, sugar, or yogurt.

Bodywork: Acupressure, *shiatsu*, reflexology.

Herbs: Eczema is best treated internally, as the cause is usually a constitutional one. Alternative remedies such as cleavers, nettle, yellowdock, or red clover may be very effective. They are often combined with relaxing herbs such as chamomile, linden flowers, or skullcap. One combination would be equal parts of cleavers, nettle, and chamomile drunk as an infusion three times a day. A stronger mixture combines the tinctures of figwort, burdock, and cleavers in equal parts. Take one teaspoonful of this mixture three times a day. To alleviate itching bathe the area with lukewarm or cold chickweed infusion. For cracked, dry, or painful skin use a salve made from calendula flowers and St. John's Wort leaves. Goldenseal applied externally may be helpful.

Homeopathy: • *Dulcamara, Rhus tox., Sulfur, Arsen alb., Graphites* • *Petroleum* and *Psorinum* must be taken alone, not in combination with other remedies.

Hydrotherapy: Heating compress: apply one time daily.

Juice Therapy: • Black currant, red grapes • Carrot, beet, spinach, cucumber, parsley • Green juices • Wheat grass

Naturopathic Medicine: While not a cure, applying zinc oxide locally often helps relieve the severe itchiness of eczema.

Reflexology: Diaphragm, liver, kidneys, intestines, adrenals, all glands, thyroid.

Mind/Body Therapy: Biofeedback, guided imagery, relaxation.

Topical Treatment: Evening Primrose oil applied directly to cracks and sore areas of the skin (folds such as elbows and behind the knee for example) may be very helpful in promoting healing.

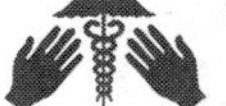

Professional Care

The following therapies should only be provided by a qualified health professional.

• Acupuncture • Environmental Medicine • Hypnotherapy • Magnetic Field Therapy • Naturopathic Medicine • Orthomolecular Medicine • Osteopathy

Detoxification Therapy: Detoxification is indicated unless the person is weakened or deficient.

Oxygen Therapy: Hydrogen peroxide therapy (IV)

Edema

Abnormal amounts of excessive fluid (commonly water and sodium), usually in subcutaneous spaces (intercellular spaces, between the cells) in the body.

Symptoms: Bloating and swelling of face, fingers, hands, legs, and in later stages, the abdomen. May be very slight, causing rings on fingers to feel tight or face to feel puffy, or may be severe enough to cause stretching and shininess of skin and overall weight gain. If fluid accumulation creates such stretching and bagginess of the skin that pressure into it creates a "pit," called pitting edema, a doctor should be consulted immediately as this may be a sign of a very serious problem.

Consider: Allergies, poor kidney excretion or secondary to problems with protein absorption, vitamin B deficiencies, or heart failure, liver, and kidney disorders.

Special Notes: Usually seen in extremities but may even occur in very slight amounts in the brain associated with allergies that cause the brain to swell and manifest as headaches, memory problems, learning disorders, or behavioral changes. Flying in airplanes, traveling to new climates, or stress can aggravate symptoms.

Small amounts of fluid buildup can occur anywhere in the body such as in the spine (causing low back pain) in the lungs (mimicking asthma/bronchitis), in the knees (mimicking arthritis), and should be a consideration in a wide variety of health problems that do not respond to the "normal" treatments.

Alternative Treatments

Refer to alternative therapy chapters for more information before evaluating or applying any treatment. Some conditions, including yours, may require a physician's care.

Diet: Whole foods diet with avoidance of foods that tend to worsen edema: caffeine, alcohol, salt, fried foods, cow's milk products, animal protein, sugar, white flour, chocolate, olives, pickles, tobacco, and soy sauce. Eating a diet of mainly processed grains and rice may lead to a vitamin B deficiency that may aggravate edema. Thus, focus on whole grains and watery vegetables such as cucumbers, apples, potatoes (whole or in soups), grapes, beets, onions, cabbage, and citrus.

Nutritional Therapy: • Vitamin B complex • Vitamin B_6 • Protein supplement (free-form amino acids) • Potassium • Vitamin C • Pantothenic acid • Alfalfa tablets

Potassium may be used with any herbal diuretic especially when taken with cornsilk tea.

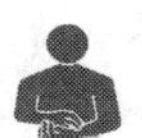

Self-Care

The following therapies can be undertaken at home under appropriate professional supervision.

• Fasting • Qigong

Aromatherapy: Juniper, rosemary, geranium, fennel.

Ayurveda: *For chronic condition:* Include diuretic foods in diet such as celery, carrot, parsley, cilantro, cranberries, pomegranate, corn, barley, rye, and adzuki beans. *Punarnava guggulu* 200 mg., generally taken twice a day after lunch and dinner.

Herbs: Competent diagnosis of the cause of water retention is essential, but diuretic herbs will address the symptom. One effective diuretic herb is dandelion leaf, also a rich source of potassium. Stimulating kidney function can remove potassium from the body, impacting a range of functions but most crucial is electrolyte balance in the heart muscle. If the diuretic is treating edema associated with congestive heart failure, any reduction in potassium will aggravate the heart symptoms. Dandelion replaces all the potassium that is flushed from the body via diuresis. Take one teaspoonful of the tincture three times a day, or an infusion of the fresh leaves three to five times a day.

Hydrotherapy: Contrast application: apply daily, repeat hot/cold, change six to eight times during treatment.

Juice Therapy: • Pears, pineapple, watermelon, cranberries • Green juices (you can add a bit of dandelion juice) • Cucumber, parsley, celery, carrot

Reflexology: Lymph system, kidneys, adrenals.

Professional Care

The following therapies should only be provided by a qualified health professional.

• Chiropractic • Craniosacral Therapy • Environmental Medicine • Magnetic Field Therapy • Naturopathic Medicine • Osteopathy • Traditional Chinese Medicine

Bodywork: Acupressure, reflexology, *shiatsu*, massage.

Detoxification Therapy: Depending on the condition of the person.

Hydrotherapy: Leon Chaitow, N.D., D.O., reports that the neutral bath (patient immersed in water at body temperature for two hours) has been effective in moving fluid from swollen tissues in cases of mild heart failure problems, swollen joints of rheumatoid patients, and fluid retention from cirrhosis of the liver.

Oxygen Therapy: Hyperbaric oxygen therapy.

Emphysema

See Respiratory Conditions chapter, page 816.

Environmental Allergies

See Allergies chapter, page 510.

Epilepsy

Recurrent episodes of disturbances in brain electrical activity that manifest as sudden brief attacks of altered consciousness, sometimes loss of consciousness, involuntary and abnormal motor function and sensation, alterations of the nervous system.

Consider: Nutrient deficiencies, thyroid disorders, stress management strategies.

Special Notes: The most common form of epilepsy is convulsive, in which the attack starts with loss of consciousness and motor control, and then the individual has extreme jerking muscular movements.

The true cause of epilepsy is unknown. Based on clinical exam and brain studies, there are four types: *1. Grand mal epilepsy:* major episodes associated with loss of consciousness. *2. Petit mal epilepsy:* milder forms usually without loss of consciousness. *3. Psychomotor epilepsy:* with different types of abnormal movements. *4. Autonomic epilepsy:* associated with flushing, whiteness of skin, rapid heartbeat, high blood pressure, abdominal symptoms, and sweating.

Emergency techniques for someone having seizure: Remain calm and do the following: move sharp objects away, do not put anything in the mouth, loosen clothing, if possible, put person on the floor or bed and try to move onto the individual's side.

Increased circulation to the brain from breathing exercises and physical exercise are very important.

Alternative Treatments

Refer to alternative therapy chapters for more information before evaluating or applying any treatment. Some conditions, including yours, may require a physician's care.

Diet: Low-fat, low-carbohydrate diet. Eliminate fried foods, salt, sugar, meat, milk, and alcohol. For long-term care follow a hypoglycemic diet. (See Hypoglycemia.) Avoid artificial sweeteners, excessive refined carbohydrates, and caffeine, and make sure bowel moves adequately (two to three times per day).

Nutritional Therapy: • L-taurine and L-tyrosine amino acids (taken 500 mg. three times daily) along with amino acid blend formulas (two times daily) • Vitamin B complex • Vitamin B_6 • Magnesium • Folic acid (Folic acid supplementation can cause decrease in B_{12} levels, and in rare cases, may aggravate epilepsy.) • Niacin (vitamin B_3) • vitamin B_5 • vitamin B_{12} • Manganese • Zinc • Calcium • Choline (start with 4 grams daily and increase to 10-12 grams within three months) • Dimethyl glycine (100 mg. two times) • Intramuscular B complex may be helpful.

Sometimes essential fatty acids aggravate symptoms.

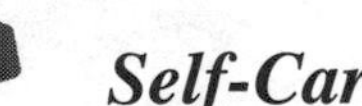

Self-Care

The following therapies can be undertaken at home under appropriate professional supervision.

• Fasting • Flower Remedies • Meditation • Yoga

Acupressure: (See Convulsions.)

Ayurveda: An herbal mixture of: *saraswati churna* 200 mg., *brahmi* 300 mg., *jatamansi* 200 mg., and *punarnava* 300 mg., one-quarter teaspoon of this mixture generally taken twice a day after lunch and dinner.

Bodywork: Massage (of abdomen after applying castor oil packs).

Herbs: For petit mal take one teaspoonful of skullcap tincture three times a day.

Hydrotherapy: • Constitutional hydrotherapy: apply two to five times weekly. • Epsom salts baths twice weekly.

Juice Therapy: Celery, carrot, and lettuce juice (three glasses daily).

Mind/Body Therapy: Biofeedback, hypnotherapy, meditation.

Reflexology: Diaphragm, colon, ileocecal, whole spine, neck area, all glands.

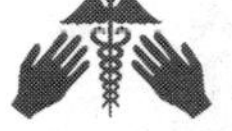

Professional Care

The following therapies should only be provided by a qualified health professional.

• Cell Therapy • Chiropractic • Craniosacral Therapy • Environmental Medicine • Magnetic Field Therapy • Naturopathic Medicine • Osteopathy • Traditional Chinese Medicine

Biological Dentistry: Hal A. Huggins, D.D.S., reports the improvement or disappearance of certain motor problems such as epilepsy and multiple sclerosis after removing toxic dental amalgams.

Bodywork: Acupressure, Feldenkrais, reflexology, Rolfing, *shiatsu.*

Detoxification Therapy: May be indicated, depending on other function.

Fainting

(See a physician immediately.)

A sudden and brief loss of consciousness, usually due to decreased flow of blood to the brain. Secondary to decreased heart output, usually due to arrhythmia (abnormal change in the beating of the heart). May also be due to heat exhaustion associated with excessive fluid loss, weakness, fatigue, anxiety, drenching sweats, and fainting.

Consider: Low blood sugar, low blood pressure (hypotension), allergies, anemia, and nutrient deficiencies such as magnesium and iron.

Alternative Treatments

Refer to alternative therapy chapters for more information before evaluating or applying any treatment. Some conditions, including yours, may require a physician's care.

Diet: Whole foods diet with adequate protein foods and fluids.

Nutritional Therapy: • Magnesium • Iron • Vitamin B • Pantothenic acid

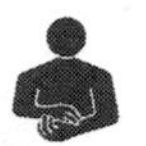

Self-Care

The following therapies can be undertaken at home under appropriate professional supervision.

Aromatherapy: Hold under nose: peppermint, neroli, basil, lavender, rosemary, black pepper.

Flower Remedies: For emotional states as appropriate. To revive someone who has fainted, put a drop of the Bach flower Rescue Remedy on the tongue.

Homeopathy: *Ignatia, Aconite, Arsen alb.*

Hydrotherapy: Constitutional hydrotherapy: apply two to five times weekly.

Practical Hints: If you feel faint, sit down and put your head between your knees until you feel better. Be sure there is plenty of fresh air.

Reflexology: Pituitary.

Traditional Chinese Medicine: Massage just under the nose to bring a person out of a faint.

Professional Care

The following therapies should only be provided by a qualified health professional.

• Environmental Medicine • Naturopathic Medicine • Oxygen Therapy

Bodywork: • Acupressure, reflexology, *shiatsu.*

Fasting: Under a doctor's supervision.

Farsightedness

See Vision Disorders chapter, page 859.

Fear

Feelings or sensations that create anxiety but are not substantiated or in proportion to the details of reality.

Symptoms: Increased frequency of breaths,

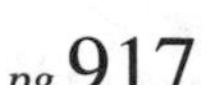

more shallow breathing, sweating, turning whitish in color, increased heart rate, feelings of weakness, and generalized discomfort.

Special Notes: There are times when fear is a normal response such as when one's well-being is threatened. However, frequent sensations of fear that are not in response to threatening situations may characterize psychological disorders or physiologic imbalances such as: nutrient deficiencies, low blood sugar, allergies, or the early stages of immune system response to infections.

According to Leon Chaitow, N.D., D.O., another word for fear is anxiety and while the above definition acknowledges the breathing connection it suggests only that breathing pattern changes are the result of fear—whereas this is a two-way street, anxiety (fear) often being the result of habitually altered breathing patterns.

It works like this:

Many people hyperventilate when afraid. They can become habituated to this pattern of breathing and this leads to a tendency for blood acid to become reduced to an excessive degree (blood needs to be slightly acid in good health) as they exhale too much carbon dioxide in relation to their physical state.

This reduces carbonic acid in the blood and alkalizes it excessively, leading to a heightened state of anxiety and excessive sensitivity of the nervous system, making them far more easily upset, aroused, alarmed—and anxious.

Breathing retraining, bodywork to relax the tense intercostal muscles, and relaxation methods can be combined to normalize this tendency, reducing a sense of fear, dread, and anxiety.

Alternative Treatments

Refer to alternative therapy chapters for more information before evaluating or applying any treatment. Some conditions, including yours, may require a physician's care.

Diet: Assess diet for excessive consumption of stressor foods such as: refined sugars, honey, maple syrup, or cow's milk products. Consume vegetable soups, broths, and a wide variety of green and yellow vegetables. Add more complex carbohydrates such as whole grains, beans, seeds, and nuts.

Nutritional Therapy: • Calcium • Magnesium • Vitamin B complex • Pantothenic acid • Adrenal glandulars • Kidney glandulars

Self-Care

The following therapies can be undertaken at home under appropriate professional supervision.

• Acupressure • Biofeedback Training • Fasting • Guided Imagery • Qigong • Yoga

Flower Remedies: Flower remedies may prove helpful. Aspen is for apprehension, foreboding, and fear of unknown origin while mimulus is for fear of known things, shyness, and timidity. Red chestnut is used for excessive fear and over caring for others. A few drops of the special extracts are taken in water.

Homeopathy: *Aconite, Actaea rac., Drosera, Calc carb., Sulfur.*

Hydrotherapy: Constitutional hydrotherapy, immersion bath, or wet sheet pack: apply two to five times weekly, neutral application as needed for sedation.

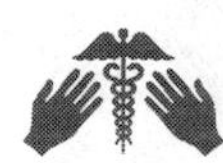

Professional Care

The following therapies should only be provided by a qualified health professional.

• Environmental Medicine • Hypnotherapy • Light Therapy • Magnetic Field Therapy • Naturopathic Medicine • Orthomolecular Medicine • Traditional Chinese Medicine

Bodywork: Rolfing may be very helpful if used in conjunction with psychotherapy.

Detoxification Therapy: Not usually indicated, unless the person's condition warrants treatment.

Female Health

See Female Health chapter, page 657.

Fever

See Children's Health chapter, page 605.

Fibrocystic Breasts

See Female Health chapter, page 674.

Flatulence

Buildup and expulsion of flatus (intestinal gas) formed by fermentation, inappropriate digestion of most commonly carbohydrates and sometimes other foodstuffs, or swallowing of air. Released by burping (eructation) through the mouth or by relieving gas through the anus.

Symptoms: Distention of abdomen,

discomfort in abdomen that may be mild or severe, chest pains that may be mild and feel like slight pressure or may be severe enough to mimic a heart attack.

Consider: Overeating, eating too quickly, excessive consumption of refined carbohydrates, excessive consumption of artificial sweeteners, food allergies, food intolerance, digestive disorders, intestinal disorders, stomach disorders, gallbladder disorders, nutrient deficiencies of B vitamins, excessive consumption of alcohol, parasites, emotional stress, and misalignment or spasm of the associated spinal vertebrae.

Alternative Treatments

Refer to alternative therapy chapters for more information before evaluating or applying any treatment. Some conditions, including yours, may require a physician's care.

Diet: Do not overeat. Overconsumption, even of healthy food, is the most common cause of flatulence. Eat simpler meals, meaning less different food items at one sitting. Chew food more slowly and thoroughly. Consume less low-fiber and more high-fiber foods. Identify and avoid allergic or intolerant foods. You may try avoiding protein and carbohydrates eaten together at meals. Try chewing a sprig of parsley after meals.

If eating beans, soaking them overnight in a quart of water containing six drops of iodine may help reduce gas.

Asafoetida powder is a powerful digestive agent. It dispels intestinal gas and when used as a spice with beans, helps to decrease gas. Try sipping lemon juice or apple cider vinegar in water with meals. Add more fermented products such as yogurt, kefir, and buttermilk to the general diet.

Leon Chaitow, M.D., D.O., suggests the European method of using super fine white, green, or yellow French clay (similar to bentonite). A teaspoon or two is dissolved in spring water and drunk, at least once a day away from mealtimes to reduce the tendency to flatulence. The clay absorbs the impurities and gas and there are no reported side effects.

Nutritional Therapy: • Vitamin B complex • Digestive enzymes such as hydrochloric acid or pancreatin • Acidophilus • Charcoal tablets • Several drops of peppermint oil in water sipped throughout the meal • vitamin B_1 • Aloe vera juice or gel • Niacin (vitamin B_3) • Lipotrophic factors (promotes the physical use of fat), may need gallbladder or bowel programs periodically.

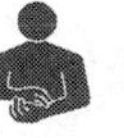

Self-Care

The following therapies can be undertaken at home under appropriate professional supervision.

• Biofeedback Training • Fasting • Qigong • Yoga

Aromatherapy: Bergamot, chamomile, fennel, juniper, lavender, peppermint, rosemary, coriander, anise.

Bodywork: Rub abdomen in clockwise direction.

Herbs: Try anise water, made by steeping one teaspoon of anise seeds in one cup of water for ten minutes. It can be taken as a tea or strained and taken as needed by the tablespoon.

Homeopathy: • *Carbo veg., Lycopodium, Argen nit., Chamomilla* • *Nux mosch* and *Cinchona*

Hydrotherapy: • Constitutional hydrotherapy unless otherwise indicated: apply two to five times weekly. • Short cold sitz baths

Juice Therapy: • One tablespoon of garlic or yellow onion juice, or mix with carrot, parsley, beet, and celery juice • Papaya juice

Naturopathic Medicine: Flatulence is almost always a sign of either maldigestion or food intolerance. When combined with bad breath and tiredness after meals, inadequate stomach acid is the typical cause.

Reflexology: Intestines, stomach, liver, gallbladder, pancreas.

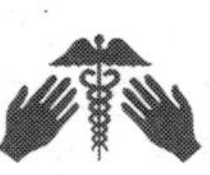

Professional Care

The following therapies should only be provided by a qualified health professional.

• Applied Kinesiology • Cell Therapy • Chiropractic • Colon Therapy • Environmental Medicine • Light Therapy • Magnetic Field Therapy • Naturopathic Medicine • Osteopathy • Traditional Chinese Medicine

Detoxification Therapy: Colon and gastrointestinal detox.

Flu

See Colds and Flu chapter, page 632.

Food Allergies

See Allergies chapter, page 511.

Food Poisoning

A term used for any health problem that is characterized by abdominal pain, associated with diarrhea, vomiting, sweating, and weakness, usually within forty-eight hours of eating a food contaminated with a virus or bacteria.

Symptoms: Symptoms vary greatly. Onset may be thirty minutes to one hour with chemical poisoning; one to twelve hours with bacterial poisoning; twelve to forty-eight hours from viral or salmonella poisoning. Stomach pain, nausea, diarrhea, and, in very severe cases, collapse and shock.

Occurrence: Many cases of diarrhea a year are probably due to food poisoning. Many go unreported as cause is not known and is usually attributed to the stomach flu.

Consider: Flu, gastrointestinal disorders, digestive enzyme deficiencies, drug interactions, stress, nutrient deficiencies, or excess (too much magnesium can cause loose stools and abdominal cramps). In infants, can also be due to intolerance to honey.

Special Notes: Usually suspect this when a number of people who ate the same food get similar symptoms. Most common forms of food poisoning are infective types such as salmonella, found usually in farm animals or passed on by food handling or flies from contaminated fecal material.

Food products most likely to cause problems are poultry such as chicken, duck, or geese, raw or partly cooked eggs, or raw fish such as clams, oysters, or sushi (Japanese raw fish dishes). Frozen poultry that is not completely thawed before being cooked is a common cause of this problem.

Other organisms such as staphylococcal bacteria can be passed from food handlers through hands, coughing, sneezing, or breathing onto the food itself. Botulism is associated with food preserved at home.

Viruses can contaminate shellfish and are often due to contaminated waters. Foods that remain at room temperature too long, such as large portions of meat prepared for restaurants and allowed to sit out at room temperature, can encourage Clostridium to grow, often referred to a the "cafeteria germ."

Other infective organisms can be giardiasis and campylobacteriosis, and may take up to one week to show symptoms. Noninfective food poisoning is caused by poisonous mushrooms, toadstools, and fresh vegetables and fruits that have been contaminated accidentally with too many chemicals and insecticides, by being stored in inappropriate containers, or from leakage of metals from the containers into the food.

If very severe vomiting and diarrhea occur, emergency medical intervention must be sought. Keep samples of food for testing if possible. If due to chemical or bacterial toxins, treatment may require pumping the stomach (gastric lavage). Milder cases can be home treated.

Usually improves within three days unless due to botulism, chemical poisoning, or mushroom poisoning.

One covert problem with infective organisms is that sometimes they do not have identifiable initial symptoms but linger in the body and may cause long-term health problems that are difficult to diagnose. May also cause constipation in addition to diarrhea.

Alternative Treatments

Refer to alternative therapy chapters for more information before evaluating or applying any treatment. Some conditions, including yours, may require a physician's care.

Diet: Stop eating all solid food, drink plenty of fluids. Immediately, take six charcoal tablets, acidophilus, bifidobacteria, *Lactobacillus bulgaricus*, and citrus seed extract. Take electrolyte replacement if needed, made by dissolving one teaspoon of salt and four teaspoons of sugar (which helps intestines absorb both) in one quart of water. Be accurate with salt or may create more dehydration. If you are traveling in areas where food poisoning is common, try eating more hot, spicy foods to encourage more gastric secretions. Avoid all drinking water except bottled water and any raw vegetables. Add high-fiber foods. Add garlic.

Nutritional Therapy: • Acidophilus • Charcoal tablets • Citrus seed extract • Garlic capsules • Vitamin C with bioflavonoids • Kelp

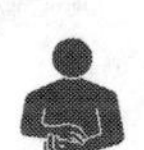

Self-Care

The following therapies can be undertaken at home under appropriate professional supervision.

• ***Fasting***

Ayurveda: For general mild food poisoning, fast and drink cumin, coriander, fennel tea.

Homeopathy: *Arsen alb., Chamomilla, Ipecac., Apis mel., Nux vom., Colchicum.*

Hydrotherapy: Constitutional hydrotherapy: apply two to five times weekly.

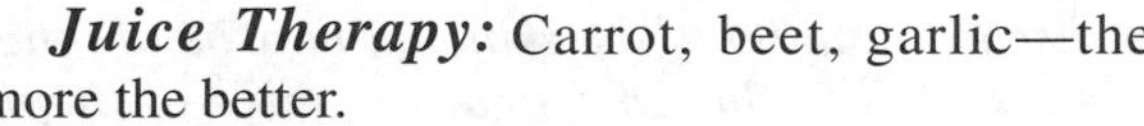

Juice Therapy: Carrot, beet, garlic—the more the better.

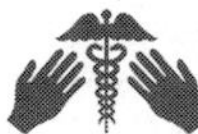

Professional Care

The following therapies should only be provided by a qualified health professional.

• Naturopathic Medicine

Oxygen Therapy: • Hydrogen peroxide therapy (IV) • Hyperbaric oxygen therapy as an adjunctive therapy is useful.

Fractures

A break in the bone.

Symptoms: There may be almost no symptoms, or mild ones such as slight swelling and tenderness with only mild aching. Or there may be severe symptoms with intense pain, discoloration, breakage of skin, severe swelling and throbbing, with possible bleeding from surrounding ruptured tissues and loss of normal movement.

Special Notes: Two main types of fractures: closed (simple: broken pieces remain beneath skin surface and there is little surrounding tissue disruption or damage) or open (compound: one or both of bone ends break through the skin). Fractures may also be classified as to the type of break: simple (broken bone does not pierce skin), compound (skin is pierced and exposed to organisms in the air), transverse (bone breaks all the way through), greenstick (only outer side of bone is broken and break is not all the way through), comminuted fracture (bone is shattered into smaller pieces).

X-rays are required to verify break. A doctor needs to properly "set" the fracture and then the following can be done to help optimize healing.

Rehabilitative exercise and manual therapy for localized and associated areas should be considered.

Alternative Treatments

Refer to alternative therapy chapters for more information before evaluating or applying any treatment. Some conditions, including yours, may require a physician's care.

Diet: Diets high in calcium from dark leafy greens, dairy products, and raw seeds and nuts. Avoid excessive consumption of caffeine, red meat, colas with phosphoric acid (most health food store colas do not have phosphoric acid). Highly processed foods also have a high phosphorus content which may lead to bone loss.

Nutritional Therapy: • Calcium • Magnesium • Vitamin C with bioflavonoids • Vitamin D • Zinc • Silicon • Vitamin K • Protein supplement (free-form amino acids)

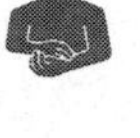

Self-Care

The following therapies can be undertaken at home under appropriate professional supervision.

• Biofeedback Training • Fasting • Guided Imagery

Bodywork: Acupressure, *shiatsu*, massage.

Herbs: • Drink an infusion of equal parts comfrey leaf and horsetail to speed the healing once the fracture has been set. • Teas: comfrey, horsetail, Solomon's seal

Homeopathy: *Calc phos., Symphytum, Ruta grav., Arnica, Aconite.*

Hydrotherapy: • Contrast application: apply daily. • Apply ice to fracture to control internal bleeding • Arm and wrist fractures: alternate hot arm bath (three minutes) and cold arm bath (thirty seconds).

Juice Therapy: Add watercress to beet and carrot juice.

Reflexology: Reflex to affected area on foot, also referral area.

Topical Treatment: • Poultice of tumeric paste mixed with a little hot water may be helpful with fractures and helps reduce swelling. • Poultice of fresh mullein leaves

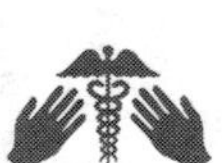

Professional Care

The following therapies should only be provided by a qualified health professional.

• Cell Therapy • Magnetic Field Therapy • Naturopathic Medicine • Reconstructive Therapy

Acupuncture: With electricity to help facilitate healing.

Chiropractic: (for fractures not requiring setting)

Oxygen Therapy: Hyperbaric oxygen therapy is useful for refractory bone fractures.

Frostbite

Excessive exposure to damp cold (temperatures around freezing) cause frostnip and immersion (trench) foot. Exposure to dry cold (temperatures that are well below freezing) cause frostbite and accidental hypothermia.

Symptoms: *Frostnip:* hardened and whitened areas on face, ears, fingers, and extremities. Peeling of skin may occur within twenty-four to seventy-two hours and recurrent bouts of milder cold sensitivity may last for life. *Immersion foot:* feet get pale, swell, cold, clammy, and numb or tingling. Infection may occur later. Swelling and pain may persist for years. *Frostbite:* area becomes extremely cold, hard, white, and difficult to feel. Upon warming up, area gets very itchy, red, swollen, blotchy, and painful. *Hypothermia:* lethargy, poor coordination, mental confusion and irritability, hallucinations, slowed respiration and heart rate, and death.

Consider: Conditions that increase risk to cold injury are: anemia, drug or alcohol excess, exhaustion and hunger, and impaired circulation secondary to other diseases. The very young or the elderly are also more at risk.

Special Notes: Hypothermia occurs when the body cannot maintain its normal temperature.

As soon as possible warm the affected areas, the hands, feet, and abdomen. Rub the area vigorously to stimulate circulation. You may even snuggle and hug the person to increase warmth.

Alternative Treatments

Refer to alternative therapy chapters for more information before evaluating or applying any treatment. Some conditions, including yours, may require a physician's care.

Nutritional Therapy: • Warm beverages • Vitamin B complex

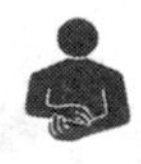

Self-Care

The following therapies can be undertaken at home under appropriate professional supervision.

• Fasting • Qigong

Herbs: To stimulate circulation: drink hot ginger tea.

Hydrotherapy: Immersion bath: neutral application to warm slowly.

Professional Care

The following therapies should only be provided by a qualified health professional.

• Naturopathic Medicine

Acupuncture: To prevent permanent nerve damage.

Oxygen Therapy: Hyperbaric oxygen therapy.

Traditional Chinese Medicine: *Dong quai* and peony formula are effective.

Fungal Infection

(See also Infections, Viral Infections, Candidiasis)

A disease, usually of the skin, but may be of other organs, that is due to fungal organisms (simple parasitic life forms including molds, mildew, and yeast), sometimes called mycoses.

Symptoms: *May be mild:* such as discoloration and swelling of the nail beds, moist, reddened patches over various parts of the body, cheesy and smelly discharge from the vagina. *May be severe:* such as infecting and disrupting normal organ functioning.

Special Notes: May be more common and/or severe in people taking long-term antibiotic medication, corticosteroids medication, immunosuppressant drugs (used to inhibit normal immune functioning), contraceptives, and in people with conditions such as obesity, AIDS, and diabetes mellitus.

Alternative Treatments

Refer to alternative therapy chapters for more information before evaluating or applying any treatment. Some conditions, including yours, may require a physician's care.

Diet: Whole foods diet with emphasis on raw food, less dairy products. Avoid foods high in yeast such as beer, and breads with yeast. Avoid sugar of all sorts (including honey and fruit juices) for some weeks while antifungal methods are being used. See Candidiasis chapter.

Nutritional Therapy: • Acidophilus • Bifidobacteria and *Lactobacillus bulgaricus* • Garlic capsules • Vitamin B complex • Pantothenic acid • Vitamins C • Vitamin E • Vitamin A • Zinc • Thymus glandular

Vitamin C to bowel tolerance. (See Orthomolecular Medicine chapter, page 402.)

Leon Chaitow, N.D., D.O., suggests taking caprylic acid capsules (extract of coconut plant) as a antifungal agent while acidophilus, etc. are being taken to repopulate sites which fungus had colonized.

Grapefruit seed extract may also be an effective remedy.

Self-Care

The following therapies can be undertaken at home under appropriate professional supervision.

• Fasting

Aromatherapy: Tea tree, patchouli, geranium.

Herbs: Fungicidal herbs are an effective topical treatment for skin infections. Examples are myrrh, tea tree, and garlic. Tea tree oil can be applied direct or diluted with calendula oil for application to sensitive skin.

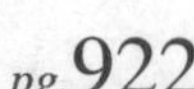

Homeopathy: *Calendula, Chamomilla, Belladonna, Merc sol., Sulfur.*

Juice Therapy: • Avoid fruit juices or dilute with water 2:1. • Add garlic to vegetable juice.

Naturopathic Medicine: Fungal infection of the nails is difficult to treat and requires patience. One therapy is to twice a day swab the infected area with tea tree or thuja oil.

Topical: To affected area: Application of some of the following: tea tree oil or gel, citrus seed extract, honey and crushed garlic, pau d'arco tea by wetting tea bag for ten minutes and then leave bag itself on the area or use gauze or cotton soaked in tea if area is too large.

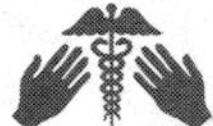

Professional Care

The following therapies should only be provided by a qualified health professional.

• Environmental Medicine • Magnetic Field Therapy • Naturopathic Medicine • Traditional Chinese Medicine

Detoxification Therapy: May be indicated, depending on the condition of the person.

Oxygen Therapy: • Hydrogen peroxide therapy (IV) • Hyperbaric oxygen therapy • Ozone/oxygen mixture may work as an effective antifungal agent. It may easily be applied externally. Methods of internal application depend upon the clinical situation.

Gallbladder Disorders

The gallbladder is a small sac-like organ that lies underneath the liver. It receives, stores, and concentrates bile made in the liver. The liver sends the bile to the gallbladder through a small tube called the cystic duct. During digestion the gallbladder contracts and sends the bile to the intestines (duodenum) to help break down (emulsify) fat that is contained in the food. The most common problem associated with the gallbladder is gallstones. Gallstones are roundish shaped combinations of cholesterol, bile, pigments, and lecithin.

Symptoms*:* Only 20 percent of people who have gallstones get symptoms (many people have gallstones that never bother them and are called "silent"). A major symptom of gallstones is usually right-sided pain in the abdomen that may be associated with right-sided shoulder pain. The shoulder pain may occur by itself without the abdominal pain.

There may be centrally located upper abdominal pain over the breastbone. The pain in general, wherever it manifests, is constant and progresses slowly, rising to a plateau, and then gradually decreases, usually within several hours after a meal, and especially after meals containing large amounts of fat. Sometimes nausea, fullness, belching, heartburn, flatulence, and vomiting are present.

If the abdomen gets extremely painful, even to the touch, and a fever starts, this may a symptom of acute cholecystitis. This is irritation and infection in the gallbladder usually due to a gallstone becoming trapped. Recurrent attacks of this are called chronic cholecystitis.

Occurrence: Women over forty years old, fair skinned, and overweight are more prone to gallstones. Women get gallstones four times as frequently as men. Twenty percent of adults over sixty-five years of age get gallstones that create problems and pain. Over half a million surgeries are performed a year to remove gallbladders due to gallbladder disorders, the most common being gallstones.

Consider: Food allergies (especially to milk products and eggs), digestive disorders (especially caused by a deficiency of HCl), intestinal diseases, excessively low-fiber diet, food intolerance, parasites, rapid weight loss, and stress.

Constipation may also be connected to gallstones.

Special Notes: Rarely does the gallbladder get inflamed without the presence of stones. Gallbladder cancer can occur, but is extremely rare (three cases per one hundred thousand people per year). This cancer usually causes jaundice (yellowing of skin), pain in upper right abdominal area, and is sometimes present with no symptoms at all.

Ultrasound may be needed for accurate diagnosis.

New surgical methods use lasers, do not need to cut into the abdomen, and heal much more quickly.

Jonathan Wright, M.D., states that most gallbladder surgeries could be easily avoided through nutritional and natural intervention, with emphasis on identification, avoidance, and treatment of food allergies.

Rule out dental implications. (See Biological Dentistry chapter, page 80.)

Alternative Treatments

Refer to alternative therapy chapters for more information before evaluating or applying any treatment. Some conditions, including yours, may require a physician's care.

Diet: Identify and avoid food allergies, especially eggs and/or cow's milk products. Cut down fat in diet, below 20 percent of total foods. Do not, however, cut out fat completely. Recent studies say that up to half of the people who try to lose weight by cutting out fat (eating less than six hundred calories and three grams of fat per day) develop gallstones[10] Especially avoid processed fats and hydrogenated fats. Eat less. Overeating is very stressful on the gallbladder. Eat regular meals, especially breakfast. It is hard on the gallbladder to go many hours without food and then suddenly have to deal with a large meal. Increase dietary fiber and decrease refined carbohydrates. Eat less animal foods and more toward a vegetarian-oriented diet. If you are overweight, lose the weight, but slowly and sensibly.

Fasting may be helpful during acute stages. Avoid animal products as much as possible during acute problems. Eat small frequent meals while having gallbladder symptoms. Black cherries, pears, beets (raw and cooked), fresh beet tops steamed with spinach leaves, or kale and yogurt are good. Increase dietary fiber. Avoid refined carbohydrates. Eat more raw foods.

First gallbladder flush: While continuing to eat, but mostly a whole foods diet with almost no animal products or processed foods: drink plenty of raw, fresh apple juice or eat apples as much as possible, in between meals, for six days. Morning of seventh day, have one-half cup of olive oil mixed with one-third cup of fresh lemon juice. Drink all at once.

Second gallbladder flush: Upon rising take three tablespoons of olive oil with three times the amount of fresh lemon juice. Or mix one-half ounce each of grapefruit juice and olive oil and take prior to meals.

Nutritional Therapy: • Multi-enzymes with bile (bile is contraindicated if ulcers coexist) • Vitamin C • Vitamin B complex • Choline inositol • Lipotrophic factors • Vitamin C • Alfalfa tablets • Lethicin • Unsaturated fatty acids • Acidophilus • L-taurine • Peppermint oil sipped in water throughout the meal may be helpful when having symptoms.

Self-Care

The following therapies can be undertaken at home under appropriate professional supervision.

• Fasting • Yoga

Herbs: In conjunction with dietary and lifestyle advice. Combine the tinctures of wild yam, fringetree bark, milk thistle, and balmony in equal parts and take one teaspoonful of this mixture three times a day. An infusion of chamomile or lemon balm may be drunk regularly throughout the day.

Hydrotherapy: Constitutional hydrotherapy: apply two to five times weekly. Hot pack to abdomen and low back: apply ten to fifteen minutes several times daily for relief of colic pain, follow each hot application with a short period of cold application.

Juice Therapy: • Carrot, beet, cucumber (add a little garlic, radish or fresh dandelion roots) • Grape, pear, grapefruit, lemon

Topical Treatment: Castor oil packs on gallbladder.

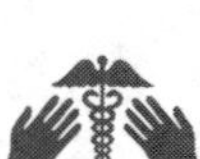

Professional Care

The following therapies should only be provided by a qualified health professional.

• Cell Therapy • Colon Therapy • Environmental Medicine • Magnetic Field Therapy • Naturopathic Medicine • Neural Therapy • Osteopathy

Acupuncture: For inflammation.

Detoxification Therapy: Detoxification is indicated, unless the person is in a weakened state.

Gastritis

See Gastrointestinal Disorders chapter, page 683.

Gastrointestinal Disorders

See Gastrointestinal Disorders chapter, page 680.

German Measles

See Children's Health chapter, page 607.

Glaucoma

See Vision Disorders chapter, page 860.

Gonorrhea

See Sexually Transmitted Diseases chapter, page 830.

Gout

See Arthritis chapter, page 531.

Hair Loss

Partial or complete loss of hair, called alopecia, which usually occurs on the scalp, but can occur anywhere on the body such as the extremities and even eyebrows, and can fall out or disappear in various patterns.

The most common pattern of hair loss is called male pattern baldness or hereditary alopecia. In this condition, hair is lost from the crown and temples, and is often replaced by a more fine, downy type of hair. This pattern of hair loss is also called androgenic alopecia, meaning it is more common in males, and is usually inherited. It may also affect women. When it does it is called female-pattern baldness, and occurs especially after menopause.

Alopecia areata is a sudden loss of very circumscribed areas of hair for no apparent reason or secondary to systemic disease. Alopecia universallis is loss of hair all over the entire body, has a poor reversal rate if occurs during childhood, but usually corrects itself but is prone to recurrences, if it begins in adulthood. Trichotillomania, hair pulling, is a neurotic disorder that usually occurs in children, may correct itself, and may be secondary to psychological problems or even physical ones such as heavy metal toxicity. Scarring alopecia is hair loss secondary to scarring due to localized trauma such as burns, physical injury, or x-rays, and often the hair cannot regrow through the scarred tissue.

Symptoms: Loss of hair in various patterns.

Occurrence: More common in men but can occur in women and is on the rise in women.

Consider: Low thyroid functioning, poor digestion, parasites, nutrient deficiencies such as iron or biotin deficiency, hormonal problems, aging, secondary to trauma, post-pregnancy, skin disease, diabetes mellitus, chemotherapy, and stress.

Special Notes: If large amounts of hair are lost it is important to see a doctor to rule out an underlying disease.

Circulation to the scalp is important. Increase exercise, scalp massage, and try lying on a slant board for fifteen minutes a day.

Minoxidol, a drug used daily to prevent hair loss, may create heart problems and perhaps female problems. The hair it grows is very fine and only on the top of the head, and the hair may fall out again soon after the drug is stopped. It is a very expensive drug, costing about one hundred dollars per month for daily treatment. Very little testing has been done on its long-term effects on women.

Alternative Treatments

Refer to alternative therapy chapters for more information before evaluating or applying any treatment. Some conditions, including yours, may require a physician's care.

Diet: Whole foods diet high in the outer coverings of plants such as potato skins, green and red peppers, sprouts, and cucumbers. These are high in silicon, which gives strength to hair and nails. Foods high in iron such as some lean meats and raisins are also important. Sea vegetables such as kelp are good for the hair and thyroid. Drink goat's milk instead of cow's milk.

Nutritional Therapy: • Flaxseed oil • Biotin • Zinc • Protein supplements such as amino acid blends • Vitamin B complex • Iron • Trace minerals

For dull, lifeless hair: Evening Primrose oil, flaxseed oil, and vitamin E. *Lost hair color:* PABA, pantothenic acid, biotin, iodine or thyroid glandular, desiccated liver. Poor liver functioning may play a role. Consider liver supplementation. High levels of copper can lead to brittle hair and split ends, and low copper levels can result in hair loss.

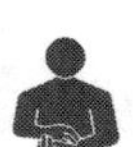

Self-Care

The following therapies can be undertaken at home under appropriate professional supervision.

• Fasting • Yoga

Aromatherapy: *For temporary or severe hair loss:* lavender, rosemary, thyme, sage.

Ayurveda: The Ayurvedic herbs *ashwagandha* and *amla* are reputed to stimulate hair growth. Apply warm *bhringaraj* oil or *brahmi* oil to the scalp regularly.

Herbs: Massage the scalp nightly with an oil made of one part rosemary oil and two parts almond oil. Internal treatment will depend upon the cause of the hair loss.

Homeopathy: *Sepia, Arnica, Acidum nit.*

Juice Therapy: Carrot, beet, spinach, nettle,

alfalfa. Add a little onion juice to the vegetable juices.

Topical Treatment: • Massage scalp with fingers daily. • Use double-strength herbal sage tea as a hair rinse or apply to scalp every day as a tonic. • Rub vitamin E oil into scalp nightly. • For two nights rub castor oil into scalp for ten minutes, then apply hot damp towel for thirty minutes. Put on plastic shower cap on overnight and wash out the following morning. The next two nights use olive oil, then use wheat germ oil for two nights. Rest one night and repeat seven-day cycle. • Apple cider vinegar used as a hair rinse may stimulate hair growth.

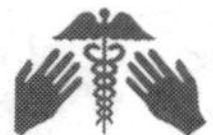

Professional Care

The following therapies should only be provided by a qualified health professional.

• Acupuncture • Cell Therapy • Magnetic Field Therapy • Naturopathic Medicine

Traditional Chinese Medicine: Kidney tonics.

Hangover

Feelings of discomfort the morning after drinking alcohol in excess the preceding night.

Alternative Treatments

Refer to alternative therapy chapters for more information before evaluating or applying any treatment. Some conditions, including yours, may require a physician's care.

Diet: Avoid bingeing on alcoholic beverages. Eat a piece of dry whole grain bread before drinking or as a remedy afterward. Drink a glass of orange juice or tomato juice the next morning. Since excessive consumption of alcohol tends to dehydrate, drink several glasses of water before bed and on rising, and preferably with juice of lemon if available.

Nutritional Therapy: Before bed, after having drank to excess: • Vitamin B complex • Vitamin C (1 gram) • Lipotrophic formula (that contains, among other elements, cysteine, and folic acid for liver, and optional, one aspirin). If possible take formula before bed and repeat first thing in morning.

According to Leon Chaitow, N.D., D.O., supplementation with the amino acid glutamine has been shown to dramatically reduce the craving for alcohol in nine out of ten patients so supplemented (with 2 grams daily in divided doses away from mealtimes).

Self-Care

The following therapies can be undertaken at home under appropriate professional supervision.

• Acupressure • Fasting

Aromatherapy: Rosemary, rose, fennel.

Herbs: Many commercially available mixtures of bitter herbs may help clear a hangover if taken first thing in the morning or last thing the "night before." Take one-quarter teaspoonful of a tincture combination of digestive bitters. Alternatively combine gentian, mugwort, and dandelion root tinctures and take one-quarter teaspoonful. An infusion is preferable but extremely bitter. Please refer to Addictions chapter for more suggestions.

Homeopathy: *Nux vom., Arsen alb., Aconite, Sulfur, Lachesis.*

Hydrotherapy: Hot spray/shower followed by cold rinse. Also, since alcohol causes dehydration: drink one quart water.

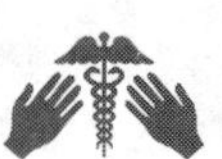

Professional Care

The following therapies should only be provided by a qualified health professional.

• Environmental Medicine • Magnetic Field Therapy • Naturopathic Medicine • Traditional Chinese Medicine

Bodywork: Reflexology, Rolfing, *shiatsu.*

Oxygen Therapy: Hyperbaric oxygen therapy is anecdotally very effective, but has no hard scientific proof of its usefulness.

Liquid oxygen drops taken in a glass of water may be effective.

Hay Fever

See Respiratory Conditions chapter, page 813.

Headache

See Headache chapter, page 691.

Head Lice

See Children's Health chapter, page 609.

Hearing and Ear Disorders, Hearing Loss

See Hearing Disorders chapters page 701.

Heart Attack, Heart Disease

See Heart Disease chapter, page 711

Heavy Metal Toxicity

Metals that have no safe amount in the human system, may accumulate within the body (fat cells, central nervous system, bones, brain, glands, and hair) and may have negative health effects. Any level of these toxic metals is not normal. The levels usually need to rise above the established safety ranges to actually manifest in health problems. However, there is individual variation, and high normal levels may aggravate one person and not another.

Symptoms*:* Wide variety of possible symptoms. In general, a harmful (above safety index range) amount of any toxic metal is a stress on the entire body and can manifest in a wide array of seemingly confusing symptoms or in the individual's weakest physical link. Symptoms that manifest depend on the type of metal toxicity, the age of the individual (children are more susceptible to toxic metal damage), the extent of the exposure, and the presence of antagonist/protective elements that inhibit absorption, binding, and effects of the toxic metals. For example, calcium deficiency aggravates lead toxicity, and the more normal levels of calcium that are in the body act to protect the system against lead toxicity.

The most common heavy metal toxicities are lead, cadmium, mercury, and nickel. Aluminum is not a heavy metal, and is absorbed and removed from the body by different mechanisms. All may be associated with a metallic taste in the mouth. Possible side effects of each are the following.

Lead: Lead toxicity may be associated with poor bone growth and development, learning disabilities, fatigue, poor task performance, irritability, anxiety, high blood pressure, weight loss, increased susceptibility to infection, ringing in the ears, decreased cognitive functioning and concentration and spelling skills, headaches, gastrointestinal problems, constipation, muscle and joint pain, tremors, and overall general decreased immune functioning.

Cadmium: Cadmium toxicity may be associated with fatigue, irritability, headaches, high blood pressure, benign (noncancerous) enlargement of the prostate (male sex) gland, increased risk for cancer, hair loss, learning disabilities, kidney disorders, liver disorders, skin disorders, painful joints, and decreased immune functioning.

Mercury: Mercury toxicity may be associated with cognitive problems, memory problems, irritability, fatigue, insomnia, gastrointestinal disorders, decreased immune response, irrational behavior, numbness, tingling, muscular weakness, impaired vision and hearing, allergic conditions, asthma, and multiple sclerosis related to dental amalgams.

Nickel: Nickel toxicity may be associated with fatigue, respiratory illnesses, heart conditions, skin rashes, psoriasis, fatigue, and headaches.

Aluminum: Aluminum toxicity may be associated with headaches, cognitive problems, learning disabilities, poor bone density (osteoporosis), ringing in the ears, gastrointestinal disorders, colic, hyperactivity in children, and ataxia (an abnormal walking pattern). It's possible role in poor memory or Alzheimer's disease is speculative at this time but also worth noting.

Possible routes of exposure to and contamination from the above metals:

Lead: Cigarette smoke exposure, eating paint that is lead based (in children especially in poor housing or older housing), eating and cooking foods in ceramic glazes that are lead based, leaded gasoline, eating liver that may be contaminated with lead, living in the inner city that may have elevated lead air levels, contaminated water, canned foods (especially fruit in which the lead-soldered cans may leach out into the food), certain bone meal supplements, and insecticides.

Cadmium: Possible contamination from cigarette and pipe smoke, instant coffee and tea, nickel-cadmium batteries, contaminated water, some soft drinks, refined grains, fungicides, pesticides, and some plastics.

Mercury: Possible contamination from mercury-based dental amalgam fillings, laxatives that contain calomel, some hemorrhoidal suppositories, inks used by some printers and tattooers, some paints, some cosmetics, and many products that may contain small amounts of mercury such as fabric softeners, wood preservatives, solvents, drugs, and some plastics and contaminated fish.

Nickel: Many pieces of jewelry have nickel

and wearing next to skin creates some absorption. Some metal cooking utensils have some nickel added to them, even stainless steel which is mostly a problem when cooking acidic foods. Cigarette smoke, hydrogenated fats (as nickel is the catalyst for the reaction to create them), some refined foods, and fertilizers contain nickel.

Aluminum: Aluminum-containing antacids, many over-the-counter drugs and douches that contain aluminum such as, to name a few, Amphojel, Maalox, Mylanta, Gelusil, Arthritis Pain Formula, Bufferin, Massengil, Summer's Eve, aluminum cookware and aluminum foil, especially when preparing and storing acidic foods, aluminum containing underarm antiperspirants, most commercial baking powders, and contaminated water.

Antagonist/protective minerals for each toxic metal:

Lead: Calcium, vitamin C, amino acids (L-lysine, L-cysteine, and L-cystine), iron, zinc.

Cadmium: Zinc, vitamin C, amino acids (L-methionine, L-cysteine, and L-lysine).

Mercury: Selenium, vitamin C, amino acids (L-glutathione, L-methionine, L-cysteine, and L-cystine).

Nickel: Iron, zinc, vitamin C.

Aluminum: Calcium, magnesium, vitamin B complex, vitamin C .

Alternative Treatments

Refer to alternative therapy chapters for more information before evaluating or applying any treatment. Some conditions, including yours, may require a physician's care.

Diet: Whole foods diet with emphasis on apples, applesauce, garlic, onions, beans, seeds, whole grains other than wheat, fresh fruits and vegetables, and lots of filtered water, at least eight glasses a day, throughout the detoxifying process. Fermented products such as yogurt and kefir are also very good.

William L. Cowden, M.D., recommends a diet of organic vegetables, fruits, seeds, grains, and nuts. He adds that a small percentage of the population whose ancestors lived in the very Northern latitudes cannot tolerate this diet. Symptoms of intolerance would be fatigue, sometimes muscle weakness, difficulty with memory and concentration, and feeling low-grade flulike symtpoms. If these symptoms occur as a result of the dietary changes, test for urine pH (acid-base balance). If urine is too alkaline, add some organic meats and/or dairy products if no allergies to dairy are present.

Nutritional Therapy: • Detoxification program with vitamin C to bowel tolerance; detox products should contain the amino acids mentioned on previous page. • Folic acid • Liver glandular • Protective nutrients as mentioned in prevoius paragraphs per metal in question • Vitamin B complex • Multivitamin

If metal toxicity and symptoms are severe, detox can occur with intravenous chelation program at a doctor's along with this oral program.

Self-Care

The following therapies can be undertaken at home under appropriate professional supervision.

• Fasting

Ayurveda: *Pancha karma* for seven days, *dashamoola basti, yasti madhu vaman, brahmi ghee nasya, shatavari rasayana,* aloe vera gel two tablespoons three times a day, *tikta ghee*, one-half teaspoon three times a day on an empty stomach.

Juice Therapy: To support liver, kidneys, and skin: carrot, celery, burdock, beet, garlic, and flaxseed or currant oils.

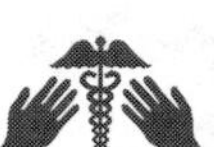

Professional Care

The following therapies should only be provided by a qualified health professional.

• Homeopathy • Naturopathic Medicine • Orthomolecular Medicine • Traditional Chinese Medicine

Oxygen Therapy: Ozone therapy in conjunction with intravenous chelation therapy has proven to be effective in treating heavy metal toxicity.

Chelation Therapy: Chelation therapy can be an effective way of clearing the system of accumulated metals.

Hemorrhoids

Veins in the lining of the anus that have become distended. Internal hemorrhoids are near the beginning of the anus and external hemorrhoids are at the opening of the anus and when they protrude outside the anus they are called prolapsing hemorrhoids.

Symptoms: Bleeding (usually bright red fresh blood that shows up on the toilet paper after wiping), protrusion of tissues, sometimes itching, mucous, discomfort and pain upon evacuating fecal material and sometimes even sitting. Any bleeding should be checked to rule out other more serious conditions. Proctoscopy (examination of the rectum through a tube) is needed to rule out cancer or polyps (small growths).

Occurrence: The frequency of hemorrhoid occurrences in both children and adults leads some doctors to consider them normal.

Regular toilet habits of sitting at the same time each day to try to evacuate bowels and to avoid straining is very helpful.

Alternative Treatments

Refer to alternative therapy chapters for more information before evaluating or applying any treatment. Some conditions, including yours, may require a physician's care.

Diet: Whole foods diet with emphasis on high-fiber foods, citrus fruits (including the inner whitish rind), drinking plenty of fluids. Especially good are whole grains such as buckwheat and millet. One tablespoon of cold processed vegetable oil a day, on food or taken alone.

For bleeding hemorrhoids: eat foods rich in vitamin K: alfalfa, kale, dark green leafy vegetables.

Nutrition: First in importance: increase whole fiber foods and raw fruits and vegetables in diet. Vitamin C with bioflavonoids (3-6 grams daily of each) and rutin (1 gram daily), vitamin A (10-25,000 IU daily), folic acid (400-800 mcg. daily), vitamin B complex two times daily, essential fatty acids (three to four on empty stomach on rising and before bed). Consider bowel cleanse and rejuvenation program as the anus is the last portion of the intestinal tract, and like the mouth, acts as a barometer of the inner health. Zinc, beta-carotene, linseed oil to soften stools.

Apply combination of zinc oxide, vitamin E, and aloe vera gel or olive oil to affected area.

Self-Care

The following therapies can be undertaken at home under appropriate professional supervision.

• Fasting • Guided Imagery • Qigong • Yoga

Aromatherapy: Cypress, juniper, frankincense, niaouli.

Ayurveda: • Drink one-half cup of aloe vera juice three times daily until condition has cleared. • The Ayurvedic compound *triphala* is recommended for hemorrhoids. • A confection of one part sesame seeds (black seeds if possible), one-half part *shatavari* (if available). Add ginger and raw sugar to taste. Take one ounce daily. • *Triphala guggulu* 200 mg., generally taken twice a day after lunch and dinner. Local application of castor oil for *vata* type, *tikta ghee* for *pitta* type.

Herbs: In Europe there is nothing to match the aptly named pilewort. The United States' equivalent is collinsonia. Combine the tinctures of collinsonia, cranesbill, and ginkgo in equal parts and take one teaspoonful of this mixture three times a day. A topical application is used to alleviate the symptoms and compliment the internal treatment. Mix 10 ml. of collinsonia tincture with 80 ml. of distilled witch hazel and apply this combination after every bowel motion and as needed. Salves may also be used containing any of the possible herbs, such as calendula, St. John's Wort, aloe, or plantain.

Homeopathy: *Aloe, Hamamelis, Nux vom., Berberis, Acidum fluor., Thuja.*

Hydrotherapy: Sitz bath: warm sitz applied daily, follow with short cold.

Juice Therapy: • Carrot, parsley • Carrot, spinach • Carrot, spinach, celery, parsley • Carrot, watercress • Beets, if they don't speed up the gastrointestinal tract.

Topical Treatment: • Epsom salts packs • Apply witch hazel frequently to hemorrhoids to shrink blood vessels. • Calendula ointment for pain and itching • Use a peeled garlic clove as a suppository for hemorrhoids.

Reflexology: Diaphragm, adrenals, rectum, sigmoid, lower spine; also chronic area up the back of the heel.

Professional Care

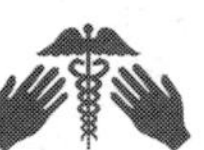

The following therapies should only be provided by a qualified health professional.

• Acupuncture • Applied Kinesiology • Cell Therapy • Light Therapy • Magnetic Field Therapy • Naturopathic Medicine • Osteopathy • Reconstructive Therapy

Body Work: • Myotherapy.

Detoxification Therapy: May be indicated. (Usually caused by congestive disorder—constipation, liver problems, etc.)

Hepatitis

Inflammation of the liver that is associated with damage or death of liver cells. There is acute hepatitis (attack that eventually heals) or chronic (ongoing liver problems).

Symptoms*:* In early stage there is usually loss of appetite, fatigue, weight loss, fever, nausea, and vomiting. Extreme fatigue is a key sign. Rashes and pain in the joints may occur. In three to ten days dark urine may manifest, and this may be followed by the skin turning yellow (jaundice). Jaundice usually takes one to two weeks to build up and then two to four weeks to fade. The liver is usually enlarged and tender to the touch. However, symptoms can occur in a wide range from mild flulike symptoms to severe liver failure and brain coma.

Occurrence: Twenty to thirty cases per one hundred thousand people in the United States.

Special Notes: Most common cause is contamination with a virus, Type A or Type B or non-A, or non-B. There can be other causes that lead to hepatitis, such as excessive alcohol consumption, drug abuse (including medical drugs, such as acetaminophen, the common over-the-counter Tylenol), overexposure to certain chemicals (such as dry cleaning fluids), and, sometimes, as a rare reaction to normal levels of therapeutic drugs.

The American Liver Foundation identifies five different viruses (termed A, B, C, D, and E) which cause hepatitis. Type C is a frequent cause of post-transfusion hepatitis. Recently, a test has been developed which can identify individuals infected with the hepatitis C virus. In general, individuals with the hepatitis C virus are identified either because they have abnormal liver tests or because a hepatitis C antibody test was obtained when they went to donate blood.

A positive test does not mean that you have a serious form of liver disease. Individuals infected with the hepatitis C may have no liver disease, a mild form of hepatitis (termed chronic persistent), or a more serious form of hepatitis (termed chronic active) that may progress over a number of years to cirrhosis. The usual indications for treatment are a positive antibody test for the hepatitis C virus, abnormal liver tests for more than six to twelve months, and a liver biopsy that shows chronic active hepatitis. Estimates are that approximately 20 percent of patients chronically infected with the hepatitis C virus will go on to develop cirrhosis.

Infectious hepatitis can spread easily the two weeks before and one week after jaundice appears. The feces contain the virus and so very strict toilet hygiene and hand and cloth washing should be observed during this time.

Alternative Treatments

Refer to alternative therapy chapters for more information before evaluating or applying any treatment. Some conditions, including yours, may require a physician's care.

Diet: Jonathan Wright, M.D., recommends a diet low in protein to minimize stress on the liver. Whole foods diet that follows a hypoglycemic regime, of small meals throughout the day, avoiding stressor foods such as refined sugars, alcohol, and caffeine. Consume plenty of filtered water. Drinking fresh lemon juice water every morning and evening followed by vegetable juice is one of the most therapeutic regimes for the liver. Do this consistently for two to four weeks and then several mornings a week for several months and whenever liver symptoms reoccur. Have lots of vegetables each day. Ideal is at least one salad and one meal of steamed or lightly sauteed vegetables per day. Grains that are easily digestible, such as millet, buckwheat, and quinoa, are very good.

Nutritional Therapy: • Vitamin C (should be to bowel tolerance to support liver) • Beta-carotene (100,000 IU daily for two weeks then reduce to 25,000-50,000) • Liver glandulars (three to four times daily) • Milk thistle extract • Vitamin B complex • Adrenal glandular • Lipotropic factor • Pantothenic acid • Protein (free-form amino acids) • Betaine HCl • Multi-enzymes • If needed, multiminerals • Evening Primrose oil

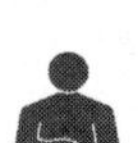

Self-Care

The following therapies can be undertaken at home under appropriate professional supervision.

• Fasting • Guided Imagery • Qigong

Aromatherapy: Rosemary.

Ayurveda: *Acute hepatitis:* Avoid hot, sour, spicy, and salty foods, meat, fish, cheese, oils, fried foods, and concentrated sweets. Try a mono-diet of mung beans for one week to strengthen liver. Add basmati rice and liver-cleansing spices such as coriander and tumeric. Take complete rest and avoid vigorous exercise. *Chronic hepatitis:* Take tonics such as aloe gel, *shatavari,* and the formula *Chyavan prash. Hepatitis B:* An herbal mixture of *kutki* 200 mg., *guduchi* 300 mg., and *shanka pushpi* 400 mg., generally taken twice a day after lunch and dinner. For all types, fresh sugarcane juice, one cup three times a day. One-half cup fresh homemade yogurt with a pinch of baking soda twice a day and *brahmi ghee nasya.*

Enemas: • Three warm enemas daily • Chlorophyll enema (one pint for fifteen minutes)

Herbs: As a range of pathologies are potentially present, competent diagnosis is essential. The liver-cell regenerative properties of herbs such as milk thistle and licorice can be helpful. Combine the glycerates of milk thistle, dandelion root, liquorice, and wahoo in equal parts and take one-half teaspoonful of this mixture three times a day. The wahoo can be replaced by fringetree bark if unobtainable. Refer to Cirrhosis for more dosage information on milk thistle.

Phyllanthus amarus (for hepatitis B): Encouraging results were found in a preliminary study in which carriers of hepatitis B virus were treated with a preparation from the plant *Phyllanthus amarus* for thirty days. Fifty-nine percent of those treated had lost the hepatitis B antigen when tested fifteen to twenty days after treatment and few or no toxic side effects were reported. *Phyllanthus amarus* has centuries of documented use in Ayurveda and may be a breakthrough in treatment of hepatitis B when used in conjunction with plants such as tumeric and milk thistle.[11]

Hydrotherapy: • Constitutional hydrotherapy: apply two to five times weekly. *Acute infectious hepatitis:* alternate hot compress (one minute) and cold compress (five minutes) over liver for one hour. Repeat three times a day. *Chronic hepatitis:* cold compress on liver every night for a few weeks. Then, reduce to one week per month for six months.

Juice Therapy: • Short juice fast using beet, carrot, and wheat grass juices • Garlic, burdock, flax, black currants

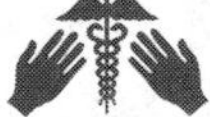

Professional Care

The following therapies should only be provided by a qualified health professional.

• Cell Therapy • Colon Therapy • Magnetic Field Therapy • Naturopathic Medicine

Oxygen Therapy: • Hydrogen peroxide therapy (IV) • Ozone may inactivate the hepatitis viruses. .

Detoxification Therapy: Depending on the condition of the person.

Herpes

See Sexually Transmitted Diseases chapter, page 831.

Hiatal Hernia

Hiatal hernia is a disorder caused when the opening in the diaphragm where the stomach and esophagus meet becomes stretched, allowing the upper end of the stomach to push up into the chest cavity. The esophageal sphincter, which normally acts as a one-way valve to allow food to travel down into the stomach, now is unable to prevent the contents of the stomach, including gastric acids, from traveling upward.

Symptoms*:* Most people have no symptoms. Sometimes there is chest pain or heartburn. The heartburn can be worse on bending over, especially after eating, worse at night, or worse with lying down. Sometimes the pain of hiatal hernia can mimic other health problems such as stomach ulcers or heart attacks.

Occurrence: More frequently in people who are overweight, who smoke, and sometimes occurs in newborns.

Special Notes: Sometimes in association with a hiatal hernia there is some material from the stomach that gets pushed upward into the esophagus. This is called esophageal reflux and may cause the heartburn.

According to Leon Chaitow, N.D., D.O., there is a mechanical aspect to hiatal hernia which can involve extreme tension in two large muscles which merge with the diaphragm—the psoas and quadratus lumborum. If either of these is chronically tense (very common) a stress will be imposed on the diaphragm which can result in the hernia. Osteopathic techniques can be applied to normalize these muscles.

Alternative Treatments

Refer to alternative therapy chapters for more information before evaluating or applying any treatment. Some conditions, including yours, may require a physician's care.

Diet: Strictly avoid overeating. Observe eating the following to see if they aggravate the problem, and if so, avoid: spicy foods, fried foods, coffee, tea, carbonated drinks, citrus juices, alcohol, whipped cream, milk shakes, peppermint, green and red peppers, and onion. Avoid eating large meals and then lying down or bending over. Avoid drinking too much with meals or drinking much after dinnertime. Eat numerous small meals throughout the day. Try to reduce stress by eating in pleasant, relaxing settings. Avoid eating foods or food combinations which cause excess gas formation. Eat sufficient fiber.

Nutritional Therapy: • Digestive enzymes if needed (pancreatin and HCl) • Vitamin B complex (one teaspoon liquid chlorophyll at dinner for two weeks) • Aloe vera juice • Multivitamin/mineral formula

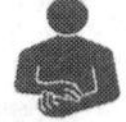

Self-Care

The following therapies can be undertaken at home under appropriate professional supervision.

• Biofeedback Training • Fasting

Breathing Exercises: Deep breathing exercises to strengthen the muscles of the diaphragm and to expand the lungs.

According to Dr. Chaitow, many people with hiatal hernia have been shown to have breathing restrictions, and to have a habit of swallowing air more frequently than the average. This leads to excessive air reaching the stomach putting great stress on the diaphragmatic aperture through which the esophagus passes and exacerbating hiatal hernia problems.

Breathing retraining and behavior modification methods can be used to help slow down the rate of swallowing to more normal levels.

Exercises and Lifestyle Hints: • Sit in armchair. Breathe in and hold your breath. Lift legs up toward your chest. Lower, and then exhale. Repeat several times. *For shortness of breath or food hung up in esophagus:* drink two (eight-ounce) glasses of water and bounce on your heels twelve times. • Sleep with your upper body in an elevated position to keep the chest cavity above the stomach. This will prevent the stomach from rising into the chest cavity. Put blocks under the head of the bed (four to eight inches high) or sleep with a wedge-shaped bolster.

Herbs: The main herbal goal is to reduce the inflammation and symptoms of reflux. Make an infusion with equal parts of comfrey root, marshmallow root, and meadowsweet and drink this often during the day. Have a cup last thing at night, keeping some by the bed to sip if needed.

Homeopathy: *Calc carb., Hepar sulph., Ferrum phos.*

Hydrotherapy: Contrast application: apply to abdomen daily.

Reflexology: Diaphragm, stomach, adrenals.

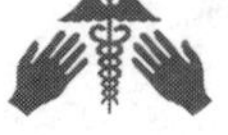

Professional Care

The following therapies should only be provided by a qualified health professional.

• Applied Kinesiology • Chiropractic • Colon Therapy • Magnetic Field Therapy • Naturopathic Medicine • Traditional Chinese Medicine

Detoxification Therapy: May be indicated, including diet changes and cleansing programs.

Osteopathy: Osteopathic muscle energy techniques to normalize tight postural muscles if these are involved.

Hiccups

A sound, sometimes called a hiccough, made by the vocal chords suddenly closing in response to the diaphragm suddenly contracting. A cluster of these is called an attack of the hiccups. This is extremely common and not serious.

Symptoms: Hiccup sounds vary from person to person.

Special Notes: Prolonged hiccup attacks that do not go away are very rare and require medication or surgery as they cause severe exhaustion.

There are numerous folk remedies to "cure" hiccups and their effectiveness varies from person to person.

Alternative Treatments

Refer to alternative therapy chapters for more information before evaluating or applying any treatment. Some conditions, including yours, may require a physician's care.

Diet: Chew a piece of very dry or charred toast, very slowly. Sip a glass of water while walking slowly but continuously, until hiccups stop.

Nutrition: Chew charcoal tablets or chewable papaya enzymes. Continue chewing tablets at least once an hour, and in extreme cases, continuously.

Self-Care

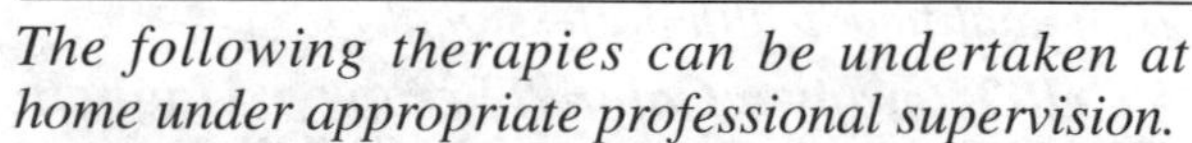

The following therapies can be undertaken at home under appropriate professional supervision.

• Biofeedback Training • Fasting

Acupressure: Place your middle and index fingers behind each earlobe. Apply light to firm pressure on these tender points, TW17 and SI17 (for an illustration of these point numbers please see the acupressure chart on page 875) for two minutes as you concentrate on breathing slowly and deeply.

Ayurveda: • Mix honey (two parts) and castor oil (one part). Take one teaspoon. • A pinch of *mayur chandrika bhasma* with one-half teaspoon

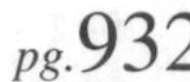

honey. Alternate nostril breathing with inner retention. (See Yoga chapter.)

Bodywork: Massage any painful areas around vertebrae at level of diaphragm.

Herbs: Combine the tinctures of black cohosh, skullcap, and vervain and take ten drops of this mixture in a little hot water. Alternatively sip a warm infusion of chamomile tea.

Homeopathy: *Nux vom., Mag phos., Ignatia, Lycopodium, Ginseng, Acidum sulf.*

Juice Therapy: Remember to chew your juices (swish around before swallowing).

Reflexology: Diaphragm, stomach.

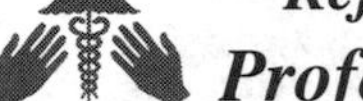

Professional Care

The following therapies should only be provided by a qualified health professional.

• Chiropractic • Environmental Medicine • Hypnotherapy • Magnetic Field Therapy • Naturopathic Medicine • Osteopathy

Bodywork: Reflexology.

Traditional Chinese Medicine: Especially effective if the hiccups have lasted for days.

High Blood Pressure

See Hypertension chapter, page 725.

Hives (Urticaria)

A skin condition characterized by itchy wheals (raised white bumps surrounded by reddish area).

Symptoms: Rashes of wheals appearing on the arms, legs, or trunk but can appear anywhere on the body. Wheals usually last for several hours.

Special Notes: Most common cause is a histamine reaction due to allergies, especially to certain foods, such as strawberries, shellfish, peanuts, milk, and eggs, and sometimes to different drugs such as penicillin or to different chemicals such as laundry soap.

Alternative Treatments

Refer to alternative therapy chapters for more information before evaluating or applying any treatment. Some conditions, including yours, may require a physician's care.

Diet: Identify allergic foods and avoid. Most common offending foods are berries, fish (sometimes even just the fumes are sufficient to create an allergic episode), soy, beef, citrus, and peanuts. Usually, if there are some foods that cause this full-blown allergic reaction, there are other foods that constantly "stress" the system but with more subtle and confusing symptoms. Eat a varied diet without repeating foods in excess, especially any food suspicious of being an allergen (causing an allergic reaction).

Hydrochloric acid secretions in the stomach are found to be low in most people with hives. It is this deficiency which seems to relate to the B complex vitamin deficiency also commonly observed in these patients.

Nutritional Therapy: *Topically:* Mix calamine lotion with beta-carotene liquid. Vitamin A capsule squeezed together with some zinc oxide ointment can be placed over the affected area.

Orally: • Pancreatic enzymes (four, four times daily on empty stomach during initial attack) • Bromelain and vitamin C taken away from meals (three to four times per day) • Vitamin B complex (two to four times daily with lots of water, then reduce to two times daily within two to three days)

After attack, on daily prevention basis take: • Bioflavonoids and pantothenic acid (1-2 grams) • Vitamin B complex • Essential fatty acids • Vitamin B_6 • Practice a varied whole foods diet.

Sometimes two Alka Seltzer Gold Tablets in water sipped every fifteen minutes for one to two hours is also helpful.

If you do not have calamine liquid try using unflavored yogurt.

Alan R. Gaby, M.D., had found that acute or chronic hives respond well to an intravenous injection of a "cocktail" composed of magnesium chloride hexahdydrate, calcium glycerophosphate, hydroxocobalamin, pyridoxine hydrochloride, dexpanthenol, B complex, and vitamin C. (This is a modification of the nutrient cocktail popularized by John Myers, M.D.)

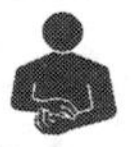

Self-Care

The following therapies can be undertaken at home under appropriate professional supervision.

• Biofeedback Training • Enemas • Fasting • Guided Imagery • Qigong

Aromatherapy: Chamomile, tagetes.

Herbs: Parsley, peppermint oil.

Homeopathy: *Apis mel., Nat mur., Urtica Urens.*

Hydrotherapy: Add oatmeal to bath.

Light Therapy: Chronic urticaria: Ultraviolet light therapy.

Topical Treatment: • Fresh coriander juice applied externally for itch and inflammation.

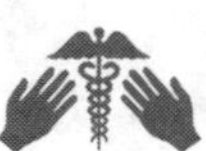

Professional Care

The following therapies should only be provided by a qualified health professional.

• Acupuncture • Applied Kinesiology • Environmental Medicine • Light Therapy • Magnetic Field Therapy • Naturopathic Medicine • Neural Therapy • Orthomolecular Medicine • Osteopathy • Traditional Chinese Medicine

Detoxification Therapy: Not indicated, unless to control the allergic state.

Oxygen Therapy: Hydrogen peroxide therapy (IV)

Hyperactivity

See Children's Health chapter, page 610.

Hypertension

See Hypertension chapter, page 725.

Hyperthyroidism

Overproduction of thyroid hormone by thyroid gland.

Symptoms*:* There are many forms of overactive thyroid, but the symptoms are similar for all of them. Rapid heartbeat, enlarged thyroid (goiter), moist skin, trembling (tremors), widened pulse pressure (lower and higher end numbers), fatigue, anxiety, weight loss, bulging eyes, excessive sweating, increased appetite, extremely low tolerance to heat, diarrhea, chest pain, and gastrointestinal disturbances. In older persons with this condition, the symptoms may be the opposite.

Occurrence: Much more rare than under active thyroid (Hypothyroidism).

Special Notes: Hyperthyroidism may be associated with and often is called Graves' disease (toxic diffuse goiter): hyperthyroidism combined with enlarged thyroid, eyes that bulge, rash and swelling in front of the lower leg that may appear before or after the condition, or thyrotoxicosis.

The thyroid is a "master" gland meaning that it is very influential on the overall health of most of the cells of the body. The thyroid gland sits at the base of the neck. If you wore a tie, it would lie somewhere behind the big knot in the tie. It consists of two lobes, one on each side of the windpipe (trachea). The thyroid is a gland that combines and concentrates iodine with tyrosine into active thyroid hormone. These reactions are controlled and influence by the pituitary gland. The thyroid gland has many physiologic effects on all the cells of the body. The two major ones are to help form protein RNA (building blocks of life) for every cell, and to increase oxygenation consumption by most cells. Thus, the thyroid greatly effects overall body metabolism.

Alternative Treatments

Refer to alternative therapy chapters for more information before evaluating or applying any treatment. Some conditions, including yours, may require a physician's care.

Diet: Whole foods diet. Eat foods which naturally and gently suppress thyroid hormone production (broccoli, brussels sprouts, cabbage, cauliflower, kale, mustard greens, rutabagas, spinach, turnips, soybeans, peaches, and pears). Avoid dairy products, excessive and repetitive consumption of wheat products, coffee, tea, and caffeinated soft drinks.

Nutritional Therapy: • Must see a qualified practitioner or orthomolecular physician. • High dosages of vitamin A and choline (under doctor's supervision) • Vitamin B complex with extra thiamine (vitamin B_1) and amino acid supplements both three times daily as increased metabolism increases demand • Multivitamin/mineral complex • Vitamin C • Iodine or kelp • Calcium • Magnesium

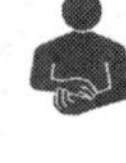

Self-Care

The following therapies can be undertaken at home under appropriate professional supervision.

• Biofeedback Training • Qigong

Hydrotherapy: Ice packs: apply repeatedly as needed to reduce thyroid function.

Juice Therapy: • Carrot, celery, spinach, parsley • Cabbage, watercress, and spinach

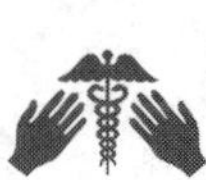

Professional Care

The following therapies should only be provided by a qualified health professional.

• Magnetic Field Therapy • Naturopathic Medicine • Traditional Chinese Medicine

Homeopathy: *Thyroidinum.*

Hypoglycemia

An abnormally low level of blood sugar (glucose), or abnormal fluctuations of blood sugar levels, secondary to an oversecretion of insulin by the pancreas (insulin acts to help clear blood of glucose).

Symptoms: Symptoms may vary from mild to severe, from once in a while to almost after every meal. They include: anxiety, weakness, sweating, rapid heart rate, extreme hunger, dizziness, poor or double vision, headache, irritability, irrational behavior, problems with memory, cognitive focus, and learning, and digestive problems. Most common time of symptoms to occur is in the afternoon around 2:00 to 3:00 P.M.

The symptoms of hypoglycemia mimic many other health problems. It may be that the symptoms are only similar or it may be that hypoglycemia is coexisting in the body with these other conditions, or is occurring secondary to these other health problems.

Occurrence: Classic hypoglycemia, the only type recognized by allopathic medicine, occurs in people with insulin dependent diabetes mellitus. However, in the alternative and orthomolecular fields, hypoglycemia is considered a well-established condition that occurs during the early stages of adrenal stress and blood sugar imbalance problems. It is associated with many other conditions than diabetes, can exist by itself, and may be the early stages of pancreatic and diabetic problems.

Consider: Excess consumption of simple sugars and refined carbohydrates, food allergies, low thyroid, nutrient deficiencies, especially of those that increase insulin sensitivity, such as vitamin B_6, chromium, zinc, essential fatty acids and some amino acids (such as alanine), excessive exercise, stress, missing meals or irregular eating habits, excessive alcohol, drug, or cigarette consumption, poor protein digestion, insufficient protein, poor digestion due to other factors, low digestive enzymes, and an excessively refined and processed diet.

Special Notes: Causes of hypoglycemia may be abnormal fluctuations of glucose and insulin and perhaps even abnormal reaction to normal fluctuations of glucose and insulin. These fluctuations or reactions may be secondary to many other factors, such as food allergies, lifestyle, nutrient levels, hereditary predisposition, etc. There is much controversy as to exactly what causes hypoglycemia, what it is, who gets it, why they get it, and what to do.

Cigarette smoking greatly aggravates stability of blood sugar. So does skipping breakfast, drinking more caffeinated beverages in the morning than is healthy for the body's pancreatic and adrenal response, eating a diet low in fiber and high in sugar. All these morning activities may create periods of low blood sugar in the mid to late afternoon, and are the most common cause of fatigue, poor concentration, and irritability at this time.

Alternative Treatments

Refer to alternative therapy chapters for more information before evaluating or applying any treatment. Some conditions, including yours, may require a physician's care.

Diet: Smaller more frequent meals (five to six) throughout the day to help keep blood glucose levels up and to help heal the pancreas and adrenals. Whole foods diet low in stressor foods such as caffeine, refined sugars, and alcohol. Focus on whole grains, seeds, nuts, fermented dairy products, and lean meats and fish.

If you cannot eat frequently enough, carry around raw seeds and nuts mixed with dried fruits or roasted tamarind nuts for flavor and munch these. Or try carrying some nut butter to eat on crackers. Identify and avoid food allergies. Avoid processed foods, dehydrated powders, and white flour products.

Eating high fiber also helps stabilize the possible fluctuations in the blood sugar. Thus, if you are having a hypoglycemic attack, take some high fiber food product with a small glass of fruit juice immediately. Eating some fiber, such as a whole grain cracker or a few bites of brown rice, one-half hour before meals with a few amino acid tablets, will often calm down reactions that tend to occur after eating or several hours after eating.

Nutrition: Chromium (100 mcg. three times daily), niacinamide, pantothenic acid, adrenal glandular, vitamin C with bioflavonoids, vitamin B complex, vitamin B_6, zinc, protein supplements (amino acids), calcium, magnesium, multi-trace minerals.

If due to malabsorption: HCl and/or digestive enzymes.

Vitamin B injections may be helpful; see an orthomolecular physician.

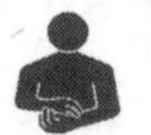

Self-Care

The following therapies can be undertaken at home under appropriate professional supervision.

• Biofeedback Training • Qigong

Herbs: Licorice, burdock, dandelion.

Hydrotherapy: Constitutional hydrotherapy: apply two to five times weekly.

Juice Therapy: If reactive then dilute all juices—carrot, beet with burdock, Jerusalem artichoke, garlic.

Reflexology: Pancreas, all glands, liver.

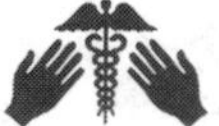

Professional Care

The following therapies should only be provided by a qualified health professional.

• Applied Kinesiology • Cell Therapy • Chiropractic • Magnetic Field Therapy • Naturopathic Medicine • Orthomolecular Medicine • Traditional Chinese Medicine

Environmental Medicine: According to Marshall Mandell, M.D., hypoglycemia is a commonly made misdiagnosis which can be applied to addictive food allergies. The withdrawal symptoms from a recent exposure to an addicting food are relieved by eating that particular food. On the surface it would seem that the relieving food has caused an increased level of blood sugar, but this is not so. The prompt relief is actually the result of an exposure to an addicting substance that relieves the withdrawal symptoms it was causing.

It takes between forty-five and sixty minutes for a protein food such as chicken, beef, nuts, or cheese to be broken down into amino acids: with the remaining portion converted into liver starch (glycogen). The glycogen is then broken down and released from the liver as blood sugar—glucose. The fact that protein foods can very rapidly give relief of "hypoglycemic" symptoms within five to ten minutes suggests that the mere introduction of these protein substances into the body will eliminate symptoms which cannot be related to blood sugar levels because there simply isn't enough time for the forty-five-to sixty-minute conversion to have taken place.

Fasting: In this condition the transition phase from beginning a fast to a state of health could be rougher than in other conditions. If juice fasting, dilute juices; if water fasting, see a physician.

Osteopathy: According to Michael Lesser, N.D., D.O., chronic muscular tensions brought about by stress throughout the body, particularly in the spinal regions, are a prime cause of hypoglycemia since when tense these tissues are burning fuel at a high rate, creating a constant requirement for glucose which the person may try to meet through sugar-rich snacks and stimulants.[12]

Hypothyroidism

Insufficient thyroid hormone, either by decreased production or increased breakdown, which is known as hypothyroidism.

Symptoms: Fatigue, weight gain, slowed heart rate, constipation, irritability, sensitivity to cold, mental depression, slowness or slurring of speech, drooping and swollen eyes, swollen face, recurrent infections, increase in allergic reaction, headaches, hair loss, brittleness of hair, female problems such as heavy menstrual flow, painful periods, and premenstrual tension, decreased immune functioning, and calcium metabolism problems. In childhood hypothyroidism can cause a retardation of normal growth and development.

Occurrence: This is a very common health problem. Hypothyroidism is recognized by medical doctors. However, unusual cases of hypothyroidism, such as borderline cases of underactive thyroid, or individuals who have normal laboratory levels of thyroid hormone, but, in their personal case, respond best and function optimally when supplemented with either thyroid nutrients or thyroid itself, are often unrecognized. Thus, they often go untreated. Undiagnosed thyroid problems can be the underlying cause in many reoccurring or nonresponsive health problems.

Consider: Food allergies, deficiencies of B vitamins, iron or digestive enzymes, liver disease, hormone imbalances, or parasites.

Special Notes: In Hashimoto's disease, the body becomes allergic to its thyroid gland and forms antibodies against it, causing low thyroid.

Home thyroid test: Keep basal thermometer by bedside. In the morning, before arising, lie still, and put thermometer under armpit and hold it there for fifteen minutes. A temperature below 97.5 degrees Fahrenheit may indicate a problem with the thyroid gland. Take the temperature in this manner for three days, except for the first few days of the menstrual cycle, and the middle day of the cycle, and calculate the average temperature. If it is consistently low, it is a suggestion that low thyroid may be a problem. The lower the temperature, the greater the degree of hypothyroidism.

Alternative Treatments

Refer to alternative therapy chapters for more information before evaluating or applying any treatment. Some conditions, including yours, may require a physician's care.

Diet: Consume foods that are naturally high in iodine such as fish, kelp, vegetables, and root vegetables such as potatoes. Avoid foods that naturally slow down the functioning of the thyroid such as: cabbage, brussels sprouts, mustard greens, broccoli, turnips, kale, spinach, peaches, and pears. Avoid sulfa drugs and antihistamines which aggravate this problem. If you are on thyroid medication, increase calcium supplementation, as studies show that the drug increases bone loss significantly. Also, increase daily consumption of foods high in vitamin B complex such as whole grains and raw nuts and seeds, and of vitamin A rich foods which are dark green and yellow vegetables, avoiding repetitive consumption of the ones mentioned above.

Nutritional Therapy: • Thyroid glandular • Tyrosine amino acid • Iodine • Vitamin B • Calcium/magnesium • Essential fatty acids • Vitamin A • Zinc

Self-Care

The following therapies can be undertaken at home under appropriate professional supervision.

• Biofeedback Training • Fasting • Qigong • Yoga

Herbs: Mild cases sometimes respond to herbal bitters such as gentian or mugwort. Kelp has been used in the past, but is only specifically helpful where an iodine deficiency is present. Associated constipation may be alleviated with yellowdock, butternut, or *cascara sagrada*. The antidepressant herb St. John's Wort can be helpful.

Homeopathy: *Calc carb.* 1M is effective in treating hypothyroidism and improving thyroid function.

Hydrotherapy: Contrast application: apply daily to stimulate thyroid function.

Juice Therapy: Never juice raw cabbage, broccoli, kale, cauliflower.

Lifestyle: Aerobic exercise is important.

Naturopathic Medicine: A commonly unrecognized cause of hypothyroidism is excessive consumption of brassica (cabbage) family foods. A component of the cabbage binds to iodine, making it unavailable to the thyroid gland for thyroid hormone production. Half a head of cabbage or the equivalent amount of broccoli, brussels sprouts, etc., can be as effective in binding iodine as the medical drug thiouracil used to treat hyperthyroidism, according to Joseph Pizzorono, N.D.

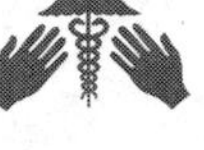

Professional Care

The following therapies should only be provided by a qualified health professional.

• Acupuncture • Cell Therapy • Magnetic Field Therapy • Naturopathic Medicine • Osteopathy • Traditional Chinese Medicine

Environmental Medicine: According to Marshall Mandell, M.D., hypothyroidism has been associated with the presence of allergies and correcting the underactive thyroid has been helpful to varying degrees.

Homeopathy: *Iodum*. Consult a physician.

Impotence

See Male Health chapter, page 733.

Infection

Growth of disease-causing organisms (bacteria, viruses, fungi) anywhere in the body. The organisms grow in colonies which are invasive, reproduce, and multiply. They can damage cells through a variety of routes, such as directly, through release of toxins, or through allergic reaction. Many of the symptoms of the infection are usually a result of the immune system mounting a response to these foreign colonies.

Symptoms: Redness, inflammation, pain, swelling, and formation of pus-filled pockets (abscess) at the site of the infection. If fever and painful joints occur, this may be a sign of an infectious disease that is spreading throughout the body and a doctor must be seen at once.

Alternative Treatments

Refer to alternative therapy chapters for more information before evaluating or applying any treatment. Some conditions, including yours, may require a physician's care.

Diet: Increase dietary garlic and unflavored yogurt. Increase diluted orange juice, apples and apple juice, grapes and grape juice, cranberries, blueberries, strawberries, raspberries, peaches, plums, figs, cabbage, onion, kelp, and raw honey. During infection and recovery time avoid refined sugar as this may depress natural immune response. Drink plenty of filtered water.

Nutritional Therapy: According to Garry Gordon, M.D., the following can be effectively used as an antibiotic replacement, particularly if used at the first sign of any cold or flu or other infectious process: • Vitamin A (400,000 IU daily for five days) • Liquid garlic extract (up to two four-ounce bottles a day) or the equivalent in high quality garlic in capsules or tablets (at least thirty to eighty daily) • Vitamin C to bowel tolerance (See Orthomolecular Medicine chapter, page 402.)

This protocol is to be used only under a physician's guidance. The dosages are for an average 175-pound adult and should be scaled down proportionately according to weight. The vitamin A should be taken for a period of at least three days, but no more than five.

Caution: *Vitamin A at such high doses can cause headaches in about 1 percent of those using it. Should this occur, either decrease the dose or use a natural remedy like feverfew or a homeopathic remedy for headaches.*

Bacterial: Vitamin C bowel tolerance technique of Robert F. Cathcart, M.D. (See Orthomolecular Medicine chapter, page 402.)

Alan R. Gaby, M.D., has found that acute infections respond well to an intravenous injection of a "cocktail" composed of magnesium chloride hexahydrate, calcium glycerophosphate, hydroxocobalamin, pyridoxine hydrochloride (vitamin B_6), dexpanthenol, B complex, and vitamin C. (This is a modification of the nutrient cocktail popularized by John Myers, M.D.)

Self-Care

The following therapies can be undertaken at home under appropriate professional supervision.

• Guided Imagery

Aromatherapy: *Fungicidal infections:* cedarwood. *Infected wounds:* frankincense, tea tree, patchouli.

Fasting: Leon Chaitow, N.D., D.O., suggests a water-only fast for twenty-four to thirty-six hours at the onset of any infection as it has a dramatic effect on the immune system, enhancing natural killer cell and other defensive immune activity. This is only true if the fast is a water-only regime.

Caution: *This is not appropriate for the very frail or very young unless supervised by an expert in these methods, such as a naturopathic or alternative physician.*

Herbs**:** Herbs such as echinacea, goldenseal, and garlic can prevent and treat infection. In small amounts taken regularly they boost resistance. Larger doses combat specific infections. Stress must be treated as it has a direct impact on immunity. In addition to working with a stress management program, use adaptogenic herbs such as Siberian ginseng. Also select the appropriate herb(s) most suited for the particular sight of infection: Garlic for the lungs, bearberry for bladder infections, myrrh topically for the skin. Echinacea can be taken internally as a tea or used externally as a poultice or wash on infectious sores.

Hydrotherapy: Constitutional hydrotherapy: apply one to two times daily depending on severity of infection.

Juice Therapy: Carrot, celery, beet, also cantaloupe.

Naturopathic Medicine: In general, goldenseal is the most useful herb for bacterial infections and licorice root the most useful herb for viral infections.

Reflexology: Adrenals, lymph system, region or area affected.

Professional Care

The following therapies should only be provided by a qualified health professional.

• Cell Therapy • Craniosacral Therapy • Environmental Medicine • Magnetic Field Therapy • Naturopathic Medicine • Traditional Chinese Medicine

Detoxification Therapy: May be indicated, depending on the person's condition. Control infection first.

Oxygen Therapy: • Hydrogen peroxide therapy (IV) • Hyperbaric oxygen therapy is a powerful antibiotic. • Ozone is a wide spectrum antibacterial, antiviral, and antifungal agent at concentrations which spare normal tissues.

Inflammation

Redness, swelling, pain, and heat, in localized areas of the body, due to tissue injury secondary to disease process, or trauma from physical, infectious, or chemical insult.

Symptoms*:* Any part of the body can be affected, internal or external.

Special Notes: Elevate and if necessary splint the affected area. Apply heat and or ice alternating, or herbal poultices, rest, take necessary antibiotics if bacterial infection, and consume a whole foods diet with emphasis on raw foods, plenty of fresh juices and filtered water, and rest, if the inflammation is severe.

According to Leon Chaitow, N.D., D.O., inflammation is a natural and potentially beneficial response of the body to factors which are irritating or damaging it. The use of anti-inflammatory drugs against arthritis has shown that over a period of years people using this medication have worse damage to their joints than people not having any treatment at all. This is because, unpleasant as it may be, the inflammation of the joints in arthritis actually precedes a degree of normalization of the damaged surface.

When inflammation is excessive or chronic it is useful to modify it, but always by methods which cause no further problems and always in the knowledge that the inflammation can be a useful and natural response to whatever is causing damage to the body.

Alternative Treatments

Refer to alternative therapy chapters for more information before evaluating or applying any treatment. Some conditions, including yours, may require a physician's care.

Diet: Whole foods diet or 75 percent raw foods diet. If there is chronic inflammation, you may consider a simple mono-diet for two to four days, eating fresh fruits and vegetables and whole grains only, with lots of filtered water. Cut down or avoid sugar, white flour, junk foods, colas. Drink plenty of fluids. Increase dietary garlic and yogurt. Glass of water with one teaspoon of fresh lemon and one teaspoon of liquid chlorophyll on rising and before bed. At least one glass of fresh vegetable juice or green drink a day with lots of homemade soups containing many vegetables and potatoes. One teaspoon of honey taken once a day and even applied locally is excellent as it has antiseptic, antimicrobial, and antibiotic characteristics. Use only raw honey for this purpose.

Nutrition: Vitamin C with bioflavonoids (3 grams first hour and then 1 gram every two hours for first few days and then keep to 3-6 grams per day), zinc (30-60 mg. daily), beta-carotene (100,000 IU first three days then reduce to 25,000 IU for several weeks). evening primrose oil, garlic capsules, vitamin A and E emulsion, silicea, mineral complex with calcium.

Proteolytic enzymes are often effective for severe or chronic inflammations and may be taken even if antibiotics are used. (Four, four times daily for several days to one week, taken away from meals in larger than normal dosages to act as anti-inflammatory agents.) If proteolytic enzymes bother gastrointestinal tract try Bromelain in large dosages such as 1 gram, but still take on empty stomach away from meals.

Dr. Leon Chaitow's nutritional strategy is as follows:

Inflammation as a phenomenon depends upon the presence of substances called leukotrienes which the body manufactures from arachidonic acid (an essential fatty acid). The vast majority of arachidonic acid in the body derives from animal proteins and fats, and a simple nutritional strategy which reduces or eliminates these from the diet can markedly reduce inflammation when it is excessive or chronic.

Another way of helping this to take place is to eat oily fish (mackerel, herring, salmon) and/or to take supplementally eicosapentaenoic acid (EPA) capsules derived from such fish. EPA reduces the production of leukotrienes.

Cutting out red meat and poultry skin, as well as full-fat dairy products, and eating fish can improve the levels of inflammation being experienced.

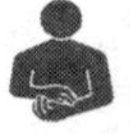

Self-Care

The following therapies can be undertaken at home under appropriate professional supervision.

• Fasting • Guided Imagery • Reflexology

Aromatherapy: Chamomile, lavender, frankincense, myrrh.

Herbs: A range of anti-inflammatory herbs are available and should be selected depending upon the site of the inflammation. For example in the lining of the digestive system use herbs such as chamomile, lemon balm, licorice, or meadowsweet. For the skin use calendula, St. John's Wort, or plantain. For rheumatic or arthritic problems use willow bark, meadowsweet, or wild yam.

Homeopathy: *Aconite, Belladonna, Ferrum phos., Sulfur.*

Hydrotherapy: • Contrast application: apply daily. *In early stages of inflammation:* place ice bag over inflamed area or immerse in ice water.

Juice Therapy: • Currents, black/red grapes, flaxseed oil added to combined vegetable juices • Pineapple

Professional Care

The following therapies should only be provided by a qualified health professional.

• Cell Therapy • Craniosacral Therapy • Light Therapy • Pancreatic Enzyme

Therapy • Naturopathic Medicine

Acupuncture: Increases endorphin levels in joints and other regions of the body, and therefore may be highly effective in treating inflammatory disease conditions.[13]

Detoxification Therapy: Inflammation is usually a congested condition, but detox depends on the specifics of the situation, in other words, what is the problem in the body?

Light Therapy: Cold (soft) laser photo stimulation therapy.

Magnetic Field Therapy: Exposure to negative magnetic field may help reduce inflammation.

Oxygen Therapy: • Hydrogen peroxide therapy • Hyperbaric oxygen may be helpful in some cases.

Insect Bites

Allergic reactions to stings from insects from the order Hymenoptera. The most common sting problems are from yellow jackets and honeybees. Other insects are hornets, bumblebees, ants, wasps, and spiders.

Symptoms: Swelling, redness, pain, dizziness, loss of breath, anxiety.

Special Notes: Though it takes the venom of one hundred bees to create a fatal dose for most adults, one bee sting may cause a fatal allergic reaction in a hypersensitive individual. In the United States, there are three to four times more deaths from bee stings than snake bites. The venom in these cases causes the heart to collapse. People with known hypersensitivities should carry a kit containing antihistamine and epinephrine when in areas likely to hold risk.

Desensitization can be carried out by qualified supervision in a manner very similar to other allergic desensitization techniques.

If you are experiencing symptoms such as flushing, generalized hives, swelling around the neck or tongue, difficulty breathing, faintness, or loss of consciousness or diarrhea, immediately consult your personal physician or go to the emergency room, as this may indicate a severe reaction to the sting.

Alternative Treatments

Refer to alternative therapy chapters for more information before evaluating or applying any treatment. Some conditions, including yours, may require a physician's care.

Nutritional Therapy: • Vitamin C as soon as possible (5 grams) with vitamin B_5 (1 gram) • Continue to take 1 gram of vitamin C and 500 mg. of B_5, every hour until pain and swelling go down. • Vitamin E (apply oil to sting)

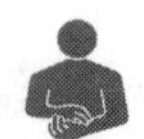

Self-Care

The following therapies can be undertaken at home under appropriate professional supervision.

Aromatherapy: According to Jean Valnet, M.D., basil, cinnamon, garlic, lavender, lemon, onion, sage, savory, and thyme are effective due to their antitoxic and antivenomous properties. Lavender may be effective in treating itching from stings.

Ayurveda: • Drink cilantro juice. • Apply sandalwood paste to sting.

Flower Remedies: Rescue Remedy.

Herbs: Apply the fresh bruised leaf, or juice, of plantain to the sting. Aloe gel can also be applied.

Homeopathy: *Immediately: Aconite, Lachesis, Apis mel., Hypericum, Urtica Urens. Insect bites: Ledum, Hypericum, Calendula. Wasp stings: Apis mel., Calendula.*

Hydrotherapy: Cold compress as needed to reduce pain and swelling.

Practical Hints: If you have a severe allergy to insect stings you should take preventive measures when outdoors. Wear slacks, footwear, and gloves while gardening and avoid cosmetics, perfumes, and hairsprays if you are going to be outdoors.

Topical Treatment: According to Leon Chaitow, N.D., D.O., apply vinegar or lemon juice or paste made of bicarbonate of soda as soon as possible to neutralize the venom. The pulped heads and buds of marigolds (calendula) make a tincture (preserved in alcohol) which may be applied to stings and other surface injuries. The pulped fresh (marigold) flower may also be applied directly to a sting and bandaged in place.

• Crush a charcoal tablet on a cotton ball, place over sting, and cover with bandage to reduce pain and swelling. • Use ice packs to relieve pain and swelling and to keep the poison from spreading. • *Wasp stings:* apply vinegar immediately. • To remove a bee stinger, try to scrape and lift it out with the dull edge of a knife or a credit card. • After removing stinger treat with a strong cold solution of three parts baking soda and one part water. If there is no access to any of the above listed items, mud applied to the sting will help draw out toxins as it dries. • To help deactivate the toxin from the stinger apply a deodorant containing aluminum.

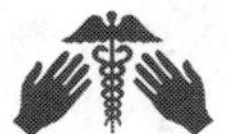

Professional Care

The following therapies should only be provided by a qualified health professional.

• Environmental Medicine • Light Therapy • Naturopathic Medicine • Orthomolecular Therapy

Insomnia

See Sleep Disorders chapter, page 838.

Irritable Bowel Syndrome

See Gastrointestinal chapter, page 685.

Jaundice

Yellowing of the skin, the whites of the eyes (sclerae), and other tissues, which is not a disease itself but usually a major signal of disease within the liver and biliary (gallbladder) system.

Symptoms: Sometimes jaundice is the only sign. Other symptoms may accompany yellowing, such as darkening of the urine, nausea, vomiting, abdominal pain, pale colored feces, holding fluid in the trunk of the body, digestive problems, generalized rashes, and severe fatigue. All these symptoms mean a doctor must be seen immediately.

Special Notes: The yellowing is due to increased circulation in the body of bilirubin in the blood. This is a yellow-brown pigment, thus the color. Normally, bilirubin should be cleared from the blood by the liver and excreted in the feces as bile, which partly gives feces the dark brownish color. When this process is not happening normally, the brownish bilirubin builds up in the blood and decreases in the stools.

Jaundice usually signals the following disorders: hepatitis, cirrhosis of the liver, breakdown of blood (hemolysis), problems in gallbladder or bile ducts (due to stones, inflammation, tumor or infection), and pernicious anemia (secondary to B_{12} deficiency). Neonatal jaundice (at birth) is common and usually is not a serious health problem.

With any of the above symptoms, blood tests need to be run right away. Other tests may also be needed, such as liver biopsy or ultrasound scanning of the liver.

Alternative Treatments

Refer to alternative therapy chapters for more information before evaluating or applying any treatment. Some conditions, including yours, may require a physician's care.

Diet: Raw diluted vegetable juice fasting or consuming mainly raw foods may be beneficial during acute stage (first several weeks). Continue to consume largely raw food diet with lots of fruits and vegetables for one month after this. *To help liver and biliary system (bile-conveying structures):* Upon arising take a glass of warm water with juice of one-half lemon. Eat plenty of raw apples and pears or grate together with yogurt and raw seeds or seed and nut butter. Consume plenty of raw green vegetables and sprouts to help cleanse blood. Try drinking barley water throughout day. (One cup of barley in three quarts of water. Simmer for three hours.) Avoid all hydrogenated and processed fats and deep fried foods.

Nutritional Therapy: • Lipotrophic formula • Liver glandular • Digestive enzymes with bile if stools are pale • Vitamin C • Vitamin B complex • Protein supplements • Essential fatty acids

Neonatal: Apply vitamin E oil to breast nipple at least three times a day.

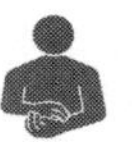

Self-Care

The following therapies can be undertaken at home under appropriate professional supervision.

• Fasting • Qigong

Aromatherapy: Geranium, rosemary, lemon.

Ayurveda: *Acute hepatitis:* Avoid hot, sour, spicy, and salty foods, meat, fish, cheese, oils, fried foods, and concentrated sweets. Try a mono-diet of mung beans for one week to strengthen liver. Add basmati rice and liver-cleansing spices such as coriander and tumeric. Take complete rest and avoid vigorous exercise. *Chronic hepatitis:* Take tonics such as aloe gel, *shatavari,* and the formula *chyavan prash.* • An herbal mixture of: *kutki* 200 mg., *guduchi* 300 mg., and *shanka pushpi* 400 mg., generally taken twice a day after lunch and dinner. For all types, fresh sugarcane juice, one cup three times a day, one-half cup fresh homemade yogurt with a pinch of baking soda twice a day, and *brahmi ghee nasya.*

Enemas: Alternate coffee and water enemas daily.

Herbs: • Jaundice can be a symptom of different conditions and so these suggestions do not replace competent diagnosis. Combine the glycerites (herb mixed in a glycerin solution) of milk thistle, dandelion root, fringetree bark, and boldo in equal parts and take one-half a teaspoonful of this mixture three times a day. An infusion of chickweed or distilled witch hazel applied topically will reduce itching. • Aloe vera gel, barberry, chamomile, dandelion, gentian root, goldenseal, neem, parsley, rose hips, yellowdock

Homeopathy: *Bryonia, Cinchona, Merc sol., Chelidonium, Nat phos., Kali bich., Chamomilla* (babies), *Phosphorus, Nux vom.*

Hydrotherapy: • Constitutional hydrotherapy: apply daily. • Foot and hand baths with a handful each of celandine leaves, artichoke leaves, dog's tooth roots, and a half-handful each of chicory leaves and dandelion flowers in two quarts water.

Juice Therapy: • Carrot and beet juice with a little radish and/or dandelion root juice added • Grapes, pear, lemon • Carrot, celery, parsley • Carrot, beet, cucumber

Reflexology: Liver.

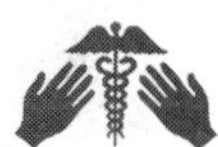

Professional Care

The following therapies should only be provided by a qualified health professional.

• Colon Therapy • Cell Therapy • Magnetic Field Therapy • Naturopathic Medicine • Osteopathy • Traditional Chinese Medicine

Detoxification Therapy: Not indicated. Evaluate the state of the body and the cause of the jaundice, and then detox may be helpful.

Light Therapy: Neonatal jaundice may be treated with exposure to full-spectrum light or blue light.

Kidney Stones

Stones anywhere in the entire urinary tract (kidney, bladder, ducts between and elsewhere [ureters]), may become blocked with stones (renal or urinary calculi).

Symptoms*:* May have no symptoms (called "silent"), or have a variety of symptoms, depending on where the stone is located and its size. Possible symptoms are: sudden severe and excruciating back pain which may come and go (intermittent), and often radiates from the back across the abdomen and into the genital area or inner thighs. This pain may be associated with nausea, vomiting, abdominal bloating, possible blood in urine, pain on urination, and chills and fever. Stones in the urinary tract can be one of the most painful conditions known to human kind, similar to the pain of childbirth.

Occurrence: One in every one thousand adults per year is hospitalized for urinary tract stones. One percent of autopsies reveals urinary stones. Stones tend to reoccur. About 60 percent of stone formers will have another stone episode within seven years.

Special Notes: The stones are formed from precipitation from a number of mineral salt solutions in the urine. In the United States the most common component (70 percent) of stones is calcium (oxalate) and/or phosphate that has come out of solution. Higher than normal levels of oxalate in the urine, related to a high dietary intake of oxalic containing foods, such as rhubarb, spinach, leafy vegetables, and coffee, may promote stone formation. Stones that are high in calcium may be one of the first signals of the body that there is a condition called hyperparathyroidism (excessive secretion of parathyroid hormone).

Research shows that soft drinks containing phosphoric acid encourage the recurrence of kidney stones in some persons.[14]

Consider: Stones are more common during the summer. This may be due to concentrated urine secondary to increased sweating and insufficient fluids to make up for this. Mild chronic dehydration may play a role in the development of stones. High levels of dietary refined carbohydrates may also encourage stone formation as the sugar stimulates the pancreatic release of insulin. This stimulates, in turn, increased calcium excretion through the urine. Other factors that also cause increased calcium excretion in the urine (hypercalciuria) and may promote stone formation are increased dietary levels of coffee, colas, acid-forming diets, such as high protein and grains with insufficient alkalinizing vegetables and fruits, insufficient fluids such as water, excessive salt consumption, stress, and insufficient amounts of magnesium which helps keep calcium in solution.

Diet alone cannot get rid of the stones. You must see a doctor.

This condition may be genetically influenced. If one parent was a stone former there is an increased risk in the children.

Cadmium toxicity may also play a role in stone formation and needs to be assessed.

Alternative Treatments

Refer to alternative therapy chapters for more

information before evaluating or applying any treatment. Some conditions, including yours, may require a physician's care.

Diet: The four most important dietary actions are: increase fluids, increase fiber, increase green vegetables, and reduce refined sugar consumption.

Must increase filtered water to at least eight glasses or more per day. Increase to point where two to three quarts of urine are produced daily. Increase green vegetables which are high in magnesium. Vegetarian-oriented diets may be helpful to prevent reoccurrences. Studies have shown that vegetarians have a 40 to 60 percent decreased risk of stones and that meat intake is correlated with calcium oxalate stone formation.[15] Foods that are helpful in decreasing stone formation are: cranberries, black cherries, rice bran, kombucha tea. It is helpful to reduce the following in the diet: salt, sugar, dairy products, caffeine, alcohol, refined carbohydrates, nuts, chocolate, pepper. Limit protein intake.

Many experts believe that if stones are of the calcium kind dairy, produce, and other rich sources of calcium should be reduced. New research shows that this may not be necessary, and that normal dietary levels of calcium do not in and of themselves encourage stones, and may actually be protective.[16] A safe strategy would be to keep calcium intake at normal levels (any supplementation should be of citrate, gluconate, lactate, or carbonate forms which alkalize the urine reducing calcium secretion) while dealing with the other factors which are known to encourage stone formation—reducing meat intake, high sugar consumptions, and making sure of adequate levels of magnesium in the diet, along with optimal fluid intake and potassium rich foods such as fruit and vegetables.

If, however, you are a stone former and you have consumed large amounts of dairy products, consider limiting dairy products and boiling water for ten minutes before drinking as this lowers calcium content by precipitating calcium carbonate.

If the stones are high in oxalates avoid foods containing or producing oxalic acid such as spinach, beets, parsley, Swiss chard, cabbage, rhubarb, and coffee. Also avoid vitamin C over 6 grams per day, which may increase oxalate excretion. Asparagus contains "asparagine" which helps in breaking up oxalate crystals. Option: Take one spoonful lemon juice each half hour for two days to help take "rough edge" off kidney stones and flush them out.

Nutritional Therapy: • Magnesium (200 mg. two times daily) • Vitamin B_6 (50 mg. three times daily) • Vitamin C (over 6 grams per day may be harmful for this condition by increasing oxalate formation) • Vitamin A • Proteolytic enzymes (away from meals) • Raw kidney glandular • Fat-soluble chlorophyll • Lysine (deficiency may increase calcium excretion in the urine)

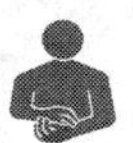

Self-Care

The following therapies can be undertaken at home under appropriate professional supervision.

• Fasting

Aromatherapy: Hyssop, juniper.

Ayurveda: Drink well-cooked barley soup with a pinch of *dugdapachan bhasma* or one-quarter teaspoon of *gokshura* and two pinches *mutral churna* or one-quarter teaspoon of *punarnava*, generally taken one cup three times a day.

For general kidney disorders, an herbal mixture of: *punarnava* 500 mg., *gokshura* 300 mg., *kamadudha* 200 mg., and *jatamansi* 200 mg. generally taken twice a day after lunch and dinner. *Punarnava guggulu* 200 mg. or *gokshura guggulu* 200 mg., generally taken two times a day after lunch and dinner. Cumin, coriander, fennel tea, generally taken one cup three times a day.

Herbs: Combine the tinctures of gravel root, cornsilk, wild yam, blackhaw in equal parts and take one teaspoonful of this mixture three times a day. Drink one cup of an infusion of nettle three times a day.

Homeopathy: *Berberis, Sarsaparilla.*

Hydrotherapy: Constitutional hydrotherapy: apply two to five times weekly, or hot pack to abdomen and low back (apply ten to fifteen minutes several times daily for relief of colicky pain).

Juice Therapy: • Lemon juice • Carrot, beet, and cucumber juice (add some garlic and/or horseradish to carrot) • Cranberry, watermelon

Mind/Body Therapy: Relaxation.

Reflexology: Ureter tubes, kidneys, bladder, diaphragm, parathyroid.

Professional Care

The following therapies should only be provided by a qualified health professional.

Detoxification Therapy: Detoxification may

be indicated. Take fluids and control mineral balance. Usually the person is congestive.

Nonsurgical Alternatives: Lithotripsy therapy: In this treatment kidney stones are shattered by ultra short sound waves, allowing the fragments to be passed in the urine.

Laryngitis

Inflammation of the larynx (the voice box: upper part of the windpipe, below root of tongue [pharynx] and at top of trachea [windpipe]).

Symptoms: Hoarseness of the voice, loss of voice, rawness, constant urge to clear throat, tickling sensation at the back of the throat, pain, possible fatigue, difficulty swallowing, and fever.

Consider: Viral, candidiasis/yeast, and bacterial infections (viral is most common and is not helped by antibiotics), excessive use of voice, screaming, rage, allergies and/or low-grade chronic allergies, inhalation of irritating substances, and secondary to illnesses such as flu, bronchitis, measles, diphtheria, and pneumonia.

Alternative Treatments

Refer to alternative therapy chapters for more information before evaluating or applying any treatment. Some conditions, including yours, may require a physician's care.

Diet: Whole foods diet with plenty of fluids, raw fruits, and vegetables. Decrease or avoid intake of refined carbohydrates.

Nutritional Therapy: • Vitamin A (100,000 IU for first three days) • Vitamin C • Garlic capsules • Zinc lozenges • Use acidophilus if taking antibiotics.

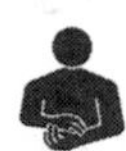

Self-Care

The following therapies can be undertaken at home under appropriate professional supervision.

• ***Guided Imagery***

Aromatherapy: Inhalations with benzoin, lavender, frankincense, thyme, and sandalwood.

Herbs: A gargle made from an infusion of red sage and yarrow will alleviate the discomfort. Do not swallow. Alternative herbs would be chamomile or cranesbill. Internally take thirty drops of echinacea tincture every hour for two days. • Gargle with bayberry or sage tea.

Hydrotherapy: Contrast application: apply one to two times daily to neck and throat, or heating compress (apply one to two times daily to neck and throat).

Homeopathy: *Aconite, Hepar sulph., Phosphorus, Spongia, Causticum, Belladonna, Kali bich., Drosera, Carbo veg.*

Juice Therapy: • Carrot, pineapple • Carrot, apple • Carrot, celery • Carrot, beet, cucumber, ginger

Naturopathic Medicine: Gargle with a tea made from licorice (*Glycyrrhiza glabra*) root.

Reflexology: Throat, chest/lung, diaphragm, lymph system, all toes.

Topical Treatment: Cold compress on throat.

Professional Care

The following therapies should only be provided by a qualified health professional.

• ***Acupuncture*** • ***Environmental Medicine*** • ***Light Therapy*** • ***Magnetic Field Therapy*** • ***Naturopathic Medicine*** • ***Osteopathy*** • ***Traditional Chinese Medicine***

Detoxification Therapy: May be indicated, depending on the condition of the person. Acute infections will not be helped. Evaluate the cause.

Oxygen Therapy: • Hydrogen peroxide therapy (IV) • Ozonated water gargles may be helpful.

Longevity

To increase the duration and quality of life.

Alternative Treatments

Refer to alternative therapy chapters for more information before evaluating or applying any treatment. Some conditions, including yours, may require a physician's care.

Diet: Consume a whole foods diet with emphasis on live foods: plenty of raw fruits and vegetables, sprouts, raw nuts, raw seeds, and whole grains. Foods that the scientific literature associates with increased longevity and decreased chronic degenerative illness are: natural foods high in fiber, olive oil, garlic, fermented foods such as yogurt, kefir, sauerkraut, goat's milk products rather than cow's, grains such as millet, buckwheat, quinoa, and amaranth, and raw seeds such as sunflower and pumpkin.

Nutritional Therapy: Sufficient and wide variety of nutrients of all kinds: • Multivitamin/mineral supplements • Essential fatty acids and digestive enzymes if necessary • Vitamin A • Vitamin C • Vitamin E • Vitamin B_6 • Garlic capsules • Kelp • Super-oxide dismutase (SOD) • Green magma • Eicosapentaenoic acid (EPA) • Gamma-linolenic acid (GLA) • evening primrose oil • Coenzyme Q10.

The only consistent success in producing longevity, in all species of animal tested, results from dietary patterns which provide reduced caloric intake alongside optimal intake of all essential nutrients and decreased environmental temperature.

Self-Care

The following therapies can be undertaken at home under appropriate professional supervision.

• Fasting • Guided Imagery • Qigong

Herbs: • Ginseng, *Gingko biloba,* gotu kola.

Homeopathy: *Arsen alb., Thuja, Hydrocotyle.*

Hydrotherapy: Spray/shower: apply daily following regular hot cleansing shower.

Juice Therapy: • Fresh fruit and vegetable juices • Wheat grass juice • Apricot, lemon, lime, papaya, pineapple

Lifestyle: Exercise in fresh air.

Professional Care

The following therapies should only be provided by a qualified health professional.

• Cell Therapy • Magnetic Field Therapy • Naturopathic Medicine

Bodywork: • Acupressure, *shiatsu,* massage.

Detoxification Therapy: Detoxification may be indicated as part of the process of antiaging, long-term health, and vitality.

Oxygen Therapy: Hydrogen peroxide therapy.

Lazy Eye

See Vision Disorders chapter, page 861.

Lung Cancer

See Respiratory Conditions chapter, page 817.

Lupus

This is a chronic, inflammatory, autoimmune (the body is attacking itself) disease that affects connective tissue (tissue that binds and supports various structures of the body and also includes the blood). Discoid lupus erythematosus (DLE) is a less serious type, affecting exposed areas of the skin and sometimes the joints. Systemic lupus erythematosus (SLE) is more serious, potentially fatal, and affects more organs of the body.

Symptoms: Symptoms vary according to the severity of the illness and which organs are affected. SLE may occur very abruptly with a fever and mimic an acute infection or it may occur very slowly over months and years with only several episodes of fever and fatigue.

Most people with SLE complain of pain in various joints that mimics arthritis, or in children simulates growing pains. In adults, there is often a history of growing pains. Over time, muscular contraction may deform the joints.

Many patients have rashes on the face or other areas, such as the neck, upper chest, and elbows. In DLE, the rash starts as red, circular, thickened areas that leave scars, most often affect the face and scalp, and may cause permanent hair loss. In SLE, there is a characteristic "butterfly-shaped" rash that occurs on the cheeks and over the bridge of the nose. Rashes in SLE patients do not scar and do not cause permanent hair loss.

Ulcers on mucous membranes such as the mouth and nose are common. Rashes and swelling of the hands and fingers may occur. Sensitivity to light (photophobia) occurs in 40 percent of people with SLE. Other problems may be kidney disorders, repetitive episodes of pleurisy (inflammation of lining of the lungs), pericarditis (inflammation of the membrane surrounding the heart), iron deficiency, anemia, and pulmonary hypertension (high blood pressure). Swelling of several or more lymph nodes is common especially in children.

SLE is classified as mild if the symptoms are mainly fever, joint pain, rash, headaches, pleurisy, and pericarditis. It is considered severe if it is associated with life-threatening diseases. Mild SLE may respond well to natural therapies. Aspirin may be useful but in high dosages in people with SLE may cause liver toxicity. Antimalarials (used to treat malaria) may help in conditions where joint and rash symptoms are predominant.

Severe SLE requires immediate corticosteroid therapy.

Occurrence: Occurs mostly in young women (90 percent of cases) and in young children.

Consider: Rule out food allergies, rheumatoid arthritis, other connective tissue diseases, parasites, candidiasis, bowel problems, and digestive enzyme deficiencies that may create symptoms that mimic SLE, or worsen SLE. Rule out migraines, epilepsy, and psychoses.

Special Notes: SLE is often chronic, with periods of improvement and relapse over many years. Sometimes there are years of remission in between periods of symptoms.

Blood tests for antinuclear antibodies (ANA) and sometimes skin biopsies are diagnostic for this condition.

According to the American Rheumatoid Association there must be four of the following eight symptoms present for lupus to be diagnosed: ANA antibodies in blood, low white blood cell or platelet count or hemolytic anemia, joint pain in a number of joints (arthritis), butterfly rash on cheeks, abnormal cells in the urine, light sensitivity, mouth sores, and seizure or psychosis.

Some drugs give a false positive test (looks like SLE): hydralazine, procainamide, and beta blockers. Sometimes these drugs produce a lupus-like condition that goes away when the drug is stopped.

Birth control pills may cause flare-ups of lupus. Treatments are aimed at decreasing symptoms. Allopathic medicine does not consider there to be a cure for lupus, but naturally oriented physicians report "cures" of lupus by eliminating causes and treating the body as a whole.

Alternative Treatments

Refer to alternative therapy chapters for more information before evaluating or applying any treatment. Some conditions, including yours, may require a physician's care.

Diet: Whole foods diet. Avoid overeating (more frequent smaller meals is suggested), limit cow's milk and beef products, increase vegetables (especially green, yellow, and orange), and consume fish several times a week. Avoid alfalfa sprouts or tablets which contain L-canavanine sulfate, a substance that may aggravate lupus.

Avoid L-tryptophan supplementation which may produce substances in the body which may promote the autoimmune process.

Assess and treat for food and chemical allergies.

According to Leon Chaitow, N.D., D.O., hydrochloric acid deficiency is common in people with lupus. Supplementation of this with meals can help, or stimulation of natural production can be achieved by careful use of specific herbs such as the "Swedish bitters" combination.

Nutritional Therapy: • Vitamin C and bioflavonoids • Proteolytic enzymes (away from meals on empty stomach) • Digestive enzymes with meals if necessary • Calcium • Magnesium • Zinc • Essential fatty acids • Amino acids: L-cysteine, L-methionine, L-cystine • Beta-carotene and vitamin A for DLE • Vitamin E (1,500 IU daily) • Garlic capsules • Vitamin B complex • Vitamin B_5 • Vitamin B_{12} (intramuscular injection 1,000 mcg. IM two times weekly) • Selenium

According to Johnathan Wright, M.D.:

1) Vitamin B_6 in high doses (500 mg. three times daily) can be very useful in reducing symptoms.

2) Over 80 percent of SLE patients are severely hypochlorhydric (diminished secretion of hydrochloric acid in stomach).

3) One hundred percent of all SLE patients have food allergies and improve with appropriate identification and treatment.

4) Over 50 percent of women with SLE have levels of testosterone and DHEA lower than other women (not men) and improve with appropriate treatment.

Self-Care

The following therapies can be undertaken at home under appropriate professional supervision.

• Biofeedback Training • Fasting • Guided Imagery • Qigong

Herbs: • Mix equal parts of the tinctures of the Chinese herbs *Bupleurum falcatum,* licorice, and wild yam. Take one teaspoonful of this mixture three times a day. Drink an infusion of nettle twice a day. In addition, as this autoimmune condition can manifest with a range of symptoms, this should be treated with the relevant herbs as they arise. • Echinacea, goldenseal, pau d'arco, red clover

Hydrotherapy: Constitutional hydrotherapy: apply two to five times weekly.

Juice Therapy: Carrot, celery, can add flaxseed oil, black currant oil, garlic.

Reflexology: All glands, intestines, liver, whole spine.

Topical Treatment: PABA cream.

Professional Care

The following therapies should only be provided by a qualified health professional.

• Cell Therapy • Chelation Therapy • Environmental Medicine • Pancreatic Enzyme Therapy • Magnetic Field Therapy • Naturopathic Medicine • Rolfing • Traditional Chinese Medicine

Detoxification Therapy: May be indicated, depending on the condition of the person.

Light Therapy: PUVA therapy.

Oxygen Therapy: • Hydrogen peroxide therapy (IV) • Hyperbaric oxygen therapy

Macular Degeneration

See Vision Disorders chapter, page 861.

Male Health

See Male Health chapter, page 733.

Measles

See Children's Health chapter, page 607.

Memory and Cognition Problems

Inability to focus mentally and utilize one's mental capabilities successfully and on demand.

Symptoms: Poor mental focus, poor learning, poor memory, difficulty following information, conversation or train of thought.

Consider: Allergies, candidiasis, thyroid disorders, stroke or poor circulation to brain, amino acid imbalance, low blood sugar, poor mental habits and laziness requiring tutoring in learning techniques. (It is possible that coping strategies taught one to forget and not to think rather than to be able to concentrate.)

Alternative Treatments

Refer to alternative therapy chapters for more information before evaluating or applying any treatment. Some conditions, including yours, may require a physician's care.

Diet: Whole foods diet including fish and adequate protein. Avoidance of food allergies or other allergies that may cause cerebral allergies which may contribute to poor concentration. Consider a diet associated with hypoglycemia as low blood sugar problems may be a contributing factor. Lots of filtered water daily.

Nutritional Therapy: • Supercholine • If low blood sugar: chromium • Protein supplements or amino acids • Pantothenic Acid • Vitamin B complex. Identification of amino acid imbalance may be helpful.

Self-Care

The following therapies can be undertaken at home under appropriate professional supervision.

• Fasting • Flower Remedies • Qigong • Yoga

Herbs: • Ginkgo leaf extract • Mix one teaspoon each of skullcap and gotu kola with hot water for improved awareness.

Homeopathy: *Argen nit., Arsen alb.*

Hydrotherapy: Cold compress: apply as needed to the face and hands. Constitutional hydrotherapy: apply two to five times weekly.

Mind/Body Therapy: • Guided Imagery, biofeedback (attention deficit disorders), meditation. • Belly breathing (for enhanced relaxation and concentration): lie on your back with your knees bent and feet on the floor at hip's width. Your hands are at your side. As you breathe, focus on your belly. As you inhale, imagine it expanding in all directions like a big balloon. As you exhale, feel it contract. Allow your exhalation to eventually become twice as long as your inhalation.

Professional Care

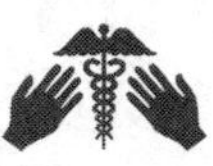

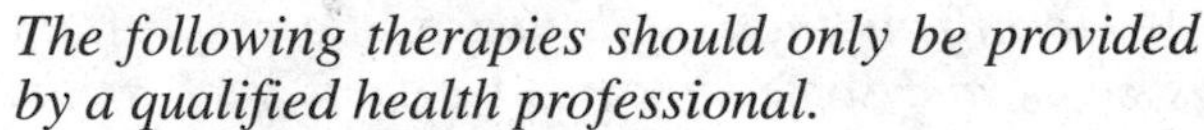

The following therapies should only be provided by a qualified health professional.

• Applied Kinesiology • Cell Therapy • Chelation Therapy • Colon Therapy • Environmental Medicine • Hypnotherapy • Light Therapy • Magnetic Field Therapy • Naturopathic Medicine • Orthomolecular Therapy • Traditional Chinese Medicine

Bodywork: Feldenkrais, Alexander technique.

Detoxification Therapy: Detoxification is not indicated unless the condition is part of a congestive disorder. May need colon cleansing, yeast treatment, or heavy metal detox.

Vision Therapy: Vision therapy may be an effective method for improving mental focus. Accuracy of aiming, speed of movement, and quality of single, clear sight are often enhanced through vision therapy even in older individuals. Increases in attention, memory, and the ability to sustain focus are often the result.

Meniere's Disease

See Hearing Disorders chapter, page 702.

Menopause, Menorrhagia, Menstrual Cramps

See Female Health chapter, page 657.

Mental Health

See Mental Health chapter, page 744.

Migraines

See Headaches chapter, page 691.

Mononucleosis

An acute (severe short-lived episode) infectious, viral disease caused usually by the Epstein-Barr virus and sometimes by the cytomegalovirus. Both of these viruses belong to the herpes group. The disease is often referred to as "mono," "sleeping sickness," or the "kissing sickness," since it is very contagious, may be transmitted by kissing, and the cardinal symptom is severe tiredness. Mono affects the lymph tissue, the respiratory system, and sometimes other organs such as the liver, spleen, and, rarely, the heart and kidneys. It presents with an increase of white abnormal blood cells and development of persistent antibodies (an immune system molecule in the blood marking exposure to a virus) to the Epstein-Barr virus and short-lived antibodies to beef, horse, and sheep red blood cells.

Symptoms: Symptoms occur four to seven weeks after exposure with severe incapacitating fatigue, headache, sometimes chills, often shortly followed by a very high fever, sore throat, with enlargement of different lymph nodes, especially the ones in the neck. It is possible for the symptoms to be varied and confusing, because the mono viruses can affect different organs such as the spleen, liver (sometimes a mild jaundice, yellowing of the skin, occurs for a short period of time), eyelids, and sometimes the heart. Ten percent of individuals develop rashes or sometimes darkened bruise-like areas in the mouth.

Occurrence: Occurs most commonly at the age when the immune system is at its peak functioning (fifteen to seventeen years old). The disease only occurs in individuals who have never had these viral antibodies before.

Consider: Mono's symptoms are very similar to the flu so that a severe flu bout must be ruled out.

Special Notes: Almost all cases improve without drugs within four to six weeks. Antibiotics do nothing for mono unless there is an associated bacterial infection. Ampicillin, an antibiotic, will often make mono worse, may cause a rash, and should be avoided. Avoid aspirin as it may create complications, in rare cases. The oral antiviral medication acyclovir is sometimes used in uncomplicated cases but natural treatments may fair as well in some responsive individuals.

Any treatment in the early stages of this disease must emphasize appropriate bed rest (for at least one month or while fever and fatigue are still present. If there is enlargement of the spleen or liver the rest may need to be prolonged, and strenuous exercise must be avoided until these organs return to normal size).

Many mono patients suffer from ongoing fatigue, depression, and varied symptoms for months to follow, but those on natural treatments seem to avoid this pit fall or recover from these reoccurrences more quickly.

Alternative Treatments

Refer to alternative therapy chapters for more information before evaluating or applying any treatment. Some conditions, including yours, may require a physician's care.

Diet: Drink plenty of filtered water, avoid excessive animal proteins, take amino acid blends or vegetable protein drinks several times per day in between meals or for a snack to help build up the organs involved and maintain better blood sugar balance. Eat four to six smaller meals throughout the day and avoid overeating at one meal at a time, eat as much raw foods as possible with emphasis on a wide variety of sprouts, seeds and nuts, and consume wholesome soups made up of a wide variety of vegetables and roots such as potatoes, turnips, yams, and beets. Avoid processed foods, soft drinks, sugar, caffeine, white flour products, and fried foods.

Before retiring, take several bites of some complex carbohydrates (crackers, potatoes, pasta, etc.) along with several bites of a protein (nut butter, yogurt, cheese, seeds, etc.) along with the last B complex for the day, some vitamin C, and a large glass of filtered water or warm herbal tea.

Nutritional Therapy: • Vitamin C to bowel tolerance (see Orthomolecular Medicine chapter page 402.) • Free-form amino acids (one-quarter to one-half teaspoon ten minutes before meals three to four times daily) • Vitamin A (50,000 IU daily for two months) • E emulsion (400-600 IU daily) • Vitamin B complex (low dose three to four times daily) • Acidophilus • Glandular tissue of organs involved (liver, spleen and/or lymph/thymus) • Chlorophyll • Multivitamin/mineral supplement

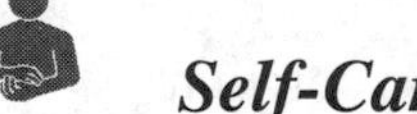

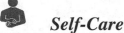

Self-Care

The following therapies can be undertaken at home under appropriate professional supervision.

• Biofeedback Training • Fasting • Qigong

Herbs: Combine the tinctures of myrrh, echinacea, wormwood, cleavers, and calendula in equal parts and take one-half teaspoonful of this mixture four times a day.

Homeopathy: *Belladonna, Merc iod., Phytolacca.*

Hydrotherapy: Constitutional hydrotherapy: apply two to five times weekly. Hyperthermia: apply one to two times weekly.

Juice Therapy: • Carrot, beet, tomato, green pepper (Add a little garlic and onion.) • Lemon, orange, pineapple • Wheat grass juice or other fresh green juices

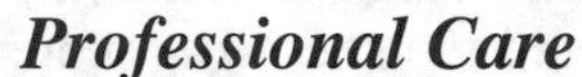

Professional Care

The following therapies should only be provided by a qualified health professional.

• Acupuncture • Cell Therapy • Magnetic Field Therapy • Naturopathic Medicine • Osteopathy • Traditional Chinese Medicine

Environmental Medicine: According to Marshall Mandell, M.D., there have been mono-like reactions in allergic people who do not have the mono infection caused by the Epstein-Barr virus.

Oxygen Therapy: Hydrogen peroxide therapy.

Motion Sickness

A disorder which manifests in some individuals experiencing motion, usually while traveling or acceleration and deceleration by other means, usually by car, train, sea, and air.

Symptoms: Mild symptoms may be uneasiness and headache, and may also include nausea. Severe symptoms may include vomiting, dizziness, excessive yawning, fatigue, weakness, inability to concentrate, excessive sweating and salivation, pallor (turning white), and severe distress. Prolonged motion sickness, such as on a long sea or air trip, may produce depression, low blood pressure, dehydration, or worsen people who are already ill due to other factors.

Special Notes: It is caused by movement on the organ of balance in the inner ear. Other factors that may play a role are: genetics, anxiety, movement immediately after eating or eating too much, and poor ventilation. There is a great variation in susceptibility of different people.

Treatment is difficult compared to prevention. Susceptible people should position themselves where there is minimal motion, focus on a point on the horizon, and try to be in a well-ventilated area. If travel is short avoid drinking or eating, move as little as possible, take preventive substances (see Nutritional Therapy) two hours before travel.

Alternative Treatments

Refer to alternative therapy chapters for more information before evaluating or applying any treatment. Some conditions, including yours, may require a physician's care.

Diet: On short trips avoid eating and drinking at all. On longer trips, try sipping small amounts of fresh lemon or lime juice, strong green tea, or ginger tea.

Nutritional Therapy: • Ginger capsules (four, taken two hours before travel and one per hour first few hours of travel) • Vitamin B complex (one) • Vitamin B_6 (50 mg.) • Magnesium (100 mg.) • Charcoal tablets (four, taken several hours before travel may be helpful if ginger capsules have not proven helpful in the past).

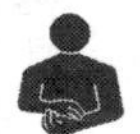

Self-Care

The following therapies can be undertaken at home under appropriate professional supervision.

• Biofeedback Training • Fasting

Acupressure: Research has shown that the nausea associated with travel sickness (and morning sickness, as well as following anaesthesia) eases dramatically following strong direct thumb pressure to acupressure point P6, (see acupressure chart, page 874) which lies on the palm side of the wrist, two thumb widths (patient's own thumb) above the main wrist crease, between the tendons, on each arm.

A minute of firm pressure to this point on one arm followed by the same to the other usually relieves motion sickness nausea for hours at a time.

Aromatherapy: A drop of peppermint oil on the tongue.

Herbs: Numerous clinical trials have shown ginger to be effective in preventing the symptoms of motion sickness.[17] It may be taken as a cup of fresh infusion, eaten as candied ginger, or as capsules of the powder. For people who do not like the taste of ginger the capsules are ideal. Usual dosage of such capsules is two to four as needed.

Homeopathy: • *Ipecac., Colchicum, Nux vom., Ignatia, Belladonna* • *Cocculus* must be taken alone, not in combination with other remedies.

Juice Therapy: Ginger.

Naturopathic Medicine: A simple, readily available therapy for nausea due to motion is to drink ginger tea. This is made by simply putting a teaspoon of ground culinary ginger into a cup of boiling water and drinking as often as needed.

Reflexology: Ear reflex, diaphragm, neck, spine.

Professional Care

The following therapies should only be provided by a qualified health professional.

• Acupuncture • Hypnotherapy • Naturopathic Medicine • Osteopathy

Environmental Medicine: According to Marshall Mandell, M.D., motion sickness often is a sensitivity reaction to the traffic fumes a person is exposed to while driving.

Traditional Chinese Medicine: Roasted ginger in capsules two to three times a day, two days before boating or flying.

Multiple Sclerosis

See Multiple Sclerosis chapter, page 755.

Mumps

See Children's Health chapter, page 608.

Muscular Cramps

Muscles are bundles of specialized cells that are able to contract and relax, creating movement. There are three types of muscles: skeletal, smooth, and cardiac (heart). Skeletal muscle has a certain level of constant contraction called muscle tone. However, excessive tone or abnormal tone can create spasms, cramps, and twitches.

Symptoms: Tightness, discomfort, pain, and sometimes tingling and burning are associated with areas in which the muscle tone has become excessive and/or the muscles are impinging on the associated tissues or nerves.

Occurrence: Everyone sometime during his or her life experiences muscle cramping. People more susceptible to this usually are sedentary (sit most of the day), do not exercise regularly, and eat too few green vegetables (magnesium-rich foods) or consume foods that reduce calcium availability to the body (acid diets higher in animal foods and grains and meats in relation to vegetables and fruits, or higher in commercial colas, caffeinated beverages, refined sugars, and highly processed foods high in phosphates).

Consider: Insufficient exercise, low thyroid, deficiency in iron (anemia), magnesium, calcium, vitamin E, folic acid, dietary imbalance, excessive coffee consumption, maladjustment of the spine or local area, residue from past injury to this area or corresponding one, stress, poor circulation secondary to heart problems, problems secondary to disease such as diabetes mellitus or arthritis, or fatigue in general.

Special Notes: The healthier the metabolism and tone of muscles (in a well-exercised and nourished individual), the less the tendency toward cramps, spasms, and twitches. The more healthy individual will be less prone to injury from trauma and will heal more quickly once injured, or will have less symptoms from small repetitive motions that may create problems in less toned individuals. Poor posture, poor or inadequate circulation, sitting habits at work, shoes, and not taking intermittent rest or exercise/stretching periods throughout the day, especially at a job that requires sustained positions, all contribute toward susceptibility to spasms.

Diuretic medication aggravates loss of minerals, particularly potassium, calcium, and magnesium, and may create worse muscle spasms.

Check for food sensitivities.

Alternative Treatments

Refer to alternative therapy chapters for more information before evaluating or applying any treatment. Some conditions, including yours, may require a physician's care.

Diet: Whole foods diet high in calcium-rich and magnesium-rich foods: leafy green vegetables, fruits (particularly apricots), yogurt, kefir, millet, sesame seeds. Also excellent are kelp, brewer's yeast, cornmeal, alfalfa, and honey. Avoid excessive consumption of citrus, meat, liver, and excess grains. The idea is to eat an alkaline diet (high in fresh vegetables and fruits) so that the overall metabolism of the body is not acidic and causes loss or imbalance of calcium. Vitamin E deficiency may also aggravate normal metabolism of muscles. Vitamin E is found in raw seeds and nuts and whole grains. Reduce phosphorous in diet, which is usually accomplished by avoiding processed foods and eating five to seven servings of vegetables and fruit per day.

Nutritional Therapy: • Magnesium (Magnesium aspartate is excellent but any magnesium should be helpful. This may be taken hourly if needed, but it may create looser stools which will stop once magnesium is reduced.) • Calcium • Vitamin E (400 IU three times daily) • Vitamin B complex with extra niacin (vitamin B_3) and thiamine (vitamin B_1) • Potassium • Vitamin C • Silicon • Niacinamide • Chlorophyll • Multimineral and trace element formula • Folic acid (500 mcg. three times daily) • Apply mixture of essential oils, evening primrose or flaxseed oil, vitamin A, and zinc oxide locally over the area (three times daily for first few days).

Some cases of muscular spasm that do not respond to the above are responsive to higher than normal dosages of folic acid, which may help improve microvascular circulation.

Alan R. Gaby, M.D., had found that acute or chronic muscle spasms respond well to an intravenous injection of a "cocktail" composed of magnesium chloride hexahydrate, calcium glycerophosphate, hydroxocobalamin, pyridoxine hydrochloride (vitamin B_6), dexpanthenol, B complex, and vitamin C. (This is a modification of the nutrient cocktail popularized by John Myers, M.D.)

If cramps are determined to be of a biochemical origin (disruption in electrolyte and trace element balance) mineral therapy with magnesium/calcium/potassium aminoethanol phosphate (AEP) may be effective.

There are many possible causes for muscular cramps, some simple, some complex. Cramps may occur in the calves due to a deficiency of sodium in the blood. Calf cramps brought on by neuralgia can also be a symptom of diabetes mellitus. Cramps may occur after long hikes, due to a slipped disk, or due to venous congestion and venous thrombosis, as during pregnancy.

Self-Care

The following therapies can be undertaken at home under appropriate professional supervision.

• Biofeedback Training • Fasting • Guided Imagery

Aromatherapy: Rosemary, lavender, marjoram, chamomile, clary sage.

Bodywork: • Acupressure, *shiatsu*, reflexology, massage, Rolfing, Feldenkrais, Hellerwork • Massage painful muscles with mixture of grated ginger juice and equal parts olive or sesame oil. • For nighttime leg cramps, soak in a warm bath before going to bed, then stretch your legs. • Regular stretching using yoga-type methods reduces likelihood of cramps, especially in main trouble areas such as the hamstring and calf muscles.

Herbs: Drink a strong decoction of cramp bark tea as needed or take one-half teaspoonful of cramp bark tincture four times a day. For temporary relief apply a mixture of equal parts tincture of lobelia and cramp bark to the effected muscles.

Hydrotherapy: • Hot pack, immersion, or sitz bath: apply as needed to relieve pain. • Take a full, hot bath for twenty to sixty minutes.

Juice Therapy: • Carrot, beet, celery, cucumber • Sweet fruit juices

Naturopathic Medicine: Quite possibly the most commonly deficient mineral, especially in men, is magnesium. As a first line of treatment for muscle cramps supplement diet with magnesium and apply local Epsom salts packs.

Reflexology: Hip/knee, hip/sciatic, lower spine, parathyroid, adrenals.

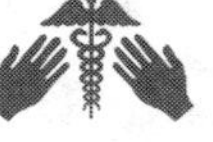

Professional Care

The following therapies should only be provided by a qualified health professional.

• Acupuncture • Applied Kinesiology • Cell Therapy • Chiropractic • Environmental Medicine • Light Therapy • Magnetic Field Therapy • Naturopathic Medicine • Orthomolecular Medicine • Osteopathy

Detoxification Therapy: May be indicated, depending on the condition of the person.

Oxygen Therapy: • Hydrogen peroxide therapy (IV) • Hyperbaric oxygen therapy

Nail Problems

Nail changes, unless due to localized trauma (usually crushing or pressure), fungus (often associated with acrylic nails for cosmetic purposes), or bacterial (tinea and candidiasis) are usually signs of métabolic and nutritional changes within the body. Nails may also be affected by skin disease or general illness.

Symptoms: *Thickened and curved nails (onychogryposis)* most often affect the big toe of elderly individuals and may signify poor circulation or a vascular system that is beginning to degenerate, or thyroid disease. *Pitting* may signify alopecia areata (hair loss or tendency toward hair loss during stress) or anemia. *Pitting together with onycholysis (separation of the nail from its normal attachment to the nail bed)* may be seen in psoriasis. *Brittle, ridged, and curved nails* may be seen in anemia secondary to iron deficiency. Brittle nails may be seen in thyroid problems, iron deficiency, kidney disorders, and/or poor circulation or be a symptom of an omega-3 fatty acid deficiency. *Vertical lines in nails* may suggest poor nutrient absorption, iron deficiency, or decreased general health or poor protein metabolism. *Horizontal lines* may occur with severe stress on the body, either emotionally, from disease and/or infection. *Flat nails* may suggest poor circulation from Raynaud's disease, nail beading (bumps) may suggest arthritis. *Nails that chip, crack, peel, and break* suggest poor mineral levels often secondary to low digestive enzymes or food allergies. *Red skin around the cuticles* may suggest poor essential fatty acid metabolism, cuticle biting and nervousness, or connective tissue disorders, such as lupus. *Nails that appear thin and brassy in color, often ridged,* suggest tendency to lose hair. *Nails that are very square and wide* may suggest tendency toward hormonal disorders. *Black splinter-like marks under the nail bed* may come from bleeding disorders or heart disease. *Greenish color* may be bacterial disease. *Whitish color* nails may suggest anemia or kidney disorders. *Whitish nails with pink color* near the tips may suggest liver disease such as cirrhosis. *Yellowish color or elevation of the ends* of the nails may suggest bronchial, lung, or lymphatic disease, or may be secondary to continual nail polish wear or nicotine staining from smoking. *Bluish color* may be iron deficiency, heart, or respiratory disease or heavy metal poisoning. *Darkening of the overall nail bed* may suggest vitamin B_{12} deficiency.

White spots on nails may signify zinc deficiency. These are sometimes called "Yom Kippur" spots as fasting for one day on the Jewish holiday of Yom Kippur is enough, in some borderline individuals, to create a zinc deficiency that shows up as transient white spots on the fingernails.

Genetics may play a role in producing poorly formed or easily injured nails that suggest joint and connective tissue problems, or may just not be significant at all. The whole person must be assessed to judge significance. Diagnosis should not be made on nail condition alone.

Alternative Treatments

Refer to alternative therapy chapters for more information before evaluating or applying any treatment. Some conditions, including yours, may require a physician's care.

Diet: Fresh carrot juice is excellent for strengthening the nails (calcium and phosphorus). Problems with nails can be due to numerous dietary factors including: excess salt intake, improper protein/calcium balance, and excess intake of citrus, lemon juice, and vinegar. In particular, assess and then consume, if appropriate, foods high in iron, quality sources of protein, whole grains, and seeds and nuts. Eat consistently, chew well, decrease stressful life circumstances and stressor foods.

Nutritional Therapy: Silicon, protein (free-form amino acids) calcium, iron, vitamin B complex, gelatin, zinc, biotin.

According to Jonathan Wright, M.D., more than 90 percent of the people with poor fingernails tested in his laboratory don't have enough stomach acid.

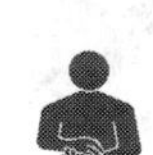

Self-Care

The following therapies can be undertaken at home under appropriate professional supervision.

• ***Fasting***

Aromatherapy: Lemon.

Ayurveda: *Fungal infection:* local application of one-half teaspoon aloe vera gel and one-quarter teaspoon of tumeric. *Brittle nails:* an herbal mixture of: *prawal panchamrit* 200 mg., and *shatavari* 500 mg. with goat's milk, generally taken twice a day after lunch and dinner. The minerals calcium, magnesium, and zinc are also beneficial. *Infected cuticles and nails:* apply *neem* oil locally.

Herbs: Drink an infusion made from equal parts of nettle and horsetail three times a day.

Homeopathy: *Calc phos., Graphites, Sulfur, Nat mur., Ferrum phos.*

Juice Therapy: Carrot, beet, celery blend.

Professional Care

The following therapies should only be provided by a qualified health professional.

• ***Magnetic Field Therapy*** • ***Naturopathic Medicine***

Oxygen Therapy: When due to fungal infection, ozone may be effective.

Traditional Chinese Medicine: Detoxifies the liver.

Narcolepsy

See Sleep Disorders chapter, page 839.

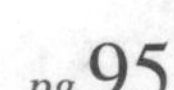

Nausea

Unpleasant sensation, that usually occurs in the higher abdominal area, and may proceed on to vomiting. It is not an illness itself but secondary to other factors such as pregnancy, inner ear disorders, overindulgence of food or alcohol, flu, or parasites.

Special Notes: If there is a deficiency of digestive enzymes, there is a need for bowel cleansing. Toxic stress in the liver or associated biliary system can also create a tendency to nausea. Anxiety and emotional stress in general may also cause nausea in some individuals.

Alternative Treatments

Refer to alternative therapy chapters for more information before evaluating or applying any treatment. Some conditions, including yours, may require a physician's care.

Diet: Eat smaller, more frequent meals, avoid fats and especially processed fats, nibble on whole grain crackers, sip liquids such as lemon water and fresh juices. Avoid aspartame (NutraSweet) and monosodium glutamate (MSG).

Nutritional Therapy: • Vitamin B complex • Vitamin B_6 • Magnesium

Excessive intake of zinc in particular or too many vitamins and minerals at one time in general may cause nausea.

Self-Care

The following therapies can be undertaken at home under appropriate professional supervision.

• Biofeedback Training • Fasting • Guided Imagery • Qigong

Acupressure: To relieve nausea firmly press P6 (for an illustration of this point number please see the acupressure chart on page 874) in the middle of the inner side of the forearm, two thumb widths (patient's own thumb) above the wrist crease. Sit comfortably as you firmly hold this point for two minutes, taking long deep breaths, making sure that the exhalation should take longer than inhalation to achieve a sense of ease and calm. Then get some fresh air and walk around, swinging your hands freely by your sides.

According to Leon Chaitow, N.D., D.O., research at Queens University, Belfast, by Professor Dundee has shown this to be effective in treating morning sickness nausea as well as the nausea associated with administration of chemotherapy and anaesthesia.

Aromatherapy: • Peppermint, rosewood • Put a drop of peppermint oil on the tongue.

Herbs: The treatment depends upon the cause. Please refer to Motion Sickness. In addition to ginger, an infusion of peppermint can be very settling.

Homeopathy: *Ipecac., Nux vom., Pulsatilla, Calc fluor., Colchicum, Arsen alb.*

Hydrotherapy: Constitutional hydrotherapy: apply two to five times weekly.

Meditation: Meditation has reduced chemotherapy associated anticipatory nausea.

Naturopathic Medicine: A simple readily available therapy for nausea due to motion or other causes (e.g., early pregnancy) is to drink ginger tea. This is made by simply putting a teaspoon of ground culinary ginger into a cup of boiling water and drinking as often as needed.

Reflexology: Liver, gallbladder, stomach, diaphragm.

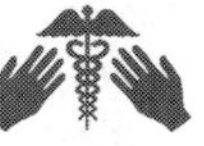

Professional Care

The following therapies should only be provided by a qualified health professional.

• Acupuncture • Colon Therapy • Craniosacral Therapy • Environmental Medicine • Hypnotherapy • Magnetic Field Therapy • Naturopathic Medicine • Neural Therapy • Osteopathy

Bodywork: Therapeutic Touch, *shiatsu.*

Nearsightedness

See Vision Disorders chapter, page 859.

Neuralgia/ Neuropathy/ Neuritis

Neuralgia: *Spasms of pain which extend along the course of a nerve. There are many types of neuralgias according to the nerve or body part affected, or to the cause (such as the disease: gouty, anemic, diabetic, syphilitic). Most common neuralgias are Bell's palsy and trigeminal neuralgia.*

Neuropathy: *A general term that signifies disturbances and pathologies in the peripheral nervous system (nerves outside of the spine), often noninflammatory in nature, and may be secondary to disease such as diabetes, pressure such as from nerve entrapment as in carpal*

tunnel syndrome in the wrist, disk lesions or due to unknown causes (usually nutritional deficiencies). When several peripheral nerves are involved it is called polyneuropathies.

Neuritis: *Inflammation of nerve or group of nerves. Symptoms are similar to above except more often include burning and may manifest with swelling and fever and in some severe cases, episodes of convulsions. Can occur anywhere in body such as sciatic nerve (buttocks or down the leg) or the optic nerve (eye).*

Symptoms: Mild or severe pain, constant or intermittent pain, burning, tingling, or stabbing forms of discomfort or pain.

Consider: Associated disease such as diabetes mellitus, thyroid disease, pressure from tumor, nutrient deficiency, metabolic imbalance, infection, gout, leukemia, alcohol abuse, heavy metal toxicity, or direct trauma.

Assessment of possible underlying disease must be made by a doctor.

Alternative Treatments

Refer to alternative therapy chapters for more information before evaluating or applying any treatment. Some conditions, including yours, may require a physician's care.

Diet: Whole foods diet, increase fluid intake, and avoid stressor and stimulating foods such as caffeinated beverages, refined sugars, cigarettes, and commercial carbonated beverages.

Nutritional Therapy: • Thiamine (vitamin B_1, 100 mg. two to three times daily) • Folic acid (500 mcg. two times daily) • Niacin (vitamin B_3) • Vitamin B complex • Vitamin B_{12} (intramuscular injections best in acute conditions) • Vitamin C and bioflavonoids • Vitamin B_6 • Pantothenic acid • Brewer's yeast • Calcium • Magnesium • Lecithin • Sometimes proteolytic enzymes on empty stomach away from meals is helpful especially in neuritis. Take at same time as vitamin C and bioflavonoids.

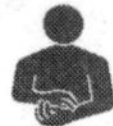

Self-Care

The following therapies can be undertaken at home under appropriate professional supervision.

• Biofeedback Training • Fasting • Relaxation • Yoga

Aromatherapy: Chamomile, eucalyptus, cedarwood, juniper, lavender.

Herbs: Combine equal parts of the tinctures of St. John's Wort, skullcap, oat, and Siberian ginseng. Take one teaspoonful of this mixture three times a day. This may be made stronger if there is much pain by the addition of valerian or Jamaican dogwood. Externally peppermint oil can be applied as a mild local anesthetic.

Homeopathy: *Belladonna, Aconite, Mag phos., Phytolacca, Chelidonium, Lycopodium, Arsen alb.*

Hydrotherapy: Contrast application: apply daily.

Juice Therapy: Parsley, celery, carrot blend.

Topical Treatment: Epsom salts packs.

Professional Care

The following therapies should only be provided by a qualified health professional.

• Acupuncture • Cell Therapy • Chiropractic • Craniosacral Therapy • Environmental Medicine • Light Therapy • Magnetic Field Therapy • Naturopathic Medicine • Neural Therapy • Osteopathy • Traditional Chinese Medicine

Detoxification Therapy: May be indicated, depending on the condition of the person.

Energy Medicine: Electro-Acuscope.

Oxygen Therapy: Hyperbaric oxygen therapy may be useful for acute conditions of neuralgia. Hydrogen peroxide therapy may also be useful for neuritis.

Night Blindness

See Vision Disorders chapter, page 861.

Nose Bleeds

Bleeding or loss of blood from the mucous membrane that lines the nose, usually from only one nostril.

Occurrence: Most commonly occur in childhood and are usually not serious.

Consider: In adults, most nosebleeds are secondary to trauma to the nose (external blows, blowing nose too strongly and rupturing of membranes, or to scratches from the fingernails), from irritating crust formations secondary to colds, infections, or the flu, very dry conditions such as high altitudes or desert areas, sudden changes in atmospheric pressure, and from nutrient deficiencies, most commonly vitamin C and/or bioflavonoids.

In adults, recurrent nose bleeds may signify underlying disease such as high blood pressure (hypertension), a tumor in the nose or sinuses, or a bleeding disorder.

What to do immediately: If nose starts to bleed

immediately after a traumatic blow to the head, this may signify a fracture in the skull and individual must proceed to a hospital immediately.

In other instances, when there is not a danger of skull fracture, do the following: sit, lean forward, blow all blood and clots out of both nostrils, open mouth and breath through mouth (avoiding blood clots obstructing air passages), pinch lower part of nose for twenty minutes, then slowly release pressure and avoid any contact or pressure with the nose.

If bleeding continues after the first twenty minutes of pressure, pack nose with gauze and apply crushed ice within a cloth against the nose and cheek. Lie back, once nose is packed and ice is applied, and refrain from any motion or activity for several hours.

If bleeding continues after twenty minutes, notify a doctor. May need to cauterize (therapeutic application of heat) and in very rare and severe cases may require surgery.

Once bleeding has stopped: Squeeze contents of vitamin E and vitamin A capsules into lining of nose. May also use zinc oxide, petroleum jelly, aloe vera gel, comfrey, or calendula ointment, and then place small gauze piece against the gel.

Blood thinners such as Coumadin or aspirin may cause nose bleeds. If this happens, notify your doctor who may alter dosage of blood thinners.

Alternative Treatments

Refer to alternative therapy chapters for more information before evaluating or applying any treatment. Some conditions, including yours, may require a physician's care.

Diet: Vitamin K which is essential for blood clotting and is found in the following foods: watercress, dark green leafy vegetables, kale, and alfalfa.

Nutritional Therapy: • Vitamin C (3 grams at start of bleeding and 1 gram every hour if bleeding continues) • Rutin and other bioflavonoids

Self-Care

The following therapies can be undertaken at home under appropriate professional supervision.

• ***Fasting***

Aromatherapy: Lemon, lavender, cypress, frankincense.

Bodywork: Acupressure, *shiatsu*, reflexology.

Herbs: Use a snuff made from finely ground oak bark. If the nosebleed is related to hypertension please refer to that section.

Homeopathy: *Hyoscyamus, Chamomilla, Rhus tox., Ipecac., Belladonna, Hamamelis.*

Hydrotherapy: Ice pack: apply over nose and to back of neck to stop bleeding.

Juice Therapy: Carrot, beet, with ginger or cayenne.

Practical Hints: Sit down with head tipped forward. Stay in cool room.

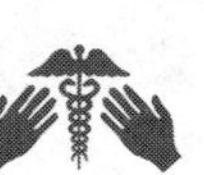

Professional Care

The following therapies should only be provided by a qualified health professional.

• ***Acupuncture*** • ***Environmental Medicine*** • ***Naturopathic Medicine*** • ***Osteopathy*** • ***Traditional Chinese Medicine***

Obesity

See Obesity and Weight Management chapter, page 762.

Osteoarthritis

See Arthritis chapter, page 530.

Osteoporosis

See Osteoporosis chapter, page 773.

Otitis Media

See Hearing and Ear Disorders chapter, page 701.

Ovarian Cysts

See Female Health chapter, page 672

Pancreatitis

Inflammation of the pancreas which may be either acute (short-lived episode that resolves [heals] completely) or chronic (irreversible, degenerative cellular changes within the pancreas which usually continue and progress even after the cause, usually alcohol, is removed).

Symptoms: Half of individuals with an acute pancreatitis attack, which usually lasts about forty-eight hours, have severe abdominal pain that radiates straight into the back. Pain usually begins suddenly, reaches a severe and maximum intensity within several minutes, and persists for hours or days. Pain is slightly relieved by sitting and worse with movement. The pain is often accompanied by nausea, vomiting, sweating, increased heart rate, dizziness, pallor (pale), and feeling very ill. During the attack, pancreatic enzymes are released into the bloodstream and diagnosis of acute pancreatitis is made by assessment of the blood levels of these enzymes. Chronic pancreatitis has similar symptoms, although the attacks usually last longer and are recurrent, becoming more severe as the disease progresses. Chronic pancreatitis is often related to gallbladder disorders or stones. In some individuals, the only sign of pancreatitis is either malabsorption (manifesting as pale-colored, bulky, and greasy stools, as the injured pancreas does not release adequate pancreatin enzymes) or diabetes mellitus (as the injured pancreas does not make enough insulin).

Recurrences may be prevented by treating the cause, such as avoiding alcohol, treating liver and gallbladder, losing weight, improving nutrition, and avoiding drugs. Chronic pancreatitis may need insulin, or nutritional and natural programs to balance blood sugar and support the pancreas, and nutrients or even drugs to reduce the pain. Rarely, after all else has been tried and failed, surgery is necessary to remove the pancreas or gallstones that are creating obstructions.

Alternative Treatments

Refer to alternative therapy chapters for more information before evaluating or applying any treatment. Some conditions, including yours, may require a physician's care.

Diet: In acute state fasting from all fluids and foods may be advised as presence of food in intestines stimulates pancreas and makes the symptoms worse. IV's given by doctors and other therapeutic interventions may be necessary. Once abdominal pain is gone, the blood level of pancreatic enzymes are normal and the appetite and feeling of well-being returns, foods can be reintroduced. Diet should follow diabetic protocol. (See Diabetes.)

Refined sugars, caffeine, and alcohol should be strictly avoided. Small, frequent meals with emphasis on complex carbohydrates, vegetables, and small amounts of fruits should be consumed. Exercise is important to stabilize blood sugar, also.

Nutritional Therapy: • Chromium (300 mcg. daily) • Pancreatin enzymes with meals • Pancreas glandular • Lipotrophic factors • Vitamin B complex with extra niacin and pantothenic acid • Vitamin C (buffered) • Try L-phenylalanine for pain reduction in chronic pancreatitis. • Acidophilus • Magnesium • Multiminerals

Self-Care

The following therapies can be undertaken at home under appropriate professional supervision.

• Fasting • Flower Remedies • Qigong

Aromatherapy: Weakness: marjoram, lemon.

Herbs: Combine equal parts of the glycerates of fringetree bark, balmony, and milk thistle. Take one teaspoonful of this three times a day.

Hydrotherapy: Constitutional hydrotherapy: apply two to five times weekly.

Juice Therapy: Carrot, Jerusalem artichoke (minimum protein intake), beet, garlic, diluted 50/50.

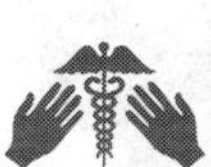

Professional Care

The following therapies should only be provided by a qualified health professional.

• Cell Therapy • Colon Therapy • Pancreatic Enzyme Therapy • Homeopathy • Magnetic Field Therapy • Naturopathic Medicine • Osteopathy • Traditional Chinese Medicine

Detoxification Therapy: Detoxification is probably indicated, unless condition may be chronic and/or due to undernourishment.

Oxygen Therapy: Hydrogen peroxide therapy (IV)

Paralysis

Total loss or partial impairment of motor function (voluntary movement) of a part of the body because one or more muscles cannot be properly contracted. Paralysis is usually classified according to the cause or to the nerve, muscle, or body part involved. It can involve a wide range of muscles, and can be permanent or temporary.

Symptoms: The affected body part manifests loss of controlled motion, either rigid or spastic muscle or possibly flaccid (soft and floppy) muscle. When all four limbs and the trunk of the body are paralyzed it is called quadriplegia. Paraplegia is when both legs and possibly part of the trunk is involved. Hemiplegia is when one half of the body is paralyzed.

Special Notes: Paralysis may be caused by spinal cord problems, brain disorders, congenital defects affecting the spine and brain, traumatic injury to the spine and brain, diseases that affect these organs, peripheral nerve disorders, and muscles diseases.

Alternative Treatments

Refer to alternative therapy chapters for more information before evaluating or applying any treatment. Some conditions, including yours, may require a physician's care.

Diet: Whole foods diet high in foods rich in magnesium, which is nature's muscle relaxant. Such foods are dark leafy greens and green drink (blended greens plus pineapple juice). Avoid foods which tend to make the blood sugar rise and drop rapidly and thus may contribute to muscular weakness or spasticity, such as excessive consumption of refined sugars, caffeinated beverages, and nutrient-poor meals which lower the body levels of minerals and trace minerals.

Nutritional Therapy: • Vitamin B_6 • Magnesium • Niacinamide • Vitamin B complex • Vitamin C • Free-form amino acids

Vitamin-mineral injections may be helpful in some individuals. Consult an orthomolecular physician.

Self-Care

The following therapies can be undertaken at home under appropriate professional supervision.

• Biofeedback Training • Fasting • Yoga

Ayurveda: *Yogaraj guggulu* 200 mg. for *vata*, *kaishore guggulu* 200 mg. for *pitta*, or *punarnava guggulu* 200 mg. for *kapha*, generally taken twice a day after lunch and dinner. For all *doshas: triphala* one-half teaspoon with warm water and *netra basti*.

Reflexology: Whole spine, brain, related reflex area.

Professional Care

The following therapies should only be provided by a qualified health professional.

• Acupuncture • Chiropractic • Craniopathy • Craniosacral Therapy • Environmental Medicine • Magnetic Field Therapy • Naturopathic Medicine • Neural Therapy • Osteopathy

Homeopathy: *Aconite, Arsen alb., Ignatia, Chamomilla, Colchicum, Conium mac.* Consult a physician..

Oxygen Therapy: Hyperbaric oxygen therapy may be useful for paralysis due to brain damage.

Parasitic Infections

See Parasitic Infections chapter, page 782.

Parkinson's Disease

A slow, progressive disorder of the central nervous system.

Symptoms: Four major symptoms: slowness of movement, muscular rigidity, resting tremor (trembling at rest or no movement), and postural instability (shuffling, unbalanced walk which progresses into uncontrollable tiny, running steps to keep from falling). This disease usually begins as a slight tremor in one hand, arm, or leg. The tremor is at its peak during rest, improves with movement, and is completely absent during sleep. The tremor gets worse with fatigue and stress. In 50 to 80 percent of individuals with Parkinson's disease, the tremor starts in one hand and resembles trying to roll a pill between the fingers, thus it is called a "pill-rolling tremor." Thc jaw, tonguc, forchcad, and cyclids may also tremble, but the voice is not shaky. Another early sign is a severe decrease in blinking of the eyes. As the disease progresses, there is more stiffness, weakness, and both sides of the body become involved, and the initial tremors may become less prominent. There may develop shaking of the head, a mask-like expression on the face in which the eyes do not blink, and a rigid, bent-over posture that is permanent. Speech becomes difficult and slow, handwriting becomes small. Depression and dementia may occur. All daily activities become difficult.

Occurrence: Fifty thousand cases a year in the geriatric population in the United States, or one in two hundred of the elderly. Men are more susceptible than women.

Special Notes: If untreated, the disease progresses over fifteen years to severe incapacitation. Modern treatment with complicated drug combinations, mobility exercises, and support groups has reduced the severity of this disease. The cause is unknown. However, an imbalance of two brain chemicals seem involved, dopamine and acetylcholine. A deficiency of dopamine in the brain may be due to underlying nutritional deficiencies, cerebral vascular disease (blockage of blood vessels in brain), side effects of antipsychotic drugs, carbon monoxide poisoning, abuse of certain designer drugs, and a rare infection (encephalitis lethargica).

Levodopa is the most commonly used drug

and cannot be taken with vitamin B_6. Using vitamin B_6 alone may be just as effective in some individuals. This drug should be taken away from protein meals, which decrease its effectiveness.

Alternative Treatments

Refer to alternative therapy chapters for more information before evaluating or applying any treatment. Some conditions, including yours, may require a physician's care.

Diet: If on the drug levodopa, must decrease the foods that are rich in vitamin B_6. These are whole grains (especially oats), raw nuts (especially peanuts), bananas, potatoes, liver, and fish. Whole foods diet with emphasis on lots of fluids, raw foods (50 to 75 percent), and sprouts. Also good are green leafy vegetables, rutabagas, sesame seeds, and sesame butter.

According to Johnathan Wright, M.D., most drug prescription for Parkinson's is done with Sinemet (trade name for a combination of levadopa and carbidopa) these days, for which one doesn't need to avoid vitamin B_6.

Nutritional Therapy: Assessment of individual amino acids is important. Consult an orthomolecular doctor. If unable to do so, take GABA (gamma-aminobutyric acid—500 mg. once daily), along with a mixed amount of free-form amino acids, calcium, and magnesium. If on levodopa, take B vitamins separately, all of them without vitamin B_6 (injectable form is optimal but high oral intake of each at about 50 mg. two times daily is good). If not on levodopa, take vitamin B complex (100 mg. three times daily), along with vitamin B_6 (300 mg. three times daily), lecithin (one teaspoon three times daily), vitamin C, evening primrose oil. Gerovital H-3 (GH-3—from Romania), multivitamin/mineral complex, DHEA (a steroid hormone produced by the adrenal glands). Consult with your doctor.

Researchers from Hahnemann University in Philadelphia report that monkeys suffering from neurological damage regained their ability to walk and climb after receiving injections of G_{M1} ganglioside, a substance that occurs naturally in nerve cells. The researchers speculate that G_{M1} ganglioside may stimulate dopamine production and stabilize injured neurons, offering hope of it becoming an effective treatment for people with Parkinson's disease.[18]

Vitamin C may help "on-off attacks" (two to five years on levadopa results in shortened positive response time to treatment) and other side effects of levadopa.

Long-term vitamin E (1,000 IU daily) supplementation may also slow the progression of Parkinson's disease.

The coenzyme nicotinamide adenine dinucleotide (NADH) in a therapeutic dose of 25-50 mg. a day produces a beneficial effect in patients with Parkinson's, with the most noticeable results occurring after intravenous rather than after intramuscular administration.[19]

A study with four patients with Parkinson's disease who were given injections of 100 mg. of neotrophin 1 (complex glycoproteins, in this case derived from snake venom) resulted in dramatic improvement after a period of six to eight weeks.[20]

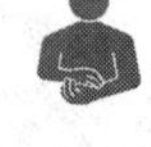

Self-Care

The following therapies can be undertaken at home under appropriate professional supervision.

• Fasting • Flower Remedies • Yoga

Herbs: Herbs work best here if used in combination with the appropriate drugs. An example of such synergistic interactions is passion flower and the drug L-dopa (levodopa). The reduction in passive tremor produced by using both L-dopa and passion flower is usually greater than the L-dopa by itself. Passion flower has only a minimal effect if used alone. Take one-half teaspoonful of passion flower tincture three times a day.

Hydrotherapy: Constitutional hydrotherapy: apply two to five times weekly.

Juice Therapy: • Carrot and spinach juice or carrot, beet, radish, garlic, and cucumber daily • Seasonal raw fruit and vegetables

Orthomolecular Medicine: Abram Hoffer, M.D., Ph.D., F.R.C.P., recommends large quantities of vitamin B_3, either niacin or niacinamide, to protect people against the tendency of L-dopa to cause psychosis. However, the vitamins in these quantities do not have much effect on the tremor.

Reflexology: Whole spine, all glands, diaphragm, chest/lung.

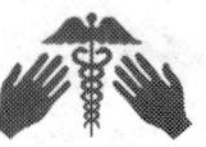

Professional Care

The following therapies should only be provided by a qualified health professional.

• Cell Therapy • Chelation Therapy • Craniosacral Therapy • Light Therapy • Magnetic Field Therapy • Naturopathic Medicine • Traditional Chinese Medicine

Bodywork: • Feldenkrais.

Detoxification Therapy: May be indicated, depending on the condition of the person.

Oxygen Therapy: Hydrogen peroxide therapy (IV)

Pellagra

Severe deficiency of niacin. Primary deficiencies usually occur in areas where maize (Indian corn) is the major constituent of the diet. Maize has a bound form of niacin that is not digestible unless it is pretreated with alkali such as in the preparation of tortillas. It also is low in tryptophan which furthers helps the body assimilate niacin. Secondary deficiencies are associated with certain disorders that promote nutrient deficiencies. These include severe diarrhea, parasites, cirrhosis of the liver, postsurgical nutrient deficiencies, stress, increased need due to genetics, and overconsumption of junk food which is very low in B vitamins and high in refined sugars which use up B vitamins in their assimilation.

Symptoms: Diarrhea, dementia, and dermatitis or, in other words, symptoms of the skin and mucous membranes, the central nervous system, and the gastrointestinal tract. Other symptoms may be redness and swelling of tongue and lips, burning of mouth, pharynx, esophagus, abdominal distention and pain or discomfort, poor digestion, vomiting, diarrhea that is possibly bloody, weakness, weight loss, poor stress coping skills, irritability, poor cold tolerance, confusion, memory impairment, and paranoia. In chronic cases, the skin that is exposed and manifests symptoms, may turn dark, become thicker, rougher, and very dry. Symptoms may appear in any combination or singly.

Occurrence: Mainly in rural and poor communities in India and South Africa, and where people subsist mainly on maize, in alcoholics, or individuals who live on junk food diets.

Consider: Rule out tongue and lip redness and swelling due to other vitamin deficiencies or diseases, and diarrhea, skin, and central nervous system disorders due to other diseases.

Special Notes: Multiple deficiencies of all the B vitamins and protein often occur together. Therefore, supplementation and dietary nutrient intervention should be balanced.

Alternative Treatments

Refer to alternative therapy chapters for more information before evaluating or applying any treatment. Some conditions, including yours, may require a physician's care.

Diet: Eat foods rich in niacin, B vitamins, protein, and the amino acid tryptophan: whole grains, bananas, raw seeds and nuts, peanuts, liver, avocados, broccoli, potatoes, tomatoes, legumes, collard greens, enriched breads and cereals, salmon, halibut, tuna, swordfish, skinless breast of chicken, and turkey. Strictly avoid refined sugars for first several weeks of therapy. Brewer's yeast is a good natural source of the B vitamins if there is no candidiasis.

Nutritional Therapy: • Niacinamide (300-1,000 mg. in divided dosages three times daily depending on severity of symptoms). This is preferable and most commonly used instead of niacin which usually creates uncomfortable flushing and chills and sometimes stomach pains. (If oral therapy cannot be taken, 100-250 mg. injectable two to three times daily.) • Vitamin B complex (100 mg. three times daily) • Protein supplements.

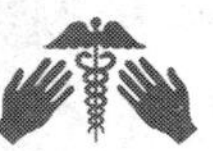

Professional Care

The following therapies should only be provided by a qualified health professional.

• Magnetic Field Therapy • Naturopathic Medicine • Orthomolecular Medicine • Traditional Chinese Medicine

Periodontal (Gum) Disease

Inflammation or degeneration of the tissue that surrounds and supports the teeth (the periodontium made up of the gingiva [gums], the bone the teeth are "set" in [alveolar bone], the supporting ligaments [periodontal ligament] and tissue that connects these structures [cementum]). The most common and often initial form of periodontal disease is inflammation of the gums, called gingivitis, which can be acute (short-lived episode), chronic (ongoing), or recurrent. Untreated gingivitis proceeds further with increasing inflammation and involvement of more tissues, such as the membranes around the bases of the teeth and possible erosion of the underlying bone. This is then called periodontitis and is the major cause of bone loss in adults.

Symptoms: Red, inflamed gum tissue that bleeds easily when exposed to very minimal injury such as with flossing or brushing the teeth, or eating hard foods such as raw apples. There is usually no pain.

Occurrence: High in individuals with poor oral hygiene (poor habits of oral brushing and flossing with a characteristic buildup of bacterial plaque [sticky deposits made up of mucous and microorganisms that grow and adhere to carbohydrate residues left on the teeth due to insufficient cleaning habits]). Increased during pregnancy and puberty which may be secondary to hormonal factors or due to increased physiologic needs for folic acid and B vitamins during these periods.

Consider: Other risk factors for periodontal disease: problems with biting surface (malocclusion), breathing through the mouth, food impaction, nutrient deficiencies especially folic acid and vitamin B complex, decreased local tissue circulation secondary to plaque buildup or consistently eating low-fiber foods and insufficient flossing, and buildup of calculus (tartar—calcified plaque mixed with saliva).

Gingivitis may be one of the first signs that there is an underlying systemic problem such as: debilitating disease such as diabetes or leukemia, heavy metal toxicity, lowered resistance, allergies, or vitamin deficiencies.

Periodontal disease may be aggravated and/or caused by hydrochloric acid deficiency, insufficient calcium in the diet or stressor foods that rob it from the system, and imbalances in the body with other minerals such as magnesium and zinc.

Special Notes: Birth control pills tend to increase the body's requirements for folic acid and if this is not met there may be an increased risk of gingivitis. Smokers are two to four times more likely to suffer periodontal disease than nonsmokers.

Best treatment is prevention with daily removal of plaque through brushing and flossing, routine cleaning by a dentist every six months (more if the disease is already occurring) not only to prevent but to monitor progress and condition of gums and supporting tissues, and eating diet high in whole foods, fiber and avoiding excessive consumption of refined carbohydrates.

Any underlying systemic problems must also be treated.

Alternative Treatments

Refer to alternative therapy chapters for more information before evaluating or applying any treatment. Some conditions, including yours, may require a physician's care.

Diet: Whole foods diet with emphasis on as many fresh fruits and vegetables as possible (five to seven servings daily), high-fiber foods, avoidance of refined sugars and carbohydrates and sufficient filtered water especially first thing in the morning and last thing in the evening, to help cleanse the mouth. Foods to emphasize are: blueberries, hawthorne berries, grapes.

Nutritional Therapy: • Floss one to two times daily and then rinse mouth (for one minute) with several mouthfuls of liquid folic acid (0.1 percent solution) and then swallow. (Sixty individuals with gingivitis rinsed for one minute two times daily and had beneficial results.[21]) • If you cannot find liquid folic acid, buy folic acid crystals in 800 mcg. capsules, empty two capsules in water and use this to gargle. • Take folic acid orally (500 mcg.—1 mg. daily depending on severity of condition) • Vitamin C (1-3 grams daily) with bioflavonoids • Vitamin A (25,000 IU daily for several months) • Calcium (650-1,500 mg. daily) • Vitamin B complex (one-two times daily) • Beta-carotene • Vitamin E • Vitamin K • Magnesium • Zinc • Vitamin B complex

"Pink toothbrush" is a syndrome caused by mild gum bleeding which causes the toothbrush to appear pink and is treated by the above.

According to Johnathan Wright, M.D., co-enzyme Q10 is widely recommended in Japan for periodontal disease.

Gum infection: Vitamin A (large dosages for first three days and then slowly reduce to maintenance over one to two weeks) with vitamin E and zinc. Or rub oil from vitamin E and A capsules along with zinc oxide cream. May add aloe vera gel when the infection is gone and gums are in last stages of healing.

If gums do not respond within several weeks of ardent adherence to flossing and program, see a dentist and/or physician. It is a good idea to get regular hygienic check-ups and know what level the pockets are at, to monitor progress and avoid periodontal disease that has gone into the bone and must be dealt with immediately to prevent further bone loss and problems.

Self-Care

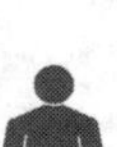

The following therapies can be undertaken at home under appropriate professional supervision.

• Fasting

Ayurveda: *Bleeding gums:* drink lemon water (juice of one-half lemon in one cup water). • Massage gums with coconut oil or goldenseal, bayberry, or myrrh. • Take 5 grams of *amla* powder in one cup water daily. • Swish a mouthful of warm sesame oil for two minutes and then massage the gums and brush the teeth with *catechu* and *neem* powder paste.

Herbs: Used both internally and topically, herbs may be most helpful. Combine equal parts of the tinctures of myrrh and echinacea and apply small amounts to the gums three times a day using a very fine paintbrush. Use a mouth wash made from an infusion of sage or chamomile. Do not swallow. Internally: combine the tinctures of echinacea, cleavers, and prickly ash in equal parts and take one teaspoonful twice a day.

Hydrotherapy: Contrast application: apply daily to face over involved areas.

Juice Therapy: Those high in beta-carotene, such as carrot or cantaloupe.

Topical Treatments: • Brush teeth with mixture of baking soda and hydrogen peroxide. • Brush tongue if coated in morning. • Massage gums with fingers. • Bleeding gums and pyorrhea (discharge of pus): morning and evening—one teaspoon apple cider vinegar in a cup of water. Use as mouthwash and drink remainder.

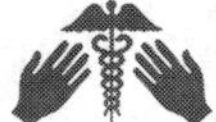

Professional Care

The following therapies should only be provided by a qualified health professional.

• Acupuncture • Environmental Medicine • Magnetic Field Therapy • Naturopathic Medicine • Traditional Chinese Medicine

Detoxification Therapy: May be indicated, depending on the condition of the person.

Oxygen Therapy: • Hyperbaric oxygen therapy • Ozonated water

Pinworms

See Children's Health chapter, page 609.

Pleurisy

Inflammation of the pleura (the membranes lining the lungs and thoracic cavity, which are constantly moist to facilitate lung movement within the chest). The inflammation is usually caused by a lung infection but in more unusual circumstances may be caused by lung cancer, rheumatoid arthritis, and pulmonary embolism (blockage of a pulmonary artery by foreign matter).

Symptoms: The symptoms of this disease come on very suddenly, with the primary characteristic being pain associated with breathing in and/or coughing. The pain may vary from vague discomfort to a severe and stabbing sensation. The pain may refer (travel) toward the shoulder of the involved side. Breathing usually becomes more rapid and shallow than usual. Motion on the side of the trunk that is involved may become limited.

Special Notes: Treatment of the underlying lung condition is paramount, along with natural analgesics for the pain and anti-inflammatories for the inflammation.

Alternative Treatments

Refer to alternative therapy chapters for more information before evaluating or applying any treatment. Some conditions, including yours, may require a physician's care.

Diet: Emphasize fresh fruits and vegetables, hearty soups, organic citrus fruits nibbling on the insides of the rinds, and using the spice tumeric very generously.

Nutritional Therapy: • Vitamin A (200,000 IU first three days, reduce to 100,000 next three days and then 50,000 IU for next two weeks) • Lung glandular (three to four, three to four times daily before meals) • Vitamin C with bioflavonoids to bowel tolerance (see Orthomolecular Medicine chapter) • Essential fatty acids (six, two times daily on empty stomach before meal containing some fat) • Proteolytic enzymes (four to six, two to four times daily on empty stomach) • Bromelain (100-200 mg. daily away from mealtimes to reduce inflammatory process without side effects)

Self-Care

The following therapies can be undertaken at home under appropriate professional supervision.

• Fasting • Qigong • Yoga

Herbs: Mix equal parts of dried mullein and pleurisy root, and drink as a hot infusion several times a day. In addition combine the tinctures of pleurisy root, elecampane and echinacea in equal parts and take one teaspoonful of this mixture three times a day. Also take either a clove or raw garlic daily or three capsules of garlic oil with each meal.

Homeopathy: *Aconite, Bryonia, Apis mel., Cantharis, Kali carb., Sulfur, Arsen alb., Phosphorus.*

Hydrotherapy: Constitutional hydrotherapy: apply daily.

Leon Chaitow, N.D., D.O., suggests alternating hot and cold applications to the rib cage many times a day to improve circulation and drainage (thirty seconds to a minute hot, followed by ten seconds cold). Repeat the alternations three to five times finishing with cold.

Juice Therapy: • Carrot, celery, parsley • Carrot, celery • Carrot, pineapple • Carrot, beet, cucumber • Garlic

Reflexology: Lymph system, adrenals, diaphragm, chest/lung.

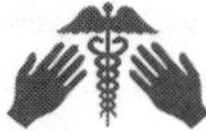

Professional Care

The following therapies should only be provided by a qualified health professional.

• Acupuncture • Cell Therapy • Environmental Medicine • Magnetic Field Therapy • Naturopathic Medicine • Osteopathy

Osteopathy and Rolfing both help to free the rib cage and thereby may promote better breathing, but cannot cure pleurisy.

Bodywork: • Rolfing.

Detoxification Therapy: May be indicated, depending on the condition of the person.

PMS (Premenstrual Syndrome)

See Female Health chapter, page 662.

Pneumonia

See Respiratory Conditions chapter, page 815.

Poison Oak/Ivy

Plants such as poison oak, ivy, sumac, ragweed, and primrose may cause a severe allergic reaction (contact dermatitis) when the oils from the leaves, bark, stems, flowers, and fruit come in contact with the skin or are inhaled. Certain species of plants are also poisonous when eaten.

Symptoms: Contact dermatitis or allergic symptoms vary greatly, and usually start with burning and itching. The skin then starts to swell, a rash spreads, and blisters form which may ooze. In severe cases, systemic symptoms may manifest, such as feeling ill in general, lethargy (fatigue), trouble sleeping, and general discomfort.

Symptoms of internal poisoning from eating plants are varied and depend on the plant. There are hundreds of different poisonous plants, the most common being the nightshades, belladonna (which produces rash, confusion, difficulty swallowing, blurred vision, and coma), foxglove (erratic heartbeat, irritation of mouth, abdominal symptoms such as pain and diarrhea), berries eaten from nightshades (black berries) or holly (red berries), with symptoms of abdominal pain, vomiting, flushing, hyperactivity, delirium, and coma.

Eating poisonous plants must be treated by pumping the stomach (gastric lavage). Death from eating poisonous plants is extremely rare.

The plants are the most poisonous in the spring and early summer but are even a problem when they are dried at other times of the year.

Occurrence: Poison ivy accounts for 350,000 cases of contact dermatitis per year. Young children are the most commonly affected from playing in patches of poisonous plants or being attracted to eating the colorful berries. Children should be taught not to eat wild plants and how to distinguish poisonous ones. Poison oak, ivy, and sumac grow as vines or bushes, and the leaves have three leaflets (ivy and oak) or a row of paired leaflets (sumac).

Special Notes: Wash any clothing that has come in contact with the plants. Sometimes cases that do not go away are due to repeated exposure through contaminated clothing. The best treatment is prevention, so if walking in areas where poisonous plants are common, know how to identify and wear protective clothing. Some sensitive individuals may react or continue to be exposed from petting animals who have run through patches of the plants, or by inhaling smoke from burning plants. In rare cases, if reaction seems so severe that there is difficulty breathing, may need to contact a physician and take corticosteroids.

Very hot water as from showering tends to spread rash and increase itching afterward.

Alternative Treatments

Refer to alternative therapy chapters for more information before evaluating or applying any treatment. Some conditions, including yours, may require a physician's care.

Nutritional Therapy: Orally: • Vitamin C (3 grams first hour then 1 gram per hour for first few days if reaction is very severe, and less if it is not) • Vitamin A (100,000 IU first two days in severe reaction and 50,000 if it is less, then reduce to 25,000 IU for next several days) • Vitamin E (1,000 IU first several days) • Zinc (50 mg. first few days) • Vitamin B complex (100 mg. of each two to three times daily first few days) • May add zinc oxide or unflavored yogurt to any of the topical treatments mentioned below.

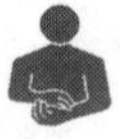

Self-Care

The following therapies can be undertaken at home under appropriate professional supervision.

• *Fasting* • *Guided Imagery*

Herbs: Apply a poultice or tincture combination of equal parts of witch hazel, mugwort, white oak bark, and plantain.

Hydrotherapy: Cold compress: apply as needed to control itching and pain.

Topical Treatment: • Rinse affected area with apple cider vinegar and goldenseal. • Frequent warm baths with apple cider vinegar or cornstarch. • Apply one of the following: aloe vera gel, witch hazel, paste of baking soda and witch hazel, paste of activated charcoal powder.

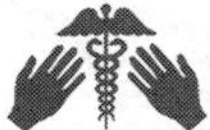

Professional Care

The following therapies should only be provided by a qualified health professional.

• *Applied Kinesiology* • *Chelation Therapy* • *Environmental Medicine* • *Magnetic Field Therapy* • *Naturopathic Medicine* • *Traditional Chinese Medicine*

Detoxification Therapy: May be indicated, depending on the condition of the person.

Oxygen Therapy: Hyperbaric oxygen therapy.

Polio

A childhood viral infection, with a wide range of manifestations from general mild illness to paralysis.

Symptoms: Symptoms may vary widely. There are two major types. *"Minor illness":* 80 to 90 percent of poliomyelitis infections, usually in very young children, may have no symptoms or mild ones such as sore throat, fatigue, fever, headache, and vomiting. Symptoms occur three to five days after exposure and last for twenty-four to seventy-two hours. *"Major illness":* In older children and adults: the two most characteristic symptoms are fever and muscular paralysis. Central nervous system symptoms occur such as deep muscle pain, tingling of skin, hypersensitivities of skin, meningitis (inflammation of the outer coverings of spinal cord and brain), severe stiff neck and backache, fever, severe headache, generalized muscle aches, and possibly widespread muscle twitching. These symptoms may occur very rapidly, culminating in severe weakness or muscular paralysis within a few hours from onset. The lower limbs are the most commonly affected. If the infection spreads to the brain there may also be difficulty in swallowing and in respiration.

Special Notes: Recovery from the minor illness, the non-paralytic polio, is total. Recovery from the major illness, the paralytic polio, occurs in half the individuals. Twenty-five percent suffer from minor residual muscle weaknesses. One in ten dies. Less than twenty-five percent are left with severe muscular disabilities. Years later, even in patients who have totally recovered, it appears that some individuals have a relapse called a "post-polio" episode, in which there is a reoccurrence of muscular weakness and pain.

Alternative Treatments

Refer to alternative therapy chapters for more information before evaluating or applying any treatment. Some conditions, including yours, may require a physician's care.

Diet: Whole foods diet with emphasis on food rich in magnesium such as dark green leafy vegetables.

Nutritional Therapy: • Magnesium (100-800 mg. daily. First, increase dosage up to the amount that creates very soft stools, then back off by 100-200 mg. and this will be daily dose. Sometimes one form of magnesium will irritate a particular individual and every dose will seem to create softer stools. You may need to explore different types of magnesium and from different companies.) • Niacinamide (taken four times daily to keep blood levels high and to increase muscular strength, motion, and to decrease pain. If not taken regularly, it will not help).

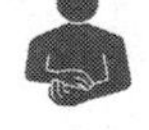

Self-Care

The following therapies can be undertaken at home under appropriate professional supervision.

• *Biofeedback Training* • *Yoga*

Juice Therapy: Carrot, beet, radish, celery.

Hydrotherapy: Constitutional hydrotherapy: apply two to five times weekly or heating compress. • Wet sock treatment: several times daily for head or chest congestion, replace socks when dry.

Whirlpool baths may improve circulation.

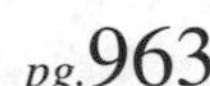

Professional Care

The following therapies should only be provided by a qualified health professional.

• *Environmental Medicine* • *Magnetic Field Therapy* • *Reconstructive Therapy* • *Traditional Chinese Medicine*

Bodywork: Treatment of post-polio syndrome: Feldenkrais.

Fasting: Under a doctor's supervision.

Pre- and Postoperative

Several weeks prior and several months to one year after surgery that requires invasion into the body, usually under a general anesthetic.

Special Notes: Nutrients and natural products taken before and after the surgical procedure may decrease healing time and pain, reduce complications, and increase quality of life during this period.

Preoperative

Alternative Treatments

Refer to alternative therapy chapters for more information before evaluating or applying any treatment. Some conditions, including yours, may require a physician's care.

Diet: Whole foods diet with avoidance of excess refined sugars, colas, and processed foods. In particular try to eat five to seven helpings of vegetables and fruits per day with unprocessed oils. Try to have at least one glass of fresh vegetable juice per day. Vary vegetables used in the juice.

Nutritional Therapy: • Zinc • Pantothenic acid • Vitamin B complex • Vitamin C • Multivitamin/mineral complex • Vitamin E • Essential fatty acids (omega-3 fatty acids) • Magnesium will help the body hold on to its potassium. • Potassium (50-100 mcg.) • Beta-carotene (100,000 units per day a few days before surgery. You may notice an orangish or yellowish skin tone.) • Alpha-ketoglutarate immediately before surgery • For cardiovascular surgery take coenzyme Q10 (200 mg.).

Do not try to follow a weight loss program before surgery, as this may cause a deficiency in amino acids, which are critical for wound healing.

To prevent blood pressure irregularities during surgery: • 10 grams vitamin C • 3 grams magnesium sulfate • 500 mg. vitamin B_6 • 50 mg. zinc sulfate

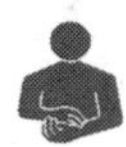

Self-Care

The following therapies can be undertaken at home under appropriate professional supervision.

• Fasting • Qigong

Flower Remedies: Rescue Remedy.

Herbs: See Postoperative. According to William L. Cowden, M.D., for preoperative anemia: yellowdock, mustard greens, turnip greens, spinach, kale. yellowdock capsules are most effective when taken with vitamin C.

Homeopathy: *Arnica.*

Hydrotherapy: Constitutional hydrotherapy: apply two to five times weekly.

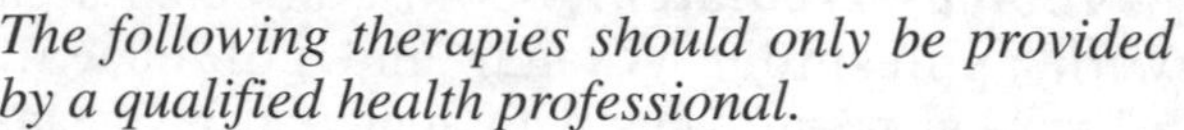

Professional Care

The following therapies should only be provided by a qualified health professional.

Oxygen Therapy: Hyperbaric oxygen therapy.

Postoperative

Alternative Treatments

Refer to alternative therapy chapters for more information before evaluating or applying any treatment. Some conditions, including yours, may require a physician's care.

Diet: Same as preoperative except, initially, consume lighter foods, such as soups, juices, broths, and pureed vegetables and fruits. Avoid refined sugars and excess consumption of fruit juices.

Nutritional Therapy: Same as preoperative except add free-form amino acids, glutamine, and extra vitamin B_6. If there is difficulty in healing or a history of difficulty in healing, taking proteolytic enzymes (on empty stomach and between meals) may hasten healing process.

• Alpha-ketoglutarate immediately after surgery. • Vitaman E and GLA can be given postoperatively by putting a teaspoon or two of flaxseed oil for GLA, and 400 units of vitamin E (puncture capsule and squirt onto skin along with flaxseed oil) onto the skin away from the incision once a day. • Sublingual co-enzymated B complex once or twice a day will help to speed up postop healing. • Arginine in very high dose. • Chromium (200-400 mcg. a day) • Selenium (50 mcg. per day) • Give aloe vera juice as soon as the patient is able to drink.

According to Alan R. Gaby, M.D., glutamine (250 mg. of body weight a day) reduced postop fall in muscle protein synthesis, and improved nitrogen balance. Glutamine requirements seem to increase after surgery to a level that isn't met by endogenous (coming from within) synthesis.

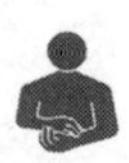

Self-Care

The following therapies can be undertaken at home under appropriate professional supervision.

Flower Remedies: Rescue Remedy.

Herbs: To facilitate postoperative healing combine herbs that help the body deal with the physiological stress of the surgery and support the healing process in the tissue, organs, and systems that experience the most trauma during the operation. A generalization can be made for all surgery as follows: combine an adaptogen with herbs to support liver detoxification, cerebral oxygen availability, and general wound healing. Combine Siberian ginseng, ginkgo, milk thistle, and hawthorn tinctures in equal amounts and take one-half teaspoonful of this mixture three times a day in the week leading up to surgery and for two weeks after. Externally apply vitamin E oil with a calendula salve to optimize healing.

Homeopathy: *Arnica.*

Hydrotherapy: Constitutional hydrotherapy: apply two to five times weekly.

Professional Care

The following therapies should only be provided by a qualified health professional.

- ***Pancreatic Enzyme Therapy***

Pregnancy

See Pregnancy and Childbirth chapter, page 790.

Premenstrual Syndrome (PMS)

See Female Health chapter, page 662.

Prostate Cancer, Prostatitis

See Male Health chapter, page 734.

Psoriasis

Common, chronic skin condition that is prone to reoccurrences.

Symptoms: Patches of skin that may be thickened and reddened and covered with silvery looking scales. It usually does not itch, but does cause discomfort and cosmetic embarrassment. Areas most commonly affected are: arms, elbows, behind the ears, scalp, back, legs, and knees.

According to Helmut Christ, M.D., of West Germany, "It has now been established that psoriasis is not a skin disorder strictly speaking, but instead an inherited metabolic disturbance which is triggered by environmental or stressful conditions, like faults in the diet, flulike conditions, the administration of penicillin, death of a family member, surgery, etc." [22]

Occurrence: Two percent of people in the United States and Europe. It occurs equally in men and women, and less in Blacks and Asians. Psoriasis usually occurs between fifteen and thirty years of age although it can manifest at any time. It does reoccur, so once it has been contracted it is always possible to return. Patients with psoriasis have a higher incidence of rheumatoid diseases than others.

Consider: Food allergies, essential fatty acid deficiencies, low digestive enzymes especially hydrochloric acid, vitamin B complex deficiencies, and emotional stress.

Special Notes: Psoriatic attacks can be encouraged by the following factors: anxiety, illness, drugs such as beta-blockers, lithium, and chloroquine, poison ivy or oak, skin damage such as cuts, lacerations, surgery, and sunburns, food allergies, nutrient deficiencies, and several infections bacterial or viral in origin. The true cause is unknown but the physiological mechanism is that the new skin is being produced ten times faster than the old skin is being shed. This creates an accumulation of the new skin which forms thickened patches with the characteristic psoriatic scales.

Mild cases of psoriasis may be helped by moderate sunlight or ultraviolet light.

Alternative Treatments

Refer to alternative therapy chapters for more information before evaluating or applying any treatment. Some conditions, including yours, may require a physician's care.

Diet: Assess and treat for food allergies. Eat a varied diet rotating foods as much as possible. Eliminate wheat and associated wheat products for several months to assess benefit. Whole foods diet as much as possible. Consume seafood high in omega-3 fatty acids: salmon, sardines, mackerel, herring. Orally, each day, take one tablespoon of a natural oil, rotating them, such as olive, flaxseed, canola, etc. Citrus foods may aggravate psoriasis in some individuals.

A good rule of thumb is: if you itch today then you ate something yesterday that your skin cannot tolerate.

Dr. Christ recommends avoiding all alcohol, nuts (except almonds), and aromatic spices (mustard, pepper, curry, etc.). He recommends eating fish, beef, venison, poultry, all kinds of fruits and vegetables, pasta, olives, olive oil, saffron, garlic, onion, herbs, and parsley. He highly recommends fresh hand-pressed fruit juices, beet juice, carrot juice, yogurt, curd, sauerkraut, and pickles without pepper.

Nutritional Therapy: • Unsaturated fatty acids (evening primrose oil—six, two times daily) • Vitamin A (75,000 IU daily for first two weeks then reduce to 50,000 IU daily for two to three months, then 25,000 daily for the rest of this year) • Folic acid (100-500 mcg. daily) • Vitamin B complex • Vitamin B_6 • Vitamin C with bioflavonoids • Zinc • Lecithin (one tablespoon with two meals a day for the first month) • Assess for hydrochloric acid deficiency. • Multimineral supplementation. • Vitamin B_{12} (by injection) may be helpful in some individuals.

Copper toxicity and low levels of zinc are characteristic of psoriasis, eczema, and acne.

European fumaric acid treatment: Dr. Christ reports success in treating psoriasis with fumaric acid monoethyl ester and fumaric acid dimethyl ester (not fumaric acid alone). He feels that psoriasis results from a metabolic error, possibly from defective fumaric acid metabolism. Fumaric acid enters into the citric acid cycle, which is the center for energy production on the cellular level. Results from clinical investigation of fumaric acid in Switzerland, West Germany, the Netherlands, and Japan are promising. Fumaric acid tablets, ointment, lotion, and scalp lotions are used in the treatment.[23]

The complete fumaric acid treatment protocol for psoriasis may be obtained from the Rheumatoid Disease Foundation.[24]

Fumaric acid may be obtained from Cardiovascular Research.[25]

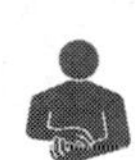

Self-Care

The following therapies can be undertaken at home under appropriate professional supervision.

• Biofeedback Training • Fasting • Guided Imagery • Yoga

Aromatherapy: Bergamot, lavender.

Bodywork: • Reflexology • Massage area with two drops calendula oil and one drop lavender oil in two tablespoons of almond oil.

Herbs: This intransigent skin condition can respond to herbs but it often takes time. The alterative herbs such as sarsaparilla[26] are used as the core of any treatment. Additional herbs can be added for associated anxiety, etc. Combine equal parts of burdock, sarsaparilla, and cleavers tinctures and take one teaspoonful three times a day. Drink an infusion of the fresh nettle or cleavers two or three times a day.

Homeopathy: *Psorinum, Sulfur, Graphites, Cuprum met., Arsen alb.*

Hydrotherapy: Heating compress: apply daily to affected areas.

According to Leon Chaitow, D.O., N.D., treatment of psoriasis in the Dead Sea region of Israel has a long history of success and has led to salt and mud from that region being marketed for home use. Dead Sea products can be used regularly on the skin or in baths to help promote healing of psoriatic lesions, as part of a comprehensive approach which also tackles dietary and allergy issues.

Dr. Chaitow recommends a neutral bath (at body temperature for profound relaxation effect) in which a pound or more of sea salt has been dissolved. Soak for forty-five minutes every day (pat dry) during acute phases.

Juice Therapy: • Apple and carrot • Beet, cucumber, and grape • No citrus • Beet, carrot, burdock, yellowdock (5 percent, i.e. two to three leaves per quart), garlic

Lifestyle: Frequent exercise, such as jogging, is recommended, in order to work up a good sweat.

Mind/Body Therapy: Deep breathing exercises, stress reduction.

Reflexology: Thyroid, adrenals, liver, diaphragm, kidneys, intestines, all glands.

Topical Treatment: • Apply sea water to skin with cotton several times daily. • Linseed or avocado oil

Professional Care

The following therapies should only be provided by a qualified health professional.

• Acupuncture • Cell Therapy • Chelation • Environmental Medicine • Hypnotherapy • Light Therapy • Magnetic Field Therapy • Naturopathic Medicine • Orthomolecular Medicine • Osteopathy

Detoxification Therapy: May be indicated, unless person is weak or deficient.

Oxygen Therapy: Hydrogen peroxide therapy (IV)

Rashes

A skin reaction that is usually temporary.

Symptoms: Most often consists of eruptions, a group of spots, or areas of redness and inflammation.

Occurrence: Everybody has rashes at some time.

Special Notes: Most rashes are not a sign of a serious problem and rashes are an element of most childhood illnesses. Skin disorders occur with rashes (allergic reactions, wide variety of dermatitises, eczema, psoriasis) and certain health disorders occur with rashes, such as liver and gallbladder problems, lupus, bleeding disorders, deficiencies of vitamins B or C, omega-3 fatty acids, or autoimmune diseases.

If rashes continue, if they form a "butterfly" shape over cheeks, if associated with a high fever and joint pains, see a doctor to rule out more serious illnesses.

Alternative Treatments

Refer to alternative therapy chapters for more information before evaluating or applying any treatment. Some conditions, including yours, may require a physician's care.

Diet: Assess and treat for food allergies. Drink plenty of filtered water. Avoid suspicious foods, the most common being citrus, berries, peanuts, shellfish, and dairy products. It is possible to suddenly develop skin reactions to foods or products (such as soaps, perfumes, jewelry) that were not reactive before. Check exposure to new products (fabric softeners, aftershaves, new clothing, etc.). Eat plenty of green, leafy vegetables and yellow vegetables such as carrots, pumpkin, sweet potatoes, and winter squash. The most important emphasis is to eat a wide variety of foods and rotate them as much as possible.

Avoid aspartame, (NutraSweet)

Nutritional Therapy: • Vitamin A (orally and topically) • Vitamin C • Vitamin E (orally and topically) • Sometimes allergic reactions can be neutralized by taking two Alka Seltzer Gold tablets or one-half teaspoon of baking soda in water every fifteen minutes three times and then every several hours until rash or reaction subsides. Do not continue this for more than a few days at a time. • Flaxseed oil or eicosapentaenoic acid (EPA) and gamma linolenic acid (GLA) taken regularly may, over time, prevent more recurrences.

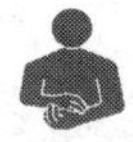

Self-Care

The following therapies can be undertaken at home under appropriate professional supervision.

• Fasting

Ayurveda: • Apply the pulp of cilantro leaf to the rash. • Drink coriander tea (one teaspoon of coriander seeds to one cup water), one-half teaspoon of *ghee* with a pinch of black pepper orally. *Neem* oil locally. Drink fresh cilantro, two tablespoons, three times a day.

Herbs: • Burdock root, gentian root • Fresh juice of coriander is good taken internally for allergies, hay fever, and skin rashes. • Take fresh aloe vera juice or gel.

Homeopathy: *Belladonna, Sulfur, Graphites, Calc carb.*

Hydrotherapy: Cold compress: apply as needed to control pain and/or itching.

According to Leon Chaitow, N.D., D.O., to relieve the irritation of most forms of skin rashes, twenty to thirty minutes in a warm alkaline (just above body heat) bath containing bicarbonate of soda (one cupful) is useful (urticaria, eczema, shingles pain, heat rash, allergic reactions to chemicals or plants, poison ivy or insect stings, sunburn).

For the same skin conditions as the alkaline bath (above) an oatmeal bath can be used. Water can be fairly warm (not very hot).

Add a few tablespoons of finely ground uncooked oatmeal powder to the bath and tie into a cloth at least a pound of coarse uncooked oatmeal. Hang this from the tap so that the water runs through it. When the bath is full remove this and use it as a sponge to gently pat areas of particular irritation. Thirty minutes in the oatmeal bath followed by patting the skin dry is indicated daily while skin is irritated.

Juice Therapy: • Drink fresh vegetable and fruit juices, especially carrot, beet, radish, and garlic. • Wheat grass juice

Naturopathic Medicine: According to Dr. Chaitow, from a naturopathic perspective skin rashes usually represent evidence of elimination of toxic wastes through the skin, or of an active immune reaction to an invading organism. Suppression of such a rash can lead to chronic disease states, and the most that should be done for the majority of rashes is to observe them, moderate any irritation they may be causing while avoiding any treatment which "makes" the rash go away.

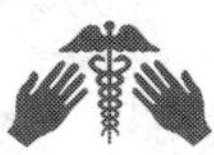

Professional Care

The following therapies should only be provided by a qualified health professional.

• Acupuncture • Naturopathic Medicine • Osteopathy • Traditional Chinese Medicine

Detoxification Therapy: May be indicated, depending on the condition of the person.

Oxygen Therapy: Hydrogen peroxide therapy.

Raynaud's Disease

Constriction and spasm of the smaller vascular system (arterioles) that most commonly occurs in the fingers and occasionally in the nose, tongue, and feet.

Symptoms: Initially, symptoms occur in response to cold and emotionally stressful situations. The fingers become white or bluish. Sometimes they also turn reddish. Tingling sensations are common. Rarely, the walls of the arteries thicken and the blood flow is permanently obstructed so that ulcers, infections, and even gangrene (death of tissue) may form around the nails.

Occurrence: More common in young women.

Consider: Rule out nutrient deficiencies, since this causes poor cold tolerance and decreased circulation.

Special Notes: A common cause is smoking which constricts the arterioles and creates poor circulation. Anything that increases circulation is helpful, such as deep breathing and biofeedback techniques.

When these symptoms develop without any known cause, this condition is labeled Raynaud's disease. When these same symptoms occur secondary to other health problems, this is then called Raynaud's phenomenon, and is usually more serious.

Some drugs produce these symptoms as a side effect, for example the beta blockers used in blood pressure treatment, as well as ergotamine used in migraine treatment, both of which may trigger Raynaud's symptoms.

Keep hands and feet as warm as possible. Exercise, stopping smoking, massage, bodywork, and manipulation are all helpful.

Alternative Treatments

Refer to alternative therapy chapters for more information before evaluating or applying any treatment. Some conditions, including yours, may require a physician's care.

Diet: Consume foods high in vitamin E such as raw seeds and nuts. Hot vegetable soups, vegetable purees, and many vegetables and fruits which are high in minerals are excellent.

According to Johnathan Wright, M.D., foods high in magnesium are recommended, as Raynaud's disease is a vasospastic condition and magnesium is a nutritional vasodilator.

Leon Chaitow, N.D., D.O., recommends avoiding coffee, as this constricts blood vessels.

Nutritional Therapy: • Vitamin E (1,000-1,500 IU daily) • Magnesium (200 mg. three times daily) • Iron (if anemic) • Vitamin B complex • Niacin (vitamin B_3) • Digestive enzymes, if necessary • Folic acid (1 gram daily) • evening primrose oil (1,000 mg.)

Take eicosapentaenoic acid (EPA) capsules (three to six daily) for at least three months, as these may decrease the viscosity of blood, allowing better circulation.

Self-Care

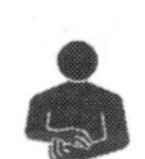

The following therapies can be undertaken at home under appropriate professional supervision.

• Biofeedback Training • Fasting • Guided Imagery • Qigong

Exercise: Rapid arm movement exercise can force blood through the tiny capillaries. Stand with arms at your side and swing them strongly round and round (like a windmill) forward and up and back and down and forward and up as high as you can, and as fast as you can (sixty to eighty swings a minute). This often relieves hand symptoms in a minute or two.

Herbs: Combine equal parts of the tinctures of ginkgo, prickly ash, and ginger and take one-half a teaspoonful of this mixture three times a day.

Homeopathy: *Arsen alb., Secale.*

Hydrotherapy: Constitutional hydrotherapy: apply two to five times weekly, begin with narrow contrast.

According to Dr. Leon Chaitow, a method by which you can condition your circulatory system is recommended by some experts, and has had success in large trials. Place two bowls with warm water in different environments. One in a warm room and one in a cold room or, outside in the cold. Dress as for indoors (lightly) and immerse the hands in the warm water indoors for between two and four minutes.

Go to the outside (or cold room) and do the same, but this time for eight to ten minutes. Go to the warm room and repeat the first immersion. This triple immersion (warm room, cold room, warm room) should be done not less than four times a day and ideally six, every other day until the symptoms of Raynaud's syndrome markedly improve. The conditioning process involves your body getting used to having warm hands in a cool atmosphere.

Juice Therapy: Fresh fruit and vegetable juices.

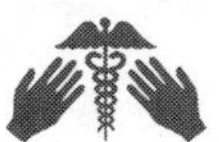

Professional Care

The following therapies should only be provided by a qualified health professional.

• Acupuncture • Cell Therapy • Chelation Therapy • Environmental Medicine • Pancreatic Enzyme Therapy • Magnetic Field Therapy • Naturopathic Medicine • Neural Therapy • Orthomolecular Medicine

Biofeedback: • According to Dr. Chaitow, one of the most useful measures for anyone with Raynaud's syndrome is application of biofeedback methods which focus on circulatory markers (temperature of the hands, etc.). • Autogenic training focuses on warmth of hands and feet as part of its methodology and may be very useful in helping to develop control over these states.

Chiropractic and Osteopathy: Osteopaths and chiropractors claim success in treating this condition by working on the neck and upper spinal structures to improve nerve and circulation supply.

Massage on a regular basis can assist in normalizing circulatory flow and relaxing tense structures in the neck and shoulder area.

Oxygen Therapy: • Hydrogen peroxide therapy • Hyperbaric oxygen therapy

Traditional Chinese Medicine: *Dong quai* and peony formula are effective.

Restless Leg Syndrome/ Periodic Leg Movement

See Sleep Disorders chapter, page 839.

Retinal Detachment, Retinopathy

See Vision Disorders chapter, page 859.

Respiratory Conditions

See Respiratory Conditions chapter, page 813.

Rheumatoid Arthritis

See Arthritis chapter, page 530.

Ringworm

Infections caused by fungi which invade "dead" tissues (from skin, hair, nails, groin, feet, and trunk).

Symptoms: The name occurs as the condition creates ring-shaped, reddish, patches that may also be scaly or blistered that spread uniformly outward leaving a circular patch of normal skin within the ring.

Alternative Treatments

Refer to alternative therapy chapters for more information before evaluating or applying any treatment. Some conditions, including yours, may require a physician's care.

Diet: According to Leon Chaitow, N.D., D.O., if ringworm is a frequent occurrence there may be benefit in treating fungus systemically as well as topically. A course involving a low-sugar diet, supplementation with garlic and probiotic substances such as *Lactobacillus acidophilus* and *Lactobacillus bifidobacteria* for several months may clear the tendency. (See Candidiasis chapter, page 587.)

Nutritional Therapy: • Vitamin A (orally and topically) • Vitamin B complex • Vitamin C with bioflavonoids • Citrus seed extract • Vitamin E (orally and topically) • evening primrose oil • Bee pollen

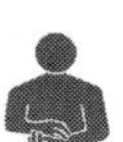

Self-Care

The following therapies can be undertaken at home under appropriate professional supervision.

• Fasting • Reflexology

Aromatherapy: Rosemary, tea tree, lavender, geranium, peppermint, thyme.

Herbs: Apply a paste made by mixing equal parts of myrrh powder and goldenseal powder mixed with a little water.

Homeopathy: *Sepia, Arsen alb., Graphites.*

Juice Therapy: Strawberry and date juice (use fresh dates).

Naturopathic Medicine: Local applications of tea tree, thuja, or thyme oils may be effective.

Topical Treatment: • Dr. Chaitow suggests that a thin slice of garlic bandaged directly over the skin lesion and left for several days has a powerful antifungal effect, and has been shown in clinical practice often to be more effective than orthodox skin creams. • Apply poultice of strong goldenseal root tea to area. Dry and dust with goldenseal root powder.

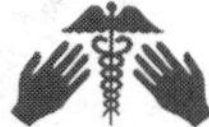

Professional Care

The following therapies should only be provided by a qualified health professional.

• Magnetic Field Therapy • Naturopathic Medicine • Traditional Chinese Medicine

Sciatica

A condition that manifests as radiating pain from the back either into the buttock and/or the lower extremity (leg) usually on the back (posterior) and outward (lateral) side. It represents pain referred somewhere along the path of the sciatic nerve.

Symptoms: Discomfort, pain, burning, tingling, stabbing, aching anywhere along the path of the sciatic nerve (from the buttock, down the leg, into the foot, although the most commonly affected areas are the buttock and thigh). In very severe cases the pain may be associated with weakness. Pain can be very severe and recurrent unless the cause is found and treated.

According to Leon Chaitow, N.D., D.O., there needs to be a clear distinction between sciatic neuralgia and sciatic neuritis. Neuritis is an active inflammatory process whereas neuralgia is an irritation of the nerve often resulting from outside mechanisms (disk, bone, muscle, distant trigger point activity).

The advice given below regarding diet, nutrients, and herbs can help neuritis more than neuralgia.

Manipulative and exercise methods are more helpful for neuralgia resulting from mechanical dysfunction. Sometimes neuralgia and neuritis coincide and both approaches are found useful.

Consider: Sometimes chronic musculoskeletal pain may be secondary to low thyroid conditions, nutrient deficiencies, old injuries in associated joints that never healed completely or correctly, referred pain from problems in internal organs, or emotional stress.

Special Notes: Treatment must include removing whatever the pressure is on the sciatic nerve (misalignment of lumbar spine), prolapsed (herniated) intervertebral disk, spasm of the buttock muscles (usually one called the piriformis), abnormal stresses on associated joints, secondary to injuries of the foot, knee, hip, or back that alter the walking gait and put abnormal and asymmetrical strain on the muscles.

Insufficient exercise and muscles which have become excessively weak and/or tense can create imbalances which are the most underappreciated causes of chronic musculoskeletal problems.

Alternative Treatments

Refer to alternative therapy chapters for more information before evaluating or applying any treatment. Some conditions, including yours, may require a physician's care.

Diet: Since thiamine (vitamin B_1) and magnesium act as natural muscle relaxants, foods that are high in these nutrients are good: dark leafy green vegetables, yellow vegetables, whole grains, and raw seeds and nuts. Avoid excess consumption of foods that drain the body of these nutrients, such as caffeinated beverages, chocolate, and refined sugars.

Nutritional Therapy: • Magnesium • Thiamine (vitamin B_1) • Vitamin B complex. • Vitamin B_{12} (injections may be helpful in some cases that are chronic and unresponsive to any other treatment) • Vitamin E • Calcium • Manganese sulfate

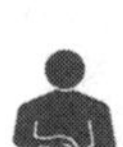

Self-Care

The following therapies can be undertaken at home under appropriate professional supervision.

• Fasting • Guided Imagery • Yoga

Acupressure: To relieve sciatica lie down on your back with your legs bent, feet flat on the floor. Place your hands underneath your buttocks (palms down) beside the base of your spine. Close your eyes and take long, deep breaths and rock your knees from side to side for two minutes to press acupressure point B48 (for an illustration of this point number please see the acupressure chart on page 875) in the buttocks. Reposition your hands for comfort and to enable different parts of the buttocks muscles to be pressed. Also try swaying your legs from side to side with your knees pulled into your abdomen and your feet off the floor.

Aromatherapy: Apply a cold press and lightly massage with chamomile or lavender, birch.

Ayurveda: *Triphala guggulu* 200 mg., generally taken one-quarter teaspoon with warm water twice a day after lunch and dinner.

Dashamoola tea *basti, mahanarayan* oil massage, and bathe with one-third cup of ginger powder and one-third cup baking soda.

Herbs: • Mix in equal parts willow bark and St. John's Wort tincture and take one-half teaspoonful three times a day. Massage with warm St. John's Wort oil will help alleviate pain. • Black cohosh, chamomile, fenugreek, juniper berries, mugwort, parsley, rosemary, skullcap

Homeopathy: *Colocynth, Viscum album, Lachesis, Rhus tox., Aconite, Arsen alb., Lycopodium, Mag phos., Ruta grav.* Dr. Chaitow recommends *Atropa Belladonna* (6X potency) for neuralgia.

Hydrotherapy: Contrast application: apply daily.

According to Dr. Chaitow a neutral bath (body temperature) has a profoundly destressing and calming effect.

Reflexology: Hip/sciatic, hip/knee, lower spine, shoulder, chronic sciatic area.

Energy Medicine: According to Dr. Chaitow, TENS is invaluable for relief of most but not all nerve pains.

Topical Treatment: According to Dr. Chaitow, for neuralgic type pain apply moist or dry heat to the affected leg(s) for an hour four times a day. This is only valid for neuralgic type pain where heat acts to relax muscles. If there is inflammation (neuritis) heat will inflame the area further. Use hot and cold alternating applications finishing with cold.

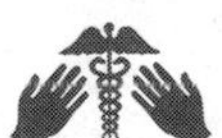

Professional Care

The following therapies should only be provided by a qualified health professional.

• Applied Kinesiology • Cell Therapy • Chiropractic • Colon Therapy • Craniosacral Therapy • Detoxification Therapy • Environmental Medicine • Magnetic Field Therapy • Naturopathic Medicine • Neural Therapy • Osteopathy • Pancreatic Enzyme Therapy • Reconstructive Therapy

Bodywork: Acupressure, reflexology, *shiatsu*, massage, Alexander technique, Feldenkrais, Trager, Rolfing, Hellerwork.

Traditional Chinese Medicine: Combination of acupuncture and herbal formulas depending upon cause of particular symptom.

Senile Dementia

See Alzheimer's Disease and Senile Dementia chapter, page 521.

Sexually-Transmitted Diseases

See Sexually Transmitted Diseases chapter, page 827.

Shingles (Herpes Zoster)

An acute (severe short-lived episode) viral [varicella-zoster virus (also causes chicken pox)] infection of the central nervous system that affects certain areas of the skin.

Symptoms: Several days (three to four) before the skin outbreaks occur, there is usually fatigue, fever, chills, and sometimes gastrointestinal upset. On the third to fourth day the skin area becomes very excessively sensitive. On the fourth or fifth day, characteristic small blisters erupt that crust and hurt along the path of a nerve so that the reddened outbreak affects a strip of skin that forms a line. This usually occurs over the ribs in the thoracic area and is usually limited to one side. Rarely, it can affect the lower part of the body or the face. The affected area is very sensitive and the pain may be very severe. The eruptions heal about five days later. Most people heal without any further problems except occasional scarring along the path of the nerve. In some individuals (about 30 percent), especially the elderly, pain may persist for long periods of time, months to years later, and sometimes be recurrent (2 percent). The older the individual and the longer the rash lasts, the more likely a lingering problem with pain will persist. One attack of herpes zoster usually gives immunity for life.

Occurrence: Can occur in any age group but is most common after fifty years of age. Several hundred cases per one hundred thousand people occur each year in the United States. It is a fairly common viral infection, but especially in those individuals whose immune systems have been severely compromised (cancer, HIV, severe trauma).

Consider: Consider chicken pox (in children), pleurisy, Bell's palsy, herpes simplex, appendicitis, colic, gallstones, colitis, trigeminal neuralgia, or contact dermatitis.

Special Notes: If the eruptions last longer than

two weeks, rule out possible underlying immune problem or cancer (particularly Hodgkin's disease). During a childhood bout of chicken pox, not all of the viral organisms are destroyed. Some lie dormant in sensory (skin) nerves for many years. When events occur that decrease the immune system, such as severe emotional stress, severe illness, or long-term usage of corticosteroids, the immune system cannot suppress the dormant organisms any longer and they become active again, causing infection along the pathway of the nerve.

See an ophthalmologist immediately if herpes zoster occurs near the eyes or on the forehead, as it can cause blindness.

Alternative Treatments

Refer to alternative therapy chapters for more information before evaluating or applying any treatment. Some conditions, including yours, may require a physician's care.

Diet: Whole foods diet with avoidance of excessive consumption of refined carbohydrates.

Nutritional Therapy: The most optimal approach if possible: • Vitamin B_{12} injections combined with adenosine monophosphate (AMP) which is usually done by an orthomolecular physician. (This along with placing plain yogurt mixed with zinc oxide, if available, along the path of the nerve [two to three times daily] often clears up herpes zoster in twenty-four to forty-eight hours, if regime is started at the first sign of the outbreak.) • L-lysine (4-5 grams initially, then 500 mg. two times daily for several weeks only) • Vitamin B_{12} (orally every hour first day) • Vitamin B complex • High doses of vitamin C plus bioflavonoids • Calcium

Dr. Cathcart's vitamin C bowel tolerance technique. (See Orthomolecular Medicine chapter, page 402.)

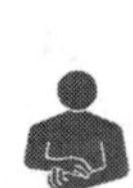

Self-Care

The following therapies can be undertaken at home under appropriate professional supervision.

• Biofeedback Training • Fasting • Qigong

Aromatherapy: Lemon, geranium, bergamot, eucalyptus, tea tree, lavender, chamomile. See Aromatherapy chapter.

Herbs: Combine equal parts of oat straw, St. John's Wort, and skullcap tinctures and take one teaspoonful of this mixture four times a day. Peppermint oil applied topically may reduce the pain through a mild local numbing effect. Do not attempt this if the skin is extremely sensitive. Colloidal oatmeal powder may be dusted on the affected skin to act as a dry lubricant, hopefully reducing pain from contact with clothes.

Homeopathy: *Arsen alb., Rhus tox., Sepia, Natrum mur., Hepar sulph., Caladium, acidum nit.*

Hydrotherapy: According to Leon Chaitow, N.D., D.O., the most calming (to the nervous system) and stress reducing bath is the neutral bath (body temperature) in which the individual soaks for thirty to sixty minutes. (Someone needs to do the topping up to keep heat at blood temperature, using a bath thermometer to check every few minutes.)

Juice Therapy: • Carrot and celery juice with one tablespoon parsley juice • Spinach, beet

Naturopathic Medicine: A gel made from licorice root appears to be an excellent topical application. Joseph Pizzorno, N.D., has seen serious pain and inflammation totally clear in just three days after application.

Reflexology: Diaphragm, all glands, whole spine.

Energy Medicine: According to Dr. Chaitow, TENS is invaluable for relief of most but not all nerve pains (in some conditions such as post-herpes neuralgia there have been both good and bad reports—bad meaning no benefit not a worsening of the condition). This method is well worth a try to see if the often intractable burning pain can be calmed in this safe manner.

Topical Treatment: • Vitamin E oil • Apply apple cider vinegar to rash.

Professional Care

The following therapies should only be provided by a qualified health professional.

• Acupuncture • Cell Therapy • Magnetic Field Therapy • Naturopathic Medicine • Neural Therapy • Orthomolecular Medicine

Energy Medicine: Light Beam Generator.

Detoxification Therapy: May be indicated, depending on the condition of the person.

Environmental Medicine: Treatment with weak dilutions of influenza vaccine can give relief to shingles.

Oxygen Therapy: Hydrogen peroxide therapy • Ozone may inactivate the herpes viruses. May be applied externally to lesions and/or internally as in autohemotherapy (withdrawal and intramuscular injection of patient's own blood).

Sinusitis

See Respiratory Conditions chapter, page 816.

Sleep Apnea, Sleep Disorders

See Sleep Disorders chapter, page 838.

Sore Throat

Inflammation in the pharynx (throat).

Symptoms: Associated with varying amounts of pain (often experienced as a rawness), usually with swallowing or speaking, accompanied by dryness, feelings of constantly needing to clear throat, and congestion of mucous membranes. Postnasal drip, enlargement of lymph nodes in the neck, and fever may also be present. Slight loss of normal voice, or hoarseness, often accompanies a sore throat and is usually not serious.

Consider: Usually caused by viral infections. But, may also be caused by bacterial infections, tonsillitis (secondary to inflammation of the tonsils), overuse of the voice, irritating substances such as smoking, allergic reactions, infections within the mouth, bacterial exposure because of too old toothbrushes (change every month), or associated with many illnesses as part of the symptom picture.

Special Notes: Viral infections do not respond to antibiotics and bacterial infections do. It is difficult to differentiate between the two merely by observation.

Sore throats are rarely serious, but often are the first symptom of many other health problems, such as the flu, herpes simplex, mononucleosis, and many childhood illnesses. Rarely, a sore throat occurs before the manifesting of a serious medical problem. If the sore throat does not resolve within two weeks, see a doctor. If any sore throat occurs with a rash, see a doctor.

Waking up with a chronic tickle in the throat may be a sign of food allergies, smoking, or environmental irritants or allergies.

A sore throat caused by a streptococcal infection (often called strep throat) must be identified and treated, or else it could create rheumatic fever or acute glomerulonephritis (disease of the glomerulus [network of blood capillaries]) of the kidney.

Alternative Treatments

Refer to alternative therapy chapters for more information before evaluating or applying any treatment. Some conditions, including yours, may require a physician's care.

Diet: Increase fluid intake including lots of filtered water, hot herbal teas, diluted fruit juices, and broths. Especially good is sipping warm water mixed with powdered vitamin C plus lemon and honey. Avoid refined sugars.

Nutritional Therapy: • Vitamin C with bioflavonoids • Vitamin A (high dose first few days) • Beta-carotene (high dose first few days) • Zinc lozenges (One every two hours unless nausea occurs, in which case more zinc than was needed was consumed. Decrease dosage.)

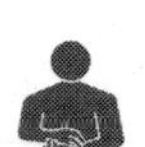

Self-Care

The following therapies can be undertaken at home under appropriate professional supervision.

• Fasting • Guided Imagery • Yoga

Aromatherapy: Inhalations with benzoin, lavender, thyme, eucalyptus, geranium, lavender, clary sage, sandalwood.

Ayurveda: • Gargle with a mixture of hot water and a quarter teaspoon of *tumeric* powder and a pinch of salt. • Gargle with other astringent herbs such as alum, sumac, sage, and bayberry.

Herbs: • If due to an infection, chew a small piece of osha root (*Ligusticum porteri*) as needed to alleviate the symptoms. Alternatively gargle with an infusion of sage or licorice. For a sore throat due to smoke or pollution irritation gargle with an infusion of lavender or hyssop. • Ginger tea or slippery elm tea are used for sore throats. • Echinacea and goldenseal are also sore throat remedies. • Take one-eighth teaspoon ground black pepper mixed with a teaspoon of honey.

Homeopathy: *Lachesis, Ignatia, Arnica, Aconite, Hydrastis, Gelsemium, Merc sol., Phytolacca.*

Hydrotherapy: Contrast application: apply one to two times daily to neck and throat. Heating compress: apply one to two times daily to neck and throat.

Juice Therapy: • Juice of red potato • Pineapple

Reflexology: Lymph system, all toes, great toes, adrenals, cervicals.

Topical Treatment: Gargle several times a day with either apple cider vinegar, hot water and one teaspoon of salt, or hot water with a teaspoon each lemon juice and honey.

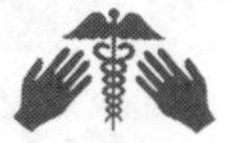

Professional Care

The following therapies should only be provided by a qualified health professional.

• Acupuncture • Cell Therapy • Environmental Medicine • Light Therapy • Pancreatic Enzyme Therapy • Magnetic Field Therapy • Naturopathic Medicine • Neural Therapy • Traditional Chinese Medicine

Detoxification Therapy: May be indicated, depending on the condition of the person. Detoxification may be helpful with chronic low-grade infection or allergies.

Energy Medicine: Light Beam Generator.

Light Therapy: Monochromatic red light therapy.

Sports Injuries

Any type of injury that occurs while performing sports or during general exercise. The most common injuries are soft tissue ones such as strains (overexercise to a harmful degree, overexertion or overstretching of the soft tissues [muscles, ligaments, and tendons]), sprains (injury to joint so that some of the soft tissues are actually torn or ruptured but the overall continuity of the joint itself is still intact), and other muscular injuries. Also, common are joint dislocations, fractures, and head injuries, all of which need to be seen by a doctor.

Symptoms: A wide variety of symptoms depending on the sport, the body parts, and joints involved and the degree of injury to that part.

Occurrence: Widespread. On the increase as exercise is on the rise.

Special Notes: The better "overall shape" muscles are in, the more adequate the stretch and warm-up time, the better the overall nutrient status of the individual, the less emotionally stressed the individual is, the better the equipment that is utilized, the less the likelihood injuries.

Equally important is cool down time in which the muscles are allowed to slowly return to a neutral nonactive state. This helps circulation and removes acidic products which result from exertion, preventing subsequent stiffness.

Both warm-up and cool down can effectively be helped by what is called "performance" massage, which anyone can learn to apply to themselves or their friends, but which is best applied by a licensed massage therapist with certification in sports massage.

It is very important to approach sports activities and exercise with common sense and information. Reinjuries are even more difficult to heal and may create more stubborn residual problems. Thus, it is important to contact a sports medicine practitioner, an exercise physiologist, or a personal trainer when embarking on a new program. Even if it is only for a one-time consultation to make sure you are on a safe path with a sensible program, it is worth it to avoid injuries down the road. Often, when you are unknowingly doing something that makes you vulnerable to injury, it will not show up or occur for several weeks to several months, until enough repetition has occurred. Thus, prevention and education is the paramount guideline when exercising or starting new sports.

Alternative Treatments

Refer to alternative therapy chapters for more information before evaluating or applying any treatment. Some conditions, including yours, may require a physician's care.

Diet: Whole foods diet especially adequate in natural carbohydrates and complex carbohydrates (60 to 70 percent of diet) and quality nonprocessed fats (no more than 20 to 25 percent of diet). Especially important to limit fat intake and excessive calories of any kind, as both can contribute to excess body fat. Excess fat will infiltrate muscles and cause them to be metabolically "out of shape" and more prone to injury. If there is inadequate complex carbohydrates, especially in the face of increased demand due to increased sport's activities, the body will go into its protein reserves and burn muscle, defeating the purpose of the exercise and making the individual actually weaker. Thus, it is not realistic to increase protein consumption because of increased exercise output. It is more important to increase quality carbohydrates, such as fresh fruits and vegetables, whole grains, potatoes, and other root vegetables.

Don't eat solid foods immediately before exercising, limit it to one and a half to two hours before or after exercise, unless you already have a habit of doing this and it does not seem to disagree with you. After all, there are no set rules except the ones that work best for each person.

Also, if you are only lightly or moderately exercising, the rules for food and exercise are not important as if you are heavily exercising or performing in competition. However, if you are prone toward allergic food reactions, especially avoid eating any allergic foods around times of athletic performance as exercise may enhance allergic reactions substantially.

Magnesium is one of the most important minerals for quality soft tissue tone. Green leafy vegetables are the best source. Foods that tend to "rob" the body of magnesium should be avoided in excess. They are caffeinated beverages, commercial sodas, excess refined sugars, and diets too high in animal protein and acid foods and too low in fresh fruits and vegetables.

Drink adequate fluids an hour or so before heavy exercising, even if you do not feel thirsty. Dehydration is a stress on the body and decreases performance capabilities.

Nutritional Therapy: *Prevention:* • Vitamin E (orally and topically) may help protect against muscle damage from exercise. • Vitamin C levels in body may help heal micro and macro injuries. • Magnesium keeps muscles flexible but toned and less susceptible to injury. • Free-form amino acids. *Acute injury:* • Calcium • Magnesium and valerian root may help reduce pain and muscle spasm when injured. • Manganese sulfate may help repair ligamentous tissue and must be taken every hour with vitamin C. • Magnesium and calcium for first two days when injured • Proteolytic enzymes (on an empty stomach, six every hour for first three hours then four times daily in between meals) for several days. If prone to injury, taking three, three times daily in between meals, for one week before competition may reduce injury rate and speed up healing time if injured. • Free-form amino acids. • *Bone fracture:* • Microcrystalline hydroxyapatite • Vitamin B_6 • Vitamin B complex • Essential fatty acids • Zinc

Recent studies reveal that antioxidant vitamins (A, C, E) offer protection against exercise-induced muscle injury in athletes.[27]

According to Leon Chaitow, N.D., D.O., healing following injury is speeded up when the amino acids arginine and glycine are supplemented (away from mealtimes).

Self-Care

The following therapies can be undertaken at home under appropriate professional supervision.

• Fasting • Biofeedback Training • Guided Imagery • Massage • Qigong

Aromatherapy: Everlast.

Herbs: Siberian ginseng.

Homeopathy: *Arnica* ointment for overuse, tendinitis, and post-traumatic inflammation. *Arnica* in an oral form may be useful until the acute inflammatory phase has passed.

Hydrotherapy: If acute; ice pack: apply twenty minutes out of each hour for the first twenty-four to thirty-six hours.

Juice Therapy: Raw fresh vegetable juices.

Naturopathic Medicine: A combination of bromelain (the enzyme from the green pineapple) and curcumin (from the spice turmeric) makes a very good oral anti-inflammatory therapy for sports injuries.

Topical Treatment: According to Johnathan Wright, M.D., dimethyl sulfoxide (DMSO) used topically is often useful.

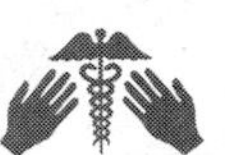

Professional Care

The following therapies should only be provided by a qualified health professional.

• Acupuncture • Applied Kinesiology • Cell Therapy • Chiropractic • Pancreatic Enzyme Therapy • Magnetic Field Therapy • Naturopathic Medicine • Neural Therapy • Osteopathy • Traditional Chinese Medicine

Bodywork: Feldenkrais, Rolfing.

Energy Medicine: Electro-Acuscope, Light Beam Generator.

Light Therapy: • Monochromatic red light therapy • Cold (soft) laser photo stimulation therapy

Massage: Skilled sports massage to injuries in important to help prevent fibrosis and scar tissue from developing at injury sites. It is also effective in reducing the chances of injury.

Oxygen Therapy: • Hydrogen peroxide therapy (IV) • Hyperbaric oxygen therapy

Reconstructive Therapy: William J. Faber, D.O., reports that relief for tennis elbow, wrist pain, chronic shoulder dislocation, rotator cuff tears, pain after severe injury, ankle weakness, and chronic and acute knee problems can be provided through reconstructive therapy.

Sprains

When a joint is overstretched or injured beyond its normal capacity the ligaments which connect bone to muscle may be injured without tearing, or may tear partially or completely. The capsule that surrounds the joint, made up of fibrous tissue, may also be injured.

Symptoms: Sprains may be *Grade 1*: mild, minimal sprain, without any ligamentous tearing, with possible mild tenderness and swelling of the area. *Grade 2:* partial tearing of ligament with very obvious swelling, bruising (black, blue, and yellow) and difficulty trying to use joint normally such as in weight bearing. *Grade 3*: a complete tear with much swelling, extreme bruising with hemorrhaging under the skin, joint instability, and inability to use the joint at all. Muscle spasms (muscle contractions that are not voluntary) may be associated with all grades of sprains, may be primary as part of the injury, or may be secondary due to the compensatory use of associated muscles because of the injury. Pain due to sprains usually increases when attempts are made to move the involved join.

Special Notes: *Grade 1:* require supportive elastic bandages, tape, or therapeutic splinting to create immobilization, elevation, followed by very gentle exercise. Optional: assessment by manual practitioner. *Grade 2:* requires immobilization for three weeks. Needs manual medicine and rehabilitation. *Grade 3:* requires casting or, rarely, surgery. Requires manual medicine and rehabilitation.

X-rays are usually necessary to rule out fractures.

Initially, for all sprains, ice (twenty minutes: optimal is to alternate with ice and moist heat, twenty minutes each, starting and ending with ice), elevate joint, immobilize, and take something for swelling, pain, and healing. When joint no longer hurts after use, and all swelling, bruising, and associated spasm is gone, gentle mobilization exercises should be initiated.

Alternative Treatments

Refer to alternative therapy chapters for more information before evaluating or applying any treatment. Some conditions, including yours, may require a physician's care.

Diet: Whole foods diet with plenty of fresh fruits, vegetables, nuts, seeds, and whole grains.

Nutritional Therapy: • Take proteolytic enzymes (such as bromelain from the pineapple plant) away from meal times on an empty stomach. *Grade 1:* six initially then three, three times daily. *Grade 2:* six initially then four, four times daily. *Grade 3:* six initially then six, four times daily for longer periods of time. Take until joint swelling is gone and pain is almost gone, decrease dosage as healing improves. • Take enzymes with vitamin C and bioflavonoids. (Increase bioflavonoids depending on amount of bruising. Initially, take with one buffered aspirin to help with reduction of pain and swelling.) • Increase calcium, magnesium, and valerian with more muscle spasm involved.

According to Leon Chaitow, N.D., D.O., healing following injury is speeded up when the amino acids arginine and glycine are supplemented (away from mealtimes).

Self-Care

The following therapies can be undertaken at home under appropriate professional supervision.

• Biofeedback Training • Fasting • Guided Imagery

Aromatherapy: Make a cold compress with camphor, lavender, chamomile, eucalyptus, or rosemary.

Herbs: Combine equal parts of the tinctures of horsetail, nettle, and willow bark and take one teaspoonful of this mixture three times a day. Apply comfrey to the affected area.

Homeopathy: *Ruta grav.*

Hydrotherapy • Contrast application: apply daily, if acute. Ice pack: apply twenty minutes out of each hour for the first twenty-four to thirty-six hours. • Ice and contrast

Juice Therapy: Raw fresh vegetable juices, including beet, radish, garlic (can dilute with comfrey tea).

Reflexology: Work reflex area on foot, referral area to affected area.

Topical Treatment: According to Jonathan Wright, M.D., dimethyl sulfoxide (DMSO) used topically is often useful.

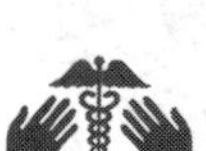

Professional Care

The following therapies should only be provided by a qualified health professional.

• Acupuncture • Applied Kinesiology • Cell Therapy • Chiropractic • Craniosacral Therapy • Energy Medicine • Magnetic Field Therapy • Naturopathic Medicine • Neural Therapy • Reconstructive Therapy

Bodywork: Massage, Feldenkrais, Rolfing.

Osteopathy: Specialized soft tissue techniques called "strain-counterstrain" were developed by osteopathic physician Laurence Jones, D.O. These relieve acute pain and spasm following strains and sprains rapidly.

Sties

An acute (short-lived) pus-filled infection (abscess), usually due to staphylococci, of one or more glands of the eye, normally located near the eye lashes.

Symptoms: Initially pain and redness occur, followed by a small, swollen, roundish area on the margin of the eyelid. A small yellowish spot in the center indicates pus. When the abscess breaks open and the pus is discharged, the pain is relieved. Swelling can occur around the whole area.

Special Notes: Do not attempt to squeeze the lump with your fingers as this may spread the infection into the blood stream and can become extremely serious.

Sties tend to reoccur.

Alternative Treatments

Refer to alternative therapy chapters for more information before evaluating or applying any treatment. Some conditions, including yours, may require a physician's care.

Diet: Whole foods diet high in garlic. Avoid refined sugars.

Nutritional Therapy: • Vitamin A (100,000 IU first two days then reduce to 50,000 next two days and then 25,000 daily for next week) • Vitamin C • Beta-carotene (50,000 IU daily for first few days)

Self-Care

The following therapies can be undertaken at home under appropriate professional supervision.

• Fasting

Detoxification: According to Leon Chaitow, N.D., D.O., if sties are recurrent consider a detoxification program (including periodic short fasts) followed by remodelling of lifestyle and dietary habits.

Herbs: • Use an eyewash made with a fresh and well-filtered infusion of eyebright and goldenseal. • Red raspberry tea

Homeopathy: *Pulsatilla, Hepar sulph., Sulfur, Graphites.*

Hydrotherapy: Contrast application: apply daily over the face and eyes.

Reflexology: Eye reflex, neck area, all toes.

Topical Treatment: Eyebath of chamomile (use flower tops) or red raspberry tea.

Hot compresses should be applied for ten minutes two to four times daily.

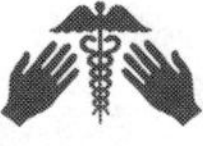

Professional Care

The following therapies should only be provided by a qualified health professional.

• Applied Kinesiology • Light Therapy • Naturopathic Medicine • Traditional Chinese Medicine

Stomach Ache

See Children's Health chapter, page 602.

Strep Throat

See Children's Health chapter, page 604.

Stroke

A sudden and severe episode in which there is some kind of blockage of blood to the brain resulting in damage to that part of the brain. When the symptoms from a stroke last for twenty-four hours or less, followed by full recovery of lost functions, the episode is called a transient ischemic attack (TIA).

In case of stroke: Get the individual to a hospital immediately.

Symptoms: Stroke symptoms may develop within a few minutes to over several days. Symptoms are: Loss and/or impairment of movement, sensation and specific functions controlled by the part of the brain that is damaged, not necessarily the specific artery that is affected. For example, damage to the speech center of the brain results in loss or slurring of speech. Also associated are: headaches, dizziness, confusion, difficulty swallowing, and visual problems. About 30 percent of cases of stroke are fatal; about 30 percent result in partial loss of function; and about 30 percent completely recover. Many people who become paralyzed by a stroke, learn to walk again. However, loss of intellectual functioning tends to not recover as well. TIA's usually last only several minutes and are warning signals.

Occurrence: Two hundred cases per one hundred thousand people in the United States per year. Higher in the elderly and in males.

Special Notes: Strokes are the most common cause of neurological damage in the industrialized Western world, and are a leading cause of death in these countries. The most common cause of strokes is secondary to arteriosclerosis (thickening of lining of arteries), high blood pressure (hypertension), or both. Other risk factors are: old age, smoking, a recent heart attack, elevated blood fats (hyperlipidemia), diabetes mellitus, blood platelet stickiness associated with a raised levels of red cells (polycythemia) or low levels of nutrients that prevent stickiness such as vitamin B_6, irregular heart beats (atrial fibrillation), oral contraceptives in women under fifty years of age, and history of a damaged heart valve.

Important: According to David Hughes, Ph.D., hyperbaric oxygen therapy done within the first six hours of a stroke may significantly improve the stroke victim's condition.

Alternative Treatments

Refer to alternative therapy chapters for more information before evaluating or applying any treatment. Some conditions, including yours, may require a physician's care.

Diet: A whole foods diet with emphasis on garlic, onions, Vitamin B_6 (all three tend to prevent platelets from sticking together) and unprocessed fats. Limit fats to 10 to 15 percent of total diet, avoid deep fried foods, animal fats, semi-solid fats, and concentrate on fresh fruits and vegetables. Especially good are raw nuts and seeds, whole grains, fresh vegetables such as broccoli, sprouts, and kelp. Limit foods that are natural plant sources of estrogens, such as soy beans and peanuts. Avoid alcoholic beverages and especially alcoholic binges (four drinks or more in short period of time). Consume more fish, especially fresh water.

Nutritional Therapy: • Vitamin E (high dosages) • Omega-3 fatty acids (fish oils) • Vitamin B_6 • Vitamin B complex • Magnesium • Vitamin C • *Ginkgo biloba* • Superoxide dismutase (SOD)

According to Leon Chaitow, N.D., D.O., well-researched studies show that taking garlic (raw or as a deodorized oil capsule) dramatically reduces platelet adhesiveness allowing improved circulatory function.

Vitamin C to bowel tolerance. (See Orthomolecular Medicine chapter, page 402)

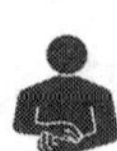

Self-Care

The following therapies can be undertaken at home under appropriate professional supervision.

• Biofeedback Training • Flower Remedies • Guided Imagery • Massage • Meditation • Qigong • Yoga

Aromatherapy: *For muscular paralysis:* • Lavender • Rub spinal column and paralyzed part with mixture of one quart of rubbing alcohol, and one ounce each of essence of lavender, essence of rosemary, and essence of basil.

Herbs: *To improve circulation to extremities:* elder flowers, hyssop, rosemary, yarrow. *To nourish nervous system:* damiana, lavender, rosemary, Siberian ginseng. Consult a trained herbalist.

Hydrotherapy: • Constitutional hydrotherapy: apply two to five times weekly. • Swimming exercise to restore strength.

Reflexology: Tip of great toe (opposite side from paralysis), other toes, reflexes to affected areas.

Professional Care

The following therapies should only be provided by a qualified health professional.

• Chelation Therapy • Hypnotherapy • Light Therapy • Magnetic Field Therapy • Naturopathic Medicine • Osteopathy • Sound Therapy • Traditional Chinese Medicine

Bodywork: • Feldenkrais.

Reconstructive Therapy: Pain after stroke.

Vision Therapy: Vision therapy may be an important ingredient in rehabilitation. Victims suffer aim, focus, and eye movement impairment as well as visual field and perceptual defects. Without evaluation by a behavioral optometrist these can be overlooked and recovery hindered. Therapy includes awareness training, visual/motor exercises and lenses and prisms. Gross and fine movement control, hand-eye coordination, attention, memory, and learning skills improve dramatically.

Sunburn

Overexposure of the skin to ultraviolet radiation (sunlight) causing inflammation and burns of the skin. Occurs more in fair-skinned individuals.

Symptoms: Symptoms appear one to twenty-four hours after exposure. The symptoms peak at seventy-two hours, unless the burning is severe. The affected skin turns anywhere from mildly reddish to severely red and darker. Symptoms range from skin becoming mildly tender to severe pain and swelling. Blisters may appear, which then open and the outer layer of the skin peels away. Sunburn on the lower extremities is usually more painful and takes longer to heal. If a large enough portion of the skin is affected, systemic symptoms may occur such as: chills, fever, weakness, shock. Secondary infections may follow once the skin has peeled. The new skin may be very sensitive to touch and to further sunlight for several weeks.

Burns are classified into three degrees. First degree burns merely redden the skin. Second degree burns cause swelling, and more pain and blisters that fill with water. Third degree burns result in more severe damage to the skin, are more prone to infection and must be seen by a doctor.

Special Notes: The best treatment is prevention. Initial summer exposure should not exceed a half an hour during the midday sun, even in persons with darker skin. The best time for sun exposure is before 11:00 A.M. and after 3:00 P.M. Cloudy summer days and foggy winter days, especially at higher altitudes, have a greater danger of sunburn as they appear to be safer but have almost the same amount of ultraviolet exposure. Reflections off of water, metal, snow, sand, silvery objects may increase the amount of rays absorbed. In the 1950s and 1960s sun worshippers used aluminum foil reflectors to increase the suntanning effect. This may have resulted in many cases of skin cancer.

Repeated overexposure to the sun and sunburns increases aging of the skin and increases risk of skin cancers.

New research suggests that sunscreens themselves may be instrumental in causing melanoma.[28] In a controversial study, Cedric Garland, Dr.P.H., and Frank Garland, Ph.D., of San Diego, California, report that by using a sunscreen one prevents the skin from producing vitamin D, which interferes with melanoma growth and that of other cancers.

According to this study, there is no evidence that sunscreens prevent cancer in humans. They only prevent sunburn, the body's natural method of warning that the skin has received too much sun.

The Garlands also state that the rise in melanoma rates have been directly proportionate to the sales rates of sunscreens. Queensland, Australia, has the highest rate of melanoma in the world, and was also the place where sunscreens were first and most strongly recommended by the medical community.

Sunscreens: If you should choose to use a sunscreen, they are rated by the FDA's Sun Protection Factors (SPF) by numbers. One is the least protective and 15 is the most protective. In some foreign countries, their 10 is equal to 15 in the United States. Very effective sunblocker formulas contain 5 percent para-aminobenzoic acid (PABA). Put on thirty minutes before going into sun as it takes at least this length of time to bind to the skin. Use the highest protection sunscreens at first. Once a tan is achieved the lower protection numbers may be used. Reapply when going in and out of the water or with prolonged sun exposure and sweating, to be safe. Sometimes PABA produces allergic reactions. Those sensitive individuals should use benzophenone sunscreens. Opaque formulas that contain zinc oxide or titanium dioxide block the sun physically by reflecting it off the skin.

Some suntanning oils and creams do not contain sunscreen and do not offer any protection against the sun.

Patients on drugs that react when in sunlight (photosensitivity usually demonstrated by rash when in the sun) should not regard sunscreens as protection against these reactions. Also, occurs in individuals with the conditions of lupus erythematosus.

Avoid further sun, apply cold compresses, and avoid creams that contain local anesthetics such as benzocaine, which may actually aggravate the symptoms.

Alternative Treatments

Refer to alternative therapy chapters for more information before evaluating or applying any treatment. Some conditions, including yours, may require a physician's care.

Nutritional Therapy: • Vitamin E (orally and topically) • Vitamin A (depending on severity of burn) *Mild:* 50,000 IU daily for several days. *More severe:* 100,000 IU for first three days then reduce to 50,000 IU daily for several weeks. • Vitamin C (amounts of all the antioxidants depend on degree of severity) • Potassium (100 mg. one time daily for one to two weeks) • Mix together vitamins A, E, essential fatty acids, zinc oxide, and aloe gel, and place on skin. • Calcium • Magnesium

Self-Care

The following therapies can be undertaken at home under appropriate professional supervision.

• Fasting

Aromatherapy: • Spray or rub with lavender and chamomile. • Prevent blistering: Apply two to three drops of lavender oil.

Herbs: Apply cool aloe vera gel liberally to the burnt area. If badly burnt apply a salve made with St. John's Wort and calendula flowers.

Homeopathy: *Natrum mur.* (as preventative); *Urtica Urens, Rhus tox.*

Hydrotherapy: • Cold compress: apply immediately and as needed to control pain. • Bathe with apple cider vinegar or colloidal oatmeal.

Juice Therapy: Carrot juice.

Naturopathic Medicine: The gel from the freshly cut aloe vera leaf applied to sunburn combined with large oral doses of vitamin E.

Topical Treatment: • Mixture of apple cider vinegar (two parts) and olive oil (one part) • PABA cream

Professional Care

The following therapies should only be provided by a qualified health professional.

• Naturopathic Medicine

Oxygen Therapy: • Hydrogen peroxide therapy (IV) • Hyperbaric oxygen therapy

Traditional Chinese Medicine: Apply Chinese black tea externally.

Swelling

Enlargement of a localized area usually secondary to infection, injury, or holding and shifting of bodily fluids.

Alternative Treatments

Refer to alternative therapy chapters for more information before evaluating or applying any treatment. Some conditions, including yours, may require a physician's care.

Diet: Whole foods diet with a decrease in salt, commercial sodas, and refined sugars and an emphasis on increasing filtered water and herbal teas but avoiding excess caffeinated beverages and undiluted fruit juices.

Nutritional Therapy: • Proteolytic enzymes (on empty stomach) • Bromelain (on empty stomach) • Vitamin C and bioflavonoids • Vitamin B complex • Vitamin B_6

Self-Care

The following therapies can be undertaken at home under appropriate professional supervision.

• Fasting

Ayurveda: • Drink barley water (boil four parts water with one part barley and strain). • External swelling: apply mixture of tumeric (two parts) and salt (one part) to affected area. • *Punarnava guggulu* 200 mg. generally taken twice a day after lunch and dinner.

Herbs: Make a fomentation (hot pack) of ginger root. Increases circulation to an area, swelling, pain, and stiff joints.

Homeopathy: *Belladonna, Aconite, Ferrum phos., Sulfur.*

Hydrotherapy: Contrast application: apply repeatedly as needed to reduce swelling.

According to Leon Chaitow, N.D., D.O., alternating immersion of the swollen area in, or applications of hot and cold (damp towels will do nicely) to the area, reduces swelling by speeding up drainage of lymph (the clear fluid which is the medium for waste disposal following injury or inflammation) and flushing the area with fresh blood. Alternatively ice massage can be useful if the swelling relates to an acute problem.

Juice Therapy: • Fresh pineapple juice • Carrot, celery, cucumber

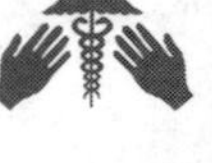

Professional Care

The following therapies should only be provided by a qualified health professional.

• Acupuncture • Environmental Medicine • Magnetic Field Therapy • Naturopathic Medicine • Traditional Chinese Medicine

Bodywork: According to Dr. Chaitow, lymphatic drainage massage and other massage techniques may help to remove swelling by opening the drainage (lymphatic) channels which might be overloaded. This may be especially useful for chronic swellings.

Osteopathy: Cranial and other osteopathic techniques exist which are aimed precisely at enhancing drainage and lymphatic flow.

Syphilis

See Sexually Transmitted Diseases chapter, page 831.

Tendonitis

A tendon is a fibrous chord that attaches a muscle to a bone or a muscle to another muscle. Inflammation can occur to the tendon itself (tendinitis) or to the lining of the tendon called the tendinous sheath (tenosynovitis). Inflammation usually occurs to both simultaneously.

If the muscle which attaches to the tendon is chronically overloaded through overuse or abuse (trauma), the tendon attachment to the bone becomes irritated, causing what is called a periosteal pain point. If this condition continues the tendon itself becomes inflamed.

Symptoms: The tendons that are involved are usually very painful and tender to the touch and are painful on motion of the involved joint. Often the joint motion becomes restricted because of the pain and the abnormal changes to the tendons themselves that affect movement. The pain can become very severe depending on the degree of inflammation. Very severe pain may radiate to the joints above and below this joint. The pain may affect daily life and make sleep difficult when the joint is moved during movements while sleeping. The involved tendons often have a "creaking" quality to them due to "friction rubs" from the inflammation itself, and may become swollen because of the inflammation or due to some fluid accumulation. Sometimes, calcium becomes deposited in the area, or the swollen tendon sheath puts extra pressure on where it inserts into the bone so that the bone enlarges at that site in response to this chronic pressure.

Occurrence: Very common in many individuals. More common in middle and older age due to decreased circulation in the tendons associated with repeated microtrauma (very small lesion). The most common cause of tendinitis is repeated or extreme trauma, excessive (not usual) exercise and strain. Certain systemic diseases have a higher incidence of tendinitis, such as rheumatoid arthritis, autoimmune disorders, gout, Reiter's syndrome (an inflammatory syndrome), when blood cholesterol levels are excessively high (hyperlipoproteinemia, Type 11), and in younger women with certain sexually transmitted diseases.

Special Notes: The most common areas to get tendinitis are the shoulder capsule (subdeltoid bursitis), the tendons of the big thumb (de Quervain's disease) and the hip capsule (trochanteric bursitis). Tendinitis and bursitis are really interchangeable terms as bursa are located near tendons.

Treatment needs to involve immobilization (splinting of the involved part), compresses with cold or heat (whatever seems to help, it varies between individuals), agents to reduce pain locally and systemically (orally and topically), and therapeutic exercise which should increase as joint becomes better and is able to tolerate increased movement.

Alternative Treatments

Refer to alternative therapy chapters for more information before evaluating or applying any treatment. Some conditions, including yours, may require a physician's care.

Diet: Avoidance of the members of the nightshade family of plants (white potato, tomato, eggplant, all peppers [except black], and tobacco), if restricted for a long time, over years, may be effective. Assessment and treatment of food allergies is imperative. Inflammation may be aggravated by food allergies in many people.

Nutritional Therapy: • Vitamin B_6 • Vitamin B complex • Vitamin C with bioflavonoids • Copper orally (2-4 mg. daily and/or wear copper bracelet. Copper is absorbed topically through the skin and may decrease chronic joint pains.[29]) • Manganese • Bromelain • Essential Fatty Acids • Cod liver oil (one tablespoon one to two hours before meals) D-phenylalanine and/or calcium/magnesium may help with pain • Vitamin E • Selenium

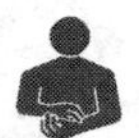

Self-Care

The following therapies can be undertaken at home under appropriate professional supervision.

• Acupressure • Biofeedback Training • Fasting • Guided Imagery • Massage • Shiatsu

Herbs: Combine equal parts of the tinctures of willow bark, cramp bark, and prickly ash and take one teaspoonful of this mixture three times a day.

Homeopathy: *Aconite, Thuja, Ruta grav., Belladonna, Apis mel.*

Hydrotherapy: • Contrast application: apply one to three times daily. If acute, ice pack: apply twenty minutes out of each hour for the first twenty-four to thirty-six hours. • Epsom salts bath. Several tablespoons of Epsom salts per bath. Soak for twenty-five to thirty minutes. Rinse and rub down with hot olive oil. Do once a week.

Osteopathic Self-Care: According to Leon Chaitow, N.D., D.O., if the tendinitis relates to chronic overload or misuse of muscles then relaxing and stretching these reduces the stress on the tendon. Osteopathic muscle energy methods can usually be safely used at home in a way which achieves this. The most successful method uses yoga-type stretches following mild painless contractions of the involved muscle.

Topical Treatment: • Rest the injured area and elevate above the level of the heart. • *Salt and vinegar therapy for stiff joints, sprains, inflammation:* soak several layers of gauze or muslin with apple cider vinegar. Place coarse, kosher salt thickly on the gauze and wrap around affected area. • *Loosening up of tendons and joints:* rub iodized salt moistened with apple cider vinegar on affected area twice a week. Be sure it is not too liquid. • Mullein hot packs. Boil three to four fresh mullein leaves in water for three minutes. Place over joint. Wrap with hot moist towel, then dry towel. Leave on for twenty minutes, three times a day.

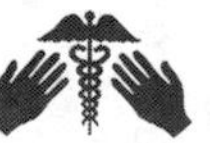

Professional Care

The following therapies should only be provided by a qualified health professional.

• Acupuncture • Cell Therapy • Chiropractic • Craniosacral Therapy • Energy Medicine • Magnetic Field Therapy • Naturopathic Medicine • Neural Therapy • Osteopathy • Reconstructive Therapy

Bodywork: Feldenkrais, Rolfing.

Detoxification Therapy: Detoxification is indicated. Treat inflammation locally.

Light Therapy: • Monochromatic red light therapy • Cold (soft) laser photo stimulation therapy

Oxygen Therapy: • Hydrogen peroxide therapy (IV) • Hyperbaric oxygen therapy

Tinnitus

See Hearing and Ear Disorders chapter, page 702.

Tonsillitis

Acute (short-lived) infection of the tonsils, usually caused by streptococcal organisms and less commonly viral.

Symptoms: Swelling and pain in the neck, pain in the throat, particularly painful on swallowing, and often the pain radiates to the ears. In very young children the main symptom may be refusal to eat. They may not complain of sore throat. Other symptoms may be: high fever, abscesses on the tonsils, temporary hearing loss, headache, hoarseness, coughing, vomiting, and general ill feelings and fatigue.

Occurrence: This is mainly a childhood condition in children, occurring most frequently in children under nine years of age. Most children experience at least one episode. It can, however, occur in older individuals but it is more rare.

Special Notes: Throat cultures (must see a doctor) are necessary to rule out strep throat and family members need to be tested at first, as they may be carriers and need to be treated along with the infected individual.

Treatment needs to include bed rest, lots of fluids, agents to reduce pain, and antibiotics if the infective organism is strep.

Alternative Treatments

Refer to alternative therapy chapters for more information before evaluating or applying any treatment. Some conditions, including yours, may require a physician's care.

Diet: Lots of fluids, especially diluted fresh fruit juices, warm broths, and light soups. *To relieve pain:* two tablespoon each of honey and glycerine with a one squeeze of lemon juice. Warm and sip slowly. If on antibiotics, consume live yogurt.

Nutritional Therapy: • Vitamin A (100,000 IU first three days, then 25,000 next week) • Zinc Lozenges (slowly dissolve in mouth every two to four hours) • Vitamin B complex • Vitamin C • If on antibiotics take acidophilus and bifidobacteria. • Garlic capsules • Ginger packs and zinc oxide should be applied externally to reduce pain.

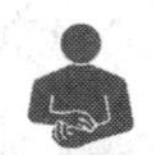

Self-Care

The following therapies can be undertaken at home under appropriate professional supervision.

• Guided Imagery • Relaxation • Yoga

Aromatherapy: Inhalations with bergamot, thyme, lavender and benzoin, tea tree, geranium, lemon (gargle, too).

Fasting: According to Leon Chaitow, N.D., O.D., there is no better approach than a pure water or diluted juice fast for the first forty-eight hours, followed by broths, etc., as recommended.

Herbs: Combine the tinctures of cleavers and echinacea in equal parts and take one teaspoonful three times a day. Drink a hot infusion made from equal parts of dried elder flower, yarrow, and peppermint throughout the day.

Homeopathy: *Belladonna, Merc sol., Phytolacca, Lachesis, Aconite.*

According to the German system of homotoxicology the tonsils are organs of excretion for toxins, and detoxification processes as well as inflammatory reactions take place in the tonsils. One theory is that many cases of chronic and recurring tonsillitis are due to the fact that the acute stage of the inflammation was quickly suppressed by powerful pharmaceutical drugs and the detoxification process was not able to occur. In treating tonsillitis one should attempt to both destroy the pathogen and also aid in the discharge of toxins.

Hydrotherapy: • Contrast application: apply one to two times daily to neck and throat. Heating compress: apply one to two times daily to neck and throat. • Gargle with hot water.

Juice Therapy: • Carrot, beet and tomato • Carrot, pineapple • Carrot, orange • Carrot, apple • Carrot, celery • Ginger

Reflexology: Great toes, lymph system, all toes, adrenals, cervical.

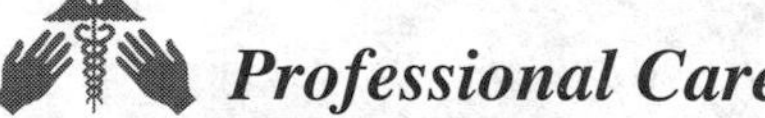

Professional Care

The following therapies should only be provided by a qualified health professional.

• Acupuncture • Cell Therapy • Magnetic Field Therapy • Naturopathic Medicine • Neural Therapy • Osteopathy • Traditional Chinese Medicine

Detoxification Therapy: May be indicated, depending on the condition of the person.

Oxygen Therapy: Hyperbaric oxygen therapy may be useful as an antibiotic.

Tuberculosis

An infection, often referred to as TB, either acute (short-lived) or chronic (long-term), which occurs as pulmonary tuberculosis (in the lungs) or extrapulmonary tuberculosis (other bodily sites), and is also classified when it occurs, in childhood or adulthood. It is caused in human beings by the bacterium Mycobacterium tuberculosis.

Symptoms: TB most commonly affects the lungs and is often asymptomatic (no symptoms) until the lung lesions (where the TB is growing on the lungs) become large enough to be seen on x-ray or to create problems. The earliest symptoms are usually coughing (usually first demonstrates as early morning cough) and flulike symptoms. Other symptoms are chest pain, difficulty breathing, coughing up blood, decreased appetite, fever, sweats (worse at night), and weight loss. Complications can occur, such as collecting fluid between the lung and the chest wall (pleural effusion), collecting air in the same space (pneumothorax), or even death. Sometimes symptoms do not occur for up to two years following initial infection. The speed of the symptoms varies widely from individual to individual.

Occurrence: In the United States, TB is responsible for 1,800 deaths per year and 20,000 new cases are reported per year. Fifteen percent of these cases are extrapulmonary TB. Most at risk are older non-white males (Africans, Hispanics, and Asians), especially if they have a history of being in physical contact with active cases (any person in a household with an active individual, especially a child, should be given an antituberculosis antibiotic drug as prevention) or people who were not appropriately treated with drugs, and in individuals from Central and South America, Africa, and Southeast Asia. People with illnesses that decrease immune competence, such as alcoholics, malnutrition, diabetics and HIV positive, are more at risk.

The major risk of catching TB from another active individual is before diagnosis is made. When individuals are on appropriate treatment, within ten to fourteen days they become noninfectious, even though the sputum (material coughed up) still has the active TB laboratory markers.

Special Notes: Prevention is the key and this has historically been done through vaccinations (Bacille Calmette-Guérin [BCG] vaccination in high-risk groups or contact tracing performed on relatives and friends of TB patients through skin testing and x-ray to rule out early stages). Vaccinations are useful where TB is still a problem. Recently, TB was so well controlled in the United States that vaccines were rarely used. However, there is now an increase in certain areas such as California and New York City. Ask your doctor for advice in this matter according to where you reside.

Diagnosis must include a chest x-ray and skin and sputum tests.

Caution: *Drugs which act as immune suppressants, i.e. corticosteroids, can retrigger tuberculosis.*

Treatment must include drugs. Two or more drugs should be used to avoid bacterial resistance to one drug. The drugs used are hard on the liver, thus, lab test monitoring the liver functions must be run regularly.

Alternative Treatments

Refer to alternative therapy chapters for more information before evaluating or applying any treatment. Some conditions, including yours, may require a physician's care.

Diet: Whole foods diet with plenty of raw foods, fluids, and lots of pears, pear juice, and pear sauce (like applesauce but made from pears) as pears may be helpful to hasten healing of the lungs. Other foods which may be helpful are: foenugreek and alfalfa sprouts, garlic, pomegranate, and all forms of fermented milk such as yogurt and kefir. Make a puree of steamed asparagus by blending in blender and keeping refrigerated, then take four tablespoons at breakfast and dinner for a few months.

Nutritional Therapy: • Vitamin A (300,000 IU for first three days, then 200,000 IU next two days, then 50,000 IU daily for several weeks) • Beta-carotene (25,000-50,000 IU) • Vitamin E (increase up to 1,000 IU daily unless a premenopausal woman with many premenstrual symptoms) • Lipotrophic formula (one daily) • Deglycerhized licorice • Citrus seed extract • Vitamin C • Lung glandular • Essential fatty acids • Vitamin B complex • Multiminerals • Zinc

Self-Care

The following therapies can be undertaken at home under appropriate professional supervision.

• Qigong

Herbs: Combine the tinctures of echinacea, elecampane, and mullein in equal parts and take one teaspoonful three times a day. Take three capsules of garlic three times a day.

Hints: Get plenty of fresh air, rest, light, exercise and relaxation.

Hydrotherapy: Constitutional hydrotherapy: apply two to five times weekly.

Juice Therapy: Raw potato juice. After juicing, allow the starch to settle and pour off the juice. Combine with an equal part of carrot juice, add one teaspoon or olive or almond oil, one teaspoon of honey, and beat until it foams. Drink three glasses daily.

Topical Treatment: • Eucalyptus oil packs • Grape packs • Alcohol packs (grain)

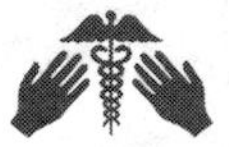

Professional Care

The following therapies should only be provided by a qualified health professional.

• Cell Therapy • Magnetic Field Therapy • Traditional Chinese Medicine

Fasting: Fasting may be indicated under a doctor's supervision.

Light Therapy: • Red Light • Sunlight

Ulcers

See Gastrointestinal Disorders, chapter page 686.

Urinary Problems

(See also Female Health [Bladder Infection], and Bedwetting)

The urinary tract is that part of the body involved in formation, concentration, and excretion (clearing) of urine. The urinary tract system includes kidneys, which make urine out of the blood and are associated with their own blood and nerve supplies, the ureters, which are tubes taking urine from the kidneys to bladder, and the urethras, which are tubes taking urine from the bladder out of the body (excretion).

Urinary problems may vary widely. They usually involve a problem anywhere along the entire urinary tract, including the kidneys.

Symptoms: Most people urinate four to six times a day, usually all during the daytime. It is not typical to get up in the middle of the night to urinate, especially two times or more, on a somewhat regular basis (unless there have been much more liquids consumed during the day). This is called nocturia (urination during the night), and is often suggestive of early diabetes, or of either kidney, heart, or liver disease. Also, it may not be associated with a serious disease, but may be secondary to other non serious bladder problems, such as obstruction.

Straining, nocturia, changes in force of stream of urine, and hesitancy are usually signs of bladder obstruction and are more common in middle-aged to older men, often secondary to an enlarged prostate due to a variety of problems, but most often not serious. *Pain or burning on urination (dysuria)* suggests inflammation or irritation of the bladder or the urethra, and is usually due to an infection from a bacteria. *Incontinence* (loss of urine not while urinating, without warning, often after sneezing, laughing, running, or coughing) is associated with many conditions such as bladder dysfunctions, cystocele (abnormal pocket formed by lax tissue) as result of stretching or aging of muscles of pelvic floor, injuries from childbirthing, fibroids on the uterus that push down on the bladder, etc. and may now be successfully treated with simple surgical procedures if the problem becomes severe enough and decreases quality of life.

Normal urine is usually clear or slightly yellowish. Certain vitamins make the urine bright yellow and have a strong odor. This is not a sign that something is wrong, it is a normal metabolic process of vitamin ingestion. This colormetric characteristic of urine while taking vitamins is often used as a mile post to help elderly patients remember to take their vitamins ("keep taking enough to keep your urine bright yellow"). Presence of other color pigments in urine usually means: red (foods such as beets, this is normal), brown, black, blue, green, or red (from certain drugs), and colors other than normal such as brownish or black may suggest the presence of diseases or blood in the urine, and must be investigated by a doctor. Cloudy urine most often is a normal precipitate of phosphate salts in alkaline urine but may suggest pus from a urinary tract infection.

Pain anywhere in the urinary tract may refer to

different areas of the body and may be the only symptom of a problem in the urinary tract, and thus be confusing. Pain from kidney disease is often referred to the low back, or between the twelfth rib and the iliac crest (hip) and sometimes to the sternum (chest bone). Bladder infections may refer pain to above the pubic area and along the urethra. Urinary problems and/or reproductive problems may create a feeling of abdominal fullness in both men and women.

Occurrence: Family history of problems in this area, especially kidney disease, may suggest a heredity predisposition (risk factor one is born with). If urinary problems occur with ear and eye disorders, this may indicate congenital (tendency towards or presence of at birth) urinary/kidney problems. Recent infections of the respiratory tract, the heart or skin may be causes for later problems in the urinary or kidney organs. History of past kidney problems, traumas (such as accidents or injuries), or other conditions such as high blood pressure or drugs taken, or history of past kidney stones or stones in primary relative (in one's personal family), all may be important information to figure out what problem an individual is having in this area.

Alternative Treatments

Refer to alternative therapy chapters for more information before evaluating or applying any treatment. Some conditions, including yours, may require a physician's care.

Diet: *Urinary infections:* Laboratory studies have shown that cranberry juice and cranberry juice cocktail may inhibit bacteria from sticking to the lining cells of the bladder and causing urinary tract infections, explaining its long history as a folk remedy. Further studies are needed to find out if this also happens in the body.[30]

Caffeine has been linked to urinary incontinence. Research shows that in people with weak bladder muscles, caffeine causes the muscles around the bladder to contract and exert additional pressure.[31]

The following foods and additives are known to irritate the bladder: coffee, tea, artificial sweeteners, carbonated beverages, tomato-based foods. Elimination of these from the diet can often result in complete relief of symptoms.

Nutritional Therapy: *Infections:* • Vitamin C • Pain and burning (acute) may be helped by cranberry juice along with vitamin C. However, in chronic cases, vitamin C may aggravate some individuals, in dosages over 1-2 grams. Instead, try alkalinizing the body by taking baking soda (one-half teaspoon) or two Alka Seltzer Gold tablets. • Vitamin B_1 (30-50 mg. two to three times per day in between meals for no more than one week, to help reduce pain, burning, and irritation) • Add mineral ascorbates with meals three times daily. • In men, if the urinary problem is secondary to prostate problems, that must be treated accordingly. (See Male Health chapter.) • Problems secondary to pelvic muscle atrophy or stretching may respond to mixed amino acids (two to three times daily, ten to fifteen minutes before meals for at least six months), along with a Kegel exercise program both for women and men (squeezing together of all the musculature around the urinary and reproductive areas accomplished by trying to squeeze everything below up towards the belly button). Repeat fifty times morning and evening as a regular part of the day, not to be discontinued once symptoms improve or go away. In other words, like other exercises, these must be kept up daily.

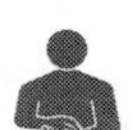

Self-Care

The following therapies can be undertaken at home under appropriate professional supervision.

• *Yoga*

Acupressure: Rub the acupressure points SP6 and ST36. (See acupressure chart, page 874.) vigorously in a circular motion for twenty to thirty seconds. Do it several times a day and before bedtime.

Aromatherapy: Tea tree oil. *Infections:* sandalwood, bergamot, juniper.

Biofeedback: May be effective in treating incontinence.

Herbs: For mild water retention and possibly mild cystitis symptoms—make an infusion of equal parts of bearberry, dandelion leaf, and nettle. Drink this hot three times a day or as needed. *Blood in urine:* comfrey. *Difficult or burning urination:* fennel, horsetail, jasmine flowers, licorice. *Cystitis, painful urination:* hibiscus. *Urinary tract infections:* buchu, burdock, coriander, cornsilk, echinacea, goldenrod, juniper berries, marshmallow root, shave grass. *Urinary incontinence:* skullcap.

Homeopathy: *Urethritis: Aconite, Apis mel., Cantharis.*

Hydrotherapy: For incontinence, use a sitz bath: apply daily with emphasis on cold. For urethritis, sitz bath: apply contrast daily.

Juice Therapy: • Carrot, parsley, celery, cucumber • Cranberry

Lifestyle: *Incontinence:* Pelvic exercises—one hundred to two hundred contractions of the bladder muscles daily—can greatly improve bladder control.

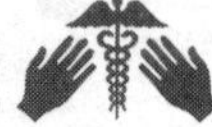

Professional Care

The following therapies should only be provided by a qualified health professional.

• Acupuncture • Magnetic Field Therapy • Naturopathic Medicine • Osteopathy

Vaginal Infections

See Female Health chapter, page 670.

Varicose Veins

Valves in the veins prevent blood from draining back into certain areas, especially the legs. When these valves are absent from birth or become incompetent, pooling of blood occurs in superficial (not deep) veins. This pooling of blood encourages the veins to become enlarged (dilated and swollen), elongated, and twist and bend more than normal (tortuous). When this happens the veins are called varicose.

Symptoms: At first the veins become more tense and stiff and this can be felt but not seen. Then, they become more enlarged and twisted and may be visualized easily as bluish, blackish prominent tubular elevations from the rest of the surrounding skin. Symptoms are not directly related to the size or degree of the varicosities. For example, very severe varicose veins may have no symptoms at all while patients with tiny varicosities may complain severely of aching, leg fatigue, itching, burning, or heat that seems relieved by elevating the legs or wearing stockings that compress the legs. Most commonly, symptoms seem to increase during the premenstrual cycle (anywhere from midcycle to onset of the period).

The most common sites for varicose veins are the back of lower leg (the calves) and along the inside of the lower and upper legs.

Occurrence: Varicose veins are very common and affect more women than men. Overall, varicose veins affect about 15 percent of adults in the United States. Varicosities do occur in families.

Special Notes: Varicosities in other parts of the body are: varicocele (varicose veins in the scrotum), hemorrhoids (varicose veins in the anus), and esophageal varices (varicose veins in the esophagus).

Risk factors for varicosities are sedentary lifestyle, obesity, smoking, standing on the legs for very long periods at a time, pregnancy, and hormonal changes at pregnancy or menopause.

If the problem of blood back sliding and pooling becomes severe enough that tissues do not get adequate nutrients and oxygen, the skin around the varicosities may become very thin, discolored, hardened, and prone to deep sores called ulcers. These need to be treated by cleaning, keeping covered, and improving the circulation and return of blood to the heart by leg compresses, elevating legs, overall exercise program, and nutrients and warm foods that increase circulation.

If a large varicosity is traumatized, such as bumping the leg or straining at the stool and bruising or lacerating a hemorrhoid, it may cause severe bleeding. Apply moderate pressure, lie down, elevate the legs, and contact a physician.

Wear support stockings. Contact an exercise physiologist or trainer and start a sensible overall exercise program (daily walking and swimming is excellent). Walking barefoot as much as possible is also excellent, along with walking on grass first thing in the morning when there is still dew on it (avoid in the colder climates during winter).

Massage area every night with almond oil with drops of myrrh oil and vitamin C crystals added, even over hemorrhoids, etc. If there is some burning discontinue, or try eliminating the vitamin C.

Alternative Treatments

Refer to alternative therapy chapters for more information before evaluating or applying any treatment. Some conditions, including yours, may require a physician's care.

Diet: Ideally, start with a bowel cleanse program or at least a few days on just fruits, vegetables, and whole grains with lots of filtered water to start cleansing the system. Whole foods diet with emphasis on the following foods: fresh fruits, including berries and cherries, and citrus fruit making sure to nibble on the inside of the rinds (organic is best when doing this), whole grains especially buckwheat (whole grain and noodles) and millet, garlic, onions, ginger, and cayenne pepper. Eat plenty of fish and cut down on red meat as much as possible. Moderately restrict fats and refined carbohydrates in diet. Foods to avoid: sugar, salt, alcohol, fried foods, processed and refined foods, animal protein, cheeses (goat is okay), and ice cream.

Nutritional Therapy: • Rutin (1 gram per day for up to one year) • Bioflavonoids (1 gram daily for same time) • Some people may have to stay on rutin and bioflavonoids permanently as their metabolism requires these to prevent reoccurrence. • Vitamin C (take throughout the day every several hours) • Vitamin B complex • Vitamin B_6 (pyridoxine: 30-100 mg. daily for several months) • Vitamin E (400 IU). *For leg cramps:* • Vitamin E • Calcium • Magnesium • Folic acid (1 gram daily for several months) • Lethicin • Vitamin D (500 mg. daily for two months)

For ulcers accompanying varicosities: • Vitamin E (orally and topically) • Zinc (orally, and topically as zinc oxide cream) • Essential fatty acids (orally and topically: squeeze one capsule on area two times daily). If ulcers do not heal try adding proteolytic enzymes (four to six, in between meals three times daily for two weeks).

Self-Care

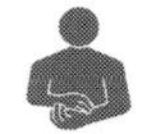

The following therapies can be undertaken at home under appropriate professional supervision.

• Fasting • Yoga

Aromatherapy: Cypress as bath oil. Lavender, juniper, rosemary (do not massage directly on top of vein), lemon.

Bodywork: Acupressure, reflexology, massage.

Herbs: Combine equal parts of the tinctures of hawthorn, ginkgo, prickly ash, and yarrow and take one teaspoonful of this mixture three times a day. A lotion for external use can be made with ten parts distilled witch hazel and one part tincture of horse chestnut.[32] This may be applied often to help ease any discomfort.

Homeopathy: *Calc fluor., Hamamelis, Pulsatilla, Calc carb., Carbo veg.*

Hydrotherapy: Cold compress or sprays/showers: apply cold application daily to affected veins (use gentle spray).

Juice Therapy: • Carrot, celery, and parsley • Carrot, spinach, and turnip • Carrot, beet, cucumber • Carrot, celery, spinach • Watercress

Reflexology: Colon, liver, adrenals. Referral area: arm.

Professional Care

The following therapies should only be provided by a qualified health professional.

• Acupuncture • Cell Therapy • Chelation Therapy • Pancreatic Enzyme Therapy • Magnetic Field Therapy • Naturopathic Medicine • Reconstructive Therapy • Traditional Chinese Medicine

Oxygen Therapy: Ozone.

Vertigo

A subjective impression of losing one's equilibrium (feeling off-balance) due to a sensation that the individual is moving around in space (subjective vertigo) or the room and objects in it are moving around the individual (objective vertigo).

True vertigo is an organic disturbance somewhere within the equilibratory system (ears, inner ear canals, the eighth cranial nerves servicing the ears, the associated brain parts, and the eyes) that may be caused by mild disturbances or secondary to specific health disorders such as middle ear infections, a herpes zoster viral infection, an inflammation of the semicircular ear canals (labyrinthitis), obstruction in an ear tube, a tumor, or a nerve inflammation.

True vertigo is contrasted to false vertigo or episodes of dizziness, faintness, or lightheadedness, which are common complaints and most often not a sign of any serious underlying problem.

Symptoms: True vertigo usually comes on very suddenly and is usually accompanied by difficulty in walking steady and feeling dizzy or faint. There may also be nausea, a generally ill sensation and pallor (losing color, turning white).

Occurrence: May occur in healthy people in specific situations such as on a roller coaster or other amusement-type rides, sailing, looking out the window of a car or watching a fast-paced movie. True vertigo associated with underlying disorders often occurs with vomiting and severe unsteadiness of gait. However, not all vertigos accompanied with these symptoms are due to underlying illness. Some people get this way by sitting on a sail boat.

Consider: Sudden attacks of vertigo, tinnitus (ringing in the ears), and losing hearing, often associated with nausea and vomiting, are symptoms of Meniere's disease. (See Hearing and Ear Disorders chapter, page 701.)

According to Johnathan Wright, M.D., some vertigo is set off by allergies.

Vertigo can be a sign for many other problems and a severe attack of it warrants a through examine of the ears, eyes, and nervous system by a doctor.

Special Notes: True vertigo is not necessarily a sign of a psychological problem. However, obsessive fear of losing one's balance or inappropriate giddiness may be a sign of depression or anxiety neurosis.

According to Leon Chaitow, N.D., D.O., anxiety itself is often the end result of hyperventilation (inappropriate breathing patterns) which is commonly associated with vertigo. Breathing retraining and appropriate manual (osteopathic, chiropractic, soft tissue manipulation, etc.) attention to spinal and thoracic restrictions, as well as postural reintegration and stress reduction are often needed to normalize such problems.

Stay still. Avoid rapid body movements, especially of the head.

Preventative measures: reduce stress, get bodywork, especially reflexology and/or chiropractic, and practice routine and adequate sleep habits.

Alternative Treatments

Refer to alternative therapy chapters for more information before evaluating or applying any treatment. Some conditions, including yours, may require a physician's care.

Diet: Avoid caffeine, especially cappucinos and chocolates, salt, fried foods, nicotine, drugs and alcohol, and aspartame (NutraSweet).

Nutritional Therapy: • Vitamin B complex (one, two times daily) • Vitamin B_6 (100 mg. daily) • Niacin (B_3—30 mg. three times daily) • Vitamin C plus bioflavonoids and rutin • *Ginkgo biloba* extract (120 mg. daily) • Ginger capsules *Prevention of acute attack:* six tablets several hours before suspected episode. *During:* three to six, two to three times daily on empty stomach. *Prevention in general in prone individual:* two tablets, two times daily on empty stomach, not to be taken for more than one month. Consult an orthomolecular physician before taking if there is a history of female problems or estrogen related tumors. • Choline (500 mg. two times daily) • Calcium • Adrenal • Vitamin E

Self-Care

The following therapies can be undertaken at home under appropriate professional supervision.

• Fasting • Qigong

Ayurveda: • Mix sesame oil with small amounts of camphor, cardamom, and cinnamon and apply to head. • The Ayurvedic herb *amla* is used for vertigo. • An herbal mixture of: *shatavari* 500 mg., *kamadudha* 200 mg., ginger 100 mg., and *brahmi* 300 mg., generally taken twice a day after lunch and dinner. *Brahmi ghee nasya.*

Herbs: Ginkgo[33] and ginger[34] may help with the symptom of vertigo, but competent diagnosis is essential. Take one 40 mg. tablet of ginkgo or two capsules of ginger three times a day.

Homeopathy: *Gelsemium, Phosphorus, Cocculus, Aconite, Nat. mur., Sulfur, Silicea, Lycopodium, Belladonna.*

Reflexology: Ear reflex, neck, cervicals, great toes.

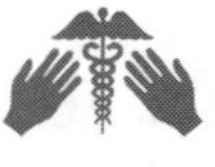

Professional Care

The following therapies should only be provided by a qualified health professional.

• Cell Therapy • Chiropractic • Craniosacral Therapy • Environmental Medicine • Hypnotherapy • Magnetic Field Therapy • Naturopathic Medicine • Osteopathy • Traditional Chinese Medicine

Viral/Bacterial Infections (Children)

See Children's Health chapter, page 606.

Viral Infections

Infection by a virus. A virus is a minute infectious agent, consisting of a nucleic acid core (either DNA or RNA: which is the basic infectious material), with a protein shell (capsid), which is often multilayered with fats. It is this capsid that is very difficult for many drugs to penetrate, thus requiring antiviral drugs to be very aggressive.

Symptoms: Viral infections classically demonstrate fever, generalized aches, chills, fatigue, and symptoms that are specific for that virus. For example, the cold virus usually produces mucous in the nose and throat, the mononucleosis virus produces severe fatigue and sometimes liver enlargement, and the polio virus produces paralysis.

Occurrence: Viruses that occur mainly in human beings are spread by themselves most commonly through respiratory routes and physiologic fluids (such as blood and semen). There are several hundred different viruses that may potentially infect man. Many are just being recognized and new ones may form or mutate, so that their physiologic expression, their interrelationships, their symptoms and assessments and their prevention and treatment are not fully known. Some viruses do not produce overt symptoms or disease. Others do and are very important to understand for the health and longevity of the human race.

Viruses vary tremendously in their effect on the body. The common cold is an acute (short-lived) viral infection. Some viruses cause cancer and terminal diseases. Some viruses incubate over a long period before the expression of the physiologic problems they cause. These are called "slow" viruses meaning they have a prolonged incubation period, such as the HTLV type III virus, which has been linked to AIDS. Exposure to it may take one year before it shows up in the blood and many years before symptoms show up in the individual.

Special Notes: A virus is the smallest of parasites as it is totally dependent on cells (plant, animal, or bacterial) for reproduction. Viruses stimulate host antibody production. Thus, identification of infection by a virus is often performed in the laboratory by measuring the blood level of antibodies to that virus.

Viruses do not respond to antibiotics. Thus, viral infections or diseases do not respond to antibiotics. However, viral infections may cause individuals that are susceptible to bacterial infections to become infected with both, and thus, sometimes, antibiotics are given for some viral infections for treatment or to prevent complications. This is a controversial treatment regime, and overuse of antibiotics is not beneficial for most individuals.

Viruses may be controlled, the symptoms may be reversed, but up until now, the viruses have not been successfully eradicated out of the body. Modern medicine is trying to change this.

Alternative Treatments

Refer to alternative therapy chapters for more information before evaluating or applying any treatment. Some conditions, including yours, may require a physician's care.

Diet: Whole foods diet with as little stressor foods as possible.

Nutritional Therapy: • Vitamin C to bowel tolerance. According to Robert Cathcart, M.D., this is an effective way to deal with viral problems, *but the protocol must be strictly adhered to.* (See Orthomolecular Medicine chapter, page 402.)

• Zinc • Proteolytic enzymes (four to six, three times daily on empty stomach in between meals) • Acidophilus • Vitamin A • Raw thymus glandular • Vitamin B complex • Pantothenic Acid (1-3 grams, two to three times daily) • Garlic capsules • Lysine • L-cysteine

An amino acid screen assessment by an orthomolecular physician may be beneficial.

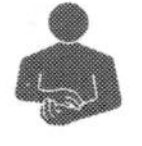

Self-Care

The following therapies can be undertaken at home under appropriate professional supervision.

• Fasting • Guided Imagery

Herbs: Combine equal parts of the tinctures of echinacea, goldenseal, and myrrh and take one teaspoonful of this mixture three times a day.

Homeopathy: *Calendula, Chamomilla, Belladonna, Merc sol., Sulfur.*

Hydrotherapy: Constitutional hydrotherapy: apply two to five times weekly. Hyperthermia: apply one to two times weekly.

Juice Therapy: Carrot, celery, beet, garlic.

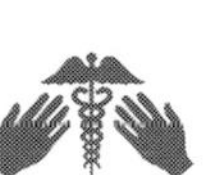

Professional Care

The following therapies should only be provided by a qualified health professional.

• Cell Therapy • Environmental Medicine • Pancreatic Enzyme Therapy • Magnetic Field Therapy • Naturopathic Medicine

Detoxification Therapy: Detoxification may be indicated unless the person is weak or deficient. Lighter diet is often recommended.

Oxygen Therapy: • Hydrogen peroxide therapy (IV) • Hyperbaric oxygen therapy • Ozone inactivates lipid enveloped viruses (herpes, mumps, measles, retroviruses—HIV, hepatitis, polio, echo virus, coxsackievirus).

Vomiting

The forceful and involuntary (unless it is self-induced as in eating disorders) expulsion of contents of the stomach out through the mouth.

Symptoms: Upset stomach, nausea, sweating, turning white, general ill feelings all usually precede the desire or urgency to vomit. Sometimes vomiting brings a sensation of relief. The dry heaves occur when vomiting continues, even after being unable to expel any more food, so that the stomach is empty and what is brought up is liquid, whitish and sour, and nausea continues.

Occurrence: Most people vomit several times throughout their lives. It rarely means anything serious unless it continues without a good reason.

Some examples of normal events that may produce vomiting are: pregnancy, eating "tainted" food, emotional disgust, an alcoholic binge, after anesthesia, and exercising excessively after eating too much food. Vomiting also needs to be induced in some cases of poisoning.

Consider: Nausea and vomiting may be symptoms of gastric disease (ulcers or inflammation), appendicitis, reaction to microbial toxins, drugs (chemotherapeutics, and hormones such as estrogens), minerals (most commonly zinc and iron), radiation, motion (motion sickness), obstruction somewhere in the gastrointestinal tract, or, a metabolic disorder such as diabetes or liver disease. It may also be symptomatic of psychological disorders such as eating disorders and bulimia (self-induced vomiting).

Vomiting blood (hematemesis) means that there is bleeding somewhere in the digestive tract, and a physician must be contacted at once. Depending on the cause of the blood, the extent of bleeding and how much it is mixed together with the contents of the stomach, the vomited blood may appear as coffee grounds (mixed with stomach acid), streaked, totally bloody, dark red, brown, or black.

Special Notes: Vomiting is a well orchestrated physiologic phenomenon. Vomiting occurs when the center in the brain for vomiting is activated. Once this occurs, messages are send to the diaphragm (muscular sheet separating the abdomen from the chest) to strongly press downward on the stomach, for the top of the stomach and esophagus (food pipe) to relax, and for the lower valve of the stomach that connects it to the rest of the intestine to strongly close. This acts like a device to extract food forcibly out of the stomach, up through the mouth, and out of the body. The brain also sends messages, at the same time, to close off the valve to the windpipe so that the food is not at risk of entering the lungs and causing suffocation.

Alternative Treatments

Refer to alternative therapy chapters for more information before evaluating or applying any treatment. Some conditions, including yours, may require a physician's care.

Diet: Continue to drink fluids but avoid solid food, and especially dairy. After vomiting has subsided: Start with a light vegetable broth and well toasted whole grain bread. If digestion occurs, move to yogurt, potatoes, soups, brown rice and steamed vegetables. After two to three days resume a normal diet.

Nutritional Therapy: Wait one day after the vomiting has stopped to take supplements. Take very light supplements for the first few days. • Folic acid (400-500 mcg. two to three times daily) • Vitamin A (10,000 IU) • Deglycerrhized licorice • Acidophilus and Vitamin B_1 (50 mg. one time) In a few days, you may add more of your regular supplements.

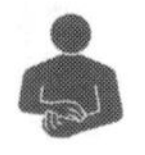

Self-Care

The following therapies can be undertaken at home under appropriate professional supervision.

• Fasting • Relaxation • Yoga

Acupressure: According to Leon Chaitow, N.D., D.O., if vomiting is associated with nausea resulting from travel or motion sickness, or from pregnancy (morning sickness) or due to anaesthesia or medication (chemotherapy), then strong thumb pressure on the point on the inner surface of the forearm, two thumb widths above the wrist crease, in the center, between the tendons will usually reduce or eliminate vomiting. (P6: see acupressure chart, page 874.)

Aromatherapy: Massage or place compress over stomach: black pepper, chamomile, fennel, camphor, lavender, peppermint, rose.

Herbs: Treatment depends upon the cause. Please refer to Motion Sickness. In addition to ginger, an infusion of peppermint can be very settling.

Homeopathy; *Ipecac., Phosphorus, Arsen alb., Nux vom.*

Hydrotherapy: Constitutional hydrotherapy: apply two to five times weekly.

Juice Therapy: Any vegetable juice with ginger.

Professional Care

The following therapies should only be provided by a qualified health professional.

• Acupuncture • Colon Therapy • Craniosacral Therapy • Environmental Medicine • Hypnotherapy • Magnetic Field Therapy • Naturopathic Medicine • Osteopathy • Therapeutic Touch • Traditional Chinese Medicine

Detoxification Therapy: May be indicated, to handle the problem.

Warts

True warts are very common, contagious skin tumors (benign [noncancerous]), "bumps," or "growths" which are caused by at least thirty-five different viruses (human pappillomavirus). Some warts can turn into cancerous tumors. However, this term, wart, is loosely used for many benign, skin, "wartlike" structures that are not caused by a virus, such as a raised, darkened skin tumor, common in the elderly, called a senile wart or verrucae, that is actually nonviral and more related to aging.

Symptoms: Warts may occur singly or in clusters. Their appearance and size varies tremendously depending on where they erupt on the body and the degree of irritation or trauma they receive through daily wear of the skin. The most common wart *(Verrucae vulgaris)* is a very well-defined, rough surfaced, roundish, or irregular growth that may be light gray, brown, grayish-black, or yellow, and is usually firm to the touch. This wart most commonly appears on the knees, elbows, fingers, face, and scalp.

Periungual warts occur around the nail beds. Plantar warts occur on the sole of the foot, are very common, and often appear flattened due to the pressure of walking on them. They are distinguished from other foot growths (corns, calluses) by the fact that when they are scratched they "pinpoint" bleed. They may be incredibly painful but this does not necesarily indicate something serious. When there are several plantar warts close together, they form a plague-like appearance called mosaic warts.

Warts that appear on a stalk (pedunculated) are common as humans age, particularly around the neck, chest, face, scalp, and armpits. Warts that are common on the face (eyelids, lips, neck) may appear as yellowish long, narrow, small growths.

Warts usually go away on their own without any treatment, within several months. However, in some individuals, they may continue for years or reoccur at the same or different parts of the body.

Occurrence: The most common wart (*Verruca vulgaris*) is universal, occurs in almost everyone, and is usually not serious. Warts in general are more common in older children and usually do not occur in elderly individuals. However, the elderly are prone to other nonviral skin growths such as "aging spots," moles, and mole changes.

Special Notes: Mole is a "loose" term applied to almost any pigmented skin blemish or "growth" that is not viral in origin and may be congenital (from birth) or not. They are usually not serious unless irritated constantly or change color, turn darker, or start to bleed.

Moles are not warts and should not be treated as such.

It is possible that immune functioning has something to do with healing and immunity to future warts since immunosuppressed (poor immune functioning secondary to serious illness such as diabetes or AIDS) individuals are much more susceptible to a wide variety of viral infections, such as warts.

Natural healing of warts may require one to two months of care, with the wart disappearing suddenly in one to three days.

Alternative Treatments

Refer to alternative therapy chapters for more information before evaluating or applying any treatment. Some conditions, including yours, may require a physician's care.

Diet: Diet is mainly an issue here if warts reoccur or do not regress, indicating the immune system may be slightly compromised. The more whole foods that are consumed, the better possible enhancement of immune functioning. Thus, avoid stressor foods as much as possible. Foods good to emphasize are those high in vitamin A, such as dark green and yellow vegetables, cold water fish, and eggs. Sulfur-containing foods such as onions, garlic, brussels sprouts, cabbage, and broccoli are also excellent. Consume adequate fermented milk products such as yogurt. Excess protein and fats may be discharged in the form of warts, moles, callouses, acne, and boils.

Nutritional Therapy: • Vitamin A (100,000 IU for five days then reduce to 25,000 IU for one month) • Beta-carotene (50,000 IU for several weeks) • Vitamin C • L-cysteine (500 mg. two times daily, for one month with amino acid blend one time daily as "back-up") • Vitamin B complex. • Zinc • Vitamin E

Apply two times daily for ten days mixture of: garlic oil, Vitamin E, castor oil, Vitamin A (squeeze these oils from capsules onto the skin) with a drop of zinc oxide cream and paste from one garlic clove crushed. Be careful not to get onto surrounding areas and cover well after applying. If surrounding skin seems to get irritated then try eliminating the fresh garlic paste.

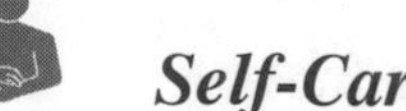

Self-Care

The following therapies can be undertaken at home under appropriate professional supervision.

• ***Fasting* • *Guided Imagery***

Aromatherapy: Lemon.

Herbs: Apply the milky latex from the stem of dandelions to the wart morning and night.

Homeopathy: *Thuja, Causticum, Calc carb., Ruta grav., Graphites.*

Naturopathic Medicine: Persistent local application of thuja oil is often an effective way of removing warts. However, equally effective is belief that the remedies will work.

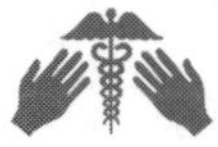

Professional Care

The following therapies should only be provided by a qualified health professional.

• ***Naturopathic Medicine***

Hypnotherapy: The worst case of warts reported by Joseph Pizzorno, N.D. (over one hundred on both hands, face, and arms) did not respond to either thuja oil or the standard medical approach of removal with liquid nitrogen. However, after only two sessions with a hypnotist, the warts were gone within a month and never returned.

Traditional Chinese Medicine: Direct moxibustion.

Weight Disorders

See Obesity and Weight Management chapter, page 762.

Whooping Cough

An acute (short-lived) bacterial disease (Bordetella pertussis), that is distinguished by a spasmodic cough that ends in a specific long, high-pitched "crowing" sound (on inhalation it sounds like a "whoop," thus, its name). It is highly contagious.

Symptoms: The bacteria invades the body and takes one to three weeks to start showing symptoms. The whole respiratory tract may be affected. The entire symptom stage takes about six weeks but may extend to three months. Initially, catarrh (mucous) is produced, along with fatigue, sneezing, coughing (starts first at night with a hacking sound without the whooping component and then begins to occur all day long), tearing of the eyes, and poor appetite. Usually, there is no accompanying fever. The second stage, ten to fourteen days after symptoms start to appear, produces a spasmodic cough consisting of about five, to sometimes over fifteen, rapid coughs, followed by a "characteristic whooping" sound produced on the last several inhalations. Large amounts of mucous are produced. Gagging and even vomiting may occur after the whooping sounds. Infants may tend to "choke" rather than whoop. The last stage (convalescent) starts at around four weeks with all the symptoms decreasing while the individual is generally starting to feel improved.

The spasmodic coughing may return at different times, for a period following the disease, especially if the upper respiratory tract is irritated or reinfected, even by a cold.

Consider: Bronchitis, pneumonia, flu, smoker's cough, and inhalant allergies.

Alternative Treatments

Refer to alternative therapy chapters for more information before evaluating or applying any treatment. Some conditions, including yours, may require a physician's care.

Diet: Drink plenty of liquids. Especially good is: one to two tablespoons honey, one tablespoon apple cider vinegar, one tablespoon fresh lemon juice, one teaspoon each of horehound and licorice extracts, one-eighth teaspoon cayenne pepper, and vitamin C powder. Add warm water and sip all day long, drinking at least three to six cups per day. Light foods can be taken between fits of coughing. During acute stage avoid, in particular, all dairy products. Eat fruits, vegetables, brown rice, clear vegetable soups, potatoes, and whole grain toast.

Add one clove of finely sliced garlic to four ounces of raw honey. Cover and let sit overnight. Add one teaspoon of mixture per cup of warm water. Sip throughout the day.

Nutritional Therapy: • Zinc lozenges (every two hours unless it causes nausea) • Vitamin C (every hour to bowel tolerance) • Vitamin A (200,000 IU first three days then 100,000 IU next three days then 25,000 IU for several months) • Beta-carotene (50,000 IU daily for one month then reduce to 25,000 IU daily) • Lung glandulars • Garlic capsules • Acidophilus

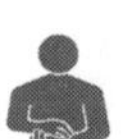

Self-Care

The following therapies can be undertaken at home under appropriate professional supervision.

Aromatherapy: Steam with tea tree, basil, chamomile, camphor, eucalyptus, peppermint, rose, lavender, thyme.

Herbs: The herbal tradition proposes a number of herbs as possible remedies, but they are not dramatically effective. These herbs include the antimicrobial and antispasmodic remedies sundew, thyme, butterbur, and wild cherry bark. One approach is to combine dried sundew, wild cherry bark, and anise in equal parts and make an infusion with one teaspoonful of this to a cup of water. This should be consumed several times a day.

Homeopathy: *Drosera, Pertussinum, Cuprum met., Mag phos.*

Hydrotherapy: Constitutional hydrotherapy: apply two to five times weekly or heating compress. Wet sock treatment: several times daily for head or chest congestion, replace socks when dry.

Juice Therapy: • Orange, lemon • Carrot, watercress

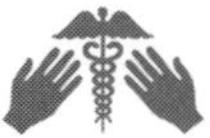

Professional Care

The following therapies should only be provided by a qualified health professional.

• Light Therapy • Magnetic Field Therapy • Naturopathic Medicine • Neural Therapy • Traditional Chinese Medicine

Osteopathy: According to Leon Chaitow, N.D., D.O., osteopathic manipulative attention can reduce the severity of the cough dramatically and make the patient far more comfortable.

Oxygen Therapy: Hydrogen peroxide therapy (IV)

Worms

In general, worms are parasites that may commonly invade the intestinal tract, and uncommonly invade other parts of the body. There are many types of worms such as tapeworms, roundworms, hookworms, pinworms, whipworms, and flukeworms.

Symptoms: Symptoms may vary depending on the worm. *Pinworms (Enterobius vermicularis)* are characterized by itching around the anus. Sometimes there are no symptoms at all. However, symptoms may include abdominal pain, joint pain, insomnia, convulsions and many other widely varying signs. The *whipworm (trichiura)* may not cause symptoms, or if there is a heavy infection, it may cause mild to severe abdominal pain and diarrhea, along with weight loss, anemia, appendicitis and, in women and children, rectal prolapse. *Tapeworm* may cause mild to severe abdominal symptoms such as cramping all the way up to abdominal obstruction. Systemic symptoms may be fever, coughing, wheezing, and if the worms enter the lungs (they may travel through the lymphatic system), there may also be severe lung problems. Adult worms may even create problems in the appendix, the liver or gall bladder or the pancreas. *Hookworms* are usually asymptomatic (no symptoms) but may develop a rash at the site where they invaded the body, may migrate to the lungs and cause pulmonary problems, or may cause severe stomach pains or anemia. Severe blood loss may create other severe problems such as heart failure.

In general, worms may be associated with overall fatigue, flulike symptoms, and vitamin and mineral deficiencies. Often, there are intestinal symptoms, poor digestive symptoms such as gas and burping, fatigue, joint pains, lowered resistance and even mood changes and depression.

Incidence: Universal.

Consider: Low digestive enzymes, food allergies, nutrient deficiencies, fungal infections, or severe stress reactions.

Special Notes: Prevention: proper hygiene, proper elimination of human waste, avoid walking barefoot on soil that may be contaminated, and avoid eating improperly cooked meat.

Worms may actually come out of the anus at night, when in bed, due to the warmth. Thus, especially children, may be checked, while sleeping.

Worms are very contagious. Check all members of household if one has been diagnosed. Be very careful with personal hygiene. Keep toilet seats cleaned well and after every use for several days at beginning of treatment.

For severe infections, use bowel cleanse programs with high colonics or home enemas, for first few weeks.

Alternative Treatments

Refer to alternative therapy chapters for more information before evaluating or applying any treatment. Some conditions, including yours, may require a physician's care.

Diet: Fasting under a doctor's supervision can be helpful. (Adults, on fresh juice, or mono-diet of one fruit or brown rice and vegetables for four days, children for only one). While fasting or just eating whole foods diet, do the following for the first four days: four times daily chew small amounts of mixture of pumpkin seeds, papaya seeds, papaya pulp, unsweetened yogurt, one tablespoon wormwood tea, one tablespoon chaparral tea and one tablespoon peppermint tea. Take with filtered water and two garlic capsules. On the fifth day: mix four cups of mixture of senna and peppermint teas, plus two tablespoons castor oil, drink all at once, with eight garlic capsules and six charcoal capsules taken all together.

Continue to consume a small amount of the original mixture one time daily for two weeks. Do not be scared if you see and remove the worms from your anus.

Other alternatives: Fig juice may kill roundworms. Before meals, try pepsin and glycerine in hot water. Upon arising and at bedtime try one clove peeled garlic followed by a glass of hot tea with lemon, no sweetener. Children with pinworms may try a heavily salted diet for one to two weeks. Tapeworms may respond to fasting on raw pineapple for three days. (Bromelain in pineapple kills the worms.)

Nutritional Therapy: • Garlic capsules • Vitamin C • Zinc • Vitamin A • Beta-carotene • Deglycerrhized licorice (two to three times daily on empty stomach)

• Aloe vera juice or gel (two times daily on empty stomach, does come flavored) • Acidophilus

Self-Care

The following therapies can be undertaken at home under appropriate professional supervision.

• Fasting

Aromatherapy: • Bergamot, chamomile, camphor, lavender, peppermint, melissa • Ringworm: tea tree, thyme

Ayurveda: • *Neem* may be effective in eliminating ringworm and parasites. • *Pippali* or Indian long pepper *(Piper longum)* is often used for worms. • As a "broad spectum antibiotic": a herbal mixture of *vidanga* 300 mg., *trikatu* 300 mg., *chitrak* 200 mg., and *kutki* 200 mg., generally taken twice a day after lunch and dinner. *Triphala* one-half teaspoon with warm water one-half hour before sleep at night.

Herbs: Make an infusion of fresh pumpkin seeds, one ounce of crushed seeds to a pint of boiling water. Drink a cup three times a day for six days a week for three weeks. Eat one ounce of pumpkin seeds a day as well. Other herbs are specific for certain worms but can be toxic.

Professional Care

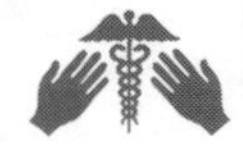

The following therapies should only be provided by a qualified health professional.

• Acupuncture • Magnetic Field Therapy
• Naturopathic Medicine

Colon Therapy: For severe cases.

Detoxification Therapy: May be indicated, depending on the condition of the person.

Oxygen Therapy: Hyperbaric oxygen therapy

Wounds

Any damage to or break of the skin and/or underlying tissues. The damage may be caused by accidents, incisions from surgery, or other traumas. Open wounds demonstrate broken skin and/or mucous membranes, whereas closed wounds do not (such as an abrasion or contusion).

Symptoms: There are many types of wounds: *abrasion*, skin scraped away; *contusion,* underlying tissues are damaged and there is much darkening or yellowing of the upper surfaces of the skin; *incised*, clean cut from scalpel from surgical procedure; *laceration*, skin is irregularly torn such as from bits of glass or a bite from an animal; *penetrating*, from a violent stab or gunshot; and *cuts*, minor breaking of the skin.

Special Notes: Any type of wound is susceptible to infection and must be properly cleaned, covered, and watched. Complications of infections may create severe health problems and, if they occur, will require treatment by a physician.

Alternative Treatments

Diet: The extent of the wound depends on how strict a whole foods diet should be adhered to. Most wounds will do well with sensible dietary habits. Severe wounds will benefit from avoiding stressor foods that may decrease immune function and healing, such as refined sugars, excess caffeine, and alcoholic beverages. The skin is made up of essential fatty acids and vitamin A and zinc are needed for repair. Foods high in these are excellent, such as green and yellow vegetables, eggs, cold water fish, raw seeds and nuts, and oysters. Fresh fruits and vegetables are high in vitamin C and also excellent. Avoid excess saturated and processed fats and consume vegetable oils or take one teaspoon daily of a quality cold processed oil so that the body gets a higher ratio of essential fatty acids in the diet.

Nutritional Therapy: • Vitamin A (50,000 IU daily for several weeks) • Zinc (30-60 mg.) • Pantothenic acid (B_5—500 mg. two times daily) • Vitamin C • Vitamin B complex

When first wounded, apply vitamin E, vitamin A, essential fatty acids all squeezed from capsules, along with a little zinc oxide cream, directly onto the area. When healing is well underway, may add aloe vera gel. Apply several times per day, keep clean and covered.

According to Leon Chaitow, N.D., D.O., healing following injury is speeded up when the amino acids arginine and glycine are supplemented (away from mealtimes). Bromelain, from the pineapple plant, taken away from meal times on an empty stomach, helps reduce inflammatory processes if these seem excessive (inflammation is part of the healing process).

Self-Care

The following therapies can be undertaken at home under appropriate professional supervision.

• Fasting • Guided Imagery

Aromatherapy: Lavender, myrrh, benzoin, bergamot, chamomile, tea tree, eucalyptus, juniper, rosemary.

Ayurveda: • The Ayurvedic rejuvenative herb *ashwagandha* is used externally on wounds and sores. • For minor cuts: aloe vera gel with tumeric applied locally, or *tikta ghee* • Apply a paste made of fresh aloe vera gel or plain *ghee,* coconut oil, licorice *ghee*, or *tikta ghee*.

Herbs: • Bathe the wound with an infusion of calendula. A diluted tincture is also used. Applying distilled witch hazel may stop bleeding and promote healing. Goldenseal may speed healing when applied as a powder or salve. Alternatively use a poultice of plantain or comfrey leaf. • Echinacea ointment

Juice Therapy: High beta-carotene, including carrot, plus choices of beet, celery, garlic.

Homeopathy: *Calendula, Hepar Sulf., Hypericum, Ledum.*

Hydrotherapy: Ice pack: apply to the arterial trunk that supplies the area.

Topical Treatment: Undiluted, unprocessed honey may help disinfect wounds and sores, and may actively promote wound healing.

Professional Care

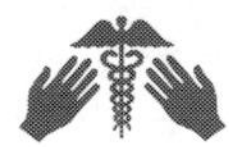

The following therapies should only be provided by a qualified health professional.

• Cell Therapy • Magnetic Field Therapy • Neural Therapy • Naturopathic Medicine

Oxygen Therapy: • Hydrogen peroxide therapy (IV) • Hyperbaric oxygen therapy

Light Therapy: • Monochromatic red light therapy • Cold (soft) laser photo stimulation therapy.

Traditional Chinese Medicine: Pseudo-ginseng *(yun nan pai yao)* externally.

Glossary

Abscess: a swollen or inflamed area of body tissue in which pus gathers.
Acid/Alkaline balance: see pH balance.
Acid pH: see pH balance.
Acidosis: an excessive acidity of body fluids due to either an accumulation of acids or a loss of bicarbonate (the hydrogen ion concentration is increased and thus the pH is decreased). See pH balance.
Acupoints: acupuncture points throughout the body, along the meridians, which correspond to specific organs. See Meridian.
Acute: in medicine: having rapid onset, severe symptoms and short duration. Opposite of chronic.
Adaptogen: a substance with qualities which increase resistance and resilience to stress, enabling the body to adapt around the problem and to avoid reaching collapse. Adaptogens work through support of the adrenal glands.
Alkaline pH: see pH balance.
Allergens: substances that cause manifestations of allergy (these may or may not be antigens). See Antigen.
Alterative: a substance with properties that gradually restore proper functioning of the body, increasing health and vitality.
Alveoli: the air cells of a lung.
Amino acids: the building blocks of which proteins are constructed, and the end product of protein digestion.
Anaerobic: pertaining to an organism, the ability to live without oxygen.
Analgesic: a pain-relieving substance.
Angina: there are many kinds of angina, the most common being an inflammatory disease of the throat, accompanied by spasms, choking, and difficulty breathing.
Angina pectoris: a heart disease involving severe pain and a feeling of pressure in the chest. Sometimes the pain radiates to the left shoulder and arm.
Angioplasty: altering the structure of a vessel by surgical procedure or by dilating the vessel using a balloon.
Anthelmintic: a substance with the property to destroy or expel intestinal worms.
Antibacterial: a substance which has the property of destroying or stopping the growth of bacteria.
Antibiotics: any of a variety of natural or synthetic substances that inhibit the growth of, or destroy, microorganisms.
Antigen: a protein, carbohydrate, or fat carbohydrate complex with the ability to identify cells as harmless and belonging to the body, or as foreign cells to be destroyed. Antigens stimulate the production of antibodies which can neutralize or destroy invading organisms. Antigens on the body's own cells are called autoantigens. Antigens on all other cells are called foreign antigens.
Anti-inflammatory: a substance which soothes inflammation or reduces the inflammatory response of the tissue directly. Anti-inflammatories work in a number of different ways, but rarely inhibit the natural inflammatory reaction.
Antimicrobial: antimicrobials help the body destroy or resist pathogenic (disease-causing) microorganisms by helping the body strengthen its own resistance to infective organisms.
Antispasmodic: antispasmodics ease cramps in smooth and skeletal muscles. They alleviate muscular tension and, as many are also nervines, ease psychological tension as well.
Antiviral: any substance which bears the properties of opposing the action of a virus.
Arterial occlusion: a closing or blockage of an artery.
Arteriosclerosis: used interchangeably with the term atherosclerosis: to describe a condition affecting the arteries. See Atherosclerosis.
Astringent: astringents have a binding action on mucous membranes, skin, and other tissue. They reduce irritation and inflammation, and create a barrier against infection that is helpful to wounds and burns.
Atherosclerosis: term applied to a variety of conditions where there is thickening, hardening, and/or loss of elasticity of the artery walls resulting in altered function of tissues and organs.
Autoimmune disease: a disease produced when the body's normal tolerance of its own antigenic markers on cells disappears. Autoantibodies are produced by B lymphocytes and attack normal cells, whose surface contains a "self" antigen or autoantigen, causing destruction of tissue. Includes diseases such as: rheumatoid arthritis, multiple sclerosis, and Graves' disease.
Autonomic nervous system: the part of the nervous system that is concerned with the control

of involuntary bodily functions. It regulates the function of glands, especially the salivary, gastric, and sweat glands, and the adrenal medulla; smooth muscle tissue, and the heart. The autonomic nervous system may act on these tissues to reduce or slow activity or to initiate their function.

Bile: stored in both the liver and gallbladder, it is important as a digestive juice due to its emulsifying action which facilitates the digestion of fats in the intestines, as well as stimulating peristalsis.

Bioaccumulation: a buildup in the body of foreign substances.

Blood clotting: see Platelet Aggregation.

Blood sugar: sugar in the form of glucose present in the blood, normally 60 to 100 milligrams/100 milliliters of blood. It rises after a meal to as much as 150 milligrams/100 milliliters of blood, but this may vary.

Bowel tolerance: the maximum amount a person can take in of a substance before experiencing loose stools or diarrhea.

Bowel toxemia: a condition in which poisonous products of bacteria growing in the bowels produce severe virus-like symptoms such as fever, diarrhea, and vomiting.

Bronchioles: a subdivision of the bronchial tubes.

Bronchodilators: chemicals that relax or open the air passages in the lungs.

Bruxism: grinding of the teeth during sleep. If untreated, bruxism can damage teeth and the temporomandibular joint.

Bulimia: the activity of bingeing on large amounts of food, followed by self-induced vomiting.

Bypass surgery: creating an alternate route for blood to pass an obstruction (commonly used to describe heart surgery to bypass the coronary artery).

Candida albicans: small, oval budding fungus or yeast that is the primary disease causing organism of the infection moniliasis candidiasis, commonly referred to as candida.

Capillaries: any of the minute blood vessels, averaging 0.008 millimeter in diameter, carrying blood and forming the capillary system. Capillaries connect the ends of the smallest arteries with the beginnings of the smallest veins.

Carbohydrate: a chemical compound that contains only carbon, hydrogen, and oxygen. Found in plants, carbohydrates—which include all sugars, starches, and celluloses—constitute a major class of animal food and are a basic source of human energy.

Carcinogens: cancer-producing agents.

Cardiac arrhythmia: irregular beating of the heart.

Cardiovascular: relating to or involving the heart and blood vessels.

Carminative: plants that are rich in aromatic volatile oils. They stimulate the digestive system to work properly and with ease; soothe the gut wall; reduce any inflammation that might be present; ease gripping pains and help with the removal of gas from the digestive tract.

Cartilage: a translucent, elastic tissue that composes most of the skeleton of embryonic and very young vertebrates and is for the most part converted into bone in the higher vertebrates.

Cell membranes: the membrane that encloses the cell. Composed of proteins, lipids, and carbohydrates.

Cellular acidosis: excessive acidity of body fluids due to an accumulation of acids, as in diabetic acidosis or renal disease.

Cellular edema: a condition in which the cells contain an excessive amount of fluid, which causes swelling of the cell membrane.

Cerebrospinal fluid: the fluid that surrounds the brain and spinal cord.

Cervix: the narrow outer end of the uterus.

Chi: see *Qi*.

Cholesterol: a steroid alcohol present in animal cells and body fluids, important in physiological processes, and implicated experimentally as a factor in atherosclerosis.

Chromosomes: present in the nucleus of cells and containing the DNA which transmits genetic information, chromosomes contain the genes or hereditary determiners. The normal number of chromosomes for a human being is forty-six in all somatic cells.

Chronic: a disease or illness of long duration showing little change or of slow progression. Opposite of acute.

Circadian rhythm: pertains to events that occur at approximately twenty-four-hour intervals, such as certain physiological phenomena.

Circulating Immune Complexes (CIC): also known as antigen-antibody complexes.

Coenzyme: an enzyme activator. A diffusible, heat-stable substance of low molecular weight that, when combined with an inactive protein called apoenzyme, forms an active compound or a complete enzyme called holoenzyme.

Colic: spasm, obstruction, or twisting in any hollow or tubular soft organ accompanied by pain.

Collagen: a structural protein of the connective tissues.

Congestive heart failure: a condition characterized by weakness, breathlessness, abdominal discomfort, and edema in lower portions of body, resulting from venous stasis and reduced outflow of blood from the left side of the heart.

Conjunctiva: the mucous membrane that lines the eye and eyelid.

Coronary artery disease: a narrowing of the coronary arteries which prevents adequate blood supply to the myocardium. Narrowing is usually caused by atherosclerosis, and may progress to the point where the heart muscle is damaged due to lack of blood supply.

Cortisol: an adrenocortical hormone, usually referred to pharmaceutically as hydrocortisone. Closely related to cortisone in physiological effects.

Coxsackievirus: a group of viruses first isolated in 1948 from two children in Coxsackie, New York. Most coxsackievirus infections in humans are mild, but the viruses do produce a variety of illnesses including aseptic meningitis (inflammation of the meninges not due to microorganisms), herpangina (a benign infectious disease of children), epidemic pleurodynia (disease characterized by pain of sharp intensity in the chest accompanied by fever), acute upper respiratory infection, and myocarditis of the newborn (inflammation of the middle layer of the walls of the heart), among others. It is possible that infection during the first trimester of pregnancy can cause increased incidence of congenital heart lesions in newborns.

Craniosacral system: pertaining to the cranium and sacrum, including the brain, spinal cord, cerebrospinal fluid, surrounding membranes, and bones of the spine.

Cyanosis: a bluish discoloration of the skin due to abnormal amounts of reduced hemoglobin in the blood.

Cyst: a closed sac or pouch with a definite wall, that contains fluid, semifluid, or solid material.

Cystathionine: an intermediate compound in the metabolism of methionine to cysteine.

Cysteine: (as in cysteine hydrochloride) a sulfur-containing amino acid found in many proteins. Valuable as a source of sulfur in metabolism.

Cytokines: chemical messengers that are involved in the regulation of almost every system in the body and are important in controlling local and systemic inflammatory response.

Cytomegalovirus: a virus related to the herpes virus that inhabits the salivary glands.

Cytotoxic: any substance which has the properties to harm or destroy cells.

Demulcent: an herb that is rich in mucilage and soothes and protects irritated or inflamed tissue. Demulcent herbs reduce irritation down the whole length of the bowel; reduce sensitivity to potentially corrosive gastric acids; help prevent diarrhea and reduce the muscle spasms that cause colic.

Demyelination: reduction of the fatty covering of the nerves, removal of the myelin sheath.

Dental amalgam: an alloy containing mercury, tin, silver, and copper that is used in dentistry to restore teeth.

Dermatitis: inflammation of the skin with itching, redness, and various skin lesions.

Desensitization: the treatment of allergies by repeated injections of dilute solutions containing the allergen. Slowly promotes tolerance of the antigen by the immune system.

Detoxification: the process of removing toxins from the body.

Diastolic pressure: the period of least pressure in the arterial vascular system.

Diuretic: a substance which increases the production and elimination of urine.

Diverticulitis: inflammation of a sac or pouch in the intestinal tract, most commonly in the colon region, causing stagnation of feces and pain.

Dopamine: an amino acid found in the adrenal gland. Used to treat hypotension and Parkinson's disease.

Doshas: the three basic types of biological humors in Ayurvedic medicine, which determine an individual's constitution.

Duodenal ulcer: damaged mucous membrane in a portion of the small intestine.

Dyspepsia: imperfect or painful digestion.

Edema: retention of excessive amounts of fluid by the body tissues.

Elastin: extracellular protein that makes the tissue elastic.

Electroacupuncture biofeedback: measurement of the electrical properties of acupuncture points.

Electrolyte: ionized salts in blood, tissue fluids and cells including salts of sodium and potassium.

Embryo: the developing human individual from the time of implantation to the end of the eighth week after conception. Characterized by the development of tissues and primary organs and organ systems.

Emmenagogue: a substance which stimulates menstrual flow and activity. In most herbal remedies, however, the term is used in the wider sense for a remedy that affects the female reproductive system.

Endocrine gland: a gland that secretes directly into the bloodstream.

Endorphins: natural opiates produced in the brain which function as the body's own natural painkillers.

Enkephalin: a chemical substance produced by the brain which acts as an opiate and produces analgesia to increase the threshold for pain.
Enzyme: any one of the numerous complex proteins that are produced by living cells and catalyze specific biochemical reactions.
Epidemiology: a branch of medical science that deals with the incidence, distribution, and control of disease in a population.
Essential fatty acids (EFA): unsaturated fatty acids (linoleic, linolenic, and arachidonic) which cannot by synthesized in the body and are considered essential for maintaining health.
Estrogen: female hormone responsible for stimulating the development of female secondary sex characteristics.
Expectorant: a substance that stimulates removal of mucous from the lungs. Stimulating expectorants "irritate" the bronchioles (a smaller subdivision of the bronchial tubes) causing expulsion of material. Relaxing expectorants soothe bronchial spasm and loosen mucous secretions, helpful in dry, irritating coughs.
Fascia: a fibrous membrane covering, supporting and separating muscles. Unites the skin with underlying tissue.
Fat: adipose tissue of the body which serves as an energy reserve. Also, in chemistry, a term used to describe one of a group of organic compounds or fatty acids. See Fatty acid.
Fertilization: the union of the ovum of a female with the male's spermatozoon (the male sex cell carried in the seminal discharge) resulting in the initiation of the development of a new individual.
Fetus: a term for a developing human usually ranging from three months after conception to birth.
Fibroblasts: cells that are the precursors of bone, collagen, and other connective tissue cells, commonly known as the healing cells.
Fluid retention: failure to eliminate fluids from the body because of a high level of salt in the body, or a renal, cardiac, or metabolic disease.
Free radicals: molecules containing an odd number of electrons resulting in an open bond or half bond, making them highly reactive and as a result, potentially destructive.
Fungus: a cellular organism that subsists on organic matter.
Giardia lamblia: a parasitic infection transmitted by an ingestion of cysts in fecally contaminated water or food.
Gastroenteritis: inflammation of the stomach and intestinal tract.
Gastrointestinal system: pertaining to the stomach and intestines.
Genitourinary system: pertaining to the genitals and urinary organs.
Geopathic stress: stress to the human body caused by harmful radiation from the earth.
Glucose: blood sugar; an intermediate in the metabolism of carbohydrates in the body.
Glycogen: glycogen is the form in which carbohydrates are stored in the human body for future conversion into sugar and for use in performing muscular work and distributing heat through the body. Glycogen is formed from sugar and is transformed into glucose as needed.
Glycoproteins: proteins combined with sugar.
HDL cholesterol: a cholesterol-poor, protein-rich lipoprotein of blood plasma associated with a reduced risk of atherosclerosis.
Hemiplegia: paralysis of only one side of the body.
Hemoglobin: the iron-containing pigment of the red blood cells.
Hemorrhage: heavy or uncontrollable bleeding.
Hepatic: hepatics aid the liver by toning and strengthening it and in some cases increasing the flow of bile. They are fundamental in maintaining health because of the important role the liver plays by not only facilitating digestion but also removing toxins from the body.
Hepatotoxic: any substance which is toxic to the liver.
Histamine: a substance produced by the body during an allergic reaction.
Homeostasis: a relatively stable state of equilibrium between the interdependent elements of an organism or group.
Hydrochloric acid (HCl): a strong corrosive irritating acid, normally present in dilute form in gastric juice.
Hypercalcemia: an excess of calcium in the blood.
Hyperthermia: unusually high fever often artificially induced for therapeutic purposes.
Hyperventilation: excessive or overbreathing resulting in a loss of carbon dioxide from the blood. Frequently found in diseases such as asthma or in induced states of anxiety.
Hypo-allergenic: lowered potential for causing allergic reactions.
Hypotensive: any remedies that lower abnormally elevated blood pressure.
Hypothalamus: a gland which contains neurosecretions that are of importance in the control of certain metabolic activities, such as water balance, sugar and fat metabolism, regulation of body temperature, and secretion of releasing and inhibiting hormones.
Iatrogenic: treatment-induced.
IgA: an antibody in the colon that binds food and bacterial antigens.
Immune reaction: antibody production.

Immunosuppressive: a substance which suppresses the body's natural immune response to an antigen.
Inflammation: an immune reaction that occurs in response to any type of bodily injury. Can include redness, heat, swelling, or pain.
Insulin: a hormone secreted by the pancreas essential for the metabolism of carbohydrates and used in the treatment and control of diabetes.
Interferon: a group of proteins released by white blood cells that combat a virus.
Interleukin-1: a compound produced by the body in response to infection, inflammation, or other immunologic challenges.
Intra-arterially: introduced (usually injected) within an artery.
Intra-articularly: introduced (usually injected) into a joint.
Intradermally: introduced (usually injected) within the substance of the skin.
Intradermal testing: an injection into the outer layers of the skin.
Intramuscularly: introduced (usually injected) within the muscle.
Intravenously: introduced (usually injected) into a vein.
Kapha: an Ayurvedic *dosha* which determines an individual's constitution.
Ketoacidosis: excessive acidity of body fluids due to an excess of ketones.
Ketone: an organic chemical derived by the oxidation of alcohol.
Lactose intolerant: an intolerance to milk and some dairy products, characterized by gastrointestinal symptoms.
Laxative: a substance which promotes bowel movements. Laxatives are divided into those that work by providing bulk, those that stimulate the production of bile in the liver and its release from the gallbladder, and those which directly trigger peristalsis.
LDL cholesterol: a cholesterol-rich, protein-poor blood plasma correlated with an increased risk of atherosclerosis.
Lesion: an injury, wound, or single infected patch in a skin disease.
Leukocytes: white blood cells.
Leukocytosis: an increased white blood cell count, usually caused by the presence of an infection.
Leukosis: abnormal growth of white blood cells.
Ligament: a band of fibrous connective tissue connecting bone, cartilages, and other structures and serving as support for muscles to facilitate or limit motion.
Limbic system: a group of brain structures that influences the endocrine and autonomic motor systems.
Lipids: liquid fats.
Lipoproteins: proteins composed of a simple protein and a fat component that carry fats in the blood.
Lymphatic system: a system of vessels and nodes throughout the body which carry the lymph fluid and help to remove toxins from the body.
Macrophage: cells that have the ability to recognize and ingest all foreign antigens as well as cell debris and other waste in the blood.
Macula: the central area of the retina.
Meninges: the three membranes covering the brain and spinal cord.
Meridian: the fourteen channels in the body through which *qi* runs. Acupuncture diagnoses illness by seeking blockages in the body's meridians.
Metabolism: the transformation in the body of the chemical energy of foodstuffs to mechanical energy or heat.
Metastasis: the spreading of a tumor from its site of origin to distant sites, usually through the bloodstream or the lymphatic system.
Methionine: a sulfur-bearing compound, an essential animo acid.
Mucosa: a mucous membrane or the moist tissue layer that lines a hollow organ or body cavity.
Musculoskeletal system: pertaining to the muscles and the skeleton.
Myocardiopathy: any disease of the heart muscle.
Myelin: a fatlike substance forming a sheath around the axons, or nerve fibers, of certain nerves.
Nervine: nervines help the nervous system and can be subdivided into three groups. Nervine tonics strengthen and restore the nervous system. Nervine relaxants ease anxiety and tension by soothing both body and mind. Nervine stimulants directly stimulate nerve activity.
Neurological: pertaining to the study of nervous diseases.
Neuromuscular: concerning both the nerves and muscles.
Neurotoxicity: having the capability of harming nerve tissue.
Neurotransmitters: substances that transmit nerve impulses to the brain.
Nosode: a nosode is a potentialized homeopathic remedy prepared from diseased tissue, such as bacteria, viruses, or pus, to treat the associated disease of the tissue material.
Occipital bone: a bone in the lower back part of the skull between the parietal and temporal bones.
Oxidized cholesterol: see Oxysterol.

Oxygenation: to supply or combine with oxygen.
Oxysterol: when cholesterol combines with oxygen and becomes oxidized, is then known as oxysterol.
Parasympathetic nervous system: the craniosacral division of the autonomic nervous system. Effects of parasympathetic stimulation are the constriction of the pupils, contraction of the smooth muscle of the alimentary canal, constriction of bronchioles, slowing of heart rate and increased secretion by glands, except sweat glands.
Pathogens: disease-producing microorganisms and toxins.
Peptide: a substance formed by two or more amino acids.
Periosteum: the sheath around a bone.
Peripheral nervous system: connects the central nervous system to all body tissues and voluntary muscles.
Peristalsis: wavelike contractions of the smooth muscles of the digestive tract; also, the wavelike contraction of the colon muscles that expel waste mater.
pH balance: a method of measurement used in chemistry to express the degree of acidity or alkalinity of a solution. A pH of 7 represents the neutral point where the solution is neither acid nor alkaline. Any higher alkalinity is expressed by a number greater than 7, and higher acidity, by a number less than 7. The calculations of these numbers are based on logarithms.
Phlegm: thick mucous secreted in abnormal quantity in the respiratory passages.
***Pitta*:** an Ayurvedic *dosha* which determines an individual's constitution.
Placebo: substances having no pharmacological effect.
Plaque: a localized abnormal patch on a body part or surface.
Plasma: the liquid part of the lymph and of the blood.
Plasma lipids: fats in the bloodstream.
Platelet: a round or oval disk found in the blood. Important in blood coagulation.
Platelet aggregation: the clustering of disks found in human blood that facilitate blood coagulation.
Polypeptide: a molecule resulting from the union of two or more amino acids.
Postacute: the period after the rapid and severe onset of symptoms.
Postpartum: the period after childbirth.
Prenatal: the period before childbirth.
Probiotics: substances that promote the growth of beneficial bacteria in the intestines.
Progesterone: a steroid hormone responsible for the changes in the endometrium in the second half of the menstrual cycle preparatory for implantation, development of maternal placenta and development of mammary glands. Used to treat menstrual disorders, among other problems.
Prostaglandin E-Z: hormone-like fatty acids, biologically active unsaturated fatty acids.
Prostate: gland that surrounds the neck of the bladder and urethra in males and secretes a thin fluid that forms part of the seminal fluid.
Protein: complex nitrogenous compounds that occur naturally in plants and animals and yield amino acids. Essential for the growth and repair of animal tissue
Qi: (also spelled *chi*), referred to in alternative medicine as the vital life energy which runs throughout the body.
***Qi* stagnation:** any blockage of energy in the body that interrupts the body's natural functions or the healing process.
Radiation necrosis: death of an area of tissue or bone surrounded by healthy parts.
Reflex sympathetic dystrophy: a chronic condition where pain does not subside and muscle function begins to deteriorate.
Renal insufficiency: the reduced capacity of the kidney to perform its functions.
Seasonal affective disorder (SAD): a mood disorder characterized by mental depression related to a certain season of the year, especially winter (also known as the "winter blues"). Symptoms include daytime drowsiness, fatigue, and diminished concentration. SAD usually afflicts adults and is four times more common in women than men.
Sebaceous glands: glands in the skin which help to retain body heat and prevent sweat evaporation.
Secretory IgA: promoting secretion or secreting immunoglobulin gamma A.
Serum cholesterol: cholesterol circulating in the blood.
Somnambulistic state: sleep walking.
Sperm: the male reproductive cell carried in the seminal discharge.
Stimulant: a substance which quickens and enlivens the physiological and metabolic activity of the body.
Subacute: a state between acute and chronic when symptoms have lessened in severity or duration.
Subluxations: terminology used by a chiropractor to explain misalignments of spinal vertebrae.
Sutura: thin fibrous membrane which unites the bony surfaces of the skull.
Systolic blood pressure: the period of greatest pressure in the arterial vascular system.

Tachycardia: an abnormally rapid heart rate.
T-cells: white blood cells which facilitate the immune system.
Tendon: a tough cord or band of dense white fibrous connective tissue that unites a muscle with some other part.
Thoracic: pertaining to the chest or thorax.
Thymus: a glandular structure of largely lymphoid tissue that functions in the development of the body's immune system, located in the upper chest or at the base of the neck.
Tonic: often used in Traditional Chinese Medicine and Ayurvedic medicine, tonics are often taken as a preventative measure to nurture and enliven.
Tonsillitis: inflammation of the tonsil.
Triglyceride: a combination of glycerol with three to five different fatty acids.
Tumor: an abnormal mass of tissue that is not inflammatory, arises without obvious cause from cells, and possesses no physiologic function.
Umbilical cord: a cord arising from the navel of the fetus that connects the fetus with the placenta.
Vascular system: includes the heart, blood vessels, lymphatic, pulmonary, and portal systems.
Vasodilator: a substance which causes the blood vessels to widen.
Vata: an Ayurvedic *dosha* which determines an individual's constitution.
Veins: the tubular branching vessels that carry blood from the capillaries toward the heart.
Ventricular fibrillation: rapid, ineffective contractions by the ventricles of the heart.
Vertebrae: any one of the thirty-three bony segments that make up the spinal column.
Viscosity: the thickness or stickiness of a bodily fluid (such as blood).
***Yang* deficiency:** because *yang* cannot function properly without *yin,* an imbalance in the energy systems of the body can create a *yang* deficiency, causing the *yang* organs to become stagnant. See *Qi.*
***Yang* organs:** *yang* organs are hollow, surface organs such as the intestines, spleen, gallblader, and the skin.
Yeast: unicellular fungi of the genus which reproduce by budding, and can cause infections.
Yin deficiency: because *yin* cannot function properly without *yang,* an imbalance in the energy systems of the body can create a *yin* deficiency, causing the *yin* organs to become stagnant. See *Qi.*
***Yin* organs:** *yin* organs are dense, internal organs such as the kidneys, lungs, heart, liver, and bones.

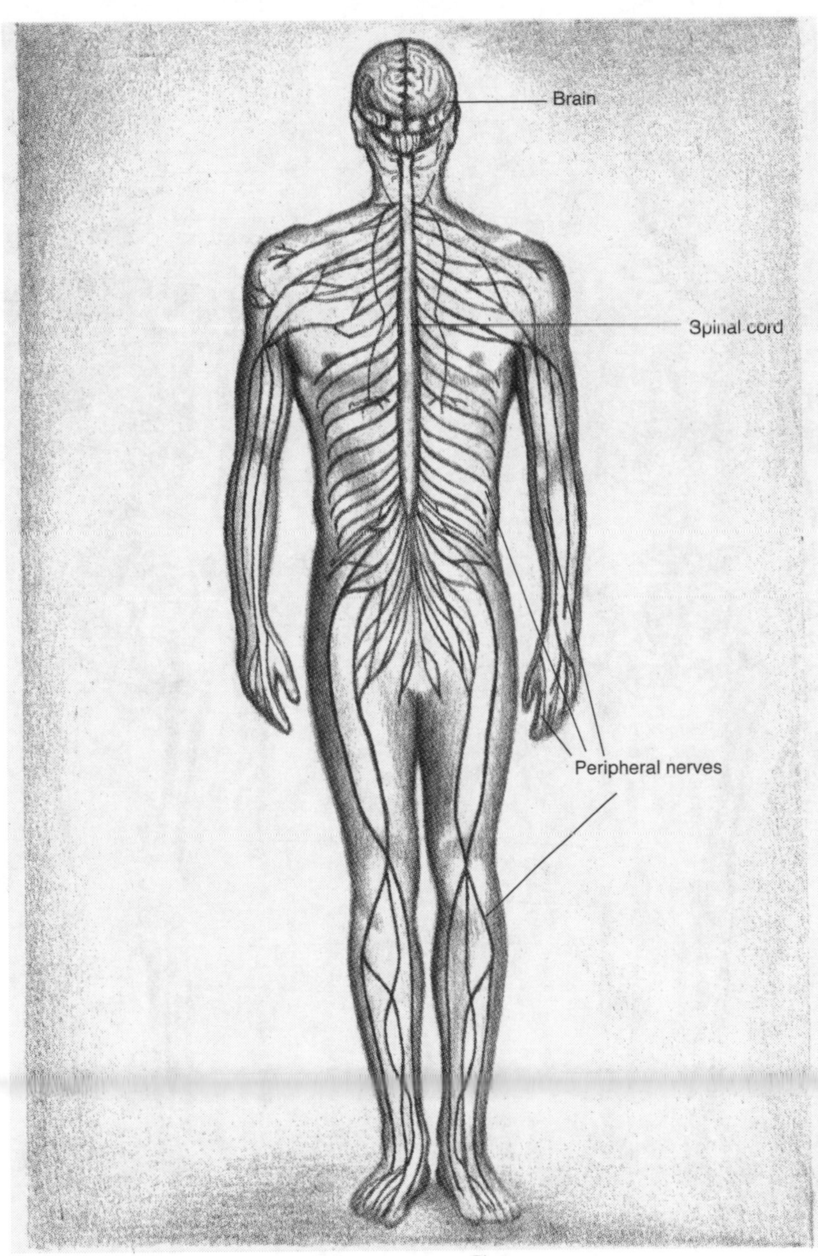

The Nervous System

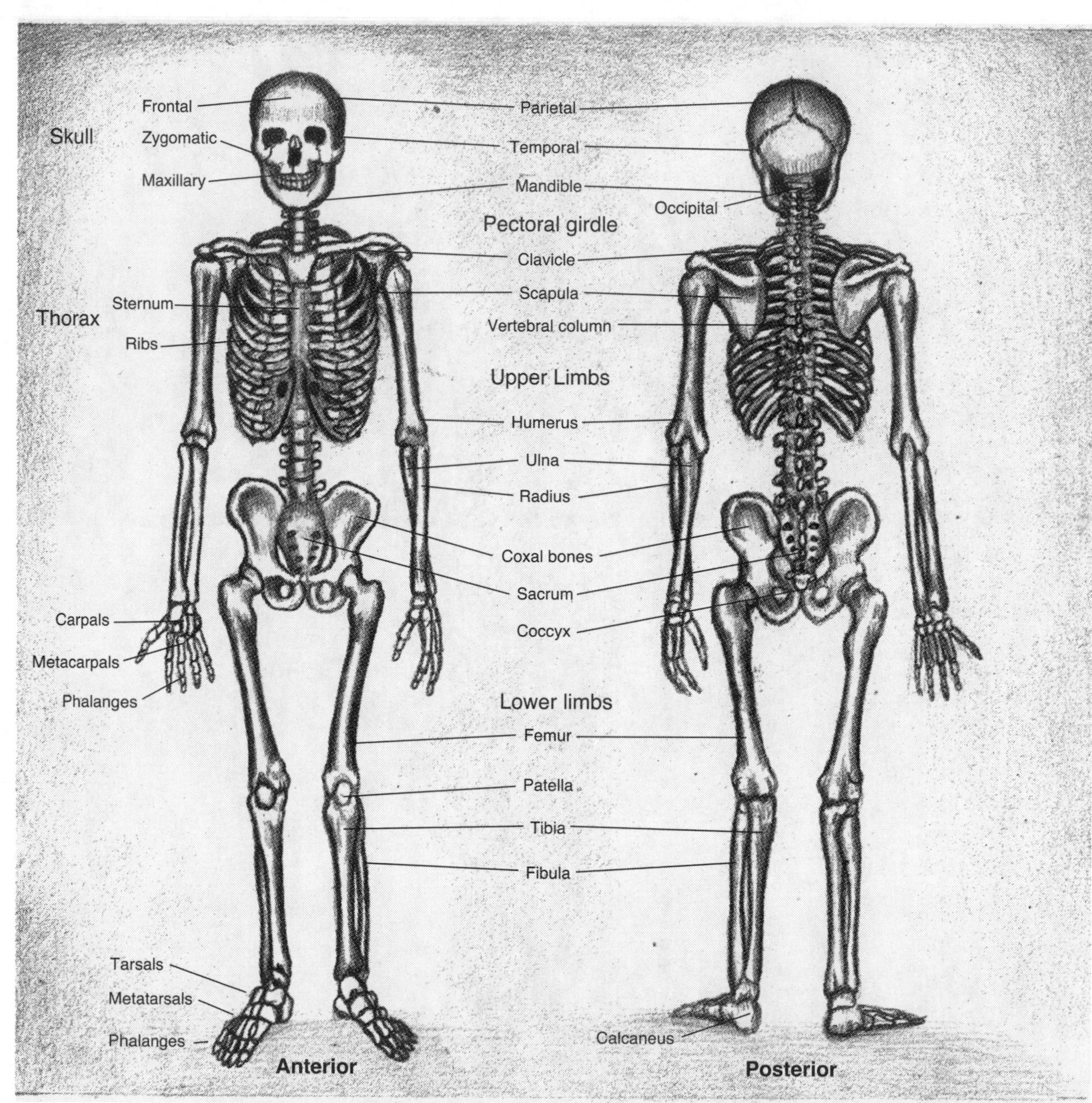

The Skeletal System

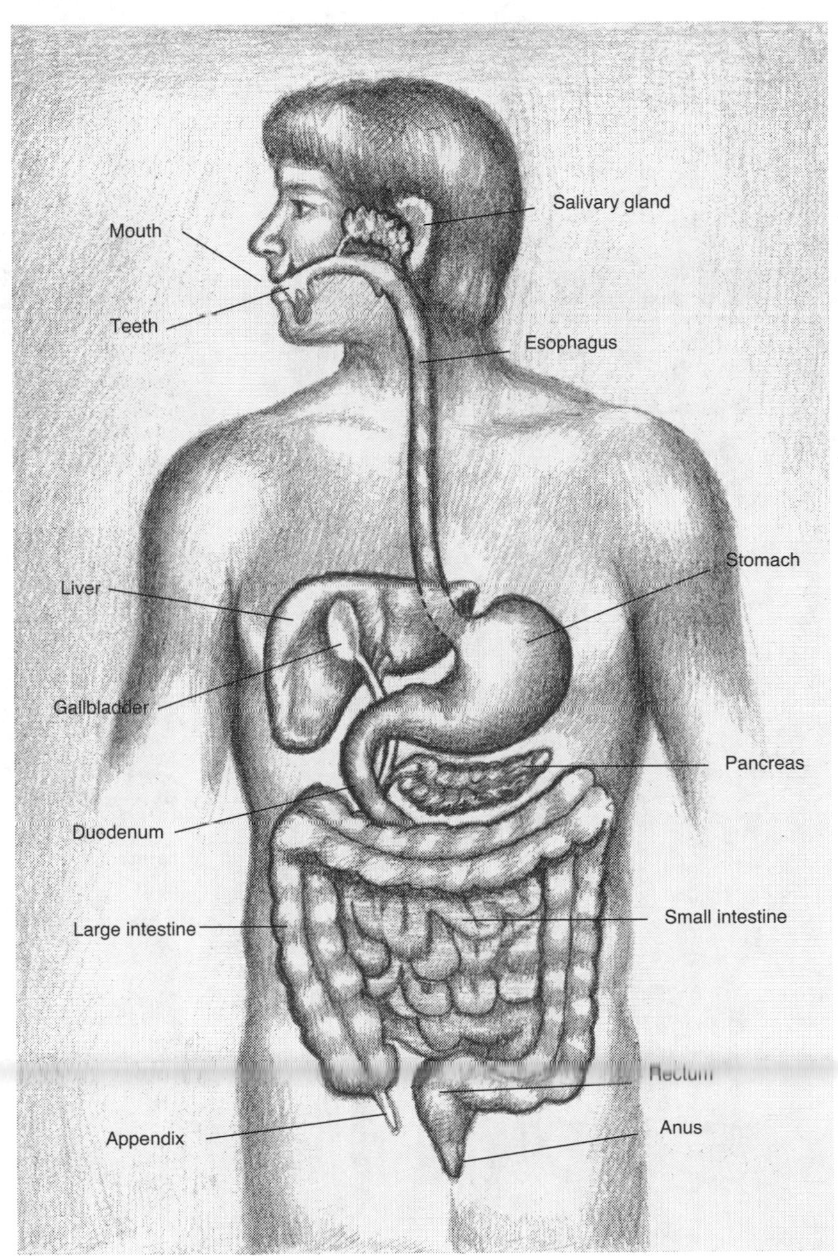

The Gastrointestinal System

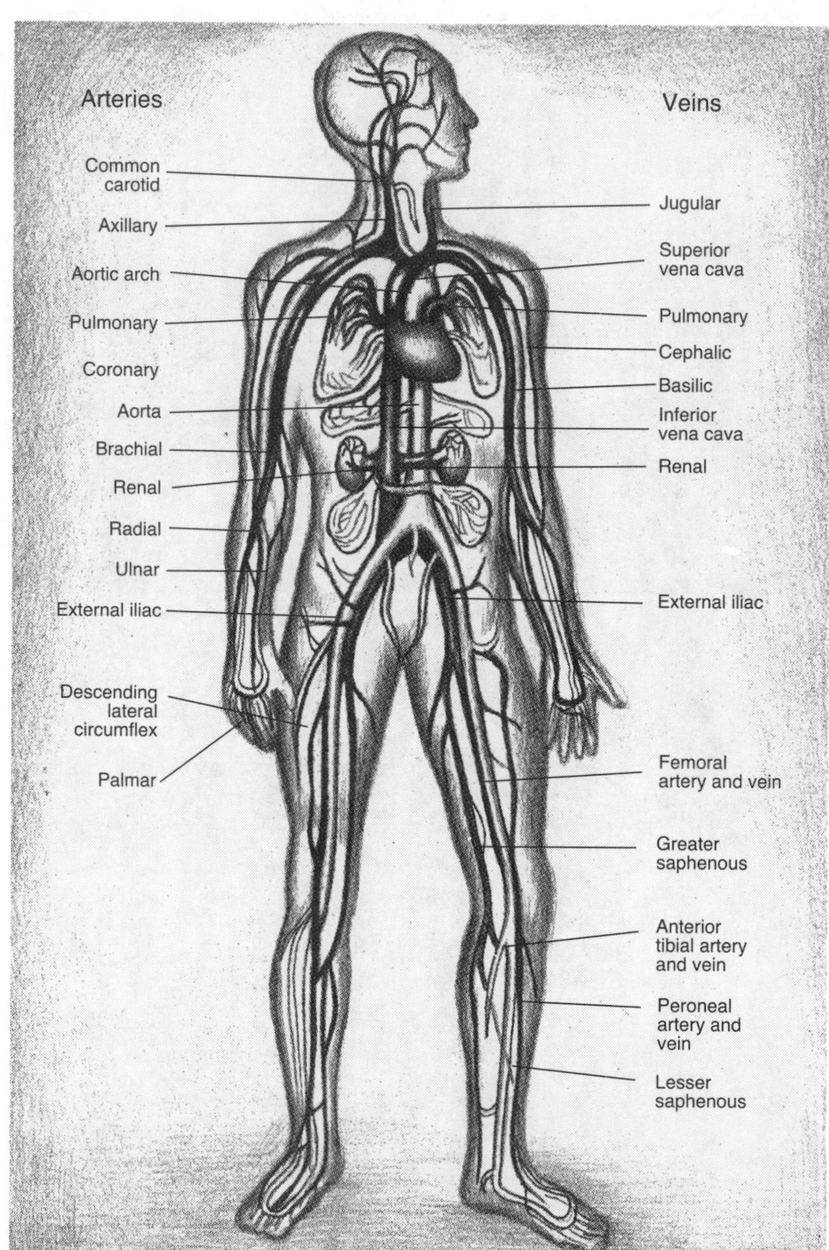
Arteries
Veins
Common carotid
Axillary
Aortic arch
Pulmonary
Coronary
Aorta
Brachial
Renal
Radial
Ulnar
External iliac
Descending lateral circumflex
Palmar
Jugular
Superior vena cava
Pulmonary
Cephalic
Basilic
Inferior vena cava
Renal
External iliac
Femoral artery and vein
Greater saphenous
Anterior tibial artery and vein
Peroneal artery and vein
Lesser saphenous

The Circulatory System

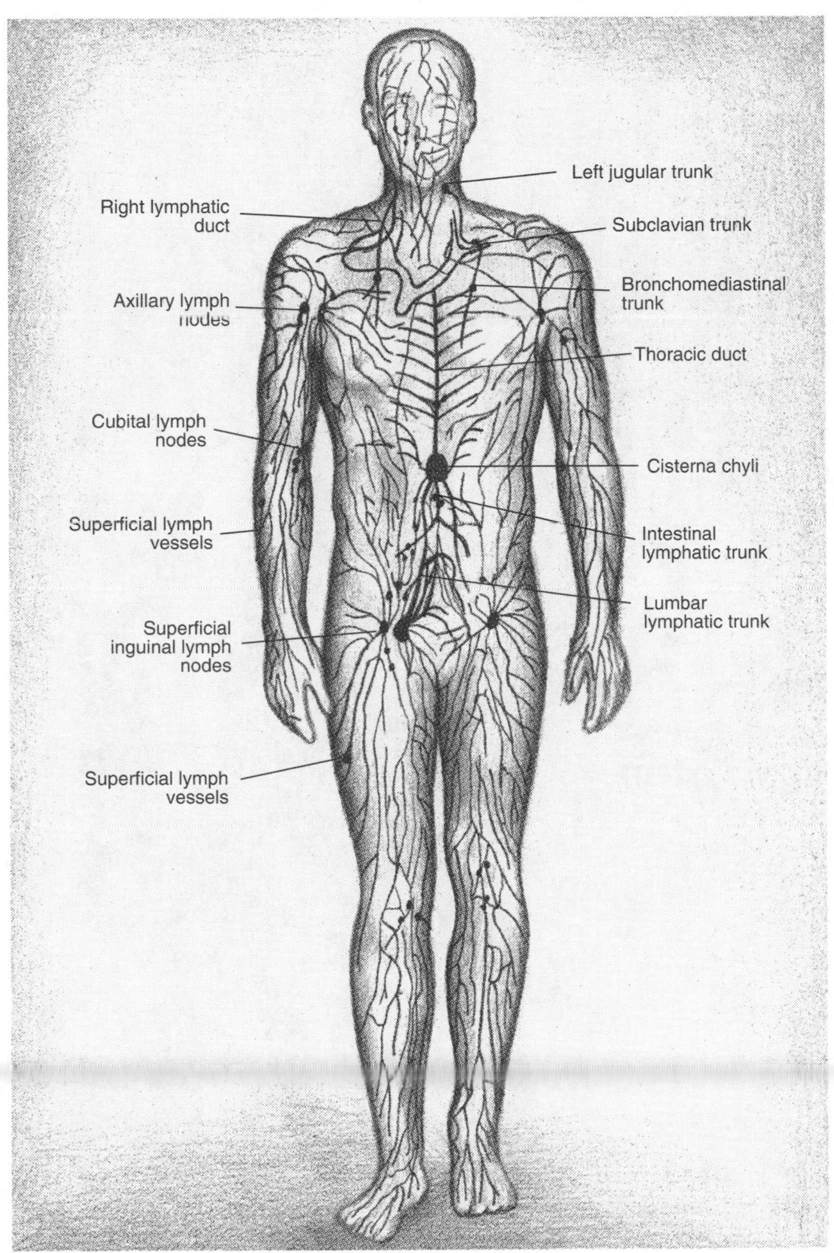
Left jugular trunk
Right lymphatic duct
Subclavian trunk
Bronchomediastinal trunk
Axillary lymph nodes
Thoracic duct
Cubital lymph nodes
Cisterna chyli
Superficial lymph vessels
Intestinal lymphatic trunk
Lumbar lymphatic trunk
Superficial inguinal lymph nodes
Superficial lymph vessels

The Lymphatic System

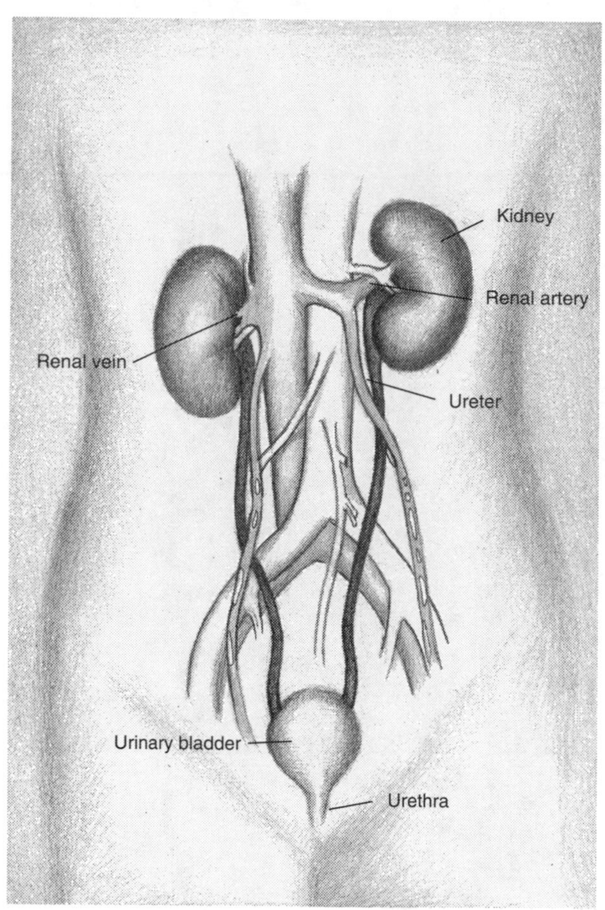

The Urinary System

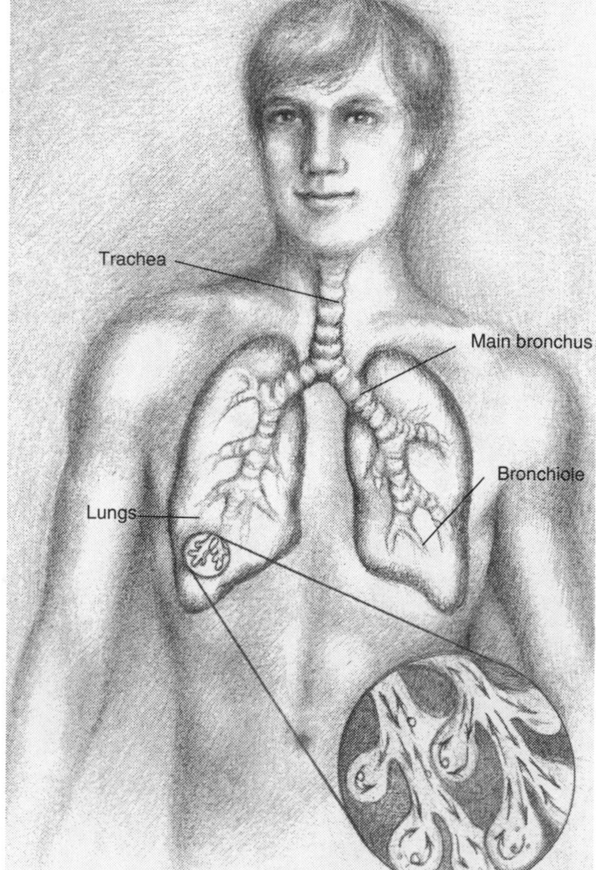

The Respiratory System

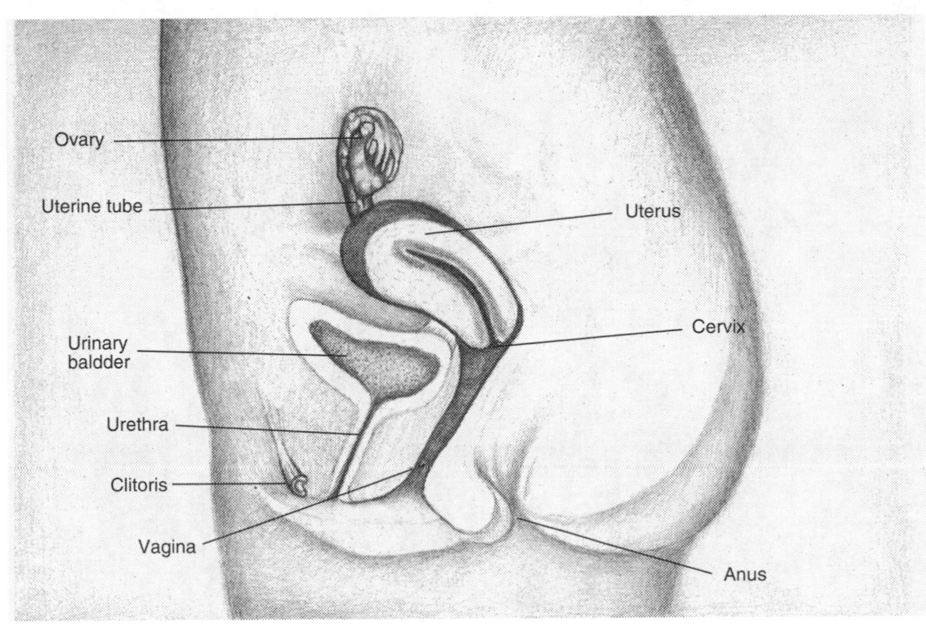

The Female Reproductive System

The Male Reproductive System

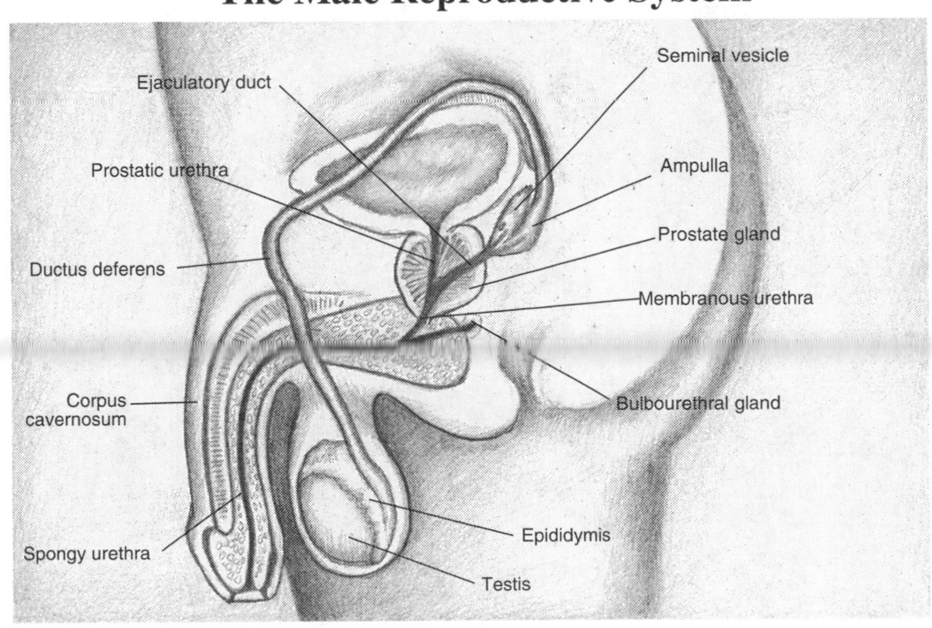

Antibiotics

The discovery of penicillin in 1928 ushered in one of the greatest changes in modern medical history—the antibiotic era. The miracles brought about by this new drug, and those that followed, thoroughly convinced physicians that infectious diseases might some day be wiped out. Indeed, antibiotics were dubbed "magic bullets" because of their seemingly precise action on the bacterial invaders that contributed to so much disease. But realities of the human condition coupled with the tenacity of the microbes has tempered such enthusiasm. The promise of antibiotics is fading as problems surface on a variety of fronts. Resistant bacteria, immune suppression, yeast colonization, superinfection, overuse and misapplication of antibiotics (including antibiotics ingested in meat and poultry), and the reemergence of diseases such as tuberculosis (once nearly eradicated from industrialized countries), have caused doctors to take a new look at these miracle drugs.

Problems Associated with the Inappropriate Use of Antibiotics

Destruction of Friendly Bacteria

The human body is home to hundreds of billions of bacteria, many of which are vital for optimum health. It is a delicately balanced system much like the rain forests of this planet. Bifidobacteria in the large intestine, and acidophilus in the small intestine and vagina protect against infection by yeast and bacteria. Likewise, "friendly" bacteria found on the skin protect against bacterial, yeast, and fungal infections. Overuse of antibiotics, especially broad-spectrum antibiotics as well as steroid drugs (such as "the pill"), can seriously disrupt the normal ecology of the body and render anyone more susceptible to subsequent bacterial, yeast, viral, and parasitic infection.

Yeast Overgrowth

Yeast overgrowth is a common side effect of antibiotic use. Women who use antibiotics often develop bowel and vaginal yeast infections. Children treated repeatedly with antibiotics for ear infections often develop yeast and fungal infections of the middle ear.[1]

Nutrient Loss

Antibiotics can contribute to nutrient loss. By disrupting the population of beneficial bacteria in the gut, antibiotics can adversely influence the availability of vitamins B_1, B_2, B_3, B_6, B_{12}, vitamin A, and folic acid. Zinc and magnesium can also be lost. When antibiotics cause diarrhea, the loss of these nutrients can be significant.

Immune Suppression

Antibiotics can in some cases hinder the immune response. For example, children given amoxicillin for chronic earaches suffer two to six times the rate of recurrent middle ear effusion than children who took a placebo.[2] According to Carol Jessop, M.D., Clinical Professor at the University of California at San Francisco, 80 percent of her patients who suffer from chronic fatigue syndrome (or chronic fatigue immunodeficiency syndrome) had a history of recurrent antibiotic treatment as a child, adolescent, or adult.[3]

Development of Food Allergies or Intolerance

Antibiotics can contribute to the development of food intolerance. According to Leo Galland, M.D., "It is no accident that the most allergic generation in history has been raised on antibiotics. Several times a week I see a new patient whose allergies appeared or became much worse after a course of antibiotics."[4]

Antibiotic Resistant Bacteria

Bacteria resistant to antibiotics is a rapidly emerging problem with potentially disastrous consequences. In 1941, only 40,000 units per day of penicillin for four days was required to cure pneumococcal pneumonia. "Today, a patient could receive 24 million units of penicillin a day and die of pneumococcal meningitis."[5] Strains of *Streptococcus pneumoniae* that are resistant to penicillin also have decreased susceptibility to broad-spectrum cephalosporin antibiotics.

A similar situation exists with regard to other antibiotics. *Haemophilus influenzae* is a bacterium responsible for ear infections, sinusitis, epiglottitis, and meningitis. In 1986, roughly 32 percent of the strains of this bacterium were resistant to ampicillin, the drug most commonly used against it.[6] In Barcelona, Spain, 50 percent of *H. influenzae* type B are resistant to five or more antibiotics, including chloramphenicol and trimethoprim-sulfamethoxazole, the most commonly used alternatives to ampicillin.[7]

Antibiotic resistance also knows no age boundaries. The bacterium *E. coli* is a common cause of bladder infection in men and women. In the United States, roughly 40 percent of the strains of *E. coli* isolated from the urine of geriatric units were resistant to trimethoprim-sulfamethoxazole. In a recent outbreak of pneumococcal pneumonia in a day care center, carriers of a penicillin-resistant strain of the bacteria were more likely to have received preventive antibiotics for recurrent ear infections.[8]

Overuse and inappropriate use of antibiotics have led to the current crisis. According to Mitchell L. Cohen of the Centers for Disease Control, "Unless currently effective antimicrobial agents can be successfully preserved and the transmission of drug-resistant organisms curtailed, the post antibiotic era may be rapidly approaching in which infectious disease wards housing untreatable conditions will again be seen."[9]

There are many ways to improve immune function so that the need for antibiotics can be reduced. By addressing diet, nutritional status, lifestyle, hygiene, genetic uniqueness, environmental factors, and psychological factors such as mood and stress, one can improve resistance to disease and minimize the chance that invading microbes will gain a foothold. What is needed is a reduced employment of these often life-saving drugs so that they work when one really needs them. This more selective use of antibiotics will also help stem the explosion of resistant organisms now appearing worldwide.

Enhancing Immune Function

The immune system is a barometer of health—and any return to a healthy state should involve immune enhancement. There are many influences on this defense mechanism.

Diet and Nutrition

In 1991, 104 children with chronic ear infections were tested for allergies to foods. Seventy-eight percent tested positive for one or more foods. After removing the offending foods for eleven weeks, 70 of the 81 children experienced significant improvement.[10]

Children with severe measles are susceptible to complications such as pneumonia, ear infections, croup, diarrhea (all commonly treated with antibiotics), and death. When such children were supplemented with vitamin A, the rate of complications was cut in half.[11]

Environment

Exposure to foreign chemicals can also diminish resistance to infection. In a study reported in *Pediatrics* (1992), 92 pregnant women had their amniotic fluid analyzed for toxic metals. A toxic risk score was calculated based on the number and amount of metals present. When the children were assessed at age three, those with the highest toxic risk scores were found to have experienced more infections (of the ear, nose, throat, and other areas), and more illness in general than those with low scores.[12] In another study, mercury amalgam fillings were found to trigger the development of bacterial resistance to several common antibiotics.[13]

Heredity

Certain genetic conditions predispose a person to infection. There is now evidence that nutrition may play a role in reversing this to some extent. For example, children with Down syndrome are highly susceptible to ear and upper respiratory infection by the bacteria *S. pneumoniae* and *H. influenzae*. In one study, when children with Down syndrome were given the trace element selenium, the production of antibodies against these bacteria increased and the rates of infectious illness went down.[14]

Lifestyle

Those who lead a sedentary life are often predisposed to respiratory infection. When sedentary women with a history of respiratory infection simply began walking for forty-five minutes each day, their rate of respiratory infection dropped dramatically.[15]

Mood, Mind, and Stress

Psychological factors have a significant impact on resistance to disease. Those who write their deepest feelings or past traumas or who share them with another person, experience an upsurge in immune function. Those who "confess" regularly in this way suffer fewer infections and make fewer trips to the doctor.[16] A study conducted at Harvard Medical School found that in people who harbored the strep bacteria in their throats, one-half of those under high stress actually became sick compared with only one-fifth of those under low stress.[17]

By addressing these and other primary factors about the way people live, doctors could sharply curtail their reliance upon antibiotics while simultaneously achieving their goal—to build immunity and direct their patients back toward health.

Natural Medicine for Immune Enhancement

Practitioners of alternative medicine or other forms of natural therapeutics already possess an arsenal of methods and substances that are helpful in promoting healing from infection.[18]

Herbal Medicine

There are numerous herbs useful in the care of infections. Some are directly antibacterial or antiviral while others are immune potentiators. Some herbs do both. Examples include goldenseal, licorice, garlic, *reishi* and *shiitake* mushrooms, and echinacea. Of these, echinacea and garlic are among the most widely used, extensively researched, and effective of all immune-building plants.

Essential Oils

Essential plant oils useful during various types of infectious illness include tea tree oil, thyme, savory, eucalyptus, inula, lavender, geranium, and citrus seed extract.

Homeopathic Medicine

Homeopathy initially gained notoriety in the United States because of its effectiveness against epidemic infectious diseases. Medicines commonly used during infection include *Apis mel., Arsen alb., Belladonna, Rhus tox., Merc iod., Hepar sulph., Lachesis,* and others.

Vitamins and Minerals

Numerous vitamins and minerals are known to be important in immune function. Among those commonly used to potentiate immune function or promote healing during infection are zinc, selenium, vitamins A, C, E, beta-carotene, coenzyme Q10, and B vitamins.

Probiotics

Supplements such as acidophilus can be used to enhance digestion and reverse many of the negative intestinal effects of prolonged antibiotic therapy. Many doctors also prescribe acidophilus (for the small intestine) and bifidobacteria (for the large intestine) concurrently whenever antibiotics must be prescribed.

Probiotics: The Friendly Bacteria

Inside each of us live vast numbers of bacteria without which we could not remain in good health. Before looking at the amazing things they do, reflect on just how many of them we house.

There are several thousand billion in each person (more than all the cells in the body) divided into over four hundred species, most of them living in the digestive tract. If they were all placed together the total weight of this "friendly" bacteria would come to nearly four pounds and, in fact, about a third of the fecal matter (water removed) which you pass consists of dead or viable bacteria.[1]

The Role of Friendly Bacteria in Health

These bacteria are not parasites. They do not just take up residence and do nothing in return, but perform many important functions in the body. We live in true symbiosis with them. As long as we provide them with a reasonable diet and as long as they remain in good health, these bacteria provide excellent service in return.

However, not all of the friendly bacteria perform the same functions, some being far more useful and plentiful than others. These are the ones presented here. Certain bacteria help to maintain good health while others have a definite value in helping us regain health once it has been upset.

These dual protective and therapeutic roles help explain why the word "probiotics" was coined since it means "for life":

- They manufacture some of the B vitamins including niacin (B_3), pyridoxine (B_6), folic acid, and biotin.[2]
- They manufacture the milk-digesting enzyme lactase which helps digest calcium-rich dairy products.[3]
- They actively produce antibacterial substances which kill or deactivate hostile disease-causing bacteria. They do this by changing the local levels of acidity, by depriving pathogenic (disease-causing) bacteria of their nutrients, or by actually producing their own antibiotic substances which can kill invading bacteria, viruses, and yeasts.[4] Naturally enough they are doing this to preserve "their" territory.
- Some bacteria (such as bifidobacteria and acidophilus) have been shown to have powerful anticarcinogenic features which are active against certain tumors.[5]
- They improve the efficiency of the digestive tract—when they are weakened, bowel function is poor.[6]
- They effectively help to reduce high cholesterol levels.[7]
- They play an important part of the development of a baby's digestive function and immune system. *Bifidobacteria infantis* is acquired from breast milk. When it is in poor supply allergies and malabsorption problems are more common.[8]
- They help protect against radiation damage and deactivate many toxic pollutants.[9]
- They help to recycle estrogen (a female hormone) which reduces the likelihood of menopausal symptoms and osteoporosis.[10]
- Therapeutically they have been shown to be useful in treatment of acne, psoriasis, eczema, allergies, migraine, gout (by reducing uric acid levels), rheumatic and arthritic conditions, cystitis, candidiasis, colitis, irritable bowel syndrome, and some forms of cancer.[11]

Types of Friendly Bacteria

Of the friendly bacteria which help the human body most are residents, while others are transient visitors, staying in your digestive tract for a few weeks before passing on. The principal forms of friendly bacteria, are as follows:[12]

Lactobacillus Acidophilus

This is the main inhabitant of the small intestine in humans and animals. It is also found in the mouth and vagina. Acidophilus manufactures lactase to digest milk sugar and produces lactic acid which suppresses undesirable bacteria and yeasts. Some strains produce natural antibiotics. They also lower cholesterol levels and kill candida yeasts, and are very susceptible to poor diet and stress conditions, pollution, and antibiotics such as penicillin.

Lactobacillus Bulgaricus

This is a transient but very important bacteria. Together with *Streptococcus thermophilus* it makes yogurt. Some strains of bulgaricus and thermophilus also produce antibiotics which kill harmful bacteria. By manufacturing lactic acid these bacteria encourage a good environment for the resident bacteria such as acidophilus and the bifidobacteria.

Bifidobacterium Bifidum and Bifidobacteriumlongum

These are the main inhabitants of the large intestine. *Bifidobacterium bifidum* is also found in the vagina and the lower part of the small intestine. In breastfed infants and adolescents these make up 99 percent of the entire flora of the bowel. There is strong evidence that the numbers and efficient working of these bacteria decline as a person ages and with any decline in our health status.

The bacteria produce a number of specialized acids and use these to prevent colonization of the large intestine by invading bacteria, yeasts, and some viruses. They also prevent potential toxicity from nitrites in food and manufacture B vitamins as well as helping detoxify bile from which they recycle estrogen in women.

Bifidobacteria Infantis

This is the main inhabitant of every infant's intestines and is found in small amounts in the vagina. Its functions are very much the same as the other bifidobacteria. In a freeze-dried form it is the only probiotic product which should be supplemented to infants without professional guidance.

What Damages the Friendly Bacteria?

Many factors influence just how healthy the flora are. While the type of friendly bacteria living in a region may seem much the same in health and disease, the tasks they perform change according to circumstances. For example, when Bifidobacteria are in a good state of health they will detoxify pollutants and carcinogens as well as manufacture various B vitamins. When in a poor state of health, however, they just cannot do these jobs as well or at all.

What Makes Friendly Bacteria Function Less Efficiently?

The level of local acidity is one major influence upon the function of the friendly bacteria and this is contributed to by diet, digestive function, and stress.[13] Another important influence is the speed of peristalsis (the wavelike contraction of the intestines) which moves food along the digestive tract. If it is too rapid (as in diarrhea, irritable bowel syndrome, or colitis) this severely reduces the efficiency of the flora. If it is too slow (as in atonic or spastic constipation) this too causes changes in their function.

The type of diet you eat is a major influence on bacterial health. The bacteria are healthier on a diet rich in complex carbohydrates (vegetables, whole grains, legumes) and low in animal fats, fatty meat, sugars, and cultured dairy products (especially "live" yogurt and cottage cheese).[14] Not surprisingly, the diet which is best for people is also ideal for healthly bacteria.

They are also influenced to a major extent by the degree of infection by yeasts and bacteria to which the bowel is subjected. Certain drugs, especially antibiotics, can severely upset this delicate balance (penicillin will kill friendly bacteria just as efficiently as it will kill disease-causing bacteria).[15] Steroids (hormonal drugs such as cortisone, ACTH, prednisone, and birth control pills) also cause great damage to the bowel flora.

Damaged friendly bacteria can regain health and efficiency by dealing with any of the factors listed above, especially diet and stress reduction, and by supplementing good quality freeze-dried bacteria such as *Lactobacillus acidophilus* or *Lactobacillus bulgaricus*.

The way products are made is important :

- When being separated from the "soup" in which they are cultured, some manufacturers spin the bacteria in a centrifuge. This damages the delicate chains of bacteria, which does not happen when a slower (and therefore more expensive) filtration process is used. This information should be on the container.
- It is preferable to take the friendly bacteria as a powder, as similar damage can occur if the bacteria are in capsule or tablet form. The bacteria should be stored in a dark glass (never plastic) container.
- Viable cultures of the particular bacteria you want, which are capable of recolonising the intestines, as a rule need to be refrigerated after the opening of their container. They should not be taken at meal times to avoid the extreme acidity of the stomach when it has food in it.

How you can be sure of the quality of supplemental friendly bacteria

There are many undesirable products on the market and it is only by insisting on the best that these can be eliminated.

Some products carry "cocktails" of bacteria which should not be together in a container and which are only minutely a part of the total flora picture, such as Bacillus laterosporus *and* Streptococcus faecium *which should be avoided.*

Even cocktails of the best friendly bacteria should not be kept in the same container since they are destined to inhabit different regions of the digestive tract and will damage each other if confined together.

- All good products should carry a guarantee of viable colonizing bacteria up to a specific expiration date.

Only a very few brands of friendly bacteria meet all these requirements.

When to Use Probiotic Supplements

Probiotics may be used in the following cases:

- Under professional guidance if there are chronic bowel problems or ongoing infections such as candidiasis.
- As a preventive against food poisoning when travelling (bifidobacteria and acidophilus kill most food-poisoning bacteria).
- After (and during) any period when antibiotics are taken.
- By all premenopausal and menopausal women to reduce chances of osteoporosis.
- By anyone with high cholesterol problems.
- By anyone with chronic health problems (acne, skin problems, allergies, arthritis, cancer, etc.) under professional guidance.
- By anyone receiving radiation treatment.
- By anyone having recurrent vaginal or bladder infections (thrush or cystitis).
- *Bifidobacteria infantis* should be given to all babies.

Which Bacteria Can the Friendly Flora Control?

Many studies prove the antibiotic effects of the friendly bacteria.

- In nineteen cases of nonspecific infection of the vagina treated with acidophilus (*Doderlein bacillus* strain) 95 percent were cured.
- In twenty-five cases of Monilia vaginitis 88 percent were cured and 12 percent relieved of symptoms. In 444 cases of trichomonas vaginitis 92 percent were cured and remained infection free up to a year later.[16]
- The acidophilin antibiotic which *Lactobacillus acidophilus* produces will kill 50 percent of twenty-seven different disease causing bacteria.[17]
- Sixteen children with salmonella poisoning and fifteen with shigella infections were cleared of all symptoms using acidophilus. *Bifidobacterium bifidum* effectively kills or controls *E. coli*, *Staphylococcus aureus* (cause of toxic shock syndrome), and shigella. Acidophilus can also control viruses such as herpes.[18]

Breast Milk and the Health of Intestinal Flora

German research shows that the state of the intestinal flora in most breastfed babies today is similar to that of formula fed babies forty years ago. The result is malabsorption and food sensitivity problems as well as increase in allergies and susceptibility to infection.[21] Further research has pointed to contamination of breast milk with pollutants such as DDT and dioxin.[22] This suggests that supplementation of all babies with *Bifidobacteria infantis* may be a helpful strategy.

The role of intestinal bacterial in rheumatoid arthritis and ankylosing spondylitis

Two major health problems, rheumatoid arthritis and ankylosing spondylitis, have been found to be associated with overgrowth in the intestines of particular harmful bacteria, proteus, and klebsiella respectively.[19] Both of these can be controlled by healthy bowel flora. The natural antibiotics manufactured by Lactobacillus bulgaricus, Lactobacillus acidophilus *and the bifidobacteria kill both of these bacteria.[20]*

British research shows that people with ankylosing spondylitis benefit if they go onto a diet low in fat and sugar and high in complex carbohydrates—the very diet that enables friendly bacteria to perform efficiently. Rheumatoid arthritis patients have been shown to benefit in recent Norwegian trials from a vegetarian diet something which also dramatically improves the health and function of the friendly bacteria.

Notes

Part One: The Future of Medicine

A New Understanding of Alternative Medicine

1 Eisenberg, D. M.; et al. "Unconventional Medicine in the United States: Prevalence, Costs, and Patterns of Use." *New England Journal of Medicine* 328 (Jan, 1993): 246-252.
2 Bergner, P. ; and Kail, K. "The U.S. Health Care Costs Crisis: A Crisis of Chronic Disease." *American Association of Naturopathic Physicians* (Sep, 1992).
3 Ibid.
4 Centers for Disease Control, Public Health Service. 1975.
5 Crook, W. G. *Chronic Fatigue Syndrome* and *The Yeast Connection*. Jackson, TN: Professional Books, 1984, 1992.
6 Alvin, L.; et al. "Electric and Magnetic Fields: Measurements and Possible Effects on Human Health from Appliances, Powerlines, and other Common Sources: What We Know, What We Don't Know in 1990." Special Epidemiological Studies Program, California Department of Health Services, 2151 Berkeley Way.
7 Sinclair, L. "Entrepreneurs Tackle Electromagnetic Fields." *Business* (Mar/Apr, 1993): 34-35.
8 Williams, R. *Biochemical Individuality*. Austin, TX: University of Texas Press, 1980.

Medical Freedom and the Politics of Health Care

1 Department of Health And Human Services, Public Health Services. Pub. no.88-50210, 1988.
2 Lynes, B. *The Healing of Cancer*. Wilmington, MA: Marcus Books, 1992.
3 Wilkes, M. S., M.D.; et. al. "Pharmaceutical Advertisements in Leading Medical Journals: Expert's Assessments." *Annals of Internal Medicine* 116 (1992): 912-919.
4 FDA (Food and Drug Administration), Department of Health and Human Services Public Health Service. Dietary Supplements Task Force Final Report." May, 1992, 2.
5 Siegel, Barry. "Faith Lost, A Doctor Turns Bitter." *Los Angeles Times*. Vol. 112, (Sep, 12, 1993): p. A1.
6 U.S. prices collected from Los Angeles, California pharmacies, June, 1993. Prices for Mexico supplied by the Farmacia Paris in Tijuana, Mexico.
7 *Physicians Desk Reference*. Oradell, NJ: Medical Economics Company, 1993.
8 Whitaker, J. "Act Now To Protect Your Health." *Health & Healing* (Sep, 1993).
9 Moss, R. *Cancer Therapy*. New York: Equinox Press, 1992, 319.
10 Kamen, J. "Hope, Heartbreak and Horror." *Omni* 15 no. 11 (Sep, 1993): insert.
Liversridge, A. "Heresy: Three Modern Galileos." *Omni* 15, No. 8, (June, 1993) 43.
11 Kamen, J. "Hope, Heartbreak and Horror." *Omni* 15 no. 11 (Sep, 1993): insert.
11 Ibid.
12 Rothstein, W. G. *American Medical Schools and the Practice of Medicine: A History*. New York: Oxford University Press 1987, 143-144.

Part Two: Alternative Therapies

Acupuncture

1 Gerber, R., M.D. *Vibrational Medicine*. Santa Fe, NM: Bear & Company, 1988.
2 De Vernejoul, P.; et al. "Study of Acupuncture Meridians using Radioactive Tracers." (In French). *Bulletin de L'Academie Nationale de Medicine* (Oct. 22, 1985): 1071-1075.
3 Zhu Zong-xiang. "Research Advances in the Electrical Specificity of Meridians and Acupuncture Points." *American Journal of Acupuncture* 9 no.3 (Jul-Sep, 1981): 203-215.
4 Becker, R. O., M.D. *Cross Currents. The Promise of Electro-Medicine. The Perils of Electropollution*. Los Angeles: Jeremy P. Tarcher, Inc., 1990.
5 Becker, R. O., M.D.; and Selden, G. *The Body Electric: Electromagnetism and the Foundation of Life*. New York: William Morrow and Company, 1985, 235.
6 Jayasuraiya, A. *Open International University's Textbook on Acupuncture*. Colombo, Sri Lanka: Open University, 1987.
7 Huard, P.; and Wong, M. *Chinese Medicine*. New York: World University Library, McGraw-Hill, 1968.
8 Hau, D. M. "Effects of Electroacupuncture on Leukocytes and Plasma Protein in the X-Irradiated Rats." *American Journal of Chinese Medicine* (1980): 354-366.
9 Chatfield, K. B. "The Treatment of Pesticide Poisoning with Traditional Acupuncture." *American Journal of Acupuncture 13* (1985):339-345.
10 Chatfield, K. B. "The Scientific Basis of Acupuncture." In *The Textbook of Natural Medicine*, ed. J. E. Pizzorno and M. T. Murray. Seattle, WA: John Bastyr College Publications, 1988.
11 Eisenberg, D., M.D.; and Wright, T. L. *Encounters With Qi: Exploring Chinese Medicine*. 2d ed. New York: Penguin Books, 1987, 77.
12 Lewith, G. T.; and Machin, D. "On the Evaluation of the Clinical Effects of Acupuncture." *Pain* 16 (Jun, 1983): 111-127.
13 Millman, B. "Acupuncture: Context and Critique." *Annual Review of Medicine* 28 (1977): 223-236.
14 Cheung, J. "Effect of Electroacupuncture on Chronic Painful Conditions in General Medical Practice—A Four-Years' Study." *American Journal of Chinese Medicine* 13 (1985): 33-38.
15 Sodipo, J. "Therapeutic Acupuncture for Chronic Pain." *Pain* 7 (1979): 359-365.
16 Bullock, M. L.; Culliton, P. D.; and Oleander, R. T. "Controlled Trial of Acupuncture for Severe Recidivist Alcoholism." *The Lancet* 1 no. 8652 (June, 1989): 1435-1439.
17 NADA Newsletter Committee. *National Acupuncture Detoxification Association Newsletter* (December 1, 1992): 1-6.
18 Wen, A. H.; and Cheung, S. Y. "How Acupuncture Can Help Addicts." *Drugs and Society* 2 (1973): 18-20.
19 Holder, J., M.D. "New Auricular Therapy Formula to Increase Retention of the Chemically Dependent in Residential Treatment." (1991) Research study funded by the State of Florida, Department of Health and Rehabilitative Services.
20 NADA Newsletter Committee. *National Acupuncture Detoxification Association Newsletter* (Dec, 1992): 1-6.
21 Eisenberg, D., M.D.; and Wright, T. L. *Encounters With Qi: Exploring Chinese Medicine*. 2d ed. New York: Penguin Books, 1987, 68-74.
22 Huard, P.; and Wong, M. *Chinese Medicine*. New York: World University Library, McGraw-Hill, 1968.
23 NADA Newsletter Committee. *National Acupuncture Detoxification Association Newsletter* (Dec, 1992): 1-6.
24 Ibid.
25 Becker, R.O., M.D. *Cross Currents: The Promise of Electromedicine. The Perils of Electropollution*. Los Angeles: Jeremy P. Tarcher, Inc., 1990.

Applied Kinesiology

1 Leisman, G.; Shambaugh, P.; and Ferentz, A. H. "Somatosensory Evoked Potential Changes During Muscle Testing." *International Journal of Neuroscience* 45 no. 1-2 (Mar, 1989): 143-151.

Aromatherapy

1 Wagner, H.; and Sprinkmeier, L. "Uber die pharmakologischen Wirkungen von Melissengeist." *Deutsche Apotheker Zeitung* 113 (1973): 1159.
2 Franchomme, P.; and Penoel, D. *Aromatherapie exactement*. Limoges: Roger Jollois, 1990.
3 Pena, E. F. "Melaeuca Alternifolia Oil. Its Use for Trichomonal Vaginitis and Other Vaginal Infections." *Obstetrics and Gynecology* 19 no. 6 (1962): 793.
4 Wolbling, R. H.; and Milbradt, R. "Klinik und Therapie des Herpes Simplex." *Therapiewoche* 34 (1984): 1193-1200.
5 Tisserand, R. B. *The Art of Aromatherapy*. Rochester, Vermont: Healing Arts Press, 1977.
6 Dodd, G. H. "Receptor Events in Perfumery." In *Perfumery. The Psychology and Biology of Fragrance*, eds. S. van Toller and G. H. Dodd. London: Chapman and Hall, 1988.
7 Steele, J. "Brain Research and Essential Oils." *Aromatherapy Quarterly* 3 (Spring, 1984): 5.
8 Lorig, T. S.; et al. "The Effects of Low Concentration Odors on EEG Activity and Behavior." *Journal of Psychophysiology* 5 (1991): 69-77.
9 Tisserand, R. B. *The Art of Aromatherapy*. Rochester, VT: Healing Arts Press, 1977.
10 Belaiche, P. *Traite de Phytotherapie et d'aromatherapie Tome I - L'aromatogramme*. Paris: Maloine S.A., 1979.
11 Woolfson, A. "Intensive Aromacare." *International Journal of Aromatherapy* 4 no. 2 (1992): 12-13.
12 Horrigan, C. "Complementing Cancer Care" *International Journal of Aromatherapy* 3 no. 4 (1991): 15-17.
13 Keller, W.; and Kober, W. "Moglickeiten der Verwendung atherischer åle zur Raundesinfektion I." *Arzneimittelforschung* 5 (1955): 224.
Keller, W.; and Kober, W. "Moglickeiten der Verwendung atherischer åle zur Raundesinfektion II." *Arzneimittelforschung* 6 (1955): 768.
14 Maruzella, J. C. "The In Vitro Antibacterial Activity of Essential Oils and Oil Combinations." *Journal of the American Pharmaceutical Association: Scientific Edition* 47 (1958): 294.
Maruzella, J. C. "Antibacterial Activity of Essential Oil Vapors." *Journal of the American Pharmaceutical Association: Scientific Edition* 49 (1960): 692.
Maruzella, J. C. "Effects of Vapors of Aromatic Chemicals on Fungi." *Journal of Pharmaceutical Science* 50 (1961): 655.
15 Wagner, H.; and Sprinkmeier, L. "Uber die pharmakologischen Wirkungen von Melissengeist." *Deutsche Apotheker Zeitung* 113 (1973): 1159.
16 Tisserand, R. B. *The Essential Oil Safety Data Manual*. Hove: The Tisserand Aromatherapy Institute, 1988.
17 Lembke, A.; and Deininger, R. "Wirkung van Bestandteilen etherischer Ole auf Bakterien, Pilze und Viren." In *Phytotherapie*, 1 Phytotherapie Kongress, Koln 1987, Hippokratos Verlag, Stuttgart (1988).
18 Valnet, J., M.D. *The Practice of Aromatherapy*. Rochester, VT: Healing Arts Press, 1980.
19 Czygan, F. C. "Essential Oils - Aspects of History of Civilization." In *Atherische åle, Analytik, Physiologie, Zusammensetzung*, ed. K. H. Kubeczka. Stuttgart, New York: Georg Thieme Verlag, 1982.
20 Valnet, J., M.D. *The Practice of Aromatherapy*. Rochester, VT: Healing Arts Press, 1980.
21 Brandt, W. "Spasmolytische Wirkung atherischer Ole." *Zeitschrift fur Phytotherapy* 9 no. 2 (1988): 33-39.
22 Wagner, H. "Zum Wirknachweis antiphlogistisch wirksamer arzneidrogen." *Zeitschrift fur Phytotherapie* 8 no. 5 (1987): 135-141.
Wagner, H. "Phlanzeninhaltsstoffe mit Wirkung aus das Komplementsystem." *Zeitschrift fur Phytotherapie* 8 no. 5 (1987): 148-149.
23 Buchbauer, G.; and Hafner, M. "Aroma Therapy"(in German). *Pharmazie in unserer Zeit* 14 no. 1 (1985): 8-18.
24 Maruzella, J. C. "The In Vitro Antibacterial

Activity of Essential Oils and Oil Combinations." *Journal of the American Pharmaceutical Association: Scientific Edition* 47 (1958): 294.
Maruzella, J. C. "Antibacterial Activity of Essential Oil Vapors." *Journal of the American Pharmaceutical Association: Scientific Edition* 49 (1960): 692.
Maruzella, J. C. "Effects of Vapors of Aromatic Chemicals on Fungi." *Journal of Pharmaceutical Science* 50 (1961): 655.
25 Gumbel, D. *Wie neugeboren Durch Heilkrauter-Essenzen*. Munich: Grafe und Unzer, 1990.
26 Ibid.
27 Franchomme, P.; and Penoel, D. "Aromatherapie exactement." ed. Roger Jollois, Limoges 1990.
28 "Aromatherapy on the Wards: Lavendar Beats Benzodiazepines." Feature Article, *International Journal of Aromatherapy* 1 no. 2 (1988): 1.
29 Rees, W. D.; Evans, B. K.; and Rhodes, J. "Treating Irritable Bowel Syndrome with Peppermint Oil." *British Medical Journal* 2 no. 6194 (Oct, 1979): 835-836.

Ayurveda

1 Bannerman, R. H.; Burton, J.; and Wen-Chieh, C., eds. *Traditional Medicine and Health Care Coverage*. Geneva: World Health Organization, 1983.
Sharma, H. M.; Triguna, B. D.; and Chopra, D. "Maharishi Ayur-veda: Modern Insights into Ancient Medicine." *Journal of the American Medical Association* 266 no.13 (1991): 2633-2637.
2 Sodhi, V. "Ayurveda: The Science of Life and Mother of the Healing Arts." In *A Textbook of Natural Medicine*., ed. J. E. Pizzorno and M. T. Murray. Seattle, WA: John Bastyr College Publications, 1989.
3 Sharma, H. M.; Triguna, B. D.; and Chopra, D. "Maharishi Ayur-veda: Modern Insights into Ancient Medicine." *Journal of the American Medical Association* 265 no. 20 (1991): 2633-2634, 2637.
Letters to the editor, Maharishi Ayur-veda. *Journal of the American Medical Association* 266 no. 13 (1991): 1769-1774.

Biofeedback Training

1 Fahrion, S. L. "Autogenic Biofeedback Treatment for Migraine." In *Research and Clinical Studies in Headache*, ed. M. E. Granger. 1978, 5, 47-71.
2 Peper, E.; and Tibbetts, V. "Fifteen-Month Follow-up with Asthmatics Utilizing EMG/ Incentive Inspirometer Feedback." *Biofeedback and Self-Regulation* 17 No. 2 (Jun,1992): 143-151.
3 Fahrion, S. L. "Hypertension and Biofeedback." *Primary Care; Clinics in Office Practice* 3 (Sep, 1991): 663-682.
4 Deputy Surgeon General Faye G. Abdellah, as quoted in Miller, N. E. "RX: Biofeedback." *Psychology Today* 19 No. 2 (Feb, 1985): 54-59.
5 Dworkin B.; et al. "Behavioral Method for the Treatment of Idiopathic Scoliosis." *Proceedings of the National Academy of Science of the United States of America* 82 (Apr, 1985): 2493-2497.
6 Deputy Surgeon General Faye G. Abdellah, as quoted in Miller, N. E. "Rx: Biofeedback." *Psychology Today* 19 No. 2 (Feb, 1985): 54-59.
7 Urinary Incontinence Guideline Panel. "Urinary Incontinence in Adults: Clinical Practice Guideline." AHCPR Pub. No. 92-0038. Rockville, MD: Agency for Health Care Policy and Research, Public Health Service, U.S. Department of Health and Human Services, Mar, 1992.
8 Werbach, M. R., M.D. *Third Line Medicine-Modern Treatment for Persistent Symptoms*. New York: Arkana Paperbacks, 1986. Reprint. Los Angeles: Third Line Press, 1986.
9 Norris, P.; and Porter, G. *Why Me? Harnessing the Healing Power of the Human Spirit*. Walpole, N.H.: Stillpoint Publishing Co., 1985.

Biological Dentistry

1 Price, W. A. *Dental Infections* Volume 1: Oral and Systemic. Cleveland, OH: Benton Publishing, 1973.
2 Neuner, O. "The Diagnosis and Therapy of Focal and Field Disorders." *Raum & Zeit* 2 no. 4 (1991): 38-42.
3 Strauss, F. G.; and Eggleston, D. W. "IgA Nephropathy Associated with Dental Nickel Alloy Sensitization." *American Journal of Nephrology* 5 (1985): 395-397.
4 "Dental Mercury Hygiene: Summary of Recommendations in 1990." *Journal of the American Dental Association* 122 (Aug, 1991): 112.
5 "Dental Amalgam: A Scientific Review and Recommended Public Health Service Strategy for Research, Education and Regulation." Final Report of the Subcommittee on Risk Management of the Committee to Coordinate Environmental Health and Related Programs. Public Health Service (Jan, 1993).
6 "Dental Mercury Hygiene: Summary of Recommendations in 1990." *Journal of the American Dental Association* 122 (Aug, 1991): 112.
7 Melillo, W. "How Safe is Mercury in Dentistry?" *The Washington Post Weekly Journal of Medicine, Science and Society*. (Sep, 1991): 4.
8 World Health Organization. *Environmental Health Criteria for Inorganic Mercury* 118. Geneva: World Health Organization, 1991.
9 Grandjean, P., M.D. et al. "Reference Intervals for Trace Elements in Blood: Significance of Risk Factors." *Scandinavian Journal of Clinical and Laboratory Investigation* 2 (Jun, 1992): 321-337.
10 Schiele, R.; et al. "Studies on the Mercury Content in Brain and Kidney Related to Number and Condition of Amalgam Fillings." Institution of Occupational and Social Medicine. University Erlangen, Nurnberg, West Germany, March 12, 1984.
11 "Dental Amalgam: A Scientific Review and Recommended Public Health Service Strategy for Research, Education and Regulation." Final Report of the Subcommittee on Risk Management of the Committee to Coordinate Environmental Health and Related Programs. Public Health Service. (Jan, 1993).
12 "Socialstyrelsen (Swedish Social Welfare and Health Administration) Stops Amalgam Use." *Svenska Dagbladet* (May, 1987): p.1.
13 Agency for Toxic Substances and Disease Registry, 1993. Division of Toxicology. Chart.
14 Taylor, J. *The Complete Guide to Mercury Toxicity from Dental Fillings*. San Diego: Scripps Publishing, 1988.
15 Ziff, S. "Consolidated Symptom Analysis of 1569 Patients." *Bio-Probe Newsletter 9* no. 2 (Mar, 1993): 7-8.
16 Huggins, H. A. *It's All in Your Head*. 4th ed. Colorado Springs, CO: Life Science Press, 1990, 103.
17 Hahn, L. J.; et al. "Dental 'Silver' Tooth Fillings: A Source of Mercury Exposure Revealed by Whole-Body Image Scan and Tissue Analysis." *Faseb* Journal 3 (1989): 2641-2646.
Hahn, L. J.; et al. "Whole-Body Imaging of the Distribution of Mercury Released from Dental Fillings into Monkey Tissues." *Faseb* Journal 4 (1990): 3256-3260.
18 Vimy, M. J.; Takahashi, Y.; and Lorscheider, F. L. "Maternal-Fetal Distribution of Mercury Released from Dental Amalgam Fillings." *American Physiological Society* 258 (1990): R939-R945.
19 Grandjean, P., M.D. "Reference Intervals for Trace Elements in Blood: Significance of Risk Factors." *Scandinavian Journal of Clinical and Laboratory Investigation* 2 (Jun, 1992): 321-337.
Schiele, R.; et al. "Studies on the Mercury Content in Brain and Kidney Related to Number and Condition of Amalgam Fillings." Institution of Occupational and Social Medicine. University Erlangen, Nurnberg, West Germany, 1984.
Vimy, M. J.; et al. "Glomerular Filtration Impairment by Mercury from Dental 'Silver' Fillings in Sheep." *The Physiologist* 33 (Aug, 1990): A 94.
Boyd, N. D.; et al. "Mercury from Dental 'Silver' Tooth Fillings Impairs Sheep Kidney Function." *American Physiological Society* 261 (1991): R1010-R1014.
20 International Labour Office. *Encyclopedia of Occupational Health and Safety*. 2d ed. New York: McGraw-Hill, 1972.
21 EPA Mercury Health Effects Update Health Issue Assessment Final Report. EPA-600/8.84.019F. (Aug, 1984) United States Environmental Protection Agency, Office of Health and Environmental Assessment.
22 Price, W. A. *Nutrition and Physical Degeneration*. La Mesa, CA: The Price-Pottinger Nutrition Foundation, Inc., 1945, 1970.
23 Wang, K. "A Report of 22 Cases of Temporomandibular Joint Dysfunction Syndrome Treated with Acupuncture and Laser Radiation." *Journal of Traditional Chinese Medicine* 12 no. 2 (Jun, 1992):116-118.
24 Grandjean, P., M.D. "Reference Intervals for Trace Elements in Blood: Significance of Risk Factors." *Scandinavian Journal of Clinical and Laboratory Investigation* 2 (Jun, 1992): 321-337.
Schiele, R.; et al. "Studies on the Mercury Content in Brain and Kidney Related to Number and Condition of Amalgam Fillings." Institution of Occupational and Social Medicine. University Erlangen, Nurnberg, West Germany, 1984.
Boyd, N. D.; et al. "Mercury from Dental 'Silver' Tooth Fillings Impairs Sheep Kidney Function." *American Physiological Society* 261 (1991): R1010-R1014.
25 Yiamouyiannis, J. A. *Fluoride—The Aging Factor*. 2d ed. Delaware, OH: Health Action Press, 1986, 74-75.
26 Mukherjee, R. N.; and Sobels, F. H. "The Effect of Sodium Fluoride and Iodoacetamide on Mutation Induction by X-Irradiation in Mature Spermatozoic of Drosophila." *Mutation Research* 6 no.2 (1968): 217-225.
27 Black, D. *Fluoridation, How Wise Is It?* Springville, UT. Tapestry Press, 1990, 1.
28 Kopf, C. "Doctor Who Advocated Fluoridation Now Calls it 'A Fraud.'" *The Forum Health Freedom News* 11 no. 6 (Jul/Aug, 1992): 28.
29 Danielson, C.; et al. "Hip Fractures and Fluoridation in Utah's Elderly Population." *Journal of the American Medical Association* 268 no. 6 (Aug, 1992): 746-748.
30 Yiamouyiannis, J. A.; and Burk, D. "Fluoridation and Cancer Age-Dependence of Cancer Mortality Related to Artificial Fluoridation." *Fluoride* 10 no. 3 (1977): 102-123.

Bodywork

1 The Bodywork KnowledgeBase is an abstracted collection of the world literature on massage compiled by Richard Van Why, available from the American Massage Therapy Association.
2 Yates, J. *A Physician's Guide to Therapeutic Massage*. Canada: Massage Therapist's Association of British Columbia, 1990.
3 The Bodywork KnowledgeBase is an abstracted collection of the world literature on massage compiled by Richard Van Why, available from the American Massage Therapy Association.
4 Quebec Task Force on Spinal Disorders. "Scientific Approach to the Assessment and Management of Activity-Related Spinal Disorders. A Monograph for Clinicians. Report of the Quebec Task Force on Spinal Disorders." *Spine* 12 no. 7 Suppl. (Sep, 1987): S1-59.
5 Beard, G. *Beard's Massage*. Philadelphia: W. B. Saunders Company, 1974. Reprint. 3d ed. 1981.
6 Barlow, W. *The Alexander Technique*. New York: Alfred A. Knopf, 1973.
7 Jones, F. P. "Body Awareness in Action." In Murphy, M. *The Future of the Body*. Los Angeles: Jeremy P. Tarcher, Inc., 1992.
8 Feldenkrais, M. *Awareness through Movement*. New York: Harper & Row, 1972. Reprint. 1977.
9 Ibid.
10 Feitis, R. *Ida Rolf Talks About Rolfing and Physical Reality*. Boulder, CO: Rolf Institute, 1978.
11 Rolf, I. P. *Structural Integration: Gravity, An Unexplored Factor in a More Human Use of Human Beings*. Boulder, CO: Rolf Institute, 1962. New ed. San Francisco, CA: Guild for Structural Integration, 1962.
12 Rolf, I. *Rolfing: The Integration of Human Structures*. New York: Harper and Row, 1977.
13 Connolly, L. "Ida Rolf." *Human Behavior* 6 no. 5 (May 1977): 17-23.

14 Cottingham, J.; Porges, S; and Richmond, K. "Shifts in Pelvic Inclination Angle and Parasympathetic Tone Produced by Rolfing Soft Tissue Manipulation." *Physical Therapy* 68 no. 9 (Sep, 1988): 1364-1370.
15 Franklin, N. "My Favorite Bodywork." *Medical Self-Care* 24 Spring, 1984: 53.

16 Richardson, N. "Aston-Patterning." *Physical Therapy Forum* 6 no. 43 (1987): 1-3.
17 Hellerwork Pearlsoft Research Study; Oct, 1982-Mar, 1983. Conducted by Body of Knowledge, Inc., 406 Berry St., Mt. Shasta, CA 96067.
18 Trager and Mentastics and the dancing cloud logo are all registered service marks of the Trager Institute.
19 Juhan, D. "The Trager Approach." *The Trager Journal* 2 (Fall, 1987): 1-3.
20 Prudden, B. *Pain Erasure*. New York: Ballantine Books, 1980.
21 Byers, D. C. *Better Health with Foot Reflexology—The Original Ingham Method*. Rev. ed., 4th print. St. Petersburg, FL: Ingham Publishing, 1983.
22 Flocco, B. "Reflexology and Premenstrual Syndrome Research Study." A paper given at the International Council of Reflexologists Conference: *Reflexology Around the World*. Virginia Beach, VA: 1991. (The paper is printed in a transcript of that conference, ed. C. Issel): 35-49.
23 Krieger, D. *Accepting Your Power to Heal*. Santa Fe, NM: Bear and Co. Publishing, 1993.
Krieger, D. "Therapeutic Touch: An Ancient but Unorthodox Nursing Intervention." *Journal of the New York State Nurses Association* 6 no. 2 (Aug, 1975): 6-10.
24 Heidt, P. "Effect of Therapeutic Touch in Anxiety Levels of Hospitalized Patients." *Nursing Research* 30 (1981): 32.
Quinn, J. F. "Therapeutic Touch as Energy Exchange: Testing the Theory." *Advances in Nursing Science* 2 (Jan, 1984): 42-49.
Krieger, D. *The Therapeutic Touch*. Englewood Cliff, NJ: Prentice-Hall, 1979.
Samerel, N. "The Experience of Receiving Therapeutic Touch." *Journal of Advances in Nursing* 17 no. 6 (1992): 651-657.
25 Smith, M. J. "Enzymes are Activated By the Laying-On of Hands." *Human Dimensions* (Feb, 1973): 46-48.
Wirth, D. "The Effect of Non-contact Therapeutic Touch on the Healing of Full Thickness Dermal Wounds." *Subtle Energies* 1 (1990): 1-20.
26 Bogusalawski, M. "The Use of Therapeutic Touch in Nursing." *The Journal of Continuing Education in Nursing* (Oct, 1979): 9-15.
Glick, M. S. "Caring Touch and Anxiety in Myocardial Infarction Patients in the Intermediate Cardiac Care Unit." *Intensive Care Nursing* 2 no.2 (1986): 61-66.
27 Bzdek, V.; and Keller, E. "Effects of Therapeutic Touch on Tension Headache Pain." *Nursing Research* 35 (1986): 101-106.
28 Krieger, D. *Accepting Your Power to Heal*. Santa Fe, NM: Bear and Co. Publishing, 1993.
Krieger, D. *The Personal Practice of Therapeutic Touch*. Santa Fe, NM: Bear and Co., 1993.
Krieger, D. *The Therapeutic Touch*. Englewood Cliff, NJ: Prentice-Hall, 1979.
29 Krieger, D. "Therapeutic Touch During Childbirth Preparation by the Lamaze Method and Its Relation to Marital Satisfaction and State of Anxiety in the Married Couple." Nursing Research Emphasis Grant for Doctoral Programs, U.S. Public Health Service #NU-00833-02. Proceedings of the Research Day of Sigma Theta Tau, Epsilon Chapter. New York University, Nov 7, 1984.
30 Murphy, M. *The Future of the Body*. Los Angeles: Jeremy P. Tarcher, Inc., 1992.

Cell Therapy

1 Spencer, D. D., M.D.; et al. "Unilateral Transplantation of Human Fetal Mesencephalic Tissue into the Caudate Nucleus of Patients with Parkinson's Disease." *New England Journal of Medicine* 327 (Nov, 1992): 1541-1548.
2 Kment, A. "Die Verteilung Trittium Markierung Herz, Leber, Nieren und Zellen bei alten Ratten." *Die Therapiewoche*. 1955: 152.
3 Schmid, F.; and Stein, J. *Zelifroschunguno Zell Therapy*. Bern and Stutgard: Hans Huber Verlag, 1963.
4 Aksenova, N. N.; et al. "Effect of Ribonuclease on Anti-Tumor Activity of Ribonuclease Acid from Normal Tissues." *Nature* 207 no. 3 (Jul, 1965): 40-42.
Alexander, P.; et al. "Effect of Nucleic Acids from Immune Lymphocytes on rat sarcomata." *Nature* 213 (Feb, 1967): 569-572.
5 Molnar, E. M. *Forever Young*. West Hartford, CT: Witkower Press, 1985.
6 Schmid, F. *Cell Therapy—A New Dimension of Medicine*. Thoune, Switzerland: Ott Publishers, 1983.
7 Ibid.
8 Ibid.

Chelation

1 Olszewer, E.; and Carter, J. P. "EDTA Chelation Therapy in Chronic Degenerative Disease." *Medical Hypotheses* 27 no. 1 (Sep, 1988): 41-49.
2 Cranton, E. M., M.D. "Protocol of the American College of Advancement in Medicine for the Safe and Effective Administration of Intravenous EDTA Chelation Therapy." In *A Textbook on EDTA Chelation Therapy*, ed. E. M. Cranton, M.D. Special Issue, *Journal of Advancement in Medicine* 2 Nos. 1-2, New York: Human Sciences Press, 1989, 269-305.
3 Farr, C. H., M.D.; White, R.; and Schachter, M., M.D. "*Chronological History of EDTA Chelation Therapy*." Presented to the American College of Advancement in Medicine, Houston, TX., May, 1993.
4 Walker, M.; and Gordon, G. *The Chelation Answer: How to Prevent Hardening of the Arteries and Rejuvenate Your Cardiovascular System*. New York: M. Evans and Company, Inc., 1982.
5 Strauts, Z., M.D. "Correspondence Re: Berkeley Wellness Letter and Chelation Therapy." *Townsend Letter for Doctors* 106 (May, 1992): 382-383.
6 Chappel, T. L., M.D. "Preliminary Findings From the Meda Analysis Study of EDTA Chelation Therapy." From a paper presented at the American College of Advancement in Medicine meeting May 5-9, 1993, in Houston, TX.
7 Walker, M.; and Gordon, G. *The Chelation Answer*. New York: M. Evans and Company, Inc., 1982, 175.
8 Olszewer, E., M.D.; and Carter, J. P., M.D. "EDTA Chelation Therapy: A Retrospective Study of 2,870 Patients." In *A Textbook on EDTA Chelation Therapy*, ed. E. M. Cranton, M.D. Special Issue, *Journal of Advancement in Medicine* 2 Nos. 1-2, New York: Human Sciences Press, 1989, 183.
9 Walker, M. *Chelation Therapy*. Stamford, CT: New Way of Life, Inc., 1984. Currently out of print.
10 Olszewer, E., M.D.; and Carter, J. P., M.D. "EDTA Chelation Therapy: A Retrospective Study of 2,870 Patients." In *A Textbook on EDTA Chelation Therapy*, ed. E. M. Cranton, M.D. Special Issue, *Journal of Advancement in Medicine* 2 Nos. 1-2, New York: Human Sciences Press, 1989, 197-211.
11 Olszewer, E., M.D.; and Carter, J. P., M.D. "EDTA Chelation Therapy: A Retrospective Study of 2,870 Patients." In *A Textbook on EDTA Chelation Therapy*, ed. E. M. Cranton M.D. Special Issue, *Journal of Advancement in Medicine* 2 Nos. 1-2, New York: Human Sciences Press, 1989, 197-211.
12 McDonagh, E. W.; Rudolph, C. J.; and Cheraskin, E., M.D. "An Oculocerebrovasculometric Analysis of the Improvement in Arterial Stenosis Following EDTA Chelation Therapy." In *A Textbook on EDTA Chelation Therapy*, ed. E. M. Cranton, M.D. Special Issue, *Journal of Advancement in Medicine* 2 Nos. 1-2, New York: Human Sciences Press, 1989, 155-166.
13 Alsleben, H. R., M.D.; and Shute, W. E., M.D. *How to Survive the New Health Catastrophes*. Anaheim, CA: Survival Publications, Inc., 1973.
14 McDonagh, E. W.; Rudolph, C. J.; and Cheraskin, E., M.D. "An "oculocerebrovasculometric Analysis of the Improvement in Arterial Stenosis Following EDTA Chelation Therapy." In *A Textbook on EDTA Chelation Therapy*, ed. E. M. Cranton, M.D. Special Issue, *Journal of Advancement in Medicine* 2 Nos. 1-2, New York: Human Sciences Press, 1989, 155-166.
15 Casdorph, H. R., M.D. "EDTA Chelation Therapy: Efficacy in Brain Disorders." In *A Textbook on EDTA Chelation Therapy*, ed. E. M. Cranton, M.D. Special Issue, *Journal of Advancement in Medicine* 2 Nos. 1-2, New York: Human Sciences Press, 1989, 131-153.
16 Alsleben, H. R., M.D.; and Shute, W. E., M.D. *How to Survive the New Health Catastrophes*. Anaheim, CA: Survival Publications, Inc., 1973.
17 Blumer, W., M.D.; and Cranton, E. M., M.D. "Ninety Percent Reduction in Cancer Mortality After Chelation Therapy with EDTA." In *A Textbook on EDTA Chelation Therapy*, ed. E. M. Cranton, M.D. Special Issue, *Journal of Advancement in Medicine* 2 Nos. 1-2, New York: Human Sciences Press, 1989, 183.
18 Alsleben, H. R., M.D.; and Shute, W. E., M.D. *How to Survive the New Health Catastrophes*. Anaheim, CA: Survival Publications, Inc., 1973.
19 Ibid.
20 Blumer, W., M.D.; and Cranton, E. M., M.D. "Ninety Percent Reduction in Cancer Mortality after Chelation Therapy with EDTA". In *A Textbook on EDTA Chelation Therapy*, ed. E. M. Cranton, M.D. Special Issue, *Journal of Advancement in Medicine* 2 Nos. 1-2, New York: Human Sciences Press, 1989, 183-188.
21 Trowbridge, J. P., M.D.; and Walker, M., *The Healing Powers of Chelation Therapy*. Stamford, CT: New Way of Life, Inc. 1992.

Chiropractic

1 Meade, T. W.; et. al. "Low Back Pain of Mechanical Origin: Randomised Comparison of Chiropractic and Hospital Outpatient Treatment." *British Medical Journal* 300 no 6737 (Jun, 1990): 1431-1437.
2 Rand Corporation. "The Appropriateness of Spinal Manipulation for Low Back Pain: Indications and Ratings by a Multidisciplinary Expert Panel." Los Angeles: *Rand Corporation Study*, 1991.
3 Jarvis, K. B.; Phillips, R. B.; and Morris, E. K. "Cost Per Case Comparison of Back Injury Claims: Chiropractic versus Medical Management for Conditions with Identical Diagnosis Codes." *Journal of Occupational Medicine* 33 no. 8 (Aug, 1991): 847-852.
4 Altman, N. *Everybody's Guide to Chiropractic Health Care*. Los Angeles: Jeremy P. Tarcher, Inc., 1990. Out of print.
5 Ibid.
6 Wood, K. "Resolution of Spasmodic Dysphonia via Chiropractic Manipulative Management." *Journal of Manipulative and Physiological Therapeutics* 14 no. 6 (Jul-Aug, 1991): 376-378.
7 Berkson, D. L. "Osteoarthritis, Chiropractic, and Nutrition: Osteoarthritis Considered as a Natural Part of a Three Stage Subluxation Complex: Its Reversibility: Its Relevance and Treatability by Chiropractic and Nutritional Correlates." *Medical Hypotheses* 36 (1991): 356-367.

Colon Therapy

1 Rooney, P. J.; Jenkins, R. T.; and Buchanan, W. W. "A Short Review of the Relationship between Intestinal Permeability and Inflammatory Joint Disease." *Clinical and Experimental Rheumatology* 8 (1990): 75-83.
Mielants, H.; et al. "Intestinal Mucosal Permeability in Inflammatory Rheumatic Diseases. II. Role of Disease." *Journal of Rheumatology* 18 no. 3 (1991): 394-400.
Smith, M. D.; Gibson, R. A.; and Brooks, P. M. "Abnormal Bowel Permeability in Ankylosing Spondylitis and Rheumatoid Arthritis." *Journal of Rheumatology* 12 no. 2 (1985): 299-305.
Lahesmaa-Rantala, R.; et al. "Intestinal Permeability in Patients with Yersinia Triggered Reactive Arthritis." *Annals of the Rheumatic Diseases* 50 no. 2 (February 1991): 91-94.
Mielants, H. "Reflections on the Link Between Intestinal Permeability and Inflammatory Joint Disease." *Clinical Experimental Rheumatology* 8 no. 5 (Sep-Oct, 1990): 523-524.
2 Donovan, P. "Bowel Toxemia, Permeability and Disease— New Information to Support an Old Concept." In *A Textbook of Natural Medicine*, ed. J. E. Pizzorno and M. T. Murray. Seattle, WA: John Bastyr College Publications, 1989.
3 Thakkur, C. *Ayurveda: The Indian Art and Science of Medicine*. New York: ASI Publications, 1974.
4 Kellogg, J. H. "Should the Colon be Sacrificed or May It Be Reformed?" *Journal of the American Medical Association* 68 no.26 (1917): 1957-1959.
5 Rooney, P. J.; Jenkins, R. T.; and Buchanan, W.

W. "A Short Review of the Relationship between Intestinal Permeability and Inflammatory Joint Disease." *Clinical and Experimental Rheumatology* 8 (1990): 75-83.
Mielants, H.; et al. "Intestinal Mucosal Permeability in Inflammatory Rheumatic Diseases. II. Role of Disease." *Journal of Rheumatology* 18 no. 3 (1991): 394-400.
Smith, M. D.; Gibson, R. A.; and Brooks, P. M. "Abnormal Bowel Permeability in Ankylosing Spondylitis and Rheumatoid Arthritis." *Journal of Rheumatology* 12 no. 2 (1985): 299-305.
Lahesmaa-Rantala, R.; et al. "Intestinal Permeability in Patients with Yersinia Triggered Reactive Arthritis." *Annals of the Rheumatic Diseases* 50 no. 2 (February 1991): 91-94.
Mielants, H. "Reflections on the Link Between Intestinal Permeability and Inflammatory Joint Disease." *Clinical Experimental Rheumatology* 8 no. 5 (Sep-Oct, 1990): 523-524.

Craniosacral Therapy

1 Fryman, V. M. "A Study of the Rhythmic Motions of the Living Cranium." *Journal of the American Osteopathic Association* 70 (May, 1971): 928-945.
Michael, D. K.; and Retzlaff, E. W. "A Preliminary Study of Cranial Bone Movement in the Squirrel Monkey." *Journal of the American Osteopathic Association.* 74 (May, 1975): 866-869.
Retzlaff, E. W.; Michael, D.K.; and Roppel, R. M. "Cranial Bone Mobility." *Journal of the American Osteopathic Association* 74 (1975): 869-873.
2 Weil, A., M.D. *Natural Health, Natural Medicine: A Comprehensive Guide to Wellness and Self-Care.* Boston, MA: Houghton Mifflin, 1990.
3 Upledger, J. E. *Your Inner Physician and You, Craniosacral Therapy SomatoEmotional Release.* Berkeley, CA: North Atlantic, 1992.
4 Ibid.

Detoxification Therapy

1 Environmental Protection Agency. "EPA Data Show Steady Progress in Cleaning Nation's Air." *Environmental News* (Oct, 1992). As reported in "Did You Know" *Our Toxic Times* 3 no. 12 (Dec, 1992):5.
2 Environmental Protection Agency. "130 Cities Exceed Lead Levels for Drinking Water." *Environmental News* (Oct, 1992). As reported in "Did You Know" *Our Toxic Times* 3 no. 12 (Dec, 1992):3.
3 Saifer, P., M.D. *Detox.* Los Angeles: Jeremy P. Tarcher, Inc., 1984.
4 Schnare, D. W. *The Unpolluting of Man.* Los Angeles: Foundation Essay Series Foundation for Advancements in Science and Education, n.d. Video.
5 Schnare, D. W.; et al. "Evaluation of a Detoxification Regimen for Fat Stored Xenobiotics."*Medical Hypotheses* 9 no. 3 (1982): 265-282.
6 Ibid.
7 Ibid.
8 Gard, Z., M.D.; and Brown, E. "Literature Review and Comparison Studies of Sauna/Hyperthermia in Detoxification." *Townsend Letter for Doctors* 107 (Jun, 1992): 470-478.
9 Shields, J. W., M.D. "Lymph, lymph glands, and homeostasis." *Lymphology* 25 no. 4 (Dec, 1992): 147-153.

Diet

1 Steinman, D. *Diet for a Poisoned Planet.* New York: Ballantine Books, 1990, 4.
2 Ibid., page 11.
3 Winter, R. *A Consumer's Dictionary of Food Additives.* New York: Crown Publishing, 1984, 3d ed., rev., 1989.
4 *Quarterly Report on Adverse Reactions Associated with Aspartame Ingestion.* Washington, D.C.: Center for Food Safety and Nutrition, U.S. Food and Drug Administration, April 1, 1988.
5 Winter, R. *A Consumer's Dictionary of Food Additives.* New York: Crown Publishing, 1984.
6 Steinman, D. *Diet for a Poisoned Planet.* New York: Ballantine Books, 1990, 355.
7 Jansson, E. *Medical, Environmental, and Economic Information on: Nitrates, Nitrites, and Nitroso-Compounds. Why American Exposure to Nitrates, Nitrites, and Nitroso-Compounds Needs to be Reduced by More than 50 Percent.* Washington, D.C.: National Network to Prevent Birth Defects, August 1, 1987.
8 *Reexamination of the GRAS Status of Sulfiting Agents.* Springfield, VA: National Technical Information Service, U.S. Department of Commerce, January 1985.
9 Steinman, D. *Diet for a Poisoned Planet.* New York: Ballantine Books, 1990, 195.
10 Winter, R. *A Consumer's Dictionary of Food Additives.* New York: Crown Publishing, 1984, 3d ed., rev., 1989.
11 Ibid.
12 Weinstock, C. P. "Doubt Prisoners' Calm Behavior Linked to Diet Sans Sugar and Bread." *Medical Tribune* (Jan, 1985): 32.
13 Weissman, J. D. *Choose to Live.* New York: Grove Press,1988.
14 Schoenthaler, S.; Doraz, W.; and Wakefield, J., Jr. "The Impact of a Low Food Additive and Sucrose Diet on Academic Performance in 803 New York City Public Schools." *International Journal of Biosocial Medical Research* 8 no. 2 (1986): 185-195.
Schoenthaler, S.; Doraz, W.; and Wakefield, J., Jr. "Testing of Various Hypotheses as Explanations for the Gains in National Standardized Academic Test Scores in the 1978-83 New York City Nutrition Policy Modification Project." *International Journal of Biosocial Medical Research* 8 no. 2 (1986): 196-203.
15 Report by Donald W. Thayer, USDA Eastern Regional Research Center, on Wholesomeness Studies of Chicken, March 19, 1984.
16 Friedman, M., ed. *Nutritional and Toxicological Consequences of Food Processing.* New York: Plenum Press, 1991.
17 Ibid.
18 *The Surgeon General's Report on Nutrition and Health.* Washington, D.C.: U.S. Department of Health and Human Services, Public Health Service, DHH (PHS) Publication No. 88-50210, 1988.
19 Wynder, E. L.; et al. "Nutrition and Metabolic Epidemiology of Cancers of the Oral Cavity, Esophagus, Colon, Breast, Prostate, and Stomach." In *Nutrition and Cancer: Etiology and Treatment* ed. G. R. Newell and N. M. Ellison. New York: Raven, 1981, 11-48.
20 Steinman, D. *Diet for a Poisoned Planet.* New York: Ballantine Books, 1990, 74.
21 Fein, G. G.; et al. "Prenatal Exposure to Polychlorinated Biphenyls: Effects on Birth Size and Gestational Age." *Journal of Pediatrics* 105 no. 2 (Aug, 1984): 315-320.
22 Ross, A. C. "Vitamin A Status: Relationship to Immunity and the Antibody Response." *Proceedings of the Society for Experimental Biology and Medicine* 200 no. 3 (Jul, 1992): 303-20.
Dennert, G. "Retinoids and the Immune System: Immunostimulation by Vitamin A" In *The Retinoids*, ed. M. B. Sporn; A. B. Roberts; and D. S. Goodman; Orlando, FL: Academic Press, 1984, 373-390.
Cohen, B. E.; et al. "Reversal of Postoperative Immunosuppression in Man by Vitamin A." *Surgery, Gynecology and Obstetrics* 149 no 5 (Nov, 1979): 658-662.
23 Ornish, D. *Stress, Diet and Your Heart.* New York: Holt, Rinehart, and Winston, 1982, 1983.
24 Unauthored Paper: Position of the American Dietetic Association: Vegetarian Diets. "Journal of the American Dietetic Association: *ADA Reports, Journal of the American Dietetic Association* 88 no. 3 (Mar, 1988): 351-355.
25 Walford, R. L.; Harris, S. B.; and Gunion, M. W. "The Calorically Restricted Low-Fat Nutrient-Dense Diet in Biosphere 2 Significantly Lowers Blood Glucose, Total Leukocyte Count, Cholesterol, and Blood Pressure in Humans." *Proceedings of the National Academy of Sciences of the United States of America* 89 no. 23 (Dec, 1992): 11533-11537.
26 Walford, R. L.; and Crew, M. "How Dietary Restriction Retards Aging: An Integrative Hypothesis." *Growth, Development, and Aging* 53 no. 4 (Winter, 1989):139-140.
27 Geiselman, P. J.; and Novin, D. "Sugar Infusion Can Enhance Feeling." *Science* 218 no. 4571 (Oct, 1982):490-491.
28 Liebman, B. "Crying Over Milk." *Nutrition Action* (Dec, 1992): 1, 6-7.
29.Ibid.
30 Ursin, G.; et al. "Milk Consumption and Cancer Incidence: A Norwegian Prospective Study." *British Journal of Cancer* 61 no. 3 (Mar, 1990): 456-459.
31 Liebman, B. "Crying Over Milk." *Nutrition Action* (Dec, 1992): 1, 6-7.
32 Bonanome, A.; and Grundy, S. M. "Effect of Dietary Stearic Acid on Plasma Cholesterol and Lipoprotein Levels." *New England Journal of Medicine* 318 no 19 (May, 1988): 1244-1248.
33 Trevisan, M.; et al. "Consumption of Olive Oil, Butter and Vegetable Oils and Coronary Heart Disease Risk Factors." The Research Group ATS-RF2 of the Italian National Research Council. *Journal of the American Medical Association* 263 no. 5 (Feb, 1990): 688-692.
34 Simopoulos, A. P. "Omega-3 Fatty Acids in Health and Disease and in Growth and Development." *American Journal of Clinical Nutrition* 54 no. 3 (Sep, 1991): 438-463.
35 Steinman, D. *Diet for a Poisoned Planet.* New York: Ballantine Books, 1990, 158-159.
36 Statistics received from chart. References: Canola Oil: Data on file, Procter and Gamble. All others: Reeves, J. B.; and Weihrauch, J. L. *Composition of Foods, Agriculture Handbook.* No. 8-4 Washington D.C.: United States Department of Agriculture, 1979.
37 Hennig, B. "Dietary Fat and Macronutrients: Relationships to Atherosclerosis." *Journal of Optimal Nutrition* 1 no. 1 (1992): 21-23.
38 Jope, R. S.; and Johnson, G. V. "Neurotoxic Effects of Dietary Aluminum." *Ciba Foundation Symposium* 169 (1992) : 254-267.
39 Liukkonen-Lilja, H.; and Piepponen, S. "Leaching of Aluminum from Aluminum Dishes and Packages." *Food Additives and Contaminants* 9 no. 3 (May/Jun 1992): 213-223.
40 Miller, B. J.; Billedeau, S. M.; and Miller, D. W. "Formation of N-nitrosamines in Microwaved Versus Skillet-Fried Bacon Containing Nitrite." *Food and Chemical Toxicology* 27 no. 5 (May, 1989): 295-299.
41 Quan, R., M.D.; et al. "Effects of Microwave Radiation on Anti-Infective Factors in Human Milk." *Pediatrics* 89 no. 4 (Apr, 1992): 667-669.
42 Lubec, G.; Wolf, C.; and Bartosch, B. "Aminoacid Isomerisation and Microwave Exposure." *The Lancet* 2 no. 8676 (Dec, 1989): 1392-1393.
43 Environmental Protection Agency. "819 Cities Exceed Lead Level for Drinking Water." *EPA Environmental News* Publication no. A-107 (May 11, 1993):R110.
44 Steinman, D. *Diet for a Poisoned Planet.* New York: Ballantine Books, 1990, 203.
45 Woltgens, J. H.; Etty, E. J.; and Nieuwland, W. M. "Prevalence of Mottled Enamel in Permanent Dentition of Children Participating in a Fluoride Programme at the Amsterdam Dental School." *Journal de Biologie Buccale* 17 no. 1 (Mar, 1989): 15-20.
46 Danielson, C.; et al. "Hip Fractures and Fluoridation in Utah's Elderly Population." *Journal of the American Medical Association* 268 no. 6 (Aug, 1992): 746-748.

Energy Medicine

1 Zhu Zong-xiang. "Research advances in the Electrical Specificity of Meridians and Acupuncture Points." *American Journal of Acupuncture* 9 no. 3 (Jul/Sep 1981): 203-215.
2 Tucker, D. Position Paper on Electroacupuncture Biofeedback ratified by the California Acupuncture Association, Included in California Acupuncture Association *Completed Scope of Practice.* Mar. 14, 1993.
3 Ibid.
4 Zacharski, J. A. "*Therapeutic Connection Between Cervical Problems and TMJ Dysfunction.*" Pamphlet, Self-Published. Menomonee, WI: 1985.
5 Lucero, K. M. "The Electro-Acuscope/Myopulse System." *Rehab Management: The Journal of Therapy and Rehabilitation* 4 no. 3 (Apr/May

1991).
6 Ibid.
7 Rein, G. *"Effect of Non-Hertzian Scalar Waves on the Immune System"*. The U.S. Psychotronics Association Journal. 1989.
8 Tsuei, J. J.; et al. "Study on Bioenergy in Diabetic Mellitus Patients." *American Journal of Acupuncture* 17 no. 1 (1989): 31-38.
9 Tsuei, J. J.; et al. "Food Allergy Study Utilizing the EAV Acupuncture Technique." *American Journal of Acupuncture* 12 no. 2 (Jun, 1984): 105-116.
10 Sullivan, S. G. "Evoked Electrical Conductivity on Lung Acupuncture Points in Healthy Persons and Lung Cancer Patients." *American Journal of Acupuncture* 13 no. 3 (1985): 261.
11 Smith, C. W.; and Best, S. *Electromagnetic Man: Health and Hazard in the Electrical Environment*. London: J. M. Dent and Sons, Ltd., 1989, 88.
12 Madill, P. "Electroacupuncture: A True and Legitimate Preventive Medicine." *American Journal of Acupuncture* 7 no. 4 (Dec, 1979): 279-292.

Environmental Medicine

1 Randolph, T. G. *Human Ecology and Susceptibility to the Chemical Environment*. Springfield, IL: C.C. Thomas, 1981.
2 Crook, W. "Food Allergy: The Great Masquerader." *Pediatric Clinic of North America* 22 no. 1 (Feb, 1975): 227-238.
3 Bioecologic medicine incorporates the differences in individual's nutritional needs due to metabolic variations.
4 Miller, J. B., M.D. "Intradermal Provocative/Neutralizing Food Testing and Subcutaneous Food Extract Injection Therapy." In *Food Allergy and Intolerance*, eds. J. Brostoff and S. Challacombe, London: Bailliere Tindall Publishers, 1987, 932-947.
5 Dickey, L., ed. "History and Documentation of Coseasonal Antigen Therapy: Intracutaneous Serial Dilution Titration, Optimal Dosage, and Provocative Testing." In *Clinical Ecology*, ed. L. Dickey. Springfield, IL: Charles C. Thomas, 1976, 18-25.
6 Rea, W.; et al. "Elimination of Oral Food Challenge Reaction by Injection of Food Extracts. A Double-Blind Evaluation." *Archives of Otolaryngology* 110 no.14 (Apr, 1984): 248-252.
Of related interest, see Scadding, G. K.; and Brostoff, J. "Low Dose Sublingual Therapy in Patients with Allergic Rhinitis Due to House Dust Mite." *Clinical Allergy* 16 no. 5 (Sep, 1986): 483-491. Several other studies have confirmed the same results found by Drs. Rea and Brostoff.
7 Egger, J.; et al. "A Controlled Trial of Oligoantigenic Diet Treatment in the Hyperkinetic Syndrome." *The Lancet* 1 no. 8428 (1985): 540-545.
8 Egger, J.; et al. "A Controlled Trial of Hyposensitisation in Children with Food-induced Hyperkinetic Syndrome." *The Lancet* 339 no. 8802 (1992): 1150-1153.
9 Schoenthaler, S.; et al. "The Impact of a Low Food Additive and Sucrose Diet on Academic Performance in 803 New York City Public Schools." *International Journal of Biosocial Research* 8 no. 2 (1986): 185-195.
10 Ashford, N. A.; and Miller, C. S. *Chemical Exposures: Low Levels and High Stakes*. New York: Van Nostrand Reinhold, 1990.
11 "Pesticides and Groundwater: A Health Concern for the Midwest." Proceedings of the Freshwater Foundation Conference, Oct. 16-17, 1986, Navarre, Minnesota.
12 Ashford, N. A.; and Miller, C. S. *Chemical Exposures: Low Levels and High Stakes*. New York: Van Nostrand Reinhold, 1990.
13 Steinman, D.; and Epstein, S., M.D. *The Safe Shopper's Bible*. New York: Macmillan: 1994.
14 Schnare, D. W.; et. al. "Body Burden Reductions of PCBs, PBBs and Chlorinated Pesticides in Human Subjects." *Ambio: A Journal of the Human Environment* 13 no. 5-6 (1984): 378-380.
15 Schnare, D. W. *The Unpolluting of Men*. Los Angeles: Foundation Essay Series, Foundation for Advancements in Science and Education, n.d. Video.
16 Saifer, P., M.D.; and Zellerbach, M. *Detox*. Los Angeles: Jeremy P. Tarcher, Inc. 1984.
17 "Chemicals Identified in Human Biological Media, A Data Base." *United States Environmental Protection Agency. EPA* 560/13-80-036B. (U.S. EPA, Washington, D.C., October, 1980).
18 Rea, W.; et al. "Pesticides and Brain Function Changes in a Controlled Environment." *Clinical Ecology* 2 no. 3 (Summer, 1984): 145-150.
Baker, E. L.; Smith, T. J.; and Landrigan, P. J. "The Neurotoxicity of Industrial Solvents: A Review of the Literature." *American Journal of Industrial Medicine* 8 no. 3 (1985): 207-217.
Feldman, R.; Mayer, R.; and Taub, A. "Evidence for Peripheral Neurotoxic Effect of Trichloroethylene." *Neurology* 20 no.6 (1970): 599-606.
Gregersen, P.; et al. "Neurotoxic Effects of Organic Solvents in Exposed Workers: An Occupational, Neuropsychological and Neurological Investigation." *American Journal of Industrial Medicine*. 5 no. 3 (1984): 201-225.
Karlsson, J. E.; et al. "Effects of Low-Dose Inhalation of Three Chlorinated Aliphatic Organic Solvents on Deoxyribonucleic Acid in Gerbil Brain. *Scandinavian Journal of Work, Environment and Health* 13 no. 5 (Oct, 1987.): 453-458.
Seppalainen, A. M. "Neurophysiology Aspects of the Toxicity of Organic Solvents." *Scandinavian Journal of Work and Environmental Health* 11 Supplement 1 (1985):61-64.
Ecobichon, D. J.; and Joy, R. M., eds. *Pesticides and Neurological Diseases*. Boca Raton, FL: CRC Press, Inc., 1982.
Saracci, R.; et al. "Cancer Mortality in Workers Exposed to Chlorophenoxy Herbicides and Chlorophenols." *The Lancet* 338 no.8774 (Oct, 1991): 1027-1032.
19 Darlington, L.; et al. "Placebo-Controlled, Blind Study of Dietary Manipulation Therapy in Rheumatoid Arthritis." *The Lancet* 1 no. 8475 (Feb, 1986): 236-238.

Enzyme Therapy

1 Howell, E., M.D. *Food Enzymes for Health and Longevity*. Woodstock Valley, CT: Omangod Press, 1980.
2 Howell, E., M.D. *Food Enzymes for Health and Longevity*. Woodstock Valley, CT: Omangod Press, 1980.
Howell, E., M.D. *Enzyme Nutrition: The Food Enzyme Concept*. Wayne, NJ: Avery Publishing Group, 1987.
3 Howell, E., M.D. *Food Enzymes for Health and Longevity*. Woodstock Valley, CT: Omangod Press, 1980.
4 Guyton, A. C., M.D. *Textbook of Medical Physiology*, 7th Edition. Philadelphia, PA: W.B. Saunders Company, 1987.
Howell, E., M.D. *Food Enzymes for Health and Longevity*. Woodstock Valley, CT: Omangod Press, 1980.
5 Howell, E., M.D. *Food Enzymes for Health and Longevity*. Woodstock Valley, CT: Omangod Press, 1980.
6 Immerman, A. "Evidence For Intestinal Toxemia-An Inescapable Clinical Phenomenon." *The American Chiropractic Association Journal of Chiropractic* 13 (Apr, 1979): S-25.
7 Wolf, M.; and Ransberger, K. *Enzyme Therapy*. New York: Vantage Press, 1972.
8 Ibid.
9 Morley, J. E.; Sterman, M. B.; and Walsh, J. H., eds. *Nutritional Modulation of Neural Function. UCLA Forum in Medical Sciences* 28. San Diego, CA: Academica Press, 1988.
10 Jaeger, C. B.; et al. "Polymer Encapsulated Dopaminergic Cell Lines as 'Alternative Neural Grafts'." *Progress in Brain Research* 82 (1990): 41-6.
11 Wolf, M.; and Ransberger, K. *Enzyme Therapy*. New York: Vantage Press, 1972.
12 Solorzano del Rio, H. E., M.D. Unpublished paper, 1992, 11.
13 Solorzano del Rio, H. E., M.D. Unpublished paper, 1992, 11. 14 Wolf, M.; and Ransberger, K. *Enzyme Therapy*. New York: Vantage Press, 1972.

Fasting

1 Cott, A. *Fasting: The Ultimate Diet*. New York: Bantam Books, 1975.
2 Chaitow, L. *The Body/Mind Purification Program*. New York: Simon and Schuster, 1990.
3 Ibid.
4 Salloum, T. K.; and Burton, A. "Fasting." In *A Textbook of Natural Medicine*, ed. M. T. Murray and J. E. Pizzorno. Seattle, WA: John Bastyr College Publications, 1989.

Flower Remedies

1 Bach E.; and Wheeler, F. J. *The Bach Flower Remedies*. New Canaan, CT: Keats Publishing Inc., 1977. Originally published by C.W. Daniel Co., Ltd., Saffron Walden, Essex, England, 1933.
2 Ibid.
3 Ibid.
4 Kaslof, L. J. *The Bach Remedies: A Self-Help Guide*. New Canaan, CT: Keats Publishing, 1988, 3.
5 Ibid., 22.
6 For more information on recommended methods of treatment, contact Ellon, USA, Inc., 644 Merrick Road, Lynbrook, NY 11563.
7 Ibid.
8 Kaslof, L. J. *The Bach Remedies: A Self-Help Guide*. New Canaan, CT: Keats Publishing, 1988, 22.
9 Ibid.,9.
10 Vlamis, G., ed. *Bach Flower Remedies to the Rescue*. Rochester, VT: Healing Arts Press, 1990.
11 Kaslof, L. J. *The Bach Remedies: A Self Help Guide*. New Canaan, CT: Keats Publishing, Inc., 1988.
12 Ibid.,

Guided Imagery

1 Sheikh, A. A.; Richardson, P.; and Moleski, L. M. "Psychosomatics and Mental Imagery." In *The Potential of Fantasy and Imagination*, eds. A. A. Sheikh and J. T. Shaffer. New York: Brandon, 1979.
Barber, T. X. "Physiologic Effects of 'Hypnotic Suggestions': A Critical Review of Recent Research,(1960-1964)." *Psychological Bulletin* 63 (Apr, 1965): 201-222.
Benson, H. *The Relaxation Response*. New York: William Morrow, 1975.
Jacobsen, E. *You Must Relax; A Practical Method of Reducing the Strains of Modern Living*. New York: McGraw-Hill, 1934.
Jevning, R.; Wallace, R. K.; and Beidebach, M. "The Physiology of Meditation: A Review. A Wakeful Hypometabolic Integrated Response." *Neuroscience & BioBehavioral Reviews* 16 no. 3 (Fall 1992): 415-424.
Schultz, J.; and Luthe, W. *Autogenic Training: A Psychophysiologic Approach in Psychotherapy*. New York: Grune and Stratton, 1959.
Pelletier, K. *Mind As Healer, Mind As Slayer: A Holistic Approach to Preventing Stress Disorders*. New York: Delacorte Press/St. Lawrence, 1977.
Levine, J.; Gordon, N. C.; and Fields, H. L. "The Mechanism of Placebo Analgesia." *The Lancet* 2 no. 8091 (Sep, 1978): 654-657.
2 Rosen, G.; Kleinman, A.; and Katon, W. "Somatization in Family Practice: a Biopsychosocial Approach." *Journal of Family Practice* 14 no. 3 (Mar,1982): 493-502.
Stoeckle, J. D.; Zola, I. K.; and Davidson, G. E. "The Quantity and Significance of Psychological Distress in Medical Patients: Some Preliminary Observations about the Decision to Seek Medical Aid." *Journal of Chronic Disease* 17 (Oct, 1964): 959-970.
3 Simonton, C.; and Matthews, S. *Getting Well Again*. Los Angeles: Jeremy P. Tarcher, 1978.
4 Ibid.
5 Norris, P.; and Porter, G. *Why Me? Harnessing the Healing Power of the Human Spirit*. Walpole NH: Stillpoint Publishing, 1985.
6 Achterberg, J. *Imagery in Healing: Shamanism and Modern Medicine*. New York: Random House, 1985.

Herbal Medicine

1 Farnsworth, N. R.; et. al. "Medicinal Plants in Therapy." *Bulletin of the World Health Organization* 63 no. 6 (1985): 965-981. Reprinted in

Classic Botanical Reprint 212, Austin, Texas: American Botanical Council.
2 Ibid.
3 Herb Trade Association. *Definition of "Herb"*. Austin, TX: Herb Trade Association, 1977.
4 Blumenthal, M. "Focus on Rain Forest Remedies." *HerbalGram* 27 (1992): 8-10. Quoting N.R. Farnsworth in Eisner, R., "Botanists Ply Trade in Tropics, Seeking Plant-Based Medicinals." *The Scientist* 4 (Jun,1991): 1, 4, 5, 25.
5 Weil, A., M.D. "A New Look at Botanical Medicine." *Whole Earth Review* 64 (1989): 3-8. Reprinted in Classic Botanical Reprint 210.
6 Farnsworth, N. R.; et al. "Medicinal Plants in Therapy." *Bulletin of the World Health Organization* 63 no. 6 (1985): 965-981. Reprinted in Classic Botanical Reprint 212, Austin, TX: American Botanical Council.
Akerele, O. "Summary of WHO Guidelines for the Assessment of Herbal Medicines." *HerbalGram* 28 (1992): 13-16. Available as Classic Botanical Reprint 234.
7 Akerele, O. "Summary of WHO Guidelines for the Assessment of Herbal Medicines." *HerbalGram* 28 (1992): 13-16. Available as Classic Botanical Reprint 234.
Akerele, O. "Guidelines for the Assessment of Herbal Medicines." *HerbalGram* 28 (1992): 17-20. Available as Classic Botanical Reprint 234.
8 Blumenthal, M. "FDA Declares 258 OTC Ingredients Ineffective: Many Herbs Included." HerbalGram 23 (1990): 32-35.
9 British Herbal Medicine Association. *British Herbal Pharmacopoeia*, Vol. I. Bournemouth, Dorset: British Herbal Medicine Association, 1990.
10 Blumenthal, M. "German MDs Required to Pass Herb Exam." *HerbalGram* 26 (1992): 45.
11 Blumenthal, M. "European Scientific Cooperative for Phytotherapy Symposium: European Harmony in Phytotherapy." *HerbalGram* 24 (1990): 41-45.
12 Murphy, M. T.; and Pizzorno, J. E. *Encyclopedia of Natural Medicine* Rocklin, CA: Prima Publishing, 1991: 83.
13 Hoffmann, D. *The New Holistic Herbal*. Rockport, MA: Element, Inc., 1991, 28.
14 German Ministry of Health. *Senna*. Commission E. Monographs for Phytomedicines. Bonn, Germany: German Ministry of Health, 1984.
15 Henry, C. J.; and Emery, B. "Effect of Spiced Food on Metabolic Rate." *Human Nutrition. Clinical Nutrition.* 40 No. 2 (Mar, 1986): 165-168.
16 Glatzel, H. "Treatment of Dyspeptic Disorders with Spice Extracts." *Hippokrates* 40 No. 23 (Dec, 1969): 916-919.(Published in German).
17 Glatzel, H. "Blood Circulation Effectiveness of Natural Spices." *Med Klin* 62 no. 51 (Dec, 1967): 1987-1989. (Published in German).
18 Buzzanca, G.; and Laterza, S. "Clinical Trial with an Antirheumatic Ointment. *Clin Ter* 83 no.1 (Oct, 1977): 71-83. (Published in Italian).
19 ESCOP, European Scientific Cooperative for Phytotherapy. *Valerian Root*. Meppel, The Netherlands: ESCOP, European Scientific Cooperative for Phytotherapy, 1990.
Foster, S. *Chamomile*. Botanical Series 307. Austin, TX: American Botanical Council, 1991.
20 German Ministry of Health. *Chamomile Flowers*. Commission E. Monographs for Phytomedicines. Bonn, Germany: German Ministry of Health, 1984.
21 Brantner, F. "Sexual Hormones From Plants in Female Medicine." *Ehk* 28 (1979):413.
22 Hahn, G.; et al. "Monk's Pepper." *Notabene medici* 16 (1986): 233, 236, 297-301.
23 Attelmann, H.; et al. "Investigation of the Treatment of Female Imbalances with Agnolyt." *Geriatrie* 2 (1972): 239.
24 Kayser, H. W.; and Istanbulluoglu, S. "Treatment of PMS Without Hormones." *Hippokrates* 25 (25): 717.
25 Amann, W. "Improvement of Acne Vulgaris with Agnus Castus (Agnolyt™)." *Therapie der Gegenwart* 106 (1967): 124-126.
26 Foster, S. *Echinacea: The Purple Coneflowers.* Botanical Series 301. Austin, TX: American Botanical Council, 1991.
27 German Ministry of Health, *Echinacea purpurea leaf.* Commission E. Monographs for Phytomedicines. Bonn, Germany: German Ministry of Health, 1989.
28 British Herbal Medicine Association. *British Herbal Pharmacopoeia.* Bournemouth, Dorset: British Herbal Medicine Association, 1983 or 1992.
29 Hobbs, C. "Valerian: A Literature Review." *HerbalGram* 21 (1989): 19-34.
30 Foster, S. *Feverfew*. Botanical Series 310. Austin, TX: American Botanical Council, 1991.
Hobbs, C. "Valerian: A Literature Review." *HerbalGram* 21 (1989): 19-34.
31 Awang, D. V. C. "The Pharmacological Activity of Commercial Plant Products." Presentation to the Annual Spring Meeting of the Nonprescription Drug Manufacturers Association of Canada, Ottowa, 1992.
Awang, D. V. C.; et al. "Parthenolide Content of Feverfew (Tanacetum Parthenium) Assessed by HPLC and H-NMR Spectroscopy." *Journal of Natural Products* 54 no. 6 (Nov.-Dec. 1991): 1516-1521.
32 Awang, D. V. C. "Feverfew Feedback." Letter. *HerbalGram* 22 (1990): 2-4, 42.
33 Foster, S. *Garlic*. Botanical Series 311. Austin, TX: American Botanical Council, 1991.
34 McCaleb, R. "Anticancer Effects of Garlic—More Proof. *HerbalGram* 27 (1992): 22-23.
You, W. C.; et al. "Allium Vegetables and Reduced Risk of Stomach Cancer." *Journal of the National Cancer Institute* 81 no. 2 (Jan, 1989): 162-164.
35 Block, E. "Antithrombotic Agent of Garlic: A Lesson from 5000 Years of Folk Medicine." In *Folk Medicine: The Art and the Science*, ed. R. P. Steiner. Washington, D.C.: The American Chemical Society, 1986.
36 Foster, S. *Garlic*. Botanical Series 311. Austin, TX: American Botanical Council, 1991.
37 Foster, S. *Garlic*. Botanical Series 311. Austin, TX: American Botanical Council, 1991.
Kleijnen, J.; Knipschild, P.; and Terriet, G. "Garlic, Onions and Cardiovascular Risk Factors. A Review of the Evidence from Human Experiments with Emphasis on Commercially Available Preparations." *British Journal of Clinical Pharmacology* 28 no. 5 (Nov, 1989): 535-544.
38 (Commission E).
39 (ESCOP, 1992).
40 Grontved, A.; et al. "Ginger Root Against Seasickness. A Controlled Trial on the Open Sea." *Acta Oto-Laryngologica* 105 no. 1-2 (Jan-Feb, 1988): 45-49.
41 Bone, M. E.; et al. "Ginger root—a New Antiemetic: The Effect of Ginger Root on Postoperative Nausea and Vomitting After Major Gynaecological Surgery." *Anaesthesia* 45 no. 8 (Aug. 1990): 669-671.
Fischer-Rasmussen, W.; et al. "Ginger Treatment of Hyperemesis Gravidarum." *European Journal of Obstetrics & Gynecology and Reproductive Biology* 38 no. 1 (Jan, 1991): 19-24.
42 Shoji, N.; et al. "Cardiotonic Principles of Ginger (*Zingiber officinale Roscoe*)." *Journal of Pharmaceutical Sciences* 71 no. 10 (Oct. 1982): 1174-1175.
43 Mustafa, T.; and Srivastava, K. C. "Ginger (*Zingiber officinale*) in Migraine Headache." *Journal of Ethnopharmacology* 29 no. 3 (Jul,1990): 267-273.
44 Leung, A. Y. "Fresh Ginger Juice in Treatment of Kitchen Burns." *HerbalGram* 16 (1989): 6.
45 Foster, S. *Ginkgo*. Botanical Series 304. Austin, TX: American Botanical Council, 1991.
46 Kleijnen, J.; and Knipschild, P. *Ginkgo biloba*. *Lancet* 340 no. 8828 (Nov, 1992): 1136-1139.
47 Braquet, P., ed. *Ginkgolides—Chemistry, Biology, Pharmacology and Clinical Perspectives*, Volume 1. Barcelona, Spain: J. Prous Science Publishers, 1988.
Braquet, P., ed. *Ginkgolides—Chemistry, Biology, Pharmacology and Clinical Perspectives*, Volume 2. Barcelona, Spain: J. Prous Science Publishers, 1989.
Fungfeld, E. W., ed. *Rokan: Ginkgo biloba.* New York: Springer-Verlag, 1988.
48 Shibata, S.; et al. " Chemistry and Pharmacology of Panax." *Economic and Medicinal Plant Research* 1 (1985): 217-284.
49 Brekhman, I. I.; and Dardymov, I. V. "Pharmacological Investigation of Glycosides From Ginseng and Eleutherococcus." *Lloydia* 32 (1969): 46-51.
50 Bombardelli, E.; Cirstoni, A.; and Lietti, A. "The Effect of Acute and Chronic (Panax) Ginseng Saponins Treatment on Adrenal Function; Biochemical and Pharmacological." *Proceedings 3rd International Ginseng Symposium* 1 (1980): 9-16.
Fulder, S. J. "Ginseng and the Hypothalamic-Pituitary Control of Stress." *American Journal of Chinese Medicine* 9 (1981): 112-118.
51 Feng, L. M.; Pan, H. Z.; and Li, W. W. "Anti-Oxidant Action of Panax Ginseng." *Chung Hsi I Chieh Ho Tsa Chih* 7 no. 5 (May 1987): 288-290, 262.
52 Hikino, H.; et al. "Antihepatotoxic Actions of Ginsenosides From Panax Ginseng Roots." *Planta Medica* 52 (1985): 62-64.
53 Ng, T. B.; and Yeung, H. W. "Hypoglycemic Constituents of Panax Ginseng." *General Pharmacology* 6 (1985): 549-552.
54 Huo, Y. S. "Anti-Senility Action of Saponin in Panax Ginseng Fruit in 327 Cases." *Chung Hsi I Chieh Ho Tsa Chih* 4 no. 10 (Oct, 1984): 593-596, 578.
55 Joo, C. N. "The Preventative Effect of Korean (P. Ginseng) Saponins on Aortic Atheroma Formation in Prolonged Cholesterol-Fed Rabbits." *Proceedings of the 3rd International Ginseng Symposium* (1980): 27-36.
56 Scaglione, F.; et al. "Immunomodulatory Effects of Two Extracts of Panax Ginseng C.A. Meyer." *Drugs Under Experimental Clinical Research* 16 no. 10 (1990): 537-542.
57 Yamamoto, M.; and Uemura, T. "Endocrinological and Metabolic Actions of P. Ginseng Principles." *Proceeding 3rd International Ginseng Symposium* (1980): 115-119.
58 Hoffmann, D. *The New Holistic Herbal*. Rockport, MA: Element, Inc., 1991, 204.
59 Hahn, F. E.; and Ciak, J. "Berberine." *Antibiotics and Chemotherapy* 3 (1976): 577-588.
60 Choudhry, V. P.; Sabir, M.; and Bhide, V. N. "Berberine in Giardiasis." *Indian Pediatrics* 9 no. 3 (Mar, 1972): 143-146.
61 Kumazawa, Y.; et al: "Activation of Peritoneal Macrophages by Berberine-Alkaloids in Terms of Induction of Cytostatic Activity." *International Journal of Immunopharmacology* 6 (1984): 587-592.
62 Hoffmann, D. *The New Holistic Herbal*. Rockport, MA: Element, Inc., 1991, 204.
63 Hobbs, C. "Hawthorn: A Literature Review." *HerbalGram* 21 (1990): 19-33.
64 (Commission E).
65 Ibid.
66 Armanini, D.; et al. "Affinity of liquorice derivatives for mineralocorticoid and glucocorticoid receptors." *Clinical Endocrinology* 19 (Nov, 1983): 609-612.
67 Hikino, H.; and Kiso, Y. "Natural Products for Liver Diseases." In *Economic and Medicinal Plant Research*, Vol.2, ed. H. Wagner; H. Hikino; and N. R. Farnsworth. London: Academic Press, 1988.
68 Pompei, R.; et al. "Antiviral Activity of Glycrrhizic Acid." *Experientia* 36 (Mar, 1980): 304-305.
69 Vogel, G. "Natural Substances with Effects on the Liver." In *New Natural Products and Plant Drugs with Pharmacological, Biological or Therapeutic Activity,* ed. H. Wagner and P. Wolff. Heidelberg: Springer-Verlag, 1977.
70 Hikino, H.; and Kiso, Y. "Natural Products for Liver Diseases." In *Economic and Medicinal Plant Research*, Vol. 2, ed. H. Wagner; H. Hikino; and N. R. Farnsworth. London: Academic Press, 1988.
71 Fintelmann, V. "Modern Phytotherapy and its Uses in Gastrointestinal Conditions." *Planta Medica* 57 no. 7 (1991): S48-S52.
72 Weiss, R. F. *Herbal Medicine*. Beaconsfield, England: Beaconsfield Publishers, 1988, 261.
73 Wagner, H.; Willer, F.; and Kreher, B. "Biologically Active Compounds From the Aqueous Extract of Urtica dioica." *Planta Medica* 55 no. 5 (Oct, 1989): 452-454.
74 Mittman, P. "Randomized, Double-Blind Study of Freeze-Dried Urtica dioica in the Treatment of Allergic Rhinitis." *Planta Medica* 56 no. 1 (Feb, 1990): 44-47.
75 Hoffmann, D. *The New Holistic Herbal*. Rockport, MA: Element, Inc., 1991, 218.
76 German Ministry of Health. *Passion Flower Leaves*. Commission E. Monographs for Phyto-

medicines. Bonn, Germany: German Ministry of Health, 1985.
77 Foster, S. *Passion Flower*. Botanical Series 314. Austin, TX: American Botanical Council, 1993.
78 Foster, S. *Peppermint*. Botanical Series 306. Austin, TX: American Botanical Council, 1991.
79 German Ministry of Health. *Peppermint Oil*. Commission E. Monographs for Phytomedicines. Bonn, Germany: German Ministry of Health, 1986.
80 (Commission E).
81 ESCOP, European Scientific Cooperative for Phytotherapy. *Peppermint Oil*. Meppel, The Netherlands: European Scientific Cooperative for Phytotherapy, 1992.
82 Hoffmann, D. *The New Holistic Herbal*. Rockport, MA: Element, Inc., 1991, 234.
83 Suzuki, O.; et al. "Inhibition of Monoamine Oxidase by Hypericin." *Planta Medica* 50 (1984): 272-274.
Muldner, H.; and Zoller, M. "Antidepressive Effect of a Hypericum Extract Standardized to an Active Hypericine Complex. Biochemical and Clinical Studies." *Arzneimittelforschung* 34 no. 8 (1984): 918-920.
84 Meruelo, D.; et al. "Therapeutic Agents with Dramatic Antiviral Activity and Little Toxicity at Effective Doses: Aromatic Polycyclicdiones Hypericin and Pseudohypericin." *Proceedings of the National Academy of Sciences* 85 (1988): 5230-5234.
85 Matei, I.; Gafitanu, E.; and Dorneanu, V. "Value of Hypericum Perforatum Oil in Dermatological Preparations." *Revista Medico- Chirurgicala Societatii de Medici Si Naturalisti Gin Iasi* 81 no. 1 (Jan-Mar, 1977): 73-74.
86 Melzer, R.; Fricke, U.; and Holzl, J. "Vasoactive Properties of Procyanidins from Hypericum Perforatum L. in Isolated Porcine Coronary Arteries." *Arzneimittelforschung* 41 no. 5 (May, 1991): 481-483.
87 Champault, G.; Patel, J. C.; and Bonnard, A. M. "A Double-Blind Trial of an Extract of the Plant Serenoa Repens in Benign Prostatic Hyperplasia." *British Journal of Clinical Pharmacology* 18 (1984): 461-462.
Boccafoschi, C.; and Annoscia, S. "Comparison of Serenoa Repens Extract with Placebo by Controlled Clinical Trial in Patients with Prostatic Adenomatosis." *Urologia* 50 (1983): 1257-1268.
88 Duvia, R.; Radice, G. P.; and Galdini, R. "Advances in the Phytotherapy of Prostatic Hypertrophy." *Med Praxis* 4 (1983): 143-148.
89 ESCOP, European Scientific Cooperative for Phytotherapy. *Valerian Root*. Meppel, The Netherlands: European Scientific Cooperative for Phytotherapy, 1990.
German Ministry of Health. *Senna*. Commission E. Monographs for Phytomedicines. Bonn, Germany: German Ministry of Health, 1984-.
90 German Ministry of Health. *Senna*. Commission E. Monographs for Phytomedicines. Bonn, Germany: German Ministry of Health, 1984-.
91 Berdyshev, V. V. "Effect of the Long-Term Intake of Eleutherococcus on the Adaptation of Sailors in the Tropics." *Voenno Meditsinskii Zhurnal* 5 (May, 1981): 57-58. (Published in Russian).
92 Kupin, V. I.; and Polevaia, E. B. "Stimulation of the Immunological Reactivity of Cancer Patients by Eleutherococcus Extract." *Voprosy Onkologii* 32 no. 7 (1986): 21-26. (Published in Russian).
93 Medon, P. J.; Ferguson, P. W.; and Watson, C. F. "Effects of Eleutherococcus Senticosus Extracts on Hexobarbital Metabolism In Vivo and In Vitro." *Journal of Ethnopharmacology* 10 no. 2 (Apr, 1984): 235-241.
94 German Ministry of Health. *Valerian*. Commission E. Monographs for Phytomedicines. Bonn, Germany: German Ministry of Health, 1985.
95 ESCOP, European Scientific Cooperative for Phytotherapy. *Valerian Root*. Meppel, The Netherlands: European Scientific Cooperative for Phytotherapy, 1990.
96 Hobbs, C. "Valerian: A Literature Review." *HerbalGram* 21 (1989): 19-34.
97 Congress of writers. "Drug Therapy of Hemorrhoids. Proven Results of Therapy with a Hamamelis Containing Hemorrhoid Ointment. Results of a Meeting of Experts. Dresden, 30 August 1991." *Fortschritte der Medizin* 109 Suppl 116 (1991): 1-11.
98 Bernard, P.; et al. "Venitonic Pharmacodynamic Value of Galenic Preparations with a Base of Hamamelis Leaves." *Journal de Pharmacie de Belgique* 27 no. 4 (Jul-Aug, 1972): 505-512.

Homeopathy

1 Bannerman, R. H.; Burton, J.; and Wen Chieh, C.; eds. *Traditional Medicine and Health Care Coverage*. Geneva, Switzerland: World Health Organization, 1983.
2 Lange, A. "Homeopathy." In A *Textbook of Natural Medicine*, eds. J. E. Pizzorno and M. T. Murray. Seattle WA: John Bastyr College Publications, 1989.
3 Hahnemann, S. *Organon of Medicine*. Translated by W. Boericke, M.D. New Dehli: B. Jain Publishing,1992.
4 Smith, R. B., Jr.; and Boericke, G. W. "Changes Caused by Succussion on N.M.R. Patterns and Bioassay of Bradykinin Triacetate (BKTA) Successions and Dilution." *Journal of the American Institute of Homeopathy* 61 (Nov/Dec 1968): 197-212.
5 Del Giudice, E.; and Preparata, G. "Superradiance: A New Approach to Coherent Dynamical Behaviors of Condensed Matter." *Frontier Perspectives* 1 no. 2 (Fall/Winter 1990) Philadelphia: Temple University, Center for Frontier Sciences.
6 Rubik, B. "Frontiers of Homeopathic Research." *Frontier Perspectives* 2 no. 1 (Spring/Summer 1991) Philadelphia: Temple University, Center for Frontier Sciences.
7 Gerber, R., M.D. *Vibrational Medicine*. Santa Fe, NM: Bear & Company, 1988, 84.
8 Leviton, R. "Homeopathy." *Yoga Journal* no. 85 (Mar/Apr 1989): 42-51,97-98,100,105.
9 Vithoulkas, G. "Homeopathy." In *Traditional Medicine and Health Care Coverage*, eds. R. H. Bannerman; J. Burton; and C. WenChieh. Geneva: World Health Organization, 1983.
10 Kleignen, J.; et al. "Clinical Trials of Homeopathy." *British Medical Journal* 302 (Feb, 1991): 316-323.
11 Gibson, R. G.; et al. "Homeopathic Therapy in Rheumatoid Arthritis: Evaluation by Double-Blind Clinical Therapeutic Trial." *British Journal of Clinical Pharmacology* 9 (May, 1980): 453-459.
Shipley, M.; et al. "Controlled Trial of Homeopathic Treatment of Osteoarthritis." *The Lancet* 1 (1983): 97-98.
Scofield, A. M. "Experimental Research in Homeopathy—A Critical Review." *British Homeopathic Journal* 73 (1984): 161-266.
12 Ferley, J. P.; et al. "A Controlled Evaluation of a Homeopathic Preparation in the Treatment of Influenza-like Syndromes." *British Journal of Clinical Pharmacology* 27 (Mar, 1989): 329-335.
13 Reilly, D. T.; et al. "Is Homeopathy a Placebo Response: Controlled Trial of Homeopathic Potency, with Pollen in Hayfever as Model." *Lancet* 2 no. 8512 (Oct, 1986): 881-886.
14 Albertini, H.; et al. "Homeopathic Treatment of Neuralgia Using Arnica and Hypericum: A Summary of 60 Observations." *Journal of the American Institute of Homeopathy* 78 (Sep, 1985): 126-128.
15 Gerhard, W. "The Biological Treatment of Migraines, Based on Experience." *Biological Therapy* 5 no 3 (Jun, 1988): 67-71.
16 Zenner, S.; and Metelmann, H. "Therapeutic Use of Lymphomyosot—Results of a Multicenter Use Observation Study on 3,512 Patients." *Biological Therapy* 8 no. 3 (Jun, 1990): 49; Biological Therapy 8 no. 4 (Oct, 1990): 79.
17 Coulter, H. L. *Divided Legacy: A History of the Schism in Medical Thought, Vol. 2*. Washington, D.C.: Wehawken Book Co., 1973-1977.
18 Ullman, D. *Homeopathy: Medicine for the 21st Century*. Berkeley, CA: North Atlantic Books, 1988, 126. Reprint. *Discovering Homeopathy: Medicine for the 21st Century*. Rev. ed. Berkeley, CA: North Atlantic Books, 1991.
19 Coulter, H. L. *Divided Legacy: A History of the Schism in Medical Thought, Vol. 2*. Washington, D.C.: Wehawken Book Co., 1973-1977.
20 Cook, T. *Samuel Hahnemann: the Founder of Homeopathic Medicine*. Wellingborough, Northhamptonshire, England: Thorsons, 1981.
21 Coulter, H. L. *Divided Legacy: A History of the Schism in Medical Thought, Vol. 2*. Washington, D.C.: Wehawken Book Co.,1973-1977.
22 McAuliffe, S. "Homeopathy Goes Mainstream: New Treatments for Old Ills." *Longevity* 4 no.12 (Nov, 1992):62.

Hydrotherapy

1 Chaitow, L. *The Body/Mind Purification Program*. New York: Simon and Schuster, 1990.
2 Boyle, W.; and Saine, A. *Lectures in Naturopathic Hydrotherapy*. East Palestine, OH: Buckeye Naturopathic Press, 1991.
3 Weatherburn, H. "Hyperthermia and Aids Treatment." *British Journal of Radiology* 61 (Sep, 1988): 862-863.
4 Chaitow, L. *The Body/Mind Purification Program*. New York: Simon and Schuster, 1990.
5 Airola, P. *How to Get Well*. Sherwood, OR: Health Plus Publishers, 1990.
6 Thrash, A., M.D.; and C.L. Jr., M.D. *Home Remedies: hydrotherapy, massage, charcoal, and other simple treatments*. Groveland, CA: *New Life Books, 1981*.
7 Buchman, D. D. *The Complete Book of Water Therapy*. New York: Dutton, 1979.
8 Airola, P. *How to Get Well*. Sherwood, OR: Health Plus Publishers, 1990.

Hyperthermia

1 Tyrrell, D.; Barrow, I.; and Arthur, J. "Local Hyperthermia Benefits Natural and Experimental Common Colds." *British Medical Journal* 298 (1989): 1280-1283.
2 Spire, B.; et al. "Inactivation of Lymphadenopathy-Associated Virus by Heat, Gamma Rays, and Ultraviolet Light." *Lancet* 1 no. 8422 (Jan, 26, 1985): 188-189.
3 Thrash, A., M.D.; and C.L. Jr., M.D. *Home Remedies: hydrotherapy, massage, charcoal, and other simple treatments*. Groveland, CA: New Life Books, 1981.
4 Standish, L.; et al. "One Year Open Trial of Naturopathic Treatment of HIV Infection Class IV-A in Men." *Journal of Naturopathic Medicine* 3 no. 1 (1992): 42-64.
5 Weatherburn, H. "Hyperthermia and Aids Treatment." *British Journal of Radiology* 61, No. 729 (Sep, 1988): 862-863.
6. Konings, A. W. T. "Membranes as Targets for Hyperthermic Cell Killing." *Recent Results in Cancer Research* 109 (1988): 9-21.
Toffoli, G.; et al. "Effect of Hyperthermia on Intracellular Drug Accumulation and Chemosensitivity in Drug-Sensitive and Drug-Resistant P388 Leukaemia Cell Lines." *International Journal of Hyperthermia* 5 no. 2 (1989): 163-172.
7 Park, M. M.; et al. "The Effect of Whole Body Hyperthermia on the Immune Cell Activity of Cancer Patients." *Lymphokine Research* 9 no. 2 (1990): 213-223.
8 Neville, A. J.; and Sauder, D. N. "Whole Body Hyperthermia (41 to 42 Degrees C) Induces Interleukin-1 in Vivo." *Lymphokine Research* 7 no. 3 (Fall, 1988): 201-206.
9 Tyrrell, D.; Barrow, I.; and Arthur, J. "Local Hyperthermia Benefits Natural and Experimental Common Colds." *British Medical Journal* 298 (1989): 1280-1283.
10 Guyton, A. C., M.D. *Textbook of Medical Physiology*, sixth ed. Philadelphia: W. B. Saunders Company, 1986.
11 Gard, Z. R., M.D.; and Brown, E. J. "Literature Review and Comparison Studies of Sauna/Hyperthermia in Detoxification." *Townsend Letter for Doctors* no. 107 (Jun, 1992): 470-478.
12 Ibid.
13 Harvey, M. A.; McRorie, M. M.; and Smith, D. W. "Suggested Limits to the Use of the Hot Tub and Sauna by Pregnant Women." *Canadian Medical Association Journal* 125 (Jul, 1981): 50-53.
14 Sawtell, N. M.; and Thompson, R. L. "Rapid in Vivo Reactivation of Herpes Simplex Virus in Latently Infected Murine Ganglionic Neurons after Transient Hyperthermia." *Journal of Virology* 66 no. 4 (Apr, 1992): 2150-2156.
15 Skibba, J. L.; et al. "Oxidative Stress as a

Precursor to the Irreversible Hepatocellular Injury Caused by Hyperthermia." *International Journal of Hyperthermia* 7 no. 5 (Sep/Oct 1991): 749-761.
16 From the Centers for Disease Control. "Self-Induced Malaria Associated with Malariotherapy for Lyme Disease—Texas." *Journal of the American Medical Association* 266 no. 16 (Oct, 1991): 2199.

Hypnotherapy

1 Findlay, S.; Podolsky, D.; and Silberner, J. "Wonder Cures From the Fringe." *U.S. News and World Report* 3 no. 13 (Sep 23, 1991): 68-74.
2 Tinterow, M. M., M.D. "Hypnotherapy for Chronic Pain." *Kansas Medicine* 88 no. 6 (Jun 1987): 190-192, 204.
3 Tinterow, M. M., M.D. "The Use of Hypnotic Anesthesia for Major Surgical Procedure." *The American Surgeon* 26 (Nov, 1960): 732-737.
4 Tinterow, M. M., M.D. "Hypnotherapy for Chronic Pain." *Kansas Medicine* 88 no. 6 (Jun, 1987): 190-192, 204.
5 Barrios, A. A. "Hypnotherapy: A Reappraisal" *Psychotherapy: Theory, Research and Practice* 7 no. 1 (Spring, 1970): 2-7.
6 Bannerman, R. H.; Burton, J.; and Wen Chieh, C., eds. *Traditional Medicine and Health Care Coverage*. Chapter 13: Hypnosis. Geneva, Switzerland: World Health Organization, 1983.
7 Olsen, K. G. "Hypnosis and Hypnotherapy." *The Encyclopedia of Alternative Health Care*. New York: Pocket Books, 1989, 1990.
8 Pratt, G. J.; Wood, D. P.; and Alman, B. M. *A Clinical Hypnosis Primer*. La Jolla, CA: Psychology and Consulting Associates Press, 1984.

Juice Therapy

1 Siegenberg, D.; et al. "Ascorbic Acid Prevents the Dose-Dependent Inhibitory Effects of Polyphenols and Phytates on Nonheme-Iron Absorption." *American Journal of Clinical Nutrition* 53 (Feb, 1991): 537-541.
2 Carper, J. *The Food Pharmacy: Dramatic New Evidence that Food is Your Best Medicine*. New York: Bantam, 1988.
3 Ofek, I.; et al. "Anti-Escherichia Coli Adhesin Activity of Cranberry and Blueberry Juices." *New England Journal of Medicine* 324 (May, 1991): 1599.
4 Cheney, G. "Anti-Peptic Ulcer Dietary Factor (Vitamin U) in Treatment of Peptic Ulcer."*Journal of the American Dietetic Association* 26 (Sep, 1950): 668-672.
5 Altman, R.; et al. "Identification of Platelet Inhibitor Present in the Melon (Cucurbitacea Cucumis Melo)." *Thrombosis and Haemostatis* 53 no. 3 (Jun, 1985): 312-313.
6 Adetumbi, M. A.; and Lau, B. H. "Allium Sativum (Garlic): A Natural Antibiotic." *Medical Hypothesis* 12 no. 3 (Nov, 1983): 227-237.
Lau, B. H. "Anticoagulant and Lipid Regulating Effects of Garlic (Allium Sativum)." In *New Protective Roles for Selected Nutrients*, eds. G. A. Spiller and J. Scala. New York: Alan R. Liss Inc, 1989.
7 Srivastava, K. C.; and Mustafa, T. "Ginger (Zingiber Officinale) and Rheumatic Disorders." *Medical Hypothesis* 29 no. 1 (May, 1989): 25-28.
Al-Yahya, M. A.; et al. "Gastroprotective Activity of Ginger Zingiber Officinale Rosc., in Albino Rats." *American Journal of Chinese Medicine* 17 nos. 1-2 (1989): 51-56.
8 Mustafa, T.; and Srivastava, K. C. "Ginger in Migraine Headache." *Journal of Ethnopharmacology* 29 no. 3 (Jul, 1990): 267-273.
Grontved, A.; and Hentzer E. "Vertigo-Reducing Effect of Ginger Root." *Journal of Oto-Rhino-Laryngology and Its Related Specialties* 48 no. 5 (1986): 282-286.
9 Murray, M. T.; and Pizzorno, J. E. *Encyclopedia of Natural Medicine*. Rocklin, CA: Prima Publishing, 1990.
Taussig, S. J. "The Mechanism of the Physiological Action of Bromelain." *Medical Hypotheses* 6 no. 1 (Jan,1980): 99-104.
10 Wattenberg, L. W. "Inhibition of Carcinogenesis by Minor Anutrient Constituents of the Diet." *Proceedings of the Nutrition Society* 49 no. 2 (Jul, 1990): 173-183.
Beyers, T., M.D.; LaChance, P. A.; and Pierson, H. F. "New Directions: The Diet-Cancer Link." *Patient Care* 24 (Nov. 30, 1990): 34-48.
Fenwick, G.; Heaney, R. K.; and Mullin, W. J. "Glucosinolates and Their Breakdown Products in Food and Food Plants." *Critical Reviews in Food Science and Nutrition* 18 no. 2 (1983): 123-201.
Wattenberg, L. W. "Inhibition of Neoplasia by Minor Dietary Constituents." *Cancer Research* 43 (1983): 2448S-2453S.
Shills, M. E., M.D. "Nutrition and Diet in Cancer." In *Modern Nutrition in Health and Disease,* eds. M. E. Shills, M.D. and V. R. Young. 7th Ed. Philadelphia: Lea and Febiger, 1988.
Shills, M. E., M.D. "Nutrition and Diet in Cancer." In *Modern Nutrition in Health and Disease,* eds. M. E. Shills, M.D. and V. R. Young. 7th Ed. Philadelphia: Lea and Febiger, 1988.
11 Shills, M. E., M.D. "Nutrition and Diet in Cancer." In *Modern Nutrition in Health and Disease,* eds. M. E. Shills, M.D. and V. R. Young. 7th Ed. Philadelphia: Lea and Febiger, 1988.
12 Weisburger, J. H. "Nutritional Approach to Cancer Prevention with Emphasis on Vitamins, Antioxidants, and Carotenoids." *American Journal of Clinical Nutrition* 53 no. 1 (Jan, 1991): 226S-237S.
Wattenberg, L. W. "Inhibition of Carcinogenesis by Minor Anutrient Constituents of the Diet." *Proceedings of the Nutrition Society* 49 no. 2 (Jul, 1990): 173-183.
13 Beyers, T.; LaChance, R. A.; and Pierson, H. E. "New Directions: The Diet-Cancer Link." *Patient Care* 24 (Nov. 30, 1990): 34-48.
14 Shills, M. E., M.D. "Nutrition and Diet in Cancer." In *Modern Nutrition in Health and Disease,* eds. M. E. Shills, M.D. and V. R. Young. 7th Ed. Philadelphia: Lea and Febiger, 1988.
15 Wilcox, G.; et al. "Oestrogenic Effects of Plant Foods in Post-Menopausal Women." *British Medical Journal* 301 no. 6757 (Oct,1990): 905-906.

Light Therapy

1 Ott, J. "Color and Light: Their Effects on Plants, Animals and People." *The International Journal of Biosocial Research* 7-10, (1985-1988): 1-131.
2 Roos, P. A. "Light and Electromagnetic Waves: The Health Implications." *Journal of the Bio-Electro-Magnetics Institute* 3 no. 2 (Summer 1991): 7-12.
3 Ott, J. *Health and Light*. Old Greenwich, CT: The Devin-Adair Co., 1973.
4 *National Institute of Health Report*. Sent to Ott, J. N., by Jaffe, R. M., M.D., Commander, United States Health Service, National Institutes of Health, Dec, 1978.
5 Roos, P. A. "Light and Electromagnetic Waves: The Health Implications." *Journal of the Bio-Electro Magnetics Institute* 3 no. 2 (Summer 1991): 7-12.
6 Garland, F. C.; et al. "Occupational sunlight exposure and melanoma in the U.S. Navy." *Archives of Environmental Health* 45 (1990): 261-267.
7 Editorial. "Excessive Sunlight Exposure, Skin Melanoma, Linked to Vitamin D." *International Journal of Biosocial and Medical Research* 13 no. 1 (1991): 13-14.
8 Ibid.
9 Garland, F. C.; et al. "Occupational sunlight exposure and melanoma in the U.S. Navy. *Archives of Environmental Health* 45 (1990): 261-267.
10 Kime, Z. R. *Sunlight*. Penryn, CA: World Health Publications: 1980.
11 Ott, J. "The Effect of Color and Light: Part 3." *The International Journal of Biosocial Research* 9 (1987): 71-107.
12 Hyman, J. W. *The Light Book*. New York: Ballantine Books, 1991.
13 Editorial. "Winter Blues? Try a Little Morning Light." *Bioenergy Health Newsletter* (Dec, 1987): 7.
14 Gutfeld, G. "The New Science of Rays and Rhythms- Cutting Edge Light Therapies that Can Brighten Your Health." *Prevention* 45 no. 2 (Feb, 1993): 67-71; 116-123.
15 Editorial. "Winter Blues? Try a Little Morning Light." *Bioenergy Health Newsletter* (Dec, 1987): 7.
16 Walker, M. *The Power of Color: The Art & Science of Making Colors Work for You*. Garden City Park, NY: Avery Publishing Group, 1991.
17 Laycock, K. A.; et al. "Characterization of a Murine model of recurrent herpes simplex viral keratitis induced by Ultraviolet B radiation." *Investigative Opthamology and Visual Science* 32 no. 10 (Sep, 1991) : 2741-2746.
Taylor, H. R. "Ultraviolet radiation and the eye: an epidemiologic study." *Transactions of the American Opthalmological Society* 87 (1990): 802-853.
Taylor, H. R. "The Biologic Effects of UV-B on the Eye." *Photochemistry and Photobiology* 50 no. 4 (Oct, 1989): 489-492.
18 Kravkov, S. V. "Color, Vision and the Autonomic Nervous System." *Journal of the Optical Society of America* 31 (Apr, 1944): 335-337.
19 Lieberman, J. *Light: Medicine of the Future*. Santa Fe, NM: Bear and Co., 1991.

Magnetic Field Therapy

1 Becker, R. O., M.D. *Cross Currents. The Promise of Electromedicine. The Perils of Electropollution.* Los Angeles: Jeremy P. Tarcher, 1990.
2 Davis, A. R.; and Rawls, W. C. *Magnetism and Its Effects on the Living System*. New York: Exposition Press, 1974.
3 Becker, R. O., M.D. *Cross Currents. The Promise of Electromedicine. The Perils of Electropollution.* Los Angeles: Jeremy P. Tarcher, 1990, 187.
4 Nakagawa, K., M.D. "Magnetic Field Deficiency Syndrome and Magnetic Treatment." *Japan Medical Journal* 2745 (Dec, 1976).(In Japanese).
5 Wertheimer, N.; and Leeper, E. "Electrical Wiring Configurations and Childhood Cancer." *American Journal of Epidemiology* 109 (1979): 273-284.
6 Wolpay, J. *Biological Effects of Power Line Fields*. New York State Power-Lines Project Scientific Advisory Panel, 1987.
7 Speers, M.; Dobbins, J.; and Miller, V. "Occupational Exposures and Brain Cancer Mortality: A Preliminary Study of East Texas Residents." *American Journal of Industrial Medicine* 13 (1988): 629-638.
8 Becker, R. O., M.D. *Cross Currents. The Promise of Electromedicine. The Perils of Electropollution.* Los Angeles: Jeremy P. Tarcher, 1990, 208.
9 Smith, C.; and Best, S. *Electromagnetic Man: Health and Hazard in the Electrical Environment.* London: J.M. Dent and Sons, Ltd., 1989.
10 Murphy, J. C.; et al. "International Commission for Protection Against Environmental Mutagens and Carcinogens. Power Frequency Electric and Magnetic Fields: A Review of Genetic Toxicology." *Mutation Research* 296 no. 3 (Mar, 1993): 221-240.
11 Becker, R. O., M.D. *Cross Currents. The Promise of Electromedicine. The Perils of Electropollution.* Los Angeles: Jeremy P. Tarcher, 1990, 210.
12 Fontenot, J.; and Levine, S. A. "Melatonin Deficiency: Its Role in Oncogenesis and Age-Relative Pathology." *Journal of Orthomolecular Medicine* 5 no. 1 (1st Quarter, 1990): 22-24.
13 Philpott, W.; and Taplin, S. *Biomagnetic Handbook*. Choctaw, OK: Enviro-Tech Products, 1990.

Meditation

1 Miller, N. "Learning of Visceral and Glandular Responses." *Science* 163 no. 866 (Jan, 1969): 434-445.
Anand, B. K.; Chhina, G.; and Singh, B. "Some Aspects of Electroencephalographic Studies in Yogis." *Electroencephalography and Clinical Neurophysiology* 13 no. 3 (Jun, 1961): 452-456.
2 Rodin, J. "Aging and Health: Effects of the Sense of Control." *Science* 233 no. 4770 (Sep, 1986): 1271-1276.
3 Shapiro, D. H.; and Walsh, R. N. *Meditation: Classic and Contemporary Perspectives*. New York: Aldine, 1984.
4 Ornish, D., M.D. *Dr. Dean Ornish's Program for Reducing Heart Disease: the Only System Scientifically Proven to Reverse Heart Disease Without Drugs or Surgery*. New York: Random House,

1990.
5 Chalmers, R. A.; et al., eds. *Scientific Research on Maharishi's Transcendental Meditation and TM-Sidhi Program:* Collected papers, Volume 2-4. Vlodrop, the Netherlands: Maharishi Vedic University Press, 1989.
Orme-Johnson, D. W.; and Farrow, J. T.; eds. *Scientific Research on the Transcendental Meditation Program:* Collected papers, Volume 1. Rheinweiler, West Germany: Maharishi European Research University Press, 1977.
Wallace, R. K.; Orme-Johnson, D. W.; and Dillbeck, M. C., eds. *Scientific Research on Maharishi's Transcendental Meditation Program:* Collected papers, Volume 5. Fairfield, IA: Maharishi International University Press, in press.
6 Wallace, R. K. "Physiological Effects of Transcendental Meditation." *Science* 167 (1970): 1751-1754.
Wallace, R. K.; et al. "A Wakeful Hypometabolic Physiologic State." *American Journal of Physiology* 221 (1971): 795-799.
Wallace, R. K.; et al. "The Physiology of Meditation." *Scientific American* 226 (1972): 84-90.
Dillbeck, M. C.; and Orme-Johnson, D. W. "Physiological Differences Between Transcendental Meditation and Rest." *American Physiologist* 42 (1987): 879-881.
Jevning, R.; Wallace, R. K.; and Beiderbach, M. "The Physiology of Meditation: A Review. A Wakeful Hypometabolic Integrated Response." *Neuroscience and Biobehavioral Reviews* 16 (1992): 415-424.
Jevning, R.; Wilson, A. F.; and Davidson, J. M. "Adrenocortical Activity During Meditation." *Hormones and Behavior* 10 no. 1 (1978): 54-60.
Jevning, R.; et al. "Forearm Blood Flow and Metabolism During Stylized and Unstylized States of Decreased Activation." *American Journal of Physiology* 245 (Regulatory, Integrative and Comparative Physiology 14) (1983): R110-R116.
Jevning, R.; et al. "Metabolic Control in a State of Decreased Activation: Modulation of Red Cell Metabolism." *American Journal of Physiology* 245 (Cell Physiology 14) (1983): C457-C461.
Jevning, R.; et al. "Modulation of Red Cell Metabolism by States of Decreased Activation: Comparison Between States." *Physiology and Behavior* 35 (1985): 679-682.
Jevning, R.; et. al. "Plasma Thyroid Hormones, Thyroid Stimulating Hormone, and Insulin During Acute Hypometabolic States in Man." *Physiology and Behavior* 40 (1987): 603-606.
O'Halloran, J. P.; et. al. "Hormonal Control in a State of Decreased Activation: Potentiation of Arginine Vasopressin Secretion." *Physiology and Behavior* 35 (1985): 591-595.
Wilson, A. F.; Jevning, R.; and Guich, S. "Marked Reduction of Forearm Carbon Dioxide Production During States of Decreased Metabolism." *Physiology and Behavior* 41 (1987): 347-352.
Farrow, J. T.; and Hebert, J. R. "Breath Suspension During the Transcendental Meditation Technique." *Psychosomatic Medicine* 44 no. 2 (1982): 133-153.
7 Banquet, J. P. "Spectral Analysis of the EEG in Meditation." *Electroancephalography and Clinical Neurophysiology* 35 (1973): 143-151.
Banquet, J. P.; and Sailhan, M. "EEG Analysis of Spontaneous and Induced States of Consciousness." *Revue d'lectroenc phalographie et de Neurophysiologie Clinque* 4 (1974): 445-453.
Banquet, J. P.; and Les vre, N. "Event-Related Potentials in Altered States of Consciousness." *Motivation, Motor and Sensory Processes of the Brain, Progress in Brain Research* 54 (1980): 447-453.
Levine, P. H. "The Coherence Spectral Array (COSPAR) and its Application to the Study of Spatial Ordering in the EEG." In *Proceedings of the San Diego Biomedical Symposium* 15 ed. J. I. Martin. New York: Academic Press, Inc., 1976, 237-247.
Badawi, K.; et. al. "Electrophysiologic Characteristics of Respiratory Suspension Periods Occurring During the Practice of the Transcendental Meditation Program." *Psychosomatic Medicine* 46 no. 3 (1984): 267-276.
Orme-Johnson, D. W.; and Haynes, C. T. "EEG Phase Coherence, Pure Consciousness, Creativity, and TM-Sidhi Experiences." *International Journal of Neuroscience* 13 (1981): 211-217.
Dillbeck, M. C.; Orme-Johnson, D. W.; and Wallace, R. K. "Frontal EEG Coherence, H-Reflex Recovery, Concept Learning, and the TM-Sidhi Program." *International Journal of Neuroscience* 15 (1981): 151-157.
Nidich, S. I.; et al. "Kohlbergian Cosmic Perspective Responses, EEG Coherence, and the Transcendental Meditation and TM-Sidhi Program." *Journal of Moral Education* 12 no. 3 (1983): 166-173.
Alexander, C. N.; et al. "Transcendental Consciousness: A Fourth State of Consciousness Beyond Sleep, Dreaming, and Waking." In *Sleep and Dreams: A Sourcebook,* ed. J. Gackenback. New York: Garland Publishing, Inc., 1986, 282-315.
8 Cranson, R. W.; et al. "Transcendental Meditation and Improved Performance on Intelligence-Related Measures: A Longitudinal Study." *Personality and Individual Differences* 12 (1991): 1105-1116.
Dillbeck, M. C. "Meditation and Flexibility of Visual Perception and Verbal Problem-Solving." *Memory and Cognition* 10 no. 3 (1982): 207-215.
Tjoa, A. "Meditation, Neuroticism and Intelligence: A follow-up." *Gedrag: Tijdacrift voor Psychologie (Behavior: Journal of Psychology)* 3 (1975): 167-182.
Travis, F. "Creative Thinking and the Transcendental Meditation Technique." *The Journal of Creative Behavior* 13 no. 3 (1979): 169-180.
Gelderloos, P.; and Van Den Berg, W. P. "Marharishi's TM-Sidhi Program: Participating in the Infinite Creativity of Nature to Enliven the Totality of the Cosmic Psyche in all Aspects of Life." *Modern Science and Vedic Science* 2 no. 4 (1989): 373-412.
Jedrczak, A.; Beresford, M.; and Clements, G. "The TM-Sidhi Program, Pure Consciousness, Creativity and Intelligence." *The Journal of Creative Behavior* 19 no. 4 (1985): 270-275.
Pelletier, K. R. "Influence of Transcendental Meditation upon Autokinetic Perception." *Perceptual and Motor Skills* 39 (1974): 1031-1034.
Dillbeck, M. C.; et. al. "Longitudinal Effects of the Transcendental Meditation and TM-Sidhi Program on Cognitive Ability and Cognitive Style." *Perceptual and Motor Skills* 62 (1986): 731-738.
Gelderloos, P.; Lockie, R. J.; and Chuttoorgoon, S. "Field Independence of Students at Maharishi School of the Age of Enlightenment and a Montessori School." *Perceptual and Motor Skills* 65 (1987): 613-614.
Jedrczak, A. "The Transcendental Meditation and TM-Sidhi Program and Field Independence." *Perceptual and Motor Skills* 59 (1984): 999-1000.
9 Orme-Johnson, D. "Medical Care Utilization and the Transcendental Meditation Program." *Psychosomatic Medicine* 49 no. 1 (1987): 493-507.
Alexander, C. N.; et. al. "Transcendental Meditation, Mindfulness, and Longevity: An Experimental Study with the Elderly." *Journal of Personality and Social Psychology* 57 no. 6 (Dec, 1989): 950-964.
Schneider, R. H.; et al. "Stress Management in Elderly Blacks: A Preliminary Report." *Proceedings of the 2nd International Conference on Race, Ethnicity and Health: Challenges in Diabetes and Hypertension.* Salvador, Brazil: July, 1991.
Schneider, R. H.; Alexander, C. N.; and Wallace, R. K. "In Search of an Optimal Behavioral Treatment for Hypertension: A Review and Focus on Transcendental Meditation." In *Personality, Elevated Blood Pressure and Essential Hypertension,* eds. E. H. Johnson; W. D. Gentry; and S. Julius. Washington, D.C.: Hemisphere Publishing Corporation. In press.
Cooper, M. J.; and Aygen, M. M. "Transcendental Meditation in the Management of Hypercholesterolemia." *Journal of Human Stress* 5 no. 4 (1979): 24-27.
10 Gelderloos, P.; et. al. "Effectiveness of the Transcendental Meditation Program in Preventing and Treating Substance Misuse: A Review." *International Journal of Addictions* 26 no. 3 (Mar, 1991): 293-325.
Alexander, C. N.; Robinson, P.; and Rainforth, M. "Treating Alcoholism and Drug Addiction Through Transcendental Meditation." *Alcoholism Treatment Quarterly.* In Press.
Dillbeck, M. C.; and Abrams, A. I. "The Application of the Transcendental Meditation Program to Correction." *International Journal of Comparative and Applied Criminal Justice* 11 no. 1 (1987): 111-132.
Bleick, C. R.; and Abrams, A. I. "The Transcendental Meditation Program and Criminal Recidivism in California." *Journal of Criminal Justice* 15 (1987): 211-230.
Abrams, A. I.; and Siegel, L. M. "The Transcendental Meditation Program and Rehabilitation at Folsom State Prison: A Cross Validation Study." *Criminal Justice and Behavior* 5 no. 1 (1978): 3-20.
11 Eppley, K. R.; Abrams, A. I.; and Shear, J. "The Effects of Meditation and Relaxation Techniques on Trait Anxiety: A Meta-Analysis." Also: Eppley, K. R.; Abrams, A. I.; and Shear, J. "Differential Effects of Relaxation Techniques on Trait Anxiety: A Meta-Analysis." *Journal of Clinical Psychology* 45 no. 6 (1989). 957-974.
Alexander, C. N.; Rainforth, M. V.; and Gelderloos, P. "Transcendental Mediation, Self Actualization and Psychological Health: A Conceptual Overview and Statistical Meta-Analysis." *Journal of Social Behavior and Personality* 6 no. 5 (1991): 189-247.
Alexander, C. N.; Druker, S. M.; and Langer, E. J. "Introduction: Major Issues in the Exploration of Adult Growth." In *Higher Stages of Human Development: Perspectives on Adult Growth,* eds. C. N. Alexander and E. J. Langer. New York: Oxford University Press, 1990, 3-32.
Alexander, C. N.; et. al. "Growth of Higher Stages of Consciousness: Maharishi's Vedic Psychology of Human Development. A Summary of a Chapter appearing in *Higher Stages of Human Development: Perspective on Adult Growth,* eds. C. N. Alexander and E. J. Langer. New York: Oxford University Press, 1990.
12 Gelderloos, P.; et al. "Effectiveness of the Transcendental Meditation Program in Preventing and Treating Substance Misuse: A Review." *International Journal of the Addictions* 26 no. 3 (Mar, 1991): 293-325.
13 Smith, G. R. "Psychological Modulation of the Human Immune Response to Varicella Zoster." *Archives of Internal Medicine* 145 no. 11 (1985): 2110-2112.
14 Alexander, C. N.; et. al. "Transcendental Meditation, Mindfulness, and Longevity. An Experimental Study with the Elderly." *Journal of Personality and Social Psychology* 57 no.6 (1989): 950-964.
15 Begley, S.; Hager, M.; and Murr, A. "Search for the Fountain of Youth." *Newsweek* (Mar, 1990): 44-48.
16 Shapiro, D. H. "A Preliminary Study of Long Term Meditators: Goals, Effects, Religious Orientation, Cognitions." *Journal of Transpersonal Psychology* 24 no. 1 (1992):23-39.
17 Kabat-Zinn, J. *Full Catastrophe Living: Using the Wisdom of Your Body and Mind to Face Stress, Pain, and Illness.* New York: Delacorte Press, 1990.
18 Meares, A. "What Can the Cancer Patient Expect from Intensive Meditation?" *Australian Family Physician* 9 no. 5 (May, 1980): 322-325.
19 Kutz, I.; Borysenko, J. Z.; and Benson, H. "Meditation and Psychotherapy: A Rationale for the Integration of Dynamic Psychotherapy, the Relaxation Response, and Mindfulness Meditation." *American Journal of Psychiatry* 142 no. 1 (Jan, 1985): 1-8.
20 Shapiro, D. H. "A Preliminary Study of Long Term Meditators: Goals, Effects, Religious Orientation, Cognitions." *Journal of Transpersonal Psychology* 24 no. 1 (1992):23-39.

Mind/Body Medicine

1 Idler, E. L.; Kasl, S. V.; and Lemke, J. H. "Self-Evaluated Health and Mortality Among the Elderly in New Haven, Connecticut, and Iowa and Washington Counties, Iowa, 1982-1986." *American Journal of Epidemiology* 131 no. 1 (Jan, 1990):

91-103.
2 Antoni, M. H.; et al. "Cognitive-Behavioral Stress Management Intervention Buffers Distress Responses and Immunologic Changes Following Notification of HIV-1 Seropositivity." *Journal of Consulting and Clinical Psychology* 59 no. 6 (Dec, 1991): 906-915.
Antoni, M. H.; et. al. "Pyschological and Neuroendocrine Measures Related to Functional Immune Changes in Anticipation of HIV-1 Serostatus Notification." *Psychosomatic Medicine* 52 no. 5 (Sep-Oct, 1990): 496-510.
Benson, H.; et al. "Decreased Blood Pressure in Borderline Hypertensive Subjects Who Practiced Meditation." *Journal of Chronic Diseases* 27 no. 3 (Mar, 1974): 163-169.
Chesney, M. A.; et. al. "Nonpharmacologic Appraches to the Treatment of Hypertension." *Circulation* 76 no. 1 Part 2 (Jul, 1987): I104-I109.
Caudill, M.; et al. "Decreased Clinic Use by Chronic Pain Patients: Response to Behavioral Medicine Intervention." *Clinical Journal of Pain* 7 no. 4 (Dec, 1991): 305-310.
3 Healy, D. L.; et al. "The Thymus-Adrenal Connection: Thymosin has Corticotropin-Releasing Activity in Primates." *Science* 222 no. 4630 (1983): 1353-1355.
4 Ader, R.; and Cohen, N. "Behaviorally Conditioned Immunosuppression." *Psychosomatic Medicine* 37 no. 4 (Jul-Aug, 1975): 333-340.
Ghanta, V. K.; et al. "Neural and Environmental Influence on Neoplasia and Conditioning of NK Activity." *Journal of Immunology* 135 2 Suppl. (Aug, 1985): 848S-852S.
5 Moyers, B. *Healing and the Mind.* New York: Doubleday, 1993.
6 Borysenko, J. *Minding the Body, Mending the Mind.* New York: Bantam Books, 1988.
7 Basmajian, J. V. "Learned Control of Single Motor Units." In *Biofeedback: Theory and Research,* eds. G. Schwartz and J. Beatty New York: Academic Press, 1977, 415-431.
8 Murphy, M. *The Future of the Body.* Los Angeles: Jeremy P. Tarcher, Inc., 1992.
9 Green, E., M.D.; and Green, A. "The Ins and Outs of Mind-Body Energy," *Science Year, 1974.* Chicago IL: World Book Science Annual Field Enterprises Educational Corp., 1973, 137-147.
10 Moyers, B. *Healing and the Mind.* New York: Doubleday, 1993, 200-201.
11 Ibid., pages 206-207.
12 Chopra, D. *Quantum Healing: Exploring the Frontiers of Mind/Body Medicine.* New York: Bantam Books, 1989.
Dossey, L. *Space, Time, & Medicine.* Boulder, CO: Shambala, 1982.
Kunz, D. *The Personal Aura.* Wheaton, IL: Theosophical Publishing House, 1991.
13 Williams, R. J. *Nutrition Against Disease: Environmental Prevention.* New York: Bantam Books, 1972.
14 Selye, H., M.D. *Stress Without Distress.* New York: Penguin, 1975.
15 Seedhouse, D.; and Cribb, A., eds. *Changing Ideas in Health Care.* New York: John Wiley & Sons, 1990.
16 Benson, H., M.D. *The Relaxation Response.* New York: William Morrow & Co., 1975.
17 LeShan, L. *Cancer As A Turning Point: A Handbook for People with Cancer, their Families and Health Professionals.* New York: Plume, 1990.
18 Seligman, M. E. *Learned Optimism.* New York: A. A. Knopf, 1991.
19 Visintainer, M. A.; Volpicelli, J. R.; and Seligman, M. E. "Tumor Rejection in Rats After Inescapable or Escapable Shock." *Science* 216 no. 4544 (Apr,1982): 437-439.
20 Talbot, M. *The Holographic Universe.* New York: Harper Collins Publishers, 1991, p. 98-99.
21 Achterberg, J. *Imagery in Healing: Shamanism and Modern Medicine.* Boston MA: Shambala, 1985.
22 Cousins, N. *Head First: The Biology of Hope and the Healing Power of the Human Spirit.* New York: Penguin Books, 1989.
23 Becker, R. O., M.D.; and Murray, D. G. "The Electrical Control System Regulating Fracture Healing in Amphibians." *Clinical Orthopedics and Related Research.* 73 (Nov-Dec, 1970): 169-198.
Becker, R. O., M.D.; and Selden, G. *The Body Electric: Electromagnetism and the Foundation of Life.* New York: William Morrow and Company, Inc., 1985.
Becker, R. O., M.D. *Cross Currents. The Promise of Electromedicine. The Perils of Electropollution.* Los Angeles: Jeremy P. Tarcher, Inc., 1990.
24 Woolridge, D. E. *The Machinery of the Brain.* New York: McGraw- Hill Book Co., Inc., 1963.
25 Krieger, D. *Accepting Your Power To Heal: The Personal Practice of Therapeutic Touch.* Santa Fe, NM: Bear & Co. Publishing, 1993.
26 Quinn, J. F. "Therapeutic Touch as Energy Exchange: Testing the Theory." *Advances in Nursing Science* 6 no. 2 (Jan, 1984): 42-49.
27 Krieger, D. *The Therapeutic Touch: How to Use Your Hands to Help or Heal.* Englewood Cliffs, NJ: Prentice-Hall, 1979.
28 Samarel, N. "The Experience of Receiving Therapeutic Touch." *Advanced Nursing* 17 no. 6 (Jun, 1992), 651-657.
29 Montagu, A. *Touching: The Human Significance of the Skin.* New York: Harper and Row, 1978.
30 Weininger, O. "Physiological Damage Under Emotional Stress as a Function of Early Experience." *Science* 119 (Feb, 1954): 285-286.
31 Ornish, D., M.D. *Dr. Dean Ornish's Program for Reversing Heart Disease: the Only System Scientifically Proven to Reverse Heart Disease Without Drugs or Surgery.* New York: Random House, 1990.
32 Kobasa, S. C.; Maddi, S. R.; and Kahn, S. "Hardiness and Health: A Prospective Study." *Journal of Personality and Social Psychology* 42 no. 1 (Jan, 1982): 168-177.
33 Spiegel, D.; et al. "Effect of Psychosocial Treatment on Survival of Patients With Metastatic Breast Cancer." *Lancet* 2 no. 8668 (Oct, 1989): 888-891.
34 Berkman, L. F.; and Syme, S. L. "Social Networks, Host Resistance, and Mortality: A Nine-Year Follow-Up Study of Alameda County Residents." *American Journal of Epidemiology* 109 No. 2 (Feb, 1979): 186-204.
35 Achterberg, J. "Ritual: The Foundation for Transpersonal Medicine." *ReVision* 14 no. 3 (1992): (158-164).
36 Kellner, R.; et al. "Changes in Chronic Nightmares After One Session of Desensitization or Rehearsal Instructions." *American Journal of Psychiatry* 149 no. 5 (May, 1992): 659-663.
37 House, J. S.; Landis, K. R.; and Umberson, D. "Social Relationships and Health." *Science* 241 no. 4865 (Jul, 1988): 540-545.
38 Achterberg, J. *Imagery in Healing: Shamanism and Modern Medicine.* Boston MA: Shambala, 1985.
39 van Dixhoorn, J.; et al. "Cardiac Events After Myocardial Infarction: Possible Effects of Relaxation Therapy." *European Heart Journal* 8 no. 11 (Nov, 1987): 1210-1214.
40 Peper, E.; and Tibbetts, V. "Fifteen-Month Follow Up With Asthmatics Utilizing EMG/ Incentive Inspirometer Feedback." *Biofeedback and Self Regulation* 17 no. 2 (Jun, 1992): 143-151.

Naturopathic Medicine

1 From the preamble to the Constitution of the World Health Organization.
2 Banneman, R. H.; Burton, J.; and WenChieh, C. *Traditional Medicine and Health Care Coverage.* Geneva: World Health Organization, 1983.

Neural Therapy

1 Klinghardt, D. K., M.D.; and Wolfe, B., M.D., *Advanced Neural Therapy Workshop.* Santa Fe, NM. December 5-6, 1992.
Dosch, J. P., M.D. *Facts About Neural Therapy According to Huneke: Regulation Therapy- Brief Summary For Patients.* Portland, OR: Medicina Biologica, 1985.
2 Gleditsch, J., M.D.; and Hopfer, F., M.D. *Neural Therapy, Reflex Zones and Somatopies.* Carmel Valley, CA: American Academy of Biological Dentistry.
3 Klinghardt, D. K., M.D.; and Wolfe, B., M.D., *Advanced Neural Therapy Workshop.* Santa Fe, NM. December 5-6, 1992.
4 Ibid.
5 Dosch, J. P., M.D. *Facts About Neural Therapy According to Huneke: Regulation Therapy- Brief Summary For Patients.* Portland, OR: Medicina Biologica, 1985.
6 Ibid.
7 Pischinger, A. *Matrix and Matrix Regulation: Basis for a Holistic Theory in Medicine.* Brussels: Haug International, 1991.

Neuro-Linguistic Programming

1 Dilts, R.; Hallbom, T.; and Smith, S. *Beliefs: Pathways to Health and Well Being.* Portland, OR; Metamorphous Press, 1990, 1-2.
2 Ibid., 3-4.
3 Andreas, C. and S. *Heart of the Mind.* Moab, UT: Real People Press, 1989, 213-215.

Nutritional Supplements

1 Pao, E. M.; and Mickle, S. "Problem Nutrients in the United States." *Food Technology* (Sep, 1981):58-79.
2 Dietary Intake Source Data: U.S. 1976-1980. Data from the National Health Survey, Series 11, #231. DHHS Publication (PHS) 8361 (Mar, 1983).
3 Brin, M. "Erythrocyte as a Biopsy Tissue for Functional Evaluation of a Thiamine Adequacy." *Journal of the American Medical Association* 187 (1964): 762-766.
Brin, M. "Example of Behavioral Changes in Marginal Vitamin Deficiency in the Rat and Man." In *Behavioral Effects of Energy and Protein Deficits.* U.S.D.H.E.W., National Institutes of Health Publication No. 79-1906 (Aug, 1979):272-277.
Brin, M. "Drugs and Environmental Chemicals in Relation to Vitamin Needs." In *Nutrition and Drug Interrelations,* ed. J. Hathcock. New York: Academic Press, 1978, 131-150.
4 Machlin, L. J.; and Brin, M. "Vitamin E." In *Human Nutrition— A Comprehensive Treatise,* Vol. 3, eds. R. Alfin-Slater and D. Kritchevsky. New York: Plenum Press, 1980.
5 Horrobin, D. F. "Fatty Acid Metabolism in Health and Disease." *American Journal of Clinical Nutrition* 57 Suppl. (1993):7335.
6 Simpson, L. O. "The Etiopathogenisis of Premenstrual Syndrome as a Consequence of Altered Blood Rheology: A New Hypothesis." *Medical Hypotheses* 25 no. 4 (Apr, 1988):189-195.
7 Benton, D.; and Roberts, G. "Effect of Vitamin and Mineral Supplementation on Intelligence of a Sample of School Children." *Lancet* 1 no.8578 (Jan, 1988): 140-143.
8 Tucker, D. M.; et al. "Nutritional Status and Brain Function in Aging." *American Journal of Clinical Nutrition* 52 (1990):93-102.
9 Enstrom, J. E.; Kamin, L. E.; and Klein, M. A. "Vitamin C Intake and Mortality Among a Sample of the United States Population." *Epidemiology* 3 (1992):194-202.
10 Cathcart, R., M.D. "Vitamin C, Titrating to Bowel Tolerance, Anascorbemia, and Acute Induced Scurvy." *Medical Hypotheses* 7 (1981):1359-1376.
11 Stahelin, H. B.; et al. "Beta-Carotene and Cancer Prevention: The Basel Study." *American Journal of Clinical Nutrition* 53 Suppl.1 (Jan, 1991):265S-269S.
12 Street, D. A.; et al. "A Population-Based Case Control Study of the Association of Serum Antioxidants and Myocardial Infarction." *American Journal of Epidemiology* 131 (1991): 719-720.
13 Harvard Physicians Study. Ongoing.
14 Berge, K. G.; and Canner, P. L. "Coronary Drug Project: Experience with Niacin. Coronary Drug Project Research Group." *European Journal of Clinical Pharmacology* 40 Suppl.1 (1991): S49-S51.
15 Packer, L. "Protective Role of Vitamin E in Biological Systems." *American Journal of Clinical Nutrition* 53 no.4 (Apr, 1991): 1050S-1055S.
16 Factor, S. A. "Retrospective Evaluation of Vitamin E Therapy in Parkinson's Disease." Presented at: "Vitamin E: Biochemistry and Health Implications." New York Academy of Sciences Meeting, New York, Nov, 1988.
17 Braverman, E. R., M.D.; and Pfeiffer, C., M.D. *The Healing Nutrients Within: Facts, Findings, and New Research on Amino Acids.* New Canaan, CT:

Keats Publishing, 1987.

18 Shambaugh, G. E., jr., M.D. "Zinc: the Neglected Nutrient." *The American Journal of Otology* 10 no.2 (Mar, 1989):156-160.

19 Lewin, S. *Vitamin C: Its Molecular Biology and Medical Potential.* New York: Van Nostrand Reinhold Co., 1973.

20 Fujioka, T.; et al. "Clinical Study of Cardiac Arrhythmias Using 24-Hour Continuous Electrocardiographic Recorder (5th Report): Antiarrhythmic Addiction of Coenzyme Q10 in Diabetics." *Tohoku Journal of Experimental Medicine* 141 Suppl. (1983):453-463.

21 Rosenbaum, M. E., M.D.; and Bosco, D. *Super Fitness Beyond Vitamins: The Bible of Super Supplements.* New York: New American Library, 1987.

22 Preston, A. M. "Cigarette Smoking—Nutritional Implications." *Progress in Food and Nutrition Science* 15 no. 4 (1991):183-217.

23 Fulghum, D. D. "Ascorbic Acid Revisited." *Archives of Dermatology* 113 no. 1 (1977): 91-92.

24 Mustafa, M. G. "Biochemical Basis of Ozone Toxicity." *Free Radical Biology and Medicine* 9 no. 3 (1990): 245-265.

25 Haas, E. M., M.D. *Staying Healthy with Nutrition.* Berkeley, CA: Celestial Arts, 1992, 741.

26 Yankelovich; Clancy; and Schulman. "Survey for Nutritional Health Alliance 1992." *Whole Foods Magazine* 16 no. 3 (Mar, 1993): 55.

Orthomolecular Medicine

1 Kunin, R. A., M.D. "Orthomolecular Psychiatry." In *The Roots of Molecular Medicine: a tribute to Linus Pauling,* ed. R. P. Heumer, M.D. New York: W. H. Freeman & Co., 1986, 180-213.

2 Kunin, R. A., M.D. "Principles that Identify Orthomolecular Medicine: A Unique Medical Specialty." *Journal of Orthomolecular Medicine* 2 no. 4 (1987): 203-206.

3 Loomis, D. C. "Which Is Safer: Drugs or Vitamins?" *Townsend Letter for Doctors* 105 (April, 1992): 219.

4 Cathcart, R. F. "The Method of Determining Proper Doses of Vitamin C for the Treatment of Disease by Titrating to Bowel Tolerance." *Orthomolecular Psychiatry* 10 no. 2 (1981): 125-132.

5 Stahelin, H. B.; et al. "Beta-carotene and Cancer Prevention: the Basel Study." *American Journal of Clinical Nutrition* 53 (Jan, 1991): 265S-269S.

6 M R C Vitamin Study Research Group. "Prevention of Neural Tube Defects: Results of the Medical Research Council Vitamin Study." *Lancet* 338 no. 8760 (Jul, 1991): 131-137.

7 Whitehead, N.; Reyner, F.; and Lindenbaum, J. "Megaloblastic Changes in the Cervical Epithelium. Association with Oral Contraceptive Therapy and Reversal with Folic Acid." *Journal of the American Medical Association* 226 no. 12 (Dec, 1973): 1421-1424.

8 Kitay, D.; and Wentz, W. B. "Cervical Cytology in Folic Acid Deficiency of Pregnancy." *American Journal of Obstetrics and Gynecology* 104 no. 7 (Aug, 1969): 931-938.

9 Woods, K.; et al. "Intravenous Magnesium Sulfate in Suspected Acute Myocardial Infarction: Results of the Second Leicester Intravenous Magnesium Intervention Trial (LIMIT-2)." *Lancet* 339 no. 8809 (Jun, 1992): 1553-1558.

10 Evans, G. W. "The Effect of Chromium Picolinate on Insulin Controlled Parameters in Humans." *International Journal of Biosocial Medical Research* 11 no. 2 (1989): 163-180.

11 Anderson, R. A.; et al. "Effects of Supplemental Chromium on Patients with Symptoms of Reactive Hypoglycemia." *Metabolism: Clinical and Experimental* 36 no. 4 (Apr, 1987): 351-355.

12 Leaf, A.; and Weber, P. C. "Cardiovascular Effects of n-3 Fatty Acids." *New England Journal of Medicine* 318 no. 9 (Mar, 1988): 549-557.

13 Kojima, T.; et al. "Long-term Administration of Highly Purified Eicosapentaenoic Acid Provides Improvement of Psoriasis." *Dermatologica* 182 no. 4 (1991): 225-230.

14 van der Tempel, H.; et al. "Effects of Fish Oil Supplementation in Rheumatoid Arthritis." *Annals of the Rheumatic Diseases* 49 no. 2(Feb, 1990): 76-80.

15 Wright, J. V., M.D. *Dr. Wright's Guide To Healing With Nutrition.* New Canaan, CT: Keats Publishing, Inc., 1990.

Osteopathy

1 Lesser, M., M.D. *Nutrition and Vitamin Therapy.* New York: Bantam, 1981. Out of Print.

2 Korr, I. M. *Neurobiological Mechanisms in Manipulative Treatment.* New York: Plenum Press, 1979.

Korr, I. M. "The Spinal Cord as Organizer of the Disease Processes: IV Axonal Transport and Neurotrophic Function in Relation to Somatic Dysfunction." *Journal of American Osteopathic Association* 80 no. 7 (March, 1981): 451-459.

3 Purse, F. M. "Clinical Evaluation of Osteopathic Manipulative Therapy in Measles." *Journal of American Osteopathic Association* 61 (Dec, 1961): 274-276.

4 Purse, F. M. "Manipulative Therapy of Upper Respiratory Infections in Children." *Journal of American Osteopathic Association* 65 no. 9 (May, 1966): 964-972.

5 Fryett, H. H. *Principles of Osteopathic Technique.* Carmel, CA: American Academy of Osteopathy, 1970.

6 Still, A. T. *Philosophy of Osteopathy.* Colorado Springs, CO: American Academy of Osteopathy, 1975.

7 Chaitow, L. *Osteopathy: A Complete Health Care System.* London: Thorsons, 1982.

Oxygen Therapy

1 Warburg, O. "The Prime Cause and Prevention of Cancer," Revised lecture at the meeting of theNobel-laureates on June 30, 1966. National Cancer Institute, Bethesda, MD, 1967.

2 Perrin, D. Study in Britain, unpublished. Great Britain, 1993.

3 Farr, C. H. Presented at the Fourth International Conference on Bio-Oxidative Medicine. Reston, VA., April 1-4, 1993.

4 Farr, C. H. "Workbook on Free Radical Chemistry and Hydrogen Peroxide Metabolism Including Protocol for the Intravenous Administration of Hydrogen Peroxide." Contains 32 citations with references in the workbook, and 123 in the Protocol. Available from the International Bio-Oxidative Medicine Foundation. P.O. Box 13205, Oklahoma City, OK, 73113, 1992.

5 Farr, C. H. "The Therapeutic Use of Intravenous Hydrogen Peroxide." Genesis Medical Center, Oklahoma City, OK 73139, Jan, 1987.

6 Farr, C. H. "Workbook on Free Radical Chemistry and Hydrogen Peroxide Metabolism Including Protocol for the Intravenous Administration of Hydrogen Peroxide." Contains 32 citations with references in the workbook, and 123 in the Protocol. Available from the International Bio-Oxidative Medicine Foundation. P.O. Box 13205, Oklahoma City, OK, 73113, 1992.

7 Farr, C. H. "The Use of Dilute Hydrogen Peroxide to Inject Trigger Points, Soft Tissue Injuries and Inflamed Joints," International Bio-Oxidative Medicine Foundation, P.O. Box 13205 Oklahoma City, OK, 73113, 1992.

8 Farr, C.H. "Rapid Recovery from Type A/Shanghai Influenza Treated with Intravenous Hydrogen Peroxide." Geneses Medical Center, Oklahoma City, OK.

9 Haskell, R. "Case History: Multiple Sclerosis Patient." Proceedings of the First International Conference on Bio-oxidative Medicine. Dallas, TX (Feb. 17-19, 1989): 13.

10 Wells, K.H.; Latino, J.; Gavalchin, J.; Poiesz, P. "Inactivation of Human Immunodeficiency Virus Type I by Ozone In Vitro." Blood, 78(7) 1882-90, 1991.

11 Sweet, F.; Ka, M.; Lee, S. "Ozone Selectively Inhibits Growth of Human Cancer Cells." *Science.* 2009(72)931, 1990.

12 Forest, W. "Aids, Cancer Cured by Hyperbaric Oxygenation." *Townsend Letter for Doctors*, 105 (April, 1992): 231-238.

13 "Immunomodulating Effect of Great Masses of Ozone among Patients Presenting and Acquired Dysimmunity of Viral Origin." Proceedings, *Ninth Ozone World Congress*, Volume 3, New York, 1989. Sponsored by the International Ozone Association.

14 The off-the-record source states that, "When medical ozone use is discontinued, T-cell counts can drop quickly and steeply." "Therefore," he states, "a person should have another way of supporting T-cell levels before he stops ozone."

15 Schulz, S. "Effekte von Ozon/O_2 bei der Clindamycin-induzierten Enterocolitis beim sibirischem Zweghamster," *OzoNachrichten* 3 (1984): 2-16.

Qigong

1 Eisenberg, D., M.D. *Encounters With Qi.* New York: W.W. Norton and Co., 1985.

2 Chang, S., M.D. *The Complete System of Self-Healing: Internal Exercises.* San Francisco, CA: Tao Publishing, 1986.

3 Lee, R. H., ed. *Scientific Investigations into Chinese Qi-Gong.* San Clemente, CA: China Healthways Institute, 1992.

4 Li-da, F. "The effects of external Qi on bacterial growth patterns." *China Qi Gong* 1 (1983): 36.

5 Lee, R. H., ed. *Scientific Investigations into Chinese Qi-Gong.* San Clemente, CA: China Healthways Institute, 1992.

6 Jahnke, R. *The Self Applied Health Enhancement Methods.* Santa Barbara, California: Health Action Books, 1991.

Reconstructive Therapy

1 Hackett, G. *Ligament and Tendon Relaxation (skeletal disability) Treated by Prolotherapy (fibro-osseus proliferation).* 3d ed. Springfield, IL: Charles C. Thomas, 1958.

2 Maynard, J.; et al. "Morphological and Biochemical Effects of Sodium Morrhuate on Tendons." *Journal of Orthopaedic Research* 3 no. 2 (1985): 236-248.

3 Ongley, M. J.; et al. "A New Approach to the Treatment of Chronic Low Back Pain." *Lancet* 2 no. 8551 (Jul 18, 1987): 143-146.

4 Klein, R. G.; et al. "A Randomized Double-Blind Trial of Dextrose-Glycerine-Phenol Injections for Chronic, Low Back Pain." *Journal of Spinal Disorders* 6 no. 1 (Feb, 1993): 23-33.

5 Liu, Y. K.; et al. "An In Situ Study of the Influence of a Sclerosing Solution in Rabbit Medial Collateral Ligaments and Its Junction Strength." *Connective Tissue Research*, 11 nos. 2 and 3 (1983): 95-102.

Sound Therapy

1 Soibelman, D. *Therapeutic and Industrial Uses of Music: a Review of the Literature.* New York: Columbia University Press, 1948.

2 Wigram, T. "The Physical Effects of Sound." *British Society for Musical Therapy Bulletin* 7 (Autumn, 1989):15.

3 Black, D. *Healing With Sound.* Springville, UT: Tapestry Press, 1991.

4 Glass, L.; and Mackey, M. C. *From Clocks to Chaos: The Rhythms of Life.* Princeton, NJ: Princeton University Press, 1988.

5 Black, D. *Healing With Sound.* Springville, UT: Tapestry Press, 1991.

6 Campbell, D., ed. *Music Physician for Times to Come: An Anthology.* Wheaton, IL: Quest Books, 1991.

7 Spintge, R.; and Droh, R. "Towards Research Standards in Musicmedicine/Music Therapy: A Proposal For a Multimodal Approach." In *MusicMedicine.* eds. R. Sprintge and R. Droh. St. Louis: MMB Music, 1992, 345-349.

8 Lee, R. H., ed. *Scientific Investigations into Chinese Qui-Gong.* San Clemente, CA: China Healthways Institute, 1992, 18.

9 Stevens, K. M. "My Room— Not Theirs! A Case Study of Music During Childbirth." *Journal of the Australian College of Midwives* 5 no. 3 (Sep, 1992):27-30.

10 Gardner, W. J.; Licklider, J. C. R.; and Weisz, A. Z. "Suppression of pain by sound." *Science* 132 (Jul, 1960):32-33.

11 Kryter, K. D. *The Effects of Noise on Man*, 2d ed. New York: Academic Press, 1985, 449.

12 Podolsky, E., ed. *Music Therapy.* New York: Philosophical Library, 1954.

13 Lee, R.H., ed. *Scientific Investigations into Chinese Qui-Gong*. San Clemente, CA: China Healthways Institute, 1992, 18.
14 Manners, P. G. *Techniques and Theories for the Emerging Pattern of Current Research*. Monograph. Bretforton Hall Clinic. Bretforton, Vale of Worcestershire, WR 11 5JH, England.

Traditional Chinese Medicine

1 A Proposed Standard International Acupuncture Nomenclature: Report of a World Health Organization Scientific Group. Geneva, Switzerland: World Health Organization, 1991.
2 Kaptchuk, T. J. *The Web that Has No Weaver*. Chicago, IL: Congdon & Weed, 1983.
3 It would be impossible to cite every study from every journal around the world that might be relevant. A sampling of a few articles include:
Tani, T. "Treatment of Type I Allergic Disease with Chinese Herbal formulas: Minor Blue Dragon Combination and Minor Bupleurum Combination." *International Journal of Oriental Medicine* 14 no. 3 (Sep, 1989): 155-166.
Chen, A., M.D. "Effective Acupuncture Therapy for Migraine: Review and Comparison of Prescriptions with Recommendations for Improved Results." *American Journal of Acupuncture* 17 no. 4 (1989): 305-316.
Chen, G. S. "The Effect of Acupuncture Treatment on Carpal Tunnel Syndrome." *American Journal of Acupuncture* 18 no. 1 (1990): 5-10.
Chen, K.; and Liang, H. "Progress of Geriatrics Research in Chinese Medicine." *International Journal of Oriental Medicine* 14 no. 1 (Mar, 1989): 49-56.
4 Zhuang, H.; et al. "Effects of Radix Salviae Miltiorrhizae Extract Injection on Survival of Allogenic Heart Transplantation." *Journal of Traditional Chinese Medicine* 10 no. 4 (Dec, 1990): 276-281.
Lu, W. "Treatment of AIDS by TCM and Materia Medica." *Journal of Traditional Chinese Medicine* 11 no. 4 (Dec, 1991): 249-252.
Di Concetto, G., M.D.; and Sotte, L. "Treatment of Headaches by Acupuncture and Chinese Herbal Therapy: Conclusive Data Concerning 1000 patients." *Journal of Traditional Chinese Medicine* 2 no. 3 (Sep, 1991): 174-176.
5 Liu, F. "Application of Traditional Chinese Drugs in Comprehensive Treatment of Primary Liver Cancer." *Journal of Traditional Chinese Medicine* 10 no. 1 (Mar, 1990): 54-60. This study showed that TCM diagnosis could enhance the prognosticative accuracy of survival of patients with primary liver cancer and that Chinese herbal medicine allowed patients to recuperate to a point where they could successfully undergo surgery and complete regimens of chemotherapy, thus prolonging survival.

Veterinary Medicine

1 Stefanatos, J. *Holistic Pet Care*. Las Vegas, NV: Agape Video Systems, 1991.
2 Pitcairn, R. H.; and Pitcairn, S. H. *Natural Health for Dogs and Cats*. Emmaus, PA: Rodale Press, 1982.
3 Jerkins, C. P. "Acupuncture for Pets," *Animals* (Sep./Oct, 1988): 8.
4 Pitcairn, R. H.; and Pitcairn, S. H. *Natural Health for Dogs and Cats*. Emmaus, PA: Rodale Press, 1982.
5 Day, C. *The Homeopathic Treatment of Small Animals: Principles and Practice*. Essex, England: Saffron Walden, The C. W. Daniel Company Ltd., 1990.
6 Ibid.

Yoga

1 Studies include:
Telles, S.; and Desiraju, T. "Oxygen Consumption During Pranayamic Type of Very Slow-Rate Breathing." *Indian Journal of Medical Research* 94 (Oct, 1991): 357-363.
Singh, V.; et al."Effect of Yoga Breathing Exercises (Pranayama) on Airway Reactivity in Subjects With Asthma." *Lancet* 335 no. 9702 (Jun, 1990): 1381-1383.
2 Goleman, D. *The Meditative Mind*. Rev. ed. Los Angeles: Jeremy P. Tarcher, Inc. 1988.
3 Ibid.
4 Borysenko, J. *Minding the Body, Mending the Mind*. New York: Bantam Books, 1988.
5 Studies include:
Nespor, K. "Pain Management and Yoga." *International Journal of Psychosomatics* 38 no. 1-4 (1991):76-81.
Stancak, A., jr.; et al. "Observations on Respiratory and Cardiovascular Rhythmicities During Yogic High-Frequency Respiration." *Physiological Research* 40 no. 3 (1991): 345-354.
Brownstein, A. H.; and Dembert, M. L. "Treatment of Essential Hypertension With Yoga Relaxation Therapy in a USAF Aviator: A Case Report." *Aviation Space and Environmental Medicine* 60 no. 7 (Jul, 1989): 684-687.
6 Herzog, H.; et al. "Changed Pattern of Regional Glucose Metabolism During Yoga Meditative Relaxation." *Neuropsychobiology*, 23 no. 4 (1990-1991): 182-187.
7 Studies include:
Nespor, K. "Pain Management and Yoga." *International Journal of Psychosomatics,* 38 no. 1-4 (1991):76-81.
Stancak, A., Jr.; et al. "Observations on Respiratory and Cardiovascular Rhythmicities During Yogic High-Frequency Respiration." *Physiological Research* 40 no. 3 (1991): 345-354.
Brownstein, A. H.; and Dembert, M. L. "Treatment of Essential Hypertension With Yoga Relaxation Therapy in a USAF Aviator: A Case Report." *Aviation Space and Environmental Medicine* 60 no. 7 (Jul, 1989): 684-687.
8 Funderburk, J. *Science Studies Yoga: a Review of Physiological Data*. Honesdale, PA: Himalayan International Institute of Yoga Science & Philosophy of USA, 1977, 36-41.
9 Ibid., pages 93.
10 Ibid., pages 47-72.
11 Ibid., page 42.
12 Ibid., page 45.
13 Ibid., page 75.
14 Ibid., pages 73-74.
15 Ibid., page 21.
16 Uma, K.; et al. "The Integrated Approach of Yoga: A Therapeutic Tool for Mentally Retarded Children: A One Year Controlled Study." *Journal of Mental Deficiency Research* 33 no. 5 (Oct, 1989): 415-421.

Part Three: Health Conditions

Addictions

1 Wurtman, R. J. "Ways That Foods Can Affect the Brain." *Nutrition Reviews* 44 suppl. (May, 1986): 2-6.
2 Stephen, D., M.D. *Nutritional Medicine*. London: Pan Books, 1987.
3 Pizzorno, J. E.; and Murray, M. T. *A Textbook of Natural Medicine*. Seattle, WA: John Bastyr College Publications, 1985.
4 Ibid.
5 Bullock, M. L.; Culliton, P. D.; and Oleander, R. T. "Controlled Trial of Acupuncture for Severe Recidivist Alcoholism." *Lancet* 1 no. 8652 (Jun, 1989): 1435-1439.
NADA Newsletter Committee. *National Acupuncture Detoxification Association Newsletter* (December 1, 1992): 1-6.
6 Holder, J., M.D. "New Auricular Therapy Formula to Increase Retention of the Chemically Dependent in Residential Treatment." (1991) Research study funded by the State of Florida, Department of Health and Rehabilitive Services.
7 Editorial Staff. "Replacing Addiction with a Coping Skill." *Health and Wellness* 1 no.1 (Dec, 1991).

AIDS

1 Duesberg, P. H. "AIDS Acquired by Drug Consumption and other Noncontagious Risk Factors." *Pharmacological Therapy* 55 (1992): 2101-2177.
2 France, A. J. "Changing Case-Definition for AIDS." *Lancet* 340 no. 8832 (Dec, 1992): 1414.
Stewart, G. T. "Changing Case-Definition for AIDS." *Lancet* 340 no. 8832 (Dec, 1992): 1414.
3 Duesberg, P. H. "AIDS Acquired by Drug Consumption and other Noncontagious Risk Factors." *Pharmacological Therapy* 55 (1992): 2109.
4 Farber, C. "Fatal Distraction." *SPIN Magazine* 8 no. 3 (May, 1992): 36.
5 Farber, C. "AIDS: Words from the Front." *SPIN Magazine* (June, 1988): 73.
6 Ibid, 4.
7 Ibid.
8 Ibid, 36.
9 Guccione, B. "Interview with Peter Duesberg." *SPIN Magazine* (Sep, 1993).
10 Farber, C. "Fatal Distraction." *SPIN Magazine* 8 no. 3 (May, 1992): 36.
11 Reported by Doctors Jorge Eichberg and Krishna Murthy, of the Southwest Foundation for Biomedical Research.
12 "Report." *General Practitioner* 7 (Sep, 1987).
13 Chaitow, L.; and Simon, S. *A World Without AIDS*. London: Thorsons, 1989.
14 Learmont, J.; et al. "Long-Term Symptomless HIV-1 Infection in Recipients of Blood Products From a Single Donor." *Lancet* 340 no. 8824 (Oct, 1992): 863-867.
15 Farber, C. "Fatal Distraction." *SPIN Magazine* 8 no. 3 (May, 1992): 36.
Kolata, G. "Doctors Stretch Rules on AIDS Drug: Some Give Possibly Toxic AZT Before Syptoms Develop." *New York Times* 137 (Dec 21, 1987): A1. Dr. Douglas Dietrich, of the New York Medical Center, told *Times* reporter Gina Kolata, "I've followed patients who've had T-cell counts of less then 10 for a year, and nothing happened to them."
16 Cohen, S. S. "Antiretroviral Therapy for AIDS." *New England Journal of Medicine* 317 no. 10 (Sep, 1987): 629.
Dournon, E.; et al. "Effects of Zidovudine in 365 Consecutive Patients with AIDS and ARC." *Lancet* 2 no. 8623 (1988):1297-1302.
Duesberg, P. "AIDS Epidemiology." *PNAS* 88 (1991):1575.
Gill, P.; et al. "Azydomythmidine Associated with Bone Marrow Failure in Anti-Immune Deficiency Syndrome." *Annals of Internal Medicine* 107 no. 4 (1987): 502-505.
Richman, D.; et al. "Toxicity of AZT in Treating AIDS and ARC. The AZT Working Group." *New England Journal of Medicine* 317 (1987):192.
Smothers, K. "Pharmacology and Toxicology of AIDS Therapies." *The AIDS Reader* 1 (1991): 29.
Volberding, P. "Zidovudine in Asymptomatic Human Immunodeficiency Virus Infection." *New England Journal of Medicine* 322 (1990): 941.
Yarchoan, R.; et al. "Anti-Retroviral Therapy for AIDS." *New England Journal of Medicine* 317 (1987): 630.
17 Standish, L.; et al. "One Year Open Trial of Naturopathic Treatment of HIV Infection Class IV-A in Men." *Journal of Naturopathic Medicine* 3 no.1 (1992): 42-64.
18 Fischl, M.; et al. "Safety and Efficacy of AZT in Treatment of Subjects Mildly Symptomatic HIV Type 1 Infection." *Annals of Internal Medicine* 112 (1990): 727-737.
Volberding, P.; et al. "AZT in Asymptomatic HIV Infection : A Controlled Trial in Patients with Fewer than 500 CD4-Positive Cells per Cubic Millimeter." *New England Journal of Medicine* 322 (1990): 941.
19 Chaitow, L.; and Simon, S. *A World Without AIDS*. London: Thorsons, 1989, 91.
Campbell, D. "Living Positively." *New Statesman* 29 (Jan, 1989).
20 Campbell, D. "AIDS: The Race Against Time." *New Statesman* 6 (Jan, 1989).
Gavrzer, B. "Why Do Some People Survive AIDS." *Daily Breeze* (Sep 18, 1988).
Elliott, M. V. "AIDS— the Unheard Voices." BBC Television, November, 1987 (Meditel productions).
21 Standish, L.; et al. "One Year Open Trial of Naturopathic Treatment of HIV Infection in Class IV-A in Men." *Journal of Naturopathic Medicine* 3 no. 1 (1992): 42-64.
22 Brayton, R.; et al. "Effect of Alchohol and Various Diseases on Leukocyte Mobilization, Phagocytosis and Intracellular Bacterial Killing."

New England Journal of Medicine 2 no. 3 (1970): 123-128.
Saxena, A.; et al. "Immunomodulating Effects of Caffeine in Rodents." *Indian Journal of Experimental Biology* 22 no. 6 (1984): 293-301.
23 Crook, W. *The Yeast Connection.* Jackson, TN: Professional Books, 1984.
24 Chaitow, L.; and Trenev, N. *Probiotics.* New York: HarperCollins, 1990.
25 Mantera-Tienza, E.; et al. "Low Vitamin B6 in HIV Infection." *Fifth International Conference on AIDS* (Jun, 1989): 468.
26 Herbert, V. "Vitamin B12, Folate and Lithium in AIDS."
27 Harriman, G.; et al. "Vitamin B12 Malabsorption in AIDS." *Archives Internal Medicine* 149 no. 9 (1989): 2039-2041.
28 Dworkin, B.; et al. "Selenium Deficiency in AIDS." *Journal of Parenteral and Enteral Nutrition* 10 no. 4 (1986): 405-407.
29 Fabris, N.; et al. "AIDS, Zinc Deficiency and Thymic Hormone Failure." *Journal of the American Medical Association* 259 (1988): 839-840.
30 Pulse, T.; et al. "A Significant Improvement in a Clinical Pilot Study Utilizing Nutritional Supplements, Essential Fatty Acids, and Stabilized Aloe Vera Juice in 29 HIV Seropositive, ARC and AIDS Patients." *Journal for the Advancement of Medicine* 3 no. 4 (1990): 209-230.
31 Guitierrez, P. "Influence of Ascorbic Acid on Free Radical Metabolism of Xenobiotics." *Drug Metabolism Review* 18 nos. 3 and 4 (1989): 319-343.
Blakeslee, J.; et al. "Human T-cell Leukaemia Virus: Inhibition by Retinoids, Ascorbic Acid and Vitamin E." *Cancer Research* 45 (1985): 3471-3476.
Bouras, P.; et al. "Monocyte Locomotion - In Vivo Effect of Ascorbic Acid." *Immunopharmocology and Immunotoxicity* 11 no. 1 (1989): 119-129.
32 Cathcart, R., M.D. "Vitamin C in the Treatment of AIDS." *Medical Hypotheses* 14 (1984): 432-433
33 Sun, Y.; et al. "Preliminary Observation on the Effects of Chinese Herbs." *Journal of Biological Response Modifier* 2 (1983): 227-237.
34 Walker, M. "Carnivora Therapy for Cancer and AIDS." *Explore* 3 no. 5 (1992): 10-15.
Walker, M. "Carnivora and AIDS." *Townsend Letter for Doctors* (May, 1992): 351-359.
35 Stimpel, M.; et al. "Macrophage Activation and Induction of Cytotoxicity by Purified Polysaccharide Fractions from Echinacea Purpurea." *Infection and Immunity* 46 (1984): 845-849.
Wacker, A.; et al. "Virus Inhibition by Echinacea Purpurea." *Planta Medica* 36 Abe, N.; et al. "Interferon Induction by Glycyrrhizin." *Microbiology and Immunology* 26 no. 6 (1982): 535-539.
37 Sharma, R.; et al. "Berberine Tannate in Acute Diarrhea." *Indian Pediatrics Journal* 7 (1978).
Choudray, V.; et al. "Berberine in Giardiasis." *Indian Pediatrics Journal* 9 (1979): 143-146.
Sack, R.; et al. "Berberine Inhibits Intestinal Secretory Response in Vibrio Cholerae, E. Coli Enterotoxins." *Infection and Immunity* 35 no. 2 (1982): 471-475.
38 Adetumbi, M.; et al. "Allium Sativum: a Natural Antibiotic." *Medical Hypotheses* 12 (1983): 227-237.
Vahora, S.; et al. "Medicinal Use of Indian Vegetables." *Planta Medica* 23 (1973): 381-393.
"Garlic in Cryptococcal Meningitis." *Chinese Medical Journal* 93 (1980): 123-126.
39 Sharma, R.; et al. "Berberine Tannate in Acute Diarrhea." *Indian Pediatrics Journal* 7 (1978).
40 Brekhmann, E. *Man and Biologically Active Substances*. London: Pergamon Press 1980.
Takada, A.; et al. "Restoration of Radiation Injury by Ginseng." *Journal of Radiation* 22 (1981): 323-325.
41 Meruelo, D.; et al. "Therapeutic Agents with Dramatic Retroviral Activity." *Proceedings of National Academy of Sciences* 85 (1988): 5230-5234.
Someya, H. "Effect of a Constituent of Hypericum on Infection and Multiplication of Epstein Barr Virus." *Journal of Tokyo Medical College* 43 no. 5 (1985): 815-826.
Barbagallo, C.; et al. "Antimicrobial Activity of Three Hypericum Species." *Fitoteripia* LVIII no. 3 (1987): 175-177.
42 Zhang, Q. C. "Preliminary Report on the Use of Momordica Charantia Extract by HIV Patients." *Journal of Naturopathic Medicine* 3 no. 1 (1992): 65-69.
Baker, R. "MAP30: Momordica Anti-HIV Protein Research Notes." *BETA* (1991): 14.
Hierholzer, J.; et al. "In Vitro Effects of Monolaurin Compounds on Enveloped RNA and DNA Viruses." *Journal of Food Safety* 4 no. 1 (1982).
Sands, J.; et al. "Extreme Sensitivity of Enveloped Viruses to Long Chained Unsaturated Monoglycerides and Alcohols." *Antimicrobial Agents and Chemotherapy* 15 no. 1 (1979): 67-73.
Aoki, T.; et al. "Antibodies to HTLV-1 and HTLV-III in Sera from Two Japanese Patients." *The Lancet* 20 (Oct, 1984): 936-937.
43 Dharmaananda, S. "Chinese Herbal Therapies for the Treatment of Immunodeficiency Syndromes." *Oriental Healing Arts International Bulletin* 12 no. 1 (Jan, 1987): 24-38.
44 Orman, D.; and Margetis, D. "Effectiveness of Acupuncture and Chinese Phytomedicinals in the Treatment of HIV and AIDS." *Journal of Naturopathic Medicine* 3 no. 1 (1992): 80-82.
45 Smith, M., M.D.; and Rabinowitz, N., M.D. "Acupuncture Treatment of AIDS." Lincoln Hospital Acupuncture Clinic, New York City, March, 1985.
Smith, M., M.D. "Research in Use of Acupuncture with AIDS." *American Journal of Acupuncture* 16 no. 2 (April-June, 1988).
46 Chaitow, L.; and Martin, S. *A World Without AIDS.* London: Thorsons, 1989, 131.
47 Zhang, Q. C. "Preliminary Report on the Use of Momordica Charantia Extract by HIV Patients." *Journal of Naturopathic Medicine* 3 no. 1 (1992): 65-69.
48 Spire, B.; et al. "Inactivation of Lymphadenopathy-Associated Virus by Heat, Gamma Rays, and Ultraviolet Light." *The Lancet* 1 no. 8422 (Jan, 1985): 188-189.
49 Weatherburn, H. "Hyperthermia and AIDS Treatment." *British Journal of Radiology* 61 no. 729 (Sep, 1988): 862.
50 Standish, L.; et al. "One Year Open Trial of Naturopathic Treatment of HIV Infection Class IV-A in Men." *Journal of Naturopathic Medicine* 3 no. 1 (1992):42-64.
51 Nault, K. "AIDS, Cancer - An Answer (Ozone Therapy)." Report in *Crosswinds.* Santa Fe, NM, December, 1988, based on Associated Press wire services report October 28, 1988.
52 Well, K.; et al. "Inactivation of Human Immunodeficiency Virus Type 1 by Ozone in Vitro." *Blood* 78 (1991): 1882-1890.
53 Vallancien, B.; and Winkler, J. M. "Immunomodulating Effect of Ozone Among Patients with AIDS." *Conference Report*. New York:1989.
54 Solomon, G. "The Emerging Field of Psychoneuroimmunology." *Institutes for the Advancement of Health* 2 no. 1 (1985): 6-19.
55 Chaitow, L.; and Martin, S. *A World Without AIDS.* London: Thorsons, 1989, 131.
56 Chaitow, L. *Soft Tissue Manipulation.* Rochester, VT: Healing Arts Press, 1989.
57 Report in *Journal of Alternative and Complementary Medicine* (UK), December, 1992.

Allergies

1 Karjalainen, J.; et al. "A Bovine Albumin Peptide as a Possible Trigger of Insulin-Dependent Diabetes Mellitus." *New England Journal Of Medicine* 327 no. 5 (Jul,1992): 302-307.
2 Mansfield, J., M.D. *Arthritis: the Allergy Connection*. San Francisco, CA: Thorsons, 1990.
3 Lesser, M., M.D. *Nutrition and Vitamin Therapy.* Berkeley, CA: Parker House, 1982.
4 Eaton, S. B., M.D.; and Konner, M. "Palaeolithic Nutrition. A Consideration of its Nature and Current Implications." *New England Journal of Medicine* 312 no. 5 (Jan, 1985): 283-289.
5 Cathcart, R. F. III, M.D. "The Vitamin C Treatment Of Allergy And The Normally Unprimed State of Antibodies." *Medical Hypotheses* 21 no. 3 (Nov, 1986): 307-32.
6 Yanick, P., Jr. "Immune Disorders- Allergy." *Townsend Letter for Doctors* 118 (May, 1993): 498-500, 502.

Alzheimer's Disease and Senile Dementia

1 Evans, D. A., M.D. "Estimated Prevalence of Alzheimer's Disease in the United States." *Millbank Quarterly* 68 no. 2 (1990): 267-289.
2 Evans, D. A., M.D.; et al. "Prevalence of Alzheimer's Disease in a Community Population of Older Persons: Higher than Previously Reported." *Journal of the American Medical Association* 262 no. 18 (Nov, 1989): 2551-2556.
3 Mann, D. M.; and Esiri, M. M. "The Pattern of Acquisition of Plaques and Tangles in the Brains of Patients Under 50 Years of Age with Down's Syndrome." *Journal of the Neurological Sciences* 89 nos. 2-3 (Feb,1989):169-79.
4 Zatta, P.; et al. "Alzheimer Dementia and the Aluminum Hypothesis." *Medical Hypotheses* 26 (1988):139-142.
5 Editorial Staff. "Growing Evidence for Aluminum/Alzheimer's Link." *Clinical Psychiatry News* (Dec, 1988): 2.
6 Thompson; et al. Research study from the Sanders-Brown Center on Aging at the University of Kentucky Medical Center, Lexington, KY, published in *Neurotoxicology* 9 (1988):1.
7 Shiele, R.; et al. "Studies on the Mercury Content in Brain and Kidney Related to Number and Condition of Dental Fillings." Institution of Occupational and Social Medicine. University Erlangen, Nurnberg, West Germany. March 12, 1984.
8 Werbach, M. R, M.D. *Nutritional Influences on Mental Illness*. Tarzana, CA: Third Line Press, 1993.
Martin, D. C. "B_{12} and Folate Deficiency Dementia." *Clinics in Geriatric Medicine* 4 no. 4 (Nov, 1988): 841-52.
Thomas, D. E.; et al. "Tryptophan and Nutritional Status of Patients with Senile Dementia." *Psychological Medicine* 16 no. 2 (May,1986):297-305.
Keatinge, A. M.; et al. "Vitamin B_1, B_2, B_6 and C Status in the Elderly." *Irish Medical Journal* 76 (Dec, 1983): 488-90.
Gibson, G. E.; et al. "Reduced Activities of Thiamine-dependent Enzymes in the Brains and Peripheral Tissues of Patients with Alzheimer's Disease." *Archives of Neurology* 45 no. 8 (Aug, 1988):836-40.
Cole, M. G.; and Prchal, J. F. "Low Serum B_{12} in Alzheimer-Type Dementia." *Age and Ageing* 13 no. 2 (Mar,1984): 101-5.
Burns, A; and Holland, T. "Vitamin E Deficiency." *Lancet* 1 no. 8484 (Apr, 1986): 805-6.
Deary, I. J.; et al. "Serum Calcium Levels in Alzheimer's Disease: A Finding and an Aetiological Hypothesis." *Personality and Individual Differences* 8 no. 1 (1987):75-80.
Torizumi, K.; et al. "Relationship Between Parathyroid Hormone and Magnesium in Sera of Dementia Patients." *Radioisotopes* 37 no. 4 (Apr, 1988): 203-208.
Ward N. I.; and Mason, J. A. "Neutron Activation Analysis Techniques for Identifying Elemental Status in Alzheimer's Disease." *Journal of Radioanalytic Nuclear Chemistry* 113 no. 2 (1987): 515-26.
9 Imagawa, M.; et al. "Coenzyme Q10, Iron, and Vitamin B6 in Genetically Confirmed Alzheimer's Disease." *Lancet* 340 no. 8820 (Sep, 1992): 671.
10 *Journal of Nutrition Research* 1 :259-266.
11 *Physician's Desk Reference.* Oradell, NJ: Medical Economics Co., 1993.
12 Gautherie, M.; et al. "Vasodilator Effect of Gingko Biloba Extract Determined by Skin Thermometry and Thermography." *Therapie* 27 no. 5 (Sep-Oct, 1972):881-892.
Warburton, D. M. "Clinical Psychopharmacology of Gingko Biloba Extract." *Presse Medicale* 15 no. 31 (Sep, 1986):1595-1604.
Allard, M. "Treatment of the Disorders of Aging with Ginkgo Biloba Extract. From Pharmacology to Clinical Medicine." *Presse Medicale* 15 no. 31 (Sep, 1986): 1540-1545.
13 Crook, W. G., M.D. *Detecting Your Hidden*

Allergies. Jackson, TN: Professional Books, 1988.
14 McDonagh, E.; Rudolph, C.; and Cheraskin, E. "An Oculocerebrovasculometric Analysis of the Improvement in Arterial Stenosis Following EDTA Chelation Therapy." In *A Textbook on EDTA Chelation Therapy*, ed. E. Cranton. Special Issue, *Journal of Advancement in Medicine* 2 nos. 1-2. New York: Human Sciences Press, 1989, 155.
Casdorph, H. R. "EDTA Chelation Therapy: Efficacy in Brain Disorders." In *A Textbook on EDTA Chelation Therapy*, ed. E. Cranton. Special Issue, *Journal of Advancement in Medicine* 2 nos. 1-2. New York: Human Sciences Press, 1989, 131-153.
15 Warren, T. *Beating Alzheimer's.* Garden City Park, NY: Avery Publishing, 1991.
16 Ibid.

Arthritis

1 National Institutes of Health. "How to Cope With Arthritis." U.S. Department of Health and Human Services Public Health Service, NIH Publication no. 82-1092 (Oct, 1991).
2 National Institutes of Health. "1993 Research Highlights. Arthritis, Rheumatic Diseases, and Related Disorders." U.S. Department of Health and Human Services Public Health Service, NIH Publication no. 93-3413 (Jan, 1993).
3 "Briefing Paper for the Government Affair." *Arthritis Foundation Agenda* (Mar 19, 1993).
4 Pizzorno, J. E.; and Murray, M. T. *Encyclopedia of Natural Medicine.* Rocklin, CA: Prima Publishing, 1991.
5 Decker, J. L. "Arthritis." In *Medicine for the Layman*, U.S. Department of Health and Human Services, Public Health Service, National Institutes of Health Publication no. 83-1945 (Dec, 1982): 9-10.
6 di Fabio, A. *Gouty Arthritis.* Franklin, TN: The Rheumatoid Disease Foundation, 1989.
7 Pizzorno, J. E.; and Murray, M. T. *Encyclopedia of Natural Medicine.* Rocklin, CA: Prima Publishing, 1991.
8 Peat, R. F. "Hormone Balancing: Natural Treatment." *The Journal of the Rheumatoid Disease Medical Association* 1 no. 1 (1986).
9 Truss, C. O., M.D. *The Missing Diagnosis.* Birmingham, AL: C. Orion Truss, 1982.
Crook, W. G., M.D. *The Yeast Connection.* 3d ed. Jackson, TN: Professional Books, 1986.
Crook, W. G., M.D.; and Stevens, L. *Solving the Puzzle of Your Hard-To-Raise Child.* Jackson, TN: Professional Books, 1987.
10 Decker, J. L. "Arthritis." In *Medicine for the Layman*, U.S. Department of Health and Human Services, Public Health Service, National Institutes of Health Publication no. 83-1945 (Dec, 1982): 11.
11 di Fabio, A. *Treatment and Prevention of Osteoarthritis, Parts I and II.* Franklin, TN: The Rheumatoid Disease Foundation, 1989.
12 Decker, J. L. "Arthritis." In *Medicine for the Layman*, U.S. Department of Health and Human Services, Public Health Service, National Institutes of Health Publication no. 83-1945 (Dec, 1982): 11.
13 di Fabio, A. *The Art of Getting Well.* Franklin, TN: The Rheumatoid Disease Foundation, 1987.
di Fabio, A. *Treatment and Prevention of Osteoarthritis, Parts I and II.* Franklin, TN: The Rheumatoid Disease Foundation, 1989.
14 Pizzorno, J. E.; and Murray, M. T. *Encyclopedia of Natural Medicine.* Rocklin, CA: Prima Publishing, 1991.
15 Ibid.
16 Ibid.
17 di Fabio, A. *Treatment and Prevention of Osteoarthritis, Parts I and II.* Franklin, TN: The Rheumatoid Disease Foundation, 1989.
18 Pizzorno, J. E; and Murray, M. T. *Encyclopedia of Natural Medicine.* Rocklin, CA: Prima Publishing, 1991, 449.
19 Lee, T. H.; et al. "Effect of Dietary Enrichment with Eicosapentaenoic and Docosahexaenoic Acids on In Vitro Neutrophil and Monocyte Leukotriene Generation and Neutrophil Function." *New England Journal of Medicine* 312 no. 19 (May, 1985): 1217-1224.
20 Pizzorno, J. E; and Murray, M. T. *Encyclopedia of Natural Medicine.* Rocklin, CA: Prima Publishing, 1991, 494.
21 Bingham, R., M.D. *Fight Back Against Arthritis.* Franklin, TN: The Rheumatoid Disease Foundation, 1985.
22 This report is based solely on product labeling as published by PDR (R). Copyright (C) 1993 by Medical Economics Data, a division of Medical Economics Company, Inc. All rights reserved. There is no affiliation between Medical Economics Company, Inc., and Future Medicine Publishing, Inc.
23 Pauling, L. *How To Live Longer and Feel Better.* New York: Avon Books, 1987.
24 di Fabio, A. *The Art of Getting Well.* Franklin, TN: The Rheumatoid Disease Foundation, 1988.
25 Kaufman, W., M.D. "The Use of Vitamin Therapy to Reverse Certain Concomitants of Aging." *Journal of the American Geriatrics Society* 3 no. 11 (Nov, 1955): 927-936.
Kaufman, W., M.D. "Niacinamide: A Most Neglected Vitamin." *Journal of the International Academy of Preventive Medicine* 8 no. 1 (Winter, 1983).
Kaufman, W., M.D. *The Common Form of Joint Dysfunction: Its Incidence and Treatment.* Brattleboro, VT: E. L. Hildreth & Co., 1949.
26 Pizzorno, J. E.; and Murray, M. T. *A Textbook of Natural Medicine.* 2 vols. Seattle, WA: John Bastyr College Publications, 1989.
27 di Fabio, A. *The Art of Getting Well.* Franklin, TN: The Rheumatoid Disease Foundation, 1988.
28 Pizzorno, J. E.; and Murray, M. T. *A Textbook of Natural Medicine.* 2 vols. Seattle, WA: John Bastyr College Publications, 1989.
29 Pizzorno, J. E.; and Murray, M. T. *Encyclopedia of Natural Medicine.* Rocklin, CA: Prima Publishing, 1991, 337.
30 Ibid, 340.
31 Pizzorno, J. E.; and Murray, M. T. *A Textbook of Natural Medicine.* 2 vols. Seattle, WA: John Bastyr College Publications, 1989.
32 Ibid.
33 Bingham, R., M.D. "Yucca Extract," *The Journal of the Academy of Rheumatoid Diseases* 2 no. 1 (1990): 20.
34 Ibid.
35 Walker, M. "Biochemical Components of Sea Cucumber for Human Benefit." *EXPLORE!* 3 no. 6 (1992): 12-17.
36 Pizzorno, J. E.; and Murray, M. T. *A Textbook of Natural Medicine.* 2 vols. Seattle, WA: John Bastyr College Publications, 1989.
37 Heimlich, J. *What Your Doctors Won't Tell You.* New York: Harper Perennial, 1990.
38 Ibid.
39 Randolph, T. G., and Moss, R. W. *An Alternative Approach to Allergies* New York: Bantam, 1982.
40 Lane, I. W., M.D. "Shark Cartilage and the Pain of Arthritis." *EXPLORE!* 3 no. 6 (1992):23.
41 Ibid.
42 Ibid.
43 Ibid.
44 Rolf, I. *Rolfing: The Integration of Human Structures.* New York: Harper & Row Publishers, 1977.

Autism

1 Knivsberg, A.; et al. "Dietary Intervention in Autistic Syndrome." *Brain Dysfunction* 3 (1990):315-27.
2 Nanson, J. L. "Autism in Fetal Alcohol Syndrome: a Report of Six Cases." *Alcoholism, Clinical and Experimental Research* 16 no. 3 (1992):558-565.
3 Hashimoto, T.; et al. "Reduced Brainstem Size in Children with Autism." *Brain and Development* 14 no. 2 (1992):94-97.
4 Cohen, D. J.; Johnson, W. T.; and Caparulo, B. K. "Pica and Elevated Blood Lead Level in Autistic and Atypical Children." *American Journal of Diseases of Children* 130 no. 1 (Jan,1976):47-8.
Lesser, M. *Vitamin Therapy.* Berkeley, CA: Parker House, 1980.
Accardo, P.; et al. "Autism and Plumbism. A Possible Association." *Clinical Pediatrics* 27 no.1 (Jan, 1988):41-44.
5 McClelland, R. J.; et al. "Central Conduction time in Childhood Autism." *British Journal of Psychiatry* 160 (May, 1992):659-63.
6 George, M. S.; et al. "Cerebral Blood Flow Abnormalities in Adults with Infantile Autism." *Journal of Nervous and Mental Disease* 180 no. 7 (Jul, 1992):413-17.
7 Markowitz, P. I. "Autism in a Child with Congenital Cytomegalovirus Infection." *Journal of Autism and Developmental Disorders* 13 no. 3 (Sep, 1983):249-53.
8 Werbach, M. R., M.D. *Nutritional Influences on Mental Illness.* Tarzana, CA: Third Line Press, 1991,75.
9 Ibid.
10 Coulter, H. L. *Vaccination, Social Violence, and Criminality: The Medical Assault on the American Brain.* Berkeley, CA: North Atlantic Books, 1990.
11 Crook, W. G., M.D.; and Stevens, L. *Solving the Puzzle of Your Hard to Raise Child.* Jackson, TN: Professional Books, 1987.
12 Ibid.
13 Tollbert, L. C. "Ascorbic Acid: Therapeutic Trial in Autism." Presentation at the Autism Society of America Annual Conference, Indianapolis, IN, July 10-13, 1991.
14 Knivsberg, A.; et al. "Dietary Intervention in Autistic Syndrome." *Brain Dysfunction* 3 (1990): 315-27.
15 Crook, W. G., M.D.; and Stevens, L. *Solving the Puzzle of Your Hard to Raise Child.* Jackson, TN: Professional Books, 1987.
16 Philpott, W. H.; and Kalita, D. K. *Brain Allergies. The Psycho-Nutrient Connection.* New Canaan, CT: Keats Publishing, 1980.
17 Upledger, J. *Your Inner Physician and You, Craniosacral Therapy SomatoEmotional Release.* Berkeley, CA: North Atlantic, 1992.

Back Pain

1 Schatz, M. P., M.D. *Back Care Basics: A Doctor's Gentle Yoga Program for Back and Neck Pain Relief.* Berkeley, CA: Rodmell Press, 1992.
2 Ibid.
3 Foster, D. N.; and Fulton, M. N. "Back Pain and the Exercise Prescription." *Clinics in Sports Medicine* 10 no. 1 (Jan, 1991):197-209.
4 Feldenkrais, M. *Body and Mature Behavior: A Study of Anxiety, Sex, Gravitation, and Learning.* New York: International Universities Press, 1970.
5 Koes, B. W.; et al. "Randomized Clinical Trial of Manipulative Therapy and Physiotherapy for Persistent Back and Neck Complaints: Results of One Year Follow Up." *British Medical Journal* 304 no. 6827 (Mar, 1992): 601-605.
6 Meade, T. W.; et al. "Low Back Pain of Mechanical Origin: Randomised Comparison of Chiropractic and Hospital Outpatient Treatment." *British Medical Journal* 300 no. 6737 (Jun, 1990):1431-1437.
7 Shekelle, P.; et al. "Spinal Manipulation for Low Back Pain." *Annals of Internal Medicine* 117 no. 7 (Oct, 1992): 590-598.
8 Jarvis, K. B.; Phillips, R. B.; and Morris, E. K. "Cost per Case Comparison of Back Injury Claims: Chiropractic versus Medical Management for Conditions with Identical Diagnostic Codes." *Journal of Occupational Medicine* 33 no. 8 (Aug, 1991):847-852.
9 Schatz, M. P., M.D. *Back Care Basics: A Doctor's Gentle Yoga Program for Back and Neck Pain Relief.* Berkeley, CA: Rodmell Press, 1992.

Cancer

1 American Cancer Society. "Cancer Facts & Figures-1993."
2 Epstein, S. S. "Evaluation of the National Cancer Program and Proposed Reforms." *International Journal of Health Services* 23 no. 1 (1983): 15-44.
3 Kabelitz, D. "Modulation of Natural Killing by Tumor Promoters. The Regulatory Influence of Adherent Cells Varies with the Type of Target Cell." *Immunobiology* 169 no. 4 (May, 1985) : 436-446.
4 American Cancer Society. "Leading Sites of Cancer Incidence and Deaths-1993 Estimates." In "Cancer Facts & Figures - 1993."
5 Cleaver, J. E.; and Bootsma, D. "Xeroderma Pigmentosum: Biochemical and Genetic Characteristics." *Annual Review of Genetics* 9 (1975): 19-38.
Fialkow, P. J. "Clonal Origin and Stem Cell Evolution of Human Tumors." In *Genetics of Human Cancer*, eds. J. J. Mulvihill; R. W. Miller;

and J. F. Fraumeni, Jr. New York: Raven Press, 1977, 439-453.

Knudson, A. G. "Mutation and Human Cancer." *Advanced Cancer Research* 17 (1973): 317-352.

Knudson, A. G. "Genetics and Etiology of Human Cancer." *Advanced Human Genetics* 8 : 1-66.

6 Dreher, H. *Your Defense Against Cancer.* New York: Harper & Row, 1988, 18.

7 Ibid, 27.

8 Zakour, R. A., Kunkel, T. A.; and Loeb, L. A. "Metal-Induced Infidelity of DNA Synthesis." *Environmental Health Perspectives* 40 (Aug, 1981): 197-205.

9 American Institute for Cancer Research. "The Cancer Process." Washington, D.C., 1991.

10 Committee on Diet, Nutrition, and Cancer. Assembly of Life Sciences, National Research Council. *Diet, Nutrition and Cancer.* Washington, D.C.: National Academy Press, 1982.

11 Ibid.

12 Simone, C. B., M.D. *Cancer and Nutrition.* Garden City Park, NY: Avery Publishing Group Inc., 1992, 15.

13 Enig, M. G.; et al. "Dietary Fat and Cancer Trends." *Federal Proceedings* 37 (1978): 2215-2220.

14 Simone, C. B., M.D. *Cancer and Nutrition.* Garden City Park, NY: Avery Publishing Group Inc., 1992, 99.

15 Ibid, 50.

16 Bristol, J. B. "Colorectal Cancer and Diet: a Case-Control Study with Special Reference to Dietary Fibre and Sugar." *Proceedings of the American Association of Cancer Research* 26 (Mar, 1985): 206.

Bristol, J. B.; et al. "Sugar, Fat and the Risk of Colorectal Cancer." *British Medical Journal Clinical Research Edition* 291 no. 6507 (Nov, 1985): 1467-1470.

17 Letter. "Body Iron Stores and the Risk of Cancer." *New England Journal of Medicine* 320 no. 15 (Apr, 1990): 1012-1014.

18 Committee on Diet, Nutrition, and Cancer. Assembly of Life Sciences, National Research Council. *Diet, Nutrition and Cancer.* Washington, D.C.: National Academy Press, 1982.

19 Simon, D.; Yen, S.; and Cole, P. "Coffee Drinking and Cancer of the Lower Urinary System." *Journal of the National Cancer Institute* 54 no. 3 (Mar, 1975): 587-591.

20 Mulvehill, J. J. "Caffeine as Teratogen and Mutagen." *Teratology* 8 no. 1 (Aug, 1973): 69-72.

Weinstein, D.; Mauer, I.; and Solomon, H. M. "The Effects of Caffeine on Chromosomes of Human Lymphocytes: In Vivo and In Vitro Studies." *Mutation Research* 16 no. 4 (Dec, 1972):391-399.

21 Sandler, R. S. "Diet and Cancer: Food Additives, Coffee, and Alcohol." *Nutrition and Cancer* 4 no. 4 (1983): 273-278.

Editorial Staff. "Beer Drinking and the Risk of Rectal Cancer." *Nutrition Reviews* 42 no. 7 (Jul, 1984): 244-247.

Potter, J. D.; and McMichael, A. J. "Alcohol, Beer and Lung Cancer: a Meaningful Relationship?" *International Journal of Epidemiology* 13 no. 2 (Jun, 1984): 240-242.

22 Dreher, H. *Your Defense Against Cancer.* New York: Harper & Row, 1988, 113.

23 American Cancer Society. "Cancer Facts & Figures-1993."

Dreher, H. *Your Defense Against Cancer.* New York: Harper & Row, 1988, 149-150.

24 Abramson, R. "EPA Officially Links Passive Smoke, Cancer." *Los Angeles Times* 112 (Jun 8, 1993): A27.

25 Dreher, H. *Your Defense Against Cancer.* New York: Harper & Row,1988, 149.

26 Weinstein, A. L. ; et al. "Breast Cancer Risk and Oral Contraceptives Use: Results from a Large Case-Control Study." *Epidemiology* 2 no. 5 (Sep, 1991): 353-358.

27 Kushi, M., *The Cancer Prevention Diet.* New York: St. Martin's Press, 1983.

28 Wasserman, M.; et al. "Organochlorine Compounds in Neoplastic and Adjacent Apparently Normal Breast Tissue." *Bulletin of Environmental Contaminants and Toxicology* 15 (1976): 478-484.

29 Westin, J.; and Richter, E. "Israeli Breast Cancer Anomaly." *Annals of the New York Academy of Science* 609 (1990): 269-279.

30 Lowengart, R. A.; et al. "Childhood Leukemia and Parents' Occupational and Home Exposures." *Journal of the National Cancer Institute* 79 no. 1 (Jul, 1987): 39-46.

31 Davis, J. R., et al. "Family Pesticide Use and Childhood Brain Cancer." *Archives of Environmental Contamination and Toxicology* 24 no. 1 (Jan, 1993): 87-92.

32 "No Pest Strip Insecticide Poses an Unacceptably High Risk of Cancer in People and Pets." *Journal of Pesticide Reform* (Spring 1988): 29.

33 Ibid.

34 Simone, Charles B., M.D. *Cancer & Nutrition.* Garden City Park, New York: Avery Publishing Group Inc., 1992, 18, 21.

35 Steinman, D. *Diet For A Poisoned Planet.* New York: Ballantine Books, 1992, 265.

36 Maugh, T. H., II. "Experts Downplay Cancer Risk of Chlorinated Water." *Los Angeles Times* (July 2, 1992).

37 Yiamouyiannis, J.; and Burk, D. "Fluoridation and Cancer. Age-Dependence of Cancer Mortality Related to Artificial Fluoridation. " *Fluoride* 10 no. 3 (1977): 102-123.

38 Maugh, T. H., II. "Studies Stir Fears over Cancer Risks for Children." *Los Angeles Times* 111 (Nov 8, 1992): A1.

39 Recer, P. "EPA Studies Report Linking Power Lines, Some Cancer." *The Associated Press.*

40 Ezzell, C. "Power-Line Static. Debates Rage Over the Possible Hazards of Electromagnetic Fields." *Science News* 140 (Sep, 1991): 202-203.

41 Ibid.

42 Gardner, M. J., et al. "Results of Case-Control Study of Leukemia and Lymphoma Among Young People near Sellafield Nuclear Plant in West Cumbria." *British Medical Journal* 300 no. 6722 (1990):423-429.

43 Wing, S.; et al. "Mortality Among Workers at Oak Ridge National Laboratory: Evidence of Radiation Effects in Follow-Up Through 1984." *Journal of the American Medical Association* 265 no. 11 (1991): 1397-1402.

44 Simone, C. B., M.D. *Cancer and Nutrition.* Garden City Park, NY: Avery Publishing Group Inc., 1992, 20-21.

45 Ibid, 190.

46 Kinsella, A. R.; and Radman, M. "Tumor Promoter Induces Sister Chromatid Exchanges." *Proceedings of the National Academy of Sciences* 75 (1978): 6149-6153.

47 Bird, C. *The Divining Hands.* New York: Dutton, 1979.

48 United States Department of Health, Education, and Welfare. "Geomagnetism, Cancer, Weather, and Cosmic Radiation". Salt Lake City, UT, 1979.

49 Warburg, O. "On the Origin of Cancer Cells." *Science* 123 (1956): 309-315.

50 Walters, R. "Enderlein Therapy: a Cancer Therapy that Promotes Gentle Self-healing." *Raum & Zeit* 3 no. 1 (1991): 24.

51 Ader, R., ed. *Psychoneuroimmunology.* New York: Academic Press, 1981.

52 Bloom, B. L.; Asher, S. J.; and White, S. W. "Marital Disruption as a Stressor: A Review and Analysis." *Psychological Bulletin* 85 no. 4 (1978): 867-894.

Fox, B. H. "Premorbid Psychological Factors as Related to Cancer Incidence." *Journal of Behavioral Medicine* 1 no. 1 (1978):45-133.

53 Bloom, B. L.; Asher, S. J.; and White, S. W. "Marital Disruption as a Stressor: A Review and Analysis." *Psychological Bulletin* 85 no. 4 (1978): 867-894.

LeShan, L. L. "An Emotional Life History Pattern Associated with Neoplastic Disease." *Annals of the New York Academy of Sciences* 125 no. 3 (1966):780-793.

Ernster, B. L.; et al. "Cancer Incidence by Marital Status: U.S. Third National Cancer Survey." *Journal of the National Cancer Institute* 63 no. 3 (1979): 567-585.

54 Greer, S.; and Morris, T. "Psychological Attributes of Women Who Develop Breast Cancer: A Controlled Study." *Journal of Psychosomatic Research* 19 no. 2 (Apr, 1975):147-153.

Horne, R. L.; and Picard, R. S. "Psychosocial Risk Factors for Lung Cancer." *Psychosomatic Medicine* 41 no. 7 (Nov, 1979): 503-514.

Paykel, E. S. "Recent Life Events in the Development of Depressive Disorders." In *The Psychobiology of the Depressive Disorders*, ed. R. A. Depue. New York: Academic Press, 1979.

55 Rogentine, G. N., Jr; et al. "Psychological Factors in the Prognosis of Malignant Melanoma: A Prospective Study." *Psychosomatic Medicine* 41 (1979): 647-655.

Greer, S.; and Morris, T. "Psychological Attributes of Women Who Develop Breast Cancer: A Controlled Study." *Journal of Psychosomatic Research* 19 (1975):147-153.

56 Dreher, H. *Your Defense Against Cancer.* New York: Harper & Row, 1988, 246-247.

57 Ibid, 200-209.

58 Brown, R. K., M.D. *AIDS, Cancer and the Medical Establishment.* New York: Robert Speller Publishers, 1986, 93-95, 97-99.

59 Walters, R. "Enderlein Therapy: a Cancer Therapy that Promotes Gentle Self-Healing." *Raum & Zeit* 3 no. 1 (1991): 24.

60 Ibid.

62 Brown, R. K., M.D. *AIDS, Cancer and the Medical Establishment.* New York: Robert Speller Publishers, 1986, 92.

62 Committee on Diet, Nutrition, and Cancer. Assembly of Life Sciences, National Research Council. *Diet, Nutrition and Cancer.* Washington, D.C.: National Academy Press, 1982.

63 Dreher, H. *Your Defense Against Cancer.* New York: Harper & Row, 1988, 38.

64 Committee on Diet, Nutrition, and Cancer. Assembly of Life Sciences, National Research Council. *Diet, Nutrition and Cancer.* Washington, D.C.: National Academy Press, 1982.

65 Goldin, B. R.; et al. "Estrogen Excretion Patterns and Plasma Levels in Vegetarian and Omnivorous Women." *New England Journal of Medicine* 307 (1982): 1542-1547.

66 Committee on Diet, Nutrition, and Cancer. Assembly of Life Sciences, National Research Council. *Diet, Nutrition and Cancer.* Washington, D.C.: National Academy Press, 1982.

67 Enig, M. G.; et al. "Dietary Fat and Cancer Trends." *Federal Proceedings* 37 (1978): 2215-2220.

68 Dreher, H. *Your Defense Against Cancer.* New York: Harper & Row, 1988, 113.

69 Bristol, J. B. "Colorectal Cancer and Diet: a Case-Control Study with Special Reference to Dietary Fibre and Sugar." *Proceedings of the American Association of Cancer Research* 26 (Mar, 1985): 206.

Bristol, J. B.; et al. "Sugar, Fat and the Risk of Colorectal Cancer." *British Medical Journal* 291 no. 6507 (Nov, 1985): 1467-1470.

70 Simon, D.; Yen, S.; and Cole, P. "Coffee Drinking and Cancer of the Lower Urinary System."*Journal of the National Cancer Institute* 54 no. 3 (Mar, 1975): 587-591.

Mulvehill, J. J. "Caffeine as Teratogen and Mutagen." *Teratology* 8 no. 1 (Aug, 1973): 69-72.

Weinstein, D.; Mauer, I.; and Solomon, H. M. "The Effects of Caffeine on Chromosomes of Human Lymphocytes: In Vivo and In Vitro Studies." *Mutation Research* 16 no. 4 (Dec, 1972): 391-399.

71 Sandler, R. S. "Diet and Cancer: Food Additives, Coffee and Alcohol." *Nutrition and Cancer* 4 no. 4 (1983): 273-279.

Editorial Staff. "Beer Drinking and the Risk of Rectal Cancer." *Nutrition Reviews* 42 no. 7 (Jul, 1984): 244-247.

Potter, J. D.; and McMichael, A. J. "Alcohol, Beer and Lung Cancer: a Meaningful Relationship?" *International Journal of Epidemiology* 13 no. 2 (1984): 240-242.

72 Smith, B. "Organic Foods vs. Supermarket Foods: Element Level." *Journal of Applied Nutrition* 45 no. 1 (1993): 35-39.

73 "Study Finds Vitamins Cut Cancer Deaths." *Los Angeles Times* (Sep 15, 1993).

74 Colditz, G. A.; et al. "Increased Green and Yellow Vegetable Intake and Lowered Cancer Deaths in an Elderly Population." *American Journal of Clinical Nutrition* 41 (1985): 32-36.

75 La Vecchia, C.; et al. "Dietary Vitamin A and the Risk of Invasive Cervical Cancer." *Interna-*

tional Journal of Cancer* 34 no. 3 (Sep,1984): 319-322.
76 Menkes, M. S.; et al. "Serum Beta-Carotene, Vitamins A, and E, Selenium and the Risk of Lung Cancer." *New England Journal of Medicine* 315 (1986): 1250.
77 "Dietary Aspects of Carcinogenesis." (Sep, 1983).
78 Ramaswamy, P.; and Natarajan, R. "Vitamin B-6 Status in Patients with Cancer of the Uterine Cervix." *Nutrition and Cancer* 6 (1984): 176-180.
79 Stahelin, H. B.; et al. "Cancer, Vitamins, and Plasma Lipids: Prospective Basel Study." *Journal of the National Cancer Institute* 73 (1984): 1463-1468.
80 Ibid.
81 Willett, W. C.; and MacMahon, B. "Prediagnosistic Serum Selenium and the Risk of Cancer." *Lancet* 2 no. 8342 (Jul, 1983): 130-134.
82 Butterworth, C. E.; et al. "Improvement in Cervical Dysplasia Associated with Folic Acid Therapy in Users of Oral Contraceptives." *American Journal of Clinical Nutrition* 35 no. 1 (Jan, 1982): 73-82.
82 Slattery, M. L.; Sorenson, A. W.; and Ford, M. H. "Dietary Calcium Intake as a Mitigating Factor in Colon Cancer." *American Journal of Epidemiology* 128 no. 3 (Sep, 1988): 504-514.
83 Stadel, V. W. "Dietary Iodine and the Risk of Breast, Endometrial, and Ovarian Cancer." *Lancet* 1 no. 7965 (Apr, 1976): 890-891.
85 Blondell, J. M. "The Anticarcinogenic Effect of Magnesium." *Medical Hypotheses* 6 no. 8 (Aug, 1980): 863-871.
86 Whelen, P.; Walker, B. E.; and Kelleher, J. "Zinc, Vitamin A and Prostatic Cancer." *British Journal of Urology* 55 no. 5 (Oct, 1983): 525-528.
87 Kroning, F. "Garlic as an Inhibitor for Spontaneous Tumors in Mice." *Acta Unio. Intern. Contra Cancrum.* 20 no. 3 (1964): 855.
88 Wynder, E. L.; Rose, D. P.; and Cohen, L. A. "Diet and Breast Cancer in Causation and Therapy." *Cancer* 58 no. 8 suppl. (Oct, 1986): 1804-183l.
89 Greenward, P.; and Lanza, E. "Dietary Fiber and Colon Cancer." *Contemporary Nutrition* 11 no. 1 (1986).
90 Committee on Diet, Nutrition, and Cancer. Assembly of Life Sciences, National Research Council. *Diet, Nutrition and Cancer*. Washington, D.C.: National Academy Press, 1982.
91 Steinman, D.; and Epstein, S. S. *The Safe Shopper's Bible*. New York: Macmillan Publishing Group, 1994 (In Press).
92 Ibid.
93 Berkman, L. F., and Syme, S. L. "Social Networks, Host Resistance, and Mortality: a Nine-Year Follow-Up Study of Alameda County Residents." *American Journal of Epidemiology* 109 no. 2 (Feb, 1979): 189-204.
94 Spiegel, D.; et al. "Effect of Psychosocial Treatment on Survival of Patients with Metastatic Breast Cancer." *Lancet* 2 no. 8668 (Oct, 1989): 888-891.
95 Derogatis, L. R. et al. "Psychological Coping Mechanisms and Survival Time in Metastatic Breast Cancer." *Journal of the American Medical Association* 242 no. 14 (Oct, 1979):1504-1508.
96 Miller, A. B. "War on Breast Cancer Screening." *Cancer Forum* 1 no. 3 (Mar, 1988).
97 Dardick, G. "Breast Self-Examine: A New Program Makes Early Detection Easier." *East-West* (Jul/Aug, 1991): 32-36.
98 Epstein, S. S.; and Steinman, D. *New Hope: Everything You Wanted to Know About Breast Cancer Prevention But The Cancer Establishment Never Told You: A Guide for Dramatically Reducing Your Risk.* New York: Macmillan Publishing Group, 1993. (In Press.)
99 Lynes, B. *The Healing Of Cancer.* Queensville, Ontario, Canada: Marcus Books, 1989, 10.
100 Cairns, J., M.D. "The Treatment of Diseases and the War Against Cancer." *Scientific American.* (Nov, 1985).
101 Fisher, B.; et al. "Five-Year Results of a Randomized Clinical Trial Comparing Total Mastectomy and Segmental Mastectomy With or Without Radiation in the Treatment of Breast Cancer." *New England Journal of Medicine* 11 (Mar, 1985): 312.
102 Curtis, R. E.; et al. "Risk of Leukemia Associated With the First Course of Cancer Treatment: an Analysis of the Surveillance, Epidemiology, and End Results Program Experience." *Journal of the National Cancer Institute* 72 no. 3 (Mar, 1984): 531-544.
103 Burzynski, S., M.D. "Antineoplastons." From a lecture presented at the October 7, 1990 World Research Foundation Congress, Los Angeles, CA.
104 Burzynski, S., M.D. "Synthetic Antineoplastons and Analogs." *Drugs Of The Future* 11 no. 8 (1986): 679.
105 Ibid.
106 Burzynski, S., M.D. "Antineoplastons." From a lecture presented at the October 7, 1990 World Research Foundation Congress, Los Angeles, CA.
107 Moss, R. *The Cancer Industry*. New York: Paragon House, 1991.
108 "Is There A Body Defense Parallel To The Immune System?: Differentiation Inducers in the Treatment of Cancer and Viral Infections." A symposium presented at the 18th International Congress of Chemotherapy, Stockholm, Sweden, July 1, 1993.
109 Burzynski, S., M.D. "Antineoplastons." From a lecture presented at the October 7, 1990 World Research Foundation Congress, Los Angeles, CA.
110 The National Cancer Institute, Cancer Information Service, January 6, 1992. (The statement reads: "The National Cancer Institute reviewed 7 cases of primary brain tumors that were treated by Dr. Burzynski with antineoplastons A10 and AS2-1 and concluded that antitumor responses occurred.")
111 Burzynski, S., M.D. "Antineoplastons." From a lecture presented at the October 7, 1990 World Research Foundation Congress, Los Angeles, CA.
112 Walters, R. *Options: The Alternative Cancer Therapy Book*. Garden City Park, NY: Avery Publishing Group, Inc. 1993, 26.
113 "Special Hearing on Alternative Medicine." Subcommittee of the Committee on Appropriations, United States Senate. June 24, 1993, 36-41.
114 Naessens, G. "714X: A Highly Promising Non-Toxic Treatment for Cancer and Other Immune Deficiencies." In *Patrons of Writers Enterprise & Research Institutional Review Board.* 10th ed. January, 1993.
115 "Special Hearing on Alternative Medicine." Subcommittee of the Committee on Appropriations, United States Senate. June 24, 1993, 104.
116 Filov, V.; et al. "Results of Clinical Study of the Preparation Hydrazine Sulfate." *Voprosy Onkologii* 36 no. 6 (1990):721-726.
117 Chlebowski, R. T., et al. "Hydrazine Sulfate in Cancer Patients with Weight Loss: A Placebo-Controlled Clinical Experience." *Cancer* 59 no. 3 (Feb, 1987):406-410.
Chlebowski, R. T.; et al. "Influence of Hydrazine Sulfate on Abnormal Carbohydrate Metabolism in Cancer Patients with Weight Loss." *Cancer Research* 44 no. 2 (Feb, 1984):857-861.
Chlebowski, R. T.; et al. "Hydrazine Sulfate Influence on Nutritional Status and Survival in Non-Small Cell Lung Cancer." *Journal of Clinical Oncology* 8 no. 1 (Jan, 1990): 9-15.
118 Lane, W.I. and Cormac, L. *Sharks Don't Get Cancer.* Garden City Park, NY: Avery Publishing, 1992, p. 47.
119 Maugh, T. H., II. "Angiogenesis Inhibitors Link Many Diseases." *Science* 212 no. 4501 (Jun, 1981): 1374- 1375.
120 Lane, W. I. and Cormac, L. *Sharks Don't Get Cancer.* Garden City Park, NY: Avery Publishing, 1992, p. 47.
121 Standish, L.; et al. "One Year Open Trial of Naturopathic Treatment of HIV Infection in Class 1V-A Men." *The Journal of Naturopathic Medicine* 3 no. 1 (1992): 42-64.
122 Williams, D. G. "The Final Results of the First Cuban Study." *Alternatives Newsletter* 4 no. 20 (Feb, 1993).
123 Duarte, A. *Jaws for Life: The Story of Shark Cartilage.* Grass Valley, CA, Duarte, 1993.
124 "Special Hearing on Alternative Medicine." Subcommittee of the Committee on Appropriations, United States Senate. June 24, 1993, 69.
125 Duarte, A. *Jaws for Life: The Story of Shark Cartilage.* Grass Valley, CA, Duarte, 1993.
126 Manner, H. W.; et al. "Amygdalin, Vitamin A and Enzyme Induced Regression of Murine Mammay Adenocarcinomas." *Journal of Manipulative and Physiological Therapeutics* 1 no. 4 (Dec, 1978): 246-248.
127 Ibid.
128 Ericson, R. *Cancer Treatment: Why So Many Failures?* Memorial Park Ridge, IL: GE-PS Cancer Memorial, 1979, 68.
129 Ibid, 62-67.
130 Cheraskin, E. *Vitamin C: Who Needs It?* Birmingham, AL: Arlington Press, 1993, 81.
131 Ibid.
132 Ibid.
133 Hoffer, A.; Pauling, L.; and Jones, H. "Biostatistical Analysis of Mortality Data for Cohorts of Cancer Patients with a Large Fraction Surviving at the Termination of the Study and a Comparison of Survival Times of Cancer Patients Receiving Large Regular Oral Doses of Vitamin C and other Nutrients with Similar Patients Not Receiving Those Doses." *Journal of Orthomolecular Medicine* 5 no. 3: 142-149.
134 Dr. Lawrence Burton, as told to Taffi McCallum on the Taffi McCallum Radio Show, WINZ, Miami, Florida, 1987.
135 Ibid.
136 Ibid.
137 From a taped lecture by Dr. Livingston given at the Cancer Control Convention, Pasadena, California, 1988.
138 Walters, R. *Options: The Alternative Cancer Therapy Book,* Garden City, NY: Avery Publishing Group, 1993, 75.
139 Livingston-Wheeler, V., M.D. *The Conquest of Cancer: Transcript From A Videotape Program.* Waterside Productions. San Diego, CA, 1984, 25.
140 Ibid, 26, 29.
141 Duerksan, S. "Skeptical Scientists Test Alleged 'Cancer Vaccine'." *Townsend Letter for Doctors* 47 (May, 1987).
142 *Cancer: A Healing Crisis*. Cancer Resource Center, Los Angeles, California, 1980, xiii.
143 Ibid.
144 Houston, R. G. *Repression and Reform in the Evaluation of Alternative Cancer Therapies*. Washington, D.C.: Project Cure, 1987, 33.
145 "Special Hearing on Alternative Medicine." Subcommittee of the Committee on Appropriations, United States Senate. June 24, 1993, 180-182.
146 Ibid, 181.
147 Gerson, M., M.D. *A Cancer Therapy: Results of Fifty Cases*. 5th ed. Bonita, CA: Gerson Institute,1990.
148 Wolf, M.; and Ransberger, K. *Enzyme Therapy*. Los Angeles, CA: Regent House, 1972, 135-146.
149 James, W. "Nutrition and Cancer: The Gonzales Story." *World Research Foundation News* 3rd & 4th Quarter(1990): 5.
150 Ibid, 4.
151 "Special Hearing on Alternative Medicine." Subcommittee of the Committee on Appropriations, United States Senate. June 24, 1993, 65.
152 Hoxey, H. *You Don't Have To Die*. New York: Milestone Books, 1956.
153 Ausubel, K. "The Troubling Case of Harry Hoxsey." *New Age Journal* (Jul/Aug, 1988): 79.
154 *Cancer Chronicles* 2 no. 2 (Aug, 1990): 5.
155 Kazuyoshi, M.; Tsunero, K.; and Namiki, M. "A Desmutagenic Factor Isolated From Burdock (*Arctium lappa linne*)." *Mutation Research* 129 (1984): 25-31.
156 Hoxey, H. *You Don't Have To Die*. New York: Milestone Books, 1956.

Candidiasis

1 Rosenbaum, M., M.D.; and Susser, M., M.D. *Solving the Puzzle of Chronic Fatigue Syndrome.* Tacoma, WA: Life Sciences Press, 1992.
2 Marshall, R. "Resistant Polysystemic Candidiasis and Coincident Immuno-Suppressant Factors." *Journal of Alternative and Complementary Medicine* (May/Jun, 1993).

3 Editorial Staff. "Contributions of Micro-Organisms to Foods and Nutrition." *Nutrition News* 38 no. 4 (1975).
Speck, M. "Natural Antibiotic Activity of Lactobacillus Acidophilus and Bulgaricus." *Cultured Dairy Products Journal* 18 no. 2 (Jul, 1983).
4 Bland, J., ed. *Medical Application of Clinical Nutrition.* New Canaan, CT: Keats Publishing, 1983.
5 Truss, C. O. *Journal of Orthomolecular Psychiatry* 13 no. 2 (1984).
6 Pizzorno, J. E.; and Murray, M. T. *A Textbook of Natural Medicine.* 2 vols. Seattle, WA: John Bastyr College Publications, 1989.
7 Sehnert, K. W., M.D.; and Mathews-Larson, J. *International Journal of Biosocial and Medical Research* 13 no. 1 (1991): 67-76.
8 Ibid.
9 Pizzorno, J. E.; and Murray, M. T. *A Textbook of Natural Medicine.* 2 vols. Seattle, WA: John Bastyr College Publications, 1989.
10 Rosenbaum, M., M.D.; and Susser, M., M.D. *Solving the Puzzle of Chronic Fatigue Syndrome.* Tacoma, WA: Life Sciences Press, 1992, 131.
11 Trowbridge, J.; and Walker, M. *The Yeast Syndrome.* New York: Bantam Books, 1986.
12 Pizzorno, J. E.; and Murray, M. T. *A Textbook of Natural Medicine.* 2 vols. Seattle, WA: John Bastyr College Publications, 1989.
13 Chaitow, L. *Post Viral Fatigue Syndrome.* London: Dents, 1989.
14 Pizzorno, J. E.; and Murray, M. T., eds. *A Textbook of Natural Medicine.* Seattle, WA: John Bastyr College Publications, 1988-89.

Children's Health

1 Dees, S. C.; and Lefkowitz, D., III. "Secretory Otitis Media in Allergic Children." *American Journal of Diseases of Children* 124 no. 3 (Sep, 1972): 364-368.
2 Ruokonen, J.; Paganus, A.; and Lehti, H. "Elimination Diets in the Treatment of Secretory Otitis Media." *International Journal of Pediatric Otorhinolaryngology* 4 no. 1 (Mar, 1982): 39-46.
3 Cantekin, E. I.; McGuire, T. W.; and Griffith, T. L. "Antimicrobial Therapy for Otitis Media with Effusion." *Journal of the American Medical Association* 266 no. 23 (Dec. 18, 1991): 3309-3317.
4 Diamant, M.; and Diamant, B. "Abuse and Timing of Use of Antibiotics in Acute Otitis Media." *Archives of Otolaryngology* 100 no. 3 (Sep, 1974): 226-32.
5 Coulter, H. L.; and Fisher, B. L. *DPT— A Shot in the Dark.* San Diego, CA: Harcourt Brace Jovanovich, 1985.
Coulter, H. L. *Vaccination, Social Violence, and Criminality: The Medical Assault on the American Brain.* Berkeley, CA: North Atlantic Books, 1990.
6 Berkow, R., M.D.; and Fletcher, A. J., eds. *The Merck Manual of Diagnosis and Therapy.* 16th ed. Rahway, NJ: Merck & Co., 1992, 2167.
7 Miller, N. Z. *Vaccines: Are They Really Safe and Effective.* Santa Fe, NM: New Atlantean Press, 1992.
8 Kalokerinos, A., M.D.. *Every Second Child.* New Canaan, CT: Keats Publishing, Co., 1981.
9 Food and Drug Administration. Press Release in *Adverse Events Associated with Childhood Vaccines: Evidence Bearing on Causality.* Vienna, VA: National Academy Press, Sep, 1993.
10 Bluestone, C. D., M.D. "Eustachian Tube Function and Allergy in Otitis Media." *Pediatrics* 61 no. 5 (May, 1978): 753-760.
11 Saarinen, U. M. "Prolonged Breast Feeding as Prophylaxis for Recurrent Otitis Media." *Acta Paediatrica Scandinavica* 71 no. 4 (Jul, 1982): 567-571.
Backon, J. "Prolonged Breast Feeding as a Prophylaxis for Recurrent Otitis Media: Relevance of Prostaglandins." *Medical Hypotheses* 13 no. 2 (Feb, 1984): 161.
12 "Breast Feeding Prevents Otitis Media." *Nutrition Reviews* 41 no. 8 (Aug, 1983): 241-242.
13 Kellogg, J. H., M.D. *Rational Hydrotherapy.* Philadelphia: F. A. Davis Publishing, 1902.
14 Jones, T. W.; et al. "Independent Effects of Youth and Poor Diabetes Control on Responses to Hypoglycemia in Children." *Diabetes* 40 no. 3 (Mar, 1991): 358-363.
15 Rapoport, J. L. "Diet and Hyperactivity." *Nutrition Reviews* 44 suppl. (May, 1986): 158-162.
16 Department of Health and Human Services, Public Health Service. "More Than You Ever Thought You Would Know About Food Additives." FDA Publication, Revised 1982, #82.2160. Out of Print.
17 Egger, J.; et al. "Controlled Trial of Oligoantigenic Treatment in the Hyperkinetic Syndrome." *Lancet* 1 no. 8428 (Mar, 1985) 540-545.
18 Harley, J. P.; et al. "Hyperkinesis and Food Additives: Testing the Feingold Hypothesis." *Pediatrics* 61 no. 6 (1978): 818-828.
19 Consensus Conference: "Defined Diets and Childhood Hyperactivity." *Journal of the American Medical Asssociation* 248 no. 3 (Jul, 1982): 29029-2.
20 Egger, J.; Stolla, A.; and McEwen, L. M. "Controlled Trial of Hyposensitisation in Children with Food-Induced Hyperkinetic Syndrome." *Lancet* 339 no. 8802 (May, 1992): 1150-1153.

Chronic Fatigue Syndrome

1 Straus, S., M.D. "Chronic Fatigue Syndrome." U.S. Department of Health and Human Services, Public Health Service, NIH Publication no. 90-3059 (Jun, 1990): 5.
2 Ibid.
3 Rosenbaum, M., M.D.; and Susser, M., M.D. *Solving the Puzzle of Chronic Fatigue Syndrome.* Tacoma, WA: Life Sciences Press, 1992.
4 Chaitow, L. *Post Viral Fatigue Syndrome.* London: Dents, 1989.
5 Cunha, B. A.; M.D. *Infectious Disease News* 5 no. 11 (Nov, 1992): 8-9.
6 Straus, S., M.D. "Chronic Fatigue Syndrome." U.S. Department of Health and Human Services, Public Health Service, NIH Publication no. 90-3059 (Jun, 1990): 5.
7 Rosenbaum, M., M.D.; and Susser, M., M.D. *Solving the Puzzle of Chronic Fatigue Syndrome.* Tacoma, WA: Life Sciences Press, 1992, 22.
8 Ibid.
9 Editorial. "Depression, Stress and Immunity." *Lancet* 1 no. 8548 (Jun, 1987): 1467-1488.
10 Hodgkinson, N. "'Yuppie Flue'— Is it All in the Mind Say Doctors." *Sunday Times London* (July 17, 1988).
11 This report is based solely on product labeling as published by PDR (R). Copyright (C) 1993 by Medical Economics Data, a division of Medical Economics Company, Inc. All rights reserved. There is no affiliation between Medical Economics Company, Inc., and Future Medicine Publishing, Inc.
12 Cox, I. M.; Campbell, M. J.; and Dowson, D. "Red Blood Cell Magnesium and Chronic Fatigue Syndrome." *Lancet* 337 no. 8744 (Mar, 1991): 757-760.
13 Simpson, L. "M. E. and B_{12}." *JRS Medicine* (Oct, 1991): 633.

Chronic Pain

1 Office of Scientific and Health Reports, National Institute of Neurological Disorders and Stroke. "Chronic Pain—Hope Through Recovery." U.S. Dept. of Health and Human Services Public Health Service, National Institutes of Health, NIH Publication no. 90-2406 (Nov, 1989): 2.
2 Melzack, R.; and Scott, T. "The Effects of Early Experience on the Response to Pain." *Journal of Physiology and Comparative Psychology* 50 (1957): 971.
3 Bresler, D.; and Katz, R. "Chronic Pain: Alternative to Neural Blockade." In *Neural Blockade in Clinical Anesthesia and Management of Pain*, eds. M. Cousins and P. Bridenbaugh. Philadelphia: Lippincott, 1980.
4 Sternbach, R., *Pain: A Psychophysiological Analysis.* New York: Academic Press, 1968.
5 Murphy, M. *The Future of the Body.* Los Angeles: Jeremy P. Tarcher, 1992.
6 Bresler, D.; and Katz, R. "Chronic Pain: Alternative to Neural Blockade." In *Neural Blockade in Clinical Anesthesia and Management of Pain*, eds. M. Cousins and P. Bridenbaugh. Philadelphia: Lippincott, 1980.
7 Jellinek, E. "Clinical Tests on Comparative Effectiveness of Analgesic Drugs." *Biometrics Bulletin* 2 (1946):87.
8 Lasagna, L.; et al. "A Study of the Placebo Response." *American Journal of Medicine* 16 (1954): 770.
9 Sternbach, R., *Pain: A Psychophysiological Analysis.* New York: Academic Press, 1968.
10 Lucero, K. M. "The Electro-Acuscope/Myopulse System." *Rehab Management: Journal of Therapy and Rehabilitation.* 4 no. 3 (Apr/May, 1991).

Colds and Flu

1 Cheraskin, E., M.D. *Vitamin C: Who Needs It.* Birmingham, AL: Arlington Press, 1993.
2 Ibid, 4.
3 Ibid.
4 Pizzorno, J. E.; and Murray, M. T. *A Textbook of Natural Medicine.* 2 vols. Seattle, WA: John Bastyr College Publications, 1989.
5 This report is based solely on product labeling as published by PDR (R). Copyright (C) 1993 by Medical Economics Data, a division of Medical Economics Company, Inc. All rights reserved. There is no affiliation between Medical Economics Company, Inc., and Future Medicine Publishing, Inc.
6 Pizzorno, J. E.; and Murray, M. T. *A Textbook of Natural Medicine.* 2 vols. Seattle, WA: John Bastyr College Publications, 1989.
7 Cohen, S.; Tyrell, D. A. J.; and Smith, A. P. "Psychological Stress and Susceptibility to the Common Cold." *New England Journal of Medicine* 325 no. 9 (Aug, 1991): 606-612.
8 Cohen, S.; Tyrell, D. A. J.; and Smith, A. P. "Psychological Stress and Susceptibility to the Common Cold." *New England Journal of Medicine* 325 no. 9 (Aug, 1991): 606-612.
9 Pizzorno, J. E.; and Murray, M. T. *A Textbook of Natural Medicine.* 2 vols. Seattle, WA: John Bastyr College Publications, 1989.
10 Pizzorno, J. E.; and Murray, M. T. *A Textbook of Natural Medicine.* 2 vols. Seattle, WA: John Bastyr College Publications, 1989.
11 Cheraskin, E., M.D. *Vitamin C: Who Needs It.* Birmingham, AL: Arlington Press, 1993, 2.
12 Ibid, 9.
13 Pizzorno, J. E.; and Murray, M. T. *A Textbook of Natural Medicine.* 2 vols. Seattle, WA: John Bastyr College Publications, 1989.
14 Pizzorno, J. E.; and Murray, M. T. *A Textbook of Natural Medicine.* 2 vols. Seattle, WA: John Bastyr College Publications, 1989.
Weiss, R.F. *Herbal Medicine.* Beaconsfield, England: Beaconsfield Publishers, 1988.
15 Pizzorno, J. E.; and Murray, M. T. *A Textbook of Natural Medicine.* 2 vols. Seattle, WA: John Bastyr College Publications, 1989.
16 Pizzorno, J. E.; and Murray, M. T. *Encyclopedia of Natural Medicine.* Rocklin, CA: Prima Publishing, 1991, 228.

Constipation

1 Subak-Sharpe, G. J. ed.; with Bogdonoff, M.; and Bressler, R., medical eds. *The Physicians' Manual for Patients.* New York: Times Books, 1984.
2 Petrakis, N.; and King, E. "Cytological Abnormalities in Nipple Aspirates of Breast Fluid from Women with Severe Constipation." *Lancet* 2 no. 8257 (Nov, 1981): 1203-1204.
3 American Cancer Society. "Cancer Facts and Figures— 1993."
4 Taylor, R. " Management of Constipation. 1. High Fibre Diets Work." *British Medical Journal* 300 no. 6731 (Apr, 1990): 1063-1064.
5 Pizzorno, J. E.; and Murray, M. T. *A Textbook of Natural Medicine.* 2 vols. Seattle, WA: John Bastyr College Publications, 1989.
6 Ibid.
7 This report is based solely on product labeling as published by PDR (R). Copyright (C) 1993 by Medical Economics Data, a division of Medical Economics Company, Inc. All rights reserved. There is no affiliation between Medical Economics Company, Inc., and Future Medicine Publishing, Inc.
8 Pizzorno, J. E.; and Murray, M. T. *A Textbook of Natural Medicine.* 2 vols. Seattle, WA: John Bastyr College Publications, 1989.

9 Cummings, J.; et al. "Colonic Response to Dietary Fibre from Carrot, Cabbage, Apple, Bran." *Lancet* 1 no. 8054 (Jan, 1978): 5.

Diabetes

1 Forsham, P. H., M.D. "Treatment of Type I and Type II Diabetes." Townsend Letter for Doctors 53 (Dec, 1987): 390-393.
2 "Diabetes in America." Pamphlet. Bethesda, MD: National Institute of Health, 1985.
3 Jovanovic-Peterson, L.; and Peterson, C. M. "Is Exercise Safe or Useful for Gestational Diabetic Women?" *Diabetes* 40 suppl. 2 (Dec, 1991):179-181.
4 Pizzorno, J. E.; and Murray, M. T. "Diabetes Mellitus." In *A Textbook of Natural Medicine*, eds. J. E. Pizzorno and M. T. Murray. Seattle, WA: John Bastyr College Publications, 1988.
5 Philpott, W. H. "Diabetes - a Reversible Disease." Unpublished paper obtainable through Philpott Medical Services, 17171 S.E. 29th St., Choctaw, OK, 73020.
6 Karljalainen, J.; et al. "Bovine Albumin Peptide as a Possible Trigger of Insulin-Dependent Diabetes Mellitus." *New England Journal of Medicine* 327 no. 5 (1992):302-307.
7 Pizzorno, J. E.; and Murray, M. T. "Diabetes Mellitus." In *A Textbook of Natural Medicine*, eds. J. E. Pizzorno and M. T. Murray. Seattle, WA: John Bastyr College Publications, 1988.
8 Forsham, P. H. "Treatment of Type I and Type II Diabetes." *Townsend Letter for Doctors* 53 (Dec, 1987): 390-393.
9 Zimmet, P. Z. "Kelly West Lecture 1991—Challenges in Diabetes Epidemiology— From West to the Rest." *Diabetes Care* 15 no. 2 (Feb, 1992):232-252.
10 Satter, D. "Diabetes Called Sure Fate for Obese People." *Los Angeles Times*, (Sunday, Feb 13): 1972, Section C.
11 King, H.; and Rewers, M. "Diabetes in Notes is Now a Third World Problem." *Bulletin of the World Health Organization* 69 no. 6 (1991): 643-648.
12 Editorial Staff. "The Prevention and Natural Treatment of Diabetes." *Prevention* 30 no.10 (Oct, 1978):108-113.
13 Philpott, W. H.; and Kalita, D. K. *Victory Over Diabetes*. New Canaan, CT: Keats Publishing,1983.
14 Weil, A. *Natural Health, Natural Medicine: A Comprehensive Manual for Wellness and Self-Care*. Boston: Houghton Mifflin, 1990, 279.
15 Chen, M. S.; et al. "Prevalence and Risk Factors of Diabetic Retinopathy among Non-Insulin Dependent Diabetic Subjects." *American Journal of Opthamology* 114 no. 6 (Dec, 1992): 723-730.
Marshall, G.; et al. "Factors Influencing the Onset and Progression of Diabetic Retinopathy in Subjects with Insulin- Dependent Diabetes Mellitus." *Opthamology* 100 no. 8 (Aug, 1993): 1133-1139.
Mandarino, L. J. "Current Hypotheses for the Biochemical Basis of Diabetic Retinopathy." *Diabetes Care* 15 no. 12 (Dec, 1992): 1892-1901.
16 Weil, A. *Natural Health, Natural Medicine: A Comprehensive Manual for Wellness and Self-Care*. Boston: Houghton Mifflin, 1990, 279.
17 Maugh, T. H. III. "New Method to Fight Diabetes Found Effective." *Los Angeles Times* (Jun 14, 1993):1.
18 Anderson, J. W.; and Sieling, B. "High Fiber Diets for Diabetics: Unconventional but Effective." *Geriatrics* 36 no. 5 (May, 1981): 64-72.
19 Ibid.
20 Berger, S. M., M.D. *What Your Doctor Didn't Learn in Medical School & What You Can Do About It*. New York: Avon Books, 1989, 179-200.
21 Philpott, W. H.; and Kalita, D. K. *Victory Over Diabetes*. New Canaan, CT: Keats Publishing,1983.
22 Potts, J. "Avoidance Protective Food Testing in Assessing Diabetes Responsiveness." *Journal of Diabetes* 26 suppl. 1 (1977).
Potts, J. "Value of Specific Testing for Assessing Insulin Resistance." *Journal of Diabetes* 29 suppl. 2 (1980).
Potts, J. "Blood Sugar-Insulin Responses to Specific Foods Versus GTT." *Journal of Diabetes* 30 suppl. 1 (1981).
Potts, J. "Insulin Resistance Related to Specific Food Sensitivity." *Journal of Diabetes* 35 suppl. 1 (1986).
23 Searcy, R. L., M.D. *Diagnostic Biochemistry*. New York: McGraw-Hill, 1969.
24 Albert, E, M.D. "Current Concepts in Diabetes Mellitus." *New York State Journal of Medicine* 53 no. 22 (Nov, 1953): 2607-2610.
25 Ellis, J. M., M.D. *Vitamin B6, The Doctor's Report*. New York: Harper & Row, 1973.
26 Jones, C. L.; and Gonzalez, V., M.D. "Pyroxidine Deficiency: a New Factor in Diabetic Neuropathy."*Journal of American Podiatry Association* 68 no. 9 (Sep, 1978): 646-653.
27 Pizzorno, J. E.; and Murray, M. T. *A Textbook of Natural Medicine*. John Bastyr College Publications, Seattle WA: John Bastyr College Publications, 1988, 14.
28 Koutsikos, D.; Agroyannis, B.; and Tzanatos-Exarchou, H. "Biotin for Diabetic Peripheral Neuropathy." *Biomedicine and Pharmacotherapy* 44 no. 10 (1990): 511-514.
29 Devamanoharan, P. S.; et al. "Prevention of Selenite Cataract by Vitamin C." *Experimental Eye Research* 52 no. 5 (May, 1991): 563-568.
30 Philpott, W. H.; and Kalita, D. K. *Victory Over Diabetes*. New Canaan, CT: Keats Publishing, 1983.
31 Shute, W. E.. *Vitamin E for Ailing and Healthy Hearts*. New York: Pyramid House, 1969.
32 Colette, C.; et al. "Platelet Function in Type I Diabetes: Effects of Supplementation with Large Doses of Vitamin E." *American Journal of Clinical Nutrition* 47 no. 2 (Feb, 1988): 256-261.
33 Stuart, M. J. "Vitamin E Deficiency: its Effect on Platelet-Vascular Interaction in Various Pathological States." *Annals of the New York Academy of Sciences* 393 (1982): 277-288.
Watanabe, J., et al. "Effect of Vitamin E on Platelet Aggregation in Diabetes Mellitus." *Thrombosis and Haemostasis* 51 (1984): 313-316.
34 Editorial Staff. "Chromium Enrichment of Foods Urged." *Medical World News* 15 no. 7 (Oct, 1974): 33-35.
35 Toepfer, E. W.; et al."Chromium in Foods Related to Biological Activity." *Journal of Agricultural Food Chemistry* 21 no.1 (1973): 69-73.
36 Pizzorno, J. E.; and Murray, M. T. *A Textbook of Natural Medicine*. Seattle, WA: John Bastyr College Publications, 1988, 10-11.
37 Merz, W.; and Schwarz, K. 'Relation of Glucose Tolerance Factor to Impaired Intravenous Glucose Tolerance of Rats on a Stock Diet." *American Journal of Physiology* 196 no. 3 (1959): 614-618.
38 Hambidge, K. M. "Chromium Nutrition in Man." *American Journal of Clinical Nutrition* 27 no. 5 (May, 1974): 505-514.
39 Sjogren A.; et al. "Magnesium, Potassium, and Zinc Deficiencies in Subjects with Type II Diabetes." *Acta Medica Scandinavica* 224 (1988): 461-463.
40 Sheehan, J. "Importance of Magnesium Chloride Repletion after Myocardial Infarction." *American Journal of Cardiology* 63 no. 14 (Apr, 1989): 35G-38G.
41 Reinhart, R. A. "Clinical Correlates of the Molecular and Cellular Actions of Magnesium on the Cardiovascular System." *American Heart Journal* 121 no. 5 (May, 1991): 1513-1521.
42 Norbiato, G.; et al. "Effects of Potassium Supplementation on Insulin Binding and Insulin Action in Human Obesity: Protein-modified Fast and Refeeding" *European Journal of Clinical Investigation* 14 no. 6 (Dec, 1984): 414-419.
43 Underwood, E. J., M.D. *Trace Elements in Human and Animal Nutrition*. Orlando, FL: Academic Press, 1986-1987.
44 Keeton, K. *Longevity: The Science of Staying Young*. New York: Viking, 1992.
45 Weil, A. *Natural Health, Natural Medicine: A Comprehensive Manual of Wellness and Self-Care*. Boston: Houghton Mifflin, 1990, 279.
46 Philpott, W. H., M.D.; and Kalita, D. K. *Victory Over Diabetes*. New Canaan, CT: Keats Publishing, 1983.
47 Riccardi, G.; and Rivallese, A. A. "Effects of Dietary Fiber and Carbohydrate on Glucose and Lipoprotein Metabolism in Diabetes Patients." *Diabetes Care* 14 (Dec, 1991): 1115-1125.
48 Williams, D. *DMSO The Complete Up-To-Date Guidebook*. Ingram, TX: Mountain Home Publishing, 1987.
49 Ivorra, M. D.; Paya, M.; and Villar, A. "A Review of Natural Products and Plants as Potential Anti-Diabetic Drugs." *Journal of Ethnopharmacology* 27 no. 3 (Dec, 1989): 243-275.
Atta-ur-Rahman; and Zaman, K. "Medical Plants with Hypoglycemic Activity." *Journal of Ethnopharmacology* 26 no. 1 (Jan, 1989): 1-55.
50 Cutler, P., M.D. "Deferoxamine Therapy in High-Ferritin Diabetes." *Diabetes* 38 (Oct, 1989): 1207-1210.

Female Health

1 Kalo-Klein, A.; and Witkin, S. S. "Candida Albicans: Cellular Immune System Interactions During Different Stages of the Menstrual Cycle." *American Journal of Obstetrics and Gynecology* 161 no. 5 (Nov, 1989):1132-1136.
2 Ibid.
3 Edelstam, G. A.; et al. "Cyclic Variation of Major Histocompatibility Complex Class II Antigen Expression in the Human Fallopian Tube Epithelium." *Fertility and Sterility* 57 no. 6 (Jun,1992):1225-29.
4 The Boston Women's Health Book Collective. *The New Our Bodies, Ourselves: a Book by and for Women*. New York: Simon and Schuster, 1992, 278.
5 Huffman, S. L.; et al. "Suckling Patterns and Post-Partum Amenorrheoea in Bangladesh." *Journal of Biosocial Science* 19 no. 2 (Apr, 1987):171-179.
6 Kennedy, K. I.; and Visness, C. M. "Contraceptive Efficiency of Lactational Amenorrhoea." *Lancet* 339 no. 8787 (Jan, 1992): 227-230.
7 Campbell, P. "Efficacy of Female Condom." *Lancet* 341 no. 8853 (May, 1993): 1155.
8 Lytle, C. D.; et al. "Virus Leakage Through Natural Membrane Condoms." *Sexually Transmitted Diseases* 17 no. 2 (Apr-Jun, 1990): 58-62.
9 Carey, R. F.; et al. "Effectiveness of Latex Condoms as a Barrier to Human Immunodeficiency Virus-Sized Particles Under Conditions of Simulated Use." *Sexually Transmitted Diseases* 19 no. 4 (Jul/Aug, 1992): 230-234.
10 Braus, P. "Facing Menopause." *American Demographics* 15 no. 3 (Mar, 1993): 44-49.
11 Follingstad, A. H. "Estriol, the Forgotten Estrogen?" *Journal of the American Medical Association* 239 no. 1 (Jan, 1978): 29-30.
12 Dawood, M. Y. "Current Concepts in the Etiology and Treatment of Primary Dysmenorrhea." *Acta Obstetricia et Gynecologica Scandinavica* 138 suppl. (1986): 7-10.
13 Lark, S. M., M.D. *Menstrual Cramps. A Self-Help Program*. Los Altos, CA: Westchester Publishing Compnay, 1993.
14 Pizzorno, J. E.; and Murray, M. T., eds. *A Textbook of Natural Medicine*. Seattle, WA: John Bastyr College Publications, 1988-1989.
15 Lark, S. M., M.D. *Menstrual Cramps. A Self-Help Program*. Los Altos, CA: Westchester Publishing Compnay, 1993.
16 Taymor M. L.; et al. "The Etiological Role of Chronic Iron Deficiency in Production of Menorrhagia." *Journal of the American Medical Association* 187 no. 5 (1964):323-327.
17 Cohen, J. D., M.D.; and Rubin, H. W., M.D. "Functional Menorrhagia: Treatment with Bioflavonoids and Vitamin C." *Current Therapeutic Research* 2 no. 11 (Nov,1960): 539-542.
Lithgow, D. M.; and Poltizer, W. M. "Vitamin A in the Treatment of Menorrhagia." *South African Medical Journal* 51 no. 7 (Feb, 1977):191-193.
18 Abraham, G. E.; and Lubran, M. M. "Serum and Red Cell Magnesium Levels in Patients with Premenstrual Tension." *The American Journal of Clinical Nutrition* 34 no. 11 (Nov, 1981): 2364-2366.
19 John, T. M. "Premenstrual Syndrome as a Western Culture-Specific Disorder." *Culture,*

Medicine and Psychiatry 11 no. 3 (Sep, 1987): 337-56.
20 Lark, S. M., M.D. *PMS Self-Help Book: A Woman's Guide*. Berkeley, CA: Celestial Arts, 1984, 26-27.
21 Abraham, G. E.; and Lubran, M. M. "Serum and Red Cell Magnesium Levels in Patients with Premenstrual Tension." *The American Journal of Clinical Nutrition* 34 no. 11 (Nov, 1981): 2364-2366.
22 Stewart, A. "Clinical and Biochemical Effects of Nutritional Supplementation on the Premenstrual Syndrome." *Journal of Reproductive Medicine* 32 no. 6 (Jun, 1987): 435-441.
23 Larsson, B.; Jonasson, A.; and Fianu, S. "Evening Primrose Oil in the Treatment of Premenstrual Syndrome." *Current Therapeutic Research* 46 no. 1 (Jul, 1989): 58-63.
24 Salonen, J. T.; et al. "High Stored Iron Levels are Associated with Excess Risk of Myocardial Infarction in Eastern Finnish Men." *Circulation* 86 no. 3 (Sep, 1992): 803-811.
Hite, S. *The Hite Report*. NY: Macmillan Publishers Co., 1976, 351.
25 Kronenberg, F. "Hot Flashes: Epidemiology and Physiology." *Annals of the New York Academy of Sciences* 592 (1990): 52-86; discussion 123-133.
26 Ibid.
27 Adlercreutz, H.; et al. "Urinary Excretion of Lignans and Isoflavonoid Phytoestrogens in Japanese Men and Women Consuming a Traditional Japanese Diet." *American Journal of Clinical Nutrition* 54 no. 6 (1991):1093-1100.
28 Cohen, J. D., M.D.; and Rubin, H. W., M.D. "Functional Menorrhagia: Treatment with Bioflavonoids and Vitamin C." *Current Therapeutic Research* 2 no. 11 (Nov,1960):539-542.
29 Adam, J. B. "Human Breast Cancer: Concerted Role of Diet, Prolactin and Adrenal C19-Delta-5 Steroids in Tumorigenesis." *International Journal of Cancer* 50 no. 6 (Apr, 1992): 854-858.
30 Prince R. L.; et al. "Prevention of Postmenopausal Osteoporosis. A Comparative Study of Exercise, Calicium Supplementation, and Hormone-Replacement Therapy." *New England Journal of Medicine* 325 no. 17 (Oct, 1991): 1189-1195.
31 Wilcox, G.; et al. "Oestrogenic Effects of Plant Foods in Postmenopausal Women." *British Medical Journal* 301 no. 6757 (Oct, 1990): 905-906.
32 Adlercreutz, H.; et al. "Dietary Phyto-Oestrogens and the Menopause in Japan." *Lancet* 339 no. 8803 (May, 1992):1233.
33 Adlercreutz, H.; et al. "Urinary Excretion of Lignans and Isoflavonoid Phytoestrogens in Japanese Men and Women Consuming a Traditional Japanese Diet." *American Journal of Clinical Nutrition* 54 no. 6 (1991):1093-1100.
34 Lark, S. M., M.D. *Dr. Susan Lark's The Menopause Self Help Book: a Woman's Guide to Feeling Wonderful the Second Half of Her Life*. Berkeley, CA: Celestial Arts, 1990, 107.
35 Haynes, S. G.; and Feinleib, M. "Women, Work and Coronary Heart Disease: Prospective Findings from the Framingham Heart Study." *American Journal of Public Health* 70 no. 2 (Feb, 1980): 133-141.
36 Lark, S. M., M.D. *Dr. Susan Lark's The Menopause Self-Help Book: a Woman's Guide to Feeling Wonderful the Second Half of Her Life*. Berkeley, CA: Celestial Arts, 1990.
37 Bernstein, S. J.; et al. "The Appropriateness of Hysterectomy. A Comparison of Care in Seven Health Plans. Health Maintenance Organization Quality of Care Consortium." *Journal of the American Medical Association* 269 no. 18 (May, 1993):2398-2402.
38 Heron, S. "Botanical Treatment of Infertility, Endometriosis and Symptoms of Menopause." Presented to the American Association of Naturopathic Physicians in Convention, *Botanical Pharmaceuticals*. Sedona, AZ, Nov 3, 1989.
39 Eschenbach, D. "Vaginal Infection." *Clinical Obstetrics and Gynecology* 26 no. 1 (Mar, 1983): 186-202.
40 Pizzorno, J. E.; and Murray, M. T., eds. *A Textbook of Natural Medicine*. Seattle, WA: John Bastyr College Publications, 1988-1989.
41 Ibid.
42 Ibid.
43 National Institutes of Health. National Cancer Institute. *What You Need to Know About Cancer of the Uterus*. Pub. no. 93-1562, Aug, 1991.
44 Stuart, F. H. *My Body, My Health: the Concerned Woman's Book of Gynecology*. New York: Wiley & Sons, 1979, 422.
45 Bernstein, J. S.; et al. "Hysterectomy: A Literature Review and Rating of Appropriateness." Santa Monica, CA: Rand, Publication no. JR-04, 1992, 7-8.
46 Heron, S. "Botanical Treatment of Infertility, Endometriosis and Symptoms of Menopause." Presented to the American Association of Naturopathic Physicians in Convention, *Botanical Pharmaceuticals*. Sedona, AZ, Nov 3, 1989.
47 Hufnagel, V. G., M.D.; and Golant, S. K. *No More Hysterectomies*. NY: Penguin Books, 1989.
48 National Institutes of Health. National Cancer Institute. *What You Need to Know About Cancer of the Uterus*. Pub. no. 93-1562, Aug, 1991.
49 Hargrove, J. T.; et al. "Menopausal Hormone Replacement Therapy with Continuous Daily Oral Micronized Estradiol and Progesterone." *Obstetrics and Gynecology* 73 no. 4 (Apr, 1989): 606-612.
50 Gambrell, R. D., Jr.; et al. "Use of the Progestogen Challenge Test to Reduce the Risk of Endometrial Cancer." *Obstetrics and Gynecology* 55 no. 6 (Jun, 1980): 732-738.
51 Colditz, G. A.; et al. "Family History, Age, and the Risk of Breast Cancer. Prospective Data from the Nurses' Health Study." *Journal of the American Medical Association* 270 no. 3 (Jul, 1993): 338-343.
52 National Women's Health Network Position Paper. "Mammography in Women Before Menopause." Washington, D.C.: National Women's Health Network, April, 1993.
53 Pizzorno, J. E.; and Murray, M. T., eds. *A Textbook of Natural Medicine*. Seattle, WA: John Bastyr College Publications, 1988-1989.
54 Shreeve, C. M., M.D. *The Alternative Dictionary of Symptoms and Cures*. London: Century Hutchinson Publishing, 1986.

Gastrointestinal Disorders

1 Pizzorno, J. E.; and Murray, M. T. *Encyclopedia of Natural Medicine*. Rocklin, CA: Prima Publishing, 1991, 239.
2 Ibid, 240.
3 Young, P. "Asthma and Allergies, An Optimistic Future." National Institues of Health, NIH Publication no. 80-388, March 1980.
4 Pizzorno, J. E.; and Murray, M. T. *Encyclopedia of Natural Medicine*. Rocklin, CA: Prima Publishing, 1991, 239.
5 This report is based solely on product labeling as published by PDR (R). Copyright (C) 1993 by Medical Economics Data, a division of Medical Economics Company, Inc. All rights reserved. There is no affiliation between Medical Economics Company, Inc., and Future Medicine Publishing, Inc.
6 Pizzorno, J. E.; and Murray, M. T. *Encyclopedia of Natural Medicine*. Rocklin, CA: Prima Publishing, 1991, 395.
7 Ibid, 397.
8 Ibid, 399.
9 Ibid.
10 Ibid, 400.
11 Ibid, 289.
12 Ibid, 343.
13 Ibid, 344.
14 Ibid.

Headache

1 Pizzorno, J. E.; and Murray, M. T., eds. *A Textbook of Natural Medicine*. Seattle, WA: John Bastyr College Publications, 1988-1989.
2 Egger, J.; et al. "Is Migraine Food Allergy? A Double-Blind Controlled Trial of Oligoantigenic Diet Treatment." *Lancet* 2 no. 8355 (Oct, 1983): 865-869.
3 Rudolph, C. J.; et al. "An Observation of the Effect of EDTA Chelation and Supportive Multivitamin Trace Mineral Supplementation of Blood Platelet Volume: A Brief Communication." *Journal of Advancement in Medicine* 3 no. 3 (Fall, 1990).
Morgenstern, E.; and Stark, G. "Morphometric Analysis of Platelet Ultra-Structure in Norma and Experimental Conditions. *Platelets* (1975): 37-42.
4 Johnson, E. S.; et al. "Efficacy of Feverfew as Prophylactic Treatment of Migraine." *British Medical Journal* 291 no. 6495 (Aug, 1985): 569-573.

Hearing Disorders

1 Black, D. *Healing With Sound*. Springville, UT: Tapestry Press, 1991.
2 Bluestone, C. D. "Otitis Media in Children: To Treat or Not to Treat?" *New England Journal of Medicine* 306 no. 23 (Jun, 1982):1399-1404.
3 Pizzorno, J. E.; and Murray, M. T. *A Textbook of Natural Medicine*. Seattle, WA: John Bastyr College Publications, 1988-1989.
4 Saarinen, U. M. "Prolonged Breast Feeding as Prophylaxis for Recurrent Otitis Media." *Acta Paediatrica Scandinavica* 71 no. 4 (Jul, 1982): 567-571.
5 Hagerman, R. J.; and Falkenstein, A. R. "An Association Between Recurrent Otitis Media in Infancy and Later Hyperactivity." *Clinical Pediatrics* 76 no. 5 (May, 1987): 253-257.
6 Toufexis, A. "Now Hear This— If You Can." *Time* 138 no. 5 (Aug, 1991): 50-51.
7 Dees, S. C.; and Lefkowitz, D., III. "Secretory Otitis Media in Allergic Children." *American Journal of Diseases of Children* 124 no. 3 (Sep,1972): 364-368.
8 Ruokonen, J.; Paganus, A.; and Lehti, H. "Elimination Diets in the Treatment of Secretory Otitis Media." *International Journal of Pediatric Otorhinolaryngology* 4 no. 1 (Mar, 1982): 39-46.
9 Asman, B. J.; and Fireman, P. "The Role of Allergies in the Development of Otitis Media with Effusion." *International Pediatrics* 3 no. 3 (1988): 231-233.
10 Editorial Staff. "Antibiotic Use: Adult Prescriptions Fall as Pediatric Prescriptions Soar." *Medical World News* 28 no. 21 (Nov, 1987): 8-10.
11 Diamant, M.; and Diamant, B. "Abuse and Timing of Use of Antibiotics in Acute Otitis Media." *Archives of Otolaryngology* 100 no. 3 (Sep,1974): 226-32.
12 Cantekin, E I; McGuire, T. W.; and Griffith, T. L. "Antimicrobial Therapy for Otitis Media with Effusion (Secretory Otitis Media)." *Journal of the American Medical Association* 266 no. 23 (Dec, 1991): 3309-3317.
13 Adlington, P.; and Hooper, W. K. "Virus Studies in Secretory Otitis Media." *Journal of Laryngology and Otology* 94 no. 2 (Feb, 1980): 191-196.
Arola, M.; Ziegler, T.; and Ruuskanen, O. "Respiratory Virus Infection as a Cause of Prolonged Symptoms in Acute Otitis Media." *Journal of Pediatrics* 116 no. 5 (May, 1990) :697-701.
14 Cohen, S. R.; and Thompson, J. W. "Otitic Candidiasis in Children: an Evaluation of the Problem an Effectiveness of Ketoconazole in 10 Patients." *Annals of Otology, Rhinology, and Laryngology* 99 no. 6 pt. 1 (Jun, 1990): 427-31.
15 Crook, W. G., M.D. "Ear Infections: Is the Treatment Part of the Problem?" *Environmental Physician* (Winter, 1992-1993).
16 van Buchen, F. L.; Dunk, J. H.; and van Hof, M. A. "Therapy of Acute Otitis Media: Myringotomy, Antibiotics, or Neither? A Double-Blind Study in Children." *Lancet* 2 no. 8252 (Oct, 1981): 883-887.
17 Bondestam, M.; Foucard, T.; and Gebre-Medhin, M. Subclinical Trace Element Deficiency in Children with Undue Susceptibility to Infections. *Acta Paediatrica Scandinavica* 74 no. 4 (Jul, 1985): 515-520.
18 Jung, T. T. "Prostaglandins, Leukotrienes, and Other Arachidonic Acid Metabolites in the Pathogenesis of Otitis Media." *Laryngoscope* 98 no. 9 (Sep, 1988): 980-993.
19 Lewis, M.; et al. "Prenatal Exposure to Heavy Metals: Effects on Childhood Cognitive Skills and Health Status." *Pediatrics* 89 no. 6 pt. 1 (Jun, 1992):1010-1015.
20 Campos, F. A.; Flores, H.; and Underwood, B. A. "Effect of an Infection on Vitamin A Status of

Children as Measured by the Relative Dose Response (RDR)." *American Journal of Clinical Nutrition* 46 no. 1 (Jul, 1987): 91-94.
Hussey, G. D.; and Klein, M. "A Randomized, Controlled Trial of Vitamin A in Children with Severe Measles." *New England Journal of Medicine* 323 no. 3 (Jul, 1990):160-164.
21 Bendich, A. "Vitamin E Status of U.S. Children." *Journal of the American College of Clinical Nutrition* 11 no. 4 (Aug, 1991): 441-444.
22 Anonymous. "Says Food Allergy Seems Important Cause of Otitis Media." *Family Practice News* 21 no. 5 (1991):14.
23 Hurst, D. S. "Allergy Management of Refractory Serous Otitis Media." *Otolaryngology and Head and Neck Surgery* 102 no. 6 (Jan, 1990): 664-669.
24 Strome, M.; Topf, P.; and Vernick, D. M. "Hyperlipidemia in Association with Childhood Sensorineural Hearing Loss." *Laryngoscope* 98 no. 2 (Feb, 1988): 165-169.
25 Spencer, J. T., Jr. "Hyperlipoproteinemia, Hyperinsulinism and Meniere's Disease." *Southern Medical Journal* 74 no. 10 (Oct, 1981): 1194-1197.
26 Cohen, S. R.; and Thompson, J. W. "Otitic Candidiasis in Children: an Evaluation of the Problem an Effectiveness of Ketoconazole in 10 Patients." *Annals of Otology, Rhinology, and Laryngology* 99 no. 6 pt. 1 (Jun, 1990): 427-431.
27 Fiocchi, A.; et al. "A Double-Blind Clinical Trial for the Evaluation of the Therapeutical Effectiveness of a Calf Thymus Derivative (Thymomodulin) in Children with Recurrent Respiratory Infections." *Thymus* 8 no. 6 (1986): 331-339.
Genova, R.; and Guerra, A. "Thymomodulin in Management of Food Allergy in Children." *International Journal of Tissue Reactions* 8 no. 3 (1986):239-242.
Cazzola, P.; Mazzanti, P.; and Bossi, G. "In Vivo Modulating Effect of a Calf Thymus Acid Lysate on Human T Lymphocyte Subsets and CD4+/CD8+ Ration in the Course of Different Diseases." *Current Therapeutic Research* 42 no. 6 (Dec, 1987): 1011-1017.
28 Pizzorno, J. E.; and Murray, M. T., eds. *A Textbook of Natural Medicine*. Seattle, WA: John Bastyr College Publications, 1988-1989,1-4.
29 Meyer, B. "A Multicenter Randomized Double-blind Study of Gingko Biloba Extract versus Placebo in the Treatment of Tinnitus." In *Rokan (Gingko Biloba) — Recent Results in Pharmacology and Clinic*, ed. Funfgeld. New York: Springer-Verlag, 1988, 245-250.

Heart Disease

1 Privitera, J. R., M.D. "Clots: Lifes's Biggest Killer." Covina, CA: 1992. Unpublished manuscript.
2 Petersdorf, R. G.; et al. *Harrison's Principles of Internal Medicine*. 10th ed. New York: McGraw Hill, 1983.
3 Ibid.
4 Werbach, M. R., M.D. *Nutritional Influences on Illness*. New Canaan, CT: Keats Publishing, 1988.
5 Weiss, R. F. *Herbal Medicine*. Gothenburg, Sweden: A. B. Arcanum, 1988.
6 Robbins, S. L.; Cotran, R. S.; and Kumar, V., eds. *Pathological Basis of Disease*. New York: W.B. Saunders, 1984.
7 U. S. Department of Health and Human Services. Public Health Service, National Institutes of Health. *Heart Attacks*. Pub. no.86-2700, Sep, 1986.
8 U. S. Department of Health and Human Services. Public Health Services, National Institutes of Health. *Stroke: Hope Through Research*. Pub. no. 83-2222, Aug, 1983.
9 National Institute of Neurological Disorders and Stroke. National Institutes of Health. *Stroke Research Highlights, 1990.*
10 U. S. Department of Health and Human Services. Public Health Service, National Institutes of Health. *Stroke: Hope Through Research*. Pub. no. 83-2222, Aug, 1983.
11 Jaffe, D.; et al. "Coronary Arteries in Newborn Children: Intimal Variations in Longitudinal Sections and Their Relationships to Clinical and Experimental Data." *Acta Paediatrica Scandinavica* Supp. 219 (1971):3-28.
12 Morin, R. J.; and Peng, S. K. "The Role of Cholesterol Oxidation Products in the Pathogenesis of Atherosclerosis." *Annals of Clinical and Laboratory Science* 19 no. 4 (Jul-Aug, 1989): 225-237.
13 Hattersley, J. G. "Acquired Atherosclerosis: Theories of Causation, Novel Therapies." *Journal of Orthomolecular Medicine* 6 no. 2 (1991): 83-98.
14 Peng, S. K.; and Taylor, C. B. "Cholesterol Autooxidation, Health and Arteriosclerosis." *World Reviews of Nutrition and Diet* 44 (1984): 117-154.
15 Malinow, M. R. "Risk for Arterial Occlusive Disease. Is Hyperhomocysteinemia an Innocent Bystander?" *Canadian Journal of Cardiology* 17 (1989): X-XI.
Stampfer, M. J.; et al. "A Prospective Study of Plasma Homocysteine and Risk of Myocardial Infarction in U.S. Physicians." *Journal of the American Medical Association* 268 no. 7 (Aug, 1992): 877-881.
16 McCully, K. S. "Homocysteine Theory of Arteriosclerosis: Development and Current Status." *Atherosclerosis Reviews* 11 (1983): 157-246.
17 Morris, R. D.; et al. "Chlorination, Chlorination Byproducts, and Cancer: A Meta-Analysis." *American Journal of Public Health* 82 no. 7 (Jul, 1992): 955-963.
Yiamouiannis, J. *Fluoride: The Aging Factor: How to Recognize and Avoid the Devestating Effects of Fluoride*. Delaware, OH: Health Action Press, 1986.
18 McCully, K. S. "Homocysteine Theory of Arteriosclerosis: Development and Current Status." *Atherosclerosis Reviews* 11 (1983): 157-246.
19 Kostner, G. M.; et al. "The Interaction of Human Plasma Low Density Lipoproteins with Glycosamino-Glycans: Influence of the Chemical Composition." *Lipids* 20 no. 1 (Jan, 1985): 24-28.
20 Morris, R. D.; et al. "Chlorination, Chlorination Byproducts, and Cancer: A Meta-Analysis." *American Journal of Public Health* 82 no. 7 (Jul, 1992): 955-963.
21 Ornish, D., M.D *Dr. Dean Ornish's Program for Reversing Heart Disease: the Only System Scientifically Proven to Reverse Heart Disease Without Drugs or Surgery*. New York: Ballantine, 1990.
22 Ibid.
23 Gruberg, E. R.; and Raymond, S. A. *Beyond Cholesterol: Vitamin B6, Arteriosclerosis, and Your Heart*. New York: St.Martin's Press, 1981.
24 This report is based solely on product labeling as published by PDR (R). Copyright (C) 1993 by Medical Economics Data, a division of Medical Economics Company, Inc. All rights reserved. There is no affiliation between Medical Economics Company, Inc., and Future Medicine Publishing, Inc.
25 Olszewski, A. J.; and McCully, K. S. "Fish Oil Decreases Serum Homocysteine in Hyperlipemic Men." *Coronary Artery Disease* 4 (1993): 53-60.
26 Kromhout, D.; Bosschieter, E. B.; and de Lezzene Coulander, C. "The Inverse Relation Between Fish Consumption and 20-Year Mortality From Coronary Heart Disease." *New England Journal of Medicine* 312 no.19 (May, 1985): 1205-1209.
27 Renaud, S.; and Nordy, A. "'Small is Beautiful': Alpha-Linoleic Acid and Eicosapentaenoic Acid in Man." *Lancet* 1 no. 8334 (May, 1983): 1169.
28 Olszewski, A. J.; et al. "Reduction of Plasma Lipid and Homocysteine Levels by Pyridoxine, Folate, Cobalamin, Choline, Riboflavin, and Troxerutin in Atherosclerosis." *Atherosclerosis* 75 no. 1 (Jan, 1989): 1-6.
29 Hattersley, J. G. "Heart Attacks and Strokes." *Townsend Letter for Doctors* 104 (Feb/Mar, 1992).
30 Mudd, S. H.; et al. "The Natural History of Homocystinuria Due to Cystathionine Beta-Synthose Deficiency." *American Journal of Human Genetics* 37 no. 1 (Jan, 1985): 1-31.
31 Editorial. "Is Vitamin B6 an Antithrombotic Agent?" *Lancet* 1 no. 8233 (Jun, 1981):1299-1300.
32 Suzman, M. M. "Effect of Pyridoxine and Low Animal Protein Diet in Coronary Artery Disease." *Circulation* suppl. no. IV-254 (Oct, 1973), Abstracts of the 46th Scientific Sessions.
33 Ibid.
34 McCully, K. S. "Homocysteine Theory of Arteriosclerosis: Development and Current Status." *Atherosclerosis Reviews* 11 (1983): 157-246.
35 Ibid.
36 Brattstrom, L.; et al. "Higher Total Plasma Homocysteine Due to Cystathionine Beta-Synthase Deficiency." *Metabolism: Clinical and Experimental* 37 no. 2 (Feb, 1988): 175-178.
37 Ibid.
38 Olszewski, A. J.; et al. "Reduction of Plasma Lipid and Homocysteine Levels by Pyridoxine, Folate, Cobalamin, Choline, Riboflavin, and Troxerutin in Atherosclerosis." *Atherosclerosis* 75 no. 1 (Jan, 1989):1-6.
39 Brattstrom, L.; et al. "Impaired Homocysteine Metabolism in Early-Onset Cerebral and Peripheral Occlusive Artery Disease." Effects of Pyridoxine and Folic Acid Treatment." *Atherosclerosis* 81 no.1 (1990): 51-60.
Olszewski, A. J.; et al. "Reduction of Plasma Lipid and Homocysteine Levels by Pyridoxine, Folate, Cobalamin, Choline, Riboflavin, and Troxerutin in Atherosclerosis." *Atherosclerosis* 75 no. 1 (Jan, 1989): 1-6.
40 Rimm, E.; et al. "Vitamin E Consumption and the Risk of Coronary Heart Disease in Men." *New England Journal of Medicine* 328 no. 20 (May, 1993): 1450-1456.
Stampfer, M. J.; et al. "Vitamin E Consumption and the Risk of Coronary Heart Disease in Women." *New England Journal of Medicine* 328 no. 20 (May, 1993): 1444-1449.
41 Jialal, I.; and Grundy, S. M. "Effect of Dietary Supplementation with Alpha-Tocopherol on the Oxidative Modification of Low Density Lipoprotein." *Journal of Lipid Research* 33 no. 6 (Jun, 1992):899-906.
Steiner, M. "Influence of Vitamin E on Platelet Function in Humans." *Journal of the American College of Nutrition* 10 no. 5 (Oct, 1991): 466-473.
42 Boscoboinik, D.; Szewczyk, A.; and Azzi, A. "Alpha-Tocopherol (Vitamin E) Regulates Vascular Smooth Muscle Cell Proliferation and Protein Kinase C Activity." *Archives of Biochemistry and Biophysics* 286 no. 1 (Apr, 1991): 264-269.
Hennig, B.; et al. "Protective Effects of Vitamin E in Age-Related Endothelial Cell Injury." *International Journal of Vitamin and Nutrition Research* 59 (1989):273-279.
43 Rimm, E.; et al. "Vitamin E Consumption and the Risk of Coronary Heart Disease in Men." *New England Journal of Medicine* 328 no. 20 (May, 1993): 1450-1456.
Stampfer, M. J.; et al. "Vitamin E Consumption and the Risk of Coronary Heart Disease in Women." *New England Journal of Medicine* 328 no. 20 (May, 1993): 1444-1449.
44 Stampfer, M.; et al. "Vitamin E and Heart Disease Incidence in the Nurses Health Study." American Heart Association Annual Meeting. New Orleans, LA, Nov 18, 1992.
45 Rimm, E.; et al. "Vitamin E and Heart Disease Incidence in the Health Professionals Study." American Heart Association Annual Meeting. New Orleans, LA, Nov 18, 1992.
46 Gey, K. F.; et al. "Inverse Correlation Between Plasma Vitamin E and Mortality from Ischemic Heart Disease in Cross-Cultural Epidemiology." *American Journal of Clinical Nutrition* 53 suppl. 1 (Jan, 1991): 326S-334S.
47 McCully, K. S. Homocysteine Metabolism in Scurvy, Growth, and Arteriosclerosis." *Nature* 231 no. 5302 (Jun, 1971): 391-392.
48 Rath, M.; and Pauling, L. "Hypothesis: Lipoprotein(a) is a Surrogate for Ascorbate." *Proceedings of the National Academy of Sciences of the U.S.A.* 87 no.16 (Aug, 1990):6204-6207.
49 Rath, M.; and Pauling, L. "Solution to the Puzzle of Human Cardiovascular Disease: Its Primary Cause is Ascorbate Deficiency Leading to the Deposition of Lipoprotein(a) and Fibrinogen/Fibrin in the Vascular Wall." *Journal of Orthomolecular Medicine* 6 (1991):125-134.
50 Ginter, E. R.; et al. "Vitamin C in the Control of Mypercholesterolemia in Man." *International Journal for Vitamin and Nutrition Research* suppl. 23 (1982):137-52.
51 Rath, M.; and Pauling, L. "Solution to the Puzzle of Human Cardiovascular Disease: Its

Primary Cause is Ascorbate Deficiency Leading to the Deposition of Lipoprotein(a) and Fibrinogen/Fibrin in the Vascular Wall." *Journal of Orthomolecular Medicine* 6 (1991):125-134.

52 Rath, M.; and Pauling, L. "Hypothesis: Lipoprotein(a) is a Surrogate for Ascorbate." *Proceedings of the National Academy of Sciences of the U.S.A.* 87 no.16 (Aug, 1990): 6204-6207.

53 Hanaki, Y.; Sugiyama, S.; and Ozawa, T. "Ratio of Low-Density Lipoprotein Cholesterol to Ubiquinone as a Coronary Risk Factor." *New England Journal of Medicine* 325 no. 11 (Sep, 1991): 814-815.

Frei, B.; Kim, M. C.; and Ames, B. N. "Ubiquinol-10 is an Effective Lipid-Soluble Antioxidant at Physiological Concentrations." *Proceedings of the National Academy of Sciences of the U.S.A.* 87 no.12 (1990): 4879-4883.

54 Salonen, J. T., et al. "Interactions of Serum Copper, Selenium and Low Density Lipoprotein Cholesterol in Atherogenesis." *British Medical Journal* 302 no. 6779 (Mar, 1991): 756-760.

55 Stead, N. W.; et al. "Effect of Selinium Supplementation on Selenium Balance in the Dependent Elderly." *American Journal of the Medical Sciences* 290 no. 6 (Dec, 1985):228-233.

56 Wood, D. A.; et al. "Adipose Tissue and Platelet Fatty Acids and Coronary Heart Disease in Scottish Men." *Lancet* 2 no. 8395 (Jul, 1984):117-121.

57 Seelig, M. S.; and Heggtveit, H. A. "Magnesium Interrelationships in Ischemic Heart Disease. A Review." *American Journal of Clinical Nutrition* 27 no. 1 (Jan, 1974):59-79.

Davis, W. H.; et al. "Monotherapy with Magnesium Increases Abnormally Low Density Lipoprotein Cholesterol: A Clinical Assay." *Current Therapeutic Research* 36 no. 2 (Aug, 1984): 341.

58 Berge, K. G.; and Canner, P. L. "Coronary Drug Project: Experience with Niacin. Coronary Drug Project Research Group." *European Journal of Clinical Pharmacology* 40 supplM.1 (1991): S49-S51.

Luria, M. H. "Effect of Low-Dose Niacin on High-Density Lipoprotein Cholesterol and Total Cholesterol/High-Density Lipoprotein Ratio." *Archives of Internal Medicine* 148 no.11 (Nov, 1988): 2493-2495.

59 Canner, P. L.; et al. "Fifteen Year Mortality in Coronary Drug Project Patients; Long-Term Benefit with Niacin." *Journal of the American College of Cardiology* 8 no. 6 (Dec, 1986): 1245-1255.

60 Karanja, N.; et al. "Plasma Lipids and Hypertension: Response to Calcium Supplementation." *American Journal of Clinical Nutrition* 45 no. 1 (Jan, 1987): 60-65.

61 Press, R. I.; Geller, J.; and Evans,G. W. "The Effect of Chromium Picolinate on Serum Cholesterol and Apolipoprotein Fractions in Human Subjects." *Western Journal of Medicine* 152 no. 1 (Jan, 1990): 41-45.

62 Urberg, M.; Benyi, J.; and John, R. "Hypercholesterolemic Effects of Nicotinic Acid and Chromium Supplementation." *Journal of Family Practice* 27 no. 6 (Dec, 1988): 603-606.

63 Simonoff, M; et al. "Low Plasma Chromium in Patients with Coronary Artery and Heart Diseases." *Biological Trace Elements Research* 6 no. 5 (Oct, 1984): 431-9.

Newman, H. A.; et al. "Serum Chromium and Angiographically Determined Coronary Artery Disease." *Clinical Chemistry* 24 no. 4 (Apr, 1978):541-544.

64 Northeast Center for Environmental Medicine Health Letter, Fall 1992.

65 Weiss, R. F. *Herbal Medicine*. Gothenburg, Sweden: A. B. Arcanum, 1988.

66 Barrie, S. A.; Wright, J. V., M.D.; and Pizzorno, J. E. "Effect of Garlic Oil on Platelet Aggregation, Serum Lipids and Blood Pressure in Humans," *Journal of Orthomolecular Medicine* 2 no. 1 (1987):15-21.

67 Srivastava, K. C. "Effects of Aqueous Extracts of Onion, Garlic and Ginger on Platelet Aggregation and Metabolism of Arachidonic Acid in the Blood Vascular System." *Prostaglandins Leukotrienes and Medicine* 13 (1984): 227-235.

68 Kostner, G. M.; et al. "HMG CoA Reductase Inhibitors Lower LDL Cholesterol Without Reducing Lp(a) Levels." *Circulation* 80 no. 5 (1989): 1313-1319.

69 Strandberg, T. E.; et al. "Long-term Mortality After 5-year Multi-Factorial Primary Prevention of Cardiovascular Diseases in Middle-Aged Men." *Journal of the American Medical Association* 266 no. 9 (Sep, 1991):1225-1229.

70 Folkers, K.; et al. "Lovastatin Decreases Coenzyme-Q Levels in Humans." *Proceedings of the National Academy of Sciences of the United States of America* 87 no. 22 (Nov, 1990): 8931-8934.

70 *New England Journal of Medicine* 312: 1250-1259, 1985

72 *Atherosclerosis* 63: 137-143, 1987.

Hypertension 4 (Supp.): III-34, 1982.

73 Farr, C. H. "The Therapeutic Use of Intravenous Hydrogen Peroxide." Monograph. Oklahoma City, OK: Genesis Medical Center, 1987.

Baker, E. *The Unmedical Miracle— Oxygen*. Indianola, WA: Drelwood Communications, 1991.

74 Walker, M.. "The Biological Therapies of Harvey Bigelsen, M.D." *Explore!* 4 no. 2 (1993): 50-53.

75 Farr, C, H., M.D.; White, R.; and Schachter, M., M.D. "Chronological History of EDTA Chelation Therapy." Presented to the American College of Advancement in Medicine, Houston, TX, May, 1993.

76 Olszewer, E.; and Carter, J. "EDTA Chelation Therapy: A Retrospective Study of 2,780 Patients." In *A Textbook on EDTA Chelation Therapy*, ed. E. M. Cranton, M.D. Special Issue, *Journal of Advancement in Medicine* 2 nos. 1-2, New York: Human Sciences Press, 1989, 209.

77 McDonagh, E.; Rudolph, C.; and Cheraskin, E. "An Oculocerebrovasculometric Analysis of the Improvement in Arterial Stenosis Following EDTA Chelation Therapy." In *A Textbook on EDTA Chelation Therapy*, ed. E. M. Cranton, M.D. Special Issue, *Journal of Advancement in Medicine* 2 nos. 1-2, New York: Human Sciences Press, 1989, 155.

78 Farr, C. H. "The Therapeutic Use of Intravenous Hydrogen Peroxide." Monograph. Oklahoma City, OK: Genesis Medical Center, 1987.

79 Ibid.

80 Ornish, D., M.D.; et al. "Can Lifestyle Changes Reverse Coronary Heart Disease? The Lifestyle Heart Trial." *Lancet* 336 no. 8708 (Jul, 1990): 129-133.

81 Chung san i hsueh yuan. "Treatment of 103 Cases of Coronary Diseases with *Ilex pubescens*." Hook, et Arn. *Chinese Medical Journal* 1 (1973): 64.

82 CASS Principal Investigators and Associates. "Myocardial Infarction and Mortality in the Coronary Artery
Surgery Study (CASS) Randomized Trial." *New England Journal of Medicine* 310 no. 12 (Mar, 1984): 750-758.

83 Peltz, J. "Insurer to Reimburse Cost of Non-Surgical Heart Care." *Los Angeles Times* (Jul 8, 1993): 1.

Hypertension

1 Havlik, R. J.; et al. "Weight and Hypertension." *Annals of Internal Medicine* 98 no. 5 pt. 2 (May, 1983): 855-859.

2 Egan, K. J.; et al. "The Impact of Psychological Distress on the Control of Hypertension." *Journal of Human Stress* 9 no. 4 (Dec, 1983): 4-10.

3 Gruchow, H. W.; Sobocinski, K. A.; and Barboriak, J. J. "Alcohol, Nutrient Intake, and Hypertension in US adults." *Journal of the American Medical Association* 253 no.11 (Mar, 1985): 1567-1570.

4 Pizzorno, J. E.; and Murray, M. T., eds. *A Textbook of Natural Medicine*. Chapter VI: "Hypertension." Seattle, WA: John BAstyr Publications, 1988.

5 Chow, H. Y.; Wang, J. C.; and Cheng, K. K. "Cardiovascular Effects of Gardenia Florida L. (Gardenise Fructus) Extract." *American Journal of Chinese Medicine* 4 no. 1 (1976): 47-51.

Brewer, G. J. "Molecular Mechanisms of Zinc Action on Cells." *Agents and Actions* suppl. 8 (1981): 37-49.

Bennett, A. E.; Doll, R.; and Howell, R. W. "Sugar Consumption and Cigarette Smoking." *Lancet* 1 (May,1970): 1011-1014.

Kershbaum, A.; et al. "Effects of Smoking and Nicotine on Adrenocortical Secretion." *Journal of the American Medical Association* 203 no. 4 (Jan, 1968): 275-278.

Fortmann, S. P.; et al. "The Association of Blood Pressure and Dietary Alcohol: Differences by Age, Sex and Estrogen Use." *American Journal of Epidemiology* 118 no. 4 (Oct, 1983): 497-507.

6 Pizzorno, J. E.; and Murray, M. T., eds. *A Textbook of Natural Medicine*. Chapter VI: "Hypertension." Seattle, WA: John BAstyr Publications, 1988.

7 He, J.; et al. "Effect of Migration on Blood Pressure: the Yi People Study." *Epidemiology* 2 no. 2 (Mar, 1991): 88-97.

Poulter, N. R; et al. "The Kenyan Luo Migration Study: Observations on the Initiation of a Rise in Blood Pressure." *British Medical Journal* 300 no. 6730 (Apr, 1990): 967-972.

Salmond, C. E; Prior, I. A; and Wessen, A. F. "Blood Pressure Patterns and Migration: a 14-Year Cohort Study of Adult Tokelauans." *American Journal of Epidemiology* 130 no. 1 (Jul, 1989): 37-52.

8 Meneely, G. R.; and Battarbee, H. D. "High Sodium-Low Potassium Environment and Hypertension." *American Journal of Cardiology* 38 no. 6 (Nov, 1976): 768-785.

Resnick, L. M.; Gupta, R. K.; and Laragh, J. H. "Intracellular Free Magnesium in Erythrocytes of Essential Hypertension: Relationship to Blood Pressure and Serum Divalent Cations." *Proceedings of the National Academy of Sciences of the United States of America* 81 no. 20 (Oct, 1984): 6511-6515.

9 Lang, T.; et al. "Relation Between Coffee Drinking and Blood Pressure: Analysis of 6,321 Subjects in the Paris Region." *American Journal of Cardiology* 52 no. 10 (Dec, 1983): 1238-42.

10 Fortmann, S. P.; et al. "The Association of Blood Pressure and Dietary Alcohol: Differences by Age, Sex and Estrogen Use." *American Journal of Epidemiology* 118 no. 4 (Oct, 1983): 497-507.

Gruchow, H. W.; Sobocinski, K. A.; and Barboriak, J. J. "Alcohol, Nutrient Intake, and Hypertension in US Adults."*Journal of the American Medical Association* 253 no. 11 (Mar, 1985): 1567-1570.

11 Bennett, A. E.; Doll, R.; and Howell, R. W. "Sugar Consumption and Cigarette Smoking." *Lancet* 1 (May,1970): 1011-1014.

12 Schroeder, K. L.; and Chen, M. S., Jr. "Smokeless Tobacco and Blood Pressure." *New England Journal of Medicine* 312 no.14 (Apr, 1985): 919.

Hampson, N. B. "Smokeless is Not Saltless." *New England Journal of Medicine* 312 no.14 (Apr, 1985): 919-920.

13 Pirkle, J. L.; et al. "The Relationship Between Blood Lead Levels and its Cardiovascular Risk Implications." *American Journal of Epidemiology* 121 no. 2 (Feb, 1985): 246-258.

14 Glauser, S. C.; Bello, C. T.; and Gauser, E. M. "Blood-Cadmium Levels in Normotensive and Untreated Hypertensive Humans." *Lancet* 1 (Apr, 1976): 717-718.

15 Resnick, L. M.; Gupta, R. K., and Laragh, J. H. "Intracellular Free Magnesium in Erythrocytes of Essential Hypertension: Relationship to Blood Pressure and Serum Divalent Cations." *Proceedings of the National Academy of Sciences of the United States of America* 81 no. 20 (Oct, 1984): 6511-6515.

16 Foushee, D. B.; Ruffin, J.; and Banerjee, U. "Garlic as a Natural Agent for the Treatment of Hypertension: a Preliminary Report." *Cytobios* 34 nos. 135-136 (1982): 145-152.

Petkov, V. "Plants with Hypotensive, Antiatheromatous and Coronary Dilating Action." *American Journal of Chinese Medicine* 7 no. 3 (1979): 197-236.

17 Namba, K.; et al. "Effect of Taurine Concentration on Platelet Aggregation in Gestosis Patients with Edema, Proteinuria, and Hypertension." *Acta Medica Okayama* 46 no. 4 (Aug,1992): 241-7.

Ceriello, A.; et al. Anti-Oxidants Show an Anti-

Hypertensive Effect in Diabetic and Hypertensive Subjects." *Clinical Science* 81 no. 6 (Dec,1991): 739-42.
Maxwell, S. R. "Can Anti-Oxidants Prevent Ischemic Heart Disease?" *Journal of Clinical Pharmacy and Therapeutics* 18 no. 2 (Apr, 1993): 85-95.
18 Skrabal, F.; Aubock, J.; and Hortnagl, H. "Low Sodium/High Potassium Diet for Prevention of Hypertension: Probable Mechanisms of Action." *Lancet* 2 no. 8252 (Oct, 1981): 895-900.
19 Armstrong, B.; et al. "Urinary Sodium and Blood Pressure in Vegetarians." *American Journal of Clinical Nutrition* 32 no.12 (Dec, 1979): 2472-2476.
Rouse I. L.; et al. "Vegetarian Diet and Blood Pressure." *Lancet* 2 no. 8352 (1983): 742-743.
20 Henry, H. J.; et al. "Increasing Calcium Intake Lowers Blood Pressure. The Literature Reviewed." *Journal of the American Dietetic Association* 85 no. 2 (Feb, 1985): 182-185.
Belizam, J. M.; et al. "Reduction of Blood Pressure with Calcium Supplementation in Young Adults." *Journal of the American Medical Association* 249 no. 9 (Mar, 1983): 1161-1165.
21 McCarron, D. A.; Morris, C. D.; and Cole, C. "Dietary Calcium in Human Hypertension." *Science* 217 no. 4556 (1982): 267-269.
22 Dyckner, T.; and Wester, P. O. "Effect of Magnesium on Blood Pressure." *British Medical Journal* 286 no. 6381 (Jan, 1983): 1847-1849.
23 Werbach, M. R., M.D. *Nutritional Influences on Illness*. Tarzana, CA: Third Line Press, 1991.
24 Gordon, N. F.; and Scott, C. B. "Exercise and Mild Essential Hypertension." *Primary Care; Clinics in Office Practice* 18 no. 3 (Sep, 1991): 683-694.
25 Goldstein, I. B.;et al. "Home Relaxation Techniques for Essential Hypertension." *Psychosomatic Medicine* 46 no. 5 (Sep-Oct, 1984): 398-414.
Brassard, C.; and Couture, R. T. "Biofeedback and Relaxation for Patients with Hypertension." *Canadian Nurse* 89 no. 1 (Jan, 1993): 49-52.
Whyte, H. M. "NHMRC Workshop on Non-Pharmacological Methods of Lowering Blood Pressure." *Medical Journal of Australia* 2 no. 1 suppl. (Jul, 1983): S13-S16.
Blanchard, E.B.; et al. "Preliminary Results from a Controlled Evaluation of Thermal Biofeedback as a Treatment for Essential Hypertension." *Biofeedback and Self Regulation* 9 no. 4 (Dec, 1984): 471-495.
26 The 1988 Report of the Joint National Committee of the American Medical Association. "The Joint National Committee on Detection, Evaluation, and Treatment of High Blood Pressure." *Archives of Internal Medicine* 148 (1988): 1023-1038.
27 McGrady, A.; Nadsady, P. A.; and Schumann-Brzezinski, C. "Sustained Effects of Biofeedback-Assisted Relaxation Therapy in Essential Hypertension." *Biofeedback and Self-Regulation* 16 no. 4 (Dec, 1991): 399-411.
28 Aivazyan, T. A.; et al. "Efficacy of Relaxation Techniques in Hypertensive Patients." *Health Psychology* 7 suppl. (1988): 193-200.
29 Petkov, V. "Plants with Hypotensive, Antiatheromatous and Coronary Dilating Action." *American Journal of Chinese Medicine* 7 no. 3 (1979): 197-236.
30 Ivanov, S. G.; et al. "The Magnetotherapy of Hypertension Patients." *Terapevticheskii Arkhiv* 62 no. 9 (1990): 71-4.

Male Health

1 Silverstein, J. I.; Baldini, G.H.; and Smith, A. D. "Management of Benign Prostatic Hypertrophy." *Clinical Geriatric Medicine* 6 69-84.
2 Hook, E. W. III, M.D., and Holmes, K. K., M.D. "Gonococcal Infections." *Annals of Internal Medicine* 102 no. 2 (Feb, 1985): 229-243.
Stamm, W. E., M.D.; et. al. "Chlamydia Trachamotis Urethral Infections in Men. Prevalence, Risk Factors, and Clinical Manifestations." *Annals of Internal Medicine* 100 no. 1 (Jan, 1984): 47-51.
3 Pizzorno, J. E.; and Murray, M. T. *A Textbook of Natural Medicine*. 2 vols. Seattle, WA: John Bastyr College Publications, 1989.
4 Pizzorno, J. E.; and Murray, M. T. *A Textbook of Natural Medicine*. 2 vols. Seattle, WA: John Bastyr College Publications, 1989.
Dyerberg, J.; et al. "Eicosapentaenoic Acid and Prevention of Thrombosis and Atherosclerosis." *Lancet* 2 no. 8081 (Jul, 1978): 117-119.
5 American Cancer Society. "Cancer Facts and Figures— 1993."
6 Ibid.
7 Blaivas, J., M.D. *Prostatism and Prostatic Cancer*. Virginia Geriatric Education Center, 1990.
8 Smith, D. R., M.D. *General Urology*. 11th ed. Los Altos, CA: Lange Medical Publications, 1984.
Abrams, W. B.; and Berkow, R.; eds. *The Merck Manual of Geriatrics*. Rahway, N.J.: Merck, Sharp and Dohme Research Labs, 1990.
Blaivas, J., M.D. *Prostatism and Prostatic Cancer*. Virginia Geriatric Education Center, 1990.
9 "Vasectomy Linked to Tripled Risk of Prostate Cancer." *Medical World News* (Sep 25, 1989).
10 Mavligit, G., M.D.; et al. "Chronic Immune Stimulation by Sperm Alloantibodies - Support for the Hypothesis That Spermatozoa Induce Immune Dysregulation in Homosexual Males." *Journal of the American Medical Association* 251 no. 2 (Jan, 1984): 237-241.
11 Smith, D. R., M.D. *General Urology*. 11th ed. Los Altos, CA: Lange Medical Publications, 1984.
Kruzel, T. "What is the Prostate and Why is it Doing This to Me?" *Health Review Newsletter* (Aug, 1991).
12 Ibid.
13 Smith, D. R., M.D. *General Urology*. 11th ed. Los Altos, CA: Lange Medical Publications, 1984.
14 This report is based solely on product labeling as published by PDR (R). Copyright (C) 1993 by Medical Economics Data, a division of Medical Economics Company, Inc. All rights reserved. There is no affiliation between Medical Economic Company, Inc., and Future Medicine Publishing, Inc.
15 Smith, D. R., M.D. *General Urology*. 11th ed. Los Altos, CA: Lange Medical Publications, 1984.
16 Dyerberg, J.; et al. "Eicosapentaenoic Acid and Prevention of Thrombosis and Atherosclerosis." *Lancet* 2 no. 8081 (Jul, 1978): 117-119.
17 Lewis, A. E. "Glandular Therapy: Historical Background and Emerging Scientific Status." *PHP Technical Information Series* (Feb, 1990).
18 Morales, A.; Surridge, D. H.; Marshall, P. "Yohimbine for Treatment of Impotence in Diabetes." *New England Journal of Medicine* 305 no. 20 (Nov, 1981): 1221.
Reid, K.; et al. "Double Blind Trial of Yohimbine in Treatment of Psychogenic Impotence." *Lancet* 2 no. 8556 (Aug, 1987): 421-423.
Morales, A.; et al. "Nonhormonal Pharma-cological Treatment of Organic Impotence." *Journal of Urology* 128 no. 1 (Jul, 1981): 45-47.
19 Brown, D. J. "Literature Review - Ginkgo Biloba; Phytotherapy Review & Commentary." *Townsend Letter for Doctors* (Dec, 1991).
20 Felter, H. W., M.D. *The Eclectic Materia Medica, Pharmacology and Therapeutics*. Portland, OR: Eclectic Medical Publications, 1983.
21 Stamey, T. A.; et al. "Prostate Specific Antigen as a Serum Marker for Adenocarcinoma of the Prostate." *New England Journal of Medicine* 317 no. 15 (Oct, 1987): 909-916.
Ellingwood, F., M.D. *American Materia Medica, Therapeutics and Pharmacognosy*. Portland, OR: Eclectic Medical Publications, 1983.
Brinker, F. *An Introduction to the Toxicology of Common Botanical Medicinal Substances*. Portland, OR: NCNM Publications, 1983.
Funk, E., M.D. *Potter's Therapeutics Materia Medica and Pharmacy*. 13th ed. Philadelphia: P. Blankiston's Son & Co., 1917.
Scudder, J. M., M.D. *Specific Medication and Specific Medicines*. 4th Rev., 15th ed. Cincinnati, OH: J. M. Scudder, 1880.
22 Farnsworth, N.; et al. "Eleuthrococcus Senticosus: Current Status as an Adaptogen." *Economic and Medicinal Plant Research* 1 (1985): 156-215.
Brekhman, I. I.; and Dardymov, I. V. "Pharmacological Investigation of Glycosides from Ginseng and Eleuthrococcus." *Lloydia* 32 no. 1 (Mar, 1969): 46-51.
23 Walker, M. "Serenoa Repens Extract (Saw Palmetto) Relief for Benign Prostatic Hypertrophy." *Townsend Letter for Doctors* (Feb/Mar, 1991).
Murray, M. "Liposterolic Extract of Serenoa Repens in the Treatment of Benign Prostatic Hyperplasia." *Phyto-Pharmica Review* 1 no. 5 (Aug, 1988).
24 Lange, J.; and Bordeaux, M. "Clinical Experimentation with V1326 in Prostatic Disorders." *Bordeaux Medical* 3 no. 11 (Nov, 1970): 2807-2808. In French.
Viollet, G. "Clinical Experimentation of a New Treatment for Prostatic Adenoma." *Vie Medicale* 23 (1970): 3457.
Kruzel, T. "What is the Prostate and Why is it Doing This to Me?" *Health Review Newsletter* (Aug, 1991).
25 Felter, H. W., M.D. *The Eclectic Materia Medica, Pharmacology and Therapeutics*. Portland, OR: Eclectic Medical Publications, 1983.
26 Felter, H. W., M.D. *The Eclectic Materia Medica, Pharmacology and Therapeutics*. Portland, OR: Eclectic Medical Publications, 1983.
Ellingwood, F., M.D. *American Materia Medica, Therapeutics and Pharmacognosy*. Portland, OR: Eclectic Medical Publications, 1983.
Culbreth, D. M. R., M.D. *A Manual of Materia Medica and Pharmacology*. Portland, OR: Eclectic Medical Publications, 1983.
Funk, E., M.D. *Potter's Therapeutics Materia Medica and Pharmacy*. 13th ed. Philadelphia: P. Blankiston's Son & Co., 1917.
Brinker, F. *An Introduction to the Toxicology of Common Botanical Medicinal Substances*. Portland, OR: NCNM Publications, 1983.
27 Felter, H. W., M.D. *The Eclectic Materia Medica, Pharmacology and Therapeutics*. Portland, OR: Eclectic Medical Publications, 1983.
Ellingwood, F., M.D. *American Materia Medica, Therapeutics and Pharmacognosy*. Portland, OR: Eclectic Medical Publications, 1983.
Culbreth, D. M. R., M.D. *A Manual of Materia Medica and Pharmacology*. Portland, OR: Eclectic Medical Publications, 1983.
Funk, E., M.D. *Potter's Therapeutics Materia Medica and Pharmacy*. 13th Ed. Philadelphia: P. Blankiston's Son & Co., 1917.
28 Farnsworth, N.; et al. "Eleuthrococcus Senticosus: Current Status as an Adaptogen." *Economic and Medicinal Plant Research* 1 (1985): 156-215.
Brekhman, I. I.; and Dardymov, I. V. "Pharmacological Investigation of Glycosides from Ginseng and Eleuthrococcus." *Lloydia* 32 no. 1 (Mar, 1969): 46-51.
29 Funk, E., M.D. *Potter's Therapeutics Materia Medica and Pharmacy*. 13th ed. Philadelphia: P. Blankiston's Son & Co., 1917.
Brinker, F. *An Introduction to the Toxicology of Common Botanical Medicinal Substances*. Portland, OR: NCNM Publications, 1983.
30 Brinker, F. *An Introduction to the Toxicology of Common Botanical Medicinal Substances*. Portland, OR: NCNM Publications, 1983.
31 Khwaja; T. A.; Dias, C. B.; and Pentecost, S.; et al. "Recent Studies on the Anticancer Activities of Mistletoe (Viscum album) and its Alkaloids." *Oncology* 43 suppl. 1 (1986): 42-50.
Bloksma, N.; et al. "Stimulation of Humoral and Cellular Immunity by Viscum Preparations." *Planta Medica* 46 no. 4 (Dec, 1982): 221-227.
32 Ellingwood, F., M.D. *American Materia Medica, Therapeutics and Pharmacognosy*. Portland, OR: Eclectic Medical Publications, 1983.
Brinker, F. *An Introduction to the Toxicology of Common Botanical Medicinal Substances*. Portland, Oregon: NCNM Publications, 1983.
Scudder, J. M., M.D. *Specific Medication and Specific Medicines*. Rev., 15th ed. Cincinnati, OH: The Scudder Brothers Co., 1903.
33 Ibid.
34 Felter, H. W., M.D. *The Eclectic Materia Medica, Pharmacology and Therapeutics*. Portland OR: Eclectic Medical Publications, 1983.
35 Mose, J. "Effect of Echinacin on Phagocytosis and Natural Killer Cells." *Medizinische Welt* 34 no. 51-52 (Dec, 1983): 1463-1467.

Wacker, A.; and Hilbig, W. "Virus Inhibition by Echinacea Purpurea." *Planta Medica* 33 (1978): 89-102. In German.
36 Martin, W. "Treatment of Prostate and Breast Cancer." *Townsend Letter for Doctors* (May, 1990).
37 Felter, H. W., M.D. *The Eclectic Materia Medica, Pharmacology and Therapeutics*. Portland OR: Eclectic Medical Publications, 1983.
Ellingwood, F., M.D. *American Materia Medica, Therapeutics and Pharmacognosy*. Portland, OR: Eclectic Medical Publications, 1983.
Brinker, F. *An Introduction to the Toxicology of Common Botanical Medicinal Substances*. Portland, OR: NCNM Publications, 1983.
38 Farnsworth, N.; et al. "Eleuthrococcus Senticosus: Current Status as an Adaptogen." *Economic and Medicinal Plant Research* 1 (1985): 156-215.
39 Dharmananda, S. *Your Nature, Your Health - Chinese Herbs in Constitutional Therapy*. Portland, OR: Institute for Traditional Medicine and Preservation of Health Care, 1986.
40 Martin, W. "Treatment of Prostate and Breast Cancer." *Townsend Letter for Doctors* (May, 1990).
Trattler, R. *Better Health Through Natural Healing: How to Get Well Without Drugs or Surgery*. New York: McGraw-Hill, 1985.
Schmid, R. *Traditional Foods Are Your Best Medicines*. Stratford, CT: Ocean View Publications, 1987.
41 Schmid, R. *Traditional Foods Are Your Best Medicines*. Stratford, CT: Ocean View Publications, 1987.
42 Schmid, R. *Traditional Foods Are Your Best Medicines*. Stratford, CT: Ocean View Publications, 1987.
43 Boyle, W.; and Saine, A. *Lectures in Naturopathic Hydrotherapy*. East Palestine, OH: Buckeye Naturopathic Press, 1991.

Mental Health

1 Regier, D. A.; et al. "The De Facto U.S. Mental and Addictive Disorders Service System." *Archives of General Psychiatry* 50 (Feb, 1993): 85.
2 Clayman, C. B., ed. *The American Medical Association Encyclopedia of Medicine*. New York: Random House, 1989.
3 Breggin, P. R. *Toxic Psychiatry: Why Therapy, Empathy and Love Must Replace the Drugs, Electroshock, and Biochemical Therapies of the "New Psychiatry"*. New York: St. Martin's Press, 1991.
4 Pizzorno, J. E.; and Murray, M. T. *A Textbook of Natural Medicine*. 2 vols. Seattle, WA: John Bastyr College Publications, 1989.
5 Lozoff, B.; Jimenez, E.; and Wolf, A., "Long-Term Developmental Outcome of Infants with Iron Deficiency." *New England Journal of Medicine* 325 (Sep, 1991): 687-694.
6 Pfeiffer, C. *Mental and Elemental Nutrients: A Physician's Guide to Nutrition and Health Care*. New Canaan, CT: Keats Publishing, 1975.
7 Schoenthaler, S.; Doraz, W.; and Wakefield, J., Jr. "The Impact of a Low Food Additive and Sucrose Diet on Academic Performance in 803 New York City Public Schools." *International Journal of Biosocial Research* 8 no. 2 (1986): 185-195.
8 Feingold, B. *Why Your Child is Hyperactive*. New York: Random House, 1975.
9 Pizzorno, J. E.; and Murray, M. T. *A Textbook of Natural Medicine*. 2 vols. Seattle, WA: John Bastyr College Publications, 1989.
10 Egger, J., et. al. "Controlled Trial of Oligoantigenic Treatment in the Hyperkinetic Syndrome." *Lancet* 1 no. 8428 (Mar, 1985): 540-545.
O'Shea, J.; and Porter, S. "Double-Blind Study of Children with Hyperkinetic Syndrome Treated with Multi-Allergen Extract Sublingually." *Journal of Learning Disabilities* 14 no. 1 (Apr,1981): 189-191.
11 Schrauzer, G.; and Shrestha, K. "Lithium in Drinking Water and Incidences in Crimes, Suicides and Arrests Related to Drug Addictions." *Biological Trace Element Research* 25 no. 2 (May, 1990): 105-113.
Wickham, E.; and Reed, J. "Lithium for the Control of Aggressive and Self-Mutilating Behavior." *International Clinical Psycho-pharmacology* 2 no. 3 (Jul, 1987): 181-190.
12 Perry, F.; et al. "Environmental Power-Frequency Magnetic Fields and Suicide." *Health Physics* 41 no. 2 (Aug, 1981): 267-277.
13 Perry, F.; and Pearl, L. "Health Effects of ELF Fields and Illness in Multistory Blocks." *Public Health* 102 no. 1 (Jan, 1988): 11-18.
14 Dowson, D. I.; and Lewith, G. T. "Overhead High Voltage Cables and Recurrent Headache and Depressions." *The Practitioner* 232 no. 1447 (Apr, 1988): 435-436.
15 Pizzorno, J. E.; and Murray, M. T. *A Textbook of Natural Medicine*. 2 vols. Seattle, WA: John Bastyr College Publications, 1989.
16 Walsh, W. "Biochemical Treatment of Behavior, Learning & Mental Disorders." *Townsend Letter for Doctors* (Aug/Sep, 1992): 299.
17 Pizzorno, J. E.; and Murray, M. T. *A Textbook of Natural Medicine*. 2 vols. Seattle, WA: John Bastyr College Publications, 1989.
18 Ott, J. "Color and Light: Their Effects on Plants, Animals and People." *The International Journal of Biosocial Research* 7-10 (1985-1988): 1-131.
19 Ott, J. *Health And Light*. Old Greenwich, CT: The Devin-Adair Co., 1973.
20 Roos, P. A. "Light and Electromagnetic Waves: The Health Implications." *Journal of the Bio-Electro-Magnetics Institute* 3 no. 2 (Summer, 1991): 7-12.
21 *Harvard Mental Health Letter* 8 no. 7 (Jan, 1992).
22 Ibid.
23 Lazarus, R. S.; and Folkman, S. *Stress, Appraisal, and Coping*. New York: Springer Publishing, 1984.
24 Nixon, P. G. "Human Functions and the Heart." In *Changing Ideas in Health Care*, eds. D. Seedhouse and A. Cribb. New York: John Wiley & Sons, 1989.
25 Achterberg, J. "Ritual: The Foundation for Transpersonal Medicine." *ReVision* 14 no. 3 (1992): 158-164.
26 Simonton, C.; and Matthews, S. *Getting Well Again*. Los Angeles: Jeremy P. Tarcher, 1978.
27 *Harvard Mental Health Letter* 8 no. 8 (Feb, 1992).
28 Berkman, L. F.; and Syme, S. L. "Social Networks, Host Resistance, and Mortality: a Nine-Year Follow-Up Study of Alameda County Residents." *American Journal of Epidemiology* 109 no. 2 (Feb, 1979): 186-204.
29 Spiegel, D.; et al. "Effect of Psychosocial Treatment on Survival of Patients with Metastatic Breast Cancer." *Lancet* 2 no. 8668 (Oct, 1989): 888-891.
30 Cohen, S.; Tyrrell, A.; and Smith, A. "Psychological Stress and Susceptibility to the Common Cold." *New England Journal of Medicine* 325 no. 9 (Aug, 1991): 606-612.
31 *Harvard Mental Health Letter* 8 no. 7 (Jan, 1992).
32 Healy, D., et. al. "The Thymus-Adrenal Connection: Thymosin Has Corticotropin-Releasing Activity in Primates." *Science* 222 no. 4630 (1983): 1353-1355.
33 Moyers, B. *Healing and the Mind*. New York: Doubleday, 1993.
34 Ibid.
35 This report is based solely on product labeling as published by PDR (R). Copyright (C) 1993 by Medical Economics Data, a division of Medical Economics Company, Inc. All rights reserved. There is no affiliation between Medical Economics Company, Inc., and Future Medicine Publishing, Inc.
36 Muldner, V.; and Zoller, M. "Antidepressive Effect of a Hypericum Extract Standardized to an Active Hypericine Complex: Biochemical and Clinical Studies." *Arzneimittel Forschung* 34 no. 8 (1984): 918-920. In German.
37 Hoffer, A., M.D.; Osmond, H.; and Smythies, J. "Schizophrenia: a New Approach. II. Results of a Year's Research." *Journal of Mental Science* 100 no. 418 (Jan, 1954): 29-45.
38 Hoffer, A. "Chronic Schizophrenic Patient Treated Ten Years or More." *Journal of Orthomolecular Medicine* 8 (1993).
39 Johnstone, E.; et al. "Disabilities and Circumstance of Schizophrenic Patients - a Follow-Up Study." *The British Journal of Psychiatry* 159 suppl. 13. (1991): 3-46.
40 Werbach, M. R., M.D. *Nutritional Influences on Mental Illness*. Tarzana, CA: Third Line Press, 1991.
41 Beasley, J. D. *The Betrayal of Health: the Impact of Nutrition, Environment, and Lifestyle on Illness in America*. New York: Times Books, 1991.
42 Walsh, W. "Biochemical Treatment of Behavior, Learning and Mental Disorders." *Townsend Letter for Doctors* (Aug/Sep, 1992): 299.
43 Ibid.
44 Knivsberg, A., et. al. "Dietary Intervention in Autistic Syndromes." *Brain Dysfunction* 3 (Nov/Dec, 1990): 315-327.
45 Braud, L.; Lupin, M.; and Braud, W. "The Use of Electromyographic Biofeedback in the Control of Hyperactivity." *Journal of Learning Disabilities* 8 no. 7 (1975).
Lupin, M.; et al. "Children Parents, and Relaxation Tapes." *Academic Therapy* 12 no. 1 (1976).
46 Chaitow, L. *The Stress Protection Plan*. San Francisco: Harper, 1992.
47 Berquier, A.; and Ashton, R. "Characteristics of the Frequent Nightmare Sufferer." *Journal of Abnormal Psychology* 101 no. 2 (May, 1992): 246-250.
48 Kellner, R.; et. al. "Changes in Chronic Nightmares After one Session of Desensitization or Rehearsal Instructions." *American Journal of Psychiatry* 149 no. 5 (May, 1992): 659-663.
49 Philpott, W.; and Taplin, S. *Biomagnetic Handbook*. Choctaw, OK: Enviro-Tech Products, 1990.

Multiple Sclerosis

1 Agranoff, B. W.; and Goldberg, D. "Diet and the Geographical Distribution of Multiple Sclerosis." *Lancet* 2 no. 7888 (Nov, 1974): 1061-1066.
2 Swank, R. L. "Multiple Sclerosis: Chronicle of its Incidence with Dietary Fat." *American Journal of Science* 220 no. 2 (Oct, 1950): 421-430.
Sinclair, H. M. "Deficiency of Essential Fatty Acids and Atherosclerosis, etcetera." *Lancet* 270 no. 1 (1956): 381-383.
Alter, M.; Yamoor, M.; and Harshe, M. "Multiple Sclerosis and Nutrition." *Archives of Neurology* 31 no. 4 (Oct, 1974): 267-272.
Agranoff, B. W.; and Goldberg, D. "Diet and the Geographical Distribution of Multiple Sclerosis." *Lancet* 2 no. 7888 (Nov, 1974): 1061-1066.
Crawford, M. A.; Budowski, P.; and Hassam, A. G. "Dietary Management in Multiple Sclerosis." *Proceedings of the Nutrition Society* 38 no. 3 (Dec, 1979): 373-379.
3 Gay, D.; Dick, G.; and Upton, G. "Multiple Sclerosis Associated with Sinusitis: Case-Controlled Study in General Practice." *Lancet* 1 no. 8940 (Apr, 1986): 815-819.
4 Crook, W. G., M.D. *The Yeast Connection*. Jackson, TN: Professional Books, 1984.
5 International Labour Office. *Encyclopedia of Occupational Health and Safety*. 2d ed. New York: Mc Graw-Hill, 1972.
6 Vimy, M. J.; Takahashi, Y.; and Lorscheider, F. L. "Maternal-Fetal Distribution of Mercury Released From Dental Amalgam Fillings." *American Physiological Society* 258 (1990): R939-R945.
Lorscheider, F.L.; et al. "Mercury From Amalgam Tooth Fillings: Its Tissue Distribution and Effects on Cell Functions." *The Toxicologist* 12 (1992): 1.
7 Vimy, M.J.; et al. "Glomerular Filtration Impairment by Mercury from Dental 'Silver' Fillings in Sheep." *The Physiologist* 33 (Aug, 1990): A 94.
Boyd, N.D.; et al. "Mercury from Dental 'Silver' Tooth Fillings Impairs Sheep Kidney Function." *American Physiological Society* 261 (1991): R1010-R1014.
Ahlrot-Westerlund, B., M.D. "Mercury in Cerebrospinal Fluid in Multiple Sclerosis." *Sweden Journal of Biological Medicine* 1 (Mar, 1989): 6.
8 Williams, L. L.; Doody, D. M.; and Horrocks, L. A. "Serum Fatty Acid Proportions Are Altered During The Year Following Acute Epstein-Barr

Virus Infection." *Lipids* 23 no. 10 (Oct, 1988): 981-988.
9 Rose, J.; et al. "Genetic Susceptibility in Familial Multiple Sclerosis Not Linked to the Myelin Basic Protein Gene." *Lancet* 341 no. 8854 (May, 1993): 1179-1181.
10 Swank, R. L.; and Dugan, B. B. "Effect of Low Saturated Fat Diet in Early and Late Cases of Multiple Sclerosis." *Lancet* 336 no. 8706 (Jul, 1990): 37-39.
11 Pageler, J. *New Hope, Real Help For Those Who Have Multiple Sclerosis.*
12 Reynolds, E. H.; Linnell, J. C.; and Faludy, J. E. "Multiple Sclerosis Associated with Vitamin B12 Deficiency." *Archives of Neurology* 48 no. 8 (Aug, 1991): 808-811.
13 Nijist, T. Q.; et al. "Vitamin B12 and Folate Concentrations in Serum and Cerebrospinal Fluid of Neurological Patients with Special Reference to Multiple Sclerosis and Dementia." *Journal of Neurology, Neurosurgery, and Psychiatry* 53 no. 11 (Nov, 1990): 951-954.
14 Webster, C. J.; et al. "The Chief Scientist Reports...Hyperbaric Oxygen for Multiple Sclerosis." *Health Bulletin* 47 no. 6 (Nov, 1989): 320-331.
15 Barnes, M. P.; et al. "Hyperbaric Oxygen and Multiple Sclerosis: Short-Term Results of a Placebo-Controlled Double-Blind Trial." *Lancet* 1 no. 8424 (Feb, 1985): 287-300.
Wiles, C. M.; et al. "Hyperbaric Oxygen in Multiple Sclerosis: A Double-Blind Trial." *British Medical Journal* 292 no. 6517 (Feb, 1986): 367-371.

Obesity and Weight Management

1 NIH Technology Assessment Conference Panel. "Methods for Voluntary Weight Loss and Control." *Annals of Internal Medicine* 116 no.11 (Jun, 1992): 942-949.
2 Ibid.
3 Editorial Staff. "Body Weight, Health and Longevity: Conclusions and Recommendations of the Workshop." *Nutrition Reviews* 43 no. 2 (Feb, 1985): 61-63.
Ingram, D.; et al. "Obesity and Breast Disease: The Role of the Female Sex Hormones." *Cancer* 64 no. 5 (Sep, 1989): 1049-1053.
4 Warwick, P. M.; et al. *Recent Advances in Obesity Research II: Proceedings of the International Conference on Obesity.* London: Newman, 1978.
5 Heleniak, E. P.; and Aston, B. "Prostaglandins, Brown Fat and Weight Loss." *Medical Hypotheses* 28 no. 1 (Jan, 1989): 13-33.
6 Editorial Staff. "Alterations in Metabolic Rate after Weight Loss in Obese Humans." *Nutrition Reviews* 43 no. 2 (Feb, 1985): 41-42.
7 Porte, D., Jr.; and Woods, S. C. "Regulation of Food Intake and Body Weight by Insulin." *Diabetologia* 20 suppl. (Mar, 1981): 274-280.
8 Krause, M. V.; and Mahan, L. K. *Food, Nutrition and Diet Therapy.* 7th ed. Philadelphia: W.B. Saunders, 1984.
9 Editorial Staff. "Alterations in Metabolic Rate after Weight Loss in Obese Humans." *Nutrition Reviews* 43 no. 2 (Feb, 1985): 41-42.
10 Wadden, T. A.; Van Itallie, T. B.; and Blackburn, G. L. "Responsible and Irresponsible Use of Very-Low-Calorie Diets in the Treatment of Obesity." *Journal of the American Medical Association* 263 no. 1 (Jan, 1990): 83-85.
11 This report is based solely on product labeling as published by PDR (R). Copyright (C) 1993 by Medical Economics Data, a division of Medical Economics Company, Inc. All rights reserved. There is no affiliation between Medical Economic Company, Inc., and Future Medicine Publishing, Inc.
12 NIH Technology Assessment Conference Panel. "Methods for Voluntary Weight Loss and Control." *Annals of Internal Medicine* 116 no. 11 (Jun, 1992): 942-949.
13 Trowell, H.; Burkitt, D.; and Heaton, K. *Dietary Fibre, Fibre-Depleted Foods and Disease.* NY: Academic Press, 1985.
14 Davidson, M. H.; et al. "The Hypo-cholesterolemic Effects of Beta-Glucan in Oatmeal and Oat Bran. A Dose-Controlled Study." *Journal of the American Medical Association* 265 no. 14 (Apr, 1991): 1833-1839.
Anderson, J. W.; and Bryant, C. A. "Dietary Fiber: Diabetes and Obesity." *American Journal of Gastroenterology* 81 no. 10 (Oct, 1986): 898-906.
15 Kendall, A.; et al. "Weight Loss on a Low-Fat Diet: Consequence of the Imprecision of the Control of Food Intake in Humans." *American Journal of Clinical Nutrition* 53 no. 5 (May, 1991): 1124-1129.
16 Schutz, Y.; Flatt, J. P.; and Jequier, E. "Failure of Dietary Fat to Promote Fat Oxidation: A Factor Favoring the Development of Obesity." *American Journal of Clinical Nutrition* 50 no. 2 (Aug, 1989): 307-314.
17 Flatt, J. P., "Body Weight, Fat Storage, and Alcohol Metabolism." *Nutrition Reviews* 50 no. 9 (Sep, 1992): 267-270.
18 Flatt, J. P., "Body Weight, Fat Storage, and Alcohol Metabolism." *Nutrition Reviews* 50 no. 9 (Sep, 1992): 267-270.
Suter, P. M.; Schutz, Y.; and Jequier, E. "The Effect of Ethanol on Fat Storage in Healthy Subjects." *New England Journal of Medicine* 326 no. 15 (Apr, 1992): 983-987.
19 Morris, B. W.; et al. "The Trace Element Chromium—a Role in Glucose Homeostasis." *American Journal of Clinical Nutrition* 55 no. 5 (May, 1992): 989-991.
20 Bryce-Smith, D., and Simpson, R. I. "Case of Anorexia Nervosa Responding to Zinc Sulphate." *Lancet* 2 no. 8398 (Aug, 1984): 350.
21 Gard, Z. R., M.D.; and Brown, E. J. "Literature Review & Comparison Studies of Sauna/Hyperthermia in Detoxification-Part I." *Townsend Letter for Doctors* 107 (Jun, 1992): 470-78.
Gard, Z. R., M.D.; and Brown; E. J. "Literature Review & Comparison Studies of the Sauna and Illness-Part II." *Townsend Letter for Doctors* 108 (Jul, 1992): 650-52, 654-56, 658-60.
22 Ibid.
23 van Dale, D.; and Saris, W. H. "Repetitive Weight Loss and Weight Regain: Effects on Weight Reduction, Resting Metabolic Rate, and Lipolytic Activity Before and After Exercise and/or Diet Treatment." *American Journal of Clinical Nutrition* 49 no. 3 (Mar, 1989): 409-416.
24 Dulloo, A. G.; and Miller D. S. "The Thermogenic Properties of Ephedrine/Methylxanthine Mixtures: Animal Studies." *American Journal of Clinical Nutrition* 43 no. 3 (Mar, 1986): 388-394.
Astrup A; et al. "The Effect of Chronic Ephedrine Treatment on Substrate Utilization, the Sympathoadrenal Activity and Energy Expenditure During Glucose-Induced Thermogenesis in Man." *Metabolism: Clinical and Experimental* 35 no. 3 (Mar, 1986): 260-265.
25 Dulloo, A. G.; and Miller D. S. "The Thermogenic Properties of Ephedrine/Methylxanthine Mixtures: Animal Studies." *American Journal of Clinical Nutrition* 43 no. 3 (Mar, 1986): 388-394.
Dulloo, A. G.; and Miller, D.S. "Aspirin as a Promoter of Ephedrine-Induced Thermogenesis: Potential Use in the Treatment of Obesity." *American Journal of Clinical Nutrition* 45 no. 3 (Mar, 1987): 564-569.

Osteoporosis

1 U.S. Department of Health and Human Services Public Health Service, National Institutes of Health. "Medicine for the Layman: Osteoporosis."
2 Tolstoi L. G.; and Levin, R. M. "Osteoporosis—the Treatment Controversy." *Nutrition Today* (Jul/Aug,1992): 6-12.
3 Nelson, M. E.; et al. "A 1-Year Walking Program and Increased Dietary Calcium in the Postmenopausal Woman: Effects on Bone." *American Journal of Clinical Nutrition* 53 no. 5 (May, 1991): 1304-1311.
4 U.S. Department of Health and Human Services, Public Health Service, National Institutes of Health. "Medicine for the Layman: Osteoporosis."
5 Pemberton, C.; et al. *Mayo Clinic Diet Manual: a Handbook of Dietary Practices.* 6th ed. Philadelphia: B. C. Decker, Inc. 1988, 208-211.
6 Coats, C., M.D. "Negative Effects of a High-Protein Diet." *Family Practice Recertification* 12 no. 12 (Dec, 1990): 80-94.
7 Marsh, A.G.; et al. "Vegetarian Lifestyle and Bone Mineral Density." *American Journal of Clinical Nutrition* 48 suppl. 3 (Sep, 1988): 837-841.
8 Weed, S. M. *Menopausal Years.* New York: Ash Tree Publishing, 1992, 22.
9 Thom, J. A.; et al. "The Influence of Refined Carbohydrate on Urinary Calcium Excretion." *British Journal of Urology* 50 no. 7 (Dec, 1987): 459-64.
10 Heaney, R. P. "Calcium Bioavailability." *Boletin-Asociacion Medica del Puerto Rico* 79 no. 1 (Jan, 1987): 27-29.
Heaney, R. P.; Recker, R. R. "Effects of Nitrogen, Phosphorus and Caffeine on Calcium Balance in Women." *Journal of Laboratory and Clinical Medicine* 99 no. 1 (Jan, 1982): 46-55.
11 Kiel, D. P., et al. "Caffeine and the Risks of Hip Fracture: the Framingham Study." *American Journal of Epidemiology* 132 no. 4 (Oct, 1990): 675- 684.
12 Lees, B.; et al. "Differences in Proximal Femur Bone Density Over Two Centuries." *Lancet* 341 no. 8846 (Mar, 1993): 673-675.
13 Cooper, C.; et al. "Water Flouridation and Hip Fracture." *Journal of the American Medical Association* 19 no. 32 (Jul, 1991): 513-514.
Sowers, M. F.; et al. "A Prospective Study of Bone Mineral Content and Fracture in Communities with Differential Fluoride Exposure." *American Journal of Epidemiology* 133 no. 7 (Apr, 1991): 649-660.
14 Kung, A. W. C.; and Pun, K. K. "Bone Mineral Density in Premenopausal Women Receiving Long-Term Physiological Doses of Levothyroxine." *Journal of the American Medical Association* 265 no. 20 (1991): 2688-2691.
15 Bachrach, L. K.; et al. "Recovery from Osteopenia in Adolescent Girls with Anorexia Nervosa." *Journal of Clinical Endocrinology and Metabolism* 72 no. 3 (Mar, 1991): 602-606.
16 Nelson, M. E. "Hormone and Bone Mineral Status in Endurance-Trained and Sedentary Postmenopausal Women. *Journal of Clinical Endocrinology and Metabolism* 66 no. 5 (May, 1988): 927-933.
17 National Institutes of Health Consensus Conference: "Osteoporosis." *Journal of the American Medical Association* 252 no. 6 (Aug, 1984): 799-802.
18 U.S. Department of Health and Human Services, Public Health Service, National Institutes of Health. "Medicine for the Layman: Osteoporosis."
19 Appleton, N. *Healthy Bones: What You Should do About Osteoporosis.* Garden City Park, NY: Avery Publishing Group, 1991, 61-62.
20 Wolfe, H. L. *Menopause: A Second Spring.* Boulder, CO: Blue Poppy Press, 1990, 151.
21 Lee, J. R., M.D. "Significance of Molecular Configuration Specificity: The Case of Progesterone and Osteoporosis." *Townsend Letter for Doctors* 119 (Jun, 1993): 558-562.
22 Hargrove, J. T.; et al. "Menopausal Hormone Replacement Therapy with Continuous Daily Oral Micronized Estradiol and Gynecology." *Obstetrics and Gynecology* 73 no. 4 (Apr, 1989): 606-612.
23 Weed, S. M. *Menopausal Years.* New York: Ash Tree Publishing, 1992, 155.
24 Lindsay, R.; et al. "Bone Response to Termination of Oestrogen Treatment." *Lancet* 1 no. 8078 (Jun, 1978): 1325-1327.
25 Wolfe, S. M., M.D.; and the Public Citizen Health Research Group. *Women's Health Alert.* Reading, MA: Addison-Wesley Publishing Company, 1991, 124.
26 Pruitt, L. A.; et al. "Weight-Training Effects on Bone Mineral Density in Early Postmenopausal Women." *Journal of Bone and Mineral Research* 7 no. 2 (Feb, 1992): 179-185.
27 Ibid.

Parasitic Infections

1 Mansfield, J. M., ed. *Parasitic Diseases.* New York: Marcel Dekker, 1981.
2 Crewe, W.; and Haddock, D. R. W. *Parasites and Human Disease.* New York: Wiley Medical Publications, 1985.
3 Oxner, R. B.; et al. "Dientamoeba Fragilis: a Bowel Pathogen?" *New Zealand Medical Journal*

100 no. 817 (1987): 64-65.
Desser, S. S.; and Yang, Y. J. "Dientamoeba Fragilis in Idiopathic Gastrointestinal Disorders." *Canadian Medical Association Journal* 114 no. 4 (1976): 290-293.
Yang, J.; and Scholten, T. "Dientamoeba Fragilis: a Review with Notes on its Epidemiology, Pathogenicity, Mode of Transmission and Diagnosis." *American Journal of Tropical Medicine and Hygiene* 26 no. 1 (1977): 16-22.
4 Mahmoud, A. A. "Parasitic Protozoa and Helminths: Biological and Immunological Challenges." *Science* 246 no. 4933 (Nov, 1989): 1015-1022.
5 Susser, M., M.D.; and Rosenbaum, M., M.D. *Solving the Puzzle of Chronic Fatigue Syndrome*. Tacoma, WA: Life Sciences Press, 1992.
6 Hall, A; et al. "Intensity of Reinfection with Ascaris Lumbricoides and its Implications for Parasite Control." *Lancet 339 No. 8804 (May, 1992: 1253-1257.*
7 Leventhal, R.; and Cheadle, R. F. *Medical Parasitology: A Self-Instructional Text*. 3d ed. Philadelphia: F.A. Davis Company, 1989.
8 Ibid.
9 Spencer, M. J.; et al. "Parasitic Infections in a Pediatric Population." *Pediatric Infectious Diseases* 2 no. 2 (Mar/Apr, 1983): 110-113.
10 Todd, S. C.; et al. "Cryptosporidium and Giardia in Surface Water in and around Manhattan." Kansas, *Transactions of the Kansas Academy of Science* 94 nos. 3-4 (1991): 101-106.
11 Juranek, D. "Giardiasis." Centers for Disease Control, Division of Parasitic Infection, Atlanta, Georgia.
12 Keystone, J. S.; et al. "Intestinal Parasites in Metropolitan Toronto Day-Care Centers." *Canadian Medical Association Journal* 131 no. 7 (1984): 733-735.
13 Spencer, M. J.; et al. "Parasitic Infections in a Pediatric Population." *Pediatric Infectious Diseases* 2 no. 2 (Mar/Apr, 1983): 110-113.
14 Hollander, D.; and Tarnawski, H. "Aging-Associated Increase in Intestinal Absorption of Macromolecules." *Gerontology* 31 no. 3 (1985): 133-137.
15 Adams, K. O.; et al. "Intestinal Fluke Infestation as a Result of Eating Sushi." *American Journal of Clinical Pathology* 86 no. 5 (1986): 688-689.
Ishizuka, T.; and Ishizuka, A. "A Case of Diphyllobothriasis Due to Eating Masou-Sushi." *Medical Journal of Australia* 145 no. 2 (1986): 114.
16 Chester, A. C.; et al. "Giardiasis as a Chronic Disease." *Digestive Diseases and Science* 30 no. 3 (1985): 215-218.
17 Plorde, J. J. "Intestinal Nematodes." In *Harrison's Principles of Internal Medicine*, 8th ed., eds. G. W. Thorne; et al. New York, McGraw-Hill, 1977.
18 Galland, L., M.D.; et al. *Journal of Nutritional Medicine* 1 (1990): 27-31.
19 *New England Journal of Medicine* (Jul 21, 1986).
20 Galland, L., M.D. *Superimmunity For Kids*. New York: Dell Publishing, 1989.
21 *Journal of Advancement in Medicine* 2 (1990).
22 Casemore, D., M.D. "Foodborne Protozoal Infection." *Lancet* 336 no. 8728 (Dec, 1990): 1427-1432.
23 Bendig, D. W., M.D. "Diagnosis of Giardiasis in Infants and Children by Endoscopic Brush Cytology." *Journal of Pediatric Gastroenterology and Nutrition* 8 no. 2 (1989): 204-206.
24 *Remington's Pharmaceutical Guide*. 17th ed. Ch. 65, p. 1235

Pregnancy and Childbirth

1 Williams, R. J. *Nutrition Against Disease, Environmental Protection*. New York: Bantam Books, 1971, 57.
2 Barnes, B.; and Bradley, S. G. *Planning for a Healthy Baby*. London: Ebury Press, 1990.
3 Price, W. A. *Nutrition and Physical Degeneration*. 50th anniv. ed. New Canaan, CT: Keats Publishing, Inc., 1989.
4 Hirson, C. "Coeliac Infertility— Folic Acid Therapy." *Lancet* 1 no. 643 (Feb, 1970): 412.
Dawson, D. W.; and Sawyers, A. H. "Infertility and Folate Deficiency. Case Reports."*British Journal of Obstetrics and Gynaecology* 89 no. 8 (Aug, 1982): 678-680.
Jackson, I.; Doig, W. B.; and McDonald, G. "Pernicious Anaemia as a Cause of Infertility." *Lancet* 2 no. 527 (Dec, 1967): 1159-1160.
Pschera, H.; et al. "Fatty Acid Composition of Cervical Mucous, Lecithin and Primary Infertility." *Infertility* 2 no. 1 (1988): 123-132.
5 Cimons, M. "U.S. Advises Folic Acid to Reduce Birth Defects." *Los Angeles Times* (Sep 15, 1992): A1-A17.
MRC Vitamin Study Research Group. "Prevention of Neural Tube Defects: Results of the Medical Research Council Vitamin Study." *Lancet* 338 no. 8760 (1991): 131-137.
6 Wilcox, A.; Weinberg, C.; and Baird, D. "Caffeinated Beverages and Decreased Fertility." *Lancet* 2 nos. 8626 & 8627 (Dec, 1988): 1453-1456.
7 Zavos, P. M. "Cigarette Smoking and Human Reproduction: Effects on Female and Male Fecundity." *Infertility* 12 no. 1 (1989): 35-46.
8 Phipps, W. R.; et al. "The Association Between Smoking and Female Infertility as Influenced by Cause of the Infertility." *Fertility & Sterility* 48 no. 3 (Sep, 1987): 377-382.
9 Barnes, B.; and Bradley, S. G. *Planning for a Healthy Baby*. London: Ebury Press, 1990.
Stenchever, M. A.; Kunysz, T. J.; and Allen, M.A. "Chromosome Breakage in Users of Marijuana." *American Journal of Obstetrics and Gynecology* 118 no. 1 (Jan, 1974): 106-113.
10 Barnes, B.; and Bradley, S. G. *Planning for a Healthy Baby*. London: Ebury Press, 1990.
11 Bracken, M. B.; et al. "Association of Cocaine Use with Sperm Concentration, Motility, and Morphology." *Fertility and Sterility* 53 no. 2 (Feb, 1990): 315-322.
12 Barnes, B.; and Bradley, S. G. *Planning for a Healthy Baby*. London: Ebury Press, 1990.
13 Terreros, M.C.; De Luca, J.C.; and Dulout, F.N. "The Effect of a Hypoproteic Diet and Ethanol Consumption on the Yield of Chromosomal Damage Detected in the Bone Marrow Cells of Mice." *Journal of Veterinary Medical Science*. 55 No. 2 (Apr 1993): 191-194.
14 Samuels, M., M.D.; and Samuels, N. *The Well Pregnancy Book*. New York: Summit Books, 1986.
15 Sutton, P. R. "Acute Dental Caries, Mental Stress, Immunity and the Active Passage of Ions Through the Teeth." *Medical Hypotheses* 31 no. 1 (Jan, 1990): 17.
Cohen, S.; Tyrrell, D. A. J.; and Smith, A. P. "Psychological Stress and Susceptibility to the Common Cold." *New England Journal of Medicine* 325 no. 9 (Aug, 1991): 606-612.
Harrison, K. L.; Callan, V. J.; and Hennessey, J. F. "Stress and Semen Quality in an In Vitro Fertilization Program." *Fertility and Sterility* 48 no. 4 (Oct, 1987): 633-636.
16 De Rosis, F.; et al. "Female Reproductive Health in Two Lamp Factories: Effects of Exposure to Inorganic Mercury Vapour and Stress Factors." *British Journal of Industrial Medicine* 42 no. 7 (Jul, 1985): 488-494.
17 Editorial Staff. "Czechoslovakian Study: Unwanted Children Face Struggle." *Pregnancy and Child Birth: Brain/Mind Bulletin Collections* 15 no. 02B (1991).
18 Samuels, M., M.D.; and Samuels, N. *The Well Pregnancy Book*. New York: Summit Books, 1986.
19 Ibid.
20 Kardaun, J. W.; et al. "Testicular Cancer in Young Men and Parental Occupational Exposure." *American Journal of Industrial Medicine* 20 no. 2 (1991): 219-227.
21 Al-Hachim, G. M. "Teratogenicity of Caffeine; A Review." *European Journal of Obstetrics & Gynecology and Reproductive Biology* 31 no. 3 (Jun, 1989): 237-247.
22 Peacock, J.C.; et al. "Cigarette Smoking and Birthweight: Type of Cigarette Smoked and a Possible Threshold Effect." *International Journal of Epidemiology*. 20 No.2 (1991): 405-412.
23 Ernhart, C.B.; et al. "Alcohol Teratogenicity in the Human: A Detailed Assessment of Specificity, Critical Period, and Threshold." *American Journal of Obstetrics and Gynecology*. 156 No.1 (Jan 1987): 33-39.
24 Editorial Staff. "Aspirin-Pregnancy Link: Lowered I.Q.'s." *Pregnancy and Child Birth: Brain/Mind Bulletin Collections* 13 no. 9K (1991).
25 Editorial Staff. "Valium Inhibits Cell Fusion in Lab Tests." *Pregnancy and Child Birth: Brain/Mind Bulletin Collections* 12 no. 13D (1991).
26 O'Leary, L. M.; Hicks, A. M.; Peters, J. M.; and London, S. "Parental Occupational Exposures and Risk of Childhood Cancer: a Review." *American Journal of Industrial Medicine* 20 no. 1 (1991): 17-35.
27 Kardaun, J. W.; et al. "Testicular Cancer in Young Men and Parental Occupational exposure." *American Journal of Industrial Medicine* 20 no. 2 (1991): 219-227.
28 Editorial. "Vitamin A and Teratogenesis." *Lancet* 1 no. 8424 (Feb, 1985): 319-320.
29 Simkin, P.; Whalley, J.; and Keppler A. *Pregnancy, Childbirth and the Newborn: The Complete Guide*. New York: Meadowbrook Press, 1991.
30 Rush, D.; Stein, Z.; and Susser, M. "A Randomized Controlled Trial of Prenatal Nutritional Supplementation in New York City." *Pediatrics* 65 no. 4 (Apr, 1980): 683-697.
31 Simkin, P.; Whalley, J.; and Keppler, A. *Pregnancy, Childbirth and the Newborn: The Complete Guide*. New York: Meadowbrook Press, 1991.
32 Rush, D.; Stein, Z.; and Susser, M. "A Randomized Controlled Trial of Prenatal Nutritional Supplementation in New York City." *Pediatrics* 65 no. 4 (Apr, 1980): 683-697.
33 Baum, G.; et al. "Meclozine and Pyridoxine in Pregnancy Sickness." *Practitioner* 190 no. 1136 (1963): 251-253.
34 Kawasaki, N., et al. "Effect of Calcium Supplementation on the Vascular Sensitivity to Angiotensin II in Pregnant Women." *American Journal of Obstetrics and Gynecology* 153 no. 5 (Nov, 1985): 576-582.
35 MRC Vitamin Study Research Group. "Prevention of Neural Tube Defects: Results of the Medical Research Council Vitamin Study." *Lancet* 338 no. 8760 (Jul, 1991): 131-137.
36 Editorial Staff. "Excessive Folic Acid." *American Family Physician* 32 no. 4 (Oct, 1985): 290-291.
37 Simmer, K.; James, C.; and Thompson, R. P. "Are Iron-Folate Supplements Harmful?" *American Journal of Clinical Nutrition* 45 no. 1 (Jan, 1987): 122-125.
38 Gertner, J. M.; et al. "Pregnancy as State of Physiologic Absorptive Hypercalciuria." *The American Journal of Medicine* 81 no. 3 (Sep, 1986): 451-456.
39 Simkin, P.; Whalley, J.; and Keppler, A. *Pregnancy, Childbirth, and the Newborn: The Complete Guide*. New York: Meadowbrook Press, 1991.
40 Page, E. W.; and Page, E. P. "Leg Cramps in Pregnancy: Etiology and Treatment." *Obstetrics and Gynecology* 1 (1953): 94.
41 Jones, Carl; Goer, H.; and Simkin, P. "The Labor Support Guide—for Father, Family and Friends." Pamphlet. Seattle, WA: Pennypress, Inc., 1984.
42 Haverkamp, A. D.; et al. "The Evaluation of Continuous Fetal Heart Rate Monitoring in High-Risk Pregnancy." *American Journal of Obstetrics & Gynecology* 125 no. 3 (Jun, 1976): 310-320.
43 Lopez, N. M. "Why Natural Childbirth is Better than Medicated Childbirth." *NAPSAC News* 14 no. 1 (1989): 6-7.
44 Ibid.
45 Langendoerfer, S.; et al. "Pediatric Follow-Up of a Randomized Controlled Trial of Intrapartum Fetal Monitoring Techniques." *Journal of Pediatrics* 97 no. 1 (Jul, 1980): 103-107.
46 Pritchard, J. "Analgesia and Anesthesia." In *William's Obstetrics*.
47 Righard, L.; and Alade, M. O. "Effect of Delivery Room Routines on Success of First Breast-Feed." *Lancet* 336 no. 8723 (Nov, 1990): 1105-1107.
48 Walton, P.; and Reynolds, F. "Epidural Analgesia and Instrumental Delivery." *Anaesthesia* 39 no. 3 (Mar, 1984): 218-223.

Klein, M. C.; et al. "Does Episiotomy Prevent Perineal Trauma and Pelvic Floor Relaxation?" *Online Journal of Current Clinical Trials* (July 1, 1992).
49 Lopez, N. M. "Why Natural Childbirth is Better than Medicated Childbirth." *NAPSAC News* 14 no. 1 (1989): 6-7.
50 Klein, M. C.; et al. "Does Episiotomy Prevent Perineal Trauma and Pelvic Floor Relaxation?" *Online Journal of Current Clinical Trials* (Jul 1, 1992).
51 Seidman, D. S.; et al. "Long-Term Effects of Vacuum and Forceps Deliveries." *Lancet* 337 no. 8757 (Jun, 1991): 1583-1585.
Nuijen, S.; and Housman, R. "Fatal Forceps." *Medicine, Science, and the Law* 23 no. 4 (Oct, 1983): 254-256.
52 Ibid.
53 Nuijen, S.; and Housman, R. "Fatal Forceps." *Medicine, Science, and the Law* 23 no. 4 (Oct, 1983): 254-256.
54 Stafford, R. S. "Alternative Strategies for Controlling Rising Cesarean Section Rates." *Journal of the American Medical Association* 263 no. 5 (Feb, 1990): 683-687.
55 Barrett, J. F. et al. "Inconsistencies in Clinical Decisions in Obstetrics." *Lancet* 336 no. 8714 (Sep, 1990): 549-551.
56 Richards, L. B. "Natural Birth Following Cesareans." *NAPSAC News* 14 no. 1 (1989): 1-5.
57 Ibid.
58 Carroll, J. C.; et al. "The Influence of the High-Risk Care Environment on the Practice of Low-Risk Obstetrics." *Family Medicine* 23 no. 3 (Mar/Apr, 1991): 184-188.
59 Ibid.
60 Ibid.
61 Ibid.
62 Ibid.
63 Editorial Staff. "Home Birth Has Better Record in First Return." *Pregnancy and Child Birth: Brain/Mind Bulletin Collections* 2 no. 7G (1991).
Simkin, P.; Whalley, J.; and Keppler, A. *Pregnancy, Childbirth and the Newborn*. New York: Meadowbrook Press, 1991.
64 Barnow, F.; and Postmantur, R. "Water Birth." *PCC Sound Consumer* (Sep, 1989): 12.
65 Noble, E. *Childbirth With Insight*. Boston: Houghton Mufflin Co, 1983.
66 Ibid.
67 Ibid.
68 Odent, M. R. "Position in Delivery." *Lancet* 335 no. 8698 (May, 1990): 1166.
Carroll, J. C.; et al. "The Influence of the High-Risk Care Environment on the Practice of Low-Risk Obstetrics." *Family Medicine* 23 no. 3 (Mar/Apr, 1991): 184-188.
69 Carroll, J. C.; et al. "The Influence of the High-Risk Care Environment on the Practice of Low-Risk Obstetrics." *Family Medicine* 23 no. 3 (Mar/Apr, 1991): 184-188.
70 Ibid.
71 Simkin, P.; Whalley, J.; and Keppler, A. *Pregnancy, Childbirth and the Newborn*. New York: Meadowbrook Press, 1991.
72 Golding, J.; et al. "Childhood Cancer, Intramuscular Vitamin K, and Pethidine Given During Labour." *British Medical Journal* 305 no. 6849 (Aug, 1992): 341-346.
73 Lawler, F. H.; Bisonni, R. S.; and Holtgrave, D. R. "Circumcision: A Decision Analysis of its Medical Value." *Family Medicine* 23 no. 8 (Nov/Dec, 1991): 587-593.
74 Jason, J. "Breast-Feeding in 1991." *New England Journal of Medicine* 325 no. 14 (Oct, 1991): 1036-1038.
75 Worthington-Roberts, B. S.; Vermeersch, J.; and Williams, S. R. *Nutrition in Pregnancy and Lactation*. 3d ed. St. Louis: Times Mirror/Mosby College Publishing, 1985.
76 Hennart, P. F.; et al. "Lysozyme, Lactoferrin, and Secretory Immunoglobulin A Content in Breast Milk: Influence of Duration of Lactation, Nutrition Status, Prolactin Status, and Parity of Mother." *American Journal of Clinical Nutrition* 53 no.1 (Jan, 1991): 32-39.
77 Parmely, M. J.; Beer, A. E.; and Billingham, R. E. "In Vitro Studies on the T-lymphocyte Population of Human Milk." *Journal of Experimental Medicine* 144 no. 2 (Aug, 1976): 358-370.
78 Lawton, J. W.; and Shortridge, K. F. "Protective Factors in Human Breast Milk and Colostrum." *Lancet* 1 no. 8005 (Jan, 1977): 253.
79 Ibid.
80 Jason, J. "Breast-Feeding in 1991." *New England Journal of Medicine* 325 no. 14 (Oct, 1991): 1036-1038.
81 Lawton, J. W.; and Shortridge, K. F. "Protective Factors in Human Breast Milk and Colostrum." *Lancet* 1 no. 8005 (Jan, 1977): 253.
82 Editorial Staff. "Necrotizing Enterocolitis and Breast Milk." *American Family Physician* 43 no. 5 (1991): 1788.
83 Saarinen, U. M. "Prolonged Breast Feeding as Prophylaxis for Recurrent Otitis Media." *Acta Paediatrica Scandinavica* 71 no. 4 (Jul, 1982): 567-571.
84 Lothe, L.; and Lindberg, T. "Cow's Milk Whey Protein Elicits Symptoms of Infantile Colic in Colicky Formula-Fed Infants: a Double-Blind Crossover Study." *Pediatrics* 83 no. 2 (Feb, 1989): 262-266.
85 Halpern, S. R.; et al. "Development of Childhood Allergy in Infants Fed Breast, Soy, or Cow Milk." *Journal of Allergy and Clinical Immunology* 51 no. 3 (Mar, 1973): 139-151.
86 Lucas, A.; et al. "Breast Milk and Subsequent Intelligence Quotient in Children Born Preterm." *Lancet* 339 no. 8788 (Feb, 1992): 261-264.
87 Worthington-Roberts, B. S.; Vermeersch, J.; and Williams, S. R. *Nutrition in Pregnancy and Lactation*. 3d ed. St. Louis: Times Mirror/Mosby College Publishing, 1985.
88 Jason, J. "Breast-Feeding in 1991." *New England Journal of Medicine* 325 no. 14 (Oct, 1991): 1036-1038.
89 Worthington-Roberts, B. S.; Vermeersch, J.; and Williams, S. R. *Nutrition in Pregnancy and Lactation*. 3d ed. St. Louis: Times Mirror/Mosby College Publishing, 1985.
90 Ibid.
91 Ibid.
92 Myrabo, J. "The First Days After Birth: Care of Mother and Baby." Pamphlet. Seattle, WA: Pennypress, 1983.
93 Simkin, P.; Whalley, J.; and Kepler, A. *Pregnancy, Childbirth and the Newborn*. New York: Meadowbrook Press, 1991.
Kitzinger, S. "Sex After the Baby Comes." Pamphlet. Seattle, WA: Pennypress, 1980.
94 Short, R. V.; et al. "Contraceptive Effects of Extented Lactational Amenorrhoea: Beyond the Bellagio Consensus." *Lancet* 337 no. 8743 (Mar, 1991): 715-717.
95 Short, R. V.; et al. "Contraceptive Effects of Extented Lactational Amenorrhoea: Beyond the Bellagio Consensus." *Lancet* 337 no. 8743 (Mar, 1991): 715-717.
Huffman, S. L.; et al. "Suckling Patterns and Post-Partum Amenorrhea in Bangladesh." *Journal of Biosocial Science* 19 no. 2 (Apr, 1987): 171-179.

Respiratory Conditions

1 Cherniack, R. M. *Respiration in Health and Disease*. Philadelphia: W. B. Saunders Co., 1983,179.
2 Jaroff, L. "Allergies: Nothing To Sneeze At." *Time* (Jun 22, 1992): 54.
3 Rubenstein, E.; and Felderman; D. D., eds. *Scientific American Medicine*. New York: Scientific American Inc., 1982.
4 Ibid.
5 Austin, P. *Natural Remedies: A Manual*. Seale, AL: Yuchi Pines Institute, 1983.
6 Rubenstein, E.; and Felderman; D. D., eds. *Scientific American Medicine*. New York: Scientific American Inc., 1982.
7 Weiss, R. *Herbal Medicine*. Beaconsfield, England: Beaconsfield Publishers, 1988.
8 Ibid.
9 Kushi, M. *The Cancer Prevention Diet*. New York: St. Martin's Press,1983.
10 Abramson, R. "EPA Officially Links Passive Smoke To Cancer." *Los Angeles Times* 112 (Jun 8, 1993): A27.
11 Rubenstein, E.; and Felderman; D. D., eds. *Scientific American Medicine*. New York: Scientific American Inc., 1982.
12 Ibid.
13 Berkow, R., M.D.; and Fletcher, A. J., eds. *The Merck Manual of Diagnosis and Therapy*. 16th ed. Rahway, NJ: Merck & Co., 1992.
14 Rubenstein, E.; and Felderman; D. D., eds. *Scientific American Medicine*. New York: Scientific American Inc., 1982.
15 "Nutrition and Cancer Study." Melbourne, Australia: University of Melbourne, Department of Medicine, 1989.
16 Rubenstein, E.; and Felderman; D. D., eds. *Scientific American Medicine*. New York: Scientific American Inc., 1982.
17 *Physicians' Desk Reference*. Oradell, NJ: Medical Economics Co., 1990.
18 Pfeiffer, C. C., M.D.; and the Publications Committee of the Brain Bio Center. *Mental and Elemental Nutrients: Physician's Guide to Nutrition and Health Care*. New Canaan, CT: Keats Publishing, Inc., 1975.
19 Babcock, D. "Whomever May Have Asthma." *Townsend Letter for Doctors*.
20 John Bastyr College. *Naturopathic Treatment Notebook*. Seattle, WA: NCNM Library Reprint, 1984.
21 Austin, P. *Natural Remedies: A Manual*. Seale, AL: Yuchi Pines Institute, 1983.
22 Airola, P. *How to Get Well*. Phoenix, AZ: Health Plus Publishers,1974.
23 John Bastyr College. *Naturopathic Treatment Notebook*. Seattle, WA: NCNM Library Reprint, 1984.
24 Weiss, R. *Herbal Medicine*. Beaconsfield, England: Beaconsfield Publishers, 1988.

Sexually Transmitted Diseases

1 Zimmerman, H. L.; et al. "Epidemiologic Differences Between Chlamydia and Gonorrhea." *American Journal of Public Health* 80 no. 11 (1990): 1338-1342.
2 Potts, J. F. "Chlamydial Infection: Screening and Management Update, 1992." *Postgraduate Medicine* 91 no. 1 (1992): 120-126.
US Department of Health and Human Services. "Chlamydia Trachomatis Infections: Policy Guidelines for Prevention and Control." Atlanta: Center for Disease Control, August 1985.
3 Kumazawa, Y.; et al. "Activation of Peritoneal Macrophages by Berberine Alkaloids in Terms of Induction of Cytostatic Activity." *Internatonal Journal of Immunopharmacology* 6 no. 6 (1984): 587-592.
4 Babbar, O. P.; et al. "Effect of Berberine Chloride Eye Drops on Clinically Positive Tracoma Patients." *Indian Journal of Medical Research* 76 suppl. (1982): 83-88.
5 Krupp, M. A.; Chatton, M. J.; and Tierney L. M.; eds. *Current Medical Diagnosis & Treatment 1986*. Los Altos: Lange Medical Publications, 1986.
6 "STD training: 'Gonorrhea Notes.'" Seattle, WA: Harborview Medical Center, 1985.
7 Derman, R. J. "Counseling the Herpes Genitalis Patient." *Journal of Reproductive Medicine* 31 suppl. 5 (May, 1986): 439-444.
8 Pompei, R.; et al. "Glyccyrhizic Acid Inhibits Virus Growth and Inactivates Virus Particles." *Nature* 281 no. 5733 (Oct, 1979): 690.
9 Willmott, F.; et al. "Zinc and Recalcitrant Trichoasis." *Lancet* 1 no. 8332 (May, 1983): 1053.
10 Sebbelov, A. M.; et al. "The Prevalence of Human Papillomavirus Type 16 and 18 DNA in Cervical Cancer in Different Age Groups: A Study on the Incidental Cases of Cervical Cancer in Norway in 1983." *Gynecologic Oncology* 41 no. 2 (May, 1991): 141-148.
Kawana, T. "Human Papilloma Virus and Cervical Cancer" *Gan To Kagaku Ryoho Japanese Journal of Cancer and Chemotherapy* 17 no. 4 pt. 1 (Apr, 1990): 615-619. In Japanese.
11 Spinillo, A.; et al. "Recurrent Vaginal Candidiasis. Results of a Cohort Study of Sexual Transmission and Intestinal Reservoir." *Journal of Reproductive Medicine* 37 no. 4 (Apr, 1992): 343-347.
12 Miles M. R.; Olsen, L.; and Rogers, A. "Recurrent Vaginal Candidiasis: Importance of an Intestinal Reservoir." *Journal of the American Medical Association* 238 no. 17 (Oct, 1977): 1836-

1837.
13 Ibid.
14 Hilton, E.; et al. "Ingestion of Yogurt Containing Lactobacillus Acidophilus as Prophylaxis for Candidal Vaginitis." *Annals of Internal Medicine* 116 no. 5 (1992): 353-357.
15 Jovanovic, R.; Congema, E.; and Nguyen, H. T. "Antifungal Agents vs. Boric Acid for Treating Chronic Mycotic Vulvovaginitis." *Journal of Reproductive Medicine* 36 no. 8 (Aug, 1991): 593-597.
16 Pompei, R.; et al. "Antiviral Activity of Glycyrrhizic Acid." *Experientia* 36 no. 3 (Mar, 1980): 304.

Sleep Disorders

1 Pizzorno, J. E.; and Murray, M. T. *A Textbook of Natural Medicine*. Seattle, WA: John Bastyr College Publications, 1989.
2 Stone, B. M. "Sleep and Low Doses of Alcohol." *Electroencephalography and Clinical Neurophysiology* 48 no. 6 (Jun, 1980): 706-709.
3 Rinkel, H. J.; Randolph, T. G.; and Zeller, M. *Food Allergy*. Springfield, IL: Charles C. Thomas, 1950.
4 This report is based solely on product labeling as published by PDR®. Copyright© 1993 by Medical Economics Data, a division of Medical Economics Company, Inc. All rights reserved. There is no affiliation between Medical Economics Company, Inc., and Future Medicine Publishing, Inc.
5 Kaplan, H. I.; and Sadock, B. *The Comprehensive Textbook of Psychiatry*. 2 vols. Baltimore, MD: Williams & Wilkens, 1985, 558-574.
6 Tsoi, W. F. "Insomnia: Drug Treatment." *Annals of the Academy of Medicine, Singapore* 20 no. 2 (Mar, 1991): 269-272.
7 Lader, M. "Rebound Insomnia and Newer Hypnotics." *Psychopharmacology* 108 no. 3 (1992): 248-255.
8 Kahn, A.; et al. "Insomnia and Cow's Milk Allergy in Infants." *Pediatrics* 76 no. 6 (Dec, 1985): 880-884.
9 Pizzorno, J. E.; and Murray, M. T. *A Textbook of Natural Medicine*. Seattle, WA: John Bastyr College Publications, 1989.
10 Lader, M. "Rebound Insomnia and Newer Hypnotics." *Psychopharmacology* 108 no. 3 (1992): 248-255.
11 Mitchell, W. *Naturopathic Applications of the Botanical Remedies*. Seattle, WA: Mitchell, 1983, 66-67.
12 Abstracts of the 4th International Symposium. "Mobilizations of Endorphins as the Basis for Effectiveness of Acupuncture Therapy." *Acupuncture and Electro-Therapeutics Research International Journal* 13 no. 4 (1988): 201.
13 Tierney, L. M. Jr., M.D.; et al. eds. *Current Medical Diagnosis & Treatment*. Norwalk, CT: Appleton & Lange, Prentice Hall, 1993.
14 Ibid.
15 Ayres, S.; and Mihan; R. "Leg Cramps and 'Restless Leg' Syndrome Responsive to Vitamin E (Tocopherol)." *California Medicine* 111 no. 2 (Aug, 1969): 87-91.

Stress

1 Scofield, M. *Work Site Health Promotion*. Philadelphia: Hanley & Belfus, Inc. 1990, 459.
2 *Harvard Mental Health Letter* 8 no. 7 (Jan, 1992).
Holmes, T. H.; and Masuda, M. "Life Changes and Illness Susceptibility." Paper presented at "Separation and Depression: Clinical and Research Aspects," a symposium given in Chicago, December, 1970.
3 Soloman, G. F. "Emotions, Stress, the Central Nervous System and Immunity." *Annals of the New York Academy of Sciences* 164 no. 2 (Oct, 1969): 335-343.
Rasmussen, A. F., Jr. "Emotions and Immunity." *Annals of the New York Academy of Sciences* 164 no. 2 (Oct, 1969): 458-462.
4 Bahnson, C. B.; and Bahnson, M. B. "Cancer as an Alternative to Psychosis: A Theoretical Model of Somatic and Psychologic Regression." In *Psychosomatic Aspects of Neoplastic Disease*, eds. D. M. Kissen and L. L. LeShan. Philadelphia: J. B. Lippincott Company, 1964, 184-202.
Levenson, F. B. *The Causes and Prevention of Cancer*. New York: Stein and Day, 1985.
5 Bartrop, R. W.; et al. "Depressed Lymphocyte Function After Bereavement." *Lancet* 1 no. 8016 (Apr, 1977): 834-836.
6 Selye, H. *Stress Without Distress*. New York: New American Library, 1975.
7 Beasley, J. D.; and Swift, J. *Kellog Report— the Impact of Nutrition, Environment, and Lifestyle on the Health of Americans*. Annandale-on-Hudson, NY: Institute of Health Policy and Practice, The Bard College Center, 1989.
8 Ibid.
9 Nixon, P. G. "Human Functions and the Heart." In *Changing Ideas in Health Care*, eds. D. Seedhouse and A. Cribb. New York: John Wiley & Sons, 1989.
10 Levenson, F. B. *The Causes and Prevention of Cancer*. New York: Stein and Day, 1985.
11 Cohen, S.; Tyrrell, D. A.; and Smith, A. P. "Psychological Stress and Susceptibility to the Common Cold." *New England Journal of Medicine* 325 (Aug, 1991): 606-612.
12 *Harvard Mental Health Letter* 8 no. 7 (Jan, 1992).
13 Achterberg, J. "Ritual: The Foundation for Transpersonal Medicine." *ReVision* 14 no. 3 (1992): 158-164.
14 Benson, H., M.D. *The Relaxation Response*. New York: William Morrow, 1975.
15 Ornish, D., M.D. *Dr. Dean Ornish's Program for Reversing Heart Disease: the Only System Scientifically Proven to Reverse Heart Disease Without Drugs or Surgery*. New York: Ballantine, 1990.
16 Kabat-Zinn, J. *Full Catastrophe Living: Using the Wisdom of Your Body and Mind to Face Stress, Pain, and Illness*. New York: Delacorte Press, 1990.
17 Goleman, D. *The Meditative Mind*. Los Angeles: Jeremy P. Tarcher, Inc., 1988, 168.
18 Beary, J. F.; and Benson, H. "A Simple Psychophysiologic Technique Which Elicits the Hypometabolic Changes of the Relaxation Response." *Psychosomatic Medicine* 36 no. 2 (Mar/Apr, 1974): 115-120.
Everly, G. S., Jr; and Benson H. "Disorders of Arousal and the Relaxation Response: Speculations on the Nature and Treatment of Stress-Related Diseases." *International Journal of Psychosomatics* 36 nos. 1-4 (1989): 15-21.
19 Goleman, D. *The Meditative Mind*. Los Angeles: Jeremy P. Tarcher, Inc., 1988, 168.
20 Murphy, M. *The Future of the Body*. Los Angeles: Jeremy P. Tarcher, Inc., 1992.
21 Ibid.
22 Funderburk, J. *Science Studies Yoga: a Review of Physiological Data*. Honesdale, PA: Himalayan International Institute of Yoga Science & Philosophy of USA, 1977, 36-41.
23 Jahnke, R. "The Most Profound Medicine — Part II and Part III: Physiological Mechanisms Operating in the Human System During the Practice of QiGong and Yoga Pranayama." *Townsend Letter for Doctors* 91-92 (Jan-Feb, 1991): 124-130; 281-285.
24 Gagnon, D. O. *Healing Herbs for Your Nervous System*. Monograph. Santa Fe, NM: Santa Fe Botanical Research & Educational Project, 1992.
25 Bach, E.; and Wheeler, F. J. *The Bach Flower Remedies*. New Canaan, CT: Keats Publishing Inc., 1977. Originally Published by C. W. Daniel Co., Ltd., Saffron Walden, Essex, England, 1933.

Vision

1 Krupp, M. A.; Chatton, M. J.; and Tierney, L. M., eds. *Current Medical Diagnosis and Treatment*. Los Altos, CA: Lange Medical Publications, 1982, 77-84.
2 Pizzorno, J. E.; and Murray, M. T. *A Textbook of Natural Medicine*. Seattle, WA: John Bastyr College publications, 1989.
3 Ibid.
4 Levine, L. "Optometrically-Relevant Side Effects of the Systemic Drugs Most Frequently Prescribed in 1991." *Journal of Behavioral Optometry* 3 no. 5 (1992): 115-119.
5 *Physician's Desk Reference*. 46th ed. Montvale, NJ: Medical Economics Data, 1992.
6 Liberman, J. *Light: Medicine of the Future*. Santa Fe, NM: Bear & Co. Publishing, 1991.
Harman, D. B. *The Coordinated Classroom*. Grand Rapids, MI: American Seating Co., 1951.
7 Dart, J. K.; Stapleton, F.; and Minassian, D. "Contact Lenses and Other Risk Factors in Microbial Keratitis." *Lancet* 338 no. 8768 (Sep, 1991): 650-653.
8 Swartwout, G.; and Henahan, J. "Cataract Prevention: a Nutritional Approach." Farmington Hills, MI: The Holistic Optometrist, 1986.
9 Duarte, A. *Cataract Breakthrough*. Huntington Beach, CA: International Institute of Natural Health Sciences, 1982.
10 Gaby, A. R., M.D.; and Wright, J. V., M.D. "Nutritional Factors in Degenerative Eye Disorders: Cataract and Macular Degeneration." *Journal of Advancement in Medicine* 6 no. 1 (Spring, 1993): 27-39.
11 Ibid.
12 Peachey, G. T. "Perspectives on Optometric Visual Training." *Journal of Behavioral Optometry* 1 no. 3 (1990): 65-70.
13 Zaba, J. N.; and Johnson, R. A. "Literacy: the Vision, Learning and Volunteer Connection." *Journal of Behavioral Optometry* 3 no. 5 (1992): 128-130.
14 Solan, H. A. "Visual Perceptual Factors and Reading. Clinical Implications of Some Recent Optometric Research." *Journal of Behavioral Optometry* 1 no. 3 (1990): 59-64.
15 Bates, W. H. *The Bates Method for Better Eyesight Without Glasses*. New York: Henry Holt & Co./Owl Books, 1981.
16 *Townsend Letter for Doctors* (Nov, 1989).
17 Lebuisson; et al. "Treatment of Senile Macular Degeneration with Ginkgo Biloba Extract. A Preliminary Double-Blind, Drug Versus Placebo Study." In *Rokan (Ginkgo Biloba) - Recent results in Pharmacology and Clinic*., ed. Funfgeld. New York: Springer-Verlag, 1988.
Scharrer, A.; and Ober, M. "Anthocyanosides in the Treatment of Retinopathies." *Klinische Monatsblatter fur Augenheilkunde* 178 no. 5 (May, 1981): 386-389. In German.
18 Bykova, M. I.; and Sosnova, T.L. "The Experience in Using Eleutherococcus For Raising The Level of Color Discrimination Function in Railroad Engineers." *Gigiena i Sanitariia* 6 (Jun, 1976): 108-110.
19 Swartwout, G. *Electromagnetic Pollution Solutions*. Hilo, HI: Aerai Publishing, 1991.

Quick Reference to Additional Health Conditions.

1. Hughes, H., Brown, B.W., Lawlis, G.F., Fulton, J.E., Jr. "Treatment of acne vulgaris by biofeedback relaxation and cognitive imagery." *Journal of Psychosomatic Research* 27 no. 3 (1983): 185-91.
2 Chaitow, L. "British Research Connects Ankylosing Spondylitis to Bowel Dysbiosis." *Townsend Letter for Doctors* (Jul, 1989): 364-365.
3 Editor. "Economy Class Syndrome: Blood Clots can Form in Your Legs on Long-Distance Flights." *Mayo Clinic Health Letter* 7 no. 7 (Jul, 1989): 7.
4 Williams, R.S., Logue, E.E., Lewis H.G., Barton T., Stead, N.W., Wallace, A.G., Pizzo, S.V. "Physical conditioning augments the fibrinolytic response to venous occlusion in healthy adults." *New England Journal of Medicine* 302 no. 18 (May 1, 1980): 987-991.
Dreyer, N.A., Pizzo, S.V. "Blood coagulation and idiopathic thromboembolism among fertile women." *Contraception* 22 no. 2 (Aug, 1980): 123-135.
5 Szanto, S., Yudkin, J. "The effect of dietary sucrose on blood lipids, serum insulin, platelet adhesiveness and body weight in human volunteers." *Postgraduate Medical Journal* no. 45 (Sept, 1969): 602.
Szanto, S., Yudkin, J., Kakkar, V.V. "Sugar intake, serum insulin and platelet adhesiveness in men with and without peripheral vascular disease." *Postgraduate Medical Journal* no. 45 (Sept, 1969): 608.
6 David, T.A., M.D., Minehart, J.R., M.D., Kornblueh, I.H., M.D. "Polarized Air as an Adjunct in the Treatment of Burns." *American Journal of Physical Medicine* 39 no. 3 (Jun, 1960): 111-113.

7 Gaiduk, V.I., Skachkova, N.K., Fedorovskaia, E.A., "Effect of a Flow-frequency alternating magnetic field on the microflora and healing of burn wounds." *Vestnik Khirurhii Imeni I.I. Grekova* 134 no. 4 (Apr, 1985): 69-74.
8 Pothmann, R. and Schmitz, G. "Acupressure in the acute treatment of cerebral convulsions in children." *Journal of Alternative Medicine* 1 no.1 (1985): 63-67.
9 Fergusson, D.M., Horwood L.J., Shannon F.T., "Early solid feeding and recurrent childhood eczema: a 10-year longitudinal study." *Pediatrics* 86 no. 4 (Oct, 1990): 541-546.
10 Skerrett, P.J., "Fat May Cut Gallstone Risk in Dieters." *Medical Tribune* 34 no. 5 (Mar, 11): 15.
11 Thyagarajan S.P., Subramanian S., Thirunalasundari, T., Venkateswaran P.S., Blumberg B.S. "Effect of Phyllanthus amarus on chronic carriers of hepatitis B virus." *Lancet* 2 no. 8614 (Oct 1, 1988): 764-766.
12 Lesser, M., M.D. *Nutrition and Vitamin Therapy.* Berkeley, CA: Parker House, 1980.
13 Ehrenprets, S. "Mobilization of Endorphins as the Basis for Effectiveness of Acupuncture Therapy." *Acupuncture and Electro-Therapeutics Res., Int. J.* 13 no. 4 (1988): (201-203).
14 Shuster, J., et al "Soft drink consumption and urinary stone recurrence: a randomized prevention trial." *Journal of Clinical Epidemiology* 45 no. 8 (Aug, 1992): 911-916.
15 Robertson, W.G., Peacock, M., Marshall, D.H. "Prevalence of urinary stone disease in vegetarians." *European Urology* 8 no. 6 (1982): 334-339.
16 Curhan G.C., et al. "A prospective study of dietary calcium and other nutrients and the risk of symptomatic kidney stones." *New England Journal of Medicine* 328 no. 12 (Mar 25, 1993): 833-8.
17 Mowrey D.B., Clayson D.E., "Motion sickness, ginger, and psychophysics." *Lancet* 1 no. 8273 (Mar 20, 1982): 655-657.
Holtmann S., Clarke A.H., Scherer H., Hohn M., "The anti-motion sickness mechanism of ginger. A comparative study with placebo and dimenhydrinate." *Acta Oto-laryngol (Stockh)* 108 no. 3-4 (Sep/Oct, 1989): 168-74.
Grontved A., Brask T., Kambskard J., Hentzer E., "Ginger root against seasickness. A controlled trial on the open sea." *Acta Oto-laryngol (Stockh)* 105 no. 1-2 (Jan/Feb, 1988): 45-49.
18 Schneider, J.S., et. al. "Recovery from Experimental Parkinism in Primates with G_{M1} Ganglioside Treatment." *Science.* 256 no. 5058 (May 8, 1992): 843-846.
19 Birkmayer, W., Birkmayer, G.J. "Nicotinamidadenindinucleotide (NADH: the new approach in the therapy of Parkinson's disease." *Annals of Clinical and Laboratory Science,* 19 no. 1 (Jan-Feb, 1989): 38-43.
20 Ericsson, A.D., M.D., et al. "Neurotrophin 1: Treatment of Parkinson's Disease." *Explore* 3 no. 6 (1992): 19-22.
21 Pack, A.R. "Folate mouthwash: effects on established gingivitis in periodontal patients." *Journal of Clinical Periodontology* 11 no. 9 (Oct, 1984): 619-628.
22 di Fabio, A. "The Surprising Psoriasis Treatment." *Chapter XX Supplement to the Art of Getting Well* Franklin, TN: Rheumatoid Disease Foundation, 1989.
23 di Fabio, A. "The Surprising Psoriasis Treatment." *Chapter XX Supplement to the Art of Getting Well* Franklin, TN: Rheumatoid Disease Foundation, 1989.
24 The complete Fumaric acid treatment protocol for psoriasis may be obtained from:
Rheumatoid Disease Foundation
5106 Old Harding Road
Franklin, TN 37064
615-646-1030
25 Fumaric acid may be obtained from:
Cardiovascular Research
1061-B Shary Circle
Concord, CA 94518
800-888-4585
26 Thurman F.M., "The treatment of psoriasis with Sarsaparilla compound." *New England Journal of Medicine* 227 no. 4 (July, 1942): 128-133.
27 Editor "Radical protection for athletes (dietary supplements' effects)." *Science News* 141 no. 24 (June 13, 1992): 398.
28 Garland, C.F., Dr.P.H, F.A.C.E., Garland, F.C., Ph.D., F.A.C.E., Gorham, E.D., M.P.H. "Could Sunscreens Increase Melanoma Risk?" *American Journal of Public Health* 82 no. 4, (April, 1992): 614-615.
29 Walker, W.R., Keats, D.M. "An Investigation of the Therapeutic Value of the 'Copper Bracelet' — Dermal Assimilation of Copper in Arthritic/ Rheumatoid Conditions." *Agents and Actions* 6 no. 4 (1976): 454-459.
30 Zafriri, D., Ofek, I., Adar, R., Pocino, M., Sharon, N. "Inhibitory activity of cranberry juice on adherence of type 1 and type P fimbriated Escherichia coli to eucaryotic cells." *Anti-microbial Agents and Chemotherapy* 33 no. 1 (Jan, 1989): 92-98.
31 Creighton, S.M., Stanton, S.L. "Caffeine: does it affect your bladder?" *British Journal of Urology* 66 no. 6 (Dec, 1990)613-614.
32 Kronberger L., Golles, J., "On the prevention of thrombosis with aesculus extract." *Medizinische Klinik* 64 no. 26 (1969): 1207-1209.
33 Warburton D.M., "Clinical psychopharmacology of Ginkgo Biloba extract." *Presse Medicale* 15 no. 31 (Sep 25, 1986): 1595-1604.
34 Grontved A., Hentzer, E. "Vertigo-reducing effect of ginger root. A controlled clinical study." *Journal of Oto-rhinolaryngology and its Related Specialties* 48 no.5 (1986): 282-286.

Appendix

Antibiotics

1 Cohen, S. R.; and Thompson, J. W. "Otitic Candidiasis in Children: an Evaluation of the Problem and Effectiveness of Ketpconazole in 10 Patients." *Annals of Otology, Rhinology, and Laryngology* 99 (1990): 427-431.
2 Cantekin, E. I., McGuire, T. W.; and Griffith, T. L. "Antimicrobial Therapy for Otitis Media with Effusion (Secretory Otitis Media)." *Journal of the American Medical Association* 266 no. 23 (1991): 3309-3317.
3 Crook, W. G. *Chronic Fatigue Syndrome* and *The Yeast Connection.* Jackson, TN: Professional Books, Inc., 1992, 339-340.
4 Galland, L,; and Buchman, D. D. *Superimmunity for Kids.* New York: E. P. Dutton, 1988, 201.
5 Neu, H. C. "The Crisis in Antibiotic Resistance." *Science* 257 (1992): 1064-1073.
6 Wenger, J. D.; et al. "Bacterial Meningitis in the United States, 1988: The Report of a Multi-State Surveillance Study. The Bacterial Study Group." *Journal of Infectious Diseases* 162 No.6 (Dec 1990): 1316-1323.
7 Shales, D. M.; et al. Antimicrobial Agents and Chemotherapies 33(1989): 198.
8 Reichler, M. "Abstracts of 91st Annual Meeting of the American Society for Microbiology." Dallas, TX, 5-9 May (American Society for Microbiology, Washington, DC, 1991), p. 404.
9 Cohen, M. L.; "Epidemiology of Drug Resistance: Implications for a Post-Antimicrobial Era." *Science* 257(1992): 1050-1055.
10 Anonymous. Says food allergy seems important cause of otitis. *Family Practical News* 21 no.5 (1991) : 14.
11 Hussey, G. D., and Klein, M. A.; A Randomized, Controlled Trial of Vitamin A in Children with Severe Measles. New England Journal of Medicine 323(1990).
12 Lewis, M,; et al. "Prenatal Exposure to Heavy Metals: Effect on Childhood Cognitive Skills and Health Status. *Pediatrics* 89(1992): 1010-1015.
13 Summers, A. O.; et al. "Mercury Released from Dental 'Silver' Fillings Increases the Incidence of Multiply Resistant Bacteria in the Oral and Intestinal Normal Flora." In "Abstracts of 91st Annual Meeting of the American Society for Microbiology." Dallas, TX, 5-9 May (American Society for Microbiology." Washington, DC, 1991).
14 Anneren, G., Magnusson, C. G. M.; Nordvall, S. L. "Increase in Serum Concentrations of IgG2 and IgG4 By Selenium Supplementation in Children with Down's Syndrome. *Arch Dis Child* 65(1990): 1353-1355.
15 Neiman, D. C.; et al. "The Effects of Moderate Exercise Training on Natural Killer-Cells and Acute Upper Respiratory Tract Infections. *International Journal of Sports Medicine* 11 no. 6 (1990).
16 Seligman, M. E. P. *Learned optimism.* New York: Alfred A. Knopf, 1991 167-184.
17 Pennebaker, J. W. *Opening Up: The Healing Power of Confiding in Others.* New York: Avon, 1991.
18 Meyer, R. J., and Haggerty, R. J. "Streptococcal Infections in Families." *Pediatrics* 4 (1962): 539-549.
19 Schmidt, M. A.; Smith, L. H.; and Sehnert, K. W., *Beyond Antibiotics: Healthier Options for Families.* Berkeley, CA: North Atlantic Books, 1992.

Probiotics

1 Chaitow, L.; and Trenev, N. *Probiotics.* New York: Harper Collins, 1990.
2 Alm, L. et al. : "Effect of Fermentation on B Vitamin Content of Milk in Sweden." *Journal of Dairy Sciences* 65 : 353-359.
3 Alm, L. *Journal of Dairy Sciences* 64 no. 4 : 509-514
4 Friend, B.; and Shahani, K. "Nutritional and Therapeutic Aspects of Lactobacilli." *Journal of Applied Nutrition.* 36, 125-153
Hamdan, I. "Acidolin and Antibiotic Produced by Acidophilus." *Journal of Antibiotics* 8, 631-636.
5 Reddy, G. "Antitumour Activity of Yogurt Components." *Journal of Food Protection* 46 (1983): 8-11.
6 Shehani, K. "Role of Dietary Lactobacilli in Gastrointestinal Microecology." *American Journal of Clinical Nutrition* 33,(1980): 2248-2257.
7 Mott, G. "Lowering of Serum Cholesterol by Intestinal Bacteria Lipids." (1973): 4282-4431.
8 Rasic, J. *Bifidobacteria and Their Role.* Boston: Birkhauser Verlag, 1983.
9 Simon, G. "Intestinal Flora in Health and Disease." In *Physiology of the Intestinal Tract* ed. L. Johnson. New York: Raven Press, 1981, 1361-1380.
10 Speck, M. "Interactions Among Lactobacilli and Man." *Journal of Dairy Sciences* 59, : 338-343.
11 Chaitow, L.; and. Trenev, N. *Probiotics.* New York: HarperCollins, 1990.
12 Microbial Ecology of Intestinal Tract Published by Old Herborn University, Herborn, Germany as Seminar Monograph 1987.
13 Giannella, R.; et al. "Gastric Acid Barrier to Ingested Microorganisms in Man." *Gut* 13: 251-256.
14 Henteges, D. "Effect of High-Beef Diet on Bacterial Flora of Humans." *Cancer Research* 37: 568-571.
15 Finegold, S. "Effect of Broad Spectrum Antibiotics on Normal Bowel Flora." *Annals of New York Academy of Sciences* 145: 269-281.

Index

B

C

D

E

H

I

M

N

O

P

S

T

U

W

THIS BOOK COULD SAVE YOUR LIFE

LEARN WAYS TO REVERSE AND PREVENT CANCER

Some of the doctors in *An Alternative Medicine Definitive Guide to Cancer:*

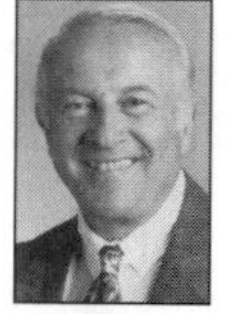

Robert Atkins, M.D.,
New York, NY
Learn about detoxification and biological support as central components in anticancer strategy.

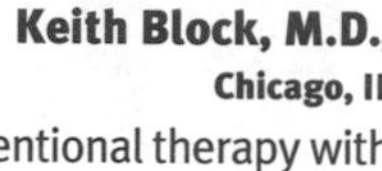

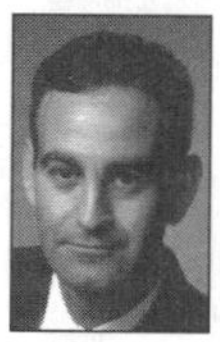

Keith Block, M.D.,
Chicago, IL
Dr. Block combines conventional therapy with immune-enhancing, detoxifying treatments to maximize cancer survival.

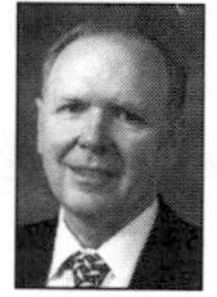

James W. Forsythe, M.D., H.M.D.,
Reno, NV
An oncologist explains his use of immune-stimulating therapies.

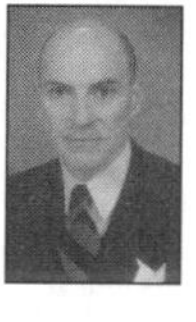

Robert A. Nagourney, M.D.,
Long Beach, CA
For those who are thinking of using chemotherapy, this oncologist can test for drug effectiveness first.

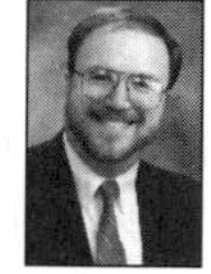

Jesse Stoff, M.D.,
Tucson, AZ
All aspects of a patient's life–body, mind, and emotions–must receive therapeutic attention. Learn how.

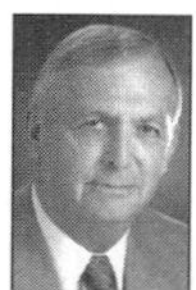

Vincent Speckhart, M.D., M.D.H.,
Norfolk, VA
An oncologist for 22 years, Dr. Speckhart explains how he reverses cancer by removing toxins and repairing the immune system.

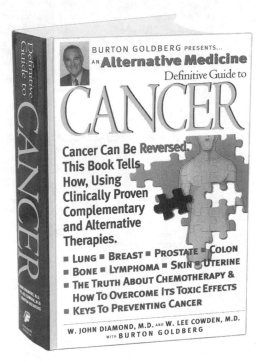

©1997 Future Medicine Publishing, Inc. Publishers of *Alternative Medicine: The Definitive Guide* and the bimonthly magazine *Alternative Medicine.*

THIS 1,116-PAGE BOOK ILLUSTRATES MANY SUCCESSFUL ALTERNATIVES TO CONVENTIONAL CARE THAT CAN REMOVE THE ROOT CAUSES OF CANCER AND RESTORE YOU TO HEALTH WITHOUT FURTHER POISONING OR DAMAGING YOUR BODY. **CALL FOR YOUR COPY TODAY. BUY A COPY FOR YOUR ONCOLOGIST AND INSIST THAT IT BE READ.**

CALL 800-333-HEAL

Valuable information featured in *An Alternative Medicine Definitive Guide to Cancer*:

- Cancer patients treated with nontoxic botanicals had twice the survival rate after one year, and four times the survival rate after two years, compared to chemotherapy patients. Readers are unlikely ever to see such results published in American medical journals, which receive their primary financial support from the pharmaceutical industry.
- The medical director of a prestigious clinic reports that in 90% of his breast cancer patients there is a dental factor.

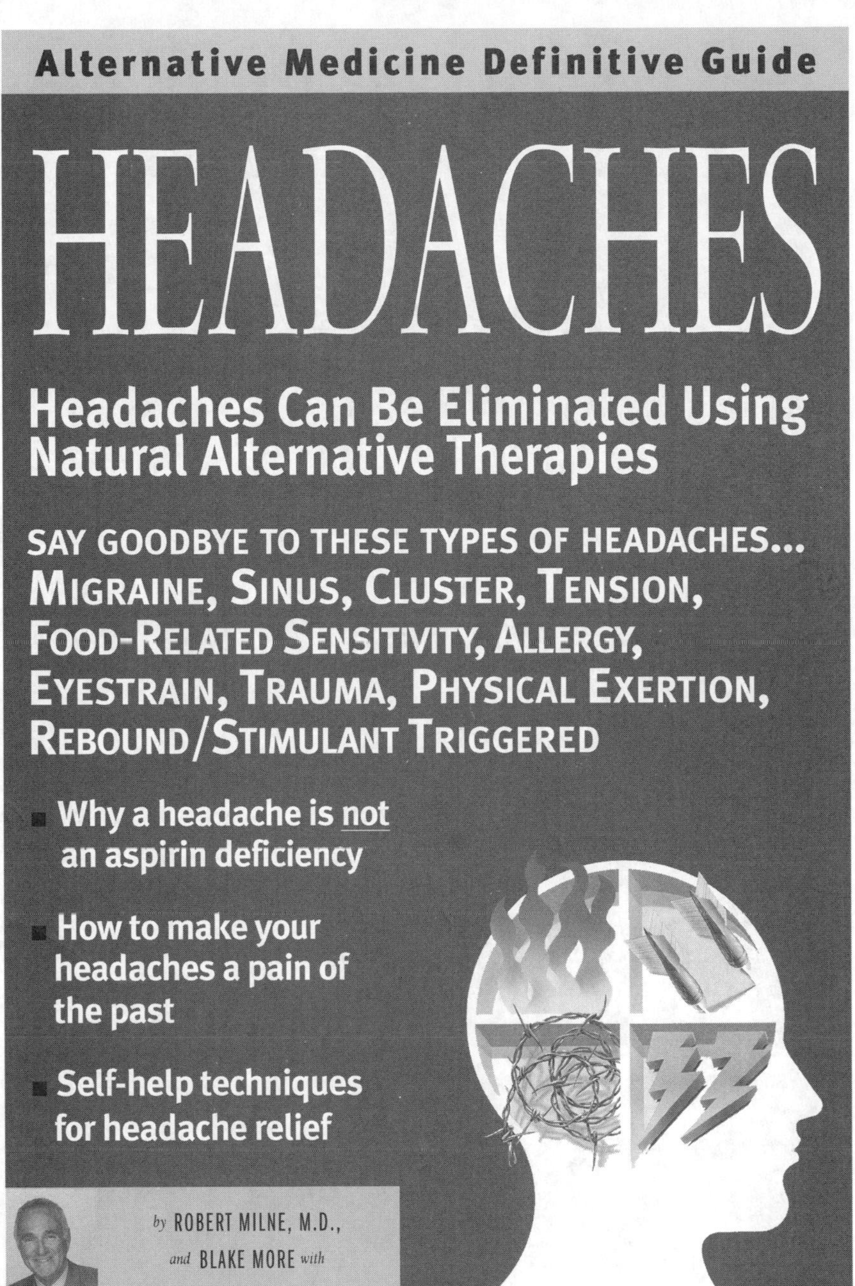
Alternative Medicine Definitive Guide
HEADACHES
Headaches Can Be Eliminated Using Natural Alternative Therapies
SAY GOODBYE TO THESE TYPES OF HEADACHES...
MIGRAINE, SINUS, CLUSTER, TENSION, FOOD-RELATED SENSITIVITY, ALLERGY, EYESTRAIN, TRAUMA, PHYSICAL EXERTION, REBOUND/STIMULANT TRIGGERED
Why a headache is not an aspirin deficiency
How to make your headaches a pain of the past
Self-help techniques for headache relief
by ROBERT MILNE, M.D., and BLAKE MORE with BURTON GOLDBERG

If you suffer from headaches, this book could change your life. It is entirely possible that with this invaluable practical information, you may well put headaches behind you as something you once suffered from, but no more.

Robert Milne, M.D., and Blake More expertly guide you through the root causes and multiple treatment options for 11 major types of headaches, from sinus to migraine, cluster to tension.

We have made every effort possible to make this book practical and user-friendly for you. For a quick reference to headache types, symptoms, treatment options, use our Master Symptom Chart. If you suffer from tension headaches, turn directly to Chapter 6; if migraines are your millstone, see Chapter 7; and if you're not sure what type of headache you have, study the symptoms list in the Master Symptom Chart until you find the clinical term that best matches your condition.

No matter what kind of headache you used to have, after reading this book your head may never pain you again.

To Order, Call 800-333-4325

website: http://www.alternativemedicine.com

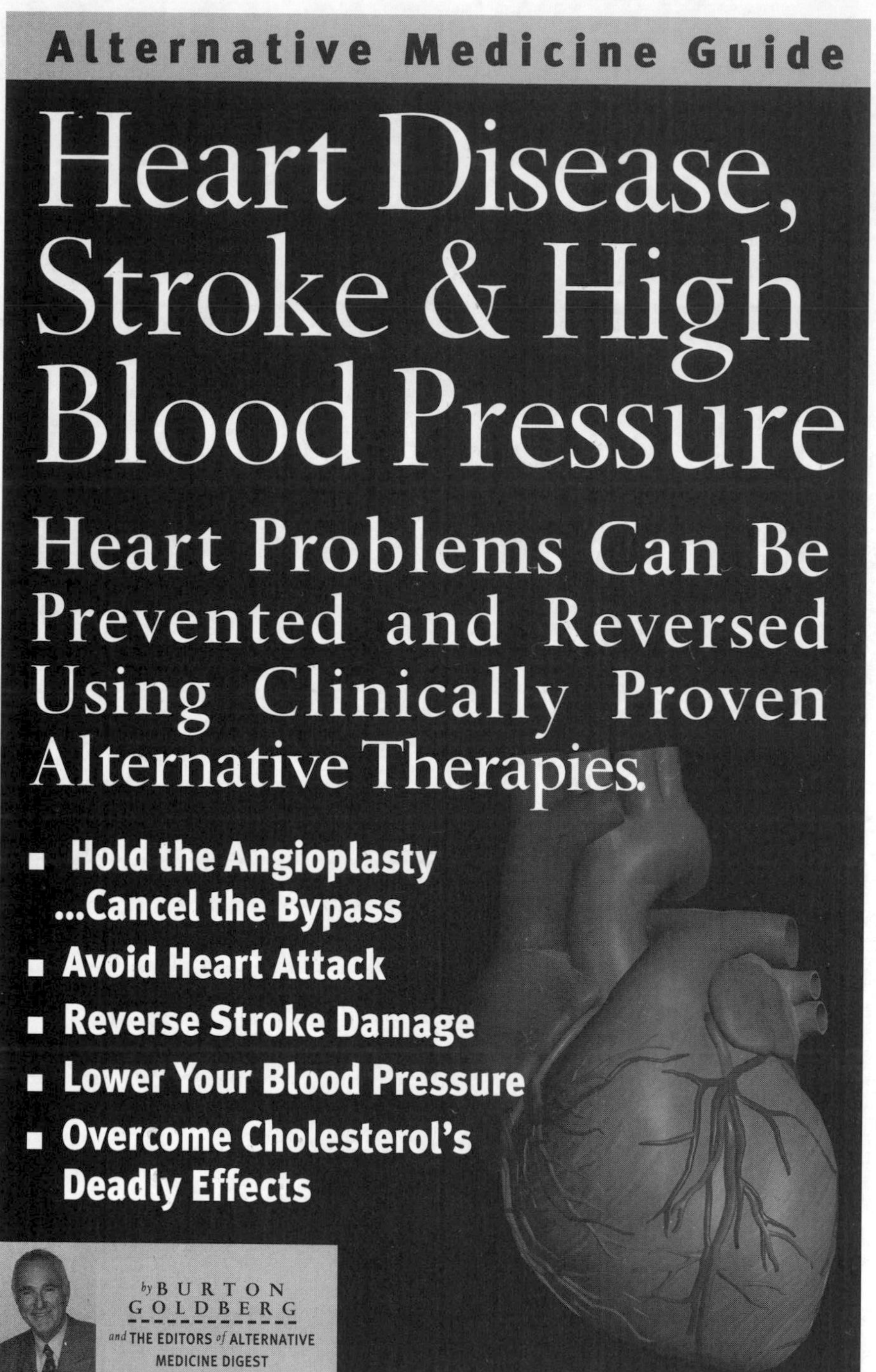

Save your heart from heart disease, attack, stroke, high blood pressure, and the dangers of angioplasty, bypass, and other invasive surgeries—12 top physicians explain their proven, safe, nontoxic, and successful heart-saving treatments.

To Order, Call 800-333-4325

website: http://www.alternativemedicine.com

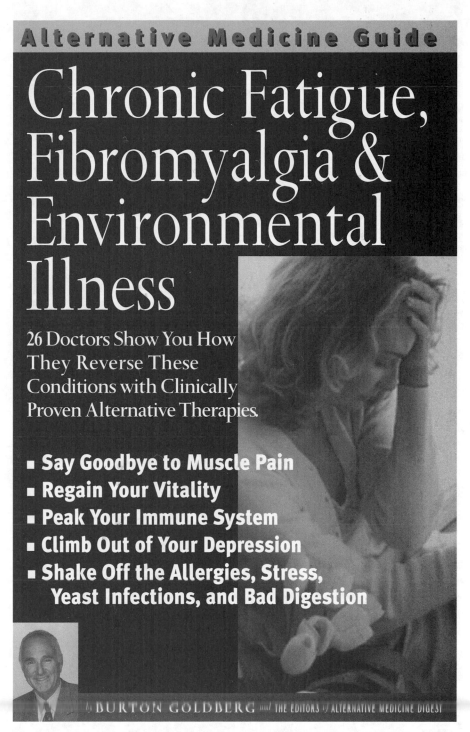

Chronic fatigue, fibromyalgia, and environmental illness can be permanently reversed using nontoxic alternative medicine treatments. In this book, 26 leading physicians explain the techniques and natural substances that brought complete recovery to their patients.

To Order, Call 800-333-4325

website: http://www.alternativemedicine.com

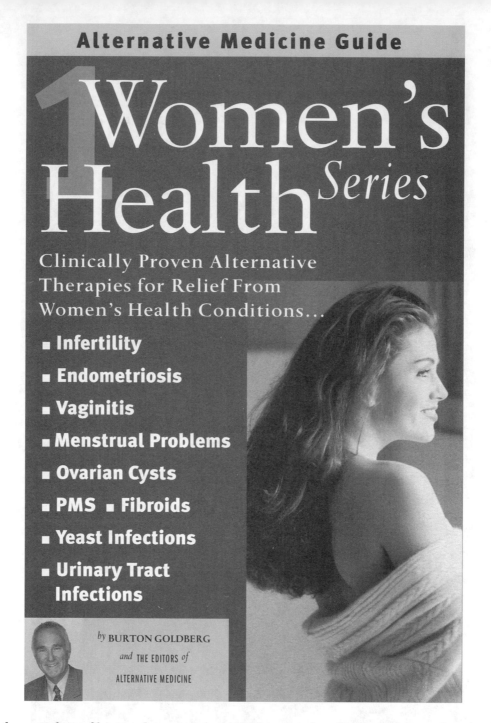

In this book, 36 leading physicians give their clinically safe and proven alternative medicine treatments for 7 major women's health conditions, complete with details on 22 actual patient success stories.

Leading practitioners explain how they use clinically proven alternative medicine therapies, such as acupuncture, herbs, nutrition and diet, supplements, homeopathy, and many other approaches, to successfully reverse women's health problems.

To Order, Call 800-333-4325

website: http://www.alternativemedicine.com

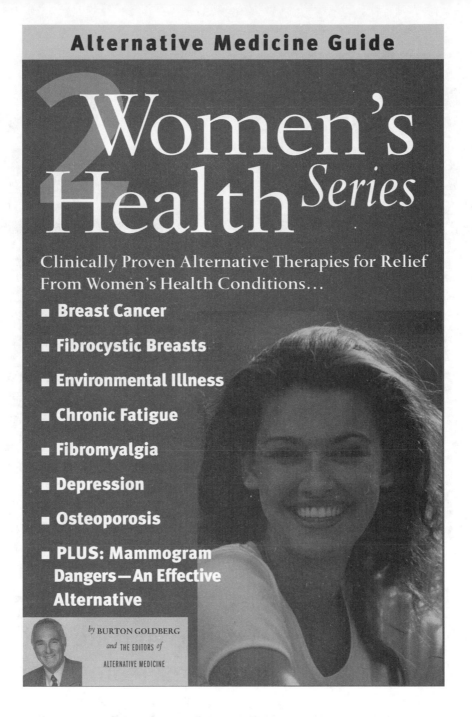

In this book, 32 leading physicians give their clinically safe and proven alternative medicine treatments for 10 major women's health conditions, complete with details on 34 actual patient success stories.

Leading practitioners explain how they use clinically proven alternative medicine therapies, such as acupuncture, herbs, nutrition and diet, supplements, homeopathy, and many other approaches, to successfully reverse women's health problems.

To Order, Call 800-333-4325

website: http://www.alternativemedicine.com

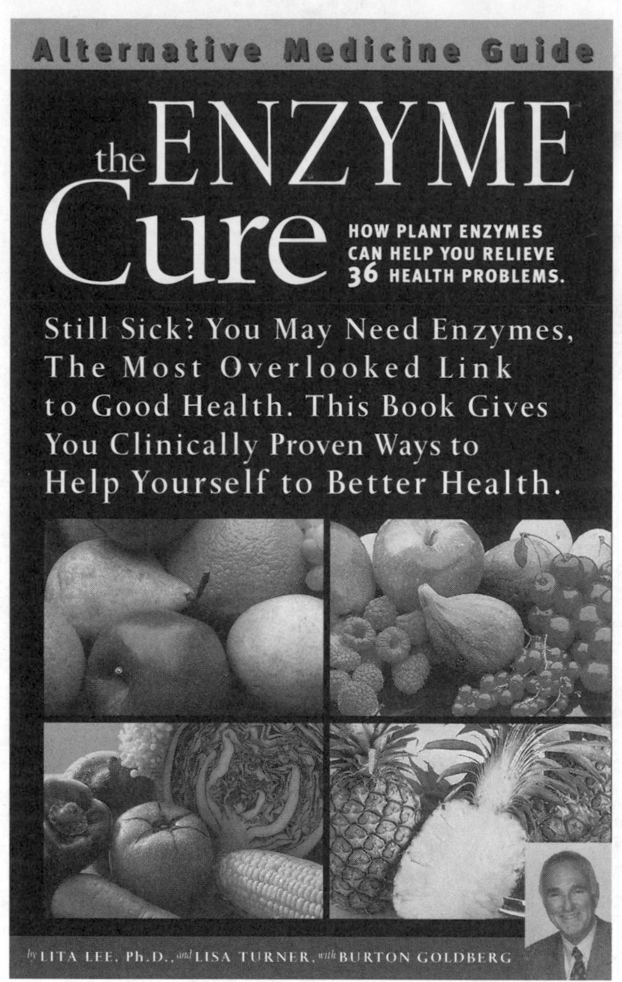

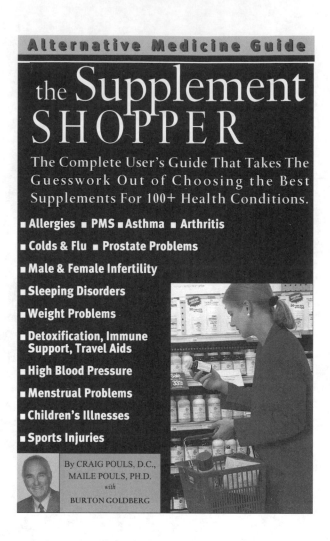

With a low-cost, self-help program, enzyme therapy can change your life for the better by rebalancing your hormones, restoring your health, and preventing illness.

At last, a single book that explains everything you need to know about selecting nutritional supplements and how to match the best brand to your exact medical problem—over 100 conditions detailed.

To Order, Call 800-333-4325

website: http://www.alternativemedicine.com

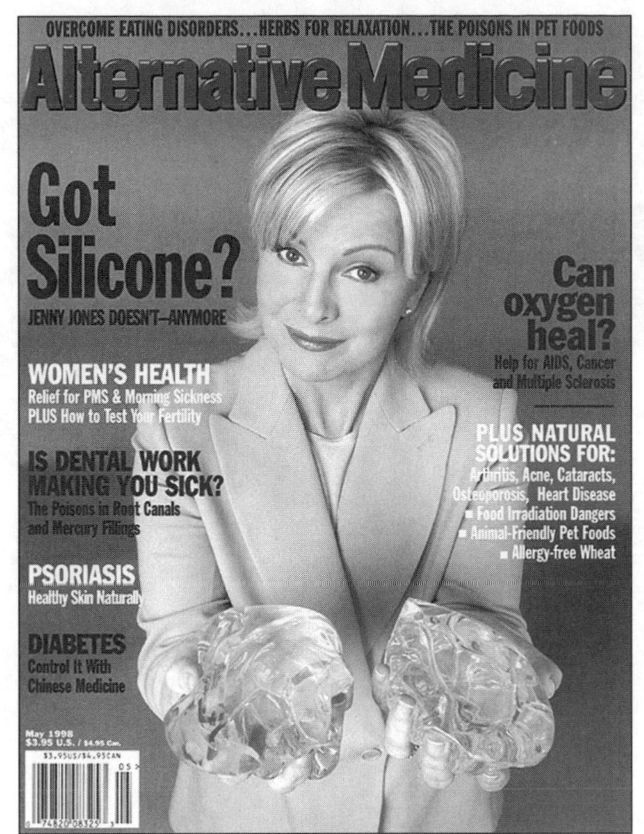

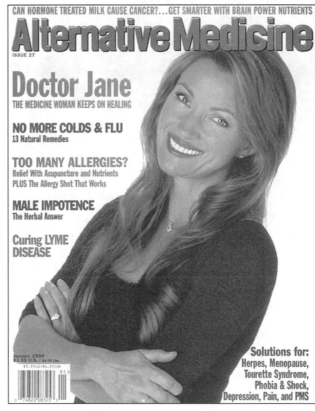

We digest it for you—*Alternative Medicine* magazine tracks the entire field—all the doctor's journals, research, conferences, and newsletters. Then we summarize what is essential for you to know to get better and stay healthy. We're your one-stop read for what's new and effective in alternative medicine.

To Order, Call 800-333-4325 or 415-435-1779

website: http://www.alternativemedicine.com

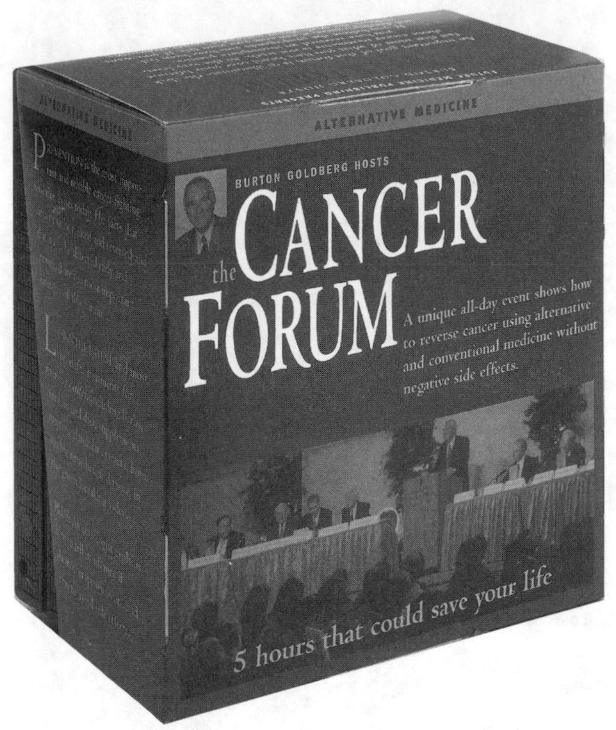

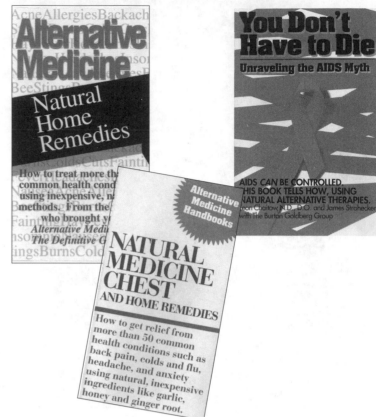

Cancer Forum Video

Let cancer experts guide you back to good health, using the best of alternative medicine. In this interactive videotaped conference, 12 of North America's prominent cancer specialists answer questions about how cancer has been reversed without toxic drugs, surgery, or radiation. This video could well be five hours of viewing that saves your life.

Alternative Medicine: Natural Home Remedies

This instructional videotape, which accompanies the informative Natural Home Remedies handbook, demonstrates how to make natural, safe remedies in your home. Our host, Jay Gordon, M.D., gives hands-on demonstrations of how to take control of your health.

Natural Medicine Chest

A concise, easy-to-use handbook that puts natural healing at your fingertips. The book lists effective yet simple remedies to help you get relief from common health conditions such as colds and flu, headaches, allergies, earaches, cramps, congestion, back pain, acne, and more. With this publication, you can build your "natural medicine chest" with products found in health food stores everywhere.

You Don't Have to Die—Unraveling the AIDS Myth

A cutting-edge publication that redefines AIDS by shattering the myths surrounding this controversial and sometimes deadly disease. Alternative therapies from around the world coupled with the latest research make this one of the most promising and compelling books on coping with AIDS today.

To Order, Call 800-333-4325

website: http://www.alternativemedicine.com